Guide to

CLINICAL

PREVENTIVE

SERVICES

SECOND EDITION

THIRD EDITION

Report of the
U.S. Preventive Services
Task Force

Guide to Clinical Preventive Services, 3rd Edition, 2000–2002

Report of the U.S. Preventive Services Task Force

The *U.S. Preventive Services Task Force* (USPSTF) was convened by the Public Health Service to rigorously evaluate clinical research in order to assess the merits of preventive measures, including screening tests, counseling immunizations, and chemoprophylaxis.

The 3rd Edition of the *Guide to Clinical Preventive Services* updates some recommendations from the 2nd Edition and evaluates additional new topics. Recommendations from the Third Task Force are being released incrementally, as they become available.

Guide to
CLINICAL
PREVENTIVE
SERVICES

SECOND EDITION
THIRD EDITION

Report of the
U.S. Preventive Services
Task Force

International Medical Publishing, Inc.

SUGGESTED CITATION: U.S. Preventive Services Task Force. Guide to Clinical Preventive Services, 2nd and 3rd eds. McLean, Virginia: International Medical Publishing, 2002

Editors:
   Carolyn DiGuiseppi, Project Director
   David Atkins
   Steven H. Woolf

Managing Editor
   Douglas B. Kamerow

Accurate indications, adverse reactions, and dosage schedules for drugs are provided in this book, but it is possible that they may change. The reader is urged to review the package information data of the manufacturers of the medications mentioned.

First Edition 1989
Second Edition - Second Printing April 1996
Second Edition - Third Printing March 1997
Second and Third Editions - First Printing July 2002
Second and Third Editions - Second Printing April 2007

If the registration slip is absent from the back of the book, you may send your name address and phone number directly to the publisher to be included in our mailing list.

International Medical Publishing, Inc.
P.O. Box 479
McLean, Virginia 22101
www.lnternationalMedicalPublishing.com
Phone: 703-734-8261
Fax: 703-734-8987

Printed in the United States of America
ISBN 978-1-1883205-13-3
Price $60.00

Foreword

It is a pleasure to present the second edition of the *Guide to Clinical Preventive Services*, a thoroughly updated and expanded version of the 1989 landmark report of the U.S. Preventive Services Task Force (USPSTF). The first edition of the *Guide* is widely regarded as the premier reference source on the effectiveness of clinical preventive services—screening tests for early detection of disease, immunizations to prevent infections, and counseling for risk reduction.

In the past six years, dramatic changes have occurred in the health care system in the United States, with an increasing emphasis on the documentation and delivery of cost-effective, high-quality care. Thanks in large part to the previous work of the USPSTF, it is no longer questioned that appropriate preventive care belongs at the top of the list of effective interventions that must be available to all Americans.

This new edition again carefully reviews the evidence for and against hundreds of preventive services, recommending a test, immunization, or counseling intervention only when there is evidence that it is effective. At a time when the leading causes of death are largely related to health-related behaviors—including tobacco use, poor diet, lack of physical activity, and alcohol use—it is particularly pertinent to highlight the importance of the health consequences of behavior. It remains extraordinarily important that physicians and other providers educate their patients about these matters.

Although the main audience for the *Guide to Clinical Preventive Services* is primary care physicians, nurse practitioners, and physician assistants, it will continue to be of great value also to policymakers, researchers, employers, and those in the health care financing community. I commend this report and its important message to all of them.

PHILIP R. LEE, M.D.
Assistant Secretary for Health
U.S. Department of Health and Human Services
Washington, DC

Preface to the Second Edition

We are gratified by the response to the first edition of the U.S. Preventive Services Task Force *Guide to Clinical Preventive Services*. The *Guide* has become an established reference source for clinicians needing evidence-based recommendations on preventive services; for managers and payers seeking information on preventive care; and for students, trainees, and researchers interested in both the process and substance of preventive service guidelines.

This second edition of the *Guide* has been completely revised. The Task Force has reevaluated each preventive service and rewritten each chapter. There are 11 new chapters in the book, bringing the total number of topics evaluated to 70. Over 6,000 citations to the literature substantiate the recommendations.

As with the first edition, the Task Force has benefitted enormously from the contributions of others. We have continued our close working relationship with our partners to the north, the Canadian Task Force on the Periodic Health Examination. Representatives of the agencies of the U.S. Public Health Service have provided wise counsel; representatives from the major primary care medical specialty societies have reviewed and commented on every chapter; and hundreds of topic experts have graciously given their time to critique specific chapters. The Task Force immensely appreciates all of this assistance; the final recommendations in the *Guide*, however, should be taken as those of the Task Force alone.

Given the revolutionary changes that are currently taking place in our health care delivery system, this edition comes out at a particularly opportune time. We know with ever-increasing certainty that health professionals can prevent many of the leading causes of death by using the proper interventions; we know that all forms of health care are now being carefully scrutinized for their effectiveness and appropriateness; and we know that managed care professionals, employers, and others are pursuing new agendas for quality in health care. The underlying philosophy of the Task Force fits the times perfectly: health professionals should recommend only those interventions for which there is convincing evidence that the benefits will outweigh the potential harms.

As before, the recommendations in the *Guide* are the beginning, not the end, of a process. The next step—implementation—is up to individual practitioners, systems of care, employers and payers, and legislative and regulatory bodies. We hope that these science-based preventive care recommendations will be helpful in all of their efforts to improve health care delivery and, ultimately, the health of the American people.

HAROLD C. SOX, JR., MD

Chairman, U.S. Preventive

Services Task Force

Joseph M. Huber Professor and Chair

Department of Medicine

Dartmouth-Hitchcock Medical Center

Lebanon, NH

J. MICHAEL McGINNIS, MD

Deputy Assistant Secretary for Health and

Director, Office of Disease Prevention

and Health Promotion

U.S. Department of Health

and Human Services

Washington, DC

Preface to the First Edition

The publication of the *Guide to Clinical Preventive Services* marks the beginning of an important new phase in the battle against premature death and disability. Abundant evidence documents that the majority of deaths among Americans below age 65 are preventable, many through interventions best provided in a clinician's office. The means are available to prevent many of these premature deaths, as well as many injuries and other types of morbidity. This *Guide*, resulting from the most comprehensive evaluation and synthesis of preventive interventions to date, offers an operational blueprint for their delivery.

Prepared under the supervision of the U.S. Preventive Services Task Force, with staff support from the U.S. Department of Health and Human Services, the *Guide* rigorously reviews evidence for over 100 interventions to prevent 60 different illnesses and conditions. The problems addressed in this report are common ones seen every day by primary care providers: cardiovascular and infectious diseases, cancers, injuries (both intentional and unintentional), alcohol and other drug abuse, and many others. Primary care clinicians have a key role in screening for many of these problems and immunizing against others. Of equal importance, however, is the clinician's role in counseling patients to change unhealthful behaviors related to diet, smoking, exercise, injuries, and sexually transmitted diseases.

The *Guide* is the culmination of over four years of literature review, debate, and synthesis of critical comments from expert reviewers. It offers the Task Force members' best judgment, based on the evidence, of the clinical preventive services that prudent clinicians should provide their patients in the course of routine clinical care. The recommendations are grouped by age, sex, and other risk factors. The quality of the evidence supporting each recommendation as well as the recommendations of other authorities are listed wherever possible, so that the reader may judge for him- or herself whether specific recommendations are appropriate.

Some will offer criticism that the recommendations go too far, expecting busy physicians and nurses to abandon their other clinical duties to become counselors or nutritionists. It is our belief that the "new morbidity" of injuries, infections, and chronic diseases demands a new paradigm for prevention in primary care—one that includes counseling about safety belt use and diet as well as giving immunizations and screening for cancer.

Others will find the Task Force recommendations too conservative. By limiting recommendations to those screening interventions, counseling maneuvers, and immunizations that have proven efficacy and effectiveness, the Task Force reaffirms the commitment to first, do no harm. All possible preventive interventions have not been examined, of course; much remains to be done as research yields new data on efficacy and effectiveness.

The *Guide* has benefitted from unprecedented cooperation—between the U.S. and Canadian Task Forces, between the Federal government and the private sector, and between the Task Force and literally hundreds of reviewers. This in itself is a gratifying accomplishment. But the real challenge lies ahead, in the offices and clinics of busy practitioners. It is our hope that the solid scientific base provided by the *Guide* will facilitate efforts to meet that challenge—to improve the health of the American people through the delivery of effective services for disease prevention and health promotion.

ROBERT S. LAWRENCE, M.D.
Chairman, U.S. Preventive
Services Task Force
Chief of Medicine, Cambridge Hospital
Director, Division of Primary Care
Harvard Medical School
Cambridge, MA

J. MICHAEL McGINNIS, M.D.
Deputy Assistant Secretary for Health and
Director, Office of Disease Prevention
and Health Promotion
U.S. Department of Health
and Human Services
Washington, DC

April 1989

U.S. Preventive Services Task Force

Harold C. Sox, Jr., M.D., Chair
Joseph M. Huber Professor and Chair
Department of Medicine
Dartmouth-Hitchcock Medical Center
Lebanon, NH

Donald M. Berwick, M.D., M.P.P., Vice Chair
Associate Clinical Professor
Department of Pediatrics
Harvard Medical School
Boston, MA

Alfred O. Berg, M.D., M.P.H.
Professor and Associate Chair
Department of Family Medicine
University of Washington
Seattle, WA

Paul S. Frame, M.D.
Tri-County Family Medicine
Cohocton, NY
Clinical Associate Professor
Department of Family Medicine
University of Rochester School of
  Medicine and Dentistry
Rochester, NY

Dennis G. Fryback, Ph.D.
Professor of Preventive Medicine and
  Industrial Engineering
Department of Preventive Medicine
University of Wisconsin–Madison
Madison, WI

David A. Grimes, M.D.
Professor and Vice Chair
Department of Obstetrics, Gynecology and
  Reproductive Sciences
UCSF/San Francisco General Hospital
San Francisco, CA

Robert S. Lawrence, M.D.
Associate Dean for Professional Education
  and Programs
Professor of Health Policy and Management
The Johns Hopkins School of Hygiene
  and Public Health
Baltimore, MD

Robert B. Wallace, M.D., M.Sc.
Professor of Preventive Medicine
Director, University of Iowa Cancer Center
University of Iowa College of Medicine
Iowa City, IA

A. Eugene Washington, M.D., M.Sc.
Professor and Chief
Department of Obstetrics, Gynecology, and
  Reproductive Sciences
UCSF/Mount Zion Medical Center
Director, Medical Effectiveness Research
  Center for Diverse Populations/UCSF
San Francisco, CA

Modena E.H. Wilson, M.D., M.P.H.
Professor of Pediatrics
Director, Division of General Pediatrics
The Johns Hopkins Children's Center
Baltimore, MD

Task Force Staff

Carolyn DiGuiseppi, M.D., M.P.H
Editor, Science Writer, and Project Director

Steven H. Woolf, M.D., M.P.H.
Editor and Science Writer

David Atkins, M.D., M.P.H.
Editor and Science Writer

Douglas B. Kamerow, M.D., M.P.H.
Managing Editor

Abigail L. Rose
Project Associate

Acknowledgments

The *Guide to Clinical Preventive Services, 2nd edition*, was prepared under the supervision of the U.S. Preventive Services Task Force, which is solely responsible for its recommendations and whose members are listed on the preceding page. Staff of the Task Force were based at and provided support by the Office of Disease Prevention and Health Promotion, U.S. Department of Health and Human Services. Support from the American College of Preventive Medicine and the Association of Teachers of Preventive Medicine for Task Force activities and staff is gratefully acknowledged. Appreciation is expressed to the members of the Canadian Task Force on the Periodic Health Examination (Richard Goldbloom, M.D., Chair), to their staff (Jennifer Dingle, M.B.A. and Patricia Randel, M.Sc.) and to Wm. Phillip Mickelson, M.D., M.A., liaison from Health Canada to the Canadian Task Force, for their collaboration, manuscript reviews, and support.

In addition to the numerous reviewers identified in Appendix B, appreciation is also expressed to the following individuals:

Specialty Society Liaisons to the U.S. Preventive Services Task Force

Edgar O. Ledbetter, M.D.
American Academy of Pediatrics
Elk Grove Village, IL

Shirley A. Shelton
American College of Obstetricians and
 Gynecologists
Washington, DC

Linda Johnson White
American College of Physicians
Philadelphia, PA

Herbert F. Young, M.D.
American Academy of Family Physicians
Kansas City, MO

Current and Former Public Health Service Liaisons to the U.S. Preventive Services Task Force

Agency for Health Care Policy
and Research
 Rockville, MD

Christine Crofton, Ph.D.
Barbara Fleming, M.D., Ph.D.
Stephen H. King, M.D.
David Lanier, M.D.

Centers for Disease Control and
Prevention
 Atlanta, GA

Alan Hinman, M.D., M.P.H.
Dixie E. Snyder, M.D., M.P.H.
William R. Taylor, M.D.
Steven Teutsch, M.D., M.P.H.

Food and Drug Administration
Rockville, MD

Freddie Ann Hoffman, M.D.
Peter H. Rheinstein, M.D., J.D., M.S.

Health Resources and Services
Administration
Rockville, MD

Colleen Kivlahan, M.D., M.S.P.H.
William A. Robinson, M.D., M.P.H.
David B. Snyder, R.Ph., D.D.S.

Indian Health Service
Rockville, MD

Craig Vanderwagen, M.D.

National Institutes of Health
Bethesda, MD

William R. Harlan, M.D.
John T. Kalberer, Jr., Ph.D.

Substance Abuse and Mental
Health Services Administration
Rockville, MD

Mary A. Jansen, Ph.D.
Elaine M. Johnson, Ph.D.
Frank J. Sullivan, Ph.D.

**Senior Advisors, U.S. Preventive
Services Task Force**

E. Harvey Estes, Jr., M.D.
North Carolina Medical Society
 Foundation, Inc.
Raleigh, NC

Jonathan E. Fielding, M.D., M.P.H.
UCLA Schools of Public Health and
 Medicine
Santa Monica, CA

Harvey V. Fineberg, M.D., Ph.D.
Harvard School of Public Health
Boston, MA

Gary D. Friedman, M.D., M.S.
Division of Research, Kaiser Permanente
Medical Care Program
Oakland, CA

Lawrence W. Green, Dr.P.H.
University of British Columbia
Vancouver, British Columbia

John C. Greene, D.M.D., M.P.H. (ret.)
University of California at San Francisco
School of Dentistry
San Rafael, CA

George A. Gross, D.O., M.P.H. (ret.)
Michigan State University
East Lansing, MI

M. Alfred Haynes, M.D.
Rancho Palos Verdes, CA

Thomas E. Kottke, M.D.
Mayo Clinic
Rochester, MN

F. Marc LaForce, M.D.
University of Rochester
Rochester, NY

Jack H. Medalie, M.D., M.P.H.
Case Western Reserve University and
 Mt. Sinai Medical Center
Cleveland, OH

F. Douglas Scutchfield, M.D.
San Diego State University
San Diego, CA

Paul D. Stolley, M.D., M.P.H.
University of Maryland
Baltimore, MD

William H. Wiese, M.D., M.P.H.
University of New Mexico
Albuquerque, NM

*Carolyn A. Williams, Ph.D., R.N.,
F.A.A.N.*
University of Kentucky
Lexington, KY

Contributing Authors

Geoffrey Anderson, M.D., Ph.D.
Sunnybrook Health Science Centre
North York, Ontario

Kathlyne Anderson, M.D., M.O.H.
Harvard School of Public Health
Boston, MA

John S. Andrews, M.D., M.P.H.
The Johns Hopkins University
Baltimore, MD

Robert Baldwin, M.D.
University of Maryland at Baltimore
Baltimore, MD

Renaldo N. Battista, M.D., Sc.D., F.R.C.P.C.
McGill University
Montreal, Quebec

Brenda L. Beagan, M.A.
Dalhousie University
Halifax, Nova Scotia

Marie-Dominique Beaulieu, M.D., M.Sc., F.C.F.P.
University of Montreal
Montreal, Quebec

Michelle Berlin, M.D., M.P.H.
University of Pennsylvania
Philadelphia, PA

Dennis Black, Ph.D.
University of California at San Francisco
San Francisco, CA

Joseph N. Blustein, M.D., M.S.
University of Wisconsin at Madison
Madison, WI

John W. Burress, M.D., M.P.H.
Harvard School of Public Health
Boston, MA

Karen J. Carlson, M.D.
Massachusetts General Hospital
Boston, MA

David Christiani, M.D., M.P.H.
Harvard School of Public Health
Boston, MA

Richard Comi, M.D.
Dartmouth-Hitchcock Medical Center
Hanover, NH

Deborah L. Craig, M.P.H.
Health Care Consultant
Halifax, Nova Scotia

Steven R. Cummings, M.D.
University of California at San Francisco
San Francisco, CA

H. Oladele Davies, M.D., M.Sc., F.R.C.P.C.
University of Calgary
Calgary, Alberta

Richard A. Deyo, M.D., M.P.H.
University of Washington
Seattle, WA

Paul Dick, M.D.C.M., F.R.C.P.C.
University of Toronto
Toronto, Ontario

Jennifer Dingle, M.B.A.
Dalhousie University
Halifax, Nova Scotia

Dennis L. Disch, M.D.
Washington University in St. Louis
St. Louis, MO

James Douketis, M.D.
McMaster University
Hamilton, Ontario

Katherine Economy, M.D.
University of California at San Francisco
San Francisco, CA

Wayne Elford, M.D., C.C.F.P., F.C.F.P.
University of Calgary
Calgary, Alberta

Virginia L. Ernster, Ph.D.
University of California at San Francisco
San Francisco, CA

Bruce Ettinger, M.D.
University of California at San Francisco
San Francisco, CA

John W. Feightner, M.D., M.Sc., F.C.F.P.
McMaster University
Hamilton, Ontario

William Feldman, M.D., F.R.C.P.C.
Hospital for Sick Children
Toronto, Ontario

Cary S. Fox, M.S.
University of California at San Francisco
San Francisco, CA

Richard Goldbloom, O.C., M.D., F.R.C.P.C.
Dalhousie University
Halifax, Nova Scotia

Deborah Grady, M.D., M.P.H.
University of California at San Francisco
San Francisco, CA

Cameron Grant, M.B.Ch.B., F.R.A.C.P.
University of Auckland
Auckland, New Zealand

Jean L. Haggerty, M.Sc.
McGill University
Montreal, Quebec

Amid I. Ismail, B.D.S., M.P.H., Dr.P.H.
Dalhousie University
Halifax, Nova Scotia

James G. Kahn, M.D., M.P.H.
University of California at San Francisco
San Francisco, CA

Amnon Lahad, M.D., M.P.H.
University of Washington
Seattle, WA

John F. Laurenzo, M.D.
University of Iowa
Iowa City, IA

Donald W. Lewis, D.D.S., D.D.P.H., M.Sc.D., F.R.C.D.C.
University of Toronto
Toronto, Ontario

Alexander G. Logan, M.D., F.R.C.P.C.
Mount Sinai Hospital
Toronto, Ontario

Sarvesh Logsetty, M.D.
Hospital for Sick Children
Toronto, Ontario

Kate Lorig, R.N., Dr.P.H.
Stanford University
Palo Alto, CA

Harriet L. MacMillan, M.D., F.R.C.P.C.
McMaster University
Hamilton, Ontario

James H. MacMillan, M.Sc.
Glaxo Canada, Inc.
Mississauga, Ontario

Alex Malter, M.D., M.P.H.
University of Washington
Seattle, WA

Anne Martell, M.A., C.M.C.
Martell Consulting Services, Ltd.
Halifax, Nova Scotia

Susan E. Moner, M.D.
University of Toronto
Toronto, Ontario

Brenda J. Morrison, Ph.D.
University of British Columbia
Vancouver, British Columbia

Lindsay E. Nicolle, M.D.
University of Manitoba
Winnipeg, Manitoba

David R. (Dan) Offord, M.D.
Chedoke-McMaster Hospitals
Hamilton, Ontario

Christopher Patterson, M.D., F.R.C.P.C.
Chedoke-McMaster Hospitals
Hamilton, Ontario

Diana B. Petitti, M.D., M.P.H.
Kaiser Permanente
Los Angeles, CA

M. Carrington Reid, M.D., Ph.D.
Yale University
New Haven, CT

Carl Rosati, M.D., F.R.C.S.C.
North York Branson Hospital
North York, Ontario

Susan M. Rubin, M.P.H.
University of California at San Francisco
San Francisco, CA

Daniel E. Singer, M.D.
Massachusetts General Hospital
Boston, MA

Steven J. Skates, Ph.D.
Massachusetts General Hospital
Boston, MA

Michael B.H. Smith, M.B., B.Ch., C.C.F.P., F.R.C.P.C.
Dalhousie University
Halifax, Nova Scotia

Walter O. Spitzer, M.D., M.P.H.
McGill University
Montreal, Quebec

Stephen R. Tabet, M.D., M.P.H.
University of Washington
Seattle, Washington

Denise Tonner, M.D.
University of Iowa
Iowa City, IA

Elaine Wang, M.D., C.M., M.Sc., F.R.C.P.C.
Hospital for Sick Children
Toronto, Ontario

Other Contributors to the U.S. Preventive Services Task Force

Hanan S. Bell, Ph.D.
American Academy of Family Physicians
Kansas City, MO

David M. Eddy, M.D., Ph.D.
Kaiser Permanente Medical Care Program
Pasadena, CA

John M. Eisenberg, M.D., M.B.A.
Georgetown University
Washington, DC

Charles M. Goldstein
National Library of Medicine
Bethesda, MD

Sheldon Greenfield, M.D.
New England Medical Center
Boston, MA

Robert S.A. Hayward, M.D., M.P.H.
McMaster University
Hamilton, Ontario

David L. Sackett, M.D., M.Sc.
University of Oxford
Oxford, England

Stephen Thacker, M.D.
Centers for Disease Control and
 Prevention
Atlanta, GA

Staff Members and Others Who Assisted in the Preparation of the *Guide*

Office of Disease Prevention and Health Promotion

James Harrell, M.A., Deputy Director

John C. Bailar III, M.D., Ph.D.

Rachel Ballard-Barbash, M.D., M.P.H.

David Baker

Karil Bialostosky, M.S.

Darla Danford, M.P.H., D.Sc.

Larry L. Dickey, M.D., M.P.H.

Martha Frazier

Walter Glinsmann, M.D.

Marthe Gold, M.D., M.P.H.

Patricia Lacey

Linda Meyers, Ph.D.

Janice T. Radak

Marilyn Schulenberg

Joanna E. Siegel, Sc.D.

Marilyn G. Stephenson, M.S., R.D.

Carla Y. Williams

Jonathan Winickoff, Summer Intern

Preventive Medicine Residents

Barbara Albert, M.D., M.S.
University of Maryland
Baltimore, MD

C. Marlo Baird, M.D., M.P.H.
The Johns Hopkins University
Baltimore, MD

Arthur R. Baker, M.D., M.P.H.
The Johns Hopkins University
Baltimore, MD

Robert Beardall, M.D., M.P.H.
The Johns Hopkins University
Baltimore, MD

Daniel Bleed, M.D., M.P.H.
The Johns Hopkins University
Baltimore, MD

Paul Denning, M.D., M.P.H.
The Johns Hopkins University
Baltimore, MD

S. Patrick Kachur, M.D., M.P.H.
The Johns Hopkins University
Baltimore, MD

Marisa Moore, M.D., M.P.H.
Mayo Clinic
Rochester, MN

Ann S. O'Malley, M.D., M.P.H.
University of Maryland
Baltimore, MD

Peter W. Pendergrass, M.D., M.P.H.
The Johns Hopkins University
Baltimore, MD

Robert Reid, M.D., M.P.H.
The Johns Hopkins University
Baltimore, MD

Donald B. Robinson, M.D., M.P.H.
The Johns Hopkins University
Baltimore, MD

Lynda Sisson, M.D., M.P.H.
Mayo Clinic
Rochester, MN

Natalie J. Smith, M.D., M.P.H.
University of California at Berkeley
Berkeley, CA

Mark S. Smolinski, M.D., M.P.H.
University of Arizona
Tucson, AZ

Craig F. Thompson, M.D., M.S.P.H.
University of Kentucky
Lexington, KY

Mary Jo Trepka, M.D., M.S.P.H.
University of Colorado
Denver, CO

American College of Preventive Medicine (Logistical and administrative support)

Hazel K. Keimowitz, M.A.
Executive Director

Rebecca Kingsley

Emily P. Slough

RII (Logistical support)

Janet E. Meleney, M.A.
Project Manager

Ola Bamgbase

Kirsten Moore

Contents

INTRODUCTION

section one
SCREENING

section three
IMMUNIZATIONS AND CHEMOPROPHYLAXIS

APPENDICES

INTRODUCTION

i. Overview

This report is intended for primary care clinicians: physicians, nurses, nurse practitioners, physician assistants, other allied health professionals, and students. It provides recommendations for clinical practice on preventive interventions—screening tests, counseling interventions, immunizations, and chemoprophylactic regimens—for the prevention of more than 80 target conditions. The patients for whom these services are recommended include asymptomatic individuals of all age groups and risk categories. Thus, the subject matter is relevant to all of the major primary care specialties: family practice, internal medicine, obstetrics-gynecology, and pediatrics. The recommendations in each chapter reflect a standardized review of current scientific evidence and include a summary of published clinical research regarding the clinical effectiveness of each preventive service.

Value of Prevention

Clinicians have always intuitively understood the value of prevention. Faced daily with the difficult and often unsuccessful task of treating advanced stages of disease, primary care providers have long sought the opportunity to intervene early in the course of disease or even before disease develops. The benefits of incorporating prevention into medical practice have become increasingly apparent over the past 30–40 years, as previously common and debilitating conditions have declined in incidence following the introduction of effective clinical preventive services. Infectious diseases such as poliomyelitis, which once occurred in regular epidemic waves (over 18,300 cases in 1954), have become rare in the U.S. as a result of childhood immunization.[1] Only three cases of paralytic poliomyelitis were reported in the U.S. in 1993, and none was due to endemic wild virus. Before rubella vaccine became available, rubella epidemics occurred regularly in the U.S. every 6–9 years; a 1964 pandemic resulted in over 12 million rubella infections, 11,000 fetal losses and about 20,000 infants born with congenital rubella syndrome.[2,3] The incidence of rubella has decreased 99% since 1969, when the vaccine first became available.[4] Similar trends have occurred with diphtheria, pertussis, and other once-common childhood infectious diseases.[1]

Preventive services for the early detection of disease have also been associated with substantial reductions in morbidity and mortality. Age-adjusted mortality from stroke has decreased by more than 50% since 1972, a trend attributed in part to earlier detection and treatment of hypertension.[5–7] Dramatic reductions in the incidence of invasive cervical cancer and in cervical cancer mortality have occurred following the implementation of screening programs using Papanicolaou testing to detect cervical dysplasia.[8] Children with metabolic disorders such as phenylketonuria and congenital hypothyroidism, who once suffered severe irreversible mental retardation, now usually retain normal cognitive function as a result of routine newborn screening and treatment.[9–16]

Although immunizations and screening tests remain important preventive services, the most promising role for prevention in current medical practice may lie in changing the personal health behaviors of patients long before clinical disease develops. The importance of this aspect of clinical practice is evident from a growing literature linking some of the leading causes of death in the U.S., such as heart disease, cancer, cerebrovascular disease, chronic obstructive pulmonary disease, unintentional and intentional injuries, and human immunodeficiency virus infection,[17] to a handful of personal health behaviors. Smoking alone contributes to one out of every five deaths in the U.S., including 150,000 deaths annually from cancer, 100,000 from coronary artery disease, 23,000 from cerebrovascular disease, and 85,000 from pulmonary diseases such as chronic obstructive pulmonary disease and pneumonia.[18] Failing to use safety belts and driving while intoxicated are major contributors to motor vehicle injuries, which accounted for 41,000 deaths in 1992.[17] Physical inactivity and dietary factors contribute to coronary atherosclerosis, cancer, diabetes, osteoporosis, and other common diseases.[19–22] High-risk sexual practices increase the risk of unintended pregnancy, sexually transmitted diseases (STDs), and acquired immunodeficiency syndrome.[23,24] Approximately half of all deaths occurring in the U.S. in 1990 may be attributed to external factors such as tobacco, alcohol, and illicit drug use, diet and activity patterns, motor vehicles, and sexual behavior, and are therefore potentially preventable by changes in personal health practices.[25]

Barriers to Preventive Care Delivery

Although sound clinical reasons exist for emphasizing prevention in medicine, studies have shown that clinicians often fail to provide recommended clinical preventive services.[26–32] This is due to a variety of factors, including inadequate reimbursement for preventive services, fragmentation of health care delivery, and insufficient time with patients to deliver the range of preventive services that are recommended.[33–35] Even when these barriers to implementation are accounted for, however, clinicians fail to perform preventive services as recommended,[28] suggesting that uncertainty among clinicians as to which services should be offered is a factor as well.

Part of the uncertainty among clinicians derives from the fact that recommendations come from multiple sources, and these recommendations often differ. Recommendations[a] relating to clinical preventive services are issued regularly by government health agencies and expert panels that they sponsor,[5,36–42] medical specialty organizations,[43–50] voluntary associations,[51–53] other professional and scientific organizations,[54,55] and individual experts.[56–59]

A second major reason clinicians might be reluctant to perform preventive services is skepticism about their effectiveness. Whether performance of certain preventive interventions can significantly reduce morbidity or mortality from the target condition is often unclear. The relative effectiveness of different preventive services is also unclear, making it difficult for busy clinicians to decide which interventions are most important during a brief patient visit. A broader concern is that some maneuvers can ultimately result in more harm than good. While this concern applies to all clinical practices, it is especially important in relation to preventive services because the individuals who receive these interventions are often healthy. Minor complications or rare adverse effects that would be tolerated in the treatment of a severe illness take on greater importance in the asymptomatic population and require careful evaluation to determine whether benefits exceed risks. This is particularly relevant for screening tests, which benefit only the few individuals who have the disorder but expose all the individuals screened to the risk of adverse effects from the test. Moreover, because recommendations for preventive services such as routine screening often include a large proportion of the population, there are potentially important economic implications.

Historical Perspective

Uncertainties about the effectiveness of clinical preventive services raise questions about the value of the routine health examination of asymptomatic persons, in which a predetermined battery of tests and physical examination procedures are performed as part of a routine checkup. The annual physical examination of healthy persons was first proposed by the American Medical Association in 1922.[60] For many years after, it was common practice among health professionals to recommend routine physicals and comprehensive laboratory testing as effective preventive medicine. While routine visits with the primary care clinician are important, performing the same interventions on all patients and performing them annually are not the most clinically effective approaches to disease prevention. Rather, both the frequency and the

---

[a]The recommendations cited here are illustrative only. Listings of recommendations made by other groups for each condition considered are cited in the relevant chapter.

content of the periodic health examination should reflect the unique health risks of the individual patient and the quality of the evidence that specific preventive services are clinically effective. This new approach to the periodic visit was endorsed by the American Medical Association in 1983 in a policy statement that withdrew support for a standard annual physical examination.[61] The individualized periodic health visit should emphasize evidence of clinical effectiveness, and thus increased attention has turned to the collection of reliable data on the effectiveness of specific preventive services.

One of the first comprehensive efforts to examine these issues was undertaken by the Canadian government, which in 1976 convened the Canadian Task Force on the Periodic Health Examination (CTFPHE). This expert panel developed explicit criteria to judge the quality of evidence from published clinical research on clinical preventive services, and the panel used uniform decision rules to link the strength of recommendations for or against a given preventive service to the quality of the underlying evidence (see Appendix A). These ratings were intended to provide the clinician with a means of selecting those preventive services supported by the strongest evidence of effectiveness. Using this approach, the CTFPHE examined preventive services for 78 target conditions, releasing its recommendations in a monograph published in 1979.[62] In 1982, the CTFPHE reconvened and applied its methodology to new evidence as it became available, periodically publishing revised recommendations and evaluations of new topics. These were updated and compiled in 1994 in *The Canadian Guide to Clinical Preventive Health Care.*[63]

A similar effort began in the U.S. in 1984 when the Public Health Service commissioned the U.S. Preventive Services Task Force (USPSTF). Like the Canadian panel, this 20-member non-Federal panel was charged with developing recommendations for clinicians on the appropriate use of preventive interventions, based on a systematic review of evidence of clinical effectiveness.[64] A methodology similar to that of the CTFPHE was adopted at the outset of the project. This enabled the U.S. and Canadian panels to collaborate in a binational effort to review evidence and develop recommendations on preventive services. The first USPSTF met regularly between 1984 and 1988 to develop comprehensive recommendations addressing preventive services. The panel members and their scientific support staff reviewed evidence and developed recommendations on preventive services for 60 topic areas affecting patients from infancy to old age, published in 1989 as the *Guide to Clinical Preventive Services.*

The Second U.S. Preventive Services Task Force

The USPSTF was reconstituted in 1990 to continue and update these scientific assessments.[65] Its charge has been to evaluate the effectiveness of clinical preventive services that were not previously examined; to reevaluate those that were examined and for which there is new scientific evidence, new technologies that merit consideration, or other reasons to revisit the published recommendations; and to produce this new edition of the *Guide*, with updated recommendations for the periodic health examination. In addition, a continuing mission of the USPSTF has been to define a research agenda by identifying significant gaps in the literature. The USPSTF has 10 members, comprising two family physicians, two internists, two pediatricians, two obstetrician-gynecologists, and two methodologists. Content experts from academic institutions and Federal agencies also joined the deliberations of the panel on an ad hoc basis. The USPSTF met quarterly between September 1990 and April 1994, with scientific support staff from the Office of Disease Prevention and Health Promotion, Public Health Service, U.S. Department of Health and Human Services, to analyze systematically scientific evidence pertaining to clinical preventive services that had been published since the first edition of the *Guide.*

The USPSTF greatly expanded its collaboration with medical specialty organizations and Federal agencies, and it has continued its close cooperation with the CTFPHE. Designated liaisons from primary care medical specialty societies (American Academy of Family Physicians, American Academy of Pediatrics, American College of Obstetricians and Gynecologists, and American College of Physicians), the agencies of the Public Health Service, and the CTFPHE attended all of the USPSTF meetings, and their respective organizations reviewed all draft recommendations. The USPSTF and the CTFPHE, which has also recently updated its analyses of the scientific evidence and recommendations,[63] shared background papers and draft chapters throughout their updating processes to avoid unnecessary duplication of effort. Seventeen chapters in *The Canadian Guide to Clinical Preventive Health Care*[63] were based in part on background papers prepared for the USPSTF, and 21 chapters in this edition of the *Guide* are based in part on papers prepared for the CTFPHE. The USPSTF also collaborated with the American College of Physicians' Clinical Efficacy Assessment Program (CEAP), which uses a similar evidence-based methodology. A liaison from the USPSTF regularly attended CEAP meetings, and several chapter updates were based on reviews prepared for CEAP.

Principal Findings of the U.S. Preventive Services Task Force

The review of evidence for the second edition of the *Guide to Clinical Preventive Services* has produced several important findings. These can be summarized as follows:

• **Interventions that address patients' personal health practices are vitally important.** Effective interventions that address personal health practices are likely to lead to substantial reductions in the incidence and severity of the leading causes of disease and disability in the U.S. Primary prevention as it relates to such risk factors as smoking, physical inactivity, poor nutrition, alcohol and other drug abuse, and inadequate attention to safety precautions holds greater promise for improving overall health than many secondary preventive measures such as routine screening for early disease.[25] Therefore, clinician counseling that leads to improved personal health practices may be more valuable to patients than conventional clinical activities such as diagnostic testing. In the past, the responsibility of the clinician was primarily to treat illnesses; the asymptomatic healthy individual did not need to see the doctor. In addition, personal health behaviors were often not viewed as a legitimate clinical issue. A patient's use of safety belts would receive less attention from the clinician than the results of a complete blood count (CBC) or a routine chest radiograph. A careful review of the data, however, suggests that different priorities are in order. Motor vehicle injuries affect nearly 3.5 million persons each year in the U.S.;[66] they account for over 40,000 deaths each year.[67] Proper use of safety belts can prevent 40–60% of motor vehicle injuries and deaths.[68–70] In contrast, there is little evidence that performing routine CBCs or chest radiographs improves clinical outcome,[71,72] and these procedures are associated with increased health care expenditures.

An important corollary of this finding is that clinicians must assist patients to assume greater responsibility for their own health. In the traditional doctor-patient relationship, the patient adopts a passive role and expects the doctor to assume control of the treatment plan. Whereas the clinician is often the key figure in the treatment of acute illnesses and injuries, the patient is the principal agent in primary prevention that addresses personal health practices. Therefore, one of the initial tasks of the clinician practicing primary prevention is shifting control to the patient. To achieve competence in the task of helping to empower patients and in counseling them to change health-related behaviors, many clinicians will need to develop new skills (see Chapter iv).

• **The clinician and patient should share decision-making.** Many preventive services involve important risks or costs that must be balanced against their possible benefits. Because not all patients weigh risks and benefits the same way, clinicians must fully inform patients about the potential consequences of proposed interventions, including the possibility of invasive follow-up procedures, tests, and treatments. Incorporating patient preferences is especially important when the balance of risks and benefits, and therefore the best decision for each patient, depends greatly on the values placed on possible outcomes (e.g., prolonged life vs. substantial morbidity from treatment). Where evidence suggested that patient values were critical to the balance of risks and benefits (e.g., screening for Down syndrome or neural tube defects, hormone prophylaxis in postmenopausal women), the USPSTF specifically recommended patient education and consideration of patient preferences in decision-making rather than a uniform policy for all patients. Shared decision-making also requires explicitly acknowledging areas of uncertainty. Patients must understand not only what is known, but also what is not yet known about the risks and benefits from an intervention, in order to make an informed decision.

• **Clinicians should be selective in ordering tests and providing preventive services.** Although certain screening tests, such as blood pressure measurement,[73–75] Papanicolaou smears,[8] and mammography,[76] can be highly effective in reducing morbidity and mortality, the USPSTF found that many others are of unproven effectiveness. Screening tests with inadequate specificity often produce large numbers of false-positive results, especially when performed routinely without regard to risk factors; these results might lead to unnecessary and potentially harmful diagnostic testing and treatment. Recognizing the cardinal importance of avoiding harm to asymptomatic patients ("primum non nocere"), the USPSTF recommended against a number of screening tests (e.g., serum tumor markers for the early detection of pancreatic or ovarian cancer) that had unproven benefit but likely downstream harms. Many tests that lack evidence that they improve clinical outcome, such as home uterine activity monitoring, have the additional disadvantage of being expensive, especially when performed on large numbers of persons in the population. In a few instances, the USPSTF found evidence that certain screening tests that have been widely used in the past (e.g., routine chest x-ray to screen for lung cancer, dipstick urinalysis for asymptomatic bacteriuria) are ineffective. Although the USPSTF did not base its recommendations on evidence of cost-effectiveness (see Chapter v), judging health benefit based on scientific evidence provides a rational basis for directing resources toward effective services and away from ineffective services and from interventions for which the balance of benefits and risks is uncertain.[65]

In addition to weighing evidence for effectiveness, selecting appropriate screening tests requires considering age, gender, and other individual risk factors of the patient in order to minimize adverse effects and unnecessary expenditures (see Chapters ii and iii). An appreciation of the risk profile of the patient is also necessary to set priorities for preventive interventions. The need for assessing individual risk underscores a time-honored principle of medical practice: the importance of a complete medical history and detailed discussion with patients regarding their personal health practices, focused on identifying risk factors for developing disease.

• **Clinicians must take every opportunity to deliver preventive services, especially to persons with limited access to care.** Those individuals at highest risk for many preventable causes of premature disease and disability, such as cervical cancer, tuberculosis, human immunodeficiency virus infection, and poor nutrition, are the same individuals least likely to receive adequate preventive services. Devising strategies to increase access to preventive services for such individuals is more likely to reduce morbidity and mortality from these conditions than performing preventive services more frequently on those who are already regular recipients of preventive care and who are often in better health. One important solution is to deliver preventive services at every visit, rather than exclusively during visits devoted entirely to prevention. While preventive checkups often provide more time for counseling and other preventive services, and although healthy individuals might be more receptive to such interventions than those who are sick, any visit provides an opportunity to practice prevention. In fact, some individuals may see clinicians only when they are ill or injured. The illness visit provides the only opportunity to reach individuals who, due to limited access to care, would be otherwise unlikely to receive preventive services.

• **For some health problems, community-level interventions may be more effective than clinical preventive services.** Important health problems that are likely to require broader-based interventions than can be offered in the clinical setting alone include youth and family violence, initiation of tobacco use, unintended pregnancy in adolescents, and certain unintentional injuries. Other types of interventions, such as school-based curricula,[77–81] community programs,[82–84] and regulatory and legislative initiatives,[85–87] might prove more effective for preventing morbidity and mortality from these conditions than will preventive services delivered in the clinical setting. There may, nevertheless, be an important role for clinicians as participants in community systems that address these types of health problems. Such a role might include becoming aware of existing community programs and encouraging patient participation and involvement; acting as a consultant for communities implementing programs or introducing legislation; and serving as an advocate to initiate and maintain effective community interventions.

A Research Agenda in Preventive Medicine

By reviewing comprehensively and critically the scientific evidence regarding clinical preventive services, the USPSTF identified important gaps in the literature and helped define targets for future clinical prevention research. Among the most important of these targets is more and better quality research evaluating the effectiveness of brief, directed counseling that can be delivered in the busy primary care practice setting. Given the importance of personal health practices, the scarcity of adequate evidence evaluating the effectiveness of brief counseling in the primary care setting is striking. The effectiveness of such counseling in reducing smoking and problem drinking is clear.[88–90] For many other behaviors, however, counseling has been tested and proven effective only in highly specialized settings (e.g., STD clinics[91–94]) or when delivered through multiple, lengthy visits with specially trained counselors (e.g., certain cholesterol-lowering interventions[95,96]). Whether the effects of these interventions can be reproduced by brief advice during the typical clinical encounter with a primary care provider is uncertain. Counseling to change some personal health practices (e.g., unsafe pedestrian behavior, drinking and driving) has received insufficient attention by researchers. Some personal health practices may not respond to brief clinician counseling in the context of routine health care. Therefore, research should also evaluate the effectiveness (and cost-effectiveness) of referring patients to allied health professionals with special counseling skills in their areas of expertise (e.g., dietitians, substance abuse counselors) and of using other modalities to educate patients in the primary care setting (e.g., videos, interactive software).

For screening interventions, randomized controlled trials are powerful in resolving controversy about the benefits and risks. Many important questions will be answered by major ongoing screening trials such as the Prostate, Lung, Colorectal, Ovarian Cancer (PLCO) Screening Trial of the National Cancer Institute,[97] and by ongoing trials evaluating the clinical efficacy of treating common asymptomatic conditions detectable by screening, such as high cholesterol levels in the elderly and moderately elevated blood lead levels in children. For unproven screening interventions, finding ways to streamline randomized controlled trials so that they can be performed efficiently and cost-effectively is essential.

Improving the Delivery of Clinical Preventive Services

This report will help resolve some of the uncertainties among primary care clinicians about the effectiveness of preventive services, thus removing one barrier to the appropriate delivery of preventive care. The USPSTF did not, however, address other barriers to implementing clinical preventive services, such as insufficient reimbursement for counseling or other preventive interventions, provider uncertainty about how to deliver recommended services, lack of patient or provider interest in preventive services, and lack of organizational/system support to facilitate the delivery of clinical preventive services. Many of these barriers are addressed by "Put Prevention into Practice," the Public Health Service prevention implementation program.[98] Programs such as "Put Prevention into Practice" can help ensure that prevention is delivered at every opportunity that patients are seen. Other publications also provide useful information on the effective delivery of clinical preventive services.[99] The increasing formation of integrated health care systems (e.g., managed care organizations) may also create new opportunities for crafting better preventive practices.

The USPSTF explored issues of prevention for a wide range of disease categories and for patients of all ages. The comprehensive and systematic approach to the review of evidence for each topic should provide clinicians with the means to compare the relative effectiveness of different preventive services and to determine, on the basis of scientific evidence, what is most likely to benefit their patients. Organizations using evidence-based methodologies to develop guidelines on clinical preventive services are finding broad agreement on a core set of preventive services of proven effectiveness that can be recommended to primary care providers and their patients.[63,100] Basing preventive health care decisions on the evidence of their effectiveness is an important step in the progress of disease prevention and health promotion in the U.S.

The draft update of this chapter was prepared for the U.S. Preventive Services Task Force by Carolyn DiGuiseppi, MD, MPH.

REFERENCES

1. Centers for Disease Control and Prevention. Summary of notifiable diseases, United States, 1993. MMWR 1994;42: 1–74.
2. Witte JJ, Karchmer AW, Case G, et al. Epidemiology of rubella. Am J Dis Child 1969;118:107–111.
3. Orenstein WA, Bart KJ, Hinman AR, et al. The opportunity and obligation to eliminate rubella from the United States. JAMA 1984;251:1988–1994.
4. Centers for Disease Control and Prevention. Rubella and congenital rubella syndrome—United States, January 1, 1991–May 7, 1994. MMWR 1994;43:391, 397–401.
5. Joint National Committee on Detection, Evaluation, and Treatment of High Blood Pressure. The fifth report of the Joint National Committee on Detection, Evaluation, and Treatment of High Blood Pressure. Bethesda: National Institutes of Health, 1993. (Publication no. 93-1088.)
6. Garraway WM, Whisnant JP. The changing pattern of hypertension and the declining incidence of stroke. JAMA 1987;258:214–217.
7. Casper M, Wing S, Strogatz D, et al. Antihypertensive treatment and U.S. trends in stroke mortality, 1962 to 1980. Am J Public Health 1992;82:1600–1606.
8. IARC Working Group. Summary chapter. In: Hakama M, Miller AB, Day NE, eds. Screening for cancer of the uterine cervix. Lyon, France: International Agency for Research on Cancer, 1986:133–144. (IARC Scientific Publication no. 76.)
9. Berman PW, Waisman HA, Graham FK. Intelligence in treated phenylketonuric children: a developmental study. Child Dev 1966;37:731–747.
10. Hudson FP, Mordaunt VL, Leahy I. Evaluation of treatment begun in first three months of life in 184 cases of phenylketonuria. Arch Dis Child 1970;45:5–12.
11. Williamson ML, Koch R, Azen C, et al. Correlates of intelligence test results in treated phenylketonuric children. Pediatrics 1981;68:161–167.
12. Azen CG, Koch R, Friedman EG, et al. Intellectual development in 12-year-old children treated for phenylketonuria. Am J Dis Child 1991;145:35–39.
13. New England Congenital Hypothyroidism Collaborative. Elementary school performance of children with congenital hypothyroidism. J Pediatr 1990;116:27–32.
14. Rovet JF, Ehrlich RM, Sorbara DL. Neurodevelopment in infants and preschool children with congenital hypothyroidism: etiological and treatment factors affecting outcome. J Pediatr Psychol 1992;17:187–213.
15. Kooistra L, Laane C, Vulsma T, et al. Motor and cognitive development in children with congenital

hypothyroidism: a long-term evaluation of the effects of neonatal treatment. J Pediatr 1994;124:903–909.

16. Fuggle PW, Grant DB, Smith I, et al. Intelligence, motor skills and behaviour at 5 years in early-treated congenital hypothyroidism. Eur J Pediatr 1991;150:570–574.

17. Kochanek KD, Hudson BL. Advance report of final mortality statistics, 1992. Monthly vital statistics report; vol 43 no 6 (suppl). Hyattsville, MD: National Center for Health Statistics, 1995.

18. Centers for Disease Control. Cigarette smoking-attributable mortality and years of potential life lost—United States, 1990. MMWR 1993;42:645–649.

19. Centers for Disease Control and Prevention. Public health focus: physical activity and the prevention of coronary heart disease. MMWR 1993;42:669–672.

20. Bouchard C, Shepard RJ, Stephens T, eds. Physical activity, fitness, and health. Champaign, IL: Human Kinetics, 1994.

21. Department of Health and Human Services. The Surgeon General's report on nutrition and health. Washington, DC: Government Printing Office, 1988. (Publication no. DHHS (PHS) 88-50210.)

22. Food and Nutrition Board, National Research Council. Diet and health: implications for reducing chronic disease. Washington, DC: National Academy Press, 1989.

23. Hatcher RA, Trussell J, Stewart F, et al. Contraceptive technology. 16th ed. New York: Irvington Publishers, 1994.

24. Institute of Medicine. AIDS and behavior: an integrated approach. Washington, DC: National Academy Press, 1994.

25. McGinnis JM, Foege WH. Actual causes of death in the United States. JAMA 1993;270:2207–2212.

26. Lewis CE. Disease prevention and health promotion practices of primary care physicians in the United States. Am J Prev Med 1988;4(suppl):9–16.

27. National Center for Health Statistics. Healthy People 2000 review, 1993. Hyattsville, MD: Public Health Service, 1994. (DHHS Publication no. (PHS) 94-1232-1.)

28. Lurie N, Manning WG, Peterson C, et al. Preventive care: do we practice what we preach? Am J Public Health 1987;77:801–804.

29. Montano DE, Phillips WR. Cancer screening by primary care physicians: a comparison of rates obtained from physician self-report, patient survey, and chart audit. Am J Public Health 1995;85:795–800.

30. Dietrich AJ, Goldberg H. Preventive content of adult primary care: do generalists and subspecialists differ? Am J Public Health 1984;74:223–227.

31. Battista RN. Adult cancer prevention in primary care: patterns of practice in Quebec. Am J Public Health 1983;73: 1036–1039.

32. Lemley KB, O'Grady ET, Rauckhorst L, et al. Baseline data on the delivery of clinical preventive services provided by nurse practitioners. Nurs Pract 1994;19:57–63.

33. Logsdon DN, Rosen MA. The cost of preventive health services in primary medical care and implications for health insurance coverage. J Ambul Care Man 1984;46–55.

34. Battista RN, Lawrence RS, eds. Implementing preventive services. Am J Prev Med 1988;4(4 Suppl):1–194.

35. Frame PS. Health maintenance in clinical practice: strategies and barriers. Am Fam Phys 1992;45:1192–1200.

36. Centers for Disease Control. Screening for tuberculosis and tuberculous infection in high-risk populations, and the use of preventive therapy for tuberculous infection in the United States: recommendations of the Advisory Committee for Elimination of Tuberculosis. MMWR 1990;39(RR-8):1–7.

37. Centers for Disease Control and Prevention. Injury control recommendations: bicycle helmets. MMWR 1995;44(RR-1):1–17.

38. Centers for Disease Control and Prevention. General recommendations on immunization: recommendations of the Advisory Committee on Immunization Practices (ACIP). MMWR 1994;43(RR-1):1–38.

39. National Institutes of Health. Early identification of hearing impairment in infants and young children. NIH consensus statement. Bethesda: National Institutes of Health, 1993;11:1–24.

40. National Cholesterol Education Program. Second report of the Expert Panel on Detection, Evaluation, and Treatment of High Blood Cholesterol in Adults. (Adult Treatment Panel II). Bethesda: National Heart, Lung, Blood Institute, National Institutes of Health, 1993.

41. Green M, ed. Bright Futures: guidelines for health supervision of infants, children and adolescents. Arlington, VA: National Center for Education in Maternal and Child Health, 1994.

42. National Cholesterol Education Program. Report of the Expert Panel on Blood Cholesterol Levels in Children and Adolescents. Bethesda: National Heart, Lung, Blood Institute, National Institutes of Health, 1991. (DHHS Publication no. (PHS)91-2732.)

43. American College of Physicians Task Force on Adult Immunization and Infectious Diseases Society of America. Guide for adult immunization. 3rd ed. Philadelphia: American College of Physicians, 1994.

44. Eddy DM, ed. Common screening tests. Philadelphia: American College of Physicians, 1991.

45. American College of Obstetricians and Gynecologists. Standards for obstetric-gynecologic services. 7th ed. Washington, DC: American College of Obstetricians and Gynecologists, 1989.

46. American Medical Association. AMA guidelines for adolescent preventive services (GAPS): recommendations and rationale. Chicago: American Medical Association, 1994.

47. American Academy of Family Physicians. Age charts for periodic health examination. Kansas City, MO: American Academy of Family Physicians, 1994. (Reprint no. 510.)

48. Peter G, ed. 1994 Red Book: report of the Committee on Infectious Diseases. 23rd ed. Elk Grove Village, IL: American Academy of Pediatrics, 1994.

49. Joint Committee on Infant Hearing. 1994 position statement. Pediatrics 1995;95:152–156.

50. American Academy of Ophthalmology. Policy statement. Frequency of ocular examinations. Washington, DC: American Academy of Ophthalmology, 1990.

51. American Cancer Society. Guidelines for the cancer-related checkup, an update. Atlanta: American Cancer Society, 1993.

52. American Diabetes Association. Screening for diabetes. Diabetes Care 1993;16:7–9.

53. American Heart Association. Statement on exercise: benefits and recommendations for physical activity programs for all Americans. Dallas, TX: American Heart Association, 1992.

54. American Optometric Association. Recommendations for regular optometric care. Alexandria, VA: American Optometric Association, 1994.

55. Consensus Development Conference: Diagnosis, prophylaxis, and treatment of osteoporosis. Am J Med 1993;94: 646–650.

56. Frame PS. A critical review of adult health maintenance. Part 1. Prevention of atherosclerotic diseases. J Fam Pract 1986;22:341–346.

57. Frame PS. A critical review of adult health maintenance. Part 2. Prevention of infectious diseases. J Fam Pract 1986;22:417–422.

58. Frame PS. A critical review of adult health maintenance. Part 3. Prevention of cancer. J Fam Pract 1986;22:511–520.

59. Frame PS. A critical review of adult health maintenance. Part 4. Prevention of metabolic, behavioral, and miscellaneous conditions. J Fam Pract 1986;23:29–39.

60. American Medical Association. Periodic health examination: a manual for physicians. Chicago: American Medical Association, 1947.

61. American Medical Association. Medical evaluations of healthy persons. Council on Scientific Affairs. JAMA 1983; 249:1626–1633.

62. Canadian Task Force on the Periodic Health Examination. The periodic health examination. Can Med Assoc J 1979;121:1194–1254.

63. Canadian Task Force on the Periodic Health Examination. Canadian guide to clinical preventive health care. Ottawa: Canada Communication Group, 1994.

64. Lawrence RS, Mickalide AD. Preventive services in clinical practice: designing the periodic health examination. JAMA 1987;257:2205–2207.

65. Sox HC Jr, Woolf SH. Evidence-based practice guidelines from the U.S. Preventive Services Task Force [editorial]. JAMA 1993;269:2678.

66. National Highway Traffic Safety Administration. Traffic safety facts 1992: a compilation of motor vehicle crash data from the Fatal Accident Reporting System and the General Estimates System. Washington, DC: Department of Transportation, 1994. (Publication no. DOT HS 808 022.)

67. National Highway Traffic Safety Administration. Traffic safety facts 1993. Washington, DC: Department of Transportation, 1994. (Publication no. DOT HS 808 169.)

68. Campbell BJ. Safety belt injury reduction related to crash severity and front seated position. J Trauma 1987;27: 733–739.

69. Cooper PJ. Estimating overinvolvement of seat belt nonwearers in crashes and the effect of lap/shoulder restraint use on different crash severity consequences. Accid Anal Prev 1994;26:263–275.

70. Department of Transportation. Final regulatory impact assessment on amendments to Federal Motor Vehicle Safety Standard 208, Front Seat Occupant Protection. Washington, DC: Department of Transportation, 1984. (Publication no. DOT HS 806 572.)

71. Tape TG, Mushlin AI. The utility of routine chest radiographs. Ann Intern Med 1986;104:663–670.

72. Shapiro MF, Greenfield S. The complete blood count and leukocyte differential count. Ann Intern Med 1987;106: 65–74.

73. Collins R, Peto R, MacMahon S, et al. Blood pressure, stroke, and coronary heart disease. Part 2, short-term reductions in blood pressure: overview of randomised drug trials in their epidemiological context. Lancet 1990;335: 827–838.

74. MacMahon SW, Cutler JA, Furberg CD, et al. The effects of drug treatment for hypertension on morbidity and mortality from cardiovascular disease: a review of randomized, controlled trials. Prog Cardiovasc Dis 1986; 29(suppl):99–118.

75. Hebert PR, Moser M, Mayer J, et al. Recent evidence on drug therapy of mild to moderate hypertension and decreased risk of coronary heart disease. Arch Intern Med 1993;153:578–581.

76. Kerlikowske K, Grady D, Rubin SM, et al. Efficacy of screening mammography: a meta-analysis. JAMA 1995;273: 149–154.

77. Hansen WB, Johnson CA, Flay BR, et al. Affective and social influences approaches to the prevention of multiple substance abuse among seventh grade students: results from Project SMART. Prev Med 1988;17:135–154.

78. Abernathy TJ, Bertrand LD. Preventing cigarette smoking among children: results of a four-year evaluation of the PAL program. Can J Public Health 1992;83:226–229.

79. Elder JP, Wildey M, de Moor C, et al. The long-term prevention of tobacco use among junior high school students: classroom and telephone interventions. Am J Public Health 1993;83:1239–1244.

80. Schinke SP, Gilchrist LD, Snow WH. Skills intervention to prevent cigarette smoking among adolescents. Am J Public Health 1985;75:665–667.

81. Botvin GJ, Dusenbury L, Tortu S, et al. Preventing adolescent drug abuse through a multi-modal cognitive-behavioral approach: results of a three-year study. J Consult Clin Psychol 1990;58:437–446.

82. Rivara FP, Thompson DC, Thompson RS, et al. The Seattle children's bicycle helmet campaign: changes in helmet use and head injury admissions. Pediatrics 1994;93:567–569.

83. Schwarz DF, Grisso JA, Miles C, et al. An injury prevention program in an urban African-American community. Am J Public Health 1993;83:675–680.

84. Davidson LL, Durkin MS, Kuhn L, et al. The impact of the Safe Kids/Healthy Neighborhoods injury prevention program in Harlem, 1988 through 1991. Am J Public Health 1994;84:580–586.

85. Erdmann TC, Feldman KW, Rivara FP, et al. Tap water burn prevention: the effect of legislation. Pediatrics 1991;88: 572–577.

86. Walton WW. An evaluation of the Poison Prevention Packaging Act. Pediatrics 1982;69:363–370.

87. Cote TR, Sacks JJ, Lambert-Huber DA, et al. Bicycle helmet use among Maryland children: effect of legislation and education. Pediatrics 1992;89:1216–1220.

88. Kottke TE, Battista RN, DeFriese GH, et al. Attributes of successful smoking cessation interventions in medical practice: a meta-analysis of 39 controlled trials. JAMA 1988;259:2882–2889.

89. Bien TH, Miller WR, Tonigan JS. Brief interventions for alcohol problems: a review. Addiction 1993;88:315–336.

90. Brief interventions and alcohol use. Bulletin 7. Leeds, UK: Effective Health Care, 1993.

91. Cohen DA, Dent C, MacKinnon D, Hahn G. Condoms for men, not women. Sex Transm Dis 1992;19: 245–251.

92. Cohen DA, MacKinnon DP, Dent C, et al. Group counseling at STD clinics to promote use of condoms. Public Health Rep 1992;107:727–731.

93. Heaton CG, Messeri P. The effect of video interventions on improving knowledge and treatment compliance in the sexually transmitted disease setting. Sex Transm Dis 1993;20:70–76.

94. Rickert VI, Gottlieb AA, Jay MS. Is AIDS education related to condom acquisition? Clin Pediatr 1992; 31:205–210.

95. Caggiula AW, Christakis G, Farrand M, et al. The Multiple Risk Factor Intervention Trial (MRFIT). IV. Intervention on blood lipids. Prev Med 1981;10:443–475.

96. The Writing Group for the DISC Collaborative Research Group. Efficacy and safety of lowering dietary intake of fat and cholesterol in children with elevated low-density lipoprotein cholesterol: the Dietary Intervention Study in Children (DISC). JAMA 1995;273:1429–1435.

97. Gohagan JK, Prorok PC, Kramer BS, et al. Prostate cancer screening in the Prostate, Lung, Colorectal, Ovarian Cancer Screening Trial of the National Cancer Institute. J Urol 1994;152:1905–1909.

98. Department of Health and Human Services, Public Health Service, Office of Disease Prevention and Health Promotion. Put Prevention into Practice education and action kit. Washington, DC: Government Printing Office, 1994.

99. Woolf SH, Jonas S, Lawrence RS, eds. Health promotion and disease prevention in clinical practice. Baltimore: Williams & Wilkins, 1995.

100. Hayward RSA, Steinberg EP, Ford DE, et al. Preventive care guidelines: 1991. Ann Intern Med 1991;114:758–783.

ii. Methodology

This report presents a systematic approach to evaluating the effectiveness of clinical preventive services. The recommendations, and the review of evidence from published clinical research on which they are based, are the product of a methodology established at the outset of the project. The intent of this analytic process has been to provide clinicians[a] with current and scientifically defensible information about the effectiveness of different preventive services and the quality of the evidence on which these conclusions are based. This information is intended to help clinicians who have limited time to select the most appropriate preventive services to offer in a periodic health examination for patients of different ages and risk categories. The critical appraisal of evidence is also intended to identify preventive services of uncertain effectiveness as well as those that could result in more harm than good if performed routinely by clinicians.

For the content of this report to be useful, and to clarify differences between the U.S. Preventive Services Task Force recommendations and those of other groups, it is important to understand the process by which this report was developed, as well as how it differs from the consensus development process used to derive many other clinical practice guidelines. First, the objectives of the review process, including the types of preventive services to be examined and the nature of the recommendations to be developed, were carefully defined early in the process. Second, the Task Force adopted explicit criteria for recommending the performance or exclusion of preventive services and applied these "rules of evidence" systematically to each topic it studied. Third, literature searches and assessments of the quality of individual studies were conducted in accordance with rigorous, predetermined methodologic criteria. Fourth, guidelines were adopted for translating these findings into sound clinical practice recommendations. Fifth, these recommendations were reviewed extensively by content experts in the U.S., Canada, Europe, and Australia. Finally, the review comments were examined by the Task Force and a final vote on recom-

---

[a] The provider of preventive services in primary care is often a physician. The term "clinician" is used in this report, however, to include other primary care providers such as nurses, nurse practitioners, physician assistants, and other allied health professionals. Although physicians may be better qualified than other providers to perform certain preventive services or to convince patients to change behavior, some preventive services may be more effectively performed by others with special training (e.g., nurses, dietitians, smoking cessation counselors, mental health professionals).

mendations was conducted. The hallmarks of this process are that it is evidence-based and explicit. Each step is examined in greater detail below.

Definition of Objectives

Systematic rules were used to select the target conditions and candidate preventive interventions to be evaluated by the Task Force.

Selection of Target Conditions. In the first edition of this report, the Task Force identified 60 of the leading causes of death and disability in the U.S. that were potentially preventable through clinical interventions. This second edition examines most of the same conditions but also reviews evidence regarding new topics that were added to the list in recent years. The new topics were selected by a rank-order process in which topics were graded on the basis of the frequency and severity of the disease and the potential impact of preventive interventions on health outcomes. In general, the Task Force judged the importance of candidate topics on the basis of two criteria:

Burden of Suffering from the Target Condition. This report examines conditions that are relatively common in the U.S. and are of major clinical significance. Thus, consideration was given to both the *prevalence* (proportion of the population affected) and *incidence* (number of new cases per year) of the condition. Conditions that were once common but have become rare because of effective preventive interventions (e.g., poliomyelitis) were included in the review.

Potential Effectiveness of the Preventive Intervention. Conditions were excluded from analysis if the panel could not identify a potentially effective preventive intervention that might be performed by clinicians.

A number of important prevention topics have not yet been examined by the Task Force due to resource and time constraints. The absence of a discussion of these topics in this report does not imply a judgment about their relative importance or effectiveness.

Selection of Preventive Services. For each target condition, the Task Force used two criteria to select the preventive services to be evaluated. First, in general, only preventive services carried out on *asymptomatic persons*[b] were

---

[b] The term "asymptomatic person" as used in this report differs from its customary meaning in medical practice. Although "asymptomatic" is often considered synonymous with "healthy," the term is used in this report to describe individuals who lack clinical evidence of the target condition. Signs and symptoms of illnesses unrelated to the target condition may be present without affecting the designation of "asymptomatic." Thus, a 70-year-old man with no genitourinary symptoms who is screened for prostate cancer would be designated asymptomatic for that condition, even if he were hospitalized for (unrelated) congestive heart failure. Preventive services recommended for "asymptomatic patients" therefore need not be delivered only during preventive checkups of healthy persons but apply equally to clinical encounters with patients being seen for other reasons (see Chapter iii).

reviewed. Thus, only primary and secondary preventive measures were addressed. In a clinical setting, *primary preventive measures* are those provided to individuals to prevent the onset of a targeted condition (e.g., routine immunization of healthy children), whereas *secondary preventive measures* identify and treat asymptomatic persons who have already developed risk factors or preclinical disease but in whom the condition has not become clinically apparent. Obtaining a Papanicolaou smear to detect cervical dysplasia before the development of cancer and screening for high blood pressure are forms of secondary prevention. Preventive measures that are part of the treatment and management of persons with clinical illnesses, such as cholesterol reduction in patients with coronary heart disease or insulin therapy to prevent the complications of diabetes mellitus, are usually considered *tertiary prevention* and are outside the scope of this report.

The second criterion for selecting preventive services for review was that the maneuver had to be performed in the *clinical setting*. Only those preventive services that would be carried out by clinicians in the context of routine health care were examined. Findings should not be extrapolated to preventive interventions performed in other settings. Screening tests are evaluated in terms of their effectiveness when performed during the clinical encounter (i.e., *case finding*). Screening tests performed solely at schools, work sites, health fairs, and other community locations are generally outside the scope of this report. Also, preventive interventions implemented outside the clinical setting (e.g., health and safety legislation, mandatory screening, community health promotion) are not specifically evaluated, although clinicians can play an important role in promoting such programs and in encouraging the participation of their patients. References to these types of interventions are made occasionally in sections of this book.

Preventive services were divided into three categories: screening tests, counseling interventions, and immunizations and chemoprophylaxis. *Screening tests* are those preventive services in which a test or standardized examination procedure is used to identify patients requiring special intervention. Nonstandardized historical questions, such as asking patients whether they smoke, and tests involving symptomatic patients are not considered screening tests in this report. *Counseling* interventions are those in which the patient receives information and advice regarding personal behaviors (e.g., diet) that could reduce the risk of subsequent illness or injury. The Task Force did not consider counseling that addresses the health-related behaviors of persons who have already developed signs and symptoms of the target condition. *Immunizations* discussed in this report include vaccines and immunoglobulins (passive immunization) taken by persons with no evidence of infectious disease. *Chemoprophylaxis* as primary prevention refers to the use of drugs or biologics taken by asymptomatic persons to reduce the risk of developing a disease.

Criteria for Determining Effectiveness

Preventive services must meet predetermined criteria to be considered effective. The criteria of effectiveness for the four categories of preventive services (Table 1) provided the analytic framework for the evaluation of effectiveness in the 70 chapters in this report. Each of these criteria must be satisfied to evaluate the "causal pathway"[1] of a preventive service, the chain of events that must occur for a preventive maneuver to influence health outcomes. Thus, a screening test is not considered effective if it lacks sufficient accuracy to detect the condition earlier than without screening or if there is inadequate evidence that early detection improves health outcomes. Similarly, counseling interventions cannot be considered effective in the absence of firm evidence that changing personal behavior can improve outcome and that clinicians can influence this behavior through counseling. Effective immunization and chemoprophylactic regimens require evidence of biologic efficacy; in the case of chemoprophylactic agents, evidence is also necessary that patients will comply with long-term use of the drug.

The methodologic issues involved in evaluating screening tests require further elaboration. As mentioned above, a screening test must satisfy two major requirements to be considered effective:

- The test must be able to detect the target condition earlier than without screening and with sufficient accuracy to avoid producing large numbers of false-positive and false-negative results (*accuracy of screening test*).
- Screening for and treating persons with early disease should improve the likelihood of favorable health outcomes (e.g., reduced disease-specific morbidity or mortality) compared to treating patients when they present with signs or symptoms of the disease (*effectiveness of early detection*).

These two requirements of screening are essential and therefore appear as headings in each of the 53 screening chapters in this report.

Table 1.
Criteria of Effectiveness

Screening tests
- Accuracy of screening tests
- Effectiveness of early detection
Counseling interventions
- Efficacy of risk reduction
- Effectiveness of counseling
Immunizations
- Efficacy of vaccine
Chemoprophylaxis
- Efficacy of chemoprophylaxis
- Effectiveness of counseling

Accuracy of Screening Tests. The "accuracy of a screening test" is used in this report to describe accuracy and reliability. *Accuracy* is measured in terms of two indices: sensitivity and specificity (Table 2). *Sensitivity* refers to the proportion of persons with a condition who correctly test "positive" when screened. A test with poor sensitivity will miss cases (persons with the condition) and will produce a large proportion of *false-negative* results; true cases will be told incorrectly that they are free of disease. *Specificity* refers to the proportion of persons without the condition who correctly test "negative" when screened. A test with poor specificity will result in healthy persons being told that they have the condition (*false positives*). An accepted reference standard ("gold standard") is essential to the empirical determination of sensitivity and specificity, because it defines whether the disease is present and therefore provides the means for distinguishing between "true" and "false" test results.

The use of screening tests with poor sensitivity and/or specificity is of special significance to the clinician because of the potentially serious consequences of false-negative and false-positive results. Persons who receive false-negative results may experience important delays in diagnosis and treatment. Some might develop a false sense of security, resulting in inadequate attention to risk-reducing behaviors and delays in seeking medical care when warning symptoms become present.

Table 2.
Definition of Terms

Term	Definition	Formula[a]
Sensitivity	Proportion of persons with condition who test positive	$\dfrac{a}{a + c}$
Specificity	Proportion of persons without condition who test negative	$\dfrac{d}{b + d}$
Positive predictive value	Proportion of persons with positive test who have condition	$\dfrac{a}{a + b}$
Negative predictive value	Proportion of persons with negative test who do not have condition	$\dfrac{d}{c + d}$

[a]Explanation of symbols

	Condition Present	Condition Absent
Positive test	a	b
Negative test	c	d

Legend:
a = true positive
b = false positive
c = false negative
d = true negative

False-positive results can lead to follow-up testing that may be uncomfortable, expensive, and, in some cases, potentially harmful. If follow-up testing does not disclose the error, the patient may even receive unnecessary treatment. There may also be psychological consequences. Persons informed of an abnormal medical test that is falsely positive may experience unnecessary anxiety until the error is corrected. Labeling individuals with the results of screening tests may affect behavior; for example, studies have shown that some persons with hypertension identified through screening may experience altered behavior and decreased work productivity.[2,3]

A proper evaluation of a screening test result must therefore include a determination of the likelihood that the patient has the condition. This is done by calculating the *positive predictive value* (PPV) of test results in the population to be screened (Table 2). The PPV is the proportion of positive test results that are correct (true positives). For any given sensitivity and specificity, the PPV increases and decreases in accordance with the prevalence of the target condition in the screened population. If the target condition is sufficiently rare in the screened population, even tests with excellent sensitivity and specificity can have low PPV in these settings, generating more false-positive than true-positive results. This mathematical relationship is best illustrated by an example (see Table 3):

> A population of 100,000 in which the prevalence of a hypothetical cancer is 1% would have 1,000 persons with cancer and 99,000 without cancer. A screening test with 90% sensitivity and 90% specificity would detect 900 of the 1,000 cases, but would also mislabel 9,900 healthy persons. Thus, the PPV (the proportion of persons with positive test results who actually had cancer) would be 900/10,800, or 8.3%. If the same test were performed in a population with a cancer prevalence of 0.1%, the PPV would fall to 0.9%, a ratio of 111 false positives for every true case of cancer detected.

Reliability (reproducibility), the ability of a test to obtain the same result when repeated, is another important consideration in the evaluation of screening tests measuring continuous variables (e.g., cholesterol level). A test with poor reliability, whether due to differences in results obtained by different individuals or laboratories (*interobserver variation*) or by the same observer (*intraobserver variation*), may produce individual test results that vary widely from the correct value, even though the average of the results approximates the true value.

Effectiveness of Early Detection. Even if the test accurately detects early-stage disease, one must also question whether there is any benefit to the patient in having done so. Early detection should lead to the implementation of clinical interventions that can prevent or delay progression of the disorder. Detection of the disorder is of little clinical value if the condition is not

Table 3.
Positive Predictive Value (PPV) and Prevalence

Testing Conditions
Size of population = 100,000
Sensitivity of test = 90%
Specificity of test = 90%

Cancer Prevalence = 1%	Cancer Present	Cancer Absent		Cancer Prevalence = 0.1%	Cancer Present	Cancer Absent
Positive test	900	9,900	Positive test		90	9,990
Negative test	100	89,100	Negative test		10	89,910
	PPV = 8.3%				PPV = 0.9%	

treatable. Thus, *treatment efficacy* is fundamental for an effective screening test. Even with the availability of an efficacious form of treatment, *early detection* must offer added benefit over conventional diagnosis and treatment if screening is to improve outcome. The effectiveness of a screening test is questionable if asymptomatic persons detected through screening have the same health outcome as those who seek medical attention because of symptoms of the disease. Studies of the effectiveness of cancer screening tests, for example, can be influenced by lead-time and length biases.

Lead-Time and Length Bias. It is often difficult to determine with certainty whether early detection truly improves outcome, an especially common problem when evaluating cancer screening tests. For most forms of cancer, 5-year survival is higher for persons identified with early-stage disease. Such data are often interpreted as evidence that early detection of cancer is effective, because death due to cancer appears to be delayed as a result of screening and early treatment. Survival data do not constitute true proof of benefit, however, because they are easily influenced by *lead-time bias*: survival can appear to be lengthened when screening simply advances the time of diagnosis, lengthening the period of time between diagnosis and death without any true prolongation of life.[4]

Length bias can also result in unduly optimistic estimates of the effectiveness of cancer screening. This term refers to the tendency of screening to detect a disproportionate number of cases of slowly progressive disease and to miss aggressive cases that, by virtue of rapid progression, are present in the population only briefly. The "window" between the time a cancer can be detected by screening and the time it will be found because of symptoms is shorter for rapidly growing cancers, so they are less likely to be found by screening. As a result, persons with aggressive malignancies will be underrepresented in the cases detected by screening, and the patients found by screening may do better than unscreened patients even if the screening itself does not influence outcome. Due to this bias, the calculated survival of persons detected through screening could overestimate the actual effectiveness of screening.[4]

Assessing Population Benefits. Although these considerations provide necessary information about the clinical effectiveness of preventive services, other factors must often be examined to obtain a broader picture of the potential health impact on the population as a whole. Interventions of only minor effectiveness in terms of *relative risk* may have significant impact on the population in terms of *attributable risk* if the target condition is common and associated with significant morbidity and mortality. Under these circumstances, a highly effective intervention (in terms of relative risk) that is applied to a small high-risk group may save fewer lives than one of only modest clinical effectiveness applied to large numbers of affected persons (see Table 4). Failure to consider these epidemiologic characteristics of the target condition can lead to misconceptions about overall effectiveness.

Potential adverse effects of interventions must also be considered in assessing overall health impact, but often these effects receive inadequate attention when effectiveness is evaluated. For example, the widely held belief that early detection of disease is beneficial leads many to advocate screening even in the absence of definitive evidence of benefit. Some may discount the clinical significance of potential adverse effects. A critical examination will often reveal that many kinds of testing, especially among ostensibly healthy persons, have potential direct and indirect adverse effects. Direct physical complications from test procedures (e.g., colonic perforation during sigmoidoscopy), labeling and diagnostic errors based on test results (see above), and increased economic costs are all potential consequences of screening tests. Resources devoted to costly screening programs of uncertain effectiveness may consume time, personnel, or money needed for other more effective health care services. To the USPSTF, potential adverse effects are considered clinically relevant and

Table 4.
Effective of Mortality Rate on Total Deaths Prevented

Reduction in Mortality with Intervention	Deaths per Year from Target Condition	Total Deaths Prevented with Intervention
50%	10	5
1%	100,000	1,000

are always evaluated along with potential benefits in determining whether a preventive service should be recommended.

Methodology for Reviewing Evidence

In evaluating effectiveness, the Task Force used a systematic approach to collect evidence from published clinical research and to judge the quality of individual studies.

Literature Retrieval Methods. Studies were obtained for review by searching MEDLARS, the National Library of Medicine computerized information system, primarily using MEDLINE (a bibliographic database of published biomedical journal articles); other MEDLARS databases such as AIDS-LINE and CANCERLIT were occasionally used. Searches for some topics involved the PSYCHINFO database and other relevant sources. Searches were generally restricted to English-language publications. Keywords used in the searches are available for most topics. The reference list was supplemented by citations obtained from experts and from reviews of bibliographic listings, textbooks, and other sources. Literature reviews for this report were generally completed by May 1995, and studies published or entered in MEDLARS subsequently are not routinely addressed.

Exclusion Criteria. Many preventive services involve tests or procedures that are not used exclusively in the context of primary or secondary prevention. Sigmoidoscopy, for example, is also performed for purposes other than screening. Thus, studies evaluating the effectiveness of procedures or tests involving patients who are symptomatic or have a history of the target condition were generally not considered admissible evidence for evaluating effectiveness in asymptomatic persons. Such tests were instead considered *diagnostic tests,* even if they were described by investigators as "screening tests." Uncontrolled studies, comparisons between time and place (ecologic or cross-cultural studies, studies with historical controls), descriptive data, and animal studies were generally excluded from the review process when evidence from randomized controlled trials, cohort studies, or case-control studies (see below) was available. *Etiologic evidence* demonstrating a causal relationship between a risk factor and a disease was considered less persuasive than evidence from well-designed *intervention studies* that measure the effectiveness of modifying the risk factor. As mentioned above, studies of preventive interventions not performed by clinicians were generally excluded from review.

Evaluating the Quality of the Evidence. The methodologic quality of individual studies has received special emphasis in this report. Although all types of evidence were considered, greater weight was given to well-designed studies. Studies that examined health outcomes (e.g., measures of morbidity or mortality) were considered more relevant to assessing effectiveness than studies that used intermediate or physiologic outcome measures to infer effectiveness. (Intermediate outcomes, such as changes in blood cholesterol levels, are often associated with, or precede, health outcomes, but their presence or absence does not necessarily prove an effect on health outcomes.) In addition, study designs were given greater weight if they were less subject to confounding (effects on outcomes due to factors other than the intervention under investigation). Three types of study designs received special emphasis: controlled trials, cohort studies, and case-control studies.

In *randomized controlled trials*, participants are assigned randomly to a study group (which receives the intervention) or a control group (which receives a standard treatment, which may be no intervention or a placebo). In this way, all confounding variables, known and unknown, should be distributed randomly and, in general, equally between the study and control groups. Randomization thereby enhances the comparability of the two groups and provides a more valid basis for inferring that the intervention caused the observed outcomes. In a *blinded* trial, the investigators, the subjects, or both (*double-blind study*) are not told to which group subjects have been assigned, so that this knowledge will not influence their assessment of outcome. Controlled trials that are not randomized are more subject to biases, including *selection bias*: persons who volunteer or are assigned by investigators to study groups may differ systematically in characteristics other than the intervention itself, thereby limiting the internal validity and generalizability of the results.

A *cohort study* differs from a clinical trial in that the investigators do not determine at the outset which persons receive the intervention or exposure. Rather, persons who have already been exposed to the risk factor or intervention and controls who have not been exposed are selected by the investigators to be followed *longitudinally* over time in an effort to observe differences in outcome. The Framingham Heart Study, for example, is a large ongoing cohort study providing longitudinal data on cardiovascular disease in residents of a Massachusetts community in whom potential cardiovascular risk factors were first measured nearly 50 years ago. Cohort studies are therefore *observational*, whereas clinical trials are *experimental*. Cohort studies are more subject to systematic bias than randomized trials because treatments, risk factors, and other covariables may be chosen by patients or physicians on the basis of important (and often unrecognized) factors that may affect outcome. It is therefore especially important for investigators to identify and correct for *confounding variables*, related factors that may be more directly responsible for health outcome than the intervention/exposure in question. For example, increased mortality among persons with low body weight can be due to the confounding variable of underlying illness. Unlike randomized controlled trials, a shortcoming of cohort studies is that one can correct only for known confounding variables.

Both cohort studies and clinical trials have the disadvantage of often requiring large sample sizes and/or many years of observation to provide adequate *statistical power* to measure differences in outcome. Failure to demonstrate a significant effect in such studies may be the result of statistical properties of the study design rather than a true reflection of poor clinical effectiveness. Both clinical trials and cohort studies have the advantages, however, of generally being *prospective* in design—the health outcome is not known at the beginning of the study and therefore is less likely to influence the collection of data—and of better collection of data to ensure the comparability of intervention and control groups.

Large sample sizes and lengthy follow-up periods are often unnecessary in *case-control studies.* This type of study differs from cohort studies and clinical trials in that the study and control groups are selected on the basis of whether they have the *disease* (cases) rather than whether they have been *exposed* to a risk factor or clinical intervention. The design is therefore *retrospective,* with the health outcome already known at the outset. In contrast to the Framingham Heart Study, a case-control study might first identify persons who have suffered myocardial infarction (cases) and those who have not (controls) and evaluate both groups to assess differences in exposure to an agent (e.g., aspirin) that purportedly reduces the risk of myocardial infarction. In case-control studies of cancer screening, prior exposure to a cancer screening test is compared between patients with cancer (cases) and those without (controls). Principal disadvantages of this study design are that important confounding variables may be difficult to identify and adjust for, health outcome is already known and may influence the measurement and interpretation of data (*observer bias*), participants may have difficulty in accurately recalling past medical history and previous exposures (*recall bias*), and improperly selected control groups may invalidate conclusions about the presence or absence of statistical associations. Both case-control and cohort studies are subject to selection biases because patients who engage in preventive behaviors (or who are selected by clinicians to receive preventive services) may differ in important ways from the general population.

Other types of study designs, such as ecologic or cross-national studies, uncontrolled cohort studies, and case reports, can provide useful data but do not generally provide strong evidence for or against effectiveness. Cross-cultural comparisons can demonstrate differences in disease rates between populations or countries, but these differences could be due to a variety of genetic and environmental factors other than the variable in question. Uncontrolled studies may demonstrate impressive treatment results or better outcomes than have been observed in the past (historical controls), but the absence of internal controls raises the question of whether the results would have occurred even in the absence of the intervention, perhaps as a result of other concurrent medical advances or changes in case selection. For further background on methodologic issues in evaluating clinical research, the reader is referred to other publications.[4-6]

In summary, claims of effectiveness in published research must be interpreted with careful attention to the type of study design. Impressive findings, even if reported to be statistically significant, may be an artifact of measurement error, the manner in which participants were selected, or other design flaws rather than a reflection of a true effect on health outcome. In particular, the p-value, which expresses the probability that a finding could have occurred by chance, does not account for bias. Thus, even highly significant p-values are of little value when the data may be subject to substantial bias. Conversely, research findings suggesting ineffectiveness may result from low statistical power, inadequate follow-up, and other design limitations. A study with inadequate statistical power may fail to demonstrate a significant effect on outcomes because of inadequate sample size rather than because of the limitations of the intervention.

The quality of the evidence is therefore as important as the results. For these reasons, the Task Force used a hierarchy of evidence in which greater weight was given to those study designs that are, in general, less subject to bias and misinterpretation. The hierarchy ranked the following designs in decreasing order of importance: randomized controlled trials, nonrandomized controlled trials, cohort studies, case-control studies, comparisons between time and places, uncontrolled experiments, descriptive studies, and expert opinion. For each of the preventive services examined in this report, the Task Force assigned "evidence ratings" reflecting this hierarchy using a five-point scale (I, II-1, etc.) adapted from the scheme developed originally by the Canadian Task Force on the Periodic Health Examination (see Appendix A).

Due to resource constraints, the Task Force generally did not perform meta-analysis or decision analysis to examine the data or to synthesize the results of multiple studies. For topics in which these techniques are appropriate, the Task Force encourages other groups to conduct such analyses. Previously published meta-analyses or decision analytic models were reviewed by the Task Force in its examination of the literature but generally did not provide the sole basis for its recommendations unless the quality of the studies and analytic model was high.

Updating the Evidence. Because the first edition of the *Guide* reviewed most of the relevant supporting evidence published before 1989, the Task Force adopted an updating process to identify important evidence and new preventive technologies to address in this edition of the report. Literature review and updating of some topics for which little new evidence had been published since 1989 were conducted off-site at academic medical centers under the supervision of Task Force members. Updating of most other topics was performed by research staff at the Office of Disease Prevention and Health Promotion.

Updating was also coordinated with the Canadian Task Force on the Periodic Health Examination, which used a similar methodology to evaluate the effectiveness of preventive services and produced a report with similar format for its Canadian audience.[7] For a number of topics in which differences in population characteristics were not important, draft chapters developed by the Canadian panel were adapted by the U.S. Task Force for inclusion in this report. The chapters on screening for ovarian cancer and hormone replacement therapy (Chapters 14 and 68, respectively) were based on reviews conducted for the American College of Physicians.

Translating Science into Clinical Practice Recommendations

Recommendations to perform or not perform a preventive service can be influenced by multiple factors, including scientific evidence of effectiveness, burden of suffering, costs, and policy concerns. The recommendations in this report are influenced largely by only one factor, scientific evidence, recognizing that the other factors often need to be considered (see below). Task Force recommendations are graded on a five-point scale (A-E), reflecting the strength of evidence in support of the intervention (see Appendix A). Interventions that have been proved effective in well-designed studies or have demonstrated consistent benefit in a large number of studies of weaker design are generally recommended in this report as "A" or "B" recommendations. Interventions that have been proved to be ineffective or harmful are generally not recommended and are assigned "D" or "E" recommendations. Even when there is no definitive evidence that a preventive service is ineffective, a "D" recommendation may be applied if there is no proven benefit and there is a known risk of complications or adverse effects from the preventive maneuver or from the diagnostic and treatment interventions that it generates. Under these conditions of uncertain benefit and known harm, the Task Force often discourages routine performance in the asymptomatic population but recognizes that future research may later establish a favorable benefit-harm relationship that supports routine performance.

For many preventive services (and much of medical practice), there is insufficient evidence that the maneuver is or is not effective in improving outcomes ("C" recommendation). *This lack of evidence of effectiveness does not constitute evidence of ineffectiveness.* A preventive service can lack evidence and receive a "C" recommendation because no effectiveness studies have been performed. In other cases, studies may have been performed but they may have produced conflicting results. Studies showing no benefit may lack adequate statistical power, making it unclear whether the maneuver would be proved effective if it were tested with a larger sample size. Studies showing a benefit may suffer from other design flaws (e.g., confounding variables) that raise questions about whether the observed effect was due to the experimental intervention or other factors.

In all of these instances, the Task Force gives the preventive service a "C" recommendation, noting that there is insufficient scientific evidence to conclude whether the maneuver should or should not be performed routinely. Practitioners and policy makers often need to consider factors other than science, however, in deciding how to proceed in the absence of evidence. The first of these considerations is potential harm to the patient. In the absence of proven benefit, many would consider the performance of potentially harmful preventive services (e.g., aspirin prophylaxis in pregnancy) to be inappropriate ("primum non nocere"). It may be entirely appropriate, however, to perform preventive services that are essentially harmless if they have a reasonable likelihood of helping the patient (e.g., patient education and counseling). Similar considerations apply to costs. Performing costly preventive services in the absence of evidence (e.g., home uterine activity monitoring for preterm labor) must be viewed differently from inexpensive maneuvers of unproven benefit (e.g., palpating the testicles in young men).

The burden of suffering from the target condition may justify the performance of preventive services, even in the absence of evidence, and similar considerations may apply to an individual patient's risk status. Unproven preventive services that are inappropriate for the general population may be appropriate to consider for individuals at markedly increased risk of the disease. Patient preferences, which are important in all clinical decisions, are essential to consider when contemplating the performance of preventive services of unproven effectiveness. The clinician's responsibility is to provide the patient with the best available information about the potential benefits and harms of the preventive service and to delineate what is known and not known about the probability of these outcomes. Patients can then make informed decisions about which option is appropriate, based on the relative importance that they assign to these outcomes.

These additional considerations account for the different language used by the Task Force in its wording of "C" recommendations. Although all preventive services in the "C" category are identified as having insufficient evidence to recommend for or against the maneuver, the Task Force often adds that arguments for or against the practice can be made on "other grounds." These include the absence of significant harm or cost, the potential of improving individual or public health, legal requirements ("other grounds" *for* performing the preventive service), and concerns that the potential harms and costs of the maneuver outweigh its potential benefits ("other grounds" for *not* performing the preventive service). In some cases, the Task Force maintains a completely neutral position, stating only that there is insufficient evidence to make a recommendation. The statement that "recommendations may be made on other grounds" is intended to call attention to factors that may help guide the clinical practice; *it does not constitute an explicit recommendation of the Task Force that these services be provided or omitted routinely in the absence of evidence of effectiveness.* Individual clinical decisions should be made on a case-by-case basis.

In selected situations, even preventive services of proven efficacy may not be recommended due to concerns about feasibility and compliance. Benefits observed under carefully controlled experimental conditions may not be generalizable to normal medical practice. That is, the preventive service may have proven *efficacy* (effects under ideal circumstances) but may lack *effectiveness* (effects under usual conditions of practice). It may be difficult for clinicians to perform the procedure in the same manner as investigators with special expertise and a standardized protocol. Even in randomized controlled trials, volunteer participants may differ in important respects from the population targeted by clinical preventive measures. The average patient, for example, may be less willing than research volunteers to comply with interventions that lack widespread acceptability. The cost of the procedure and other logistical considerations may make implementation of the recommendation difficult for the health care system without compromising quality or the delivery of other health care services.

Review Process

The Task Force initiated a review process early in the production of this edition by inviting primary care specialty societies and U.S. Public Health Service agencies to appoint liaisons to attend and participate in Task Force meetings. Representatives of the American Academy of Family Physicians, American Academy of Pediatrics, American College of Physicians, and American College of Obstetricians and Gynecologists participated in Task Force discussions and provided expert review by members of their organizations. Similarly, ex officio liaisons of U.S. Public Health Service agencies (Agency for Health Care Policy and Research, Centers for Disease Control and Prevention, National Institutes of Health, etc.) provided access to the expertise of government researchers and databases in examining Task Force documents.

Following this initial review, Task Force recommendations were reviewed by content experts in government health agencies, academic medical centers, and medical organizations in the U.S., Canada, Europe, and Australia. More than 700 experts reviewed recommendations included in this report. Recommendations were modified on the basis of reviewer comments if the reviewer identified relevant studies not examined in the report, misinterpretations of findings, or other issues deserving revision within the constraints of the Task Force methodology. The format of this report was designed in consultation with representatives of medical specialty organizations, including the American Medical Association, the American College of Physicians, the American Academy of Family Physicians, the American Academy of Pediatrics, the American College of Obstetricians and Gynecologists, the American College of Preventive Medicine, the American Dental Association, and the American Osteopathic Association.[8]

Conclusion

Recommendations appearing in this report are intended as guidelines, providing clinicians with information on the proven effectiveness of preventive services in published clinical research. Recommendations for or against performing these maneuvers should not be interpreted as standards of care but rather as statements regarding the quality of the supporting scientific evidence. Clinicians with limited time can use this information to help select the preventive services most likely to benefit patients in selected risk categories (see Chapter iii), but no recommendation can take into account all the factors that influence individual clinical decisions in individual patients. Sound clinical decisions should take into account the medical history and priorities of each patient and local conditions and resources, in addition to the available scientific evidence. Departure from these recommendations by clinicians familiar with a patient's individual circumstances is often appropriate.

The draft update of this chapter was prepared for the U.S. Preventive Services Task Force by Steven H. Woolf, MD, MPH.

REFERENCES

1. Battista RN, Fletcher SW. Making recommendations on preventive practices: methodological issues. Am J Prev Med 1988;4(suppl):53–67.
2. Lefebvre RC, Hursey KG, Carleton RA. Labeling of participants in high blood pressure screening programs: implications for blood cholesterol screenings. Arch Intern Med 1988;148:1993–1997.
3. MacDonald LA, Sackett DL, Haynes RB, et al. Labelling in hypertension: a review of the behavioural and psychological consequences. J Chronic Dis 1984;37:933–942.
4. Sackett DL, Haynes RB, Tugwell P. Clinical epidemiology: a basic science for clinical medicine. Boston: Little, Brown, 1985.

5. Fletcher RH, Fletcher SW, Wagner EH. Clinical epidemiology: the essentials. Baltimore: Williams & Wilkins, 1988.

6. Bailar JC III, Mosteller F, eds. Medical uses of statistics. 2nd ed. Boston: NEJM Books, 1992.

7. Canadian Task Force on the Periodic Health Examination. Canadian guide to clinical preventive health care. Ottawa: Canada Communication Group, 1994.

8. Centers for Disease Control. Chronic disease control activities of medical and dental organizations. MMWR 1988;37: 325–328.

iii. The Periodic Health Examination: Age-Specific Charts

The periodic health visit is an important opportunity for the delivery of clinical preventive services. Identification of specific preventive services that are appropriate for inclusion in the periodic health examination has been one of the principal objectives of the U.S. Preventive Services Task Force project. The process by which these determinations were made is discussed in detail in Chapter ii. This chapter explores the services that were evaluated by the Task Force and are recommended as part of the periodic health examination of the asymptomatic individual. It includes a series of five tables listing specific preventive services that are recommended for patients in different age groups. Conditions that are likely to benefit from early identification but that are not considered appropriate for routine screening are listed in Table 6. Disorders appearing in this table are often overlooked by clinicians due to failure to recognize suggestive signs or symptoms. For example, child abuse may not be diagnosed if physical findings suggestive of abuse are overlooked during routine or symptomatic examinations.[1]

The Task Force judged it especially important to emphasize those preventive services that have been proven to be effective in properly conducted studies, and to tailor the content of the periodic health examination to the individual needs of the patient. This approach is based on the recognition that the limited time afforded to patient encounters may be most constructively used if the clinician focuses on interventions of proven efficacy. The clinician can then choose from among these effective interventions for each patient according to the likeliest causes of illness and injury based on that individual's age, sex, and other risk factors. Thus, the two most important factors to consider are the potential effectiveness of clinical interventions in improving clinical outcomes and the leading causes of mortality and morbidity.

Clinical efforts directed toward promoting health and preventing disease are of limited value if the preventive intervention does not improve outcome. Thus, the major consideration in setting priorities is effectiveness of the intervention. Although suicide and homicide are important causes of death among adolescents, for example, the effectiveness of efforts by primary care clinicians to prevent deaths from intentional injuries has not been established (see Chapters 50 and 59). On the other hand, there are effective measures to reduce the risk of motor vehicle injuries, a leading cause of death in this age group. Proper use of safety belts has been shown to reduce the risk of injury and death from motor vehicle crashes by as much as 40–60%.[2–5] Alcohol intoxication is associated with nearly half of all fatal crashes.[6] With one of three deaths among young persons occurring in motor vehicle crashes,[7] the busy clinician seeing adolescent patients is best advised to direct attention to the use of safety belts and the dangers of driving while under the influence of alcohol, rather than to interventions of unproven effectiveness. For each recommendation in Tables 1–5, the reader is urged to refer to appropriate chapters in the text to obtain detailed information about the scientific rationale.

It is also important to consider the leading causes of morbidity and mortality for patients when establishing priorities for the periodic health examination. For example, a clinician wishing to practice prevention during the few remaining minutes of an office visit with a 56-year-old female might consider a number of different counseling interventions that are effective in changing behavior, such as counseling about reducing dietary fat or avoiding high-risk sexual behavior. A 56-year-old female is considerably more likely to die from cardiac disease than from HIV or other sexually transmitted diseases. For women age 55–64 years in the U.S. during 1993, the death rate due to heart disease was 204/100,000, making it the second leading cause of death. HIV, on the other hand, is not even among the 10 leading causes of death for women of that age group.[7] It seems clear on the basis of mortality data alone that a few minutes with such a patient might be more productively spent by discussing dietary fat. Leading causes of death by age group are provided for each table.

While more difficult to measure than mortality, leading causes of morbidity also should guide the use of preventive services. The adolescent population provides a clear example. Over 60% of gonococcal infections occur in persons under age 25.[8] The prevalence of chlamydial infection is highest among young women age 15–19.[9] Each year in the U.S., about 1 million adolescent females aged 15–19 (about 8–10% of this age group) and nearly 30,000 girls under age 15 become pregnant.[10] Thus, encounters with the adolescent population should target unintended pregnancy and sexually transmitted diseases as important causes of morbidity in this age group. Essential hypertension, neoplasms, and problem drinking account for a large number of office and outpatient department visits in older patients,[11–13] while injuries and poisonings account for 32% of emergency room visits among the general population.[14] Among elderly patients, commonly reported causes of chronic morbidity include visual and hearing impairments.[11]

Individual risk factors are also important to consider in designing the periodic health examination. The leading causes of morbidity and mortality may differ considerably for persons in special high-risk groups as compared to individuals of the same age and sex in the general population. For example, minority children in central cities are 6 times as likely as nonurban non-minority children to have elevated blood lead levels.[15] Therefore, periodic health examinations for members of this high-risk population should include activities to prevent lead exposure, including screening. Injection drug use is also uncommon in the general population, but among individuals with this history, acquired immunodeficiency syndrome (AIDS) is the leading cause of death[16] and hepatitis B is an important cause of morbidity and mortality. Thus, essential preventive interventions in the periodic health examination of an injection drug user are counseling about measures to prevent transmission of HIV and other infectious diseases and immunization against hepatitis B virus. The differences in priorities among individuals in different age groups and risk categories and the varying effectiveness of some preventive services in different populations make it impossible to recommend a uniform periodic health examination for all persons.

Many of the preventive services appearing in Tables 1–5 are recommended only for members of high-risk groups. These are listed separately in the lower half of each table and are grouped by general patient characteristics that broadly define high-risk populations. This organization will help the clinician to identify patients who might be eligible for one or more of the interventions listed. It is crucial, however, to then read the specific high-risk definition indicated by an annotated high-risk (HR) code after each intervention, because patients may share characteristics of the general high-risk grouping without actually meeting the individual high-risk definitions for every intervention within that group. For example, a 23-year-old woman whose high-risk sexual behavior is limited to having two recent sexual partners should be screened for gonorrhea and chlamydia infection, but she may not require screening for syphilis or a hepatitis A vaccine. To avoid providing unnecessary preventive services, clinicians must evaluate carefully whether patients who are potentially at risk meet the specific high-risk definitions for each potential intervention. While nonstandardized historical questions were not evaluated by the Task Force and therefore are not included in the tables, the history and physical examination can be used to identify high-risk individuals who would benefit from targeted interventions. Appropriate chapters in the text provide more detailed guidelines to help identify individuals at increased risk.

Task Force recommendations can be compared with those of other major organizations and government agencies, which are listed in each chapter under the heading *Recommendations of Other Groups*. In addition, the *Clinical Intervention* section contains detailed recommendations and, in many cases, concise information for the clinician on: conditions to remain alert for, anticipatory guidance, currently recommended techniques, drug dosages, and other specifics for performing recommended preventive services. It is not the intent of the *Guide* to supply comprehensive information on how to provide these preventive services. The interested reader is referred to the U.S. Public Health Service's prevention implementation program, "Put Prevention Into Practice,"[17] and to other published sources on the implementation of clinical preventive services.[18]

The preventive services examined in this report and appearing in Tables 1–5 include only those preventive services that might be performed by primary care clinicians on asymptomatic persons in the context of *routine* health care (see Chapter ii). Preventive measures involving persons with signs or symptoms and those performed outside the clinical setting are not within the scope of this report or its recommendations. While the Task Force did not evaluate all components of the physical examination, several specific screening maneuvers that might be performed as part of the physical examination are included if they were considered. The tables are not intended as a complete list of all that should occur during the periodic health examination. Rather, these recommendations encompass those preventive services that have been examined by the Task Force and that have been shown to have satisfactory evidence of clinical effectiveness, based on the methodology discussed in the preceding chapter.

At the same time, the preventive interventions listed are not exhaustive. The periodic health examination performed by most pediatricians, for example, includes a number of maneuvers that were not examined by the Task Force, such as screening for developmental disorders and anticipatory guidance; the interested reader can refer to the recommendations of other groups for further information on such topics.[19–21] Similarly, Task Force recommendations relating to preventive services during pregnancy should not be interpreted as comprehensive guidelines for prenatal care.

Preventive services listed in each table are not necessarily recommended at every periodic visit. For example, although sigmoidoscopy is recommended for persons age 50 and over, it is not recommended annually even though periodic visits in this age group may occur once a year. Where a specific periodicity has been proven effective (e.g., annual fecal occult blood testing in persons 50 years of age and over), this information is included in the footnotes for each table. The Task Force has not attempted to design a periodicity schedule for health supervision visits because for many interventions, evidence of an optimal periodicity is lacking. In addition, periodicity for certain interventions varies with patient characteristics (age, gender, risk factors).

Although the preventive services listed in Tables 1–5 can serve as the basis for designing periodic checkups devoted entirely to health promotion and disease prevention, they may also be performed during visits for other reasons (e.g., illness visits, chronic disease checkups) when indicated. Health maintenance needs to be considered at every visit. For patients with limited access to care, the illness visit may provide the only realistic opportunity to discuss prevention. It is recognized that busy clinicians may not be able to perform all recommended preventive services during a single clinical encounter. Indeed, it is not clear that such a grouping is either necessary or clinically effective. If a sparser, evidence-based protocol is used, health maintenance can frequently be done during acute visits. Patients suffering from an acute illness or injury, however, may not be receptive to some preventive interventions. The clinician must therefore use discretion in selecting appropriate preventive services from these tables and may wish to give special emphasis to those effective interventions aimed at the leading causes of illness and disability in the age group. Recommended preventive services that cannot be performed by the clinician at the current visit should be scheduled for a later health visit.

Immunizations appearing in Tables 1–5 are those recommended on a routine basis and do not apply to persons with special exposures to infected individuals. The reader is referred to Chapter 67 for detailed guidelines on immunizations in such circumstances.

Tables 1–5 do not include interventions for which the Task Force found insufficient evidence on which to base recommendations for or against inclusion in the periodic health examination (i.e., "C" recommendations). The Task Force recognizes that there may be other grounds on which to base a recommendation for or against an intervention when scientific evidence is not available, including patient preference, costs associated with the procedure, the likelihood of benefit or harms from the procedure, and the burden of suffering from the condition. Consideration of these other grounds can guide the clinician in making decisions about the appropriate use of these interventions. The reader is referred to Chapter ii for detailed discussion of the development of "C" recommendations. For many important causes of morbidity and mortality, evidence of effective preventive interventions is lacking. There is a great need for well-controlled, randomized studies with adequate sample sizes to evaluate the effectiveness of preventive interventions for many conditions. Such topics merit attention in the planning of future research agendas.

The draft update of this chapter was prepared for the U.S. Preventive Services Task Force by Ann O'Malley, MD, MPH, and Carolyn DiGuiseppi, MD, MPH.

Table 1. Birth to 10 Years

Interventions Considered and Recommended for the Periodic Health Examination	Leading Causes of Death
	Conditions originating in perinatal period
	Congenital anomalies
	Sudden infant death syndrome (SIDS)
	Unintentional injuries (non-motor vehicle)
	Motor vehicle injuries

Interventions for the General Population

SCREENING
Height and weight [Ch 21]
Blood pressure [Ch 3]
Vision screen (age 3–4 yr) [Ch 33]
Hemoglobinopathy screen (birth)[1] [Ch 43]
Phenylalanine level (birth)[2] [Ch 44]
T_4 and/or TSH (birth)[3] [Ch 45]

COUNSELING
Injury Prevention [Ch 57,58]
Child safety car seats (age <5 yr)
Lap-shoulder belts (age ≥5 yr)
Bicycle helmet, avoid bicycling near traffic
Smoke detector, flame retardant sleepwear
Hot water heater temperature <120–130°F
Window/stair guards, pool fence
Safe storage of drugs, toxic substances, firearms, & matches
Syrup of ipecac, poison control phone number
CPR training for parents/caretakers

Diet and Exercise
Breast-feeding, iron-enriched formula and foods (infants & toddlers) [Ch 22,56]

Limit fat & cholesterol, maintain caloric balance, emphasize grains, fruits, vegetables (age ≥2 yr) [Ch 56]
Regular physical activity* [Ch 55]

Substance Use [Ch 54]
Effects of passive smoking*
Anti-tobacco message*

Dental Health [Ch 61]
Regular visits to dental care provider*
Floss, brush with fluoride toothpaste daily*
Advice about baby bottle tooth decay*

IMMUNIZATIONS [Ch 65]
Diphtheria-tetanus-pertussis (DTP)[4]
Oral poliovirus (OPV)[5]
Measles-mumps-rubella (MMR)[6]
H. influenzae type b (Hib) conjugate[7]
Hepatitis B[8]
Varicella[9]

CHEMOPROPHYLAXIS
Ocular prophylaxis (birth) [Ch 27]

Interventions for High-Risk Populations

POPULATION	POTENTIAL INTERVENTIONS (See detailed high-risk definitions)
Preterm or low birth weight	Hemoglobin/hematocrit (HR1)
Infants of mothers at risk for HIV	HIV testing (HR2)
Low income; immigrants	Hemoglobin/hematocrit (HR1); PPD (HR3)
TB contacts	PPD (HR3)
Native American/Alaska Native	Hemoglobin/hematocrit (HR1); PPD (HR3); hepatitis A vaccine (HR4); pneumococcal vaccine (HR5)
Travelers to developing countries	Hepatitis A vaccine (HR4)
Residents of long-term care facilities	PPD (HR3); hepatitis A vaccine (HR4); influenza vaccine (HR6)
Certain chronic medical conditions	PPD (HR3); pneumococcal vaccine (HR5); influenza vaccine (HR6)
Increased individual or community lead exposure	Blood lead level (HR7)
Inadequate water fluoridation	Daily fluoride supplement (HR8)
Family h/o skin cancer; nevi; fair skin, eyes, hair	Avoid excess/midday sun, use protective clothing* (HR9)

[1]Whether screening should be universal or targeted to high-risk groups will depend on the proportion of high-risk individuals in the screening area, and other considerations (see Ch. 43). [2]If done during first 24 hr of life, repeat by age 2 wk. [3]Optimally between day 2 and 6, but in all cases before newborn nursery discharge. [4]2, 4, 6, and 12–18 mo; once between ages 4–6 yr (DTaP may be used at 15 mo and older). [5]2, 4, 6–18 mo; once between ages 4–6 yr. [6]12–15 mo and 4–6 yr. [7]2, 4, 6 and 12–15 mo; no dose needed at 6 mo if PRP-OMP vaccine is used for first 2 doses. [8]Birth, 1 mo, 6 mo; or, 0–2 mo, 1–2 mo later, and 6–18 mo. If not done in infancy: current visit, and 1 and 6 mo later. [9]12–18 mo; or older child without hx of chickenpox or previous immunization. Include information on risk in adulthood, duration of immunity, and potential need for booster doses.

*The ability of clinician counseling to influence this behavior is unproven.

HR1 = Infants age 6–12 mo who are: living in poverty, black, Native American or Alaska Native, immigrants from developing countries, preterm or low birth weight infants, or infants whose principal dietary intake is unfortified cow's milk (see Ch. 22).

HR2 = Infants born to high-risk mothers whose HIV status is unknown. Women at high risk include: past or present injection drug use; persons who exchange sex for money or drugs, and their sex partners; injection drug-using, bisexual, or HIV-positive sex partners currently or in past; persons seeking treatment for STDs; blood transfusion during 1978–1985 (see Ch. 28).

HR3 = Persons infected with HIV, close contacts of persons with known or suspected TB, persons with medical risk factors associated with TB, immigrants from countries with high TB prevalence, medically underserved low-income populations (including homeless), residents of long-term care facilities (see Ch. 25). See Ch. 25 for indications for BCG vaccine.

HR4 = Persons ≥2 yr living in or traveling to areas where the disease is endemic and where periodic outbreaks occur (e.g., countries with high or intermediate endemicity; certain Alaska Native, Pacific Island, Native American, and religious communities). Consider for institutionalized children aged ≥2 yr. Clinicians should also consider local epidemiology (see Ch. 65–67).

HR5 = Immunocompetent persons ≥2 yr with certain medical conditions, including chronic cardiac or pulmonary disease, diabetes mellitus, and anatomic asplenia. Immunocompetent persons ≥2 yr living in high-risk environments or social settings (e.g., certain Native American and Alaska Native populations) (see Ch. 66).

HR6 = Annual vaccination of children ≥6 mo who are residents of chronic care facilities or who have chronic cardiopulmonary disorders, metabolic diseases (including diabetes mellitus), hemoglobinopathies, immunosuppression, or renal dysfunction (see Ch. 66). See Ch. 66 for indications for amantadine/rimantadine prophylaxis.

HR7 = Children about age 12 mo who: 1) live in communities in which the prevalence of lead levels requiring individual intervention, including residential lead hazard control or chelation, is high or undefined; 2) live in or frequently visit a home built before 1950 with dilapidated paint or with recent or ongoing renovation or remodeling; 3) have close contact with a person who has an elevated lead level; 4) live near lead industry or heavy traffic; 5) live with someone whose job or hobby involves lead exposure; 6) use lead-based pottery; or 7) take traditional ethnic remedies that contain lead (see Ch. 23).

HR8 = Children living in areas with inadequate water fluoridation (<0.6 ppm) (see Ch. 61).

HR9 = Persons with a family history of skin cancer, a large number of moles, atypical moles, poor tanning ability, or light skin, hair, and eye color (see Ch. 12).

Table 2. Ages 11–24 Years

Interventions Considered and Recommended for the Periodic Health Examination	Leading Causes of Death
	Motor vehicle/other unintentional injuries
	Homicide
	Suicide
	Malignant neoplasms
	Heart diseases

Interventions for the General Population

SCREENING
Height & weight [Ch 21]
Blood pressure[1] [Ch 3]
Papanicolaou (Pap) test[2] (females) [Ch 9]
Chlamydia screen[3] (females <20 yr) [Ch 29]
Rubella serology or vaccination hx[4] (females >12 yr) [Ch 32]
Assess for problem drinking [Ch 52]

COUNSELING
Injury Prevention [Ch 57,58]
Lap/shoulder belts
Bicycle/motorcycle/ATV helmets*
Smoke detector*
Safe storage/removal of firearms* [Ch 50,59]

Substance Use
Avoid tobacco use [Ch 54]
Avoid underage drinking & illicit drug use* [Ch 52,53]
Avoid alcohol/drug use while driving, swimming, boating,etc.* [Ch 57,58]

Sexual Behavior [Ch 62,63]
STD prevention: abstinence;* avoid high-risk behavior;* condoms/female barrier with spermicide*
Unintended pregnancy: contraception

Diet and Exercise
Limit fat & cholesterol; maintain caloric balance; emphasize grains, fruits, vegetables [Ch 56]
Adequate calcium intake (females) [Ch 56]
Regular physical activity* [Ch 55]

Dental Health [Ch 61]
Regular visits to dental care provider*
Floss, brush with fluoride toothpaste daily*

IMMUNIZATIONS [Ch 65,66]
Tetanus-diphtheria (Td) boosters (11–16 yr)
Hepatitis B[5]
MMR (11–12 yr)[6]
Varicella (11–12 yr)[7]
Rubella[4] (females >12 yr) [Ch 32]

CHEMOPROPHYLAXIS
Multivitamin with folic acid (females planning/capable of pregnancy) [Ch 42]

Interventions for High-Risk Populations

POPULATION	POTENTIAL INTERVENTIONS (See detailed high-risk definitions)
High-risk sexual behavior	RPR/VDRL (HR1); screen for gonorrhea (female) (HR2), HIV (HR3), chlamydia (female) (HR4); hepatitis A vaccine (HR5)
Injection or street drug use	RPR/VDRL (HR1); HIV screen (HR3); hepatitis A vaccine (HR5); PPD (HR6); advice to reduce infection risk (HR7)
TB contacts; immigrants; low income	PPD (HR6)
Native Americans/Alaska Natives	Hepatitis A vaccine (HR5); PPD (HR6); pneumococcal vaccine (HR8)
Travelers to developing countries	Hepatitis A vaccine (HR5)
Certain chronic medical conditions	PPD (HR6); pneumococcal vaccine (HR8); influenza vaccine (HR9)
Settings where adolescents and young adults congregate	Second MMR (HR10)
Susceptible to varicella, measles, mumps	Varicella vaccine (HR11); MMR (HR12)
Blood transfusion between 1978–1985	HIV screen (HR3)
Institutionalized persons; health care/lab workers	Hepatitis A vaccine (HR5); PPD (HR6); influenza vaccine (HR9)
Family h/o skin cancer; nevi; fair skin, eyes, hair	Avoid excess/midday sun, use protective clothing* (HR13)
Prior pregnancy with neural tube defect	Folic acid 4.0 mg (HR14)
Inadequate water fluoridation	Daily fluoride supplement (HR15)

[1]Periodic BP for persons aged ≥21 yr. [2]If sexually active at present or in the past: q ≤ 3 yr. If sexual history is unreliable, begin Pap tests at age 18 yr. [3]If sexually active. [4]Serologic testing, documented vaccination history, and routine vaccination against rubella (preferably with MMR) are equally acceptable alternatives. [5]If not previously immunized: current visit, 1 and 6 mo later. [6]If no previous second dose of MMR. [7]If susceptible to chickenpox.

*The ability of clinician counseling to influence this behavior is unproven.

HR1 = Persons who exchange sex for money or drugs, and their sex partners; persons with other STDs (including HIV); and sexual contacts of persons with active syphilis. Clinicians should also consider local epidemiology (see Ch. 26).

HR2 = Females who have: two or more sex partners in the last year; a sex partner with multiple sexual contacts; exchanged sex for money or drugs; or a history of repeated episodes of gonorrhea. Clinicians should also consider local epidemiology (see Ch. 27).

HR3 = Males who had sex with males after 1975; past or present injection drug use; persons who exchange sex for money or drugs, and their sex partners; injection drug-using, bisexual, or HIV-positive sex partner currently or in the past; blood transfusion during 1978–1985; persons seeking treatment for STDs. Clinicians should also consider local epidemiology (see Ch. 28).

HR4 = Sexually active females with multiple risk factors including: history of prior STD; new or multiple sex partners; age under 25; nonuse or inconsistent use of barrier contraceptives; cervical ectopy. Clinicians should consider local epidemiology of the disease in identifying other high-risk groups (see Ch. 29).

HR5 = Persons living in, traveling to, or working in areas where the disease is endemic and where periodic outbreaks occur (e.g., countries with high or intermediate endemicity; certain Alaska Native, Pacific Island, Native American, and religious communities); men who have sex with men; injection or street drug users. Vaccine may be considered for institutionalized persons and workers in these institutions, military personnel, and day-care, hospital, and laboratory workers. Clinicians should also consider local epidemiology (see Ch. 66, 67).

HR6 = HIV positive, close contacts of persons with known or suspected TB, health care workers, persons with medical risk factors associated with TB, immigrants from countries with high TB prevalence, medically underserved low-income populations (including homeless), alcoholics, injection drug users, and residents of long-term care facilities (see Ch. 25). See Ch. 25 for indications for BCG vaccine.

HR7 = Persons who continue to inject drugs (see Ch. 53).

HR8 = Immunocompetent persons with certain medical conditions, including chronic cardiac or pulmonary disease, diabetes mellitus, and anatomic asplenia. Immunocompetent persons who live in high-risk environments or social settings (e.g., certain Native American and Alaska Native populations) (see Ch. 66).

HR9 = Annual vaccination of: residents of chronic care facilities; persons with chronic cardiopulmonary disorders, metabolic diseases (including diabetes mellitus), hemoglobinopathies, immunosuppression, or renal dysfunction; and health care providers for high-risk patients (see Ch. 66). See Ch. 66 for indications for amantadine/rimantadine prophylaxis.

HR10 = Adolescents and young adults in settings where such individuals congregate (e.g., high schools and colleges), if they have not previously received a second dose (see Ch. 65, 66).

HR11 = Healthy persons aged ≥13 yr without a history of chickenpox or previous immunization. Consider serologic testing for presumed susceptible persons aged ≥13 yr (see Ch. 65, 66).

HR12 = Persons born after 1956 who lack evidence of immunity to measles or mumps (e.g., documented receipt of live vaccine on or after the first birthday, laboratory evidence of immunity, or a history of physician-diagnosed measles or mumps) (see Ch. 65, 66).

HR13 = Persons with a family or personal history of skin cancer, a large number of moles, atypical moles, poor tanning ability, or light skin, hair, and eye color (see Ch. 12).

HR14 = Women with prior pregnancy affected by neural tube defect who are planning pregnancy (see Ch. 42).

HR15 = Persons aged <17 yr living in areas with inadequate water fluoridation (<0.6 ppm) (see Ch. 61).

Table 3. Ages 25–64 Years

Interventions Considered and Recommended for the Periodic Health Examination	Leading Causes of Death
	Malignant neoplasms
	Heart diseases
	Motor vehicle and other unintentional injuries
	Human immunodeficiency virus (HIV) infection
	Suicide and homicide

Interventions for the General Population

SCREENING
Blood pressure [Ch 3]
Height and weight [Ch 21]
Total blood cholesterol (men ages 35–65, women ages 45–65) [Ch 2]
Papanicolaou (Pap) test (women)[1] [Ch 9]
Fecal occult blood test[2] and/or sigmoidoscopy (≥50 yr) [Ch 8]
Mammogram ± clinical breast exam[3] (women 50–69 yr) [Ch 7]
Assess for problem drinking [Ch 52]
Rubella serology or vaccination hx[4] (women of childbearing age) [Ch 32]

COUNSELING

Substance Use
Tobacco cessation [Ch 54]
Avoid alcohol/drug use while driving, swimming, boating, etc.* [Ch 57,58]

Diet and Exercise
Limit fat & cholesterol; maintain caloric balance; emphasize grains, fruits, vegetables [Ch 56]
Adequate calcium intake (women) [Ch 56]

Regular physical activity* [Ch 55]

Injury Prevention [Ch 57,58]
Lap/shoulder belts
Motorcycle/bicycle/ATV helmets*
Smoke detector*
Safe storage/removal of firearms* [Ch 50,59]

Sexual Behavior [Ch 62,63]
STD prevention: avoid high-risk behavior;* condoms/female barrier with spermicide *
Unintended pregnancy: contraception

Dental Health [Ch 61]
Regular visits to dental care provider*
Floss, brush with fluoride toothpaste daily*

IMMUNIZATIONS [Ch 32,66]
Tetanus-diphtheria (Td) boosters
Rubella[4] (women of childbearing age)

CHEMOPROPHYLAXIS
Multivitamin with folic acid (women planning or capable of pregnancy) [Ch 42]
Discuss hormone prophylaxis (peri- and postmenopausal women) [Ch 68]

Interventions for High-Risk Populations

POPULATION	POTENTIAL INTERVENTIONS (See detailed high-risk definitions)
High-risk sexual behavior	RPR/VDRL (HR1); screen for gonorrhea (female) (HR2), HIV (HR3), chlamydia (female) (HR4); hepatitis B vaccine (HR5); hepatitis A vaccine (HR6)
Injection or street drug use	RPR/VDRL (HR1); HIV screen (HR3); hepatitis B vaccine (HR5); hepatitis A vaccine (HR6); PPD (HR7); advice to reduce infection risk (HR8)
Low income; TB contacts; immigrants; alcoholics	PPD (HR7)
Native Americans/Alaska Natives	Hepatitis A vaccine (HR6); PPD (HR7); pneumococcal vaccine (HR9)
Travelers to developing countries	Hepatitis B vaccine (HR5); hepatitis A vaccine (HR6)
Certain chronic medical conditions	PPD (HR7); pneumococcal vaccine (HR9); influenza vaccine (HR10)
Blood product recipients	HIV screen (HR3); hepatitis B vaccine (HR5)
Susceptible to measles, mumps, or varicella	MMR (HR11); varicella vaccine (HR12)
Institutionalized persons	Hepatitis A vaccine (HR6); PPD (HR7); pneumococcal vaccine (HR9); influenza vaccine (HR10)
Health care/lab workers	Hepatitis B vaccine (HR5); hepatitis A vaccine (HR6); PPD (HR7); influenza vaccine (HR10)
Family h/o skin cancer; fair skin, eyes, hair	Avoid excess/midday sun, use protective clothing* (HR13)
Previous pregnancy with neural tube defect	Folic acid 4.0 mg (HR14)

---

[1]Women who are or have been sexually active and who have a cervix: q ≤ 3 yr. [2]Annually. [3]Mammogram q1–2 yr, or mammogram q1–2 yr with annual clinical breast examination. [4]Serologic testing, documented vaccination history, and routine vaccination (preferably with MMR) are equally acceptable alternatives.

*The ability of clinician counseling to influence this behavior is unproven.

HR1 = Persons who exchange sex for money or drugs, and their sex partners; persons with other STDs (including HIV); and sexual contacts of persons with active syphilis. Clinicians should also consider local epidemiology (see Ch. 26).

HR2 = Women who exchange sex for money or drugs, or who have had repeated episodes of gonorrhea. Clinicians should also consider local epidemiology (see Ch. 27).

HR3 = Men who had sex with men after 1975; past or present injection drug use; persons who exchange sex for money or drugs, and their sex partners; injection drug-using, bisexual, or HIV-positive sex partner currently or in the past; blood transfusion during 1978–1985; persons seeking treatment for STDs. Clinicians should also consider local epidemiology (see Ch. 28).

HR4 = Sexually active women with multiple risk factors including: history of STD; new or multiple sex partners; nonuse or inconsistent use of barrier contraceptives; cervical ectopy. Clinicians should also consider local epidemiology (see Ch. 29).

HR5 = Blood product recipients (including hemodialysis patients), persons with frequent occupational exposure to blood or blood products, men who have sex with men, injection drug users and their sex partners, persons with multiple recent sex partners, persons with other STDs (including HIV), travelers to countries with endemic hepatitis B (see Ch. 66).

HR6 = Persons living in, traveling to, or working in areas where the disease is endemic and where periodic outbreaks occur (e.g., countries with high or intermediate endemicity; certain Alaska Native, Pacific Island, Native American, and religious communities); men who have sex with men; injection or street drug users. Consider for institutionalized persons and workers in these institutions, military personnel, and day-care, hospital, and laboratory workers. Clinicians should also consider local epidemiology (see Ch. 66, 67).

HR7 = HIV positive, close contacts of persons with known or suspected TB, health care workers, persons with medical risk factors associated with TB, immigrants from countries with high TB prevalence, medically underserved low-income populations (including homeless), alcoholics, injection drug users, and residents of long-term care facilities (see Ch. 25). See Ch. 25 for indications for BCG vaccine.

HR8 = Persons who continue to inject drugs (see Ch. 53).

HR9 = Immunocompetent institutionalized persons aged ≥50 yr and immunocompetent persons with certain medical conditions, including chronic cardiac or pulmonary disease, diabetes mellitus, and anatomic asplenia. Immunocompetent persons who live in high-risk environments or social settings (e.g., certain Native American and Alaska Native populations) (see Ch. 66).

HR10 = Annual vaccination of residents of chronic care facilities; persons with chronic cardiopulmonary disorders, metabolic diseases (including diabetes mellitus), hemoglobinopathies, immunosuppression, or renal dysfunction; and health care providers for high-risk patients (Ch. 66). See Ch. 66 for indications for amantadine/rimantadine prophylaxis.

HR11 = Persons born after 1956 who lack evidence of immunity to measles or mumps (e.g., documented receipt of live vaccine on or after the first birthday, laboratory evidence of immunity, or a history of physician-diagnosed measles or mumps) (see Ch. 66).

HR12 = Healthy adults without a history of chickenpox or previous immunization. Consider serologic testing for presumed susceptible adults (see Ch. 65, 66).

HR13 = Persons with a family or personal history of skin cancer, a large number of moles, atypical moles, poor tanning ability, or light skin, hair, and eye color (see Ch. 12).

HR14 = Women with previous pregnancy affected by neural tube defect who are planning pregnancy (see Ch. 42).

Table 4. Age 65 and Older

Interventions Considered and Recommended for the Periodic Health Examination	Leading Causes of Death
	Heart diseases
	Malignant neoplasms (lung, colorectal, breast)
	Cerebrovascular disease
	Chronic obstructive pulmonary disease
	Pneumonia and influenza

Interventions for the **General** Population

SCREENING
Blood pressure [Ch 3]
Height and weight [Ch 21]
Fecal occult blood test[1] and/or
   sigmoidoscopy [Ch 8]
Mammogram ± clinical breast exam[2]
   (women ≤69 yr) [Ch 7]
Papanicolaou (Pap) test (women)[3] [Ch 9]
Vision screening [Ch 33]
Assess for hearing impairment [Ch 35]
Assess for problem drinking [Ch 52]

COUNSELING

Substance Use
Tobacco cessation [Ch 54]
Avoid alcohol/drug use while driving,
   swimming, boating, etc.* [Ch 57,58]

Diet and Exercise
Limit fat & cholesterol; maintain caloric
   balance; emphasize grains, fruits,
   vegetables [Ch 56]
Adequate calcium intake (women) [Ch 56]
Regular physical activity* [Ch 55,58]

Injury Prevention [Ch 57,58]
Lap/shoulder belts
Motorcycle and bicycle helmets*
Fall prevention*
Safe storage/removal of firearms* [Ch 50,59]
Smoke detector*
Set hot water heater to <120–130°F*
CPR training for household members

Dental Health [Ch 61]
Regular visits to dental care provider*
Floss, brush with fluoride toothpaste daily*

Sexual Behavior
STD prevention: avoid high-risk sexual
   behavior;* use condoms* [Ch 62]

IMMUNIZATIONS [Ch 66]
Pneumococcal vaccine
Influenza[1]
Tetanus-diphtheria (Td) boosters

CHEMOPROPHYLAXIS
Discuss hormone prophylaxis (women)
   [Ch 68]

Interventions for High-Risk Populations

POPULATION	POTENTIAL INTERVENTIONS (See detailed high-risk definitions)
Institutionalized persons	PPD (HR1); hepatitis A vaccine (HR2); amantadine/rimantadine (HR4)
Chronic medical conditions; TB contacts; low income; immigrants; alcoholics	PPD (HR1)
Persons ≥75 yr; or ≥70 yr with risk factors for falls	Fall prevention intervention (HR5)
Cardiovascular disease risk factors	Consider cholesterol screening (HR6)
Family h/o skin cancer; nevi; fair skin, eyes, hair	Avoid excess/midday sun, use protective clothing* (HR7)
Native Americans/Alaska Natives	PPD (HR1); hepatitis A vaccine (HR2)
Travelers to developing countries	Hepatitis A vaccine (HR2); hepatitis B vaccine (HR8)
Blood product recipients	HIV screen (HR3); hepatitis B vaccine (HR8)
High-risk sexual behavior	Hepatitis A vaccine (HR2); HIV screen (HR3); hepatitis B vaccine (HR8); RPR/VDRL (HR9)
Injection or street drug use	PPD (HR1); hepatitis A vaccine (HR2); HIV screen (HR3); hepatitis B vaccine (HR8); RPR/VDRL (HR9); advice to reduce infection risk (HR10)
Health care/lab workers	PPD (HR1); hepatitis A vaccine (HR2); amantadine/rimantadine (HR4); hepatitis B vaccine (HR8)
Persons susceptible to varicella	Varicella vaccine (HR11)

[1]Annually. [2]Mammogram q1–2 yr, or mammogram q1–2 yr with annual clinical breast exam. [3]All women who are or have been sexually active and who have a cervix: q≤3 yr. Consider discontinuation of testing after age 65 yr if previous regular screening with consistently normal results.

*The ability of clinician counseling to influence this behavior is unproven.

HR1 = HIV positive, close contacts of persons with known or suspected TB, health care workers, persons with medical risk factors associated with TB, immigrants from countries with high TB prevalence, medically underserved low-income populations (including homeless), alcoholics, injection drug users, and residents of long-term care facilities (see Ch. 25). See Ch. 25 for indications for BCG vaccine.

HR2 = Persons living in, traveling to, or working in areas where the disease is endemic and where periodic outbreaks occur (e.g., countries with high or intermediate endemicity; certain Alaska Native, Pacific Island, Native American, and religious communities); men who have sex with men; injection or street drug users. Consider for institutionalized persons and workers in these institutions, and day-care, hospital, and laboratory workers. Clinicians should also consider local epidemiology (see Ch. 66, 67).

HR3 = Men who had sex with men after 1975; past or present injection drug use; persons who exchange sex for money or drugs, and their sex partners; injection drug-using, bisexual, or HIV-positive sex partner currently or in the past; blood transfusion during 1978–1985; persons seeking treatment for STDs. Clinicians should also consider local epidemiology (see Ch. 28).

HR4 = Consider for persons who have not received influenza vaccine or are vaccinated late; when the vaccine may be ineffective due to major antigenic changes in the virus; for unvaccinated persons who provide home care for high-risk persons; to supplement protection provided by vaccine in persons who are expected to have a poor antibody response; and for high-risk persons in whom the vaccine is contraindicated (see Ch. 66).

HR5 = Persons aged 75 years and older; or aged 70–74 with one or more additional risk factors including: use of certain psychoactive and cardiac medications (e.g., benzodiazepines, antihypertensives); use of ≥4 prescription medications; impaired cognition, strength, balance, or gait. Intensive individualized home-based multifactorial fall prevention intervention is recommended in settings where adequate resources are available to deliver such services (see Ch. 58).

HR6 = Although evidence is insufficient to recommend routine screening in elderly persons, clinicians should consider cholesterol screening on a case-by-case basis for persons ages 65–75 with additional risk factors (e.g., smoking, diabetes, or hypertension) (see Ch. 2).

HR7 = Persons with a family or personal history of skin cancer, a large number of moles, atypical moles, poor tanning ability, or light skin, hair, and eye color (see Ch. 12).

HR8 = Blood product recipients (including hemodialysis patients), persons with frequent occupational exposure to blood or blood products, men who have sex with men, injection drug users and their sex partners, persons with multiple recent sex partners, persons with other STDs (including HIV), travelers to countries with endemic hepatitis B (see Ch. 66).

HR9 = Persons who exchange sex for money or drugs and their sex partners; persons with other STDs (including HIV); and sexual contacts of persons with active syphilis. Clinicians should also consider local epidemiology (see Ch. 26).

HR10 = Persons who continue to inject drugs (see Ch. 53).

HR11 = Healthy adults without a history of chickenpox or previous immunization. Consider serologic testing for presumed susceptible adults (see Ch. 65, 66).

Table 5. Pregnant Women**

Interventions Considered and Recommended for the Periodic Health Examination

---

Interventions for the General Population

SCREENING

First visit
Blood pressure [Ch 3,37]
Hemoglobin/hematocrit [Ch 22]
Hepatitis B surface antigen (HBsAg)
  [Ch 24]
RPR/VDRL [Ch 26]
Chlamydia screen (<25 yr) [Ch 29]
Rubella serology or vaccination history
  [Ch 32]
D(Rh) typing, antibody screen [Ch 38]
Offer CVS (<13 wk)[1] or amniocentesis
  (15–18 wk)[1] (age ≥35 yr) [Ch 41]
Offer hemoglobinopathy screening [Ch 43]
Assess for problem or risk drinking [Ch 52]
Offer HIV screening[2] [Ch 28]

Follow-up visits
Blood pressure [Ch 3,37]
Urine culture (12–16 wk) [Ch 31]
Offer amniocentesis (15–18 wk)[1] (age ≥35
  yr) [Ch 41]

Offer multiple marker testing[1] (15–18 wk)
  [Ch 41]
Offer serum α-fetoprotein[1] (16–18 wk)
  [Ch 42]

COUNSELING
Tobacco cessation; effects of passive
  smoking [Ch 54]
Alcohol/other drug use [Ch 52,53]
Nutrition, including adequate calcium intake
  [Ch 56]
Encourage breastfeeding [Ch 22,56]
Lap/shoulder belts [Ch 57]
Infant safety car seats [Ch 57]
STD prevention: avoid high-risk sexual
  behavior;* use condoms* [Ch 62]

CHEMOPROPHYLAXIS
Multivitamin with folic acid[3] [Ch 42]

Interventions for High-Risk Populations

POPULATION	POTENTIAL INTERVENTIONS (See detailed high-risk definitions)
High-risk sexual behavior	Screen for chlamydia (1st visit) (HR1), gonorrhea (1st visit) (HR2), HIV (1st visit) (HR3); HBsAg (3rd trimester) (HR4); RPR/VDRL (3rd trimester) (HR5)
Blood transfusion 1978–1985	HIV screen (1st visit) (HR3)
Injection drug use	HIV screen (HR3); HBsAg (3rd trimester) (HR4); advice to reduce infection risk (HR6)
Unsensitized D-negative women	D(Rh) antibody testing (24–28 wk) (HR7)
Risk factors for Down syndrome	Offer CVS[1] (1st trimester), amniocentesis[1] (15–18 wk) (HR8)
Prior pregnancy with neural tube defect	Folic acid 4.0 mg,[3] offer amniocentesis[1] (15–18 wk) (HR9)

---

[1]Women with access to counseling and follow-up services, reliable standardized laboratories, skilled high-resolution ultrasound, and, for those receiving serum marker testing, amniocentesis capabilities. [2]Universal screening is recommended for areas (states, counties, or cities) with an increased prevalence of HIV infection among pregnant women. In low-prevalence areas, the choice between universal and targeted screening may depend on other considerations (see Ch. 28). [3]Beginning at least 1 mo before conception and continuing through the first trimester.

*The ability of clinician counseling to influence this behavior is unproven.

**See Tables 2 and 3 for other preventive services recommended for women of childbearing age.

HR1 = Women with history of STD or new or multiple sex partners. Clinicians should also consider local epidemiology. Chlamydia screen should be repeated in 3rd trimester if at continued risk (see Ch. 29).

HR2 = Women under age 25 with two or more sex partners in the last year, or whose sex partner has multiple sexual contacts; women who exchange sex for money or drugs; and women with a history of repeated episodes of gonorrhea. Clinicians should also consider local epidemiology. Gonorrhea screen should be repeated in the 3rd trimester if at continued risk (see Ch. 27).

HR3 = In areas where universal screening is not performed due to low prevalence of HIV infection, pregnant women with the following individual risk factors should be screened: past or present injection drug use; women who exchange sex for money or drugs; injection drug-using, bisexual, or HIV-positive sex partner currently or in the past; blood transfusion during 1978–1985; persons seeking treatment for STDs (see Ch. 28).

HR4 = Women who are initially HBsAg-negative who are at high risk due to injection drug use, suspected exposure to hepatitis B during pregnancy, multiple sex partners (see Ch. 24).

HR5 = Women who exchange sex for money or drugs, women with other STDs (including HIV), and sexual contacts of persons with active syphilis. Clinicians should also consider local epidemiology (see Ch. 26).

HR6 = Women who continue to inject drugs (see Ch. 53).

HR7 = Unsensitized D-negative women (see Ch. 38).

HR8 = Prior pregnancy affected by Down syndrome, advanced maternal age (≥35 yr), known carriage of chromosome rearrangement (see Ch. 41).

HR9 = Women with previous pregnancy affected by neural tube defect (see Ch. 42).

Table 6.
Conditions for Which Clinicians Should Remain Alert

Condition	Population	Chapter
Symptoms of peripheral arterial disease	Older persons, smokers, diabetic persons	5
Skin lesions with malignant features	General population, particularly those with established risk factors	12
Symptoms and signs of oral cancer and premalignancy	Persons who use tobacco, older persons who drink alcohol regularly	16
Subtle or nonspecific symptoms and signs of thyroid dysfunction	Older persons, postpartum women, persons with Down syndrome	20
Signs of ocular misalignment	Infants and children	33
Symptoms and signs of hearing impairment	Infants and young children (<3 yr)	35
Large spinal curvatures	Adolescents	47
Changes in functional performance	Older persons	48
Depressive symptoms	Adolescents, young adults, persons at increased risk for depression	49
Evidence of suicidal ideation	Persons with established risk factors for suicide	50
Various presentations of family violence	General population	51
Symptoms and signs of drug abuse	General population	53
Obvious signs of untreated tooth decay or mottling, inflamed or cyanotic gingiva, loose teeth, and severe halitosis	General population	61
Evidence of early childhood caries, mismatching of upper and lower dental arches, dental crowding or malalignment, premature loss of primary posterior teeth (baby molars) and obvious mouth breathing	Children	61

REFERENCES

1. Johnson CF. Inflicted injury versus accidental injury. Pediatr Clin North Am 1990;37:791–814.
2. National Highway Traffic Safety Administration. Traffic safety facts 1993: occupant protection. Washington DC: Department of Transportation, 1993.
3. Campbell BJ. Safety belt injury reduction related to crash severity and front seated position. J Trauma 1987;27: 733–739.
4. Cooper PJ. Estimating over involvement of seat belt nonwearers in crashes and the effect of lap/shoulder restraint use on different crash severity consequences. Accid Anal Prev 1994;26:263–275.
5. National Highway Traffic Safety Administration. Final regulatory impact assessment on amendments to Federal Motor Vehicle Safety Standard 208, Front Seat Occupant Protection. Washington, DC: Department of Transportation, 1984. (Publication no. DOT HS 806 572.)
6. National Highway Traffic Safety Administration. Traffic safety facts 1993. Washington DC: Department of Transportation, 1994. (Publication no. DOT HS 808 169.)
7. National Center for Health Statistics. Annual summary of births, marriages, divorces and deaths: United States, 1993. Monthly vital statistics report; vol 42 no 13 (suppl). Hyattsville, MD: Public Health Service, 1994.
8. Centers for Disease Control and Prevention. Summary of notifiable diseases, United States, 1993. MMWR 1994;42: 1–73.
9. Zimmerman HL, Potterat JJ, Dukes RL, et al. Epidemiologic differences between chlamydia and gonorrhea. Am J Public Health 1990;80:1338–1342.
10. Ventura SJ, Taffel SM, Mosher WD, et al. Trends in pregnancies and pregnancy rates, United States, 1980–88. Monthly vital statistics report; vol 41 no 6 (suppl). Hyattsville, MD: National Center for Health Statistics, 1992.
11. Benson V, Marano MA. Current estimates from the National Health Interview Survey, 1992. Vital and health statistics; series 10 no 189. Hyattsville, MD: National Center for Health Statistics, 1994.
12. Schappert SM. National Ambulatory Medical Care Survey: 1992 summary. Advance data from vital and health statistics; no 253. Hyattsville, MD: National Center for Health Statistics, 1994.
13. McCaig LF. Outpatient department summary: National Hospital Ambulatory Medical Care Survey, 1992. Advance data from vital and health statistics; no 248. Hyattsville, MD: National Center for Health Statistics, 1994.
14. McCaig LF. National Hospital Ambulatory Medical Care Survey: 1992 emergency department summary. Advance data from vital and health statistics; no 245. Hyattsville, MD: National Center for Health Statistics, 1994.
15. Brody DJ, Pirkle JL, Kramer RA. Blood lead levels in the US population. JAMA 1994;272:277–283.
16. Curran JW, Jaffe HW, Hardy AM, et al. Epidemiology of HIV infection and AIDS in the United States. Science 1988; 239:610–616.
17. Department of Health and Human Services, Public Health Service, Office of Disease Prevention and Health Promotion. Clinician's handbook of preventive services. Washington, DC: Government Printing Office, 1994.
18. Woolf SH, Jonas S, Lawrence RS, eds. Health promotion and disease prevention in clinical practice. Baltimore: Williams & Wilkins, 1995.
19. American Academy of Pediatrics. Guidelines for health supervision II. Elk Grove Village, IL: American Academy of Pediatrics, 1988.
20. American Academy of Pediatrics, Committee on Practice and Ambulatory Medicine. Recommendations for preventive pediatric health care. Pediatrics 1995;96:373–374.
21. Green M, ed. Bright Futures: guidelines for health supervision of infants, children and adolescents. Arlington, VA: National Center for Education in Maternal and Child Health, 1994.

iv. Patient Education and Counseling for Prevention

Today's major health care problems are increasingly the result of chronic and acute conditions related to individual behavior.[1] A significant proportion of coronary disease and cancer can be attributed to use of tobacco or unhealthy diets, and the majority of sexually transmitted diseases and injuries are related to patient behavior. While mortality from some of these conditions is decreasing, morbidity from most chronic diseases continues to increase.[2,3] For these conditions, prevention at all levels—primary (preventing disease), secondary (early diagnosis), and tertiary (preventing or slowing deterioration)—requires active participation by the patient with guidance and support from the clinician. The patient must take responsibility for carrying out the day-to-day preventive behaviors, accurately reporting progress to the clinician, and discussing health-related problems. Effective patient participation requires education, motivation, and counseling. While busy clinicians cannot fill all the educational needs, they can be pivotal in starting and guiding the process.

Effectiveness of Clinical Counseling

Published evidence regarding counseling's effectiveness in changing specific patient behaviors is reviewed in detail in Chapters 54 through 64. For a number of important health-related behaviors (e.g., smoking, problem drinking) there is good evidence from high-quality studies that clinicians can change patient behavior through simple counseling interventions in the primary care setting.[4-7] For many other behaviors, the effectiveness of clinician counseling has been demonstrated only over the short term[8] or in specialized settings involving relatively intensive counseling.[9-14] In many cases, the effects of counseling on specific behaviors have never been examined in appropriately designed studies. Small changes in behavior may be difficult to prove in prospective studies, yet they could have important health benefits if applied to large populations at risk. Given the safety and generally low cost of advising patients about health-related behaviors, the U.S. Preventive Services Task Force (USPSTF) recommends routinely addressing some health behaviors even when the long-term effectiveness of such counseling has not yet been definitively proven. In their updated recommendations, however, the USPSTF explicitly distinguishes between recommendations based on good evidence of the effectiveness of counseling per se (e.g., smoking cessation) and recommendations made primarily on the basis of the strong link between behavior and disease (e.g., sexually transmitted disease prevention). The USPSTF recognizes that determining the effectiveness of counseling interventions, especially ones that are feasible in the primary care setting, is a research priority. Studies that have demonstrated benefits from brief counseling (e.g., for smoking cessation) help identify critical components of clinician counseling that may apply to other target conditions. This chapter will discuss the objectives of patient education and counseling and provide strategies that can be used in day-to-day practice, offering some examples of how these strategies can be applied.

Objectives of Patient Education and Counseling for Prevention

There are two major objectives of patient education and counseling related to primary prevention: changing health behaviors and improving health status. In addition to the studies cited above, a number of other studies of patient education have demonstrated successful health behavior change in areas such as weight control,[15,16] exercise,[17-19] and contraceptive use.[20] No area of behavior change has been studied more thoroughly than compliance with medication and with other preventive or therapeutic regimens.[21-24] Several general points have emerged from these and other studies of effective counseling to change behavior, which can be incorporated into strategies for effective patient counseling (see below).

A large range of health status changes can be achieved from well-implemented patient education efforts.[25] Various programs have been reported to: lower blood pressure;[23,26] reduce mortality from hypertension,[27] melanoma,[28] hematologic malignancies,[29] and breast cancer;[30] reduce pain and disability from arthritis;[31-34] reduce the incidence of low birth weight babies;[35,36] and maintain better blood glucose levels in diabetics.[37,38] While many of these changes in health status are mediated by changes in health behaviors and better compliance with therapeutic regimens, it seems that some clinical benefits occur independent of these factors.[39] A growing body of evidence suggests that when people have confidence that they can affect their health, they are more likely to do so than those without such confidence.[40] This confidence has been termed "perceived self-efficacy."[41] Self-efficacy can be enhanced through skills mastery, modeling, reinterpreting the meaning of symptoms, and persuasion. Efficacy-enhancing strategies for use in clinical practice are included in the suggestions for patient education described below.

Patient Education/Counseling Strategies

An underlying principle of patient education and counseling is that knowledge is necessary but not sufficient to change health behaviors. If knowledge alone could accomplish changes in health behavior, there would be many fewer smokers and more exercisers. Patient education involves more than simply telling people what to do or giving them an instructional pamphlet.

Few studies compare the efficacy of different types of counseling. The following recommendations have been chosen because they each have been found to be useful in changing certain health behaviors. Most of the suggested strategies can be incorporated into the practice setting without changing existing practice patterns. Many can be implemented in brief periods of time during routine health visits.

1. **Frame the teaching to match the patient's perceptions.** When counseling patients, the clinician should consider and incorporate, where possible, the beliefs and concerns of the patient. Research suggests that people have only a few important beliefs about any one subject.[42] To persuade patients to change their behavior, it is first necessary to identify their beliefs relevant to the behavior and to provide information based on this foundation.[43] The clinician can elicit important beliefs by asking such questions as "When you think of heart disease, what do you think of?" and "What gets in the way of your eating a low-fat diet?" Once the patient's concerns and understanding of the issues are apparent, teaching can then be focused appropriately. In considering a patient's belief system, the provider is challenged to facilitate the bridging of cross-cultural gaps as well. Culturally sensitive education and counseling requires that clinicians assess their own cultural beliefs and be aware of local ethnic, regional, and religious beliefs and practices.[44] Such knowledge aids the development of culturally specific health teaching. A fixed message will not be effective for all patients. By fitting teaching and recommendations to patients' perceptions of their own health and ability to change, clinicians can enhance self-efficacy, which has been shown to improve health behaviors and health status.[41] If a patient with morbid obesity complains that he or she is not able to exercise, the clinician might reframe the patient's conception of what is meant by "exercise." One might initiate a very gentle and brief exercise program, such as 1 minute of physical activity each hour.

2. **Fully inform patients of the purposes and expected effects of interventions and when to expect these effects.** Telling the patient when to expect to see beneficial effects from the intervention may avoid discouragement when immediate benefits are not forthcoming. When rheumatologists told patients about the purposes of their medications, 79% of them were compliant 4 months later, compared with only 33% compliance for those patients who were not given clear information about the purpose of the drugs.[49] Informing patients that the beneficial effects of a low-cholesterol diet or regular physical activity may not become apparent for several months might increase the likelihood of long-term compliance. If side effects are common, the patient should be told what to

expect, and under what circumstances the intervention should be stopped or the provider consulted.

3. **Suggest small changes rather than large ones.** Patients can be asked to do slightly more than they are doing now: "It is great that you are walking 10 minutes in the morning; could you add an additional 5 minutes?" When someone is very overweight, losing 100 pounds might seem like an impossible task, whereas losing 3–4 pounds in the next month seems reachable. By achieving a small goal, the patient has initiated positive change.[41] The rationale for this suggestion comes from self-efficacy theory. Successful persuasion involves not only increasing a patient's faith in his or her capabilities, but also structuring interventions so that people are likely to experience success.[45]

4. **Be specific.** Specific and informational instructions will generally lead to better compliance.[46] For example, when suggesting a physical activity program, it is helpful to ask the patient how much he or she can comfortably do now.[47] The patient can then be asked to perform this activity 3 times a week and then add to it by 10–25% per week, until the person is doing some type of aerobic exercise 20–30 minutes 3–4 times a week. Behavior change is enhanced if the regimen and its rationale are explained, demonstrated to the patient (if appropriate), and written down for patients to take home.

5. **It is sometimes easier to add new behaviors than to eliminate established behaviors.**[48,49] Thus, if weight loss is a concern, suggesting that the patient begin moderate physical activity may be more effective than suggesting a change in current dietary patterns.

6. **Link new behaviors to old behaviors.** For example, a clinician might suggest to patients that they exercise before eating lunch, use an exercise bike while watching the evening news, or take prescribed medications twice daily when brushing the teeth.

7. **Use the power of the profession.** Patients see clinicians as health experts, and they regard what the clinician says as important. The clinician need not be afraid to tell a patient, "I want you to stop smoking," or "I want you to cut half the fat out of your diet." These direct messages are powerful, especially if they are simple and specific.[5] It is important to recognize that some patients lack confidence in their ability to make lifestyle changes. The clinician can be sympathetic and supportive while providing firm, definite messages.

8. **Get explicit commitments from the patient.** Asking patients to describe how the intended regimen will be followed encourages them to begin to think about how to integrate this new behavior into their daily schedule. Clinicians should ask patients to describe what specifically they plan to achieve this week (i.e., what, when, and how often). For example, the patient can be asked to describe what physical activity he or she will

undertake, when it will be done, and how often. The more specific the commitment from the patient, the more likely it is to be followed. After getting the commitment, the clinician can also ask the patient how sure he or she is that he or she will carry out the commitment, for example using a scale of 0 (not at all sure) to 10 (totally sure). A patient with a high degree of certainty that he or she will carry out the commitment is more likely to follow through.[41] If a patient expresses uncertainty, the clinician can explore the problems that might be encountered in carrying out the regimen. This is best done in a nonjudgmental manner, e.g., "Many people have problems starting or continuing an exercise program; do you think you may have any problems? How will you begin?" The clinician and patient can then seek solutions for potential problems.

9. **Use a combination of strategies.** Educational efforts that integrate individual counseling, group classes, audiovisual aids, written materials, and community resources are more likely to be effective than those employing a single technique.[5] Programs can be tailored to individual needs; for example, some patients will not attend group classes, and others may have inflexible work schedules. Written materials strengthen the message[50] and may be personalized by jotting pertinent comments in the margins; this will help to remind patients later of the clinician's suggestions. The clinician should ensure that printed materials are accurate, consistent with their views, and at a reading level appropriate to their patient population. Printed materials cannot, however, substitute for verbal communication with patients. Multiple studies have demonstrated that clinicians' individual attention and feedback are more useful than the news media or other communication channels in changing patient knowledge and behavior.[51]

10. **Involve office staff.** Patient education and counseling is a responsibility that is shared among physicians, nurses, clinical nurse specialists, health educators, dietitians, and other allied health professionals as appropriate. A team approach facilitates patient education. The receptionist can encourage patients to read materials that the clinician has reviewed, approved, and placed in the reception area. Staff members and the office environment can communicate consistent positive health messages.[52] Forming a patient education committee can help to generate program ideas and promote staff commitment.[52]

11. **Refer.** In a busy practice, it may not be possible to do complete patient education and counseling. In some situations, patients are best served by appropriate referrals. There are four major referral sources: community agencies, national voluntary health organizations such as the American Heart Association and the American Cancer Society, instructional references such as books and video tapes, and, finally, other patients. One of the best ways to change health behavior is to connect the patient with a role model, someone with the same problem who has made changes and is doing well.[41] An up-to-

date, written list of specific referral sources (including name, address, and telephone number) can be prepared for each of the 10 or so most common counseling topics and given to patients who need referral. Clinicians should check the credibility and appropriateness of an agency, organization, or other references before referral.

12. **Monitor progress through follow-up contact.** Scheduling a follow-up appointment or telephone call within the next few weeks—to evaluate progress, reinforce successes, and identify and respond to problems—improves the effectiveness of clinician counseling.[5,6] In one study, a monthly call to older persons with osteoarthritis reduced their reported pain and utilization of services.[53] A study in which calls were made to internal medicine patients between visits reduced visits by 19% and hospital days by 28%.[54] Provider-initiated contact may be more effective than patient-initiated phone calls.[55] Proactive calls (calls made by the provider to the patient) have been shown to reinforce behavior change effectively.[56–59] It is also important for the clinician to followup on referrals to monitor progress and support continued compliance.

Implementing Patient Counseling in the Practice Setting

As described in Chapter i, clinicians face important barriers to implementing counseling interventions, such as insufficient reimbursement, provider uncertainty about how to counsel effectively, varying interest on the part of patient or staff, and lack of organizational/system support to facilitate the delivery of patient education. Many of these barriers are addressed by "Put Prevention into Practice" (PPIP), the Public Health Service's prevention implementation program.[60] PPIP provides tools that can assist the provider in delivering appropriate counseling to change patients' personal health practices every time patients are seen. Other publications also provide useful information on the effective delivery of prevention-related education and counseling.[61]

The clinician and public health community are faced with substantial morbidity and mortality from chronic, infectious, and traumatic conditions that are related to personal behaviors. With a large and growing body of literature demonstrating its effectiveness in promoting healthier behavior, patient education and counseling has become an increasingly important part of the delivery of clinical preventive services.

The draft update of this chapter was prepared for the U.S. Preventive Services Task Force by Kate Lorig, RN, DrPH.

REFERENCES

1. McGinnis JM, Foege WH. Actual causes of death in the United States. JAMA 1993;270:2207–2212.
2. Verbrugge LM. Longer life but worsening health? Trends in health and mortality of middle-aged and older persons. Milbank Mem Fund Q 1984;62:475–519.

3. Rothenberg RB, Koplan JP. Chronic disease in the 1990's. Annu Rev Public Health 1990;2:267–296.

4. Lichtenstein EL, Glasgolo RE. Smoking cessation: what have we learned over the past decade? J Consult Clin Psychol 1992;60:518–527.

5. Kottke TE, Battista RN, DeFriese GH, et al. Attributes of successful smoking cessation interventions in clinical practice: a meta-analysis of 42 controlled trials. JAMA 1988;259:2882–2889.

6. Bien TH, Miller WR, Tonigan JS. Brief interventions for alcohol problems: a review. Addiction 1993;88:315–336.

7. Brief interventions and alcohol use. Effective Health Care Bulletin 7. Leeds, U.K.: Nuffield Institute for Health Care, University of Leeds, 1993.

8. Bass J, Christoffel K, Widome M, et al. Childhood injury prevention counseling in primary care settings. Pediatrics 1993;92:544–553.

9. Caggiula AW, Christakis G, Farrand M, et al. The Multiple Risk Factor Interventions Trial (MRFIT). IV. Intervention on blood lipids. Prev Med 1981;10:443–475.

10. The Writing Group for the DISC Collaborative Research Group. Efficacy and safety of lowering dietary intake of fat and cholesterol in children with elevated low-density lipoprotein cholesterol: the Dietary Intervention Study in Children (DISC). JAMA 1995;273:1429–1435.

11. Ramsay LE, Yeo WW, Jackson PR. Dietary reduction of serum cholesterol concentration: time to think again. BMJ 1991;303:953–957.

12. Dattilo AM, Kris-Etherton PM. Effects of weight reduction on blood lipoproteins: a meta-analysis. Am J Clin Nutr 1992;56:320–328.

13. Hopkins PN. Effects of dietary cholesterol on serum cholesterol: a meta-analysis and review. Am J Clin Nutr 1992;55:1060–1070.

14. Wood PD, Stefanick ML, Williams PT, et al. The effects on plasma lipoproteins of a prudent weight-reducing diet, with or without exercise, in overweight men and women. N Engl J Med 1991;325:461–466.

15. Brownell KD, Kramer FM. Behavioral management of obesity. Med Clin North Am 1989;73:185–201.

16. Brownell KD, Wadden TA. Etiology and treatment of obesity: understanding a serious, prevalent and refractory disorder. J Consult Clin Psychol 1992;60:505–517.

17. King AC, Blair SN, Bild DE, et al. Determinants of physical activity and interventions in adults. J Med Sci Sports Exerc 1988;24(Suppl 6):S221–S236.

18. King AC, Martin JE. Exercise adherence and maintenance. In: Painter P, ed. Resource manual for guidelines and exercise testing and prescription. 2nd ed. Philadelphia: American College of Sports Medicine 1988;93:443–454.

19. Disman RK, ed. Exercise adherence: its impact on public health. Champaign, IL: Human Kinetics, 1988.

20. Nathanson CA, Becker MH. The influence of client-provider relationships on teenage women's subsequent use of contraception. Am J Public Health 1985;75:33–38.

21. Haynes RB, Taylor DW, Sackett DL. Compliance in health care. Baltimore: Johns Hopkins University Press, 1979.

22. Roter D. Which facets of communication have strong effect on outcome: a meta-analysis. In: Stewart M, Roter D, eds. Communicating with medical patients. Newbury Park, CA: Sage Publications, 1989.

23. National Institutes of Health, Working Group on Health Education and High Blood Pressure Control. The physician's guide: improving adherence among hypertensive patients. Bethesda: National Institutes of Health, 1987.

24. Cramer JA. Optimizing long-term patient compliance. Neurology 1995;45:525–528.

25. Mazzuca SA. Does patient education in chronic disease have therapeutic value? J Chronic Dis 1982;35:521–529.

26. Levine DM, Green LW, Deeds SG, et al. Health education for hypertensive patients. JAMA 1979;241:1700–1703.

27. Morisky DE, Levine DM, Green LW. Five-year blood pressure control and mortality following health education for hypertensive patients. Am J Public Health 1983;73:153–162.

28. Fawzy FI, Fawzy NW, Hyun CS, et al. Malignant melanoma: effects of an early structured psychiatric intervention, coping and effective state on recurrence and survival 6 years later. Arch Gen Psychiatry 1993;50:681–689.

29. Richardson JL, Shelton DR, Krailo M, et al. The effect of compliance with treatment among patients with hematologic malignancies. J Clin Oncol 1990;8:356–364.

30. Spiegel D, Bloom JR, Kraemer HC, et al. Effects of psychosocial treatment on survival of patients with metastatic breast cancer. Lancet 1989;2:888–891.

31. Lorig KR, Konkol L, Tronzalez V. Arthritis patient education: a review of the literature. Patient Educ Counsel 1987;10:207–252.

32. Hirano PC, Laurent DD, Lorig KR. Arthritis patient education studies, 1987–1992: a review of the literature. Patient Educ Counsel 1994;24:9–54.

33. Mullen PD, Laville E, Biddle AK, et al. Efficacy of psychoeducational interventions on pain, depression, and disability with arthritic adults: a meta-analysis. J Rheumatol 1987;14:33–39.

34. Parker JC, Iverson GL, Smarr KL, et al. Cognitive-behavioral approaches to pain management in rheumatoid arthritis. Arthritis Care Res 1993;6:207–212.

35. Windsor RA, Cutter G, Morris J, et al. The effectiveness of smoking cessation methods for smokers in public health maternity clinics: a randomized trial. Am J Public Health 1985;75:1389–1392.

36. Klaus MK, Kennel J, Berkowitz G. Maternal assistance and support in labor: father, nurse, midwife or doula? Clin Consult Obstet Gynecol 1992;4:211–217.

37. Padgett D, Mumford E, Hynes M, et al. Meta-analysis of the effects of educational and psychosocial interventions in the management of diabetes mellitus. J Clin Epidemiol 1988;41:1007–1030.

38. Brown SA. Studies of educational interventions and outcomes in diabetic adults: a meta-analysis revised. Patient Educ Counsel 1990;16:189–215.

39. Lorig KR, Laurin J. Some notions about assumptions underlying health education. Health Educ Q 1985;12:231–243.

40. Schwarzer R. Self-efficacy, physical symptoms and rehabilitation of chronic disease. In: Schwarzer R, ed. Self-efficacy: thought control of action. Washington, DC: Hemisphere Publishing Corporation, 1992.

41. Bandura A. Social foundations of thoughts and action: a social cognitive theory. Englewood Cliffs, NJ: Prentice-Hall, 1986.

42. Miller GA. The magical number seven; plus or minus two: some limits on our capacity for processing information. Psychol Rev 1956;63:81–97.

43. Fishbein M, Ajzen I. Belief, attitude, intention, and behavior. Reading, MA: Addison-Wesley, 1975.

44. Price JL, Cordell B. Cultural diversity and patient teaching. J Continuing Educ Nurs 1994;25:163–166.

45. Bandura A. Self-efficacy mechanism: psychobiologic functioning. In: Schwarzer R, ed. Self-efficacy: thought control of action. Washington, DC: Hemisphere Publishing Corporation, 1992.

46. Daltroy LH, Katz JN, Liang MH. Doctor-patient communications and adherence to arthritis treatments. Arthritis Care Res 1992;5:S19.

47. Martin JE, Dubbert PM. Exercise applications and promotion in behavioral medicine: current status and future directions. J Consult Clin Psychol 1982;50:1004–1017.

48. Tabak ER, Mullen PD, Simons-Morton DG, et al. Definition and yield of inclusion criteria for a meta-analysis of patient education studies in clinical preventive services. Eval Health Prof 1991;14:388–411.

49. Mullen PD, Simons-Morton DG, Ramirez G, et al. A meta-analysis of studies evaluating patient education for three groups of preventive behaviors. Presented at Prevention '93. St. Louis, MO, April 17–20, 1993.

50. Bernier MJ. Developing and evaluating printed education materials: a prescriptive model for quality. Orthop Nurs 1993;12:39–46.

51. Mullen PD, Green LW, Persinger G. Clinical trials of patient education for chronic conditions: a comparative analysis of intervention types. Prev Med 1985;14:753–781.

52. Vogt HB, Kapp C. Patient education in primary care practice. Postgrad Med 1987;81:273–278.

53. Weinberger M, Tierney WM, Booher P, et al. Can the provision of information to patients with osteoarthritis improve functional status? Arthritis Rheum 1989;32:1577–1583.

54. Wasson J, Gaudette C, Whaley F, et al. Telephone care as a substitute for routine clinic follow-up. JAMA 1992;267: 1788–1793.

55. Sanson-Fisher R, Halpin S, Redman S. Notification and follow-up of Pap test results: current practice and women's preferences. Prev Med 1994;23:276–283.

56. Weinberger M, Kirkman MS, Samsa GP, et al. A nurse-coordinated intervention for primary care patients with non-insulin-dependent diabetes mellitus: impact on glycemic control and health-related quality of life. J Gen Intern Med 1995;10:59–66.

57. van Elderen-van Kemenade T, Maes S, van den Broek Y. Effects of a health education programme with telephone follow-up during cardiac rehabilitation. Br J Clin Psychol 1994;33:367–378.

58. Ahring KK, Ahring JP, Joyce C, et al. Telephone modem access improves diabetes control in those with insulin-requiring diabetes. Diabetes Care 1992;15:971–975.

59. Lerman C, Hanjani P, Caputo C, et al. Telephone counseling improves adherence to colposcopy among lower-income minority women. J Clin Oncol 1992;10:330–333.

60. Department of Health and Human Services, Public Health Service, Office of Disease Prevention and Health Promotion. "Put Prevention into Practice" education and action kit. Washington, DC: Government Printing Office, 1994.

61. Woolf SH, Jonas S, Lawrence RS, eds. Health promotion and disease prevention in clinical practice. Baltimore: Williams & Wilkins, 1995.

v. Cost-Effectiveness and Clinical Preventive Services

Documented effectiveness is—or generally should be—the most basic requirement for providing a health care service. It is a particularly important prerequisite for preventive services, where the clinician has a compelling responsibility to "do no harm" to healthy patients. The fundamental role of effectiveness for clinical decisions motivated the U.S. Preventive Services Task Force effort to evaluate the evidence of effectiveness for clinical preventive services, and the Task Force recommendations in the following chapters are reflections of this evidence.

Effectiveness alone, however, is not a sufficient basis to initiate services in most practical health care contexts. Factors other than effectiveness, reflecting the immediate trade-offs and broad implications of providing a service, are relevant to the goals and the practical constraints confronted by every decision maker. Chapter i describes several of these factors, and they are cited in the subsequent chapters when they are likely to be relevant to a clinician's decision. The present chapter focuses on a single approach, cost-effectiveness analysis, that can combine information on the health benefits, health risks, and costs of health care services. Although cost-effectiveness analysis was not the basis of recommendations in this edition of the *Guide*, this chapter should alert readers that the Task Force believes such analyses should have an increasing role in individual and public policy decisions about providing preventive services as the analytic methodology matures.

Properly used, cost-effectiveness analysis incorporates and complements evidence of effectiveness to inform recommendations on clinical preventive and other health care services. It is intended not to substitute mechanically for complex decision-making processes but rather to be used in combination with other evidence. Efforts to enable cost-effectiveness analysis to be more easily, systematically, and usefully considered in policy decisions are under way. The work of the Panel on Cost-Effectiveness in Health and Medicine (PCEHM), convened in 1993, complements the work of the Task Force in the area of cost-effectiveness analysis. The PCEHM is working to standardize methodology, provide guidelines for cost-effectiveness analysis, and resolve technical differences among studies to improve their quality and comparability. The work of this group will be an important resource for those organizations formulating policy related to clinical preventive services.

Assessing the Cost-Effectiveness of Interventions

Cost-effectiveness analysis is a method for assessing and summarizing the value of a medical technology, practice, or policy.[1,2] Underlying the methodology is the assumption that the resources available to spend on health care are constrained, whether from the societal, organizational, practitioner, or patient point of view. Cost-effectiveness information is intended to inform decisions about health care investments within this finite budget. The cost-effectiveness ratio summarizes information on cost and effect, allowing interventions to be compared on the basis of their worth and priority to the patient, society in general, or some other constituency. Although the cost-effectiveness ratio takes the form of a price—that is, a dollar cost per unit of effect—it is generally interpreted in the inverse manner, as a measure of the benefit achievable for a given level of resources.

The cost-effectiveness ratio encapsulates a defined set of information.[3] The numerator of the ratio summarizes the costs and financial savings associated with the intervention, including the costs of the intervention itself, side effects, and savings from avoided illness and disability. These costs consist of both medical costs (e.g., physician visits, hospitalization, treatment) and nonmedical costs (e.g., transportation, caretaker) associated with the intervention or the illness.

The denominator of the cost-effectiveness ratio reflects the health effect of the intervention. This feature of cost-effectiveness analysis distinguishes it from cost-benefit analysis, in which health benefits are translated into dollars. The year of life saved is probably the most commonly used measure of the health effect. Years of life saved may be adjusted for the quality of life of those years, reflecting the effects of medical interventions on morbidity as well as the length of life. Analyses that incorporate quality of life adjustment are sometimes categorized as "cost-utility" analyses.

The measurement, estimation, and valuation of the elements contained in a cost-effectiveness analysis is a complex undertaking. Chapter ii provides detail on the issues related to assessing the effect of interventions. The assessment of cost can be equally difficult. Issues include the management of indirect costs, such as hospital overhead; the identification of costs as distinct from charges, which often contain elements of profit or costs shifted among patients; and the generalizability of costs from one practice or region to other areas. The measurement of quality of life is also complex and has developed into a specialized field of study.[4]

Contexts for the Use of Cost-Effectiveness Analysis: Societal and Clinical

Cost-effectiveness analysis frequently takes a "societal" view in analyzing health care interventions. Although there is no single "societal" decision maker, various organizations and individuals make decisions that do or should reflect a range of societal goals. Public and private health insurance systems, hospitals and other providers, and government advisory and regulatory bodies set policies and develop recommendations that influence or determine aspects of clinical practice.

The standard argument for the use of cost-effectiveness analysis in these contexts is the need to allocate resources efficiently, obtaining the most desirable set of services for a given budgetary outlay. This objective should be distinguished from that of saving money—a purpose often incorrectly ascribed to cost-effectiveness analysis.[5] Although cost-effectiveness analysis is seldom used in the textbook fashion of ranking interventions and selecting the most cost-effective set, it can offer important guidance to decision makers. It can be used to screen out new procedures or technologies that are poor uses of medical resources. It can illuminate the trade-offs involved in service delivery, such as by outlining the costs and returns for more frequent screening or for applying certain treatments or preventive interventions to particular population groups.

As interest in prioritizing uses of health care resources increases, a range of public and private efforts is focusing on the development and refinement of practical cost-effectiveness applications. Several countries are developing systems for incorporating cost-effectiveness analysis into decisions whether to include drugs in government formularies or for marketing approval.[6,7] In 1993, the World Bank introduced the disability adjusted life year (DALY) in its *World Development Report: Investing in Health*, spurring interest in the use of cost-effectiveness criteria for allocating health care resources in developing countries.[8]

The clinical setting is clearly a primary location for the implementation of policies guided by cost-effectiveness analysis, but its use in this setting is controversial. Medical care policies, including those based on cost-effectiveness considerations, have the potential to constrain the clinician's traditional freedom to select among treatment alternatives. Debate also arises from the primacy of the clinician's advocacy role, which could be jeopardized if the clinician were charged with making decisions to achieve societal priorities that conflict with individual patient choices.

The degree to which the clinician can or should be responsive to general societal welfare as against individual concerns is likely to remain a topic of debate for some time. However, it is both reasonable and necessary for clinicians to consider cost-effectiveness in many cases, weighing whether the marginal benefit to an individual patient of a test, procedure, or treatment as compared to an alternative justifies its additional cost to the patient or to society as a whole.

Cost-Effectiveness Analysis as a Supplement to Information on Effectiveness

Cost-effectiveness analysis supplements information on effectiveness in two ways: by addressing the value of an intervention, and by clarifying and aggregating information related to effectiveness and cost. As noted earlier, it does not address all additional factors of interest to a decision maker. For example, neither an assessment of effectiveness nor of cost-effectiveness will address a policy's effect on the relative well-being of different socio-economic groups, so-called "distributional equity" effects.

Value. Cost-effectiveness information can be used to assess whether an intervention is a "good buy" compared to others or to some formal or informal standard. The cost-effectiveness ratio is a form of price in this sense. More technically, the incremental cost-effectiveness ratio indicates the additional quantity of resources that must be devoted to an intervention, compared to a less expensive but less effective alternative, in order to obtain a given additional benefit. It thus demonstrates the opportunity cost— the value of the foregone alternative use—of the investment.

For example, if a prostate cancer screening program is implemented, the opportunity cost incurred is the health benefit that could have been obtained had the funds been spent on a different program. Cost-effectiveness analysis summarizes the costs per unit of benefit for comparison with the alternatives, or simply for making a judgment about the overall "price" of the program's benefits.

In the clinical setting, the opportunity costs of clinicians' time and other resources are also relevant for the setting of priorities. Limits to such requisites as office space, the duration of the office visit, and the patient's ability to assimilate medical advice during a given visit are particularly evident for interventions such as counseling and patient teaching. To maximize the value of the visit to the patient, the clinician must consider the opportunity cost of various uses of the available resources and prioritize the interventions to be included.

A primary component of value is the magnitude of the benefit offered by an intervention. To be desirable, an intervention must be more than effective; its effect must be important enough to justify the risks and costs associated with it. An effective intervention may be clinically inconsequential, or it may help so few of the individuals to whom it is offered that it is not worth implementing. Cost-effectiveness analysis provides an insight to the magnitude of the benefit an intervention provides. Frequently, analyses report the magnitude of the benefit directly. In almost all cases, however, the cost-effectiveness ratio provides an indirect indication. If it imposes any meaningful cost, an intervention with minimal effectiveness will have a very high ratio of cost to effectiveness, alerting the decision maker to the need to examine the desirability of the intervention.

Aggregation of Effects. The ability of cost-effectiveness models to account for a wide range of an intervention's effects offers a particular advantage to decision makers in determining the value of a service. The full effect of health care policy decisions is difficult to assess intuitively, involving benefits and costs that accrue to different persons or groups and occur at different times. Cost-effectiveness analysis offers a systematic approach to documenting and aggregating these effects.

Cost-Effectiveness Analysis and Recommendations for Clinical Preventive Services

Cost-effectiveness analysis has direct relevance for policies concerning clinical preventive services. An example is that of screening and vaccination to prevent the complications of rubella during pregnancy (see Chapter 32). On the basis of evidence of rubella vaccine effectiveness, the Task Force recommends screening all women of childbearing age and vaccinating susceptible women or, alternatively, routine vaccination of all women in this age group.

Should this recommendation be implemented? If so, under what protocol? Preventable rubella cases occur; an average of 7 cases of congenital rubella syndrome occurred in the U.S. each year during the 1980s, and a larger number during the rubella outbreak in the early 1990s.[9] Screening and vaccination strategies could likely prevent some cases, although not all, in upcoming years.

From a broad perspective, the relevant issue is the opportunity cost of implementing this effort. If the resources available for health services were unlimited, there would be no opportunity cost and no reason to question the implementation of rubella vaccination for women of childbearing age. In fact, more intensive strategies than those the Task Force recommends, such as repeated vaccination of adult women, might be an even surer way of eliminating as many cases of rubella in pregnancy as possible. Because the level of health care spending by business, government, health care institutions, and individuals ultimately affects quality of life both directly and indirectly, however, it becomes necessary to assess whether the benefit of an intervention like rubella vaccination of adult women—or of one vaccination protocol versus another—is worth its cost.

On its face, the case of rubella vaccination prompts several questions related to cost-effectiveness. The total cost of fully implementing the Task Force recommendation would be significant because of the large population involved: some 60 million women aged 15 to 44. In addition, the attainable benefit is limited by the low incidence of preventable rubella in pregnancy. Childhood vaccination has already markedly decreased the overall incidence of the disease, and benefit is further limited in the case of a screening strategy by the occurrence of rubella infection in women with apparent immunity on screening.[10] Finally, if a rubella vaccination policy were to be implemented, a strategy or protocol would need to be chosen. Routine vaccination is presumably more effective but may be more costly than screening followed by selective vaccination. Would the added benefit justify the difference in cost?

Similar issues arise in considering many of the clinical preventive services discussed in this volume. The recommended screening of all persons over age 50 for colorectal cancer (see Chapter 8) would potentially add billions of dollars to health system costs and should be considered in light of the benefit it could provide.[11] Recommended counseling interventions for young adults would compete for time during office visits and should be prioritized in terms of their demands on practitioner and patient time and the benefit they offer. Recommended protocols—the frequency of interventions and the populations targeted to receive them—can greatly affect the outcomes and costs of an intervention and should be determined with regard for cost-effectiveness considerations.

In general, the policy questions regarding these interventions do not concern their inherent desirability. The effectiveness and risks of interventions recommended by the Task Force have been carefully evaluated. Instead, the question is whether there are likely to be other interventions that are more desirable—other uses of resources that are preferable. While the opportunity cost of a given service often is not apparent, the overall pressure of resource constraints in all domains of health care is becoming increasingly obvious. In many areas of medical technology, large additional expenditures have been shown to produce only small, marginal gains in health status or outcome at our current levels of health care technology.

Use of Cost-Effectiveness Analysis in the Absence of Data on Effectiveness

Evidence of effectiveness, although always desirable, is not always available. Research documenting effectiveness is frequently complex, time-consuming, and expensive. As a result, the effectiveness of many services remains to be established. For others, evidence of effectiveness is equivocal. Cost-effectiveness analysis cannot provide evidence of effectiveness where none exists. However, it can distinguish critical gaps in existing knowledge from questions that are less important for future research because a decision is not influenced by the existing uncertainty. Cost-effectiveness analysis can also illuminate dimensions of the trade-off between action and inaction.

For example, the Task Force has found insufficient evidence to recommend for or against providers counseling their patients to engage in physical activity (see Chapter 55). Cost-effectiveness analysis could summarize the conflicting considerations entering into a decision on this intervention, including the implications of both a decision to implement and not to implement exercise counseling.

In general, the decision to provide a service that has not been proven effective must consider the extent of potential benefit, the likelihood that the intervention is effective, and the type of evidence indicating probable effectiveness. These decisions must also weigh the costs and untoward effects of the intervention, including the societal costs of institutionalizing an unproven practice. Because of the possibility for harm and the cost, the provision of an unproven intervention to an asymptomatic and healthy population is seldom justified. When a *probably* effective intervention imposes little or no cost and is safe, its implementation may be warranted.

Cost-Effectiveness of Preventive versus Curative Services

Prevention is still commonly promoted on the basis of claims that it saves money, although screening, counseling, and other preventive services often cost more than they save, just as other medical services do. Given this tendency, efforts to document the cost-effectiveness of preventive measures may be interpreted to imply that the value of preventive services should be examined closely, while curative services are subjected to no such test.

Preventive and curative services should be held to the same basic standard of cost-effectiveness. A preventive service may be more cost-effective than many curative services and be a good use of health care funds, even if it is not as cost-effective as other preventive services.

Current Limits on Use of Cost-Effectiveness Analysis

Cost-effectiveness studies are currently available on many health care services. The weight of the cost-effectiveness evidence is convincing for a limited number of these, most of which are clearly cost-effective or clearly cost-ineffective in any realistic scenario.

A much larger group of services remains for which cost-effectiveness is not yet established. Information on costs and outcomes is inadequate for many interventions. For others, the cost-effectiveness analyses have not been done, or their quality is insufficient to provide conclusive evidence. Finally, the variation in cost-effectiveness analysis methodology often makes it difficult to take cost-effectiveness results at face value.

Decision makers today should consider cost-effectiveness results where adequate analysis has been done. Care should be taken in evaluating the methodology used. The reader should examine challenges to the study's validity, such as the choice of costs included in the analysis and the quality and representativeness of data on costs and effectiveness. In addition to providing specific information, cost-effectiveness analysis raises important questions about the opportunity costs of alternative choices that decision-makers should consider.

Cost-Effectiveness and Task Force Recommendations on Effectiveness

The Task Force recommendations in this *Guide* reflect the evidence of effectiveness of interventions. They are intended to inform clinicians about a basic and important aspect of clinical preventive services and contribute to the process of evaluating the priority of these services. The recommendations do not systematically incorporate other decision factors, such as cost-effectiveness or the ethical implications of recommendations, and therefore should not be viewed as comprehensive societal guidelines for clinical preventive services. Evidence of effectiveness should be supplemented when possible by information on cost-effectiveness in any decision-making context in which available resources can be used for multiple purposes.

The draft of this chapter was prepared for the U.S. Preventive Services Task Force by Joanna E. Siegel, ScD, and Donald M. Berwick, MD, MPP.

REFERENCES

1. Eisenberg JM. Clinical economics: a guide to the economic analysis of clinical practices, JAMA 1989;262 2879–2886.
2. Drummond MF, Stoddart GL, Torrance GW. Methods for the economic evaluation of health care programmes. New York: Oxford University Press, 1987.
3. Weinstein MC, Stason WB. Foundations of cost-effectiveness analysis for health and medical practices. N Engl J Med 1977;296:716–721.
4. Patrick DL, Erickson P. Health status and health policy: allocating resources to health care. New York: Oxford University Press, 1993.
5. Doubilet P, Weinstein MC, McNeil BJ. Use and misuse of the term "cost-effective" in medicine. N Engl J Med 1986;314:253–256.
6. Henry D. Economic analysis as an aid to subsidisation decisions: the development of Australian guidelines for pharmaceuticals. Pharmacoeconomics 1992;1:54–67.
7. Canadian Coordinating Office for Health Technology Assessment. Guidelines for economic evaluation of pharmaceuticals: Canada. 1st ed. Ottawa: CCOHTA, 1994.
8. World Bank. World Development Report 1993: investing in health. New York: Oxford University Press, 1993.
9. Centers for Disease Control. Increase in rubella and congenital rubella syndrome—United States, 1988–90. MMWR 1991;40:93–99.
10. Lee SH, Ewert DP, Frederick PD, Mascola L. Resurgence of congenital rubella syndrome in the 1990s. Report on missed opportunities and failed prevention policies among women of childbearing age. JAMA 1992;267:2616–2620.
11. Wagner J. From the Congressional Office of Technology Assessment: costs and effectiveness of colorectal cancer screening in the elderly. JAMA 1990;264:2732.

SCREENING

1. Screening for Asymptomatic Coronary Artery Disease

RECOMMENDATION

There is insufficient evidence to recommend for or against screening middle-aged and older men and women for asymptomatic coronary artery disease, using resting electrocardiography (ECG), ambulatory ECG, or exercise ECG. Recommendations against routine screening can be made on other grounds for individuals who are not at high risk of developing clinical heart disease (see *Clinical Intervention*). Routine screening is not recommended as part of the periodic health visit or pre-participation sports examination for children, adolescents, or young adults. Clinicians should emphasize proven measures for the primary prevention of coronary disease (see *Clinical Intervention*).

Burden of Suffering

Ischemic heart disease is the leading cause of death in the U.S., accounting for approximately 490,000 deaths in 1993.[1] The American Heart Association estimates that approximately 1.5 million Americans will suffer a myocardial infarction (MI) in 1995, and one third will not survive the event.[2] Atherosclerotic coronary artery disease (CAD) is the underlying cause of most ischemic cardiac events and can result in myocardial infarction, congestive heart failure, cardiac arrhythmias, and sudden cardiac death. Clinically significant CAD is uncommon in men under 40 and premenopausal women, but risk increases with advancing age and in the presence of risk factors such as smoking, hypertension, diabetes, high cholesterol, and family history of heart disease. Although mortality from heart disease has declined steadily over the past three decades in the U.S.,[2] the total burden of coronary disease is predicted to increase substantially over the next 30 years due to the increasing size of the elderly population.[3] The cost of medical care and lost economic productivity due to heart disease in the U.S. has been projected to exceed $60 billion in 1995.[2]

Angina is the most common presenting symptom of myocardial ischemia and underlying CAD, but in many persons the first evidence of

CAD may be myocardial infarction or sudden death.[4] It has been estimated that 1–2 million middle-aged men have asymptomatic but physiologically significant coronary disease, also referred to as silent myocardial ischemia.[4,5]

Accuracy of Screening Tests

There are two screening strategies to reduce morbidity and mortality from CAD. The first involves screening for modifiable cardiac risk factors, such as hypertension, elevated serum cholesterol, cigarette smoking, physical inactivity, and diet (see Chapters 2, 3, and 54–56). The second strategy is early detection of asymptomatic CAD. The principal tests for detecting asymptomatic CAD include resting and exercise ECGs, which can provide evidence of previous silent myocardial infarctions and silent or inducible myocardial ischemia. Thallium-201 scintigraphy, exercise echocardiography, and ambulatory ECG (Holter monitoring) are less commonly used for screening purposes. The efficacy of each of these tests may be evaluated by (a) its ability to detect atherosclerotic plaque, and (b) its ability to predict the occurrence of a serious clinical event in the future (acute MI, sudden cardiac death).

Several resting ECG findings (ST depression, T-wave inversion, Q waves, and left axis deviation) increase the likelihood of coronary atherosclerosis and of future coronary events. However, these findings are uncommon in asymptomatic persons, occurring in only 1–4% of middle-aged men without clinical evidence of CAD,[6,7] and they are not specific for CAD. One third to one half of patients with angiographically normal coronary arteries have Q waves, T-wave inversion, or ST-T changes on their resting ECG.[8–10] Conversely, a normal ECG does not rule out CAD. In the Coronary Artery Surgery Study, 29% of patients with symptomatic, angiographically proven CAD demonstrated a normal resting ECG.[11] Asymptomatic persons with baseline ECG abnormalities (Q waves, ST-segment depression, T-wave inversion, left ventricular hypertrophy, and ventricular premature beats) have a higher risk of future coronary events.[6,12–19] However, prospective studies lasting between 5 and 30 years have found that symptomatic CAD develops in only 3–15% of persons with these ECG findings.[6,13,18,20] Furthermore, most coronary events occur in persons without resting ECG abnormalities.[6,7,18,21,22] Thus, routine ECG testing in asymptomatic persons, in whom the pretest probability of having CAD is relatively low, is not an efficient process for detecting CAD or for predicting future coronary events.

The exercise ECG is more accurate than the resting ECG for detecting clinically important CAD. Most patients with asymptomatic CAD do not have a positive exercise ECG, however.[23–26] ECG changes often do not become apparent until an atherosclerotic plaque has progressed to the point that it significantly impedes coronary blood flow.[24,27] In addition, most asymptomatic persons with an abnormal exercise ECG result (usually defined by a specific magnitude of ST-segment depression) do not have underlying CAD.[27,28] A 1989 meta-analysis found considerable variability in the accuracy of exercise-induced ST depression for predicting CAD (sensitivity 23–100%, specificity 17–100%).[29] Although several investigators reported that adjusting the ST segment for heart rate (ST/HR slope or ST/HR index) improves the ability to predict significant CAD[30–32] and future coronary events,[25] other studies have not shown an advantage.[33–37]

The exercise ECG is also more accurate than the resting ECG in predicting future coronary events. While asymptomatic persons with a positive exercise ECG are more likely to experience an event than those with negative tests,[25,38–43] longitudinal studies following such patients from 4 to 13 years have shown that only 1–11% will suffer an acute MI or sudden death.[25,42,44,45] As with resting ECG, the majority of events will occur in those with a negative exercise test result.[24,26,44–47] The pathophysiology of acute coronary syndromes may explain the insensitivity of exercise ECG for subsequent coronary events. Unstable angina, MI, and sudden death often result from an acute, occluding thrombus precipitated by the rupture of a mild, non-flow-limiting plaque.[48–50] Among healthy men who subsequently developed symptomatic CAD after a negative screening test, 73% experienced a MI or sudden death as their initial manifestation.[24,45] In contrast, the majority of asymptomatic persons with a positive exercise ECG develop angina as their initial event.[5,24,45,51] Thus, while exercise ECG may predict the presence of more severe coronary stenosis and risk of angina in asymptomatic persons, it does not accurately predict risk of acute coronary events.

The addition of thallium-201 scintigraphy to conventional exercise testing improves its accuracy in detecting CAD, making it a useful diagnostic test in persons with symptoms of CAD.[52,53] However, the probability of CAD after a positive scan is low in asymptomatic persons, and most coronary events occur in those with a negative test result.[23,44] Because of these limitations and its expense, thallium-201 scintigraphy is not a practical screening test for asymptomatic persons.[23,44,52,54] The ambulatory ECG can detect episodes of ST-segment depression which may indicate silent ischemia in asymptomatic persons with CAD. These episodes, however, also occur commonly in healthy volunteers[55–57] and are not reliable predictors of future coronary events, even in asymptomatic or mildly symptomatic patients with documented CAD.[58,59] There have been no studies of exercise echocardiography in screening asymptomatic populations for CAD.

False-positive screening test results are undesirable for several reasons. Persons with abnormal results frequently undergo invasive diagnostic procedures such as coronary angiography. Abnormal test results may produce considerable anxiety. An abnormal ECG tracing may disqualify some patients from jobs, insurance eligibility, and other opportunities, although the extent of these problems is not known. Proposed strategies for reducing false-positive results include: performing workups in accordance with a Bayesian model;[60] using discriminant functions to interpret the stress ECG;[41] and targeting testing to high-risk groups.

Effectiveness of Early Detection

Although case-control and cohort studies show that asymptomatic persons with selected ECG findings are at increased risk of MI and cardiac death,[5,7,22,25,38–43] there is little evidence that routine screening is an effective means to reduce the incidence of acute coronary events in asymptomatic persons. Antianginal drugs such as nitroglycerin, β-adrenergic blockers, and calcium channel blockers reduce the frequency and the duration of silent ischemia.[61–63] In a recent study, atenolol reduced the incidence of cardiac events (MI, cardiac arrest, or worsening angina) in patients who had both silent ischemia and CAD documented by angiography or prior MI;[64,65] extrapolating these benefits to completely asymptomatic patients with silent ischemia on routine screening may not be justified, given their much lower risk of acute events.[46]

Both aspirin therapy and drug treatment for high cholesterol reduce the incidence of MI and cardiac mortality in patients with symptomatic coronary disease, but the balance of risks and benefits of these therapies in asymptomatic patients is not resolved (see Chapters 2 and 69). Benefits are more likely to exceed risks in asymptomatic patients with underlying coronary disease, however, due to their higher absolute risk of MI and coronary death. New diagnostic techniques may prove more sensitive than angiography in identifying the mild-to-moderate plaques that are a risk factor for developing an acute occlusive thrombus.[66,67] Their utility will remain in question, however, until appropriate trials demonstrate that early detection and treatment of small coronary plaques is more effective than treatment based on identifiable risk factors (e.g., high blood pressure or high cholesterol) in asymptomatic patients.[48,49]

Among patients with symptomatic coronary disease, coronary artery bypass grafting prolongs life compared with medical therapy in patients with left main coronary or three-vessel disease with poor left ventricular function.[11] The prevalence of high-risk coronary disease among asymptomatic persons, however, is very low; while some patients may suffer a MI or sudden cardiac death as their initial manifestation of CAD, most patients with severe coronary disease initially develop angina.[5,45] As a result, it is not clear that the benefit of identifying a small number of individuals with severe coronary disease before they develop symptoms is sufficient to justify routine screening of large populations of asymptomatic persons. Recent randomized trials have demonstrated that percutaneous transluminal coronary angioplasty (PTCA) reduces the frequency of angina in patients with symptomatic CAD, but it does not reduce the incidence of MI or cardiac death.[68,69] The value of coronary angioplasty for asymptomatic coronary stenoses is not known.

A screening ECG has been recommended to provide a "baseline" to help interpret changes in subsequent ECGs.[70] Even when important differences are noted between the baseline ECG and a subsequent tracing, these do not necessarily reflect ongoing or recent ischemia. Using the development of a new Q wave on serial ECG as a criterion, the Framingham Study reported an annual incidence of unrecognized MI of 5.4/1,000 men aged 65–74.[71] Less specific changes develop more commonly than Q waves. Baseline ECGs are often not available when needed for comparison, nor do they significantly contribute to decision making for patients being evaluated for chest pain,[72–75] especially in those with no history of cardiovascular disease.[76] One large study found that a baseline ECG was available in 55% of patients evaluated for acute chest pain.[73] The availability of a prior ECG was associated with small but significant reduction in hospitalization rates for those patients who had chest pain not due to acute MI. Only a small subset of the asymptomatic population is likely to benefit from having a baseline ECG, however: those with baseline ECG abnormalities suggestive of ischemia who subsequently develop acute noncardiac chest pain. Savings from preventing a few unnecessary hospitalizations among these patients must be weighed against the high costs of routine ECG screening in the large population of asymptomatic persons.

Another argument for ECG screening is that the early identification of persons at increased risk for CAD on the basis of ECG findings may help to modify other important cardiac risk factors such as cigarette smoking, hypertension, and elevated serum cholesterol.[70] While the efficacy of risk factor modification is well established,[22,77] no studies have evaluated whether identifying high-risk patients with abnormal ECGs improves efforts to modify risk factors or leads to better clinical outcomes.

Periodic ECG screening is often recommended for persons who might endanger public safety were they to experience an acute cardiac event at work (e.g., airline pilots, bus and truck drivers, railroad engineers). Cardiac events in such individuals are more likely to affect the safety of a large number of persons, and clinical intervention, either through medical treatment or work restrictions, might prevent such catastrophes. No studies have addressed the efficacy of ECG screening in these persons, however.

Preliminary exercise ECG testing has also been recommended for sedentary persons planning to begin vigorous exercise programs, based on evidence that strenuous exertion may increase the risk of sudden cardiac death. The usual underlying cause of sudden cardiac death during exercise is hypertrophic cardiomyopathy or congenital coronary anomalies in young persons and CAD in older persons. Cardiac events during exercise in persons without symptomatic heart disease are uncommon, however, and exercise ECG may not accurately predict those who are at risk. Among over 3,600 asymptomatic, hypercholesterolemic middle-aged men who underwent submaximal exercise ECG during the Lipid Research Clinics Coronary Primary Prevention Trial, 62 (2%) subsequently experienced an acute cardiac event during moderate or strenuous physical activity during follow-up (average 7.4 years).[78] Although men with exercise-induced ECG changes were at increased risk, only 11 of 62 events occurred in men with an abnormal baseline exercise test (sensitivity 18%). Moreover, few of the men with abnormal test results experienced an activity-related event during follow-up (positive predictive value 4%). Although the negative predictive value of baseline ECG was high (over 98%), it was no better than multivariate analysis based on clinical risk factors alone. Given the low incidence of activity-related events in middle-aged men, and the uncertain benefit of restricting activity in those with abnormal exercise tests, the potential benefits of pre-exercise testing appear small. In populations at low risk for heart disease, any benefits of detecting the rare individual with asymptomatic CAD may be offset by adverse effects of labeling and exercise restrictions for the larger number of persons with false-positive ECG results.

Recommendations of Other Groups

The routine use of resting electrocardiogram to screen for CAD in asymptomatic adults is not recommended by the American College of Physicians (ACP)[79] or the Canadian Task Force on the Periodic Health Examination.[80] The American Academy of Family Physicians (AAFP) recommends a baseline electrocardiogram for men 40 years and older with two or more cardiac risk factors and sedentary men about to begin a vigorous exercise program; this recommendation is under review.[81] A task force sponsored by the American College of Cardiology and the American Heart Association (ACC/AHA) recommends baseline testing for all persons over 40 years of age and for those about to have exercise stress testing.[82]

The AAFP recommends exercise electrocardiography for those whose jobs are linked to public safety (e.g., pilots, air traffic controllers) or that require high cardiovascular performance (e.g., police officers, firefighters).[81] The American College of Sports Medicine recommends exercise ECG testing for men over age 40, women over age 50, and other asymptomatic persons with multiple cardiac risk factors, prior to beginning a vigorous exercise program.[83] The ACC/AHA recognize that the exercise ECG is frequently used to screen asymptomatic persons in some high-risk groups but concluded that there is divergence of opinion with respect to its usefulness.[84] The ACP does not recommend exercise testing with ECG or thallium scintigraphy as a routine screening procedure in asymptomatic adults.[79,85]

Discussion

Heart disease is the leading cause of death in the U.S., and interventions that produce even modest reductions in the incidence of acute ischemic events may have substantial public health benefits. Although the resting electrocardiogram can detect evidence of coronary heart disease in asymptomatic persons and identify individuals at increased risk of future coronary events, the ECG has important weaknesses as a screening test. The large majority of asymptomatic persons with abnormal ECG results do not have CAD and are at relatively low risk for developing symptomatic heart disease in the near future. Routine screening may subject many of them to the inconvenience, expense and potential risks of follow-up testing (i.e., cardiac catheterization or radionuclide imaging) to evaluate false-positive screening results. Although exercise testing is more sensitive and specific for high-grade coronary stenoses, the exercise ECG is too time-consuming and expensive for routine use in asymptomatic persons. Finally, neither resting nor exercise ECG reliably detects the mild to moderate atherosclerotic lesions which are often responsible for acute coronary events.

A second important problem with screening for asymptomatic CAD is the lack of evidence that earlier detection leads to better outcomes. The only interventions proven to reduce coronary events in asymptomatic persons are modifications of risk factors such as smoking, high cholesterol, and elevated blood pressure. These interventions, however, should be encouraged for all patients with modifiable risk factors, not only those with screening tests suggestive of CAD. The benefits of more invasive treatments for coronary stenosis (e.g., bypass surgery, angioplasty) are unproven in asymptomatic persons. For certain occupations, such as pilots and heavy equipment operators, where sudden death or incapacitation would endanger the safety of others, considerations other than benefit to the individual patient may favor screening. Although screening cannot reliably identify all persons at risk of an acute event, it may increase the margin of safety for the public.

To minimize the potential adverse effects of false-positive test results, routine screening with ECG should be avoided in populations where the prevalence of CAD is low, including most adults under 40, and middle-aged men and women without coronary risk factors. Even in high-risk individuals, the benefits of screening to identify asymptomatic CAD are unproven. For some persons, however, identifying those at high risk of coronary mortality may help guide treatment decisions (e.g., use of aspirin or cholesterol-lowering drugs).

There are major costs associated with widespread screening with resting ECG in asymptomatic adults, and use of other screening tests (ambulatory ECG, exercise testing, and echocardiography) would be substantially more expensive.[79] The inconvenience, expense, and potential risks of routine screening might be justified if it significantly reduced the incidence of MI and sudden cardiac death, but such evidence is not yet available. Until appropriate studies demonstrate a benefit of screening for CAD, identification and treatment of major cardiac risk factors such as hypertension, elevated serum cholesterol, and cigarette smoking remain the only proven measures for reducing coronary morbidity and mortality in asymptomatic persons.

CLINICAL INTERVENTION

There is insufficient evidence to recommend for or against screening middle-aged and older men and women for asymptomatic coronary artery disease with resting electrocardiography (ECG), ambulatory ECG, or exercise ECG ("C" recommendation). Recommendations against routine screening may be made on other grounds for persons who are not at high risk of developing symptomatic CAD; these grounds include the limited sensitivity and low predictive value of an abnormal resting ECG in asymptomatic persons, and the high costs of screening and follow-up. Screening selected high-risk asymptomatic persons (e.g., those with multiple cardiac risk factors) is indicated only where results will influence treatment decisions (e.g., use of aspirin or lipid-lowering drugs in asymptomatic persons). Screening individuals in certain occupations (pilots, truck drivers, etc.) can be recommended on other grounds, including possible benefits to public safety. The choice of specific screening test for asymptomatic CAD is left to clinical discretion: exercise ECG is more accurate than resting ECG but is considerably more expensive.

Routine ECG screening as part of the periodic health visit or preparticipation sports physical is not recommended for asymptomatic children, adolescents, and young adults ("D" recommendation).

Clinicians should emphasize proven measures for the primary prevention of coronary disease in all patients (see Chapter 3, Screening for Hypertension; Chapter 2, Screening for High Blood Cholesterol; Chapter 54, Counseling to Prevent Tobacco Use; Chapter 55, Counseling to Promote Physical Activity; and Chapter 56, Counseling to Promote a Healthy Diet).

The draft update of this chapter was prepared for the U.S. Preventive Services Task Force by Dennis L. Disch, MD, and Harold C. Sox, Jr., MD.

REFERENCES

1. National Center for Health Statistics. Annual summary of births, marriages, divorces, and deaths: United States, 1993. Monthly vital statistics report; vol 42 no 13. Hyattsville, MD: Public Health Service, 1994.
2. American Heart Association. Heart and stroke facts: 1995 statistical supplement. Dallas, TX: American Heart Association, 1995.
3. Weinstein MC, Coxson PG, Williams LW, Pass TM, Stason WB, Goldman L. Forecasting coronary heart disease incidence, mortality and cost: the Coronary Heart Disease Policy Model. Am J Public Health 1987;77:1417–1426.
4. Thaulow E, Erikssen J, Sandvik L, Erikssen G, Jorgensen L, Cohn PF. Initial clinical presentation of cardiac disease in asymptomatic men with silent myocardial ischemia and angiographically documented coronary artery disease (the Oslo Ischemia Study). Am J Cardiol 1993;72:629–633.
5. Cohn PF. Silent myocardial ischemia. Ann Intern Med 1988;109:312–317.
6. Rose G, Baxter PJ, Reid DD, McCartney P. Prevalence and prognosis of electrocardiographic findings in middle-aged men. Br Heart J 1978;40:636–643.
7. Sox HC Jr, Garber AM, Littenberg B. The resting electrocardiogram as a screening test: a clinical analysis. Ann Intern Med 1989;111:489–502.
8. Kemp HG, Vokonas PS, Cohn PF, Gorlin R. The anginal syndrome associated with normal coronary arteriograms. Am J Med 1973;54:735–742.
9. Kemp HG, Kronmal RA, Vlietstra RE, Frye FL. Seven year survival of patients with normal or near normal coronary arteriograms: a CASS registry study. J Am Coll Cardiol 1986;7:479–483.
10. Cohn PF, Gorlin R, Vokonas PS, Williams RA, Herman MV. A quantitative clinical index for the diagnosis of symptomatic coronary artery disease. N Engl J Med 1972;286:901–907.
11. Coronary Artery Surgery Study (CASS). A randomized trial of coronary artery bypass surgery. Survival data. Circulation 1983;68:939–950.
12. Cedres B, Liu K, Stamler J, et al. Independent contribution of electrocardiographic abnormalities to risk of death from coronary heart disease, cardiovascular diseases and all causes: findings of three Chicago epidemiologic studies. Circulation 1982;65:146–153.
13. Multiple Risk Factor Intervention Trial Research Group. Baseline electrocardiographic abnormalities, antihypertensive treatment, and mortality in the Multiple Risk Factor Intervention Trial. Am J Cardiol 1985;55:1–15.
14. Harlan WR, Cowie CC, Oberman A, et al. Prediction of subsequent ischemic heart disease using serial resting electrocardiograms. Am J Epidemiol 1984;113:370–376.
15. Joy M, Trump DW. Significance of minor ST segment and T wave changes in the resting electrocardiogram of asymptomatic subjects. Br Heart J 1981;45:48–55.
16. Kannel WB, Gordon T, Castelli WP, Margolis JR. Electrocardiographic left ventricular hypertrophy and risk of coronary heart disease: the Framingham study. Ann Intern Med 1970;72:813–822.
17. Kannel WB. Common ECG markers for subsequent clinical coronary events. Circulation 1987;75(Suppl II):II-25–II-27.
18. Knutsen R, Knutsen SF, Curb JD, Reed DM, Kauz JA, Yano K. The predictive value of resting electrocardiograms for 12-year incidence of coronary heart disease in the Honolulu Heart Program. J Clin Epidemiol 1988;41:293–302.
19. Rabkin SW, Mathewson FL, Tate RB. The electrocardiogram in apparently healthy men and the risk of sudden death. Br Heart J 1982;47:546–552.
20. Kannel WB, Anderson K, McGee DL, et al. Nonspecific electrocardiographic abnormality as a predictor of coronary heart disease: the Framingham Study. Am Heart J 1987;113:370–376.
21. Pedoe HD. Predictability of sudden death from the resting electrocardiogram: effect of previous manifestations of coronary heart disease. Br Heart J 1978;40:630–635.
22. Multiple Risk Factor Intervention Trial Research Group. Exercise electrocardiogram and coronary heart disease mortality in the Multiple Risk Factor Intervention Trial. Am J Cardiol 1985;55:16–24.
23. Cohn PF. Clinical importance of silent myocardial ischemia in asymptomatic subjects. Circulation 1989;81:691–693.

24. Epstein SE, Quyumi A, Bonow RO. Sudden cardiac death without warning: possible mechanisms and implications for screening asymptomatic populations. N Engl J Med 1989;321:320–323.
25. Okin PM, Anderson KM, Levy D, Kligfield P. Heart rate adjustment of exercise-induced ST segment depression: improved risk stratification in the Framingham Offspring Study. Circulation 1991;83:866–874.
26. Weiner DA. Screening for latent coronary artery disease by exercise testing. Circulation 1991;83:1104–1106.
27. Detrano R, Froelicher V. A logical approach to screening for coronary artery disease. Ann Intern Med 1987;106:846–852.
28. Uhl GS, Froelicher V. Screening for asymptomatic coronary artery disease. J Am Coll Cardiol 1983;3:946–955.
29. Gianrossi R, Detrano R, Mulvihill D, et al. Exercise-induced ST depression in the diagnosis of coronary artery disease: a meta-analysis. Circulation 1989;80:87–98.
30. Elamin MS, Boyle R, Kardash MM, et al. Accurate detection of coronary heart disease by new exercise test. Br Heart J 1982;48:311–320.
31. Hollenberg M, Zoltick JM, Go M, et al. Comparison of a quantitative treadmill exercise score with standard electrocardiographic criteria in screening asymptomatic young men for coronary artery disease. N Engl J Med 1985;313:600–606.
32. Kligfield P, Ameisen O, Okin PM. Heart rate adjustment of ST segment depression for improved detection of coronary artery disease. Circulation 1989;79:245–255.
33. Bobbio M, Detrano R. A lesson from the controversy about heart rate adjustment of ST segment depression. Circulation 1991;84:1410–1413.
34. Bobbio M, Detrano R, Schmid JJ, et al. Exercise-induced ST depression and ST/heart rate index to predict triple-vessel or left main coronary disease: a multicenter analysis. J Am Coll Cardiol 1992;19:11–18.
35. Lachterman B, Lehmann KG, Detrano R, Neutel J, Froelicher VF. Comparison of ST segment/heart rate index to standard ST criteria for analysis of exercise electrocardiogram. Circulation 1990;82:44–50.
36. Morise AP, Duval RD. Accuracy of ST/heart rate index in the diagnosis of coronary artery disease. Am J Cardiol 1992;69:603–606.
37. Pryor DB. The academic life cycle of a noninvasive test. Circulation 1990;82:302–304.
38. Bruce RA, Hossack KF, DeRouen TA, Hofer V. Enhanced risk assessment for primary coronary heart disease events by maximal exercise testing: 10 years' experience of Seattle Heart Watch. J Am Coll Cardiol 1983;2:565–573.
39. Giagnoni E, Secchi MB, Wu SC, et al. Prognostic value of exercise EKG testing in asymptomatic normotensive subjects: a prospective matched study. N Engl J Med 1983;309:1085–1089.
40. Gordon DJ, Ekelund LG, Karon JM, et al. Predictive value of the exercise tolerance test for mortality in North American men: the Lipid Research Clinics Mortality Follow-up Study. Circulation 1986;74:252–261.
41. Hopkirk JAC, Uhl GS, Hickman JR Jr, Fischer J, Medina A. Discriminant value of clinical and exercise variables in detecting significant coronary artery disease in asymptomatic men. J Am Coll Cardiol 1984;3:887–894.
42. Josephson RA, Shefrin E, Lakatta EG, Brant LJ, Fleg JL. Can serial exercise testing improve prediction of coronary events in asymptomatic individuals? Circulation 1990;81:20–24.
43. Weiner DA, Becker L, Bonow R. The diagnostic and prognostic significance of an asymptomatic positive exercise test. Circulation 1987;75(Suppl II):II-20–II-21.
44. Fleg JL, Gerstenblith G, Zonderman AB, et al. Prevalence and prognostic significance of exercise-induced silent myocardial ischemia detected by thallium scintigraphy and electrocardiography in asymptomatic volunteers. Circulation 1990;81:428–436.
45. McHenry PL, O'Donnell J, Morris SN, Jordan JJ. The abnormal exercise electrocardiogram in apparently healthy men: a predictor of angina pectoris as an initial coronary event during long-term follow-up. Circulation 1984;70:547–551.
46. Cohn PF. Should silent ischemia be treated in asymptomatic individuals? Circulation 1990;82(3 Suppl):II149–II154.
47. Bodenheimer MM. Risk stratification in coronary disease: a contrary viewpoint. Ann Intern Med 1992;116:927–936.
48. Coplan NL, Fuster VF. Limitations of the exercise test as a screen for acute cardiac events in asymptomatic patients. Am Heart J 1990;119:987–990.
49. Fuster V, Badimon L, Badimon JJ, Chesebro JH. The pathogenesis of coronary artery disease and the acute coronary syndromes. N Engl J Med 1992;326:242–250, 310–318.

50. Little WC, Constantinescu M, Applegate RJ, et al. Can coronary angiography predict the site of a subsequent myocardial infarction in patients with mild-moderate coronary artery disease? Circulation 1988;78:1157–1166.
51. Hickman JR Jr, Uhl GS, Cook RL, Engel PH, Hopkirk A. A natural history study of asymptomatic coronary artery disease (abstr). Am J Cardiol 1980;45:422.
52. Kotler TS, Diamond GA. Exercise thallium-201 scintigraphy in the diagnosis and prognosis of coronary artery disease. Ann Intern Med 1990;113:684–702.
53. Diamond GA. How accurate is SPECT thallium scintigraphy? J Am Coll Cardiol 1990;16:1017–1021.
54. Schwartz RS, Jackson WG, Celio PV, Richardson LA, Hickman JR Jr. Accuracy of exercise 201-Tl myocardial scintigraphy in asymptomatic young men. Circulation 1993;87:165–172.
55. Kohli RS, Cashman PM, Lahiri A, Raftery EB. The ST segment of the ambulatory electrocardiogram in a normal population. Br Heart J 1988;60:4–16.
56. Deanfield JE, Ribiero P, Oakley K, Krikler S, Selwyn AP. Analysis of ST-segment changes in normal subjects: implications for ambulatory monitoring in angina pectoris. Am J Cardiol 1984;54:1321–1325.
57. Quyyumi AA, Wright C, Fox K. Ambulatory electrocardiographic ST segment changes in healthy volunteers. Br Heart J 1983;50:460–464.
58. Hedblad B, Juul-Moller S, Svensson K. Increased mortality in men with ST segment depression during 24 h ambulatory long-term ECG recording. Eur Heart J 1989;10:149–158.
59. Quyyumi AA, Panza JA, Diodati JG, Callahan TS, Bonow RO, Epstein SE. Prognostic implications of myocardial ischemia during daily life in low risk patients with coronary artery disease. J Am Coll Cardiol 1993;21:700–708.
60. Detrano R, Yiannikas J, Salcedo EE, et al. Bayesian probability analysis: a prospective demonstration of its clinical utility in diagnosing coronary disease. Circulation 1984;69:541–547.
61. Shell WE, Kivowitz CF, Rubins SB, et al. Mechanisms and therapy of silent myocardial ischemia: the effect of transdermal nitroglycerin. Am Heart J 1986;112:222–229.
62. Deedwania PC, Carbajal EV, Nelson JR, Hait H. Anti-ischemic effects of atenolol versus nifedipine in patients with coronary artery disease and ambulatory silent ischemia. J Am Coll Cardiol 1991;17:963–969.
63. Juneau M, Theroux P, Waters D. Effect of diltiazem slow-release formulation on silent myocardial ischemia in stable coronary artery disease. The Canadian Multicenter Diltiazem Study Group. Am J Cardiol 1992;69:30B–35B.
64. Pepine CJ, Cohn PF, Deedwania PC, et al. Effects of treatment on outcome in mildly symptomatic patients with ischemia during daily life: the Atenolol Silent Ischemia Study (ASIST). Circulation 1994;90:762–768.
65. Pepine CJ, Cohn PF, Deedwania PC, et al. The prognostic and economic implications of a strategy to detect and treat asymptomatic ischemia: the Atenolol Silent Ischemia Trial (ASIST) protocol. Clin Cardiol 1991;14:457–462.
66. Lees AM, Lees RS, Shoen FJ, et al. Imaging human atherosclerosis with 99mTc-labeled low density lipoproteins. Arteriosclerosis 1988;8:461–470.
67. Rifkin RD, Uretsky BF. Screening for latent coronary artery disease by fluoroscopic detection of calcium in the coronary arteries. Am J Cardiol 1993;71:434–436.
68. Parisi AF, Folland ED, Hartigan P. A comparison of angioplasty with medical therapy in the treatment of single-vessel coronary artery disease. N Engl J Med 1992;326:10–16.
69. RITA Participants. Coronary angioplasty versus coronary artery bypass surgery: the Randomised Intervention Treatment of Angina (RITA) trial. Lancet 1993;341:573–580.
70. Colleen MF. The baseline screening electrocardiogram: is it worthwhile? An affirmative view. J Fam Pract 1987;25:393–396.
71. Kannel WB, Abbott RD. Incidence and prognosis of unrecognized myocardial infarction: an update on the Framingham study. N Engl J Med 1984;311:1144–1177.
72. Hoffman JR, Igarash E. Influence of electrocardiographic findings on admission decisions in patients with acute chest pain. Am J Med 1985;79:699–707.
73. Lee TH, Cook F, Weisberg MC, Rouan GW, Brand DA, Goldman L. Impact of the availability of a prior electrocardiogram on the triage of the patient with acute chest pain. J Gen Intern Med 1990;5:381–388.
74. Rubenstein LZ, Greenfield S. The baseline ECG in the evaluation of acute cardiac complaints. JAMA 1980;244:2536–2539.
75. Sox HC Jr. The baseline electrocardiogram. Am J Med 1991;91:573–575.
76. Ziemba SE, Hubbell FA, Fine MJ, Burns MJ. Resting electrocardiograms as baseline tests: impact on the management of elderly patients. Am J Med 1991;91:576–583.

77. Ekelund LG, Suchindran CM, McMahon RP, et al. Coronary heart disease morbidity and mortality in hypercholesterolemic men predicted from an exercise test: the Lipid Research Clinics Coronary Primary Prevention Trial. J Am Coll Cardiol 1989;14:556–563.
78. Siscovick DS, Ekelund LG, Johnson JL, Truong Y, Adler A. Sensitivity of exercise electrocardiography for acute cardiac events during moderate and strenuous physical activity: the Lipid Research Clinics Coronary Primary Prevention Trial. Arch Intern Med 1991;151:325–330.
79. Eddy DM, ed. Common screening tests. Philadelphia: American College of Physicians, 1991:398–401.
80. Canadian Task Force on the Periodic Health Examination. The periodic health examination: 1984 update. Can Med Assoc J 1984;130:2–15.
81. American Academy of Family Physicians. Age charts for periodic health examination. Kansas City, MO: American Academy of Family Physicians, 1994. (Reprint no. 510.)
82. American College of Cardiology/American Heart Association. Guidelines for electrocardiography. A report of the American College of Cardiology/American Heart Association Task Force on Assessment of Diagnostic and Therapeutic Cardiovascular Procedures (Committee on Electrocardiography). J Am Coll Cardiol 1992;19:473–481.
83. American College of Sports Medicine. Guidelines for exercise testing and prescription. 4th ed. Philadelphia: Lea & Febiger, 1991.
84. American College of Cardiology/American Heart Association. Guidelines for exercise testing. A report of the American College of Cardiology/American Heart Association Task Force on assessment of cardiovascular procedures (Subcommittee on Exercise Testing). J Am Coll Cardiol 1986;8:725–738.
85. American College of Physicians. Efficacy of exercise thallium-201 scintigraphy in the diagnosis and prognosis of coronary artery disease. Ann Intern Med 1990;113:703–704.

2. Screening for High Blood Cholesterol and Other Lipid Abnormalities

RECOMMENDATION

Periodic screening for high blood cholesterol is recommended for all men ages 35–65 and women ages 45–65. There is insufficient evidence to recommend for or against routine screening of asymptomatic persons over age 65, but recommendations to screen healthy men and women ages 65–75 may be made on other grounds (see *Clinical Intervention*). There is also insufficient evidence to recommend for or against routine screening in children, adolescents, or young adults. Recommendations for screening adolescents and young adults with risk factors for coronary disease, and against routine screening in children, may be made on other grounds (*see* Clinical Intervention). There is insufficient evidence to recommend for or against routine screening for other lipid abnormalities. All patients should receive periodic screening and counseling regarding other measures to reduce their risk of coronary disease (*see* Chapter 3, Screening for Hypertension; Chapter 54, Counseling to Prevent Tobacco Use; Chapter 55, Counseling to Promote Physical Activity; and Chapter 56, Counseling to Promote a Healthy Diet).

Burden of Suffering

Elevated blood cholesterol is one of the major modifiable risk factors for coronary heart disease (CHD),[1] the leading cause of death in the U.S. CHD accounts for approximately 490,000 deaths each year,[2] and angina and nonfatal myocardial infarction (MI) are a source of substantial morbidity. CHD is projected to cost over $60 billion in 1995 in the U.S. in medical expenses and lost productivity.[3] The incidence of CHD is low in men under age 35 and in premenopausal women (1–2/1,000 annually),[4] but climbs exponentially during middle age for both men and women. The onset of CHD is delayed approximately 10 years in women compared with men, probably due to effects of estrogen,[5] but women account for 49% of all CHD deaths in the U.S.[2] Clinical events are the result of a multifactorial process that begins years before the onset of symptoms. Autopsy studies detected early lesions of atherosclerosis in many adolescents and young

15

adults.[6–10] The onset of atherosclerosis and symptomatic CHD is earlier among persons with inherited lipid disorders such as familial hypercholesterolemia (FH)[11] and familial combined hyperlipidemia (FCH).[12]

Serum Cholesterol and Risk of Coronary Heart Disease. Epidemiologic, pathologic, animal, genetic, and clinical studies support a causal relationship between blood lipids (usually measured as serum levels) and coronary atherosclerosis.[1,13–15] Extended follow-up of large cohorts (predominantly middle-aged men)[16–18] provides evidence that CHD risk increases in a continuous and graded fashion, beginning with cholesterol levels as low as 150–180 mg/dL;[a] this association extends to cholesterol levels measured as early as age 20 in men.[14,19] During middle age, for each 1% increase in total cholesterol, CHD risk increases by an estimated 3%.[20] High cholesterol (≥240 mg/dL) is also a risk factor in middle-aged women, but most coronary events in women occur well after menopause.[5,17,21–24] Some studies report that cholesterol alone is a weak predictor of CHD mortality in the elderly,[24a,190] but an overview of 24 cohort studies indicates that high cholesterol remains a risk factor for CHD after age 65,[23] with the strongest associations among healthier elderly populations followed over longer periods.[25–27] The association is weaker in older women than in men[23] and is not consistent for cholesterol levels measured after age 75.[28–31]

Expert panels have defined high and "borderline high" (200–239 mg/dL) cholesterol to simplify clinical decisions.[1] Because CHD is a multifactorial process, however, there is no definition of high cholesterol that discriminates well between individuals who will or will not develop CHD.[32,33] Due to nonlipid risk factors, persons with cholesterol below 240 mg/dL account for the majority of all CHD events.[34,35] Among middle-aged men, 9–12% of those with cholesterol 240 mg/dL or greater will develop symptomatic CHD over the next 7–9 years,[34,36] but most of them have multiple other risk factors for CHD.[35] The excess (i.e., absolute) risk due to high cholesterol (and the probable benefit of lowering cholesterol) increases with the underlying risk of CHD. In a 12-year study of over 316,000 men aged 35–57, the excess CHD mortality attributable to high cholesterol was greatest in men over age 45, and in those who smoked or had hypertension.[16] The increase in CHD mortality associated with a given increment in serum cholesterol was steepest at very high values (>300 mg/dL).[16] Excess risk from high cholesterol is smaller in women, who have less than half the CHD risk as do men at any given cholesterol level.[17,23,37] Although the relative risk associated with high serum choles-

---

[a]To convert values for serum total cholesterol, HDL-C, and LDL-C to mmol/L, multiply by 0.02586. Equivalent values for commonly used thresholds are 280 mg/dL = 7.2 mmol/L, 240 mg/dL = 6.2 mmol/L, 200 mg/dL = 5.2 mmol/L.

terol declines with age,[17,23,28] the excess risk generally does not, due to the much higher incidence of CHD in older persons.[31,38,39]

Other Lipid Constituents and Risk of Coronary Disease. The risk associated with high total cholesterol is primarily due to high levels of low-density lipoprotein cholesterol (LDL-C),[1] but there is a strong, independent, and inverse association between high-density lipoprotein cholesterol (HDL-C) levels and CHD risk.[40–42] Low HDL-C increases risk even when cholesterol is below 200 mg/dL,[41] a pattern present in up to 20% of men with confirmed CHD.[43] In many studies, measures of HDL-C or the ratio of total cholesterol to HDL-C are better predictors of CHD risk than is serum cholesterol alone.[5,22,23,24a,41,44] High total cholesterol in association with high HDL-C (≥60 mg/dL) is common in older women (especially those taking estrogen) but is not associated with an increased risk for CHD.[1,41] The importance of triglycerides as an independent risk factor for CHD remains uncertain.[40,45] Three large studies reported strong associations between triglyceride levels over 200–300 mg/dL (2.26–3.39 mmol/L) and cardiovascular mortality in women,[21,22,24] but other analyses found no association after controlling for obesity, fasting glucose, or low HDL-C.[46] The combination of high triglycerides and low HDL-C often occurs in association with other CHD risk factors such as hypertension and diabetes and is associated with a high risk of CHD.[46a]

Prevalence of High Cholesterol and Low HDL-C. Serum total cholesterol and LDL-C increase 1–2 mg/dL per year in men from ages 20–40, 2 mg/dL per year in women from ages 40–60,[47] and an average 18% during the perimenopausal period, due in part to age-related increases in weight.[48] The prevalence of serum cholesterol 240 mg/dL or higher increases from 8–9% in adults under age 35 to nearly 25% for men age 55 and nearly 40% for women over 65.[49] Approximately 11% of men and 3% of women over age 20 have low HDL-C (<35 mg/dL) with desirable or borderline-high total cholesterol.[49]

Accuracy of Screening Tests

Both total cholesterol and HDL-C can be measured in venipuncture or finger-stick specimens from fasting or nonfasting individuals. Due to normal physiologic variation and measurement error, a single measurement may not reflect the patient's true (or average) cholesterol level. Stress, minor illness, posture, and seasonal fluctuations may cause serum cholesterol to vary 4–11% within an individual.[50] Laboratory assays are subject to random errors, due to variation in sample collection, handling, and reagents, and to systematic errors (bias), due to methods that consistently overestimate or underestimate cholesterol values.[51] In a survey of 5,000 clinical laboratories, 93% of the measurements were within 9% of a reference standard.[52]

Desktop analyzers can produce reliable results, but some devices may not meet standards for accuracy.[53] Variation in training and operating technique can introduce additional error when instruments are used outside clinical laboratories.[54] Average bias for measurements based on capillary specimens compared to venous specimens was +4–7%.[55]

As a result of these considerations, a single measure of serum cholesterol could vary as much as 14% from an individual's average value under acceptable laboratory conditions.[50] For an individual with a "true" cholesterol level of 200 mg/dL, the 95% range of expected values is 172–228 mg/dL.[56] Some authorities therefore recommend advising patients of their "cholesterol range," rather than a single value.[56] Where more precise estimates are necessary, an average of at least two measurements on two occasions has been recommended, and a third if the first two values differ by more than 16%.[50]

Screening Children by Family History. Although cholesterol levels in childhood correlate moderately well with levels in adulthood (correlation coefficient 0.4–0.6), many children with elevated serum cholesterol (defined as serum cholesterol ≥200 mg/dL or LDL-C ≥130 mg/dL, the 90–95th percentile in U.S. children under 19 years)[57] do not have high cholesterol as adults.[58–60] Furthermore, the association between childhood cholesterol levels and CHD in adults has not been studied. Because of the familial aggregation of CHD and hypercholesterolemia,[57,61,62] some experts recommend screening for family history of either premature cardiovascular disease (age 55 or younger) or parental hypercholesterolemia (≥240 mg/dL) to identify a subset of children who are more likely to be at risk from hypercholesterolemia as adults.[57] Under this definition, only 25% of all children would be screened, but the predictive value of family history is limited: 81–90% of children with such histories have normal cholesterol.[63–66] Even when parental cholesterol has been measured and found to be elevated, most children have normal cholesterol values.[57,67,68]

Parental and childhood cholesterol levels are highest in heterozygous FH (estimated prevalence 1 in 500), which is strongly associated with premature CHD. Up to 50% of men with FH develop clinical CHD by age 50.[69,70] Screening based on family history, as defined above, does not appear to be an efficient strategy for detecting FH, however. Many children would be screened, and few of those identified and treated for high cholesterol would have FH.[71] By itself, a parental history of premature CHD is likely to detect less than half of all children with FH.[70] Tracing and screening families of index cases with FH may be more cost-effective than population screening for FH.[72]

Screening for Other Lipid Abnormalities. Measurements of HDL-C and triglycerides are less reliable than measurement of total cholesterol due to greater biologic and analytic variability.[73,74] The 95% range of expected values for an individual with HDL-C of 37 mg/dL is 29–45 mg/dL.[75] A survey of 250 laboratories found that one third of all HDL-C measurements varied more than 10% from a reference value.[76] Triglycerides must be measured on fasting specimens. Even then, intraindividual variation is greater than 20%, and a single measure is inadequate to categorize levels as high or normal.[73,74] Measurement of apolipoproteins (e.g., apoB) has been evaluated as a screening test for FH, familial coronary disease, and high LDL-C, but these assays are not yet widely available or adequately standardized.[57]

Effectiveness of Early Detection

No long-term study has compared routine cholesterol screening to alternate strategies (selective case-finding or universal dietary advice without screening) with change in cholesterol levels or CHD incidence as an outcome. The increase in cholesterol screening over the past decade in the U.S. has been accompanied by significant improvements in dietary knowledge,[77] fat consumption,[78] average cholesterol levels,[79] and CHD mortality,[14] but it is difficult to isolate the contribution of screening from other factors (e.g., public education, changes in food supply) that may account for these trends. In community- or practice-based trials, patients receiving risk-factor screening and targeted dietary advice had slightly lower average cholesterol levels (1–3%) than did unscreened controls at 1–3-year follow-up, but dietary interventions were limited.[80-82] Whether screening improves the effectiveness of routine dietary advice has been examined in two short-term studies where all subjects received counseling about diet; cholesterol screening modestly improved mean cholesterol levels in one study but had no effect in the other.[83,84] In a school-based study in which all children received similar health education, cardiovascular risk-factor screening (including cholesterol measurement) was associated with improved dietary knowledge and self-reported behavior, but changes in lipid levels were not assessed.[85]

The primary evidence to support cholesterol screening is the ability of cholesterol-lowering interventions to reduce the risk of CHD in patients with high cholesterol. These benefits are now well established for persons with preexisting atherosclerotic vascular disease. In individual trials and overviews of studies enrolling persons with angina or prior myocardial infarction (MI), cholesterol-lowering treatments slowed the progression of atherosclerosis,[86] reduced the incidence of CHD,[87,88] and reduced overall mortality.[89] In the first long-term trial of newer cholesterol-lowering drugs, treatment with simvastatin over 5.4 years reduced coronary mortality 42% and all-cause mortality 30% in 4,444 men and women with coronary disease.[90]

The absolute benefit of treating high cholesterol in persons without cardiovascular disease, however, is much smaller due to the much lower risk of death or MI (annual CHD mortality 0.1–0.3% in middle-aged men with asymptomatic high cholesterol vs. 2–10% per year in patients with symptomatic CHD).[91] The risks and benefits of lowering cholesterol in asymptomatic persons—primarily middle-aged men with very high cholesterol—have been examined in trials using medications, modified diets in institutional patients, or outpatient dietary counseling, and in overviews of these trials.

Trials of Cholesterol-Lowering Drugs in Asymptomatic Men. Three large, multicenter, placebo-controlled trials of lipid-lowering medications provide the best evidence that lowering cholesterol can reduce combined CHD incidence (fatal and nonfatal events) in asymptomatic persons. These trials enrolled hypercholesterolemic middle-aged men (age 30–59, mean cholesterol 246–289 mg/dL) and lowered total cholesterol 9–10% (and LDL-C 10–13%) over periods of 5–7 years. In the World Health Organization Cooperative Trial, treatment with clofibrate significantly reduced the incidence of nonfatal MI by 25%,[92] but this benefit was offset by significant increases in noncardiac and total mortality (40% and 30% respectively, p = 0.01).[93] The Lipid Research Clinics (LRC) Coronary Primary Prevention Trial reported a significant 19% reduction in cumulative incidence of MI and sudden cardiac death in patients treated with cholestyramine over 7 years (7.0% vs. 8.6%).[36] In the Helsinki Heart Study, treatment with gemfibrozil significantly reduced the 5-year cumulative incidence of cardiac events by 34% (2.7% vs. 4.1%).[94] Most of the benefit of gemfibrozil was confined to men with a high ratio of LDL-C to HDL-C (≥5) and triglycerides >200 mg/dL.[95] Effects on CHD mortality were not statistically significant in any of these trials. Two additional drug trials reported 1–3-year results in largely asymptomatic populations.[96,97] Roughly 30% of subjects had CHD at entry, however, and these accounted for most of the coronary events during follow-up.

Trials of Diet in Institutionalized Persons. Demonstrating a clinical benefit of modern cholesterol-lowering diets in asymptomatic persons has proven difficult. In three controlled trials in institutionalized patients, fat-modified diets reduced serum cholesterol 12–14% with generally favorable effects on CHD over periods of up to 8 years.[98–100] Each of these studies used diets high in polyunsaturated fat, which have been associated with adverse effects,[15] and none excluded patients with CHD. As a result, their findings may not be applicable to currently recommended low-fat diets in asymptomatic persons.

Trials of Dietary Advice in Outpatients. The only trials to examine the clinical benefits of a diet low in total and saturated fat in persons without CHD are multifactorial intervention trials, which offered dietary counseling, smoking cessation advice, and/or treatment of high blood pressure to middle-aged men.[101-105] Among Norwegian smokers with very high cholesterol levels (mean 320 mg/dL) and fat consumption (44% calories), dietary advice lowered cholesterol 13% and, in conjunction with smoking cessation, reduced CHD incidence by 47%.[103] The remaining trials achieved much smaller (0–5%) reductions in cholesterol and insignificant effects on CHD; the benefits of intervention in some studies may have been limited by ineffective counseling and follow-up,[101,104] lower cholesterol levels at baseline,[101] or adverse effects of other therapies.[102,105] In the most systematic test of dietary counseling in adults, 10 weekly group sessions and periodic individual counseling were provided over 6 years to over 6,000 men (mean cholesterol 253 mg/dL).[102] Average cholesterol level declined 5% in men receiving counseling, but only 2% compared to controls. Greater changes were observed in men who lost at least 5 pounds and those with higher serum cholesterol at baseline,[106] but there was no significant reduction in CHD mortality or incidence in the intervention group.[102,107]

Short-term metabolic studies and selected trials in patients with CHD indicate that reducing dietary saturated fat and/or increasing polyunsaturated fat intake can reduce elevated total and LDL-C as much as 10–20%.[108-110] Due to variable compliance, trials of diet counseling in the primary care setting have achieved much smaller and inconsistent average reductions in serum cholesterol in asymptomatic persons (0–4%).[80-82,111-116] Although larger changes have been reported in uncontrolled follow-up studies after cholesterol screening,[117,118] these results may be biased by selective or short-term follow-up and regression to the mean in persons with high cholesterol. Ongoing studies are examining the efficacy of cholesterol screening and intervention in primary care settings in the U.S.[119] More stringent diets can produce larger reductions in cholesterol,[120] but long-term data in asymptomatic persons are limited. Two trials in women at risk for breast cancer lowered total fat intake to 20% of calories and reduced total cholesterol 6–7% over 1–2 years.[121,122]

Overviews of Cholesterol-Lowering Trials. At least 10 quantitative overviews (meta-analyses) of randomized trials have attempted to resolve uncertainties about the risks and benefits of lowering cholesterol, including effects on mortality.[18,88,89,91,123-128] Three recent overviews provide the most comprehensive analyses of long-term cholesterol-lowering trials published through 1993; 35 diet and drug trials were included in one analysis,[91] 28 in the second (excluding trials that used estrogens or thyroxine),[18,89] and 22 in the third (all trials achieving at least a 4% reduction in cholesterol for at least 3 years).[128] These overviews support a dose-response relationship between change in serum cholesterol and reduction in CHD incidence (fatal and nonfatal events combined) comparable to that predicted from epidemiologic studies: after 2–5 years of treatment, each 1% reduction in serum cholesterol yields a 2–3% reduction in total CHD, for both diet and drug interventions, and in patients with or without CHD at entry.[18,89,128]

When only trials enrolling asymptomatic persons were analyzed, however, neither CHD mortality nor total mortality was significantly reduced by cholesterol lowering:[128] difference in total mortality among treated versus control subjects = +6%, 95% confidence interval (CI) –3% to +17%.[89] Moreover, noncardiac mortality was increased 20–24% among patients treated with lipid-lowering medications.[89,91,128] While observing similar effects of treatment, each overview offered distinct interpretations of these findings. Law et al. concluded that the increase in noncoronary mortality was most likely due to chance: the finding was of borderline statistical significance (p = 0.02), did not reflect any consistent cause of excess mortality among trials, and was independent of compliance with therapy.[89] Gordon attributed adverse effects to trials employing hormones or fibrate medications.[128] Davey Smith et al. concluded that lipid-lowering drugs reduced overall mortality in high-risk persons (i.e., persons with CHD), but were harmful in those at lower risk.[91] When trials were stratified by the observed CHD mortality in the control group, drug treatment was associated with a significant 20% increase in all-cause mortality in 10 trials enrolling low-risk subjects (CHD mortality <1% per year), including the WHO, LRC, and Helsinki studies.[91] A single trial (the WHO clofibrate study) accounts for nearly half of all patient-years of treatment in persons without CHD[128] and has a strong influence on results of any meta-analysis.

Due to methodologic concerns about combining results from trials employing different cholesterol-lowering drugs and diets, meta-analysis cannot prove or disprove possible harms from lipid-lowering medications.[129] These analyses, however, illustrate the importance of underlying CHD risk in determining whether expected benefits are likely to justify possible risks of treatment. Even if drugs are safe, the margin of benefit may be small for many persons with asymptomatic hypercholesterolemia. In the LRC and Helsinki trials, preventing one coronary death required treating 300–400 middle-aged men for 5–7 years.[36,94] The benefits of lipid-lowering medications on nonfatal CHD are more pronounced but must be weighed against the unpleasant and occasionally serious side effects of some drugs (see below).[92,127,130] The newest class of lipid-lowering drugs, HMG-CoA reductase inhibitors or "statins," lowers cholesterol more effectively and appears to be well-tolerated in trials lasting up to 6 years.[90,97] These drugs are more likely to have significant effects on mortality in patients without CHD, but long-term trials of these agents in asymptomatic persons have yet to report results.[131]

Cholesterol Reduction in Women. Lipid-lowering medications and diet effectively lower cholesterol in women,[132] but no trial has specifically examined the benefits of cholesterol reduction in asymptomatic women.[133] Trials that included female subjects with CHD observed qualitatively similar benefits of cholesterol reduction on angiographic or clinical endpoints in women and men.[90,99,133] In the 4S trial, simvastatin significantly reduced CHD incidence, but not mortality, in women with CHD.[90] Two trials in women without CHD, with a cumulative enrollment of more than 6,000 women, observed no effect of drug or diet treatment on CHD incidence or mortality after 1–3 years;[96,100] the short duration of follow-up may have limited the power of these studies to detect a difference.[133] Long-term data on drug therapy in women are limited, with the exception of estrogen therapy (see Chapter 68).

Cholesterol Reduction in Older Adults. The benefit of lowering cholesterol in older persons has been questioned due to the weak association between serum cholesterol and all-cause mortality after age 60.[17,28,30] Associations between cholesterol and mortality in unselected elderly populations, however, are likely to be confounded by the increasing prevalence of chronic illnesses which increase mortality and independently lower serum cholesterol.[26,134,135] Direct evidence that cholesterol reduction is beneficial in asymptomatic older persons is not yet available, but cholesterol-lowering diets and medications reduced overall mortality 26–30% in persons over 60 with clinical CHD.[90,136,137] In two trials in patients without CHD that included older subjects, however, cholesterol reduction produced significant benefits in younger but not in older patients (over age 60 or 65).[96,98] Newer cholesterol-lowering agents are efficacious and well-tolerated in older patients.[90,138] A large multicenter trial is under way to examine the effectiveness of pravastatin and various antihypertensive medications in asymptomatic persons over age 60 with hypertension and high cholesterol.[138] There are few controlled trials of dietary counseling to lower cholesterol in older patients; no significant change in cholesterol levels was observed among rural Medicare recipients offered diet counseling[139] or older patients receiving diet counseling and placebo medication.[138]

Cholesterol Reduction in Adolescents and Young Adults. Determining the benefits of lowering cholesterol in children, adolescents, and young adults is difficult, due to their low near-term risk of clinical coronary disease. The assumption that early treatment is more effective than treatment begun later in life[57] rests on observations that early atherosclerosis is present in many adolescents and young adults, is associated with lipid levels, progresses with age,[6] and is difficult to reverse in middle age.[86] New evidence, however, suggests that much of the clinical benefit of lowering cholesterol can be achieved within 2–5 years of initiating therapy.[18] These benefits have been attributed to stabilizing "lipid-rich" lesions[87] and improving endothelial function,[140] and they suggest that the additional benefits of early drug therapy for hypercholesterolemia (i.e., before middle age) may not justify the added expense and possible risks of longer treatment. Intensive diet or drug intervention for adolescents and young adults with FH, although never tested in a prospective trial, has become standard treatment due to the very high levels of LDL-C and dramatically increased risk of premature CHD in persons with FH.[11,71] Even in FH, however, most clinical events occur in middle age (i.e., after age 40), and risk is variable: MI was rare before age 30 in men in one study, and onset of CHD is later in women and nonsmokers with FH.[69,141]

Modified diets lower cholesterol in young adults, but the contribution of universal screening in motivating risk reduction in young persons is uncertain. Neither a multiple-intervention trial in Australian workers[142] nor a study of risk assessment in a general practice in the U.K.[116] demonstrated that screening and dietary advice led to long-term reduction in cholesterol levels in younger men (under age 35–40). The effectiveness of screening and dietary counseling has not been adequately studied in young adults and cannot be predicted reliably from studies in middle-aged men.

Cholesterol Reduction in Children. Dietary fat intake in children is associated with total cholesterol and LDL-C levels,[143,144] but controlled trials have not consistently demonstrated that individual dietary counseling is effective in children.[145–147] Results from the largest trial reported that children with elevated LDL-C who received intensive family-oriented dietary counseling (30 sessions over 3 years) experienced a significant but modest (3.2 mg/dL) reduction in mean LDL-C compared with controls.[148] Uncontrolled studies of dietician counseling for hyperlipidemic children and adolescents have reported larger short-term reductions in mean cholesterol and LDL-C,[149–153] but such studies are prone to bias from regression to the mean and selective follow-up. Physical activity and fitness are associated with higher levels of HDL-C in children and adolescents, but controlled and uncontrolled trials[154–159] have reported inconsistent effects of exercise interventions on lipids. Drug therapy effectively lowers cholesterol in children, but side effects limit compliance with bile-acid resins, the only therapy currently recommended for routine use in children.[57] In one study of 80 children with FH or FCH, only 13% were still compliant with resin therapy after 3 years.[160] Ongoing studies are examining the safety and efficacy of newer agents in children.

Potential Adverse Effects of Screening and Intervention. Measurement of serum cholesterol is safe and relatively inexpensive, but widespread screening may have some undesirable consequences. In populations in which the potential benefits of early detection may be small (e.g., low-risk young persons), the possibility of harm may influence decisions about universal screening.[161] Anecdotal reports have reported decreased well-being in persons diagnosed with high cholesterol (i.e., "labeling"),[162] but a prospective study did not confirm this effect.[163] Other possible adverse effects of screening include inconvenience and expense of screening and follow-up, opportunity costs to the busy clinician, misinformation due to inaccurate results, and reduced attention to diet in persons with "desirable" cholesterol levels.[164] The importance of possible adverse effects of screening has not been systematically studied.

The safety of cholesterol-lowering interventions is especially important in children and young persons. Dietary restrictions may reduce intake of calories, calcium, vitamins, and iron in children,[165–167] and failure-to-thrive due to excessively fat-restricted diets has been reported, albeit rarely, in children.[168,169] In the most comprehensive trial of dietary intervention in children, however, no adverse effects on growth, sexual development, psychological measures, iron status, or blood micronutrients were detected at 3-year follow-up.[148] Other controlled studies also support the safety of properly performed dietary intervention in children.[147,166,170] The elderly may also be at risk from modified diets if adequate intake of calories, calcium, and essential vitamins is not maintained, but these effects have not been directly examined.

The inappropriate use of drug therapy is of greater concern, especially in young persons in whom the benefit of early drug treatment may not justify the costs and possible risks.[18,161] According to a national survey of pediatricians and family physicians, one in six regularly prescribed drugs for hypercholesterolemic children, and a substantial number did so based on inappropriate criteria, or used drugs not routinely recommended for children.[171] Persons under age 40 accounted for over 1 million prescriptions for lipid-lowering drugs in 1992;[172] gemfibrozil was the second most commonly prescribed lipid-lowering drug in the U.S. in 1992,[172] despite limited indications for its use[1] and important safety concerns. Fibrate medications (e.g., clofibrate and gemfibrozil) have been associated with an increase in gallstone disease,[92] adverse trends in CHD mortality[93,173] and cancer mortality in individual trials,[93,174] and a significant increase in noncoronary mortality in a recent overview of long-term trials.[128] HMG-CoA reductase inhibitors have not been associated with important adverse effects in trials lasting up to 6 years.[90] The safety of lifelong therapy with these agents cannot yet be determined; several medications in this class have been reported to cause liver tumors in animal studies.

Early Detection of Other Lipid Abnormalities. The importance of detecting low HDL-C or high triglycerides remains unproven, especially in persons with normal serum cholesterol. Weight loss in obese subjects,[132,175] smoking cessation, exercise,[176,176a] and moderate alcohol consumption[177] can raise HDL-C and/or lower triglyceride levels. Some of these lifestyle interventions have only small effects, however, and most can be recommended independent of lipid levels. Most importantly, no trial has directly examined the benefit of raising HDL-C or lowering triglycerides.[40,45] Secondary analyses of several trials have attributed varying proportions of the clinical benefit of drug therapy to increases in HDL-C,[40,94,95] or reductions in triglycerides,[136] but all of the subjects had high total or LDL cholesterol. The benefit of drug treatment for low HDL-C and normal cholesterol has not been determined but is being studied in men with CHD.[43]

Recommendations of Other Groups

The National Cholesterol Education Program Adult Treatment Panel II, convened by the National Heart, Lung, and Blood Institute, recommends routine measurement of nonfasting total cholesterol and HDL-C in all adults age 20 or older at least once every 5 years.[1,178] The Canadian Task Force on the Periodic Health Examination concluded there was insufficient evidence to recommend routine cholesterol screening but endorsed case-finding in men 30–59 years old.[127] The American Academy of Family Physicians[179] recommends measurement of total cholesterol at least every 5 years in adults age 19 and older; these recommendations are under review. The American College of Obstetricians and Gynecologists recommends periodic screening of cholesterol in all women over age 20, and in selected high-risk adolescents.[180] In guidelines revised in 1995, the American College of Physicians (ACP) concluded that screening serum cholesterol was appropriate but not mandatory for asymptomatic men aged 35–65 and women aged 45–65; screening is not recommended for younger persons unless they are suspected of having a familial lipoprotein disorder or have multiple cardiac risk factors. The ACP concluded that evidence was not sufficient to recommend for or against screening asymptomatic persons between the ages of 65 and 75, but it recommends against screening after age 75.[181]

Selective screening of children and adolescents is recommended by the National Cholesterol Education Program Expert Panel on Blood Cholesterol Levels in Children and Adolescents,[57] the American Academy of Pediatrics (AAP),[182] the Bright Futures guidelines,[183] the American Medical Association Guidelines for Adolescent and Preventive Services (GAPS),[184] and the American Academy of Family Physicians.[179] Screening with nonfasting cholesterol in all children and adolescents who have a parental history of hypercholesterolemia, and with fasting lipid profile in those with a family history of premature cardiovascular disease, is recommended. These organizations recommend that children who have multiple risk factors for CHD (such as smoking or obesity) and whose family history cannot be ascertained be screened at the discretion of the physician.

Discussion

Elevated serum cholesterol is an important risk factor for CHD in men and women in the U.S., and there is now good evidence that lowering serum cholesterol can reduce the risk of CHD. Whereas measures that lower serum cholesterol and provide other health benefits (e.g., regular physical activity, reducing dietary fat, and maintaining a healthy weight) should be encouraged in all persons, cholesterol screening can identify high-risk individuals who are most likely to benefit from individualized dietary counseling or drug treatment. In addition, screening may help clinicians and patients identify priorities for risk factor modification and reinforce public awareness of the importance of a healthy diet.

Some important questions remain, however, about routine lipid screening in asymptomatic and low-risk persons, including when to begin screening and which constituents to measure. Overall, evidence is strongest for screening for high serum cholesterol in middle-aged men (ages 35–65), based on the reduction in coronary morbidity in trials enrolling asymptomatic men with very high cholesterol (mean 280 mg/dL). The epidemiology and pathophysiology of CHD is similar in men and women, suggesting that reducing high cholesterol levels will also reduce CHD in asymptomatic women. Extrapolations to premenopausal women may not be appropriate, given their low risk of CHD and the apparent protective effects of estrogen on CHD incidence. The optimal age to screen women is not known; the later onset of hypercholesterolemia and CHD suggests that routine screening should begin around age 45.

Direct evidence that screening and intervention is effective in persons over age 65 is not yet available, but epidemiologic studies indicate that the risks of high cholesterol extend up to age 75. Given the high risk of CHD in the elderly, and the benefits of lowering cholesterol in symptomatic older men and women, screening may be reasonable in older persons who do not have major comorbid illnesses. Since individual cholesterol levels usually plateau by age 65 in women (and earlier in men), continued screening is less important in patients who have had desirable cholesterol levels throughout middle age.

There is not yet evidence that routine lipid screening is effective in reducing cholesterol levels or CHD risk in younger populations. Universal screening is an inefficient way to identify the small number of hypercholesterolemic young persons at risk for premature CHD, most of whom have multiple nonlipid risk factors or a history suggestive of familial dyslipidemia. Most "high-risk" young persons (excluding young men with FH) have a near-term risk of CHD well below that of hypercholesterolemic middle-aged men,[185] and are not appropriate candidates for early drug therapy. Screening young persons can provide information to help stimulate lifestyle changes, but promoting a healthy lifestyle (e.g., healthy diet, regular physical activity, etc.) is important for all young persons, including the majority with "desirable" cholesterol levels. International comparisons suggest that cholesterol levels explain only part of the strong association between diet and heart disease.[186a] As a result, it is uncertain whether routine cholesterol screening in low-risk younger populations is of sufficient benefit to justify the inconvenience, costs, and possible risks of screening and treatment. In a study modeling benefits of cholesterol screening, a conservative strategy of screening only middle-aged men and others with multiple CHD risk factors produced benefits comparable to screening all adults over age 20; if interventions had adverse effects on quality of life, the more conservative strategy was preferable.[186] Should future studies demonstrate that routine screening and targeted interventions are more effective in the primary care setting than universal dietary advice in young persons, this would provide some additional justification for early screening.

The benefits of screening children are even less certain. Progression of atherosclerosis in childhood is limited, many children with high cholesterol are not hypercholesterolemic as adults, and it is uncertain whether or not reducing cholesterol levels in childhood will significantly alter the risk of CHD many years later. Given the limited effectiveness of dietary counseling, poor compliance with currently recommended drug therapy, and the potential for adverse reactions in children, widespread pediatric screening might result in more harm than good.

The benefit of measuring HDL-C or triglycerides at initial screening is unproven. Measures to lower high triglycerides or raise HDL-C (e.g., weight reduction in obese persons and exercise) have relatively modest effects and should be encouraged regardless of lipid levels. Measures of HDL-C and lipoprotein analysis improve the estimation of coronary risk and should be obtained to guide treatment decisions in patients with high total cholesterol. There is, however, no evidence that they significantly improve the management of patients who do not have high total cholesterol.

While a single cholesterol test is relatively inexpensive, the cumulative costs of screening can be substantial under protocols calling for measurement of HDL-C, periodic screening, and detailed evaluation and treatment of the large population with high cholesterol. To be effective, dietary interventions require regular follow-up and reinforcement. Under optimistic assumptions, tailored dietary therapy in middle-aged men is estimated to cost more than $20,000 per year of life gained, when costs of screening and follow-up are included.[187] Drug treatment of asymptomatic middle-aged men (assuming no important adverse effects) has been estimated to cost at least \$50,000–90,000 per year of life saved.[35,188] HMG-CoA reductase inhibitors are substantially more expensive than earlier medications, but they lower LDL-C more effectively and also raise HDL-C. These agents may improve the cost-effectiveness of drug therapy for asymptomatic hypercholesterolemia, especially in high-risk men,[189] but the long-term safety and effectiveness of these agents in persons without CHD have not yet been established.

CLINICAL INTERVENTION

Periodic screening for high blood cholesterol, using specimens obtained from fasting or nonfasting individuals, is recommended for all men ages 35–65 and women ages 45–65 ("B" recommendation). There is insufficient evidence to recommend for or against routine screening in asymptomatic persons after age 65, but screening may be considered on a case-by-case basis ("C" recommendation). Older persons with major CHD risk factors (smoking, hypertension, diabetes) who are otherwise healthy may be more likely to benefit from screening, based on their high risk of CHD and the proven benefits of lowering cholesterol in older persons with symptomatic CHD. Cholesterol levels are not a reliable predictor of risk after age 75, however. There is insufficient evidence to recommend routine screening in children, adolescents, or young adults ("C" recommendation). For adolescents and young adults who have a family history of very high cholesterol, premature CHD in a first-degree relative (before age 50 in men or age 60 in women), or major risk factors for CHD screening may be recommended on other grounds: the greater absolute risk attributable to high cholesterol in such persons, and the potential long-term benefits of early lifestyle interventions in young persons with high cholesterol. Recommendations against routine screening in children may be made on other grounds, including the costs and inconvenience of screening and follow-up, greater potential for adverse effects of treatment, and the uncertain long-term benefits of small reductions in childhood cholesterol levels.

The appropriate interval for periodic screening is not known. Periodic screening is most important when cholesterol levels are increasing (e.g., middle-aged men, perimenopausal women, and persons who have gained weight). An interval of 5 years has been recommended by experts,[1] but longer intervals may be reasonable in low-risk subjects (including those with previously desirable cholesterol levels).

There is insufficient evidence to recommend for or against routine measurement of HDL-C or triglycerides at initial screening ("C" recommendation). For high-risk persons (middle-aged persons with high cholesterol or multiple nonlipid risk factors for CHD), measurement of HDL-C

or lipoprotein analysis can be recommended to help identify individuals at highest risk of CHD, in whom individual diet or drug therapy may be indicated.

Decisions about interventions for high cholesterol should be based on at least two measures of cholesterol and assessment of the absolute risk of CHD in each individual. This assessment should take into account the age of the patient (higher risk in men over 45 and women over 55), results of lipoprotein analysis (or ratio of total cholesterol to HDL-C), and the presence and severity of other risk factors for CHD (see above).[178] More specific algorithms for risk assessment have been published.[185] Initial therapy for patients with elevated cholesterol is counseling to reduce consumption of fat (especially saturated fat) and promote weight loss in overweight persons. A two-step dietary program effective in lowering serum cholesterol has been described in detail elsewhere.[1] Benefits of drug therapy are likely to justify costs and potential risks only in persons at high risk of CHD (e.g., middle-aged men and postmenopausal women with very high cholesterol or multiple risk factors). The risks and benefits of drug therapy in asymptomatic persons over 65 have not yet been determined. In postmenopausal women with high cholesterol, estrogen therapy can lower LDL-C and raise HDL-C and is associated with lower risk of CHD in epidemiologic studies (see Chapter 68). Patients should receive information on the potential benefits, costs, and risks of long-term therapy before beginning treatment on cholesterol-lowering drugs.

All adults, adolescents, and children over age 2 years, including those with normal cholesterol levels, should receive periodic counseling regarding dietary intake of fat and saturated fat (see Chapter 56) and other measures to reduce the risk of coronary disease (see Chapters 3, 54, and 55).

The draft update of this chapter was prepared for the U.S. Preventive Services Task Force by David Atkins, MD, MPH, and Carolyn DiGuiseppi, MD, MPH.

REFERENCES

1. National Cholesterol Education Program. Second report of the Expert Panel on Detection, Evaluation, and Treatment of High Blood Cholesterol in Adults (Adult Treatment Panel II). Bethesda: National Heart, Lung, and Blood Institute, National Institutes of Health, 1993. (Publication no. 93-3095.)
2. National Center for Health Statistics. Annual summary of births, marriages, divorces, and deaths: United States, 1993. Monthly vital statistics report; vol 42 no 13. Hyattsville, MD: Public Health Service, 1994.
3. American Heart Association. Heart and stroke facts: 1995 statistical supplement. Dallas, TX: American Heart Association, 1994.
4. National Center for Health Statistics. Coronary heart disease incidence by sex—United States, 1971–87. MMWR 1992;41:526–529.
5. Bush TL, Fried LP, Barrett-Connor E. Cholesterol, lipoproteins, and coronary heart disease in women. Clin Chem 1988;34:B60–B70.

6. Pathological Determinants of Atherosclerosis in Youth (PDAY) Research Group. Relationship of atherosclerosis to serum lipoprotein cholesterol concentrations and smoking. JAMA 1990; 264:3018–3024.

7. Newman WP III, Wattigney W, Berenson GS. Autopsy studies in United States children and adolescents. Relationship of risk factors to atherosclerotic lesions. Ann NY Acad Sci 1991;623:16–25.

8. PDAY Research Group. Natural history of aortic and coronary atherosclerotic lesions in youth: findings from the PDAY study. Arterioscler Thromb 1993;131:291–298.

9. Strong JP, McGill HC Jr. The pediatric aspects of atherosclerosis. J Atheroscler Res 1969;9:251–265.

10. Stary HC. The sequence of cell and matrix changes in atherosclerotic lesions of coronary arteries in the first forty years of life. Eur Heart J 1990;11(Suppl E):E3–E19.

11. Bild D, Williams R, Brewer H, et al. Identification and management of heterozygous familial hypercholesterolemia: summary and recommendations from an NHLBI workshop. Am J Cardiol 1993;72:1D–5D.

12. Cortner JA, Coates PM, Liacouras CA, et al. Familial combined hyperlipidemia in children: clinical expression, metabolic defects, and management. J Pediatr 1993;123:177–184.

13. LaRosa JC, Hunninghake D, Bush D, et al. The cholesterol facts. A joint statement by the American Heart Association and the National Heart, Lung, and Blood Institute. Circulation 1990; 81:1721–1733.

14. Stamler J, Stamler R, Brown V, et al. Serum cholesterol. Doing the right thing. Circulation 1993;88:1954–1960.

15. Grundy SM. Cholesterol and coronary heart disease. Future directions. JAMA 1990;264:3053–3059.

16. Neaton JD, Wentworth D, for the Multiple Risk Factor Intervention Trial Research Group. Serum cholesterol, blood pressure, cigarette smoking, and death from coronary heart disease. Overall findings and differences by age for 316,099 white men. Arch Intern Med 1992;152:56–64.

17. Anderson KM, Castelli WP, Levy D. Cholesterol and mortality: 30 years of follow-up from the Framingham Study. JAMA 1987;257:2176–2180.

18. Law MR, Wald NJ, Thompson SG. By how much and how quickly does reduction in serum cholesterol lower risk of ischemic heart disease? BMJ 1994;308:367–373.

19. Klag MJ, Ford DE, Mead LA, et al. Serum cholesterol in young men and subsequent cardiovascular disease. N Engl J Med 1993;328:313–318.

20. Davis CE, Rifkind BM, Brenner H, et al. A single cholesterol measurement underestimates the risk of coronary heart disease. JAMA 1991;264:3044–3046.

21. Stensvold I, Tverdal A, Urdal P, Graff-Iversen S. Non-fasting serum triglyceride concentration and mortality from coronary heart disease and any cause in middle aged Norwegian women. BMJ 1993;307:1318–1322.

22. Bass KM, Newschaffer CJ, Klag MJ, Bush TL. Plasma lipoprotein levels as predictors of cardiovascular death in women. Arch Intern Med 1993;153:2209–2216.

23. Manolio TA, Pearson TA, Wenger NK, et al. Cholesterol and heart disease in older persons and women: review of an NHLBI workshop. Ann Epidemiol 1992;2:161–176.

24. Bengtsson C, Bjorkelund C, Lapidus L, Lissner L. Association of serum lipid concentrations and obesity with mortality in women: 20 year follow up of participants in prospective population study in Gothenburg, Sweden. BMJ 1993;307:1385–1388.

24a. Grover SA, Palmer CS, Coupal L. Serum lipid screening to identify high-risk individuals for coronary death: the results of the Lipids Research Clinics Prevalence Cohort. Arch Intern Med 1994; 154:679–684.

25. Harris T, Cook EF, Kannel WB, et al. Proportional hazards analysis of risk factors for coronary heart disease in individuals aged 65 or older: the Framingham Heart Study. J Am Geriatr Soc 1988;36: 1023–1028.

26. Harris TB, Makuc DM, Kleinman JC, et al. Is the serum cholesterol-coronary heart disease relationship modified by activity level in older persons? J Am Geriatr Soc 1991;39:747–754.

27. Shipley MJ, Pocock SJ, Marmot MG. Does plasma cholesterol concentration predict mortality from coronary heart disease in elderly people? 18 year follow up in Whitehall study. BMJ 1991;303:89–92.

28. Kronmal RA, Cain KC, Ye Z, et al. Total serum cholesterol levels and mortality risk as a function of age. Arch Intern Med 1993;153:1065–1073.

29. Zimetbaum P, Frishman WH, Ooi WL, Derman MP, et al. Plasma lipids and lipoproteins and the incidence of cardiovascular disease in the very elderly. Arterioscler Thromb 1992;12:416–423.

30. Krumholz HM, Seeman TE, Merrill SS, et al. Lack of association between cholesterol and coronary

heart disease mortality and morbidity and all-cause mortality in persons older than 70 years. JAMA 1994;272:1335–1340.

31. Hulley SB, Newman TB. Cholesterol in the elderly: is it important? JAMA 1994;272:1372–1373.

32. Wald NJ, Law M, Watt H, et al. Apolipoproteins and ischemic heart disease: implications for screening. Lancet 1994;343:75–79.

33. Toronto Working Group on Cholesterol Policy. Asymptomatic hypercholesterolemia: a clinical policy review. J Clin Epidemiol 1990;43:1029–1121.

34. Pooling Project Research Group. Relationship of blood pressure, serum cholesterol, smoking habit, relative weight and ECG abnormalities to incidence of major coronary events. Final report of the Pooling Project. J Chronic Dis 1978;31:201–306.

35. Goldman L, Gordon DJ, Rifkind BS, et al. Cost and health implications of cholesterol lowering. Circulation 1992;85:1960–1968.

36. The Lipid Research Clinics Coronary Primary Prevention Trial Results. I. Reduction in incidence of coronary heart disease. JAMA 1984;251:351–364.

37. Kannel WB, Wilson PF. Risk factors that attenuate the female coronary disease advantage. Arch Intern Med 1995;155:57–61.

38. Benafante R, Reed D. Is elevated serum cholesterol a risk factor for coronary heart disease in the elderly? JAMA 1990;263:393–396.

39. Rubin SM, Sidney S, Black DM, et al. High blood cholesterol in elderly men and the excess risk for coronary heart disease. Ann Intern Med 1990;113:916–920.

40. NIH Consensus Development Panel on Triglyceride, High-density Lipoprotein and Coronary Heart Disease. Triglyceride, high-density lipoprotein, and coronary heart disease. JAMA 1993;269:505–510.

41. Castelli WP, Garrison RJ, Wilson PW, et al. Incidence of coronary heart disease and lipoprotein cholesterol levels: the Framingham Study. JAMA 1986;256:2835–2838.

42. Gordon DJ, Probstfield JL, Garnson RJ, et al. High-density lipoprotein cholesterol and cardiovascular disease: four prospective American studies. Circulation 1989;79:8–15.

43. Rubins HB, Robins SJ, Iwane MK, et al. Rationale and design of the Department of Veterans Affairs High-Density Lipoprotein Cholesterol Intervention Trial (HIT) for secondary prevention of coronary artery disease. Am J Cardiol 1993;71:45–52.

44. Kinosian B, Glick H, Garland G. Cholesterol and coronary heart disease: predicting risk by levels and ratios. Ann Intern Med 1994;121;641–647.

45. Report of Meeting of Physicians and Scientists. Hypertriglyceridemia and vascular risk. Lancet 1993;342:781–787.

46. Criqui MH, Heiss G, Cohn R. Plasma triglyceride level and mortality from coronary heart disease. N Engl J Med 1993;328:1220–1225.

46a. Tenkanen L, Pietilä K, Manninen V. The triglyceride issue revisited. Arch Intern Med 1994;154:2714–2720.

47. Chung SJ. Formulas predicting the percentile of serum cholesterol levels by age in adults. Arch Pathol Lab Med 1990;114:869–875.

48. van Beresteijn ECH, Korevaar JC, Huijbregts PCW, et al. Premenopausal increase in serum cholesterol: a 10-year longitudinal study. Am J Epidemiol 1993;137:383–392.

49. Sempos C, Cleeman JI, Carroll MD, et al. Prevalence of high blood cholesterol levels among US adults. An update based on guidelines from the second report of the National Cholesterol Education Program Adult Treatment Panel. JAMA 1993;269:3009–3014.

50. Cooper GR, Myers GL, Smith SJ, et al. Blood lipid measurements. Variations and practical utility. JAMA 1992;267:1652–1660.

51. Laboratory Standardization Panel, National Cholesterol Education Program. Recommendations for improving cholesterol measurement. Bethesda: National Institutes of Health, National Heart, Lung and Blood Institute, 1990. (NIH Publication no. 90-2964.)

52. Ross JW, Myers GL, Gilmore BF, et al. Matrix effects and the accuracy of cholesterol analysis. Arch Pathol Lab Med 1993;117:393–400.

53. Kaufman HW, McNamara JR, Anderson KM, et al. How reliably can compact chemistry analyzers measure lipids? JAMA 1990;263:1245–1249.

54. Belsey R, Vandenbark M, Goitein RK, et al. Evaluation of a laboratory system intended for use in physicians' offices. II. Reliability of results produced by health care workers without formal or professional training. JAMA 1987;258:357–361.

55. Greenland P, Bowley NL, Meiklejohn B, et al. Blood cholesterol concentration: fingerstick plasma vs. venous serum sampling. Clin Chem 1990;36:628–630.
56. Belsey R, Baer DM. Cardiac risk classification based on lipid screening. JAMA 1990;263:1250–1252.
57. National Cholesterol Education Program. Report of the Expert Panel on Blood Cholesterol Levels in Children and Adolescents. Bethesda: National Institutes of Health, National Heart, Lung and Blood Institute, 1991. (NIH Publication no. 91-2732.)
58. Webber LS, Srinivasan SR, Wattigney WA, Berenson GS. Tracking of serum lipids and lipoproteins from childhood to adulthood. The Bogalusa Heart Study. Am J Epidemiol 1991;133:884–899.
59. Stuhldreher WL, Orchard TJ, Donahue RP, et al. Cholesterol screening in childhood: sixteen-year Beaver County Lipid Study experience. J Pediatr 1991;119:551–556.
60. Lauer RM, Clarke WR. Use of cholesterol measurements in childhood for the prediction of adult hypercholesterolemia. The Muscatine Study. JAMA 1990;264:3034–3038.
61. Mjos OD, Thelle DS, Forde OH, Vik-Mo H. Family study of high density lipoprotein cholesterol and the relation to age and sex. The Tromso Heart Study. Acta Med Scand 1977;201:323–329.
62. Croft JB, Cresanta JL, Webber LS, et al. Cardiovascular risk in parents of children with extreme lipoprotein cholesterol levels: the Bogalusa Heart Study. South Med J 1988;81:341–349.
63. Wong ND, Hei TK, Qaqundah PY, et al. Television viewing and pediatric hypercholesterolemia. Pediatrics 1992;90:75–79.
64. Bell MM, Joseph S. Screening 1140 fifth graders for hypercholesterolemia: family history inadequate to predict results. J Am Board Fam Pract 1990;3:259–263.
65. Davidson DM, Van Camp J, Iftner CA, et al. Family history fails to detect the majority of children with high capillary blood total cholesterol. J School Health 1991;61:75–80.
66. Steiner MH, Neinstein LS, Pennbridge J. Hypercholesterolemia in adolescents: effectiveness of screening strategies based on selected risk factors. Pediatrics 1991;88:269–275.
67. Shea S, Basch CE, Irigoyen M, et al. Failure of family history to predict high blood cholesterol among Hispanic preschool children. Prev Med 1990;19:443–455.
68. Benuck I, Gidding SS, Donovan M, et al. Usefulness of parental serum total cholesterol levels in identifying children with hypercholesterolemia. Prev Cardiol 1992;69:713–717.
69. Mabuchi H, Koizumi J, Shimizu M, et al. Development of coronary heart disease in familial hypercholesterolemia. Circulation 1989;79:225–232.
70. Scientific Steering Committee on behalf of the Simon Broome Register Group. Risk of fatal coronary heart disease in familial hypercholesterolemia. BMJ 1991;303:893–896.
71. Williams RR, Hunt SC, Schumacher C. Diagnosing heterozygous familial hypercholesterolemia using new practical criteria validated by molecular genetics. Am J Cardiol 1993;72:171–176.
72. Williams RR, Schumacher C, Barlow G, et al. Documented need for more effective diagnosis and treatment of familial hypercholesterolemia according to data from 502 heterozygotes in Utah. Am J Cardiol 1993; 72(suppl):18D–24D.
73. Smith S, Cooper G, Myers G, Sampson E. Biological variability in concentrations of serum lipids: sources of variation among results from published studies and composite predicted values. Clin Chem 1993;39:1012–1022.
74. Bachorik PS, Cloey TA, Finney CA, et al. Lipoprotein-cholesterol analysis during screening: accuracy and reliability. Ann Intern Med 1991;114:741–747.
75. Christenson RH, Roeback JR, Watson TE, Hla KM. Improving the reliability of total and high-density lipoprotein cholesterol measurements. Arch Pathol Lab Med 1991;115:1212–1216.
76. McQueen MJ, Henderson AR, Patten RL, et al. Results of a province-wide quality assurance program assessing the accuracy of cholesterol, triglycerides, and high-density lipoprotein cholesterol measurements and calculated low-density lipoprotein cholesterol in Ontario, using fresh human serum. Arch Pathol Lab Med 1991;115: 1217–1222.
77. Frank E, Winkleby M, Fortmann S, et al. Improved cholesterol-related knowledge and behavior and plasma cholesterol levels in adults during the 1980s. JAMA 1992;268:1566–1572.
78. National Heart, Lung and Blood Institute. Daily dietary fat and total food-energy intake—Third National Health and Nutrition Examination Survey, Phase 1, 1988–91. MMWR 1994;43:116–117, 123–125.
79. Johnson CL, Rifkind BM, Sempos CT, et al. Declining serum total cholesterol levels among US adults. The National Health and Nutrition Examination Surveys. JAMA 1993;269:3003–3008.
80. Imperial Cancer Research Fund OXCHECK Study Group. Effectiveness of health checks conducted by nurses in primary care: final results of the OXCHECK study. BMJ 1995;310:1099–1104.

81. Family Heart Study Group. Randomised controlled trial evaluating cardiovascular screening and intervention in general practice: principal results of British family heart study. BMJ 1994;308:313–320.

82. Murray D, Luepker R, Pirie P, et al. Systematic risk factor screening and education: a community-wide approach to prevention of coronary heart disease. Prev Med 1986;15:661–672.

83. Elton PJ, Ryman A, Hammer M, et al. Randomised controlled trial in northern England of the effect of a person knowing their own serum cholesterol level. J Epidemiol Community Health 1994; 48:22–25.

84. Robertson I, Phillips A, Mant D, et al. Motivational effects of cholesterol measurement in general practice health checks. Br J Gen Pract 1992;42:469–472.

85. Resnicow K, Corss D, Lacosse J, et al. Evaluation of a school-site cardiovascular risk factor screening intervention. Prev Med 1993;22:838–856.

86. Hong MK, Mintz GS, Popma JJ, et al. Limitations of angiography for analyzing coronary atherosclerosis progression or regression. Ann Intern Med 1994;121:348–354.

87. Brown BG, Zhao XQ, Sacco DE, Albers JJ. Lipid lowering and plaque progression. New insights into prevention of plaque disruption and clinical events in coronary disease. Circulation 1993;87:1781–1791.

88. Rossouw JE. The effects of lowering serum cholesterol on coronary heart disease risk. Med Clin North Am 1994;78:181–195.

89. Law M, Thompson S, Wald N. Assessing possible hazards of reducing serum cholesterol. BMJ 1994;308:373–379.

90. Scandinavian Simvastatin Survival Study Group. Randomised trial of cholesterol lowering in 4444 patients with coronary heart disease: the Scandinavian Simvastatin Survival Study (4S). Lancet 1994;344:1383–1389.

91. Davey Smith G, Song F, Sheldon TA. Cholesterol lowering and mortality: the importance of considering initial level of risk. BMJ 1993;306:1367–1373.

92. Report from the Committee of Principal Investigators. A cooperative trial in the primary prevention of ischaemic heart disease using clofibrate. Br Heart J 1978;40:1069–1118.

93. Heady JA, Morris JN, Oliver MF. WHO clofibrate/cholesterol trial: clarifications. Lancet 1992;340:1405–1406.

94. Frick MH, Elo O, Haapa K, et al. Helsinki Heart Study: primary prevention trial with gemfibrozil in middle-aged men with dyslipidemia. Safety of treatment, changes in risk factors, and incidence of coronary heart disease. N Engl J Med 1987;317:1237–1245.

95. Manninen V, Tenkanen L, Koskinen P, et al. Joint effects of serum triglyceride and LDL cholesterol and HDL cholesterol concentrations on coronary heart disease in the Helsinki Heart Study. Implications for treatment. Circulation 1992;85:37–45.

96. Dorr AE, Gundersen K, Schneider JC, et al. Colestipol hydrochloride in hypercholesterolemic patients—effect on serum cholesterol and mortality. J Chronic Dis 1978;31:5–14.

97. Bradford RH, Shear CL, Chremos AN, et al. Expanded clinical evaluation of lovastatin (EXCEL) study results. 1. Efficacy in modifying plasma lipoproteins and adverse event profile in 8245 patients with moderate hypercholesterolemia. Arch Intern Med 1991;151:43–49.

98. Dayton S, Pearce ML, Hashimoto S, et al. A controlled clinical trial of a diet high in unsaturated fat in preventing complications of atherosclerosis. Circulation 1969;40(Suppl II):1–63.

99. Miettinen M, Turpeinen O, Karvonen MJ, et al. Effect of cholesterol-lowering diet on mortality from coronary heart disease and other causes. Lancet 1972;2:835–838.

100. Frantz ID, Dawson EA, Ashman PL, et al. Test of effect of lipid lowering by diet on cardiovascular risk. The Minnesota Coronary Survey. Arteriosclerosis 1989;9:129–135.

101. World Health Organization European Collaborative Group. European collaborative trial of multifactorial prevention of coronary heart disease: final report on the 6-year results. Lancet 1986; 1:869–872.

102. Multiple Risk Factor Intervention Trial Research Group. Multiple Risk Factor Intervention Trial: risk factor changes and mortality results. JAMA 1982;248:1465–1477.

103. Hjermann I, Velve Byre K, Holme I, et al. Effect of diet and smoking intervention on the incidence of coronary heart disease. Report from the Oslo Study Group of a randomized trial in healthy men. Lancet 1981;2:1303–1310.

104. Wilhelmsen L, Berglund G, Elmfeldt D, et al. The multifactor primary prevention trial in Goteborg, Sweden. Eur Heart J 1986;7:279–288.

105. Miettinen TA, Huttunen JK, Naukkarinen V, et al. Multifactorial prevention of cardiovascular diseases in middle-aged men. Risk factor changes, incidence and mortality. JAMA 1985;254:2097–2102.

106. Caggiula AW, Christakis G, Farrand M, et al. The Multiple Risk Factor Intervention Trial (MRFIT). IV. Intervention on blood lipids. Prev Med 1981;10:443–475.

107. Multiple Risk Factor Intervention Trial Research Group. Coronary heart disease death, nonfatal acute myocardial infarction and other clinical outcomes in the Multiple Risk Factor Intervention Trial. Am J Cardiol 1986;58:1–13.

108. Hegsted DM, Ausman LM, Johnson JA, et al. Dietary fat and serum lipids: an evaluation of the experimental data. Am J Clin Nutr 1993;57:875–883.

109. Truswell AS. Review of dietary intervention studies: effect on coronary events and on total mortality. Aust NZ J Med 1994;24:98–106.

110. Denke MA. Cholesterol-lowering diets. A review of the evidence. Arch Intern Med 1995;155:17–26.

111. Ramsay LE, Yeo WW, Jackson PR. Dietary reduction of serum cholesterol concentration: time to think again. BMJ 1991;303:953–957.

112. Murray DM, Kurth C, Mullis R, et al. Cholesterol reduction through low-intensity interventions: results from the Minnesota Heart Health Program. Prev Med 1990;19:181–189.

113. Lindholm LH, Ekbom T, Dash C, et al. The impact of health care advice given in primary care on cardiovascular risk. BMJ 1995;310:1105–1109.

114. Henkin Y, Garber DW, Osterlund LC, et al. Saturated fats, cholesterol and dietary compliance. Arch Intern Med 1992;152:1167–1174.

115. Bae CY, Keenan JM, Wenz J, et al. A clinical trial of the American Heart Association Step One Diet for treatment of hypercholesterolemia. J Fam Pract 1991;33:249–254.

116. Gibbins RL, Riley M, Brimble P. Effectiveness of programme for reducing cardiovascular risk for men in one general practice. BMJ 1993;306:1652–1656.

117. Wynder E, Harris R, Haley N. Population screening for plasma cholesterol: community results from Connecticut. Am Heart J 1989;117:649–656.

118. Gemson D, Sloan R, Messeri P, Goldberg I. A public health model for cardiovascular risk reduction. Impact of cholesterol screening with brief non-physician counseling. Arch Intern Med 1990; 150:985–989.

119. Ammerman A, Caggiula A, Elmer PJ, et al. Putting medical practice guidelines into practice: the cholesterol model. Am J Prev Med 1994;10:209–216.

120. Ornish D, Brown SE, Scherwitz LW, et al. Can lifestyle changes reverse coronary heart disease? Lancet 1990;336:129–133.

121. Insull W, Henderson MM, Prentice RL, et al. Results of a randomized feasibility study of a low-fat diet. Arch Intern Med 1990;150:421–427.

122. Boyd NF, Cousins M, Beaton M, et al. Quantitative changes in dietary fat intake and serum cholesterol in women: results from a randomized, controlled trial. Am J Clin Nutr 1990;52:470–476.

123. Holme I. Relation of coronary heart disease incidence and total mortality to plasma cholesterol reduction in randomized trials. Use of meta-analysis. Eur Heart J 1993;69(suppl):S42–S47.

124. Yusuf S, Wittes J, Friedman L. Overview of results of randomized clinical trials in heart disease. II. Unstable angina, heart failure, primary prevention with aspirin and risk factor modification. JAMA 1988;260:2259–2263.

125. Muldoon MF, Manuck SB, Matthews KA. Lowering cholesterol concentrations and mortality: a quantitative review of primary prevention trials. BMJ 1990;301:309–314.

126. Ravnskov U. Cholesterol lowering trials in coronary heart disease: frequency of citation and outcome. BMJ 1992;305:15–19.

127. Canadian Task Force on the Periodic Health Examination. Canadian guide to clinical preventive health care. Ottawa: Canada Communication Group, 1994:649–669.

128. Gordon DJ. Cholesterol lowering and total mortality. In: Rifkind BM, ed. Lowering cholesterol in high-risk individuals and populations. New York: Marcel Dekker, 1995:333–348.

129. Thompson SG. Controversies in meta-analysis: the case of the trials of serum cholesterol reduction. Stat Methods Med Res 1993;2:173–192.

130. Knodel LC, Talbert RL. Adverse effects of hypolipidaemic drugs. Med Toxicol 1987;2:10–32.

131. Collins R, Keech A, Peto R, et al. Cholesterol and total mortality. Need for larger trials. BMJ 1993; 306:1689.

132. Wood PD, Stefanick ML, Williams PT, et al. The effects on plasma lipoproteins of a prudent weight-reducing diet, with or without exercise, in overweight men and women. N Engl J Med 1991;325: 461–466.

133. Moreno GT, Manson JE. Cholesterol and coronary heart disease in women: an overview of primary and secondary prevention. Coron Artery Dis 1993;4:580–587.

134. Manolio TA, Ettinger WH, Tracy RP, et al. Epidemiology of low cholesterol levels in older adults. The Cardiovascular Health Study. Circulation 1993;87:728–737.

135. Davey Smith G, Shipley MJ, Marmot MG, et al. Plasma cholesterol concentration and mortality. The Whitehall Study. JAMA 1992;267:70–76.

136. Carlson LA, Rosenhamer G. Reduction of mortality in the Stockholm Ischaemic Heart Disease Secondary Prevention Study by combined treatment with clofibrate and nicotinic acid. Acta Med Scand 1988;223:405–418.

137. Leren P. The effect of plasma cholesterol lowering diet in male survivors of MI. Acta Med Scand 1966;(Suppl 466):1–92.

138. LaRosa JC, Applegate W, Crouse JR III, et al. Cholesterol lowering in the elderly: results of the Cholesterol Reduction in Seniors Program (CRISP) pilot study. Arch Intern Med 1994;154:529–539.

139. Ives DG, Kuller LH, Traven N. Use and outcomes of cholesterol-lowering intervention in rural elderly subjects. Am J Prev Med 1993;9:274–281.

140. Levine GN, Keaney JF, Vita JA. Cholesterol reduction in cardiovascular disease. Clinical benefits and possible mechanisms. N Engl J Med 1995;332:512–521.

141. Hill JS, Hayden MR, Frohlich J, et al. Genetic and environmental factors affecting incidence of coronary artery disease in heterozygous familial hypercholesterolemia. Arterioscler Thromb 1991; 11:290–297.

142. Gomel M, Oldenburg B, Simpson JM, et al. Work site cardiovascular risk reduction: a randomized trial of health risk assessment, education, counseling, and incentives. Am J Public Health 1993; 83:1231–1238.

143. Nicklas TA, Farris RP, Smoak CG, et al. Dietary factors relate to cardiovascular risk factors in early life. Bogalusa Heart Study. Arteriosclerosis 1988;8:193–199.

144. Shea S, Basch CE, Irigoyen M, et al. Relationships of dietary fat consumption to serum total and low-density lipoprotein cholesterol in Hispanic preschool children. Prev Med 1991;20:237–249.

145. Walker R, Heller R, Redman S, et al. Reduction of ischemic heart disease risk markers in the teenage children of heart attack patients. Prev Med 1992;21:616–629.

146. Shannon BM, Tershakovec AM, Achterberg CL, et al. Cholesterol education for at-risk children. Pediatrics 1994;94:923–927.

147. Lapinleimu H, Viikari J, Jokinen E, et al. Prospective randomised trial in 1062 infants of diet low in saturated fat and cholesterol. Lancet 1995;345:471–476.

148. The Writing Group for the DISC Collaborative Research Group. Efficacy and safety of lowering dietary intake of fat and cholesterol in children with elevated low-density lipoprotein cholesterol: the Dietary Intervention Study in Children (DISC). JAMA 1995;273:1429–1435.

149. Quivers ES, Driscoll DJ, Garvey CD, et al. Variability in response to a low-fat, low-cholesterol diet in children with elevated low-density lipoprotein cholesterol levels. Pediatrics 1992;89:925–929.

150. Vartiainen E, Puska P, Pietinen P, et al. Effects of dietary fat modifications on serum lipids and blood pressure in children. Acta Paediatr Scand 1986;75:396–401.

151. Kuehl KS, Cockerham JT, Hitchings M, et al. Effective control of hypercholesterolemia in children with dietary interventions based in pediatric practice. Prev Med 1993;22:154–166.

152. Polonsky SM, Bellet PS, Sprecher DL. Primary hyperlipidemia in a pediatric population: classification and effect of dietary treatment. Pediatrics 1993;91:92–96.

153. Riggs TW, Holmes RD, Gendelman BS, Knust MM. Dietary treatment of childhood hypercholesterolemia. Ann NY Acad Sci 1991;623:457–459.

154. Linder CW, DuRant RH, Mahoney OM. The effect of physical conditioning on serum lipids and lipoproteins in white male adolescents. Med Sci Sports Exerc 1983;15:232–236.

155. Savage MP, Petratis MM, Thomson WH, et al. Exercise training effects on serum lipids of prepubescent boys and adult men. Med Sci Sports Exerc 1986;18:197–204.

156. Sasaki J, Shindo M, Tanaka H, et al. A long-term aerobic exercise program decreases the obesity index and increases the high-density lipoprotein cholesterol concentration in obese children. Int J Obesity 1987;11:339–345.

157. Widhalm K, Maxa E, Zyman H. Effect of diet and exercise upon the cholesterol and triglyceride content of plasma lipoproteins in overweight children. Eur J Pediatr 1978;127:121–126.

158. Fripp RR, Hodgson JL. Effect of resistive training on plasma lipid and lipoprotein levels in male adolescents. J Pediatr 1987;111:926–931.

159. Weltman A, Janney C, Rians CB, et al. The effects of hydraulic-resistance strength training on serum lipid levels in prepubertal boys. Am J Dis Child 1987;141:777–780.

160. Liacouras CA, Coates PM, Gallagher PR, et al. Use of cholestyramine in the treatment of children with familial combined hyperlipidemia. J Pediatr 1993;122:477–482.

161. Hulley SB, Newman TB, Grady D, et al. Should we be measuring blood cholesterol levels in young adults? JAMA 1993;269:1416–1419.

162. Brett AS. Psychologic effects of the diagnosis and treatment of hypercholesterolemia: lessons from case studies. Am J Med 1991;91:642–647.

163. Irvine MJ, Logan AG. Is knowing your cholesterol number harmful? J Clin Epidemiol 1994; 47:131–145.

164. Kinlay S, Heller R. Effectiveness and hazards of case finding for a high cholesterol concentration. BMJ 1990;300:1545–1547.

165. Shea S, Basch CE, Stein AD, et al. Is there a relationship between dietary fat and stature or growth in children three to five years of age? Pediatrics 1993;92:579–586.

166. Nicklas TA, Webber LS, Koschak ML, Berenson GS. Nutrient adequacy of low fat intakes for children: the Bogalusa Heart Study. Pediatrics 1992;89:221–228.

167. Copperman N, Schebendach J, Arden M, Jacobson MS. Nutrient adequacy of pediatric office-based dietary therapy of hyperlipidemia. Ann NY Acad Sci 1991;623:419–421.

168. Pugliese MT, Weyman-Daum M, Lifshitz F. Parental health beliefs as a cause of nonorganic failure to thrive. Pediatrics 1987;80:175–182.

169. Lifshitz F, Moses N. Growth failure: a complication of dietary treatment of hypercholesterolemia. Am J Dis Child 1989;143:537–542.

170. Fuchs GJ, Farris RP, DeWier M, et al. Effect of dietary fat on cardiovascular risk factors in infancy. Pediatrics 1994;93:756–763.

171. Kimm SYS, Payne GH, Lakatos E, et al. Primary care physicians and children's blood cholesterol. Prev Med 1992;21:191–202.

172. Editor. Use of cholesterol-lowering drugs. United States, 1992. Stat Bull Metrop Life Insur Co 1993;74:10–17.

173. Frick MH, Heinonen OP, Huttunen JK, et al. Efficacy of gemfibrozil in dyslipidemic subjects with suspected heart disease. An ancillary study in the Helsinki Heart Disease Study frame population. Ann Med 1993;25:41–45.

174. Huttunen JK, Heinonen OP, Manninen V, et al. The Helsinki Heart Study: an 8.5 year safety and mortality follow-up. J Intern Med 1994;235:31–39.

175. Dattilo AM, Kris-Etherton PM. Effects of weight reduction on blood lipids and lipoproteins: a meta-analysis. Am J Clin Nutr 1992;56:320–328.

176. Rosenson RS. Low levels of high-density lipoprotein cholesterol (hypoalphalipoproteinemia). Arch Intern Med 1993;153:1528–1538.

176a. King AC, Haskell WL, Young DR, et al. Long-term effects of varying intensities and formats of physical activity on participation rates, fitness, and lipoproteins in men and women aged 50 to 65 years. Circulation 1995; 91: 2596–2604.

177. Steinberg D, Pearson TA, Kuller LH. Alcohol and atherosclerosis. Ann Intern Med 1991; 114:967–976.

178. Expert Panel on Detection, Evaluation, and Treatment of High Blood Cholesterol in Adults. Summary of the second report of the National Cholesterol Education Program (NCEP) Expert Panel on the Detection, Evaluation, and Treatment of High Blood Cholesterol In Adults (Adult Treatment Panel II). JAMA 1993;269:3015–3023.

179. American Academy of Family Physicians. Age charts for periodic health examination. Kansas City, MO: American Academy of Family Physicians, 1994. (Reprint no. 510.)

180. American College of Obstetricians and Gynecologists. The obstetrician-gynecologist in primary preventive health care: a report of the ACOG Task Force on Primary and Preventive Health Care. Washington, DC: American College of Obstetricians and Gynecologists, 1993.

181. American College of Physicians. Serum cholesterol, high-density lipoprotein cholesterol, and triglycerides screening tests for the prevention of coronary heart disease in adults. Ann Intern Med 1996 (in press).

182. Committee on Nutrition, American Academy of Pediatrics. Statement on cholesterol. Pediatrics 1992;90:469–473.

183. Green M, ed. Bright Futures: guidelines for health supervision of infants, children and adolescents. Arlington VA: National Center for Education in Maternal and Child Health, 1994.

184. American Medical Association. Guidelines for adolescent preventive services (GAPS): recommendations and rationale. Chicago: American Medical Association, 1994.

185. Anderson KM, Wilson PWF, Odell PM, et al. An updated coronary risk profile. A statement for health professionals. Circulation 1991;83:356–362.

186. Krahn M, Naylor C, Basinski A, Detsky A. Comparison of an aggressive (U.S.) and a less aggressive (Canadian) policy for cholesterol screening and treatment. Ann Intern Med 1991;115:248–255.

186a. Verschuren WMM, Jacobs DR, Bloemberg BPM, et al. Serum total cholesterol and long-term coronary heart disease mortality in different cultures: twenty-five year follow-up of the Seven Countries Study. JAMA 1995;274:131–136.

187. Kristiansen IS, Eggen AE, Thelle DS. Cost effectiveness of incremental programmes for lowering serum cholesterol concentration: is individual intervention worth while? BMJ 1991;302:1119–1122.

188. Goldman L, Weinstein M, Goldman PA, Williams LW. Cost-effectiveness of HMG-CoA reductase inhibition for primary and secondary prevention of coronary heart diseases. JAMA 1991;265:1145–1151.

189. Hamilton VH, Racicot F-E, Zowall H, et al. The cost-effectiveness of HMG-CoA reductase inhibitors to prevent coronary heart disease. JAMA 1995;273:1032–1038.

190. Corti M-H, Guralnik JM, Salive ME, et al. HDL cholesterol predicts coronary heart disease mortality in older persons. JAMA 1995;274:539–544.

3. Screening for Hypertension

RECOMMENDATION

Screening for hypertension is recommended for all children and adults (see *Clinical Intervention*).

Burden of Suffering

Hypertension is usually defined as a diastolic blood pressure of 90 mm Hg or higher or a systolic pressure of 140 mm Hg or higher.[1] It is present in an estimated 43 million Americans and is more common in blacks and older adults.[1a] Hypertension is a leading risk factor for coronary heart disease, congestive heart failure, stroke, ruptured aortic aneurysm, renal disease, and retinopathy. These complications of hypertension are among the most common and serious diseases in the U.S., and successful efforts to lower blood pressure could thus have substantial impact on population morbidity and mortality. Heart disease is the leading cause of death in the U.S., accounting for nearly 740,000 deaths each year (287 deaths per 100,000 population), and cerebrovascular disease, the third leading cause of death, accounts for about 150,000 deaths each year (58/100,000).[2] Milder forms of hypertension predict progression to more severe elevations and development of cardiovascular disease.[1,3,4] Coronary heart disease mortality begins to increase at systolic blood pressures above 110 mm Hg and at diastolic pressures above 70 mm Hg.[5] The prevalence of unrecognized and uncontrolled hypertension, and the mortality from cardiovascular disease, have declined substantially in the U.S. in the past several decades.[1]

Treatable (also known as secondary) causes of hypertension such as aortic coarctation or renovascular disease also may be associated with severe consequences, including congestive heart failure, aortic rupture, or stroke.[6–9] There are no population data available for estimating the true prevalence of secondary hypertension. The incidence of coarctation of the aorta has been estimated at 0.2–0.6/1,000 live births and the prevalence at 0.1–0.5/1,000 children.[10–12]

Accuracy of Screening Tests

The most accurate devices for measuring blood pressure (e.g., intra-arterial catheters) are not appropriate for routine screening because of their invasiveness, technical limitations, and cost. Office sphygmomanometry (the blood pressure cuff) remains the most appropriate screening test for hypertension in the asymptomatic population. Although this test is highly accurate when performed correctly, false-positive and false-negative results (i.e., recording a blood pressure that is not representative of the patient's average blood pressure) do occur in clinical practice.[13] One study found that 21% of persons diagnosed as mildly hypertensive based on office sphygmomanometry had no evidence of hypertension when 24-hour ambulatory recordings were obtained.[14]

Errors in measuring blood pressure may result from instrument, observer, and/or patient factors.[15] Examples of instrument error include manometer dysfunction, pressure leaks, stethoscope defects, and cuffs of incorrect width or length for the patient's arm size. The observer can introduce errors due to sensory impairment (difficulty hearing Korotkoff sounds or reading the manometer), inattention, inconsistency in recording Korotkoff sounds (e.g., Phase IV vs. Phase V), and subconscious bias (e.g., "digit preference" for numbers ending with zero or preconceived notions of "normal" pressures). The patient can be the source of misleading readings due to posture and biologic factors. Posture (i.e., lying, standing, sitting) and arm position in relation to the heart can affect results by as much as 10 mm Hg.[15] Biologic factors include anxiety, meals, tobacco, alcohol, temperature changes, exertion, and pain. Due to these limitations in the test-retest reliability of blood pressure measurement, it is commonly recommended that hypertension be diagnosed only after more than one elevated reading is obtained on each of three separate visits over a period of one to several weeks.[1]

Additional factors affect accuracy when performing sphygmomanometry on children; these difficulties are especially common when testing infants and toddlers under 3 years of age.[16–18] First, there is increased variation in arm circumference, requiring greater care in the selection of cuff sizes.[19] Second, the examination is more frequently complicated by the anxiety and restlessness of the patient. Third, the disappearance of Korotkoff sounds (Phase V) is often difficult to hear in children and Phase IV values are often substituted. Fourth, erroneous Korotkoff sounds can be produced inadvertently by the pressure of the stethoscope diaphragm against the antecubital fossa. Finally, the definition of pediatric hypertension has itself been uncertain because of confusion over normal values during childhood. The definition of hypertension in childhood is essentially arbitrary, based on age-specific percentile.[18] Age-, sex-, and height-specific blood pressure nomograms for U.S. children and adolescents have been published more recently, based on data from 56,108 children aged 1–17 years.[20]

Self-measured (home) blood pressure and ambulatory blood pressure monitoring may provide useful information in special circumstances (e.g., research, persistent "white-coat" hypertension), but there is insufficient evidence at present to warrant their routine use in screening.[1,21-28]

Effectiveness of Early Detection

There is a direct relationship between the magnitude of blood pressure elevation and the benefit of lowering pressure. In persons with malignant hypertension, the benefits of intervention are most dramatic; treatment increases 5-year survival from near zero (data from historical controls) to 75%.[29] Over the past 30 years, the results of many randomized clinical trials of the effects of antihypertensive drug therapy on morbidity and mortality in adult patients (≥21 years of age) with less severe hypertension have been published.[30-32] The efficacy of treating hypertension is clear, as demonstrated in a number of older randomized controlled trials in adults with diastolic blood pressures ranging from 90 to 129 mm Hg.[33-38] For example, in the Veterans Administration Cooperative Study on Antihypertensive Agents, middle-aged men with diastolic blood pressure averaging 90 through 114 mm Hg experienced a significant reduction in "morbid" events (e.g., cerebrovascular hemorrhage, congestive heart failure) after treatment with antihypertensive medication.[34]

Persons with mild (Stage 1) to moderate (Stage 2)[1] diastolic hypertension (90–109 mm Hg) also benefit from treatment.[30,39-41] This was confirmed in the Hypertension Detection and Follow-Up Program, a randomized controlled trial involving nearly 11,000 hypertensive men and women, of whom 40% were black.[39] The intervention group received standardized pharmacologic treatment ("stepped care") while the control group was referred for community medical care. There was a statistically significant 17% reduction in 5-year all-cause mortality in the group receiving standardized drug therapy; the subset with diastolic blood pressure 90–104 mm Hg experienced a 20% reduction in mortality.[39] Deaths due to cerebrovascular disease, ischemic heart disease, and other causes were also significantly reduced in the stepped care group.[42] Similar effects on all-cause mortality and cardiovascular events have been reported in other randomized controlled trials, such as the Australian National Blood Pressure Study (initial diastolic blood pressure 95–109 mm Hg)[40] and the Medical Research Council (MRC) trial (diastolic blood pressure 90–109 mm Hg).[41] In these two trials, the relative reduction in rates of stroke or other trial endpoints with treatment was similar in those with diastolic blood pressures <95 or 95–99 mm Hg and those with higher diastolic blood pressures, although the absolute benefit was less due to smaller initial risk of stroke and other diseases at lower blood pressures. Both trials included untreated control groups and did not report a significant reduction in deaths from noncardiovascular causes in the actively treated groups, confirming that the benefit was due to antihypertensive treatment rather than to other medical care.

Earlier studies included some subjects over age 65 years, but in insufficient numbers to permit firm conclusions. Four large, randomized placebo-controlled trials have since demonstrated conclusively the benefit of antihypertensive treatment in elderly subjects (aged 60–97 years).[43–48] Three of these studies included persons with diastolic blood pressures of 90–120 mm Hg, and among them reported significant reductions in all-cause mortality,[46] cardiovascular mortality,[43,46] cardiovascular events,[47] and strokes.[46,47] The Systolic Hypertension in the Elderly Program (SHEP) trial included over 4,000 subjects ≥60 years of age with isolated systolic hypertension (systolic blood pressure ≥ 160 mm Hg, with diastolic blood pressure < 90 mm Hg), and reported significant reductions in the incidence of stroke, myocardial infarction, and left ventricular failure.[48] A meta-analysis combining these and other trials that included persons aged ≥60 years demonstrated that antihypertensive treatment in elderly persons significantly reduced mortality from all causes (–12%), stroke (–36%), and coronary heart disease (–25%), as well as stroke and coronary heart disease morbidity.[49] This meta-analysis suggested reduced benefit with increasing age, although differences were not statistically significant. A second meta-analysis of randomized controlled trials in persons over age 60 years concluded that absolute 5-year morbidity and mortality benefits derived from trials were greater for older than for younger subjects.[50] This meta-analysis calculated that 18 (95% CI, 14–25) elderly hypertensive subjects needed to be treated for 5 years to prevent one cardiovascular event.

Treatment of hypertension is associated with multiple benefits, including reduced coronary heart disease and vascular deaths, but meta-analyses suggest it produces the largest reductions in cerebrovascular morbidity and mortality.[30–32,49,50] Improved treatment of high blood pressure has been credited with a substantial portion of the greater than 50% reduction in age-adjusted stroke mortality that has been observed since 1972.[1,51,52]

Although the efficacy of antihypertensive treatment for essential (also called primary) hypertension has been well established in clinical research, certain factors may influence the magnitude of benefit from hypertension screening achieved in actual practice. Compliance with drug therapy may be limited by the inconvenience, side effects, and cost of these agents.[53,54] Serious or life-threatening drug reactions in the clinical trials were rare, but less serious side effects were common, resulting in discontinuation of randomized treatment (almost 20% by the fifth year in the MRC trial,[41] for example) or a substantial increase in patient discomfort.[34] Higher incidences of mild hypokalemia, hyperuricemia, and elevated fasting blood sugar have also been reported in treated individuals.[35] A population-based case-control study suggested an increased risk of primary cardiac arrest with certain diuretic regimens (e.g., higher doses, use without potassium-sparing therapy).[55] However, current drug regimens, including low-dose diuretics, are associated with fewer adverse effects and with favorable effects on quality of life.[55a] Newer classes of drugs (e.g., calcium channel blockers, angiotensin-converting enzyme inhibitors) have not been assessed in long-term trials with clinical endpoints. Their effects on cardiovascular morbidity and mortality may differ from the effects reported in the clinical trials cited above, which used diuretics or beta-blockers.

Whether hypertension screening is equally effective for other populations or with treatments other than drugs is less clear. The benefits of hypertension treatment are less well studied in certain population groups, such as children (see below), Native Americans, Asians and Pacific Islanders, and Hispanics. The effects of nonpharmacologic first-line therapy (i.e., weight reduction in overweight patients, increased physical activity, sodium restriction, and decreased alcohol intake) on cardiovascular morbidity and mortality are unstudied. Although these nonpharmacologic therapies can sometimes lower blood pressure in the short term,[1,56–62a] the magnitude of blood pressure reduction achieved is generally smaller than that achieved with drug therapy, and both the magnitude and duration of reduction in actual practice may be limited by biologic factors (e.g., varying responsiveness to sodium restriction) and the difficulties of maintaining behavioral changes (e.g., weight loss). Some of these interventions, such as sodium restriction, may also have adverse effects on quality of life.[63]

The detection of high blood pressure during childhood is of potential value in identifying those children who are at increased risk of primary hypertension as adults and who might benefit from earlier intervention and follow-up. Hypertensive vascular and end-organ damage may begin in childhood,[64–69] although it is unclear how strongly these pathophysiologic changes are associated with subsequent cardiovascular disease. Prospective cohort studies have shown that children with high blood pressure are more likely than other children to have hypertension as adults.[70–78] Correlation coefficients from these studies were generally less than 0.5, however, suggesting a limited role for high blood pressure in childhood as a predictor of adult hypertension. Although controlled trials in children show that short-term (up to 3 years) effects on blood pressure can be achieved with changes in diet and activity,[79–82] studies demonstrating long-term changes in blood pressure are lacking. There are no trials showing that lowering blood pressure in childhood results in reduced blood pressure in adulthood. A relationship between lowering blood pressure during childhood and improved morbidity and mortality in later life is unlikely to be demonstrated, given the difficulty of performing such studies.

A relatively high proportion of children with hypertension have secondary, potentially curable forms. Among children and adolescents whose hypertension was evaluated in primary care centers, an estimated 28% had secondary hypertension (e.g., renal parenchymal disease, coarctation of the aorta).[69] This contrasts with hypertensive adults seen in primary care settings, of whom only 7% are estimated to have secondary hypertension.[83] Screening children and adolescents may be justifiable if the morbidity of these conditions is improved by early detection and treatment. Many causes of secondary hypertension in childhood are detectable by careful history-taking (e.g., preterm birth, umbilical artery catheter, chronic pyelonephritis, renal disease, bronchopulmonary dysplasia; symptoms of cardiac, renal, endocrinologic, or neurologic disease) or physical examination (e.g., murmur, decreased femoral pulses, abdominal bruit).[69,84] Characteristic symptoms and signs, such as those of aortic coarctation, are often overlooked, however.[85–87] Numerous surgical case series suggest that delay in surgical repair of aortic coarctation increases the likelihood of irreversible hypertension,[88–94] although none of these series controlled for other differences between persons presenting early versus late in life. Uncontrolled studies indicate that some important causes of hypertension for which definitive cures are available, including coarctation and renovascular disease, may not be diagnosed until complications such as congestive heart failure, aortic rupture, or stroke occur.[6–9] Prognosis with early surgical intervention is improved compared with historical controls.[88,95]

Recommendations of Other Groups

Recommendations for adults have been issued by the Joint National Committee on Detection, Evaluation, and Treatment of High Blood Pressure,[1] and similar recommendations have been issued by the American Heart Association.[96] These call for routine blood pressure measurement at least once every 2 years for adults with a diastolic blood pressure below 85 mm Hg and a systolic pressure below 130 mm Hg. Measurements are recommended annually for persons with a diastolic blood pressure of 85–89 mm Hg or systolic blood pressure of 130–139 mm Hg. Persons with higher blood pressures require more frequent measurements. The American College of Physicians (ACP)[97] and the American Academy of Family Physicians (AAFP)[98] recommend that all adults 18 years and older be screened for hypertension every 1–2 years. The AAFP policy is currently under review. The ACP also recommends screening at every physician visit for other reasons, and that those in high-risk groups (e.g., diastolic 85–89 mm Hg, previous history of hypertension) be screened on an annual basis. The Canadian Task Force on the Periodic Health Examination recommends that all persons aged 21 years and over receive a blood pressure measurement during any visit to a physician ("case finding").[99]

The American Academy of Pediatrics (AAP),[100] the National Heart, Lung, and Blood Institute,[18] the AAFP,[98] Bright Futures,[101] the American

Medical Association,[102] and the American Heart Association[103] recommend that children and adolescents receive blood pressure measurements every 1 or 2 years during regular office visits. The Canadian Task Force found insufficient evidence to recommend for or against routine blood pressure measurement in persons under age 21 years.[99] The AAP recommends against universal neonatal blood pressure screening.[104]

Discussion

It is clear from several large randomized clinical trials that lowering blood pressure in hypertensive adults is beneficial and that death from several common diseases can be reduced through the detection and treatment of high blood pressure. Estimates suggest that an average diastolic blood pressure reduction of 5–6 mm Hg in everyone with hypertension could reduce the incidence of coronary heart disease by 14% and the incidence of strokes by 42%.[30,31] At the same time, it is important for clinicians to minimize the potential harmful effects of detection and treatment. For example, if performed incorrectly, sphygmomanometry can produce misleading results. Some hypertensive patients thereby escape detection (false negatives) and some normotensive persons receive inappropriate labeling (false positives), which may have certain psychological, behavioral, and even financial consequences.[105] Treatment of hypertension can also be harmful as a result of medical complications, especially related to drugs. Clinicians can minimize these effects by using proper technique when performing sphygmomanometry, making appropriate use of non-pharmacologic methods, and prescribing antihypertensive drugs with careful adherence to published guidelines.[1,106–108]

The diastolic blood pressure above which therapy has been proven effective (i.e., diastolic blood pressure > 90 mm Hg) is to a large extent based on the artificial cutpoints chosen for study purposes rather than on a specific biologic cutpoint defining increased risk. The coronary heart disease mortality risk associated with blood pressure occurs on a continuum that extends well below the arbitrarily defined level for abnormal blood pressure, beginning for systolic blood pressure above 110 mm Hg and for diastolic pressure above 70 mm Hg.[5] Nevertheless, many organizations outside the U.S. have been reluctant to recommend drug therapy for persons with diastolic blood pressures below 100 mm Hg who lack additional risk factors.[106,108–111] Drug treatment of mild hypertension is of particular concern for young adults: the evidence for therapeutic benefit comes primarily from several older trials[34,36,38] that included only a few individuals in their 20s, the potential adverse effects of decades of antihypertensive therapy are undefined, and the absolute benefits in young adults are likely to be limited given their small risk of stroke and coronary heart disease.

For persons with mild hypertension, most recommendations suggest including age and/or the presence of other cardiovascular disease risk factors or concomitant diseases (e.g., smoking, obesity, renal disease, peripheral vascular disease) to modify treatment decisions.[1,106,108–111]

Tracking studies and pathophysiologic evidence suggest there may be some benefit from early detection of primary hypertension in childhood, but there is insufficient evidence to support routine screening solely for this purpose. The lack of evidence is of concern because it is unclear whether a policy of routinely screening all children and adolescents to detect primary hypertension would achieve sufficient clinical benefit later in life to justify the costs and potential adverse effects of widespread testing and treatment. Potentially curable causes of hypertension, which account for a relatively large proportion of cases in young children, are often overlooked on history and physical examination, with rare but potentially catastrophic consequences. Evidence from case series and multiple time series indicate that early detection of secondary hypertension in childhood is of substantial benefit to the small number of patients affected.

CLINICAL INTERVENTION

Periodic screening for hypertension is recommended for all persons ≥21 years of age ("A" recommendation). The optimal interval for blood pressure screening has not been determined and is left to clinical discretion. Current expert opinion is that adults who are believed to be normotensive should receive blood pressure measurements at least once every 2 years if their last diastolic and systolic blood pressure readings were below 85 and 140 mm Hg, respectively, and annually if the last diastolic blood pressure was 85–89 mm Hg.[1] Sphygmomanometry should be performed in accordance with recommended technique.[1] Hypertension should not be diagnosed on the basis of a single measurement; elevated readings should be confirmed on more than one reading at each of three separate visits. In adults, current blood pressure criteria for the diagnosis of hypertension are an average diastolic pressure of 90 mm Hg or greater and/or an average systolic pressure of 140 mm Hg or greater.[1] Once confirmed, patients should receive appropriate counseling regarding physical activity (Chapter 55), weight reduction and dietary sodium intake (Chapter 56), and alcohol consumption (Chapter 52). Evidence should also be sought for other cardiovascular risk factors, such as elevated serum cholesterol (Chapter 2) and smoking (Chapter 54), and appropriate intervention should be offered when indicated. The decision to begin drug therapy may include consideration of the level of blood pressure elevation, age, and the presence of other cardiovascular disease risk factors (e.g., tobacco use, hypercholesterolemia), concomitant disease (e.g., diabetes, obesity, peripheral vascular disease), or target-organ damage (e.g., left ventricular hypertrophy, elevated creatinine).[1,106,108] Antihypertensive drugs should be prescribed in accordance with recent guidelines[1,106,108] and with attention to current techniques for improving compliance.[53,54]

Measurement of blood pressure during office visits is also recommended for children and adolescents ("B" recommendation). This recommendation is based on the proven benefits from the early detection of treatable causes of secondary hypertension; there is insufficient evidence to recommend for or against routine periodic blood pressure measurement to detect essential (primary) hypertension in this age group. Sphygmomanometry should be performed in accordance with the recommended technique for children, and hypertension should only be diagnosed on the basis of readings at each of three separate visits.[18] In children, criteria defining hypertension vary with age.[18] Age-, sex-, and height-specific blood pressure nomograms for U.S. children and adolescents have been published.[20]

Routine counseling to promote physical activity (Chapter 55) and a healthy diet (Chapter 56) for the primary prevention of hypertension is recommended for all children and adults.

The draft update of this chapter was prepared for the U.S. Preventive Services Task Force by Carolyn DiGuiseppi, MD, MPH, based in part on material prepared for the Canadian Task Force on the Periodic Health Examination by Alexander G. Logan, MD, FRCPC, and Christopher Patterson, MD, FRCPC.

REFERENCES

1. Joint National Committee on Detection, Evaluation, and Treatment of High Blood Pressure. The fifth report of the Joint National Committee on Detection, Evaluation, and Treatment of High Blood Pressure. Bethesda: National Institutes of Health, 1993. (NIH Publication no. 93-1088.)

1a. Burt VL, Whelton P, Roccella EJ, et al. Prevalence of hypertension in the US adult population: results from the Third National Health and Nutrition Examination Survey, 1988–1991. Hypertension 1995;25:305–313.

2. National Center for Health Statistics. Annual summary of births, marriages, divorces, and deaths: United States, 1993. Monthly vital statistics report; vol 42 no 13. Hyattsville, MD: Public Health Service, 1994.

3. Dawber TF. The Framingham study: the epidemiology of atherosclerotic disease. Cambridge, MA: Harvard University Press, 1980.

4. Sagie A, Larson MG, Levy D. The natural history of borderline isolated systolic hypertension. N Engl J Med 1993;329:1912–1917.

5. Neaton JD, Wentworth D. Serum cholesterol, blood pressure, cigarette smoking, and death from coronary heart disease. Overall findings and differences by age for 316,099 white men. Multiple Risk Factor Intervention Trial Research Group. Arch Intern Med 1992;152:56–64.

6. Cheitlin MD. Coarctation of the aorta. Med Clin North Am 1977;61:655–673.

7. Hiner LB, Falkner B. Renovascular hypertension in children. Pediatr Clin North Am 1993;40:123–140.

8. Rocchini AP. Cardiovascular causes of systemic hypertension. Pediatr Clin North Am 1993;40:141–147.

9. Rodd CJ, Sockalosky JJ. Endocrine causes of hypertension in children. Pediatr Clin North Am 1993;40:149–164.

10. Report of the New England Regional Infant Cardiac Program. Pediatrics 1980;65(suppl):375–461.

11. Buyse ML, ed. Birth defects encyclopedia. St. Louis, MO: Blackwell Scientific Publications, 1990:156.
12. Mustard WT, Rowe RD, Keith JD, et al. Coarctation of the aorta, with special reference to the first year of life. Ann Surg 1955;141:429–436.
13. Tifft CP. Are the days of the sphygmomanometer past? Arch Intern Med 1988;148:518–519.
14. Pickering TG, James GD, Boddie C, et al. How common is white coat hypertension? JAMA 1988;259: 225–228.
15. Perloff D, Grim C, Flack J, et al. Human blood pressure determination by sphygmomanometry. Office of Scientific Affairs, American Heart Association. Circulation 1993;88:2460–2470.
16. Uhari M, Nuutinen M, Turtinen J, et al. Pulse sounds and measurement of diastolic blood pressure in children. Lancet 1991;338:159–161.
17. Nuutinen M, Turtinen J, Uhari M. Random-zero sphygmomanometer, Rose's tape, and the accuracy of the blood pressure measurements in children. Pediatr Res 1992;32:243–247.
18. Task Force on Blood Pressure Control in Children. Report of the Second Task Force on Blood Pressure Control in Children—1987. Pediatrics 1987;79:1–25.
19. Gomez-Marin O, Prineas RJ, Rastam L. Cuff bladder width and blood pressure measurement in children and adolescents. J Hypertens 1992;10:1235–1241.
20. Rosner B, Prineas RJ, Loggie JMH, et al. Blood pressure nomograms for children and adolescents, by height, sex, and age, in the United States. J Pediatr 1993;123:871–886.
21. Hoegholm A, Kristensen KS, Madsen NH, et al. White coat hypertension diagnosed by 24-h ambulatory monitoring: examination of 159 newly diagnosed hypertensive patients. Am J Hypertens 1992;5: 64–70.
22. James GD, Pickering TG, Yee LS, et al. The reproducibility of average ambulatory, home, and clinic pressures. Hypertension 1988;11:545–549.
23. Hall CL, Higgs CMB, Notarianni L, et al. Home blood pressure recording in mild hypertension: value of distinguishing sustained from clinic hypertension and effect on diagnosis and treatment. J Hum Hypertens 1990;4:501–507.
24. Bottini PB, Carr AA, Rhoades RB, et al. Variability of indirect methods used to determine blood pressure: office vs mean 24-hour automated blood pressures. Arch Intern Med 1992;152:139–144.
25. Pearce KA, Grimm RH Jr, Rao S, et al. Population-derived comparisons of ambulatory and office blood pressures: implications for the determination of usual blood pressure and the concept of white coat hypertension. Arch Intern Med 1992;152:750–756.
26. Kleinert HD, Harshfield GA, Pickering TG, et al. What is the value of home blood pressure measurement in patients with mild hypertension? Hypertension 1984;6:574–578.
27. Berenson GS, Dalferes E Jr, Savage D, et al. Ambulatory blood pressure measurements in children and young adults selected by high and low casual blood pressure levels and parental history of hypertension: the Bogalusa Heart Study. Am J Med Sci 1993;305:374–382.
28. Harshfield GA, Alpert BS, Pulliam DA, et al. Ambulatory blood pressure recordings in children and adolescents. Pediatrics 1994;94:180–184.
29. Hansson L. Current and future strategies in the treatment of hypertension. Am J Cardiol 1988;61: 2C–7C.
30. Collins R, Peto R, MacMahon S, et al. Blood pressure, stroke, and coronary heart disease. Part 2, short-term reductions in blood pressure: overview of randomised drug trials in their epidemiological context. Lancet 1990; 335:827–838.
31. MacMahon SW, Cutler JA, Furberg CD, et al. The effects of drug treatment for hypertension on morbidity and mortality from cardiovascular disease: a review of randomized, controlled trials. Prog Cardiovasc Dis 1986; 29(suppl):99–118.
32. Hebert PR, Moser M, Mayer J, et al. Recent evidence on drug therapy of mild to moderate hypertension and decreased risk of coronary heart disease. Arch Intern Med 1993;153:578–581.
33. Veterans Administration Cooperative Study Group on Antihypertensive Agents. Effects of treatment on morbidity in hypertension: results in patients with diastolic pressures averaging 115 through 129 mm Hg. JAMA 1967; 202:1028–1034.
34. Veterans Administration Cooperative Study Group on Antihypertensive Agents. Effects of treatment on morbidity in hypertension. II. Results in patients with diastolic pressures averaging 90 through 114 mm Hg. JAMA 1970; 213:1143–1152.
35. Veterans Administration Cooperative Study Group on Antihypertensive Agents. Effects of treatment on morbidity in hypertension. III. Influence of age, diastolic pressure, and prior cardiovascular disease: further analysis of side effects. Circulation 1972;45:991–1004.

36. Wolff FW, Lindeman RD. Effects of treatment in hypertension: results of a controlled study. J Chronic Dis 1966; 19:227–240.

37. Hypertension-Stroke Cooperative Study Group. Effect of antihypertensive treatment on stroke recurrence. JAMA 1974;229:409–418.

38. Smith WM. Treatment of mild hypertension: results of a ten-year intervention trial. Circ Res 1977;40(5 Suppl 1):I98–105.

39. Hypertension Detection and Follow-Up Program Cooperative Group. Five-year findings of the Hypertension Detection and Follow-Up Program. I. Reduction in mortality of persons with high blood pressure, including mild hypertension. JAMA 1979;242:2562–2572.

40. Management Committee of the Australian National Blood Pressure Study. The Australian therapeutic trial in mild hypertension. Lancet 1980;1:1261–1267.

41. Medical Research Council Working Party. MRC trial of treatment of mild hypertension: principal results. BMJ 1985;291:97–104.

42. Medical Research Council Working Party. Persistence of reduction in blood pressure and mortality of participants in the Hypertension Detection and Follow-Up Program. JAMA 1988;259:2113–2122.

43. Amery A, Birkenhager W, Brixko P, et al. Mortality and morbidity results from the European Working Party on High Blood Pressure in the Elderly Trial. Lancet 1985;i:1349–1354.

44. Amery A, Birkenhager W, Brixko P, et al. Efficacy of antihypertensive drug treatment according to age, sex, blood pressure and previous cardiovascular disease in patients over the age of 60. Lancet 1986;ii: 589–592.

45. Staessan J, Bulpitt C, Clement D, et al. Relation between mortality and treated blood pressure in elderly patients with hypertension: report of the European Working Party on High Blood Pressure in the Elderly. BMJ 1989; 298:1552–1556.

46. Dahlof B, Lindholm LH, Hansson L, et al. Morbidity and mortality in the Swedish Trial in Old Patients with Hypertension (STOP-Hypertension). Lancet 1991;338:1281–1285.

47. MRC Working Party. Medical Research Council trial of treatment of hypertension in older adults: principal results. BMJ 1992;304:405–412.

48. SHEP Cooperative Research Group. Prevention of stroke by antihypertensive drug treatment in older persons with isolated systolic hypertension. Final results of the Systolic Hypertension in the Elderly Program (SHEP). JAMA 1991;265:3255–3264.

49. Insua JT, Sacks HS, Lau T-S, et al. Drug treatment of hypertension in the elderly: a meta-analysis. Ann Intern Med 1994;121:355–362.

50. Mulrow CD, Cornell JA, Herrera CR, et al. Hypertension in the elderly: implications and generalizability of randomized trials. JAMA 1994;272:1932–1938.

51. Garraway WM, Whisnant JP. The changing pattern of hypertension and the declining incidence of stroke. JAMA 1987;258:214–217.

52. Casper M, Wing S, Strogatz D, et al. Antihypertensive treatment and U.S. trends in stroke mortality, 1962 to 1980. Am J Public Health 1992;82:1600–1606.

53. McClellan WM, Hall WD, Brogan D, et al. Continuity of care in hypertension: an important correlate of blood pressure control among aware hypertensives. Arch Intern Med 1988;148:525–528.

54. National Institutes of Health. The physician's guide: improving adherence among hypertensive patients. Working Group on Health Education and High Blood Pressure Control. Bethesda: Department of Health and Human Services, 1987.

55. Siscovick DS, Raghunathan TE, Psaty BM, et al. Diuretic therapy for hypertension and the risk of primary cardiac arrest. N Engl J Med 1994;330:1852–1857.

55a. Neaton JD, Grimm RH Jr, Prineas RJ, et al. Treatment of mild hypertension study: final results. JAMA 1993;270:713–724.

56. National High Blood Pressure Education Program Working Group. National High Blood Pressure Education Program Working Group report on primary prevention of hypertension. Arch Intern Med 1993;153:186–208.

57. The Trials of Hypertension Prevention Collaborative Research Group. The effects of nonpharmacologic interventions on blood pressure of persons with high normal levels. Results of the Trials of Hypertension Prevention, Phase 1. JAMA 1992;267:1213–1220.

58. Langford HG, Davis BR, Blaufox MD, et al. Effect of drug and diet treatment of mild hypertension on diastolic blood pressure. Hypertension 1991;17:210–217.

59. Schotte DE, Stunkard AJ. The effects of weight reduction on blood pressure in 301 obese patients. Arch Intern Med 1990;150:1701–1704.

60. World Hypertension League. Physical exercise in the management of hypertension: a consensus statement by the World Hypertension League. J Hypertens 1991;9:283–287.

61. Cutler JA, Follmann D, Elliott P, et al. An overview of randomized trials of sodium reduction and blood pressure. Hypertension 1991;17(Suppl I):I27–I33.

62. Law MR, Frost CD, Wald NJ. By how much does dietary salt reduction lower blood pressure? III. Analysis of data from trials of salt reduction. BMJ 1991;302:819–824.

62a. Blumenthal JA, Siegel WC, Appelbaum M. Failure of exercise to reduce blood pressure in patients with mild hypertension: results of a randomized controlled trial. JAMA 1991;266:2098–2104.

63. Wassertheil-Smoller S, Oberman A, Blaufox D, et al. The Trial of Antihypertensive Interventions and Management (TAIM) study. Final results with regard to blood pressure, cardiovascular risk, and quality of life. Am J Hypertens 1992;5:37–44.

64. Newman WP, Freedman DS, Voors AW, et al. Relation of serum lipoprotein levels and systolic blood pressure to early atherosclerosis: the Bogalusa Heart Study. N Engl J Med 1986;314:138–144.

65. Schieken RM, Clarke WR, Lauer RM. Left ventricular hypertrophy in children with blood pressure in the upper quintile of the distribution. The Muscatine Study. Hypertension 1981;3:669–675.

66. Culpepper WS 3d, Sodt PC, Messerli FH, et al. Cardiac status in juvenile borderline hypertension. Ann Intern Med 1983;98:1–7.

67. Burke GL, Arcilla RA, Culpepper WS, et al. Blood pressure and echocardiographic measures in children: the Bogalusa Heart Study. Circulation 1987;75:106–114.

68. Prebis JW, Gruskin AB, Polinsky MS, et al. Uric acid in childhood essential hypertension. J Pediatr 1981;98:702–707.

69. Feld LG, Springate JE. Hypertension in children. Curr Probl Pediatr 1988;18:317–373.

70. Shear CL, Burke GL, Freedman DS, et al. Value of childhood blood pressure measurements and family history in predicting future blood pressure status: results from 8 years of follow-up in the Bogalusa Heart Study. Pediatrics 1986;77:862–869.

71. Michels VV, Bergstrahl EJ, Hoverman VR. Tracking and prediction of blood pressure in children. Mayo Clin Proc 1987;62:875–881.

72. Lauer RM, Clarke WR, Beaglehole R. Level, trend and variability of blood pressure during childhood. Circulation 1984;69:242–249.

73. Nelson MJ, Ragland DR, Syme SL. Longitudinal prediction of adult blood pressure from juvenile blood pressure levels. Am J Epidemiol 1991;136:633–645.

74. Kneisley J, Schork N, Julius S. Predictors of blood pressure and hypertension in Tecumseh, Michigan. Clin Exp Hypertens [A] 1990;12:693–708.

75. Gillman MW, Cook NR, Rosner B, et al. Identifying children at high risk for the development of essential hypertension. Pediatrics 1993;122:837–846.

76. St George IM, Williams SM, Silva PA. The stability of high blood pressure in Dunedin children: an eight year longitudinal study. NZ Med J 1990;103:115–117.

77. Nishio T, Mori C, Watanabe K, et al. Quantitative analysis of systolic blood pressure tracking during childhood and adolescence using a tracking index: the Shimane Heart Study. J Hypertens 1989; 7 (Suppl 1):S35–S36.

78. Yong L-C, Kuller LH. Tracking of blood pressure from adolescence to middle age: the Dormont High School Study. Prev Med 1994;23:418–426.

79. Hofman A, Hazebroek A, Valkenburg HA. A randomized trial of sodium intake and blood pressure in newborn infants. JAMA 1983;250:370–373.

80. Bal' LV, Shugaeva EN, Deev AA, et al. Results of a three-year trial of arterial hypertension prevention in a population of children aged 11–15 years by overweight control. Cor Vasa 1990;32:448–456.

81. Hansen HS, Froberg K, Hyldebrandt N, et al. A controlled study of eight months of physical training and reduction of blood pressure in children: the Odense schoolchild study. BMJ 1991;303:682–685.

82. Sinaiko AR, Gomez-Marin O, Prineas RJ. Effect of low sodium diet or potassium supplementation on adolescent blood pressure. Hypertension 1993;21:989–994.

83. Williams GH, Braunwald E. Hypertensive vascular disease. In: Braunwald E, et al, eds. Harrison's principles of internal medicine. New York: McGraw-Hill, 1987.

84. De Santo NG, Capasso G, Giordano DR, et al. Secondary forms of hypertension. Semin Nephrol 1989; 9:272–286.

85. Strafford MA, Griffiths SP, Gersony WM. Coarctation of the aorta: a study in delayed detection. Pediatrics 1982;69:159–163.

86. Thoele DG, Muster AJ, Paul MH. Recognition of coarctation of the aorta. A continuing challenge for the primary care physician. Am J Dis Child 1987;141:1201–1204.
87. Ward KE, Pryor RW, Matson JR, et al. Delayed detection of coarctation in infancy: implications for timing of newborn follow-up. Pediatrics 1990;86:972–976.
88. Westaby S, Parnell B, Pridie RB. Coarctation of the aorta in adults. Clinical presentation and results of surgery. J Cardiovasc Surg 1987;28:124–127.
89. Nanton MA, Olley RM. Residual hypertension after coarctectomy in children. Am J Cardiol 1976;37: 769–772.
90. Presbitero P, Demarie D, Villani M, et al. Long term results (15–30 years) of surgical repair of aortic coarctation. Br Heart J 1987;57:462–467.
91. Shinebourne EA, Tam ASY, Elseed AM, et al. Coarctation of the aorta in infancy and childhood. Br Heart J 1976;38:375–380.
92. Liberthson RR, Pennington DG, Jacobs ML, et al. Coarctation of the aorta: review of 234 patients and clarification of management problems. Am J Cardiol 1979;43:835–840.
93. Lawrie GM, DeBakey ME, Morris GC Jr, et al. Late repair of coarctation of the descending thoracic aorta in 190 patients. Arch Surg 1981;116:1557–1560.
94. Forfang K, Rostad H, Sorland S. Coarctation of the aorta. Follow-up of 218 patients operated on after 13 years of age. Acta Med Scand 1981;645:15–22.
95. Bobby JJ, Emami JM, Farmer RDT, et al. Operative survival and 40 years follow-up of surgical repair of aortic coarctation. Br Heart J 1991;65:271–276.
96. Grundy SM, Greenland P, Herd A, et al. Cardiovascular and risk factor evaluation of healthy American adults. A statement for physicians by an ad hoc committee appointed by the Steering Committee, American Heart Association. Circulation 1987;75:1340A–1362A.
97. Eddy D, ed. Common screening tests. Philadelphia: American College of Physicians, 1991.
98. American Academy of Family Physicians. Age charts for periodic health examination. Kansas City, MO: American Academy of Family Physicians, 1994. (Reprint no. 510.)
99. Canadian Task Force on the Periodic Health Examination. Canadian guide to clinical preventive health care. Ottawa: Canada Communication Group, 1994:636–648, 944–951.
100. American Academy of Pediatrics. Recommendations for preventive pediatric health care. Pediatrics 1995;96:373–374.
101. Green M, ed. Bright Futures: guidelines for health supervision of infants, children and adolescents. Arlington, VA: National Center for Education in Maternal and Child Health, 1994.
102. American Medical Association. AMA guidelines for adolescent preventive services (GAPS): recommendations and rationale. Chicago: American Medical Association, 1994.
103. American Heart Association. Integrated cardiovascular health promotion in childhood. A statement for health professionals from the Subcommittee on Atherosclerosis and Hypertension in Childhood of the Council on Cardiovascular Disease in the Young. Circulation 1992;85:1638–1650.
104. American Academy of Pediatrics. Routine evaluation of blood pressure, hematocrit, and glucose in newborns. Pediatrics 1993;92:474–476.
105. MacDonald LA, Sackett DL, Haynes RB, et al. Labelling in hypertension: a review of the behavioral and psychological consequences. J Chronic Dis 1984;37:933–942.
106. Haynes RB, Lacourciere Y, Rabkin SW, et al. Report of the Canadian Hypertension Society Consensus Conference. 2. Diagnosis of hypertension in adults. Can Med Assoc J 1993;149:409–418.
107. Ogilvie RI, Burgess ED, Cusson JR, et al. Report of the Canadian Hypertension Society Consensus Conference. 3. Pharmacologic treatment of essential hypertension. Can Med Assoc J 1993;149: 575–584.
108. Sever P, Beevers G, Bulpitt C, et al. Management guidelines in essential hypertension: report of the second working party of the British Hypertension Society. BMJ 1993;306:983–987.
109. Whitworth JA, Clarkson D, Dwyer T, et al. The management of hypertension: a consensus statement. Australian Consensus Conference 1993. Med J Aust 1994;160(suppl):S1–S16.
110. WHO/ISH Mild Hypertension Liaison Committee. 1993 guidelines for the management of mild hypertension. Memorandum from a World Health Organization/International Society of Hypertension meeting. Hypertension 1993;22:392–403.
111. Jackson R, Barham P, Bills J, et al. Management of raised blood pressure in New Zealand: a discussion document. BMJ 1993;307:107–110.

4. Screening for Asymptomatic Carotid Artery Stenosis

RECOMMENDATION

There is insufficient evidence to recommend for or against screening asymptomatic persons for carotid artery stenosis using the physical examination or carotid ultrasound. For selected high-risk patients, a recommendation to discuss the potential benefits of screening and carotid endarterectomy may be made on other grounds (see *Clinical Intervention*). All persons should be screened for hypertension (see Chapter 3), and clinicians should provide counseling about smoking cessation (see Chapter 54).

Burden of Suffering

Cerebrovascular disease is the third leading cause of death in the U.S., accounting for over 149,000 deaths in 1993.[1] Most stroke-related morbidity and mortality occur in older adults: 87% of all deaths and 74% of all hospitalizations occur in persons age 65 years or older.[2] Strokes can result in substantial neurologic deficits as well as serious medical and psychological complications. With an estimated prevalence of 3 million stroke survivors,[3] this illness places enormous burdens on family members and caretakers, often necessitating skilled care in an institutional setting. The direct and indirect costs of stroke in the U.S. have been estimated at $30 billion annually.[4] The principal risk factors for ischemic stroke are increased age, hypertension, smoking, coronary artery disease, atrial fibrillation, and diabetes.[4-7] Of these, the most important modifiable risk factors are hypertension and smoking.[8] Improved treatment of high blood pressure has been credited with the greater than 50% reduction in age-adjusted stroke mortality that has been observed since 1972 (see Chapter 3).

Population-based cohort studies have established that persons with carotid artery stenosis are at increased risk for subsequent stroke, myocardial infarction (MI), and death.[9,10] The risk of stroke is greatest for persons with neurologic symptoms such as transient ischemic attacks (TIAs), but is also increased in patients with asymptomatic lesions. The prevalence of hemodynamically significant carotid stenosis varies with age and other risk factors: population-based studies estimate that 0.5% of persons in their 50s and about 10% of those over age 80 have carotid stenosis greater than

50%.[11] The proportion of all strokes attributable to previously asymptomatic carotid stenosis seems to be small, however. In a study of 250 patients over age 60 with cerebral infarction, only 13% had ipsilateral carotid stenosis of 70% or greater.[12]

Accuracy of Screening Tests

Two methods are used to screen for carotid artery stenosis: clinical auscultation for carotid bruits and noninvasive studies of the carotid artery. Neck auscultation is an imperfect screening test for carotid stenosis. There is considerable interobserver variation among clinicians in the interpretation of the key auditory characteristics—intensity, pitch, and duration—of importance in predicting stenosis.[13] In addition, a cervical bruit can be heard in 4% of the population over age 40, but the finding is not specific for significant carotid artery stenosis. Between 40% and 75% of arteries with asymptomatic bruits do not have significant compromise in blood flow;[14] similar sounds can also be produced by anatomic variation and tortuosity, venous hum, goiter, and transmitted cardiac murmur.[13,15–17] Finally, hemodynamically significant stenotic lesions may exist in the absence of an audible bruit.[13,15,18] Using 70–99% stenosis on a carotid angiogram as a reliable standard, a carotid bruit has a sensitivity of 63–76% and a specificity of 61–76% for clinically significant stenosis.[19]

Persons with cervical bruits can be evaluated further with greater accuracy by noninvasive study of the carotid arteries. Older techniques (e.g., spectral analysis phonoangiography, continuous-wave or pulsed Doppler ultrasound, B-mode real-time ultrasound, oculoplethysmography, ophthalmodynamometry, periorbital directional Doppler ultrasound, and thermography) have been replaced largely by carotid duplex sonography which combines the capabilities of B-mode and Doppler ultrasound. A 1995 meta-analysis of 70 studies comparing the accuracy of noninvasive diagnostic tests to carotid angiography (the reference standard) concluded that carotid duplex, carotid Doppler, and magnetic resonance angiography (MRA) were equally effective in diagnosing carotid stenosis of 70% or greater: estimated sensitivity ranged from 83% to 86%, specificity from 89% to 94%.[20] Depending on the underlying population characteristics, the positive predictive value of carotid duplex ranges from 82% to 97%.[21] The performance of noninvasive tests for screening asymptomatic persons, however, has not been assessed in a prospective study. Although MRA seems to be quite sensitive and spares patients the risks of conventional angiography, it is unlikely to be a useful screening test due to costs (over $400) and inconvenience.[22]

Effectiveness of Early Detection

The rationale for testing for carotid artery stenosis is that persons with asymptomatic stenoses are not only at increased risk for cerebrovascular disease,[11,12] but that early detection can reduce morbidity due to cerebrovascular disease. According to this rationale there are several benefits to early detection of asymptomatic carotid stenosis. An awareness of the diagnosis might motivate patients to modify other risk factors (e.g., high blood pressure, smoking, physical inactivity). Performing carotid endarterectomy in some individuals might prevent subsequent cerebral infarction distal to the obstruction. Finally, antiplatelet drugs (aspirin and ticlopidine) might reduce stroke risk in asymptomatic individuals with carotid artery stenosis. No study has specifically compared a strategy of screening and early intervention in asymptomatic persons to intervening only in symptomatic patients (e.g., those with TIAs). The first symptom of carotid stenosis in some patients may be an irreversible stroke, however. A number of studies have examined whether interventions in asymptomatic persons can reduce the subsequent incidence of fatal and nonfatal stroke.

A bruit over the carotid artery is a fair indicator of vascular disease but a poor predictor that ischemic stroke will occur in its arterial distribution. The proportion of persons with asymptomatic bruits who will experience stroke is small: the annual incidence of stroke ipsilateral to a bruit and unheralded by TIAs is only 1–3%.[9,10,16,23–25] Higher grades of stenosis (assessed by sonography) are associated with increasing risk of neurologic events, rising to 5–7% per year with high-grade stenosis or total occlusion.[26,27] However, in those persons who will suffer a stroke, the degree of carotid stenosis does not always predict the risk of cerebral infarction,[16,23,28] or its location.[11,12] Carotid artery lesions may be less a predictor of atherothrombotic strokes than of generalized atherosclerotic disease; persons with carotid artery disease are considerably more likely to die from ischemic heart disease than from a cerebrovascular event.[9,10]

One of the major justifications for screening is the belief that carotid endarterectomy for high-grade, asymptomatic lesions detected through screening can prevent stroke. Three studies published before 1987 reported improved outcomes after endarterectomy. These studies provide poor quality evidence because they included previously symptomatic patients, were convenience samples derived from surgeons' practices, had inconsistent measurement criteria, or did not randomly assign patients.[17,29,30] Four more recent randomized trials have compared aspirin with endarterectomy in patients with asymptomatic carotid artery stenosis. The first study comparing aspirin alone with endarterectomy alone[31] enrolled only 71 patients before it was terminated due to excess MI in the surgical group; no conclusions could be drawn regarding the effectiveness of endarterectomy for preventing stroke.[32] The second study, the 1991 European CASANOVA trial, randomized 410 patients with moderately severe stenosis (>50% but <90%) to treatment with aspirin/dipyridamole or aspirin/dipyridamole plus surgery.[33] The protocol was complex: some patients in both groups had contralateral symptoms, patients with stenosis greater than 90% were excluded, and 72 patients received therapy appropriate for the other group (more in the group randomized to surgery). There were no differences in the numbers of neurologic events and deaths between the two groups. The power of the study, however, was insufficient to exclude a clinically important benefit in the surgical group.[33] A third study, published in 1993, randomized 444 older veterans (mean age 64) with 50% or greater carotid stenosis to aspirin plus carotid endarterectomy or aspirin therapy alone. Patients who underwent carotid endarterectomy had lower rates of ipsilateral neurologic events, the primary endpoint: the combined incidence of TIAs, transient monocular blindness, and stroke was 8% in the surgery group versus 21% with aspirin only (p < 0.001), during an average follow-up of 48 months. The two groups had similar outcomes, however, using a combined endpoint of stroke or death from any cause. The power of the study was insufficient to exclude up to a 20% reduction in stroke in the surgically treated group.[34] The generalizability of this study was limited by the lack of female subjects and by the excessive morbidity and mortality in both groups (over 40% incidence of stroke or death in both groups over the 4-year follow-up).

The Asymptomatic Carotid Artery Study (ACAS),[35] funded by the National Institutes of Health, recently reported final results that provide stronger evidence of the benefit of endarterectomy for asymptomatic stenoses.[36] This multicenter study randomized 1662 patients with asymptomatic stenoses greater than 60% (mean stenosis 73%) to endarterectomy plus aspirin or to aspirin alone. Most patients (87%) were over age 60, and more than two thirds had coronary heart disease. The trial was stopped after a median follow-up of 2.7 years. The estimated 5-year risk for ipsilateral stroke or perioperative stroke or death was 5.1% for surgical patients and 11% for medically treated patients, a reduction in cumulative risk of 53% (95% confidence interval, 22 to 72). The absolute reduction in the combined incidence of major ipsilateral stroke, major perioperative stroke, or perioperative death, however, was considerably smaller (estimated 5-year risk of 3.4% in the surgery group vs. 6% in the medical group), not statistically significant (p = 0.13), and evident only in the fifth year of follow-up. Subgroup analyses suggest that endarterectomy may be less effective in women than in men (17% vs. 66% reduction in 5-year event rate), possibly due to higher perioperative complication rates (3.6% in women vs. 1.7% in men); neither of these differences between genders was statistically significant, however. The medical centers participating in this trial had been rigorously evaluated for the quality of patient management, and only surgeons with a perioperative complication rate of less than 3% among asymptomatic patients were allowed to participate.[37] Published studies have reported a perioperative mortality ranging from 1% to 3%,[33,34,38–40] and a perioperative stroke rate ranging between 2% and

10%, depending on patient characteristics and surgical expertise.[13,33,34,39–44] In six prospective trials of endarterectomy published after 1990, perioperative complication rates (stroke and death combined) range from 3% to 8%.[38] Complication rates seem to be lower in asymptomatic patients than in symptomatic patients, however.[38,40] A fifth trial of surgery versus medical management for asymptomatic carotid artery stenosis is still in progress.[11]

Antiplatelet therapy with aspirin or ticlopidine offers a second possible intervention to reduce the risk of stroke in patients with asymptomatic carotid artery stenosis. Clinical trials have demonstrated a benefit of aspirin in reducing stroke among symptomatic patients (i.e., in persons with TIAs or stroke),[45–48] but observed no benefit on stroke in a large trial in asymptomatic physicians (prevalence of carotid disease unknown).[49] Among patients with asymptomatic carotid disease, who have a lower risk of ischemic events than do symptomatic patients, chronic aspirin therapy may not provide sufficient benefits to justify the documented risks of hemorrhagic complications (see Chapter 69). A multicenter prospective study comparing aspirin to placebo in asymptomatic patients with >50% carotid stenosis found no difference in stroke rates.[50] Ticlopidine is an alternative to aspirin in patients with risk factors for gastrointestinal hemorrhage, aspirin intolerance, and in patients who continue to have vascular events despite aspirin therapy, but its use is limited by high cost and small risk of neutropenia (approximately 1%).[51,52] The efficacy of ticlopidine in patients with asymptomatic carotid artery stenosis is not known.

Reducing serum lipids may slow the progression of carotid atherosclerosis and reduce clinical events. In a randomized trial enrolling patients with moderately elevated levels of LDL cholesterol (130–190 mg/dL) and early carotid atherosclerosis diagnosed by B-mode ultrasound, lovastatin induced regression of atherosclerosis and reduced total cardiovascular events compared to placebo.[52a] Lipid-lowering drug therapy has not been examined specifically for treatment of advanced carotid stenosis, but is generally recommended for patients with high cholesterol and symptomatic vascular disease, based on its ability to reduce coronary heart disease mortality (see Chapter 2). No controlled studies have examined changes in the behavior of patients (e.g., smoking cessation or dietary modification) on learning the results of carotid artery examinations.

Recommendations of Other Groups

Although auscultation of the carotid arteries is widely considered a routine component of the physical examination, the Canadian Task Force on the Periodic Health Examination[53] recommended against screening for bruits in asymptomatic persons, based on the poor sensitivity and specificity of cervical bruits as an indicator of significant carotid stenosis. The American

Academy of Family Physicians recommends auscultation for carotid bruits in people age 40 and older with risk factors for cerebrovascular or cardiovascular disease, those with neurologic symptoms (e.g., TIA) or those with a history of cardiovascular disease;[54] this policy is currently under review. The 1988 guidelines of the American College of Physicians recommend that patients with asymptomatic bruits should not have further diagnostic testing but should be educated about potential symptoms of a TIA in the carotid circulation.[55] In 1988, an ad hoc multidisciplinary consensus panel involved in designing the ACAS study recommended a baseline noninvasive study of the carotid arteries in persons considered at high risk for extracranial carotid arterial disease.[56] In 1992, the Ad Hoc Committee of the Joint Council of the Society for Vascular Surgery and the North American Chapter of the International Society for Vascular Surgery recommended that patients with asymptomatic carotid artery stenosis greater than 75% who are otherwise healthy and have a projected life expectancy more than 5 years should be considered for surgery if the operative morbidity and mortality rates are less than 3%.[57]

Discussion

The effectiveness of routine screening and intervention to reduce morbidity from asymptomatic carotid artery disease remains uncertain. The most effective interventions to prevent stroke are smoking cessation and the identification and treatment of hypertension. Although screening will detect some patients with asymptomatic high-grade carotid lesions who may benefit from endarterectomy, such patients account for only a small proportion of all strokes. In addition, there are several reasons to be cautious about undertaking widespread screening in asymptomatic persons on the basis of the current evidence:[11,38,58] the risk of major stroke ipsilateral to stenotic lesions is relatively low without surgery (approximately 1% per year); the absolute reduction in major stroke and death due to surgery over 5 years in ACAS was small and not conclusive; surgery may result in other nonfatal complications (cranial nerve injury, MI, etc.); and the low complication rate of the ACAS-selected surgeons is not likely to reflect the typical risk of endarterectomy in the community. If complication rates of surgery are higher or underlying risk of stroke lower than reported for the ACAS study, the risks of surgery for asymptomatic carotid artery disease may outweigh the benefits. Routine screening will also subject some patients without significant carotid disease to the risks of angiography (1% risk of stroke), due to occasional false-positive results of carotid ultrasound.

As a result, it is not yet clear whether widespread screening in the primary care setting will be an effective way to reduce morbidity and mortality from stroke. Noninvasive testing for carotid artery stenosis is expensive (over $150 for carotid duplex or Doppler ultrasound);[20] the cost of screening 50% of the population over age 60 in the U.S. has been estimated at over $7 billion.[58] Auscultation for bruits involves little direct expense and may detect a majority of patients with severe stenosis, but the costs of follow-up testing of all patients with asymptomatic bruits could be substantial. Revised cost-effectiveness analyses of various screening and treatment strategies for asymptomatic carotid disease are under way. Patients most likely to benefit from screening are older men (over age 60) who have other risk factors for stroke, no contraindications to major surgery, and access to high-quality vascular surgery centers. Evidence regarding the effectiveness of antiplatelet drugs for asymptomatic persons is not yet sufficient to make a recommendation.

CLINICAL INTERVENTION

There is insufficient evidence to recommend for or against screening asymptomatic persons for carotid artery stenosis, using physical examination or carotid ultrasound ("C" recommendation). A recommendation may be made on other grounds to discuss the potential benefits of screening with high-risk patients (e.g., persons over age 60 at high risk for vascular disease), provided that high-quality vascular surgical care is available (surgical morbidity and mortality less than 3%). These other grounds include the increased prevalence of significant carotid disease, and the possible long-term benefit of endarterectomy in patients with asymptomatic stenosis greater than 60% when performed by qualified surgeons. Patients should be screened and counseled about other risk factors for cerebrovascular disease as discussed in other chapters (see Chapters 3 and 54).

The draft update of this chapter was prepared for the U.S. Preventive Services Task Force by Stephen Tabet, MD, MPH, Alfred O. Berg, MD, MPH, and David Atkins, MD, MPH.

REFERENCES

1. National Center for Health Statistics. Annual summary of births, marriages, divorces, and deaths: United States. Monthly vital statistics report; vol 42 no 13. Hyattsville, MD: Public Health Service, 1994.
2. Centers for Disease Control. Cerebrovascular disease mortality and Medicare hospitalization—United States, 1980–1990. MMWR 1992;41:477–480.
3. Gresham GE, Duncan PW, Stason WB, et al. Post-stroke rehabilitation. Clinical practice guideline no. 16. Rockville, MD: Agency for Health Care Policy and Research, 1995. (AHCPR Publication no. 95-0662.)
4. Matchar DB, McCrory DC, Barnett HJM, et al. Medical treatment for stroke prevention. Ann Intern Med 1994;121:41–53.
5. Schoenberg BS. Epidemiology of cerebrovascular disease. South Med J 1979;72:331–336.
6. Davis PH, Dambrosia JM, Schoenberg DG, et al. Risk factors for ischemic stroke: a prospective study in Rochester, Minnesota. Ann Neurol 1987;22:319–327.
7. D'Agostino RB, Wolf PA, Belanger AJ, et al. Stroke risk profile: adjustment for antihypertensive medication. The Framingham Study. Stroke 1994;25:40–43.

8. Whisnant JP, Homer D, Ingall TJ, et al. Duration of cigarette smoking is the strongest predictor of severe extracranial carotid artery atherosclerosis. Stroke 1990;21:707–714.

9. Heyman A, Wilkinson WE, Heyden S, et al. Risk of stroke in asymptomatic persons with cervical arterial bruits: a population study in Evans County, Georgia. N Engl J Med 1980;302:838–841.

10. Wolf PA, Kannel WB, Sorlie P, et al. Asymptomatic carotid bruit and risk of stroke: the Framingham study. JAMA 1981;245:1442–1445.

11. Warlow C. Endarterectomy for asymptomatic stenosis? Lancet 1995;345:1254–1255.

12. Amarenco P, Cohen A, Tzourio C, et al. Atherosclerotic disease of the aortic arch and the risk of ischemic stroke. N Engl J Med 1994;331:1474–1479.

13. Chambers BR, Norris JW. Clinical significance of asymptomatic neck bruits. Neurology 1985;35:742–745.

14. Quinones-Baldrich WJ, Moore WS. Asymptomatic carotid stenosis: rationale for management. Arch Neurol 1985;42:378–382.

15. Caplan LR. Carotid-artery disease. N Engl J Med 1986;315:886–888.

16. Chambers BR, Norris JW. Outcome in patients with asymptomatic neck bruits. N Engl J Med 1986;315:860–865.

17. Thompson JE, Patman RD, Talkington CM. Asymptomatic carotid bruit: long-term outcome of patients having endarterectomy compared with unoperated controls. Ann Surg 1978;188:308–316.

18. Kuller LH, Sutton KC. Carotid artery bruit: is it safe and effective to auscultate the neck? Stroke 1984;15:944–947.

19. Sauvé JS, Lauoacis A, Østbye T, et al. Does this patient have a clinically important carotid bruit? JAMA 1993;270:2843–2845.

20. Blakeley DD, Oddone EZ, Hasselblad V, et al. Noninvasive carotid artery testing: a meta-analytic review. Ann Intern Med 1995;122:360–367.

21. Zwiebel WJ. Duplex sonography of the cerebral arteries: efficacy, limitations, and indications. Am J Radiol 1992;158:29–36.

22. Bosmans H, Marchal G, Van Hecke P, Vanhoenacker P. MRA review. Clin Imaging 1992;16:152–167.

23. Bogousslavsky J, Despland PA, Regli F. Asymptomatic tight stenosis of the internal carotid artery: long-term prognosis. Neurology 1986;36:861–863.

24. Meissner I, Wiebers DO, Whisnant JP, et al. The natural history of asymptomatic carotid artery lesions. JAMA 1987;258:2704–2707.

25. Hennerici M, Hulsbomer HB, Hefter H, et al. Natural history of asymptomatic extracranial arterial disease: results of a long-term prospective study. Brain 1987;110:777–791.

26. Nicholls SC, Bergelin RO, Strandness DE. Neurologic sequelae of unilateral carotid artery occlusion. J Vasc Surg 1989;10:542–548.

27. Cote R, Barnett HJ, Taylor DW. Internal carotid artery occlusion: a prospective study. Stroke 1983;14:898–902.

28. Yatsu FM, Fields WS. Asymptomatic carotid bruit: stenosis or ulceration, a conservative approach. Arch Neurol 1985;42:383–385.

29. Busuttil RW, Baker JD, Davidson RK, et al. Carotid artery stenosis: hemodynamic significance and clinical course. JAMA 1981;245:1438–1441.

30. Moneta GL, Taylor DC, Nicholls SC, et al. Operative versus nonoperative management of asymptomatic high-grade internal carotid artery stenosis: improved results with endarterectomy. Stroke 1987;18:1005–1010.

31. Mayo Asymptomatic Carotid Artery Study Group. Effectiveness of carotid endarterectomy for asymptomatic carotid stenosis: design of a clinical trial. Mayo Clin Proc 1989;64:897–904.

32. Mayo Asymptomatic Carotid Artery Study Group. Results of a randomized controlled trial of carotid endarterectomy for asymptomatic carotid stenosis. Mayo Clin Proc 1992;67:513–518.

33. The CASANOVA Study Group. Carotid surgery versus medical therapy in asymptomatic carotid stenosis. Stroke 1991;22:1229–1235.

34. Hobson RW, Weiss DG, Fields WS, et al. Efficacy of carotid endarterectomy for asymptomatic carotid stenosis. N Engl J Med 1993;328:221–227.

35. The Asymptomatic Carotid Atherosclerosis Study Group. Study design for randomized prospective trial of carotid endarterectomy for asymptomatic atherosclerosis. Stroke 1989;20:844–849.

36. Executive Committee for the Asymptomatic Carotid Atherosclerosis Study. Endarterectomy for asymptomatic carotid artery stenosis. JAMA 1995;273:1421–1428.

37. Moore WS, Vescera CL, Robertson JT, et al. Selection process for participating surgeons in the Asymptomatic Carotid Atherosclerosis Study (ACAS). Stroke 1991;22:1353–1357.

38. Barnett HJM, Eliasiziw M, Meldrum HE. Drugs and surgery in the prevention of ischemic stroke. N Engl J Med 1995;332:238–248.

39. Brott T, Labutta RJ, Kempzinski RF. Changing patterns in the practice of carotid endarterectomy in a large metropolitan area. JAMA 1986;255:2609–2612.

40. Mattos MA, Modi JR, Mansour AM, et al. Evolution of carotid endarterectomy in two community hospitals: Springfield revisited—seventeen years and 2243 operations later. J Vasc Surg 1995;21:719–726.

41. Grotta JC. Current medical and surgical therapy for cerebrovascular disease. N Engl J Med 1987;317: 1505–1516.

42. Coyle KA, Gray BC, Smith RB 3rd, et al. Morbidity and mortality associated with carotid endarterectomy: effect of adjunctive coronary revascularization. Ann Vasc Surg 1995;9:21–27.

43. Rubin JR, Pitluk HC, King TA, et al. Carotid endarterectomy in a metropolitan community: the early results after 8535 operations. J Vasc Surg 1988;7:256–260.

44. Zurbruegg HR, Seiler RW, Grolimund P, et al. Morbidity and mortality of carotid endarterectomy: a literature review of the results in the last 10 years. Acta Neurochir (Wien) 1987;84:3–12.

45. Canadian Cooperative Study Group. A randomized trial of aspirin and sulfinpyrazone in threatened stroke. N Engl J Med 1978;299:53–59.

46. Bousser MG, Eschwege E, Haguenau M, et al. AICLA controlled trial of aspirin and dipyridamole in the secondary prevention of atherothrombotic cerebral ischemia. Stroke 1983;14:5–14.

47. UK-TIA Study Group. United Kingdom transient ischemic attack (UK-TIA) aspirin trial: interim results. BMJ 1988; 296:316–320.

48. Antiplatelet Trialists Collaboration. Collaborative overview of randomized trials of anti-platelet treatment. Part 1: prevention of death, myocardial infarction and stroke by prolonged antiplatelet therapy in various categories of patients. BMJ 1994;308:81–106.

49. The Steering Committee of the Physicians' Health Study Research Group. Final report on the aspirin component of the ongoing Physicians' Health Study. N Engl J Med 1989;321:129–135.

50. Côté R, Battista RN, Abrahamowicz M, et al. Lack of effect of aspirin in asymptomatic patients with carotid bruits and substantial carotid narrowing. Ann Intern Med 1995;123:649–655.

51. Gent M, Blakely JA, Easton JD, et al. The Canadian American Ticlopidine Study (CATS) in thromboembolic stroke. Lancet 1989;1:1215–1220.

52. Hass WK, Easton JD, Adams HP. A randomized trial comparing ticlopidine hydrochloride with aspirin for the prevention of stroke in high-risk patients. N Engl J Med 1989;321:501–507.

52a. Furberg CD, Adams HP, Applegate WB, et al. Effect of lovastatin on early carotid atherosclerosis and cardiovascular events. Circulation 1994;90:1679–1687.

53. Canadian Task Force on the Periodic Health Examination. Canadian guide to clinical preventive health care. Ottawa: Canada Communication Group, 1994:692–704.

54. American Academy of Family Physicians. Age charts for periodic health examination. Kansas City, MO: American Academy of Family Physicians, 1994. (Reprint no. 510.)

55. American College of Physicians, Health and Public Policy Committee. Diagnostic evaluation of the carotid arteries. Ann Intern Med 1988;109:835–837.

56. Toole JF, Adams HJ, Dyken M, et al. Evaluation for asymptomatic carotid artery atherosclerosis: a multidisciplinary consensus statement. South Med J 1988;81:1549–1552.

57. Moore WS, Moh JP, Najafi H, et al. Carotid endarterectomy: practice guidelines. J Vasc Surg 1992;15:469–479.

58. Mayberg MR, Winn HR. Endarterectomy for asymptomatic carotid artery stenosis: resolving the controversy. JAMA 1995;273:1459–1461.

5. Screening for Peripheral Arterial Disease

RECOMMENDATION

Routine screening for peripheral arterial disease in asymptomatic persons is not recommended. Clinicians should be alert to symptoms of peripheral arterial disease in persons at increased risk (see *Clinical Intervention*) and should evaluate patients who have clinical evidence of vascular disease.

Burden of Suffering

Peripheral arterial disease (PAD) becomes increasingly common with age. An estimated 12–17% of the population over age 50 have PAD.[1–4] Increased mortality has been well documented in patients with PAD, a disease that is strongly associated with coronary artery disease and that shares many of the same risk factors.[1,2,5–9] Although only a small proportion of individuals with PAD and intermittent claudication develop skin breakdown or limb loss, pain and associated disability often restrict ambulation and the overall quality of life.[1,5] Persons at increased risk for PAD include cigarette smokers and persons with diabetes mellitus or hypertension.[1,5,9,10] Diabetic PAD is responsible for about 50% of all amputations.[1]

Accuracy of Screening Tests

There is evidence that a history of intermittent claudication and the palpation of peripheral pulses are unreliable techniques for the detection of PAD.[1,3,8,11] In one study, a battery of noninvasive tests for PAD was administered to 624 hyperlipidemic subjects aged 38–82.[7] In this population, the sensitivity and positive predictive value of a classic history of claudication were only 54% and 9%, respectively, when compared with the results of formal noninvasive testing. The sensitivity of an abnormal posterior tibial pulse was 71%, the positive predictive value was 48%, and the specificity was 91%. An abnormal dorsalis pedis pulse had a sensitivity of only 50%; this artery is congenitally absent in 10–15% of the population.[11] The authors concluded that symptoms and abnormal pulses are not pathognomonic for PAD.[7] Greater accuracy has been achieved with noninvasive testing using Doppler ankle-arm pressure ratios, measurement of reactive hyperemia after exercise, pulse reappearance time, ultrasound duplex scanning, and plethysmography.[1,5,12,13] At present, however, additional data on sensitivity, specificity, and positive predictive value of these tests in asymptomatic populations are needed before noninvasive testing can be considered for routine screening.

Effectiveness of Early Detection

Because surgery for PAD is offered only to patients with symptomatic disease, the rationale for the early detection of asymptomatic PAD is that risk factor modification following detection might lower subsequent morbidity and mortality from PAD and systemic atherosclerotic disease. By virtue of its strong association with coronary atherosclerosis and coronary events,[5] the early diagnosis of PAD might also lead to the detection of asymptomatic coronary heart disease. Evidence of these benefits is lacking, however. There has been no research to examine whether the detection and treatment of asymptomatic persons with PAD reduces the morbidity or mortality observed in symptomatic patients. It is clear that certain interventions are beneficial in symptomatic persons. There is evidence, for example, that patients who stop smoking have marked improvement in PAD symptoms and reduced overall cardiovascular mortality.[1,14] Certain antithrombotic drugs may also be of benefit.[15] It is unknown whether treatment measures used in symptomatic patients are beneficial in asymptomatic patients.[1,6] Examples include walking programs, control of weight and blood pressure, correction of elevated serum lipids and glucose, proper foot care, and certain drugs.

Recommendations of Other Groups

There are no official recommendations for physicians to screen asymptomatic persons for PAD, although inspection of the skin and palpation of peripheral pulses are often included in the physical examination of the extremities. A recent international workshop sponsored by the American Diabetes Association and American Heart Association recommends annual screening for PAD in patients with diabetes.[16]

Discussion

Evidence is lacking that routine screening for PAD in asymptomatic persons is effective in reducing morbidity or mortality from this disease. Many of the behavioral interventions that might be prescribed after detecting PAD—smoking cessation (Chapter 54), blood pressure control (Chapter 3), and exercise (Chapter 55)—can be recommended without screening and are of proven value in the prevention of other atherosclerotic conditions, such as coronary heart and cerebrovascular disease. Screening by physical examination in the general population of asymptomatic adults, where the prevalence of PAD is low, is likely to produce a substantial number of false-positive results. Positive screening results will necessitate expensive noninvasive tests and may lead to potentially hazardous invasive tests such as arteriography. At the same time, it is not known whether the early detection of PAD in asymptomatic patients will result in more effective treatment of risk factors or better outcomes.

CLINICAL INTERVENTION

Routine screening for peripheral arterial disease in asymptomatic persons is not recommended ("D" recommendation). Clinicians should screen for hypertension (see Chapter 3) and hypercholesterolemia (Chapter 2), and they should provide appropriate counseling regarding the use of tobacco products (Chapter 54), physical activity (Chapter 55), and nutritional risk factors for atherosclerotic disease (Chapter 56). Clinicians should be alert to symptoms of PAD in persons at increased risk (persons over age 50, smokers, diabetics) and evaluate patients who have clinical evidence of vascular disease.

The draft update of this chapter was prepared for the U.S. Preventive Services Task Force by Stephen Tabet, MD, MPH, and Alfred O. Berg, MD, MPH.

REFERENCES

1. Strandness DE, Didisheim P, Clowes AW, et al, eds. Vascular diseases: current research and clinical applications. Orlando, FL: Grune and Stratton, 1987.
2. Criqui MH, Fronek A, Barrett-Connor E, et al. The prevalence of peripheral arterial disease in a defined population. Circulation 1985;71:510–515.
3. Lombardi G, Polotti R, Polizzi N, et al. Prevalence of asymptomatic peripheral vascular disease in a group of patients older than 50. J Am Geriatr Soc 1986;34:551–552.
4. Fowkes FGR, Housley E, Cawood EHH, et al. Edinburgh artery study: prevalence of asymptomatic and symptomatic peripheral arterial disease in the general population. Int J Epidemiol 1991;20:384–392.
5. Vogt MT, Cauley JA, Newman AB, et al. Decreased ankle/arm blood pressure index and mortality in elderly women. JAMA 1993;270:465–469.
6. Kannel WB, McGee DL. Update on some epidemiologic features of intermittent claudication: the Framingham study. J Am Geriatr Soc 1985;33:13–18.
7. Criqui MH, Fronek A, Klauber MR, et al. The sensitivity, specificity, and predictive value of traditional clinical evaluation of peripheral arterial disease: results from noninvasive testing in a defined population. Circulation 1985; 71:516–522.
8. Criqui MH, Coughlin SS, Fronek A. Noninvasively diagnosed peripheral arterial disease as a predictor of mortality: results from a prospective study. Circulation 1985;72:768–773.
9. Krupski WC. The peripheral vascular consequences of smoking. Ann Vasc Surg 1991;5:291–304.
10. McGill HC. The cardiovascular pathology of smoking. Am Heart J 1988;115;250–257.
11. Kappert A, Winsor T. Diagnosis of peripheral vascular diseases. Philadelphia: FA Davis, 1972:26.
12. Barnes RW. Noninvasive diagnostic techniques in peripheral vascular disease. Am Heart J 1979;97:241–244.
13. Moneta GL, Strandness DE. Peripheral arterial duplex scanning. J Clin Ultrasound 1987;15:645–651.
14. Jonason T, Bergstrom R. Cessation of smoking in patients with intermittent claudication: effects on the

risk of peripheral vascular complications, myocardial infarction and mortality. Acta Med Scand 1987; 221:253–260.

15. Arcan JC, Blanchard J, Boissel JP, et al. Multicenter double-blind study of ticlopidine in the treatment of intermittent claudication and the prevention of its complications. Angiology 1988;39:802–811.

16. American Heart Association. Assessment of peripheral vascular disease in diabetes. Circulation 1993; 88:819–827.

6. Screening for Abdominal Aortic Aneurysm

RECOMMENDATION

There is insufficient evidence to recommend for or against routine screening of asymptomatic adults for abdominal aortic aneurysm with abdominal palpation or ultrasound.

Burden of Suffering

Approximately 8,700 deaths from abdominal aortic aneurysm (AAA) were reported in the U.S. in 1990,[1] but undiagnosed ruptured aneurysms are probably responsible for many additional cases of sudden death in older persons. Once rupture occurs, massive intraabdominal bleeding is usually fatal unless prompt surgery can be performed. A review of six case-series including 703 cases of ruptured aneurysm estimated that only 18% of all patients with ruptured AAA reached a hospital and survived surgery.[2] The large majority of deaths from AAA occur in older men and women; men over 60 and women over 70 accounted for 95% of all deaths from AAA in a recent report.[2] Approximately 0.8% of male deaths and 0.3% of female deaths among persons over 65 years of age in the U.S. were attributed to AAA in 1990.[1]

An aneurysm is usually defined as a focal dilation of the aorta at least 150% of the normal aortic diameter.[3] Given a normal aortic diameter in older men of 2 cm (range 1.4–3.0 cm),[4] an aortic diameter above 3 cm usually indicates an aneurysm. The pathogenesis of aneurysms is not completely understood, but well-established risk factors for AAA include increasing age, male gender, and family history of aneurysms.[3] The male to female ratio for death from AAA is 11:1 between ages 60 and 64 and narrows to 3:1 between ages 85 and 90.[5] Other possible risk factors include tobacco use, hypertension, peripheral vascular disease, and presence of peripheral arterial aneurysms.[3,6–8] In populations over age 60, estimates of prevalence range from 2% to 8% and increase with age.[8–10] A recent community study in England screened nearly 9,000 men and women aged 65–80 with ultrasound: 7% of men and 1% of women had an aneurysm at least 3 cm in diameter.[11] Among all patients, only 0.6% had aneurysms 5 cm or larger, and only 0.3% had aneurysms of 6 cm or more.[11] There are only limited data on the incidence of new aneurysms in a previously screened population. In one study, 189 men who had a normal ultrasound at age 65–66 years were rescreened 5 years later; only 2 (1%) had an aortic diameter greater than 3 cm.[12]

Few aneurysms less than 4 cm in diameter will rupture.[2,13,14] Overall, 3–6% of aneurysms greater than 4 cm in diameter will rupture annually,[14,15] but the rate of rupture is directly related to the size of the aneurysm. The natural history of most aneurysms is one of gradual enlargement; growth rates have been estimated to average 0.2 cm/year for aneurysms under 4 cm, and 0.5 cm/year for those over 6 cm.[8]

Efficacy of Screening Tests

Two tests, palpation of the abdomen during physical examination and abdominal ultrasound, have been seriously advocated as screening tests for AAA. Other tests that can detect aneurysms—plain radiographs of the abdomen, computed tomography (CT), and magnetic resonance imaging (MRI)—are either not sensitive enough or are too expensive to be practical for screening in asymptomatic populations.

The accuracy of physical examination in detecting AAA is not completely known. Large aneurysms are easier to detect than small ones, and it is easier to detect aneurysms in thin people. Estimates of the sensitivity of physical examination in detecting AAA range from 22% to 96%.[17,18] The high sensitivity obtained in series of preoperative cases probably represents the preponderance of large aneurysms in this population. Lederle reported a sensitivity of 50% and a positive predictive value of 35% in a high-risk population screened in an internal medicine clinic (9% prevalence of AAA).[19] Four of five aneurysms greater than 5 cm diameter in this series were detected by palpation. In contrast, Allen reported a 22% sensitivity, 94% specificity, and positive predictive value of 17% in a population with a 5% prevalence of aneurysms.[17] No large-scale community-based studies of screening for AAA by physical examination have been reported.

Ultrasound is an extremely sensitive and specific test for AAA of all sizes, at least in cases where the diagnosis and size of the aneurysm can be confirmed at surgery. Reported sensitivities range from 82% to 99%, with sensitivity approaching 100% in some series of patients with a pulsatile mass.[16] In a small proportion of patients, visualization of the aorta will be inadequate due to obesity, bowel gas, or periaortic disease. Although ultrasound screening is noninvasive and relatively simple, compliance with invitations to be screened has been variable (50–64% attendance) in community screening trials.[7,11] Diagnostic abdominal ultrasound is currently expensive in the U.S. ($100–$175 per examination), but screening for AAA alone could probably be performed much more quickly and cheaply.[2]

Effectiveness of Early Detection

No prospective or retrospective controlled trials of screening for AAA that include outcome data have yet been reported. A pilot trial in England that offered screening at random to older subjects has enrolled 15,000 men and women, but it may not have sufficient power to prove a benefit in mortality.[8] The difficulty of identifying all deaths caused by AAA, combined with varying compliance with screening, may make it difficult to conduct definitive controlled trials of AAA screening.[8,20]

Surgical resection and repair with an artificial graft is a very effective treatment for AAA. Among 13 large case-series of surgery for nonruptured aneurysms published since 1980, overall surgical mortality was 4% (range 1.4–6.5%); mortality during emergency surgery for rupture is much higher, averaging 49% (range 23–69%).[3] Mortality after elective surgery is often due to underlying cardiovascular disease in patients with AAA. If the patient survives the immediate postoperative period, long-term survival is comparable to similar persons without aneurysms, but late postoperative complications (graft infection, graft occlusion, and aortoenteric fistula) may result in additional deaths and morbidity.[3] The high prevalence of cardiovascular disease in patients with AAA and competing causes of morbidity and mortality in older patients may diminish the benefit of detecting asymptomatic aneurysms in older populations. Of 124 patients aged 65–80 who had large aneurysms detected in a community screening program, 27% were deemed unfit for surgery or died of other causes before surgery.[11] In recent series, up to 40% of patients undergoing surgery for nonruptured aneurysms had died within 6 years after surgery, primarily due to coronary heart disease or stroke.[3,21]

Risk of elective surgery must be balanced against the risk of rupture of an untreated aneurysm, which is directly related to aneurysm size. Most vascular surgeons currently recommend surgery for asymptomatic aneurysms 5 cm or larger, since the risk of rupture (25–41% over 5 years) is substantially higher than risks from surgery.[3] While more aggressive management of smaller aneurysms (4–5 cm) has been recommended by some,[22] others have suggested that asymptomatic, slow-growing aneurysms under 6 cm can be successfully followed by serial ultrasound.[2,11] A large community-based screening program, which employed this conservative strategy over 8 years, observed two cases of rupture among 29 subjects with aneurysms 5–5.9 cm, for a rate of 1.5%/year.[11,23] A model fitted to data from 13 studies of untreated aneurysms supports a relatively low risk of rupture in aneurysms less than 6 cm; estimated annual rates of rupture for aneurysms 4–4.9, 5–5.9, 6–6.9, and over 7 cm were 1%, 3%, 9%, and 25%, respectively.[2] These data, which are based largely on incidentally detected cases, may not reflect accurately the prognosis of asymptomatic aneurysms discovered by routine ultrasound screening. Furthermore, decisions to forgo surgery in patients with larger aneurysms were likely to have been influenced by factors (e.g., age, comorbidity, lack of symptoms) that may have independently influenced the risk of rupture. Trials are currently ongoing to determine the optimal management of patients with AAA that are 4–5.4 cm in size.[24]

Recommendations of Other Groups

The Canadian Task Force on the Periodic Health Examination[7] concluded that there was poor evidence to include or exclude screening for AAA in the periodic health examination of asymptomatic individuals. They noted that targeted physical examination may be considered prudent for men over 60, however, and that ultrasound screening could be considered in selected high-risk men over 60: smokers with other risk factors for AAA (hypertension, claudication, family history, or other vascular disease).

Discussion

No prospective or retrospective controlled trials of screening for AAA have yet been reported that include data on mortality or other clinical outcomes. At present, the only effective intervention available for patients with aneurysms is major abdominal surgery. Until further data are available from population-based screening trials, it is uncertain whether the projected benefit from preventing ruptured aneurysms is sufficient to justify the costs of widespread screening and the potential risks from increased surgery. While there is general consensus that resection is indicated for incidentally discovered, large aneurysms (6 cm or larger), these are relatively uncommon in the general population; the appropriate management of smaller (4–5 cm) aneurysms remains controversial. Data from older case series may not be a reliable guide to the natural history of asymptomatic aneurysms discovered by ultrasound. For many older patients with small aneurysms, the risk of dying from coronary heart disease or stroke is much higher than the risk from ruptured AAA.[21]

The benefits of routine screening will depend on other parameters that merit further research: the proportion of clinically important aneurysms that are detected without screening; the sensitivity and specificity of abdominal palpation for detecting AAA in the primary care setting; risk factors for rapid growth or rupture of AAA; and long-term morbidity of patients undergoing elective surgery. Patient compliance with recommendations for follow-up or surgery will also directly influence the ability of screening to prevent ruptured aneurysms.

A recent cost-effectiveness analysis compared different screening protocols in a high-risk population of men between 60 and 80 years of age.[25] The authors concluded that a single screen for AAA by abdominal palpation might be considered cost-effective, but it would be of small clinical benefit (average increase in life expectancy of 0.002 year). A single screen with ultrasound was at the high end of the cost range that might be considered cost-effective ($41,550/year of life gained), and repeat screening was not cost-effective. They noted that, due to the variable quality of the available data, screening for AAA could prove to be very cost-effective or could actually cause a net harm. If low-cost screening ultrasound were available (vs. $150 average charge for diagnostic ultrasound in the U.S.), ultrasound screening would be much more cost-effective, and preferable to physical examination.[25]

CLINICAL INTERVENTION

There is insufficient evidence to recommend for or against routine screening for abdominal aortic aneurysms with abdominal palpation or ultrasound ("C" recommendation). Recommendations against routine ultrasound screening in the general population may be made on other grounds, such as the low prevalence of clinically significant AAA and the high cost of screening. Although direct evidence that screening for AAA reduces mortality or morbidity is not available in any population, clinicians may decide to screen selected high-risk patients, due to the significant burden of disease and the availability of effective surgical treatment for large aneurysms. Men over age 60 who have other risk factors (e.g., vascular disease, family history of AAA, hypertension, or smoking) are at highest risk for AAA and death due to ruptured aneurysms. Screening is not indicated for patients who are not appropriate candidates for major abdominal surgery (e.g., those with severe cardiac or pulmonary disease). If screening is performed, it is not certain whether ultrasound or abdominal palpation is the preferred test. Abdominal palpation is less expensive but also less sensitive than ultrasound. Cost-effectiveness analysis suggests that repeat examination of individuals with a previous normal ultrasound is not indicated.[24]

The draft of this chapter was prepared for the U.S. Preventive Services Task Force by Paul S. Frame, MD, and David Atkins, MD, MPH.

REFERENCES

1. National Center for Health Statistics. Vital statistics of the United States, 1990, Volume II–Mortality, Part A. Hyattsville, MD: National Center for Health Statistics, 1994. (Publication no. NCHS 94-1101.)
2. Law MR, Morris J, Wald NJ. Screening for abdominal aortic aneurysms. J Med Screening 1994;1: 110–116.
3. Ernst CB. Abdominal aortic aneurysm. N Engl J Med 1993;328:1167–1172.
4. Collin J, Araujo L, Walton J, et al. Oxford screening program for abdominal aortic aneurysm in men aged 65 to 74 years. Lancet 1988;2:613–615.

5. Collin J. The epidemiology of abdominal aortic aneurysm. Br J Hosp Med 1988;40:64–67.
6. Ballard DF, Etchason JA, Hilborne LH, Campion ME, Kamberg CJ, Solomon DH, et al. Abdominal aortic aneurysm surgery: a literature review and ratings of appropriateness and necessity. Santa Monica, CA: Rand, 1992. (Publication JRA-04.)
7. Canadian Task Force on the Periodic Health Examination. Canadian guide to clinical preventive health care. Ottawa: Canada Communication Group, 1994:672–679.
8. Harris P. Screening for aortic aneurysm: the surgical perspective. J Med Screening 1994;1:106–109.
9. Lindholm L, Ejlertsson G, Forsberg L, Norgren L. Low prevalence of abdominal aortic aneurysm in hypertensive patients. Acta Med Scand 1985;218:305–310.
10. O'Kelly TJ, Heather BP. General practice-based population screening for abdominal aortic aneurysms: a pilot study. Br J Surg 1989;76:479–480.
11. Scott AP, Wilson NM, Ashton HA, et al. Is surgery necessary for abdominal aneurysms less than 6 cm in diameter? Lancet 1993;342:1395–1396.
12. Emerton ME, Shaw E, Poskitt K, et al. Screening for abdominal aortic aneurysm: a single scan is enough. Br J Surg 1994;81:1112–1113.
13. Cronenwett JL, Sargent SK, Wall MH, Hawkes ML, Freeman DH, Dain BJ, et al. Variables that affect the expansion rate and outcome of small abdominal aortic aneurysms. J Vasc Surg 1990;11:260–269.
14. Nevitt MP, Ballard DJ, Hallett JW. Prognosis of abdominal aortic aneurysm: a population-based study. N Engl J Med 1989;321:1009–1014.
15. Cronenwett JL, Murphy TF, Zelenock GB, Whitehouse WM, Lindenauer SM, Graham LM, et al. Actuarial analysis of variables associated with rupture of small abdominal aortic aneurysms. Surgery 1985;98:472–483.
16. Quill DS, Colgan MP, Sumner DS. Ultrasonic screening for the detection of abdominal aortic aneurysms. Surg Clin North Am 1989;69:713–720.
17. Allen PIM, Gourevitch D, McKinley J, Tudway D, Goldman M. Population screening for aortic aneurysms [letter]. Lancet 1987;2:736.
18. Nusbaum JW, Friemanis AK, Thomford NR. Echography in the diagnosis of abdominal aortic aneurysm. Arch Surg 1971;102:385–388.
19. Lederle FA, Walker JM, Reinke DB. Selective screening for abdominal aortic aneurysms with physical examination and ultrasound. Arch Intern Med 1988;148:1753–1756.
20. Lederle FA. Screening for snipers: the burden of proof. J Clin Epidemiol 1990;43:101–104.
21. Johnston KW. Nonruptured abdominal aortic aneurysm: six-year follow-up results from the multi-center prospective Canadian aneurysm study. J Vasc Surg 1994;20:163–170.
22. Katz DA, Littenberg B, Cronenwett JL. Management of small abdominal aortic aneurysms: early surgery vs. watchful waiting. JAMA 1992;268:2678–2686.
23. Scott RAP. Risk of rupture in abdominal aortic aneurysm [comment]. Lancet 1994;343:539.
24. Lederle FA, Wilson SE, Johnson GR, et al. Design of the Abdominal Aortic Aneurysm Detection and Management study: ADAM VA Cooperative Study Group. J Vasc Surg 1994;20:296–303.
25. Frame PS, Fryback DG, Patterson C. Screening for abdominal aortic aneurysm in men aged between 60 and 80 years: a cost-effectiveness analysis. Ann Intern Med 1993;119:411–416.

7. Screening for Breast Cancer

RECOMMENDATION

Routine screening for breast cancer every 1–2 years, with mammography alone or mammography and annual clinical breast examination (CBE), is recommended for women aged 50–69. There is insufficient evidence to recommend for or against routine mammography or CBE for women aged 40–49 or aged 70 and older, although recommendations for high-risk women aged 40–49 and healthy women aged ≥70 may be made on other grounds (see *Clinical Intervention*). There is insufficient evidence to recommend for or against the use of screening CBE alone or the teaching of breast self-examination.

Burden of Suffering

In the U.S. in 1995, there were an estimated 182,000 new cases of breast cancer diagnosed and 46,000 deaths from this disease in women.[1] Approximately 32% of all newly diagnosed cancers in women are cancers of the breast, the most common cancer diagnosed in women.[1] The annual incidence of breast cancer increased 55% between 1950 and 1991.[2] The incidence in women during the period 1987–1991 was 110/100,000.[2] In 1992, the annual age-adjusted mortality from breast cancer was 22/100,000 women.[3] The age-adjusted mortality rate from breast cancer has been relatively stable over the period from 1930 to the present.[1,2] For women, the estimated lifetime risk of dying from breast cancer is 3.6%.[2] Breast cancer resulted in 2.2 years of potential life lost before age 65 per 1,000 women under age 65 in the U.S. during 1986–1988.[4] This rate was surpassed only by deaths resulting from motor vehicle injury and infections. Breast cancer is the leading contributor to cancer mortality in women aged 15–54,[1] although 48% of new breast cancer cases and 56% of breast cancer deaths occur in women age 65 and over.[2] As the large number of women in the "baby boom" generation age, the number of breast cancer cases and deaths will increase substantially unless age-specific incidence and mortality rates decline.

Important risk factors for breast cancer include female gender, residence in North America or northern Europe, and older age.[5] In American women, the annual incidence of breast cancer increases with age: 127

cases/100,000 for women aged 40–44; 229/100,000 for women aged 50–54; 348/100,000 for women aged 60–64; and 450/100,000 for women aged 70–74.[2] The risk for a woman with a family history of breast cancer in a first-degree relative is increased about 2–3-fold, and for women under 50 it is highest when the relative had premenopausally diagnosed breast cancer.[6–9] Women with previous breast cancer or carcinoma in situ and women with atypical hyperplasia on breast biopsy are also at significantly increased risk.[6,7,10–12] Other factors associated with increased breast cancer risk include a history of proliferative breast lesions without atypia on breast biopsy, late age at first pregnancy, nulliparity, high socioeconomic status, and a history of exposure to high-dose radiation.[6,7,10–12] Associations between breast cancer and oral contraceptives, long-term estrogen replacement therapy, obesity, and a diet high in fat have been suggested, but causal relationships have not been established.[6,7,13,14]

Accuracy of Screening Tests

The three screening tests usually considered for early detection of breast cancer are clinical breast examination (CBE), x-ray mammography, and breast self-examination (BSE). Estimates of the sensitivity and specificity of these maneuvers depend on a number of factors, including the size of the lesion, the characteristics of the breast being examined, the age of the patient, the extent of follow-up to identify false negatives, the skill and experience of the examiner or radiographic interpreter, and (in the case of mammography) the quality of the mammogram. Because multiple clinical trials have demonstrated the effectiveness of screening, measures of screening test performance (such as sensitivity and specificity) are primarily helpful in comparing trials, screening programs, and community practice. Uniform definitions, however, are necessary for such comparisons. For example, different studies may use similar definitions of sensitivity, such as the number of screen-detected cancers compared to the total of screen-detected cancers plus interval cancers, but one may use a fixed interval (e.g., 12 months)[15] and another a variable interval (e.g., time to next screen),[16] making direct comparisons difficult. The ability to detect interval cancers may also vary and will affect such estimates.

A review[17] of the current clinical trial data, published and unpublished, summarized screening test performance for mammography using uniform definitions. Sensitivity of mammography did not dramatically differ across the trials. Estimates from three Swedish trials using mammography alone averaged about 75%, while estimates for mammography combined with CBE ranged from 75% in the Health Insurance Plan of Greater New York (HIP) to 88% in the Edinburgh trial and the Canadian National Breast Cancer Screening Study in women aged 50–59 (NBSS 2). Specificity estimates ranged from 98.5% in the HIP trial to 83% in the Canadian NBSS 2. Sensitivity estimates for mammography alone and for combined screening with CBE have generally been 10–15% lower for women aged 40–49 compared with women greater than age 50.[15,17–19] Preliminary results from two North American demonstration projects suggest improved sensitivity of mammography, especially for women in their forties, with current mammographic techniques.[20] Significant variations in interpreter performance have also been observed.[21–23] In the Canadian trials, agreement was about 50% beyond that attributable to chance between radiologists at five screening centers and a single reference radiologist.[21]

The effectiveness of CBE alone has not been evaluated directly, but comparisons of the sensitivity and specificity of this maneuver to that of mammography can be considered. The Canadian NBSS 2 was designed to assess the incremental value of mammography above a careful, thorough (5–10 minutes) CBE.[24,25] Preliminary results showing no incremental benefit highlighted the fact that higher sensitivity (88% for mammography plus CBE vs. 63% for CBE alone)[17] may not guarantee improved effectiveness. Specificity was comparable or slightly better for CBE alone. Sensitivity of CBE for women aged 40–49 (Canadian NBSS 1) was about 10% lower at initial screen compared to the estimate for women aged 50–59 (Canadian NBSS 2).[26] Specificity estimates were similarly lower for younger women.

Data regarding the accuracy of BSE are extremely limited. One report calculated an upper limit of sensitivity ranging from 12 to 25% by assuming all interval cases in the clinical trials were detected by BSE.[17] Using a similar approach, the overall sensitivity of BSE alone was estimated to be 26% in women also screened by mammography and CBE in the Breast Cancer Detection Demonstration Project (BCDDP).[27] Estimated BSE sensitivity decreased with age, from 41% for women aged 35–39 to 21% for women aged 60–74.[27] Thus, as currently practiced, BSE appears to be a less sensitive form of screening than is CBE or mammography, and its specificity remains uncertain. The sensitivity of BSE can be improved by training, as measured by the proportion of benign lumps[28] detected on human models and artificial lumps[29] on silicone breast models, although whether this improved detection on models translates into improved personal BSE performance is unknown.

Adverse effects of screening tests are an important consideration. False-positive tests, resulting from the effort to maximize disease detection, may have negative consequences including unnecessary diagnostic tests. In the Canadian trials there were 7–10% false positives from combined screening with mammography and CBE among women aged 40–49 and 4.5–8% among those aged 50–59.[24,30] In a study of the yield of a first mammographic screening among women, half as many cancers per 1,000 first screening mammograms were diagnosed in women aged 40–49 (3/1,000) compared to women aged 50–59 (6/1,000).[31] Yet, women aged 40–49 underwent twice as many diagnostic tests per cancer detected compared to women aged 50–59 (43.9 vs. 21.9). Women aged 60–69 had a higher yield from screening, with 13 breast cancers diagnosed per 1,000 first screening mammograms and 10.2 diagnostic tests performed per cancer detected.

Mammographic screening may also adversely affect psychological well-being. Increased anxiety about breast cancer after a false-positive mammogram has been reported both at short- and long-term follow-up in studies surveying groups of screened women.[32,33] No impact on compliance in obtaining future screening examinations was observed, however. Women who underwent a surgical biopsy as a result of a false-positive screening mammogram were more likely to report their workup as a stressful experience than were those who did not have a biopsy.[32]

Excess breast cancers in populations that received doses of ionizing radiation significantly greater than currently delivered by mammography, such as survivors from atomic bombing in Japan[34] and patients with benign breast disease,[35] have raised concerns about the potential radiation risk from screening mammograms. There is no direct evidence of an increased risk of breast cancer from mammographic screening, however. Assuming a mean breast dose of 0.1 rad from a mammogram and extrapolating from higher doses of radiation, modeling suggests that in a group of 100,000 women receiving annual screening from ages 50 to 75, 12.9 years would be lost due to radiogenic cancers but 12,623 years would be gained through a 20% reduction in breast cancer mortality as a result of that screening.[34]

Fewer data are available regarding adverse effects associated with CBE and BSE. A dramatic increase in false-positives was observed after instruction in BSE in a nonrandomized controlled trial evaluating performance on human models,[28] although no increase was found in a randomized controlled trial evaluating performance on silicone breast models.[29] The latter study also assessed the impact of training on variables other than detection performance on models. Adverse effects, such as unnecessary physician visits, heightened anxiety levels, or increased radiographic and surgical procedures, were not observed.[29]

Effectiveness of Early Detection

Seven randomized controlled trials[16,30,36–40] have evaluated the effectiveness of screening for breast cancer in women by either mammography alone or combined with CBE compared to no periodic screening. The age of participants at date of first invitation ranged from 40 to 74. The six trials[16,36–40] that included women aged ≥50 showed a reduction in breast cancer mortality of 20–30% in the intervention group. The reduction was statistically significant in the Health Insurance Plan of Greater New York (HIP),[37] the Swedish two-county trials,[16] an overview of the Swedish trials,[40] and two meta-analyses of the trials.[41,42]

The results of these six trials including women aged ≥50 have convincingly demonstrated the effectiveness of mammographic screening (with or without CBE) for breast cancer in women aged 50–69. The HIP trial screened women aged 40–64 with annual CBE and two-view mammography.[37] For women who were over age 50 at the time of entry into the study, mortality from breast cancer in the intervention group was more than 50% lower than in the control group at 5 years, decreasing to a 21% difference after 18 years of follow-up. The Edinburgh trial[36] screened women aged 45–64 from 84 general medicine practices with two-view mammography and CBE on the initial screen followed by annual CBE and biennial single-view mammography. Preliminary results at seven years found a relative risk of 0.80 (95% confidence interval [CI], 0.54 to 1.17) for women aged 50 and older at entry. The results from 10-year follow-up showed little change.[17] An overview pooled the data through 1989 from the four Swedish randomized controlled trials of breast cancer screening with mammography alone.[40] All women diagnosed with breast cancer before randomization were excluded and endpoints were independently reviewed. Breast cancer mortality was reduced by about 30% for women aged 50–69 at entry using an endpoint of breast cancer as the underlying cause of death. A meta-analysis that included the most recently published results of these trials reported a 23% reduction in breast cancer mortality for women aged 50 and older.[42] A meta-analysis of European case-control studies done within screening mammography programs also reported significantly reduced breast cancer mortality among women aged 50 and older.[42]

There are few data regarding the optimal periodicity of screening in this age group. Although an annual interval has been recommended by many groups, an analysis of data from the Swedish two-county study found little evidence that an annual interval would confer greater benefit than screening every 2 years for women over the age of 50.[19] This trial used mammography alone, but the reduction in breast cancer mortality was similar to that seen in the trials combining CBE with mammography.[36,37] The similar mortality reductions found in screening trials using periodicities ranging from 12 to 33 months in women aged ≥50 suggests that biennial screening intervals are as effective as annual intervals. In a meta-analysis of the trials evaluating screening mammography,[42] the estimated reduction in breast cancer mortality was the same (23%) for screening intervals of 12 months and 18–33 months in women aged 50–74.

There is limited and conflicting evidence regarding the benefit of screening women aged 70–74. The Swedish two-county trial and BCDDP time series included women up to age 74 at entry, and each found a reduction of breast cancer mortality for the intervention group as a whole.[16,44] The Swedish overview, however, reported a relative risk of 0.98 (95% CI, 0.63 to 1.53) at 12-year follow-up for the age subgroup 70–74.[40] The wide confidence interval, due to small numbers in this subgroup analysis, does not preclude the possibility of a substantial benefit from screening in this age group. No clinical trials have evaluated screening in women over 74 years of age at enrollment.

Although all six trials found a benefit of screening among the total group of enrolled women who were 40–74 years at entry,[16,36–40] there is uncertainty about the effectiveness of screening women between the ages of 40 and 49. The Canadian NBSS 1 was specifically designed to address this uncertainty.[30] This trial compared combined annual mammography and CBE to an initial CBE among women aged 40–49 at entry. At 7-year follow-up, no benefit of annual screening was observed (RR = 1.36; 95% CI, 0.84 to 2.21). This Canadian trial has been the subject of much criticism.[45–47] Possible irregularities with randomization have been refuted by its investigators.[48] An independent review is planned by the National Cancer Institute of Canada to determine whether the randomization was compromised. Although mammography quality issues have also been a concern, there is little evidence to suggest that the practices were inconsistent with the standards of the other clinical trials or community practice at the time of the study.[48] In addition, improvement in mammographic quality over the course of the study period was noted by both inside and outside observers.[48] The proportion of controls receiving mammography, 26%, can be compared to available estimates of 13% in the two-county trial, 24% in the Malmo trial (35% for women 45–49), and 24% in the Stockholm trial.[38,39,49] This contamination may nevertheless have reduced the trial's ability to detect a benefit from the screening intervention. An excess of node-positive cancers detected in the intervention group raised concerns about subject randomization.[30] While this may have been the result of chance, other contributing factors suggested by the investigators include under-ascertainment secondary to lower surgical dissection rates in the control group and incomplete breast cancer ascertainment at preliminary follow-up (although these possibilities are unlikely to account for all of the observed excess).[48] Although the effect of these factors should diminish with long-term follow-up, the results are unlikely to achieve statistical significance because sample size calculations were based on an estimated 40% reduction in breast cancer mortality, which is greater than the typical reduction in mortality observed in the other six trials that included women in this age group.[30]

Subgroup analyses of the other trials that included women under 50 have yielded conflicting evidence regarding the benefit of screening women aged 40–49. No benefit was observed in the Stockholm trial or in one arm of the two-county trial, while the remaining trials reported non-significant benefits of about 22% or more.[17,50] One meta-analysis, which pooled the results from 7-year follow-up of six published clinical trials without adjustment for variation in screening method or interval, found no reduction in breast cancer mortality for women in their forties (RR = 1.08; 95% CI, 0.85 to 1.39).[41] When the Canadian trial was excluded from the analysis, the estimate changed little (RR= 0.99; 95% CI, 0.74 to 1.32). The overview of the Swedish trials found a nonsignificant 13% reduction (RR= 0.87; 95% CI, 0.63 to 1.20) only after 8–12 years of follow-up in this age group.[40] More recent meta-analyses of published mammography trial data reported nonsignificant 8–10% reductions in breast cancer mortality in women aged 40–49.[42,43] One meta-analysis reported a significant benefit for women in this age group when unpublished data were included and the Canadian trial was excluded.[43] Longer duration of follow-up was associated with a greater reduction in mortality, although this finding may have been due to chance.[42] Thus, there is conflicting evidence from clinical trials and meta-analyses, primarily based on subgroup analyses, regarding the benefit of screening women aged 40–49. An ongoing British trial is evaluating the effectiveness of annual mammography screening in women enrolled at age 40 or 41.

A recent analysis of data by tumor size, nodal status, and stage from the BCDDP, a U.S. screening project using annual two-view mammography and CBE, suggests comparable 14-year survival rates for women 40–49 and women 50–59.[51] A similar analysis of breast cancers detected in the Swedish two-county trial confirms this finding.[52] Based on these data, time series comparisons of survival, frequency of interval cancers in the two-county trial, and subgroup analysis of available clinical trial data, some experts have suggested that annual screening intervals may be necessary to achieve a reduction in breast cancer mortality from screening for women aged 40–49.[19,20,52] In a meta-analysis of published trial results, however, the estimated mortality reduction from screening women in this age group was similar for 12- and 18–33-month screening intervals (1% and 12%, respectively).[42]

There is no direct evidence that assesses the effectiveness of CBE alone compared to no screening. Modeling studies of the HIP trial estimated that two thirds of the effectiveness of the combined screening may have been a result of CBE.[53-56] The Canadian NBSS 2 was designed to test the incremental value of annual mammography over a careful annual CBE among women aged 50–59 at study entry.[24] At 7-year follow-up, there was no difference in breast cancer mortality for the group receiving combined screening compared to CBE alone (RR = 0.97; 95% CI, 0.62 to 1.52). This result suggests that thorough CBE may be as effective as mammography for screening in this age group. The confidence interval is wide, however, and substantial benefit or harm from screening is not excluded by the preliminary data. Concerns regarding the early quality of mammography of Canadian NBSS 1 also apply to this trial.[48] Long-term follow-up and additional studies are needed to confirm this apparent lack of an incremental benefit of mammography above a careful, thorough annual CBE. It is also unclear whether CBE adds benefit to screening with mammography. A meta-analysis of mammography trial results reported similar reductions in breast cancer mortality with and without the addition of CBE.[42]

Evidence for effectiveness of BSE alone is also limited. In the United Kingdom Trial of Early Detection of Breast Cancer, a nonrandomized community trial, 40–50% of women living in two districts participated in BSE instruction that included a short film and a lecture by a specially trained health provider.[57] At 7-year follow-up, there was no reduction in breast cancer mortality in the BSE communities compared with the control districts. Baseline comparability of intervention and control districts, treatment variation by community, and contamination by other screening modalities were not assessed, however. A World Health Organization (WHO) population-based randomized controlled trial in Leningrad comparing formal BSE instruction to no intervention in women aged 40–64 has reported increases in physician visits, referrals for further screening tests, and excisional biopsies in the intervention group at 5-year follow-up.[58] Breast cancer patients in the two groups did not differ in number, size, or nodal status of their tumors. Completeness of endpoint assessment is a concern in this study, given the lack of a national tumor registry. Follow-up through 1999 is planned for reporting mortality results. In a case-control study of women who had been diagnosed with advanced stage (TNM III or IV) breast cancer, there was no association between disease status and self-reported BSE.[59] Proficiency in practicing BSE, however, was reported as poor by both cases and controls. For the small group of women reporting thorough BSE compared to all others, the relative risk was 0.54 (95% CI, 0.30 to 0.98). A meta-analysis of pooled data from 12 descriptive studies found that women who practiced BSE before their illness were less likely to have a tumor of 2.0 cm or more in diameter or to have evidence of extension to lymph nodes.[60] The studies from which these data were obtained, however, suffer from important design limitations and provide little information on clinical outcome (i.e., breast cancer mortality). Retrospective studies of the effectiveness of BSE have produced mixed results.[27,61–63]

Recommendations of Other Groups

The American Cancer Society (ACS),[64] American College of Radiology,[65] American Medical Association,[66] American College of Obstetricians and Gynecologists (ACOG),[67] and a number of other organizations[65] recommend screening with mammography every 1–2 years and annual CBE beginning at the age of 40, and annual mammography and CBE beginning at age 50.

The American Academy of Family Physicians (AAFP) recommends CBE every 1–3 years for women aged 30–39 and annually for those aged 40 and older, and mammography annually beginning at age 50;[68] these recommendations are currently under review. The American College of Physicians (ACP) recommends screening mammography every 2 years for women aged 50–74 and recommends against mammograms for women under 50 or over 75 years and baseline mammograms.[69] The ACP makes the same recommendations for high-risk women, unless the woman expresses great anxiety about breast cancer or insists on more intensive screening. The Canadian Task Force on the Periodic Health Examination recommends annual CBE and mammography for women aged 50–69 and recommends against mammograms in women under 50.[70] The National Cancer Institute states there is a general consensus among experts that routine mammography and CBE every 1–2 years in women aged 50 and over can reduce breast cancer mortality, and that randomized clinical trials have not shown a statistically significant reduction in mortality for women under the age of 50.[71]

Organizations that presently recommend routine teaching of BSE include the AAFP,[68] ACOG,[67] and ACS.[64] The recommendations of the AAFP are currently under review.

Discussion

At this time, there is little doubt that breast cancer screening by mammography with or without CBE has the potential of reducing mortality from breast cancer for women aged 50 through about 70. The benefit derived from biennial screening appears to be quite similar to the benefit derived from annual screening. Given this similarity in effectiveness, biennial screening is likely to have the added benefit of increased cost-effectiveness. The incremental value of CBE above mammography or vice versa is uncertain, although the Canadian NBSS 2[24] suggests that careful CBE may be as effective as mammography.

Evidence does not establish a clear benefit from screening in women aged 40–49. Only the Canadian NBSS 1[30] was designed to test the effectiveness of screening in this age group, however, and none of the trials had adequate power for subgroup analysis. If screening is in fact ineffective in younger women, one possible explanation is a lower sensitivity of mammography in younger women (see *Accuracy of Screening Tests*). Other possibilities include suboptimal screening intervals, differential (less aggressive) treatment offered to women with mammographically detected cancer, and varying biologic characteristics of breast tumors.[52,72] The

Swedish overview,[40] HIP,[37] and Edinburgh[36] trials suggest some benefit in women aged 40–49 after 8–12 years of follow-up, but it is possible that the delayed benefit is due to screening women in their fifties who entered the trials in their middle to late forties.[72a] The final results of the Canadian NBSS 1 may provide important information. An ongoing British trial and a proposed trial in Europe which will enroll women only in their early forties and compare mammography to no screening could also clarify this issue.[73] Until further information is available, it is unclear whether any potential improvement in breast cancer mortality achieved by screening women aged 40–49 is of sufficient magnitude to justify the potential adverse effects that may occur as a result of widespread screening.

Because breast cancer incidence increases with age, the burden of suffering due to breast cancer in elderly women is substantial. In addition, there is no evidence (as there is in younger women) that sensitivity of mammography in older women is not comparable to that in women aged 50–69. This is an age group, moreover, in which underutilization of breast cancer screening is common.[74–76] In a decision analysis of the utility of screening women over 65 for breast cancer, screening saved lives at all ages, but the savings decreased substantially with increasing age and co-morbidities.[77] In the oldest women, those aged ≥85, short-term morbidity such as anxiety or discomfort from the screening may have outweighed the small benefits. Until more definitive data become available for elderly women, it is reasonable to concentrate the large effort and expense associated with screening mammography on women in the age group for which benefit has been most clearly demonstrated: those aged 50–69. Screening women aged 70 and older might be considered on an individual basis, depending on general health and other considerations (e.g., personal preference of the patient).

The age range of 50–69 years, for which mammography has been proven effective, is to a large extent based on artificial cutpoints chosen for study purposes rather than on biologic cutpoints above or below which the ratio of benefits to risks sharply decreases. Both the incidence of breast cancer and the sensitivity of mammography increase with age. Thus, it is logical that women in their seventies, for whom only limited clinical trial experience is available, benefit from breast cancer screening. For women aged <50 years, evidence has been insufficient to establish a clear benefit from breast cancer screening. This age cutpoint may be a marker for biologic changes that occur with age, especially menopause. It is therefore plausible that women in their late forties, particularly postmenopausal women, might derive some intermediate benefit from screening. The risks and benefits of mammography and CBE may be best considered as changing on an age continuum rather than at a specific chronologic age. Guidelines for breast cancer screening should be interpreted with this in mind.

No large study has quantitated the effectiveness of breast cancer screening by either CBE or mammography for women who are at higher risk of developing breast cancer than the general population. The increased incidence of disease in high-risk women increases the positive predictive value (PPV) of screening tests used in this group. For example, in a community screening program, the PPV of mammography was increased 2–3-fold for women with a family history of breast cancer.[31] This is an especially important consideration for women under 50, in whom the benefit of screening has not been established for the general population. There may be a benefit from screening younger women in high-risk groups, but studies confirming this effect are lacking. Nevertheless, given their increased burden of suffering, screening high-risk women under age 50 may be considered on an individual basis for women who express a strong preference for such screening.

Data regarding the effectiveness of BSE are extremely limited, and the accuracy of BSE as currently practiced appears to be considerably inferior to that of CBE and mammography. False-positive BSE, especially among younger women in whom breast cancer is uncommon, could lead to unnecessary anxiety and diagnostic evaluation, although a small randomized clinical trial[29] did not find such adverse effects. A point also worth consideration is that time devoted to teaching BSE may reduce time available for prevention efforts with proven effectiveness. Given the present state of knowledge and the potential adverse effects and opportunity cost, a recommendation for or against inclusion of teaching BSE during the periodic health examination cannot be made.

CLINICAL INTERVENTION

Screening for breast cancer every 1–2 years, with mammography alone or mammography and annual clinical breast examination (CBE), is recommended for women aged 50–69 ("A" recommendation). Clinicians should refer patients to mammographers who use low-dose equipment and adhere to high standards of quality control. Such standards have recently been established by the Mammography Quality Standards Act, a federal law mandating that all mammography sites in the U.S. be accredited through a process approved by the Department of Health and Human Services.[78] There is insufficient evidence to recommend annual CBE alone for women aged 50–69 ("C" recommendation). For women aged 40–49, there is conflicting evidence of fair to good quality regarding clinical benefit from mammography with or without CBE, and insufficient evidence regarding benefit from CBE alone; therefore, recommendations for or

against routine mammography or CBE cannot be made based on the current evidence ("C" recommendation). There is no evidence specifically evaluating mammography or CBE in high-risk women under age 50; recommendations for screening such women may be made on other grounds, including patient preference, high burden of suffering, and the higher PPV of screening, which would lead to fewer false positives than are likely to occur from screening women of average risk in this age group. There is limited and conflicting evidence regarding clinical benefit of mammography or CBE for women aged 70–74 and no evidence regarding benefit for women over age 75; however, recommendations for screening women aged 70 and over who have a reasonable life expectancy may be made based on other grounds, such as the high burden of suffering in this age group and the lack of evidence of differences in mammogram test characteristics in older women versus those aged 50–69 ("C" recommendation). There is insufficient evidence to recommend for or against teaching BSE in the periodic health examination ("C" recommendation).

The draft update of this chapter was prepared for the U.S. Preventive Services Task Force by Marisa Moore, MD, MPH, and Carolyn DiGuiseppi, MD, MPH.

REFERENCES

1. Wingo PA, Tong T, Bolden S. Cancer statistics, 1995. CA Cancer J Clin 1995;45:8–30.
2. Ries LAG, Miller BA, Hankey BF, et al, eds. SEER cancer statistics review, 1973–1991: tables and graphs. Bethesda: National Cancer Institute, 1994. (NIH Publication no. 94-2789.)
3. Kochanek KD, Hudson BL. Advance report of final mortality statistics, 1992. Monthly vital statistics report; vol 43 no 6 (suppl). Hyattsville, MD: National Center for Health Statistics, 1995.
4. Centers for Disease Control and Prevention. Years of potential life lost before age 65, by race, Hispanic origin, and sex—United States, 1986–1988. MMWR 1992;41(SS-6):13–23.
5. Kelsey JL. A review of the epidemiology of human breast cancer. Epidemiol Rev 1979;1:74–109.
6. Kelsey JL, Gammon MD. The epidemiology of breast cancer. CA Cancer J Clin 1991;41:146–165.
7. Harris JR, Lippman ME, Veronesi U, et al. Breast cancer. N Engl J Med 1992;327:319–327.
8. Slattery ML, Kerber RA. A comprehensive evaluation of family history and breast cancer risk. JAMA 1993; 270:1563–1568.
9. Colditz GA, Willett WC, Hunter DJ, et al. Family history, age, and risk of breast cancer [published erratum appears in JAMA 1993;270:1548]. JAMA 1993;270:338–343.
10. London SJ, Connolly JL, Schnitt SJ, et al. A prospective study of benign breast disease and the risk of breast cancer. JAMA 1992;267:941–944.
11. Dupont WD, Page DL. Risk factors for breast cancer in women with proliferative breast disease. N Engl J Med 1985;312:146–151.
12. Bodian CA. Benign breast diseases, carcinoma in situ, and breast cancer risk. Epidemiol Rev 1993;15:177–187.
13. Grady D, Rubin SM, Petitti DB, et al. Hormone therapy to prevent disease and prolong life in postmenopausal women. Ann Intern Med 1992;117:1016–1037.
14. Kelsey JL, Gammon MD. Epidemiology of breast cancer. Epidemiol Rev 1990;12:228–240.
15. Robertson CL. A private breast imaging practice: medical audit of 25,788 screening and 1,077 diagnostic examinations. Radiology 1993;187:75–79.
16. Tabar L, Fagerberg G, Duffy SW, et al. Update of the Swedish two-county program of mammographic screening for breast cancer. Radiol Clin North Am 1992;30:187–210.

17. Fletcher SW, Black W, Harris R, et al. Report of the International Workshop on Screening for Breast Cancer. J Natl Cancer Inst 1993;85:1644–1656.
18. Peeters PH, Verbeek AL, Hendriks JH, et al. Screening for breast cancer in Nijmegen. Report of 6 screening rounds, 1975–1986. Int J Cancer 1989;43:226–230.
19. Tabar L, Faberberg G, Day NE, et al. What is the optimum interval between mammographic screening examinations? An analysis based on the latest results of the Swedish two-county breast cancer screening trial. Int J Cancer 1987;55:547–551.
20. Sickles EA, Kopans DB. Deficiencies in the analysis of breast cancer screening data [editorial]. J Natl Cancer Inst 1993;85:1621–1624.
21. Baines CJ, McFarlane DV, Wall C. Audit procedures in the National Breast Screening Study: mammography interpretation. J Can Assoc Radiol 1986;37:256–260.
22. Gadkin BM, Feig SA, Muir HD. The technical quality of mammography in centers participating in a regional breast cancer awareness program. Radiographics 1988;8:133–145.
23. Elmore JG, Wells CK, Lee CH, et al. Variability in radiologists' interpretations of mammograms. N Engl J Med 1994;331:1493–1499.
24. Miller AB, Baines CJ, To T, et al. Canadian National Breast Screening Study: 2. Breast cancer detection and death rates among women aged 50 to 59 years. Can Med Assoc J 1992;147:1477–1488.
25. Canadian National Breast Screening Study [correction]. Can Med Assoc J 1993;148:718.
26. Baines CJ, Miller AB, Bassett AA. Physical examination: its role as a single screening modality in the Canadian National Breast Screening Study. Cancer 1989;63:1816–1822.
27. O'Malley MS, Fletcher SW. Screening for breast cancer with breast self-examination. JAMA 1987;257:2197–2203.
28. Hall DC, Adams CK, Stein GH, et al. Improved detection of human breast lesions following experimental examination. Cancer 1980;46:408–411.
29. Fletcher SW, O'Malley MS, Earp JL, et al. How best to teach women breast self-examination. A randomized controlled trial. Ann Intern Med 1990;112:772–779.
30. Miller AB, Baines CJ, To T, et al. Canadian National Breast Screening Study: breast cancer detection and death rates among women aged 40 to 49 years. Can Med Assoc J 1992;147:1459–1476.
31. Kerlikowske K, Grady D, Barclay J, et al. Positive predictive value of screening mammography by age and family history of breast cancer. JAMA 1993;270:2444–2450.
32. Gram IT, Lund E, Slenker SE. Quality of life following a false positive mammogram. Br J Cancer 1990;62:1018–1022.
33. Lerman C, Trock B, Rimer BK, et al. Psychological and behavioral implications of abnormal mammograms. Ann Intern Med 1991;114:657–661.
34. Feig SA, Ehrlich SM. Estimation of radiation risk from screening mammography: recent trends and comparison with expected benefits. Radiology 1990;174:639–647.
35. Mattsson A, Ruden B, Hall P, et al. Radiation-induced breast cancer: long-term follow-up of radiation therapy for benign breast disease. J Natl Cancer Inst 1993;85:1679–1685.
36. Roberts MM, Alexander FE, Anderson TJ, et al. Edinburgh trial of screening for breast cancer: mortality at seven years. Lancet 1990;335:241–246.
37. Shapiro S, Venet W, Strax P, et al, eds. Periodic screening for breast cancer. Baltimore: Johns Hopkins University Press, 1988.
38. Andersson I, Aspegren K, Janzon L, et al. Mammographic screening and mortality from breast cancer: the Malmo mammographic screening trial. BMJ 1988;297:943–948.
39. Frisell J, Eklund G, Hellstrom L, et al. Randomized study of mammography screening—preliminary report on mortality in the Stockholm trial. Breast Cancer Res Treat 1991;18:49–56.
40. Nystrom L, Rutqvist LE, Wall S, et al. Breast cancer screening with mammography: overview of Swedish randomised trials. Lancet 1993;341:973–978.
41. Elwood JM, Cox B, Richardson AK. The effectiveness of breast cancer screening by mammography in younger women. Online Curr Clin Trials 1993;2:Doc. no. 32.
42. Kerlikowske K, Grady D, Rubin SM, et al. Efficacy of screening mammography: a meta-analysis. JAMA 1995; 273:149–154.
43. Smart CR, Hendrick RE, Rutledge JH III, et al. Benefit of mammography screening in women aged 40 to 49 years: current evidence from randomized controlled trials. Cancer 1995;75:1619–1626.
44. Morrison AS, Brisson J, Khalid N. Breast cancer incidence and mortality in the Breast Cancer Detection Demonstration Project. J Natl Cancer Inst 1988;80:1540–1547.

45. Mettlin CJ, Smart CJ. The Canadian National Breast Screening Study. An appraisal and implications for early detection policy. Cancer 1993;72:1461–1465.
46. Baines CJ, Miller AB, Kopans DB, et al. Canadian National Breast Screening Study: assessment of technical quality by external review. Am J Roentgenol 1990;155:743–747.
47. Kopans DB, Feig SA. The Canadian National Breast Screening Study: a critical review. Am J Roentgenol 1993;161:755–760.
48. Baines CJ. The Canadian National Breast Screening Study: a perspective on criticisms. Ann Intern Med 1994; 120:326–334.
49. Tabar L, Fagerberg CJ, Gad A, et al. Reduction in mortality from breast cancer after mass screening with mammography. Lancet 1985;8433:829–832.
50. Eckhardt S, Badellino F, Murphy GP. UICC meeting on breast-cancer screening in pre-menopausal women in developed countries. Int J Cancer 1994;56:1–5.
51. Smart CR, Hartmann WH, Beahrs OH, et al. Insights into breast cancer screening of younger women. Cancer 1993;72(suppl):1449–1456.
52. Tabar L, Duffy SW, Burhenne LW. New Swedish breast cancer detection results for women aged 40–49. Cancer 1993;72(suppl):1437–1448.
53. Bailar JC. Mammography: a contrary view. Ann Intern Med 1976;84:77–84.
54. Eddy DM. Screening for cancer: theory, analysis and design. Englewood Cliffs, NJ: Prentice-Hall, 1980.
55. Shapiro S. Evidence on screening for breast cancer from a randomized trial. Cancer 1977;39: 2772–2782.
56. Shwartz M. An analysis of the benefits of serial screening for breast cancer based upon a mathematical model of the disease. Cancer 1978;41:1550–1564.
57. Ellman R, Moss SM, Coleman D, et al. Breast self-examination programmes in the trial of early detection of breast cancer: ten year findings. Br J Cancer 1993;68:208–212.   .
58. Semiglazov VF, Moiseyenko VM, Bavli JL, et al. The role of breast self-examination in early breast cancer detection (results of the 5-years USSR/WHO randomized study in Leningrad). Eur J Epidemiol 1992;8:498–502.
59. Newcomb PA, Weiss NS, Storer BE, et al. Breast self-examination in relation to the occurrence of advanced breast cancer. J Natl Cancer Inst 1991;83:260–265.
60. Hill D, White V, Jolley D, et al. Self examination of the breast: is it beneficial? Meta-analysis of studies investigating breast self examination and extent of disease in patients with breast cancer. BMJ 1988;297: 271–275.
61. Locker AP, Caseldine J, Mitchell AK, et al. Results from a seven-year programme of breast self-examination in 89,010 women. Br J Cancer 1989;60:401–405.
62. Le Geyte M, Mant D, Vessey MP, et al. Breast self examination and survival from breast cancer. Br J Cancer 1992;66:917–918.
63. Kuroishi T, Tominaga S, Ota J, et al. The effect of breast self-examination on early detection and survival. Jpn J Cancer Res 1992;83:344–350.
64. American Cancer Society. Guidelines for the cancer-related checkup: an update. Atlanta: American Cancer Society, 1993.
65. Dodd GD. Screening for breast cancer. Cancer 1993;72:1038–1042.
66. Council on Scientific Affairs, American Medical Association. Mammographic screening in asymptomatic women aged 40 years and older. JAMA 1989;261:2535–2542.
67. American College of Obstetricians and Gynecologists. The obstetrician-gynecologist and primary-preventive health care. Washington, DC: American College of Obstetricians and Gynecologists, 1993.
68. American Academy of Family Physicians. Age charts for periodic health examination. Kansas City, MO: American Academy of Family Physicians, 1994. (Reprint no. 510.)
69. American College of Physicians. Screening for breast cancer (approved July 15, 1995). Ann Intern Med 1996 (in press).
70. Canadian Task Force on the Periodic Health Examination. Canadian guide to clinical preventive health care. Ottawa: Canada Communication Group, 1994 :787–795.
71. Volkers N. NCI replaces guidelines with statement of evidence. J Natl Cancer Inst 1994;86:14–15.
72. Breast cancer screening in women under 50 [editorial]. Lancet 1991;337:1575–1576.
72a. de Koning HJ, Boer R, Warmerdam PG, et al. Quantitative interpretation of age-specific mortality reductions from the Swedish breast cancer-screening trials. J Natl Cancer Inst 1995;87:1217–1223.
73. Murphy GP, Odartchenko N. Report on the UICC workshops on breast cancer screening in premenopausal women in developed countries. CA Cancer J Clin 1993;43:372–373.

74. Mammography and clinical breast examinations among women aged 50 years and older–behavioral risk factor surveillance system, 1992. MMWR 1993;42:737–741.

75. Coleman EA, Feuer EJ, the NCI Breast Cancer Screening Consortium. Breast cancer screening among women from 65 to 74 years of age in 1987–88 and 1991. Ann Intern Med 1992;117:961–966.

76. Sienko DG, Hahn RA, Mills EM, et al. Mammography use and outcomes in a community: the Greater Lansing Area Mammography Study. Cancer 1993;71:1801–1809.

77. Mandelblatt JS, Wheat ME, Monane M, et al. Breast cancer screening for elderly women with and without comorbid conditions. Ann Intern Med 1992;116:722–730.

78. Hendrick RE. Mammography quality assurance. Cancer 1993;72:1466–1474.

8. Screening for Colorectal Cancer

RECOMMENDATION

Screening for colorectal cancer is recommended for all persons aged 50 and older with annual fecal occult blood testing (FOBT), or sigmoidoscopy (periodicity unspecified), or both (see *Clinical Intervention*). There is insufficient evidence to determine which of these screening methods is preferable or whether the combination of FOBT and sigmoidoscopy produces greater benefits than does either test alone. There is also insufficient evidence to recommend for or against routine screening with digital rectal examination, barium enema, or colonoscopy, although recommendations against such screening in average-risk persons may be made on other grounds (see *Clinical Intervention*). Persons with a family history of hereditary syndromes associated with a high risk of colon cancer should be referred for diagnosis and management (see *Clinical Intervention*).

Burden of Suffering

Colorectal cancer is the second most common form of cancer in the U.S. and has the second highest mortality rate, accounting for about 140,000 new cases and about 55,000 deaths each year.[1] An individual's lifetime risk of dying of colorectal cancer in the U.S. has been estimated to be 2.6%.[2] About 60% of patients with colorectal cancer have regional or distant metastases at the time of diagnosis.[1] Estimated 5-year survival is 91% in persons with localized disease, 60% in persons with regional spread, and only 6% in those with distant metastases.[2] The average patient dying of colorectal cancer loses 13 years of life.[2] In addition to the mortality associated with colorectal cancer, this disease and its treatment—surgical resection, colostomies, chemotherapy, and radiotherapy—can produce significant morbidity. Persons at highest risk of colorectal cancer include those with uncommon familial syndromes (i.e., hereditary polyposis and hereditary nonpolyposis colorectal cancer [HNPCC]) and persons with longstanding ulcerative colitis.[3,4] Familial syndromes are estimated to account for 6% of all colorectal cancers,[3] and various genetic mutations associated with these syndromes have been identified.[4a] Other principal risk factors include a history of colorectal cancer or adenomas in a first-degree relative, a personal history of large adenomatous polyps or colorectal cancer, and a prior diagnosis of endometrial, ovarian, or breast cancer. In an analysis of two large cohorts involving over 840,000 patient-years of follow-up, a family history of colorectal cancer was associated with a significant increase in risk in younger persons (1.7–4-fold increase between ages 40 and 60), but was not associated with a significantly increased risk in persons after age 60;[4b] risk was higher in persons with more than one affected relative. The absolute increase in lifetime risk in persons with a family history was modest, however: an estimated cumulative incidence of colorectal cancer by age 65 of 4% vs. 3% in persons without a family history.[4b] Diets high in fat or low in fiber may also increase the risk of colorectal cancer.[3]

Accuracy of Screening Tests

The principal screening tests for detecting colorectal cancer in asymptomatic persons are the digital rectal examination, FOBT, and sigmoidoscopy. Less frequently mentioned screening tests include barium enema and colonoscopy, which have been advocated primarily for high-risk groups. The digital rectal examination is of limited value as a screening test for colorectal cancer. The examining finger, which is only 7–8 cm long, has limited access even to the rectal mucosa, which is 11 cm in length. A negative digital rectal examination provides little reassurance that the patient is free of colorectal cancer because fewer than 10% of colorectal cancers can be palpated by the examining finger.[3]

A second screening maneuver is FOBT. The reported sensitivity and specificity of FOBT for detecting colorectal cancer in asymptomatic persons are 26–92% and 90–99%, respectively (usually based on two samples from three different stool specimens), with the widely varying estimates reflecting differences in study designs.[5–10] Positive reactions on guaiac impregnated cards, the most common form of testing, can signal the presence of bleeding from premalignant adenomas and early-stage colorectal cancers. The guaiac test can also produce false-positive results, however. The ingestion of foods containing peroxidases,[11] and gastric irritants such as salicylates and other antiinflammatory agents,[12] can produce false-positive test results for neoplasia. Nonneoplastic conditions, such as hemorrhoids, diverticulosis, and peptic ulcers, can also cause gastrointestinal bleeding. FOBT can also miss small adenomas and colorectal malignancies that bleed intermittently or not at all.[13,14] Other causes of false-negative results include heterogeneous distribution of blood in feces,[15] ascorbic acid and other antioxidants that interfere with test reagents,[16] and extended delay before testing stool samples.[17]

As a result, when FOBT is performed on asymptomatic persons, the majority of positive reactions are falsely positive for neoplasia. The reported positive predictive value among asymptomatic persons over age 50 is only about 2–11% for carcinoma and 20–30% for adenomas.[6,5,9,18–20] Assuming a false-positive rate of 1–4%, a person who receives annual FOBT from age 50 to age 75 has an estimated 45% probability of receiving a false-positive result.[21] This large proportion of false-positive results is an important concern because of the discomfort, cost, and occasional complications associated with follow-up diagnostic tests, such as barium enema and colonoscopy.[22,23] Rehydration of stored slides can improve sensitivity, but this occurs at the expense of specificity.[24] In one study, rehydration improved sensitivity from 81% to 92%, but it decreased specificity from 98% to 90% and lowered positive predictive value from 6% to 2%. Due to the high false-positive rate, about one third of the entire screened population of asymptomatic patients underwent colonoscopy for abnormal FOBT results within a 13-year period.[5]

Other tests have been proposed to improve the accuracy of screening for fecal occult blood. Current evidence is equivocal as to whether Hemo-Quant (SmithKline Diagnostics, Sunnyvale, CA), a quantitative measurement of hemoglobin in the stool, has better sensitivity or specificity than does qualitative FOBT.[9,10,25–29] Recently developed hemoglobin immunoassays offer the promise of improved sensitivity and specificity but require further evaluation before being considered for routine screening.[30,31]

The third screening test for colorectal cancer is sigmoidoscopy. Sigmoidoscopic screening in asymptomatic persons detects 1–4 cancers per 1,000 examinations.[32,33] However, the sensitivity and diagnostic yield of sigmoidoscopy screening varies with the type of instrument: the rigid (25 cm) sigmoidoscope, the short (35 cm) flexible fiberoptic sigmoidoscope, or the long (60 cm) flexible fiberoptic sigmoidoscope. Since only 30% of colorectal cancers occur in the distal 20 cm of bowel, and less than half occur in or distal to the sigmoid colon,[34–37] the length of the sigmoidoscope has a direct effect on case detection. The rigid sigmoidoscope, which has an average depth of insertion of about 20 cm[38–44] and allows examination to just above the rectosigmoid junction,[45] can detect only about 25–30% of colorectal cancers. The 35-cm flexible sigmoidoscope, however, can visualize about 50–75% of the sigmoid colon and can detect about 50–55% of polyps. Longer 60-cm instruments have an average depth of insertion of 40–50 cm, reaching the proximal end of the sigmoid colon in 80% of examinations[46,47] with the capability of detecting 65–75% of polyps and 40–65% of colorectal cancers[48–52] Researchers have examined the feasibility of introducing a 105-cm flexible sigmoidoscope in the family practice setting,[53] but it is unclear whether the added length substantially increases the rate of detection of premalignant or malignant lesions. Barium enema studies have confirmed that some neoplasms within reach of the sigmoidoscope may not be seen on endoscopy.[54]

Sigmoidoscopy can also produce false-positive results, primarily by detecting polyps that are unlikely to become malignant during the patient's lifetime. Autopsy studies have shown that 10–33% of older adults have colonic polyps at death,[55] but only 2–3% have colorectal cancer.[56-58] Depending on the type of adenomatous polyp, an estimated 5–40% eventually become malignant,[59] a process that takes an average of 10–15 years.[60,61] It follows that the majority of asymptomatic persons with colonic polyps discovered on routine sigmoidoscopic examination will not develop clinically significant malignancy during their lifetime. For these persons, interventions that typically follow such a discovery (i.e., biopsy, polypectomy, frequent colonoscopy), procedures that are costly, anxiety provoking, and potentially harmful, are unlikely to be of significant clinical benefit.

Other potential screening tests for colorectal cancer include colonoscopy and barium enema, which appear to have comparable accuracy. About 95% of colorectal cancers are within reach of the colonoscope, and the examination has an estimated 75–95% sensitivity in detecting lesions within its reach.[20,21] Colonoscopy, which requires sedation and often involves the use of a hospital suite, is more expensive than other screening tests and has a higher risk of anesthetic and procedural complications. The estimated sensitivity and specificity of air-contrast barium enema in detecting lesions within its reach are about 80–95% and 90%, respectively, using subsequent diagnosis as a reference standard.[21] Some retrospective studies have reported a higher sensitivity of barium enema for detecting colorectal cancer (about 90–96%),[62,63] with pathologic diagnosis as the reference standard, but these estimates generally do not account for the selection bias introduced by the case-selection methods.

Effectiveness of Early Detection

Persons with early-stage colorectal cancer at the time of diagnosis appear to have longer survival than do persons with advanced disease.[2] Since there is little information on the extent to which lead-time and length biases (see Chapter ii) account for these differences, researchers in the U.S. and Europe launched large clinical trials in the late 1970s to collect prospective data on the effects of screening on co-lorectal cancer mortality.

Two of these trials[5,6] examined the effect of routine FOBT on colorectal cancer mortality. A randomized controlled trial involving over 46,000 volunteers over age 50 found that the 13-year cumulative mortality from colorectal cancer was 33% lower among persons advised to undergo annual FOBT (5.9 deaths per 1,000) than among a control group that was not offered screening (8.8 deaths per 1,000).[5] The report provided insufficient data, however, to determine to what extent observed differences in outcome were attributable to FOBT or to the large number of colonoscopies that were performed due to frequent false-positive FOBT. An analysis of the study data by other authors suggested that one third to one half of the mortality reduction was due to "chance" selection of persons for colonoscopy,[64] but the assumptions in the analysis have been disputed by the authors.[65] Another controlled trial,[6] which was not randomized, assigned over 21,000 patients to a control group that received a standard periodic health examination or to a study group that was also offered FOBT; both groups received sigmoidoscopy screening. Among new patients (first visit to the preventive medicine clinic), colorectal cancer mortality was 43% lower in the study group than in controls, a difference of borderline statistical significance ($p = 0.053$, one-tail), and there was no difference in outcomes among patients seen previously at the clinic. Recent case-control studies have also reported a 31–57% reduction in risk among persons receiving FOBT.[66,67] Three large clinical trials of FOBT screening, currently under way in Europe, are expected to report their results in the coming years.[7,68,69]

Recent case-control studies have provided important information on the effectiveness of sigmoidoscopy screening. The largest study found that 9% of persons who died of colorectal cancer occurring within 20 cm of the anus had previously undergone a rigid sigmoidoscopic examination, whereas 24% of persons in the control group had received the test.[70] The adjusted odds ratio of 0.41 (95% confidence interval, 0.25–0.69) suggested that sigmoidoscopy screening reduced the risk of death by 59% for cancers within reach of the sigmoidoscope. The investigators noted that the adjusted odds ratio for patients who died of more proximal colon cancers was 0.96. This finding added support to the hypothesis that the reduced risk of death from cancers within reach of the rigid sigmoidoscope was due to screening rather than to confounding factors. Another case-control study reported that the odds ratio for dying of colorectal cancer was 0.21 in screened subjects, and the benefit appeared to be limited to cancers within the reach of the sigmoidoscope.[71]

Older evidence of the effectiveness of sigmoidoscopy screening suffered from important design limitations. A randomized controlled trial of multiphasic health examinations, which included rigid sigmoidoscopy, reported that the study group had significantly lower incidence and mortality rates from colorectal cancer.[72–74] A subsequent analysis of the data, however, revealed that the proportion of subjects receiving sigmoidoscopy and the rate of detection or removal of polyps were similar in both the study and control groups, thus suggesting little benefit from sigmoidoscopy.[75] Two large screening programs found that persons receiving periodic rigid sigmoidoscopy had less advanced disease and better survival from colon cancer than was typical of the general population.[76–78] However, both studies lacked internal controls and used nonrandomized methods to select participants; other methodologic problems with these investigations are outlined in other reviews.[75,79]

An important consideration in assessing the effectiveness of sigmoidoscopic screening is the potential iatrogenic risk associated with the procedure. Complications from sigmoidoscopy are relatively rare in
asymptomatic persons but can be potentially serious. Perforations are reported to occur in approximately 1 of 1,000–10,000 rigid sigmoidoscopic
examinations.[20,21,32,80] Although there are fewer data available on flexible
sigmoidoscopy, the complication rate appears to be less than or equal to
that observed for rigid sigmoidoscopy. The reported risk of perforation
from colonoscopy is about one in 500–3,000 examinations,[5,81] and the risk
of serious bleeding is 1 in 1,000.[5] The estimated risk of perforation during
barium enema is 1 in 5,000–10,000 examinations.[82]

There is little useful evidence regarding the effectiveness of
colonoscopy or barium enema screening in asymptomatic persons. Several
recent studies describe colonoscopy screening of asymptomatic persons,
but they report only the anatomic distribution of polyps and do not address clinical outcomes.[48,49,83] A prospective study demonstrated a significantly lower incidence of subsequent colorectal cancer in patients with
previously diagnosed adenomas who received periodic colonoscopy and
polypectomy, but potential biases in the control groups (historical controls
and population incidence rates) prevent definitive conclusions.[84] No studies have directly examined the effectiveness of routine barium enema
screening in decreasing colorectal cancer mortality in asymptomatic persons. Modeling studies suggest its effectiveness might be comparable to a
screening strategy of periodic sigmoidoscopy.[21]

There is limited information on the optimal age to begin or end
screening and the frequency with which it should be performed. The age
groups in which screening has been shown to decrease mortality are ages
50–80 for FOBT[5] and over age 45 for sigmoidoscopy.[70] Theoretically, the
potential yield from screening should increase beyond age 50 since the incidence of colorectal cancer after this age doubles every 7 years.[2] Modeling studies suggest that beginning screening at age 40 rather than at age
50 offers no improvement in life expectancy.[21] There is little evidence
from which to determine the proper age for discontinuing screening. The
optimal interval for screening is less certain for sigmoidoscopy than for
FOBT, for which there is good evidence of benefit from annual screening.
A modeling study of sigmoidoscopy screening estimated that an interval of
10 years would preserve 90% of the effectiveness of annual screening; this
model assumes that adenomatous polyps take 10–14 years to become invasive cancers.[21] Another model suggested that an interval of 2–4 years
would allow detection of 95% of all polyps greater than 13 mm in diameter.[85] In a case-control study, the risk reduction associated with sigmoidoscopy screening did not diminish during the first 9–10 years after
sigmoidoscopy.[70] Other studies suggest that a single sigmoidoscopic

screening examination may be adequate for low-risk individuals,[86] an approach being investigated in the United Kingdom.[87]

Primary preventive measures to prevent colorectal cancer are currently under investigation. An association between colorectal cancer and dietary intake of fat and fiber has been demonstrated in a series of epidemiologic studies (see Chapter 56). Case-control and cohort studies also suggest that aspirin use may decrease the risk of colon cancer.[88–90]

Recommendations of Other Groups

The American Cancer Society recommends annual digital rectal examination for all adults beginning at age 40, annual FOBT beginning at age 50, and sigmoidoscopy every 3–5 years beginning at age 50.[91] Similar recommendations have been issued by the American Gastroenterological Association,[92] the American Society for Gastrointestinal Endoscopy,[92] and the American College of Obstetricians and Gynecologists.[93] The American College of Physicians' (ACP) guidelines, revised in 1995, recommend offering a variety of screening options to persons from age 50 to 70, depending on local resources and patient preferences: flexible sigmoidoscopy, colonoscopy, or air-contrast barium enema, repeated at 10-year intervals. The ACP recommends that annual FOBT be offered to persons who decline these screening tests, but concluded that there was relatively little benefit of continuing endoscopic screening beyond age 70 in individuals who had been adequately screened up to that age.[21] The American College of Radiology recommends screening with barium enema every 3–5 years as an equivalent alternative to periodic sigmoidoscopy.[94] The recommendations of the American Academy of Family Physicians are currently under review.[95] Most organizations recommend more intensive screening of those in high-risk groups (e.g., familial polyposis, inflammatory bowel disease) with periodic colonoscopy or barium enema. The Canadian Task Force on the Periodic Health Examination concluded that there was insufficient evidence to support screening of asymptomatic individuals over age 40 but that persons with a history of cancer family syndrome should be screened with colonoscopy.[96] An expert panel convened by the Agency for Health Care Policy and Research is expected to issue guidelines for colorectal cancer screening and surveillance in 1996.

Discussion

In summary, recent studies have provided compelling evidence of the effectiveness of FOBT and sigmoidoscopy screening, but the evidence is not definitive. At least one randomized controlled trial and several observational studies have shown that annual FOBT in persons over age 50 can reduce colorectal cancer mortality. This evidence does not, however, clarify whether the observed benefits were due to FOBT or to the effect of performing colonoscopy on a large proportion of the screened population. For sigmoidoscopy, a case-control study supports a strong association between regular screening and reduced colorectal cancer mortality from cancers within reach of the sigmoidoscope. This study was limited, however, by its small number of cases, potential selection biases, and inability to provide prospective evidence of benefit. There are additional concerns about the adverse effects, costs, and optimal frequency of screening. Studies that will help resolve these uncertainties are currently in progress; the final results of ongoing European FOBT trials will be unavailable for several years, however, and a large United States study[97] of FOBT and sigmoidoscopy screening will not be completed until the turn of the century.

An important limitation to the effectiveness of screening for colorectal cancer is the ability of patients and clinicians to comply with testing. Patients may not comply with FOBT for a variety of reasons,[68,98] but compliance rates are generally higher than for sigmoidoscopy. Recent clinical trials report compliance rates of 50–80% for FOBT among volunteers,[5-7,68,69] but lower rates (about 15–30%) have been reported in community screening programs.[99-101] Although the introduction of flexible fiberoptic instruments has made sigmoidoscopy more acceptable to patients,[102] the procedure remains uncomfortable, embarrassing, and expensive, and therefore many patients may be reluctant to agree to this test. A survey of patients over age 50 found that only 13% wanted to receive a sigmoidoscopy examination after being advised that they should receive the test; the most common reasons cited for declining the test were cost (31%), discomfort (12%), and fear (9%).[103] In a study in which sigmoidoscopy was recommended repeatedly, only 31% of participants consented to the procedure,[72-74] but this study was performed during years when rigid sigmoidoscopy was common. Compliance rates as low as 6–12% have been reported. Studies suggest that physician motivation is a major determinant of patient compliance,[104,105] and physicians may be reluctant to perform screening sigmoidoscopy on asymptomatic persons. It has been estimated that a typical family physician with 3,000 active patients (one third aged 50 or older) would have to perform five sigmoidoscopies daily to initially screen the population and two daily procedures for subsequent screening.[33] In addition, examinations using 60-cm sigmoidoscopes are more time-consuming[35-39] and require more extensive training[106-108] than do those using shorter instruments.

Another limitation to screening is its cost. Although a formal cost-effectiveness analysis of screening for colorectal cancer is beyond the scope of this chapter, the economic implications associated with the widespread performance of FOBT and sigmoidoscopy are clearly significant. A single flexible sigmoidoscopic examination costs between $100 and $200.[22,109] A policy of routine FOBT and sigmoidoscopic screening of all persons in the United States over age 50 (about 63 million persons) would cost over $1 billion per year in direct charges.[109] Others have calculated that FOBT screening alone could cost the United States and Canada between $500 million and $1.2 billion each year.[110,111] Another model predicted that performing annual FOBT on persons over age 65 would cost about $35,000 per year of life saved; adding flexible sigmoidoscopy would increase the cost to about $42,000 to $45,000 per year of life saved.[112] Mathematical models suggest that barium enema screening every 3–5 years might have comparable or superior cost-effectiveness when compared with sigmoidoscopy screening, but neither the clinical effectiveness nor acceptability of barium enema screening has been demonstrated directly in clinical studies.

The downstream effects of screening are also of concern. The logistical difficulties and costs of performing FOBT and sigmoidoscopy on a large proportion of the U.S. population are significant, due to the limited acceptability of the tests and the expense of performing screening and follow-up on a large proportion of the population. Moreover, the tests have potential adverse effects that must be considered, such as false-positive results that lead to expensive and potentially harmful diagnostic procedures. Studies that have reported reduced mortality from FOBT used rehydrated slides to increase sensitivity, thereby producing a higher proportion of false-positive results than with nonrehydrated slides; 32% of the annually screened population underwent colonoscopy during a 13-year follow-up period.[65] If this rate is extrapolated to the 63 million Americans over age 50 who would receive annual FOBT, it can be predicted that about 20 million persons would require colonoscopy.

The full implications of this "screening cascade" need to be considered, along with the scientific evidence of clinical benefits, before reaching conclusions about appropriate public policy. For example, using nonrehydrated slides rather than rehydrated slides could substantially reduce the adverse effects and costs of a national screening program. As noted earlier, data from a major screening trial suggest that using nonrehydrated slides rather than rehydrated slides could increase the positive predictive value of FOBT from 2% to 6%, subjecting far fewer screened persons to unnecessary colonoscopy. This improvement in specificity, however, comes at the expense of sensitivity, which decreased from 92% with rehydration to 81% in nonrehydrated slides. The use of nonrehydrated slides would therefore allow a much larger proportion of persons with cancer to escape detection.

The special considerations that apply to persons at increased risk of colorectal cancer are complicated by inadequate epidemiologic and effectiveness data and inconsistent disease classifications. Having a single family member with colorectal cancer does not carry the high risk associated with hereditary cancer syndromes (e.g., familial polyposis, HNPCC).[4,113] A family history that is suggestive of the latter includes a pattern of diagnoses consistent with autosomal dominant inheritance of a highly penetrant disorder. Characteristic features include a family history of colorectal cancer being diagnosed at an early age, frequent cases of multiple primary cancers, or florid adenomatous colonic polyps. Performing periodic colonoscopy to screen for cancer in these groups may be justified in light of the high risk of disease and the incidence of proximal colonic lesions, but there is no direct evidence to determine the optimal strategy in this population.

CLINICAL INTERVENTION

Screening for colorectal cancer is recommended for all persons aged 50 or over ("B" recommendation). Effective methods include FOBT and sigmoidoscopy. There is insufficient evidence to determine which of these screening methods is preferable or whether the combination of FOBT and sigmoidoscopy produces greater benefits than either test alone. Although there is good evidence to support FOBT on an annual basis, there is insufficient evidence to recommend a periodicity for sigmoidoscopy screening. A frequency of every 3–5 years has been recommended by other groups on the basis of expert opinion, and a well-designed case-control study suggests that protection remains unchanged for at least 10 years after rigid sigmoidoscopy. Current evidence suggests that at least some of the benefits of FOBT in reducing colorectal cancer mortality may be achieved through colonoscopic evaluation of abnormal results. Widespread FOBT or sigmoidoscopy screening is therefore likely to generate substantial direct and indirect costs. Appropriate public policy may require consideration of factors other than the scientific evidence of clinical benefit. The appropriate age to discontinue screening has not been determined.

Patients who are offered these tests should receive information about the potential benefits and harms of the procedures, the probability of false-positive results, and the nature of the tests that will be performed if an abnormality is detected. FOBT screening should adhere to current guidelines for dietary restrictions, sample collection, and storage. Although slide rehydration increases the sensitivity of FOBT, it also decreases specificity, and there is insufficient evidence to determine whether rehydration results in better outcomes than screening with nonrehydrated slides. Sigmoidoscopy should be performed by a trained examiner. The instrument should be selected on the basis of examiner expertise and patient comfort. Longer (e.g., 60-cm instrument) flexible sigmoidoscopes have greater sensitivity and are more comfortable than shorter, rigid sigmoidoscopes.

There is insufficient evidence to recommend for or against routine screening with digital rectal examination, barium enema, or colonoscopy

("C" recommendation). Recommendations against using these tests for screening average-risk persons may be made on other grounds (e.g., availability of alternate tests of proven effectiveness, inaccuracy of digital rectal examination, costs and risks of colonoscopy).

In persons with a single first-degree relative with colon cancer, it is not clear that the modest increase in the absolute risk of cancer justifies routine use of colonoscopy over other screening methods. The increased risk of developing cancer at younger ages may justify beginning screening before age 50 in persons with a positive family history, however, especially when affected relatives developed colorectal cancer at younger ages. Direct evidence of the benefit of screening in younger persons is not available for any group. For persons with a family history of hereditary syndromes associated with a very high risk of colon cancer (i.e., familial polyposis or HNPCC), as well as those previously diagnosed with ulcerative colitis, high-risk adenomatous polyps, or colon cancer, regular endoscopic screening is part of routine diagnosis and management; referral to specialists is appropriate for these high-risk patients.

The draft update of this chapter was prepared for the U.S. Preventive Services Task Force by Steven H. Woolf, MD, MPH.

REFERENCES

1. Wingo PA, Tong T, Bolden S. Cancer statistics, 1995. CA Cancer J Clin 1995;45:8–30.
2. Ries LAG, Miller BA, Hankey BF, et al, eds. SEER cancer statistics review, 1973–1991: tables and graphs. Bethesda: National Cancer Institute, 1994. (NIH Publication no. 94-2789.)
3. Winawer SJ, Shike M. Prevention and control of colorectal cancer. In: Greenwald P, Kramer BS, Weed DL, eds. Cancer prevention and control. New York: Marcel Dekker, 1995:537–559.
4. Rustgi AK. Hereditary gastrointestinal polyposis and nonpolyposis syndromes. N Engl J Med 1994;331: 1694–1702.
4a. Toribara NW, Sleisenger MH. Screening for colorectal cancer. N Engl J Med 1995;332:861–867.
4b. Fuchs CS, Giovannucci EL, Colditz GA, et al. A prospective study of family history and the risk of colorectal cancer. N Engl J Med 1994;331:1669–1674.
5. Mandel JS, Bond JH, Church TR, et al. Reducing mortality from colorectal cancer by screening for fecal occult blood. N Engl J Med 1993;328:1365–1371.
6. Winawer SJ, Flehinger BJ, Schottenfeld D, Miller DG. Screening for colorectal cancer with fecal occult blood testing and sigmoidoscopy. J Natl Cancer Inst 1993;85:1311–1318.
7. Kewenter J, Asztely M, Engaras B, Haglind E, Svanvik J, Ahren C. A randomised trial of faecal occult blood testing for early detection of colorectal cancer: results of screening and rescreening of 51,325 subjects. In: Miller AB, Chamberlain J, Day NE, Hakama M, Prorok PC, eds. Cancer screening. Cambridge, England: Cambridge University Press, 1991:117–125.
8. Thomas WM, Pye G, Hardcastle JD, Walker AR. Screening for colorectal carcinoma: an analysis of the sensitivity of Haemoccult. Br J Surg 1992;79:833–835.
9. Ahlquist DA, Wieland HS, Moertel CG, et al. Accuracy of fecal occult blood screening for colorectal neoplasia: a prospective study using Hemoccult and HemoQuant tests. JAMA 1993;269:1262–1267.
10. St John DJB, Young GP, McHutchison JG, Deacon MC, Alexeyeff MA. Comparison of the specificity and sensitivity of Hemoccult and HemoQuant in screening for colorectal neoplasia. Ann Intern Med 1992;117:376–382.
11. Illingworth DG. Influence of diet on occult blood tests. Gut 1965;6:595–598.
12. Rees WD, Turnberg LA. Reappraisal of the effects of aspirin on the stomach. Lancet 1980;2:410–413.

13. Crowley ML, Freeman LD, Mottet MD, et al. Sensitivity of guaiac-impregnated cards for the detection of colorectal neoplasia. J Clin Gastroenterol 1983;5:127–130.

14. Griffith CDM, Turner DJ, Saunders JH. False-negative results of Hemoccult test in colorectal cancer. BMJ 1981;283:472.

15. Rosenfield RE, Kochwa S, Kaczera Z, et al. Nonuniform distribution of occult blood in feces. Am J Clin Pathol 1979;71:204–209.

16. Jaffe RM, Kasten B, Young DS, et al. False-negative stool occult blood tests caused by ingestion of ascorbic acid (vitamin C). Ann Intern Med 1975;83:824–826.

17. Morris DW, Hansell JR, Ostrow D, et al. Reliability of chemical tests for fecal occult blood in hospitalized patients. Dig Dis 1976;21:845–852.

18. Windeler J, Kobberling J. Colorectal cancer and Haemoccult. A study of its value in mass screening using meta-analysis. Int J Colon Dis 1987;2:223–228.

19. Bang KM, Tillett S, Hoar SK, et al. Sensitivity of fecal Hemoccult testing and flexible sigmoidoscopy for colorectal cancer screening. J Occup Med 1986;28:709–713.

20. Winawer SJ, Schottenfeld D, Flehinger BJ. Colorectal cancer screening. J Natl Cancer Inst 1991;83: 243–253.

21. Eddy DM, Ferioli C, Anderson DS. Screening for colorectal cancer. Ann Intern Med 1996 (in press).

22. Brandeau ML, Eddy DM. The workup of the asymptomatic patient with a positive fecal occult blood test. Med Decis Making 1987;7:32–46.

23. Lieberman DA. Colon cancer screening: the dilemma of positive screening tests. Arch Intern Med 1990; 150:740–744.

24. Wells HJ, Pagano JF. "Hemoccult" (TM) test-reversal of false-negative results due to storage. Gastroenterology 1977;72:1148.

25. Schwartz S, Dahl J, Ellefson M, et al. The HemoQuant test: a specific and quantitative determination of heme (hemoglobin) in feces and other materials. Clin Chem 1983;29:2061–2067.

26. Ahlquist DA, McGill DB, Schwartz S, et al. HemoQuant, a new quantitative assay for fecal hemoglobin: comparison with Hemoccult. Ann Intern Med 1984;101:297–302.

27. Ahlquist DA, McGill DB, Schwartz S, et al. Fecal blood levels in health and disease: a study using HemoQuant. N Engl J Med 1985;312:1422–1428.

28. Ahlquist DA, McGill DB, Fleming JL, et al. Patterns of occult bleeding in asymptomatic colorectal cancers. Cancer 1989;63:1826–1830.

29. Joseph AM, Crowson TW, Rich EC. Cost-effectiveness of HemoQuant versus Hemoccult for colorectal cancer screening. J Gen Intern Med 1988;3:132–138.

30. St. John DJB, Young GS, Alexeyeff M, et al. Most large and medium colorectal adenomas can be detected by immunochemical occult blood tests. Gastroenterology 1990;98(suppl):A312.

31. Songster CL, Barrows GH, Jarrett DP. Immunochemical detection of fecal occult blood—the fecal smear punch-disc test: a noninvasive screening test for colorectal cancer. Cancer 1980;45:1099–1102.

32. Bolt RJ. Sigmoidoscopy in detection and diagnosis in the asymptomatic individual. Cancer 1971;28: 121–122.

33. Frame PS. Screening flexible sigmoidoscopy: is it worthwhile? An opposing view. J Fam Pract 1987;25: 604–607.

34. Cady N, Persson AV, Monson DO, et al. Changing patterns of colorectal carcinoma. Cancer 1974;33: 422–426.

35. Rhodes JB, Holmes FF, Clark GM. Changing distribution of primary cancers in the large bowel. JAMA 1977; 238:1641–1643.

36. Abrams JS, Reines HD. Increasing incidence of right-sided lesions in colorectal cancer. Am J Surg 1979; 137:522–526.

37. Greene FL. Distribution of colorectal neoplasms. A left-to-right shift of polyps and cancer. Am J Surg 1983;49:62–65.

38. Winnan G, Berci G, Panish J, et al. Superiority of the flexible to the rigid sigmoidoscope in routine proctosigmoidoscopy. N Engl J Med 1980;302:1011–1012.

39. Bohlman TW, Katon RM, Lipshutz GR, et al. Fiberoptic pansigmoidoscopy: an evaluation and comparison with rigid sigmoidoscopy. Gastroenterology 1977;72:644–649.

40. Winawer SJ, Leidner SD, Boyle C, et al. Comparison of flexible sigmoidoscopy with other diagnostic techniques in the diagnosis of rectocolon neoplasia. Dig Dis Sci 1979;24:277–281.

41. Marks G, Boggs HW, Castro AF, et al. Sigmoidoscopic examinations with rigid and flexible fiberoptic sigmoidoscopes in the surgeon's office. Dis Colon Rectum 1979;22:162–169.

42. Protell RL, Buenger N, Gilbert DA, et al. The short colonoscope: preliminary analysis of a comparison with rigid sigmoidoscopy and Hemoccult testing. Gastrointest Endosc 1978;24:208.

43. Nivatvongs S, Fryd DS. How far does the proctosigmoidoscope reach? N Engl J Med 1980;303: 380–382.

44. Nicholls RJ, Dube S. The extent of examination by rigid sigmoidoscopy. Br J Surg 1982;69:438.

45. Shatz BA, Freitas EL. Area of colon visualized through the sigmoidoscope. JAMA 1954;156:717–719.

46. Gillespie PE, Chambers TJ, Chan KW, et al. Colonic adenomas: a colonoscopic survey. Gut 1979;20: 240–245.

47. Lehman GA, Buchner DM, Lappas JC. Anatomical extent of fiberoptic sigmoidoscopy. Gastroenterology 1983; 84:803–808.

48. Lieberman DA, Smith FW. Screening for colon malignancy with colonoscopy. Am J Gastroenterol 1991;86:946–951.

49. Johnson DA, Gurney MS, Volpe RJ, Jones DM, et al. A prospective study of the prevalence of colonic neoplasms in asymptomatic patients with an age-related risk. Am J Gastroenterol 1990;85:969–974.

50. Tedesco FJ, Waye JD, Avella JR, Villalobos MM. Diagnostic implications of the spatial distribution of colonic mass lesions (polyps and cancers): a prospective colonoscopic study. Gastrointest Endosc 1980;26:95–97.

51. Shinya H, Wolff WI. Morphology, anatomic distribution and cancer potential of colonic polyps: an analysis of 7,000 polyps endoscopically removed. Ann Surg 1979;190:679–683.

52. Winawer SJ, Gottlieb LS, Stewart ET, et al. First progress report of the National Polyp Study. Gastroenterology 1983;84:1352.

53. Dervin JV. Feasibility of 105-cm flexible sigmoidoscopy in family practice. J Fam Pract 1986;23: 341–344.

54. Glick SN, Teplick SK, Balfe DM, et al. Large colonoscopic neoplasms missed by endoscopy. Am J Radiol 1989; 152:513–517.

55. Correa P, Strong JP, Reif A, et al. The epidemiology of colorectal polyps: prevalence in New Orleans and international comparisons. Cancer 1977;39:2258–2264.

56. Hughes LE. The incidence of benign and malignant neoplasms of the colon and rectum: a postmortem study. NZ J Surg 1968;38:30–35.

57. Rickert RR, Auerback O, Garfinke L, et al. Adenomatous lesions of the large bowel: an autopsy survey. Cancer 1979;43:1847–1857.

58. Williams AR, Balasooriy BAW, Day DW. Polyps and cancer of the large bowel: a necropsy study in Liverpool. Gut 1982;23:835–842.

59. Muto T, Bussey HJR, Morson BC. The evolution of cancer of the colon and rectum. Cancer 1975;36: 2251–2270.

60. Morson BC. Evolution of cancer of the colon and rectum. Cancer 1974;34:845–849.

61. Morson BC. The evolution of colorectal carcinoma. Clin Radiol 1984;35:425–431.

62. Johnson CD, Carlson HC, Taylor WF, Weiland LP. Barium enemas of carcinoma of the colon: sensitivity of double- and single-contrast studies. Am J Radiol 1983;140:1143–1149.

63. Fork FT. Radiographic findings in overlooked colon carcinoma: a retrospective analysis. Acta Radiol 1988; 29:331–336.

64. Lang CA, Ransohoff DF. Fecal occult blood screening for colorectal cancer: is mortality reduced by chance selection for screening colonoscopy? JAMA 1994;271:1011–1013.

65. Mandel JS, Ederer F, Church T, Bond J. Screening for colorectal cancer: which test is best? [letter]. JAMA 1994;272:1099.

66. Selby JV, Friedman GD, Quesenberry CP, Weiss NS. Effect of fecal occult blood testing on mortality from colorectal cancer: a case-control study. Ann Intern Med 1993;118:1–6.

67. Wahrendorf J, Robra BP, Wiebelt H, Oberhausen R, Weiland M, Dhom G. Effectiveness of colorectal cancer screening: results from a population-based case-control evaluation in Saarland, Germany. Eur J Cancer Prev 1993; 2:221–227.

68. Kronborg O, Fenger C, Sndergaard O, et al. Initial mass screening for colorectal cancer with fecal occult blood test. A prospective randomized study at Funen in Denmark. Scan J Gastroenterol 1987;22: 677–686.

69. Hardcastle JD, Thomas WM, Chamberlain J, et al. Randomised, controlled trial of faecal occult blood screening for colorectal cancer: results for first 107,349 subjects. Lancet 1989;1:1160–1164.

70. Selby JV, Friedman GD, Quesenberry CP Jr, Weiss NS. A case-control study of screening sigmoidoscopy and mortality from colorectal cancer. N Engl J Med 1992;326:653–657.

71. Newcomb PA, Norfleet RG, Storer BE, Surawicz TS, Marcus PM. Screening sigmoidoscopy and colorectal cancer mortality. J Natl Cancer Inst 1992;84:1572–1575.

72. Cutler JL, Ramcharan S, Feldman R, et al. Multiphasic checkup evaluation study. 1. Methods and population. Prev Med 1973;2:197–206.

73. Dales LG, Friedman GD, Collen MF. Evaluating periodic multiphasic health checkups: a controlled trial. J Chronic Dis 1979;32:385–404.

74. Friedman GD, Collen MF, Fireman BH. Multiphasic health checkup evaluation: a 16-year follow-up. J Chronic Dis 1986;39:453–463.

75. Selby JV, Friedman GD, Collen MF. Sigmoidoscopy and mortality from colorectal cancer: the Kaiser Permanente Multiphasic Evaluation Study. J Clin Epidemiol 1988;41:427–434.

76. Gilbertsen VA. Proctosigmoidoscopy and polypectomy in reducing the incidence of rectal cancer. Cancer 1974;34:936–939.

77. Gilbertsen VA, Nelms JM. The prevention of invasive cancer of the rectum. Cancer 1978;41: 1137–1139.

78. Hertz REL, Deddish MR, Day E. Value of periodic examinations in detecting cancer of the colon and rectum. Postgrad Med 1960;27:290–294.

79. Morrison A. Screening in chronic disease. New York: Oxford University Press, 1985.

80. Nelson RL, Abcarian H, Prasad ML. Iatrogenic perforation of the colon and rectum. Dis Colon Rectum 1982; 25:305–308.

81. Waye J, Lewis B, Yessayan S. Colonoscopy: a prospective report of complications. Gastrointest Endosc 1990; 36(suppl):A226.

82. MacCarty RL. Colorectal cancer: the case for barium enema. Mayo Clin Proc 1992;67:253–257.

83. DiSario JA, Foutch PG, Mai HD, Pardy K, Manne RK. Prevalence and malignant potential of colorectal polyps in asymptomatic, average-risk men. Am J Gastroenterol 1991;86:941–945.

84. Winawer SJ, Zauber AG, Ho MN, et al. Prevention of colorectal cancer by colonoscopic polypectomy. N Engl J Med 1993;329:1977–1981.

85. Carroll RLA, Klein M. How often should patients be sigmoidoscoped? A mathematical perspective. Prev Med 1980;9:741–746.

86. Sakamoto MS, Hara JH, Schlumpberger JM. Screening flexible sigmoidoscopy in a low-risk, highly screened population. J Fam Pract 1994;38:245–248.

87. Atkin WS, Cuzick J, Northover JMA, Whynes DK. Prevention of colorectal cancer by once-only sigmoidoscopy. Lancet 1993;341:736–740.

88. Thun MJ, Namboodiri MM, Heath CW. Aspirin use and reduced risk of fatal colon cancer. N Engl J Med 1991;325:1593–1596.

89. Kune A, Kune S, Watson LF. Colorectal cancer risk, chronic illness, operations, and medications: case control results from the Melbourne colorectal cancer study. Cancer Res 1988;48:4399–4404.

90. Rosenberg L, Ralmer JR, Zauber AG, Warshauer ME, Stolley PD, Shapiro S. A hypothesis: nonsteroidal anti-inflammatory drugs reduce the incidence of large-bowel cancer. J Natl Cancer Inst 1991;83: 355–358.

91. American Cancer Society. Guidelines for the cancer-related checkup: an update. Atlanta: American Cancer Society, 1993.

92. Fleischer DE, Goldberg SB, Browning TH, et al. Detection and surveillance of colorectal cancer. JAMA 1989; 261:580–585.

93. American College of Obstetricians and Gynecologists. Routine cancer screening. Committee Opinion no. 128. Washington, DC: American College of Obstetricians and Gynecologists, 1993.

94. Ferrucci JT. Screening for colon cancer: programs of the American College of Radiology. Am J Radiol 1993;160:999–1003.

95. American Academy of Family Physicians. Age charts for periodic health examination. Kansas City, MO: American Academy of Family Physicians, 1994. (Reprint no. 510.)

96. Canadian Task Force on the Periodic Health Examination. Canadian guide to clinical preventive health care. Ottawa: Canada Communication Group, 1994:797–809.

97. Greenwald P. Colon cancer overview. Cancer 1992;70:1206–1215.

98. Blalock SJ, DeVellis BM, Sandler RS. Participation in fecal occult blood screening: a critical review. Prev Med 1987;16:9–18.

99. Elwood TW, Erickson A, Lieberman S. Comparative educational approaches to screening for colorectal cancer. Am J Public Health 1978;68:135–138.

100. Winchester DP, Shull JH, Scanlon EF, et al. A mass screening program for colorectal cancer using chemical testing for occult blood in the stool. Cancer 1980;45:2955–2958.
101. Ahlquist DA. Occult blood screening: obstacles to effectiveness. Cancer 1992;70:1259–1265.
102. Winawer SJ, Miller C, Lightdale C, et al. Patient response to sigmoidoscopy: a randomized, controlled trial of rigid and flexible sigmoidoscopy. Cancer 1987;60:1905–1908.
103. Petravage J, Swedberg J. Patient response to sigmoidoscopy recommendations via mailed reminders. J Fam Pract 1988;27:387–389.
104. Holt WS. Factors affecting compliance with screening sigmoidoscopy. J Fam Pract 1991;32:585–589.
105. Launoy G, Veret JL, Richir B, et al. Involvement of general practitioners in mass screening: experience of a colorectal cancer mass screening programme in the Calvados region (France). Eur J Cancer Prev 1993;2:229–232.
106. Shapiro M. Flexible fiberoptic sigmoidoscopy: the long and the short of it. Gastrointest Endosc 1984; 30:114–116.
107. Griffin JW. Flexible fiberoptic sigmoidoscopy: longer may not be better for the nonendoscopist. Gastrointest Endosc 1985;31:347–348.
108. Weissman GS, Winawer SJ, Baldwin MP, et al. Multicenter evaluation of training of nonendoscopists in flexible sigmoidoscopy. CA Cancer J Clin 1987;37:26–30.
109. Clayman CB. Mass screening for colorectal cancer: are we ready? JAMA 1989;261:609.
110. Frank JW. Occult-blood screening for colorectal carcinoma: the yield and the costs. Am J Prev Med 1985;1:18–24.
111. Ransohoff DF, Lang CA. Screening for colorectal cancer. N Engl J Med 1991;325:37–41.
112. Wagner J. From the Congressional Office of Technology Assessment: costs and effectiveness of colorectal cancer screening in the elderly. JAMA 1990;264:2732.
113. Lynch HT, Watson P, Smyrk TC, et al. Colon cancer genetics. Cancer 1992;70:1300–1312.

9. Screening for Cervical Cancer

RECOMMENDATION

Routine screening for cervical cancer with Papanicolaou (Pap) testing is recommended for all women who are or have been sexually active and who have a cervix. Pap smears should begin with the onset of sexual activity and should be repeated at least every 3 years (see *Clinical Intervention*). There is insufficient evidence to recommend for or against an upper age limit for Pap testing, but recommendations can be made on other grounds to discontinue regular testing after age 65 in women who have had regular previous screenings in which the smears have been consistently normal. There is insufficient evidence to recommend for or against routine screening with cervicography or colposcopy, or for screening for human papilloma virus infection, although recommendations against such screening can be made on other grounds (see *Clinical Intervention*).

Burden of Suffering

Approximately 16,000 new cases of cervical cancer are diagnosed each year, and about 4,800 women die from this disease annually.[1] The lifetime risk of dying from cervical cancer in the U.S. is 0.3%.[1a] Although the 5-year survival rate is about 90% for persons with localized cervical cancer, it is considerably lower (about 14%) for persons with advanced (Stage IV) disease. The incidence of invasive cervical cancer has decreased significantly over the last 40 years, due in large part to organized early detection programs. Although all sexually active women are at risk for cervical cancer, the disease is more common among women of low socioeconomic status, those with a history of multiple sex partners or early onset of sexual intercourse, and smokers. The incidence of invasive cervical cancer among young white women has increased recently in the United States. Infection with human immunodeficiency virus (HIV) and certain types of human papilloma virus (HPV) also increases the risk of cervical cancer.[2]

Accuracy of Screening Tests

The principal screening test for cervical cancer is the Pap smear. Although the Pap smear can sometimes detect endometrial, vaginal, and other cancers,[3,4] its use as a screening test is intended for the early detection of cervical dysplasia and cancer. Other proposed cervical screening tests include cervicography, colposcopy, and testing for HPV infection. The role of pelvic examination, which usually accompanies the collection of the cervical specimen, is discussed in Chapter 14 in relation to ovarian cancer screening.

Precise data on the sensitivity and specificity of the Pap smear in detecting cancer and dysplasia are lacking due to methodologic problems. Depending on study design, false-negative rates of 1–80% have been reported; a range of 20–45% has been quoted most frequently, primarily in studies comparing normal test results with subsequent smears.[5–11] Studies using cone biopsy results as the reference standard have reported false-negative rates as low as 10%.[12] Although reliable data are lacking, specificity is probably greater than 90%[13] and may be as high as 99%.[6,11] The detection of precursor cervical intraepithelial neoplasia (CIN) by Pap smears may have poor specificity for cervical carcinoma, however, because a substantial proportion of CIN-1 lesions do not progress to invasive disease or may regress spontaneously. The test-retest reliability of Pap smears is influenced to some extent by variations in the expertise and procedures of different cytopathology laboratories.

A large proportion of diagnostic errors may be attributable to laboratory error. In one study of over 300 laboratories given slides with known cytologic diagnoses, false-negative diagnoses were made in 7.5% of smears with moderate dysplasia or frank malignancy, and false-positive diagnoses were made in 8.9% of smears with no more than benign atypia.[14] A survey of 73 laboratories in one state revealed a false-negative rate of 4.4% and a false-positive rate of 2.7%.[15] These data were reported in 1990, before the introduction of federal legislation designed to improve the accuracy of cytopathologic laboratory interpretation.[16] With the adoption of the Bethesda system for classification of cervical diagnoses,[17] a large proportion of benign smears are interpreted as "atypical," a finding that poses little premalignant potential but that often generates intensive follow-up testing.

Another cause of false-negative Pap smears is poor specimen collection technique. A 1991 survey of 600 laboratories found that 1–5% of specimens received were either unsatisfactory or suboptimal, generally because endocervical cells were absent from the smear.[18] Another study found that poor sampling technique accounted for 64% of false-negative results.[19] The Pap smear has traditionally been obtained with a spatula, to sample the ectocervix, and a cotton swab, to obtain endocervical cells. A 1990 survey found that about half of physicians used a spatula and cotton swab to collect Pap smears.[20] In recent years, new devices have been introduced to improve sampling of the squamocolumnar junction. Controlled studies have shown that using an endocervical brush in combination with a spatula is more likely to collect endocervical cells than using a spatula or cotton swab.[21-30] There is conflicting evidence, however, that the endocervical brush increases the detection rate for abnormal smears or affects clinical outcomes.[31-33] There is also conflicting evidence regarding the importance of collecting endocervical cells. Although some large series have reported that CIN is detected over 2 times more frequently when endocervical cells are present,[34,35] other series[36,37] have shown no association between the presence of endocervical cells and the detection rate for dysplasia. The brush is more expensive than the cotton swab, but studies suggest that this cost is easily recovered by the reduced need for repeat testing.[38] Other methods for improving the sensitivity of cervical cancer screening, such as acetic acid washes to improve the visibility of lesions, remain investigational.[39,40]

There are important potential adverse effects associated with inaccurate interpretation of Pap smears. False-negative results are significant because CIN or more invasive lesions may escape detection and progress to more advanced disease during the period between tests. The potential adverse effects of false-positive results include patient anxiety regarding the risk of cervical cancer,[41,42] as well as the unnecessary inconvenience, discomfort, and expense of follow-up diagnostic procedures. Studies have shown that the distribution of patient education materials that explain the meaning of abnormal results is associated with a reduction in patient anxiety and stress and a better patient understanding of test results.[43-45]

Other tests, such as cervicography and colposcopy, have been proposed to help improve the sensitivity of screening,[46] but their accuracy and technical requirements are suboptimal. Cervicography, in which a photograph of the cervix is examined for atypical lesions, has a sensitivity that is comparable to the Pap smear (approximately 60%) but a much lower specificity (approximately 50%); the reported positive predictive value in most studies is only 1–26%, and about 10–15% of cervigrams are unsatisfactory.[47-51] Colposcopy, in which the cervix is examined under magnification with acetic acid washing and suspicious lesions are biopsied, is widely performed on women with abnormal Pap smears but has poor sensitivity (34–43%), specificity (68%), and positive predictive value (4–13%) when used as a screening test for cervical neoplasia in asymptomatic women.[52-54] Other disadvantages of colposcopy screening include its cost, the limited availability of the equipment, the time and skills required to perform the procedure, and patient discomfort. Using a 10-point score for assessing pain, one study reported that women who underwent colposcopy gave the procedure a range of scores from 3 to 4.6.[55]

Another proposed screening strategy is testing for HPV infection, a known risk factor for cervical cancer. Of the more than 70 types of HPV that have been identified, several oncogenic forms (e.g., types 16 and 18) have a strong epidemiologic association with cervical cancer. However, the natural history of how HPV infection progresses to cancer is poorly understood.[56] One study of women infected with either HPV type 16 or 18 found that 67% of the lesions remained unchanged or regressed after a mean of 5 years, 29% progressed to a more advanced stage of dysplasia, and 3% recurred.[57] The high prevalence of HPV infection in young women also limits its predictive value. In one study, nearly half of female college students had evidence of HPV when tested by polymerase chain reaction technology.[58] The reported positive predictive value of this HPV test for CIN-2 or CIN-3 lesions and carcinoma is less than 10%.[59] HPV typing to identify women with oncogenic strains may improve the future accuracy of the test and its role in directing follow-up, but its current suitability for routine screening in asymptomatic women is limited by its poor predictive value, uncertain natural history, and, due to the absence of an effective treatment, the lack of evidence that screening affects clinical outcomes.[60]

Effectiveness of Early Detection

Early detection of cervical neoplasia provides an opportunity to prevent or delay progression to invasive cancer by performing clinical interventions such as colposcopy, conization, cryocautery, laser vaporization, loop electrosurgical excision, and, when necessary, hysterectomy.[61] There is evidence that early detection through routine Pap testing and treatment of precursor CIN can lower mortality from cervical cancer. Correlational studies in the United States, Canada, and several European countries comparing cervical cancer data over time have shown dramatic reductions in the incidence of invasive disease and a 20–60% reduction in cervical cancer mortality rates following the implementation of cervical screening programs.[62-70] Case-control studies have shown a strong negative association between screening and invasive disease, also suggesting that screening is protective.[71-75] These observational studies do not constitute direct evidence that screening was responsible for the findings,[76] and randomized controlled trials to provide such evidence have not been performed. Nonetheless, the large body of supportive evidence accumulated to date has prompted the adoption of routine cervical cancer screening in many countries and makes performance of a controlled trial of Pap smears unlikely for ethical reasons.

Observational data suggest that the effectiveness of cervical cancer screening increases when Pap testing is performed more frequently.[72] Aggressive dysplastic and premalignant lesions are less likely to escape detection when the interval between smears is short. There are, however, diminishing returns as frequency is increased.[71,77] Although studies have shown that reducing the interval between Pap smears from 10 years to 5 years is likely to achieve a significant reduction in the risk of invasive cervical cancer, case-control studies and mathematical modeling have demonstrated that increasing to a 2–3-year interval offers only slight added benefit.[71,78–80] There is little evidence that women who receive annual screening are at significantly lower risk for invasive cervical cancer than are women who are tested every 3–5 years. These findings were confirmed in a major study of eight cervical cancer screening programs in Europe and Canada involving over 1.8 million women.[81] According to this report, the cumulative incidence of invasive cervical cancer was reduced 64.1% when the interval between Pap tests was 10 years, 83.6% at 5 years, 90.8% at 3 years, 92.5% at 2 years, and 93.5% at 1 year. These estimates were for women aged 35–64 who had at least one screening before age 35, and they are based on the assumption of 100% compliance.

Recommendations of Other Groups

A consensus recommendation that all women who are or have been sexually active, or who have reached age 18, should have annual Pap smears has been adopted by the American Cancer Society, National Cancer Institute, American College of Obstetricians and Gynecologists (ACOG), American Medical Association, American Academy of Family Physicians (AAFP), and others.[82] The recommendation permits Pap testing less frequently after three or more annual smears have been normal, at the discretion of the physician. Guidelines for determining frequency based on risk factors have been issued by ACOG.[83] The consensus did not recommend an age to discontinue Pap testing. The AAFP recommends that screening can be discontinued at age 65 if there is documented evidence of previously negative smears, but its recommendations are currently under review.[84] The American College of Physicians (ACP) recommends Pap smears every 3 years for women aged 20–65, and every 2 years for women at high risk.[85] The ACP also recommends screening women aged 66–75 every 3 years if not screened in the 10 years before age 66. The Canadian Task Force on the Periodic Health Examination recommends screening for cervical cancer with annual Pap smears in women following initiation of sexual activity or age 18, and after two normal smears, screening every 3 years to age 69.[86] The Canadian Task Force recommends considering more frequent screening for women at increased risk. In their guidelines for adolescent preventive services (GAPS), the American Medical Association recommends annual screening with a Pap test for female adolescents who are sexually active or age 18 or older.[87] Bright Futures also recommends annual Pap testing for sexually active adolescent females.[88] Similar recommendations have been endorsed by the American Academy of Pediatrics.[89]

Discussion

It has been estimated that screening women aged 20–64 every 3 years with Pap testing reduces cumulative incidence of invasive cervical cancer by 91%, requires about 15 tests per woman, and yields 96 cases for every 100,000 Pap smears. Annual screening reduces incidence by 93%, but requires 45 tests and yields only 33 cases for every 100,000 tests.[81] Empirical data also support the effectiveness of a 3-year interval. A study of 25,000 Dutch women found that screening a stable population every 3 years reduced the incidence of squamous cell carcinoma of the cervix from 0.38 per 1000 to zero within 12 years.[67] There are, in addition, important economic considerations to performing Pap tests every 2–3 years, since annual testing could double or triple the total number of smears taken on over 92 million American women at risk,[90] yet provide only limited added benefit in lowering mortality.[81]

Annual testing, however, has been common. In the mid-1980s, a survey of recently trained gynecologists found that 97% recommend a Pap test at least once a year.[91] The preference of many clinicians for performing annual Pap smears is based on concerns that less frequent testing may result in more harm than good, but reliable scientific data to support these opinions are lacking. Specifically, advocates of annual testing have expressed concerns that data demonstrating little added value to annual testing are based on retrospective studies and mathematical models that are subject to biases and invalid assumptions; that an interval longer than 1 year may permit aggressive, rapidly growing cancers to escape early detection; that the public may obtain Pap smears at a lower frequency than that publicized in recommendations; that a longer interval might affect compliance among high-risk women, a group with poor coverage even with an annual testing policy; that repeated testing may offset the false-negative rate of the Pap smear; that the test is inexpensive and safe; and that a large proportion of women believe it is important to have an annual Pap test and, while visiting the clinician, may receive other preventive interventions. Definitive evidence to support these concerns is lacking.

Women who have never engaged in sexual intercourse are not at risk for cervical cancer and therefore do not require screening.[92–94] In addition, screening of women who have only recently become sexually active (e.g., adolescents) is likely to have low yield. The incidence of invasive cancer in women under age 25 is only about 1–3 per 100,000, a rate that is much lower than that of older age groups.[11] One study found that most women with CIN who had become sexually active at age 18 were not diagnosed with severe dysplasia or carcinoma in situ until age 30.[93]

Although invasive cervical cancer is uncommon at young ages, authorities have recommended since the early 1980s that screening should begin with the onset of sexual activity.[82,92,94] This policy is based in part on the concern that a proportion of young women with CIN may have an aggressive cell type that can progress rapidly and go undetected if screening is delayed to a later age. There is some evidence that adenocarcinomas are accounting for a growing proportion of new cervical cancer cases in young women,[95,96] but the exact incidence and natural history of aggressive disease in young women remain uncertain. The Pap smear is also a poor screening test for adenocarcinoma, compared with squamous cell carcinoma. Another reason given for early screening is the concern that the incidence of cervical dysplasia occurring in young women appears to be on the rise, coincident with the increasing sexual activity of adolescents. On these grounds, testing should begin by age 18, since many American teenagers are sexually active by this age. Screening in the absence of a history of sexual intercourse may be justified if the credibility of the sexual history is in question.

When screening is initiated, it is frequently recommended that the first two to three smears be obtained 1 year apart as a means of detecting aggressive tumors at a young age. There is little evidence to suggest, however, that young women whose first two tests are separated by 2 or 3 years, rather than 1 year, have a greater mortality or person-years of life lost.[78] Recommendations to perform these first tests annually are based primarily on expert opinion.

Elderly women do not appear to benefit from Pap testing if repeated cervical smears have consistently been normal.[97,78] Modeling data suggest that continued testing of previously screened women reduces the risk of dying from cervical cancer by only 0.18% at age 65 and 0.06% at age 74.[80] Many older women have had incomplete screening, however. A reported 17% of women over age 65 and 32% of poor women in this age group have never received a Pap test.[98] In a study of elderly minority women with an average age of 75 years, the mean reported number of prior Pap smears received since age 65 was 1.7.[99] Further screening in this group of older women is important[78,100] and some studies suggest that it is cost-effective.[101] Women who have undergone a hysterectomy in which the cervix was removed do not benefit from Pap testing, unless it was performed because of cervical cancer. Post-hysterectomy screening has the potential to detect vaginal cancer, but the yield and predictive value are likely to be very low. Women who had hysterectomies performed in which the cervix was left behind probably still require screening.

The effectiveness of cervical cancer screening is more likely to be improved by extending testing to women who are not currently being screened and by improving the accuracy of Pap smears than by efforts to increase the frequency of testing. Studies suggest that those at greatest risk for cervical cancer are the very women least likely to have access to testing.[102,103] Incomplete Pap testing is most common among blacks, the poor, uninsured persons, the elderly, and persons living in rural areas.[98,104–106] In addition, many women who are tested receive inaccurate results due to interpretative or reporting errors by cytopathology laboratories or specimen collection errors by clinicians. The failure of some physicians to provide adequate follow-up for abnormal Pap smears is another source of delay in the management of cervical dysplasia.[107] Finally, a large proportion of patients with abnormal smears (30% in studies of poor, elderly black women[108]) do not return for further evaluation. Various techniques may enhance physician and patient compliance with screening, follow-up of abnormal results, and patient compliance with rescreening.[109–112]

CLINICAL INTERVENTION

Regular Pap tests are recommended for all women who are or have been sexually active and who have a cervix ("A" recommendation). Testing should begin at the age when the woman first engages in sexual intercourse. Adolescents whose sexual history is thought to be unreliable should be presumed to be sexually active at age 18. There is little evidence that annual screening achieves better outcomes than screening every 3 years. Pap tests should be performed at least every 3 years ("B" recommendation). The interval for each patient should be recommended by the physician based on risk factors (e.g., early onset of sexual intercourse, a history of multiple sex partners, low socioeconomic status). (Women infected with human immunodeficiency virus require more frequent screening according to established guidelines.[113]) There is insufficient evidence to recommend for or against an upper age limit for Pap testing, but recommendations can be made on other grounds to discontinue regular testing after age 65 in women who have had regular previous screening in which the smears have been consistently normal ("C" recommendation). Women who have undergone a hysterectomy in which the cervix was removed do not require Pap testing, unless the hysterectomy was performed because of cervical cancer or its precursors. Patients at increased risk because of unprotected sexual activity or multiple sex partners should receive appropriate counseling about sexual practices (see Chapter 62).

The use of an endocervical brush increases the likelihood of obtaining endocervical cells, but there is conflicting evidence that sampling these cells improves sensitivity in detecting cervical neoplasia. Physicians should submit specimens to laboratories that have adequate quality control measures to ensure optimal accuracy in the interpretation and reporting of results. Thorough follow-up of test results should also be ensured, including repeat testing and referral for colposcopy as indicated. Physicians should consider providing patients with a pamphlet or other written information

about the meaning of abnormal smears to help ensure follow-up and minimize anxiety over false-positive results.

There is insufficient evidence to recommend for or against routine cervicography or colposcopy screening for cervical cancer in asymptomatic women, nor is there evidence to support routine screening for HPV infection ("C" recommendation). Recommendations against such screening can be made on other grounds, including poor specificity and costs.

The draft update of this chapter was prepared for the U.S. Preventive Services Task Force by Steven H. Woolf, MD, MPH.

REFERENCES

1. Wingo PA, Tong T, Bolden S. Cancer statistics, 1995. CA Cancer J Clin 1995;45:8–30.
1a. Ries LAG, Miller BA, Hankey BF, et al, eds. SEER cancer statistics review, 1973–1991: tables and graphs. Bethesda: National Cancer Institute, 1994. (NIH Publication no. 94-2789.)
2. American Cancer Society. Cancer facts and figures–1993. Atlanta: American Cancer Society, 1993.
3. Mitchell H, Giles G, Medley G. Accuracy and survival benefit of cytological prediction of endometrial carcinoma on routine cervical smears. Int J Gynecol Pathol 1993;12:34–40.
4. Sherman ME, Paull G. Vaginal intraepithelial neoplasia: reproducibility of pathologic diagnosis and correlation of smears and biopsies. Acta Cytol 1993;37:699–704.
5. Kim HS, Underwood D. Adenocarcinoma in the cervicovaginal Papanicolaou smear: analysis of a 12-year experience. Diagn Cytopathol 1991;7:199–224.
6. Soost HJ, Lange HJ, Lehmacher W, Ruffing-Kullmann B. The validation of cervical cytology: sensitivity, specificity, and predictive values. Acta Cytol 1991;35:8–14.
7. Foltz AM, Kelsey JL. The annual Pap test: a dubious policy success. Milbank Mem Fund Q 1978;56: 426–462.
8. Coppleson LW, Brown B. Estimation of the screening error rate from the observed detection rates in repeated cervical cytology. Am J Obstet Gynecol 1974;119:953–958.
9. Benoit AG, Krepart GV, Lotocki RJ. Results of prior cytologic screening in patients with a diagnosis of Stage I carcinoma of the cervix. Am J Obstet Gynecol 1984;148:690–694.
10. Jones DE, Creasman WT, Dombroski RA, et al. Evaluation of the atypical Pap smear. Am J Obstet Gynecol 1987;157:544–549.
11. Boyes DA, Morrison B, Knox EG, et al. A cohort study of cervical cancer screening in British Columbia. Clin Invest Med 1982;5:1–29.
12. Sfameni SF, Jobling TW, Trickey NRA, Havelock C. Evaluation of serial cervical cytology in the assessment of preinvasive cervical neoplasia. Aust NZ J Obstet Gynaecol 1989;29:40–43.
13. Tawa K, Forsythe A, Cove JK, et al. A comparison of the Papanicolaou smear and the cervigram: sensitivity, specificity, and cost analysis. Obstet Gynecol 1988;71:229–235.
14. Yobs AR, Swanson RA, Lamotte LC. Laboratory reliability of the Papanicolaou smear. Obstet Gynecol 1985;65:235–243.
15. DeBoy JM, Jarboe BR. Maryland's cytology labs: 1989–90 proficiency testing results. Md Med J 1991;40: 107–111.
16. Helfand M, O'Connor GT, Zimmer-Gembeck M, Beck JR. Effect of the Clinical Laboratory Improvement Amendments of 1988 (CLIA '88) on the incidence of invasive cervical cancer. Med Care 1992;30:1067–1082.
17. The 1988 Bethesda System for reporting cervical/vaginal cytologic diagnoses. Acta Cytol 1989;33: 567–574.
18. Davey DD, Nielsen ML, Rosenstock W, Kline TS. Terminology and specimen adequacy in cervico-vaginal cytology: the College of American Pathologists Interlaboratory Comparison Program experience. Arch Pathol Lab Med 1992;116:903–907.
19. Dodd LG, Sneige N, Villarreal Y, et al. Quality-assurance study of simultaneously sampled, non-correlating cervical cytology and biopsies. Diagn Cytopathol 1993;9:138–144.
20. Clement KD, Christenson PD. Papanicolaou smear cell recovery techniques used by primary care physicians. J Am Board Fam Pract 1990;3:253–258.

21. Helderman G, Graham L, Cannon D, Waters K, Feller D. Comparing two sampling techniques for endocervical cell recovery on Papanicolaou smears. Nurs Pract 1990;15:30–32.

22. Hoffman MS, Hill DA, Gordy LW, Lane J, Cavanagh D. Comparing the yield of the standard Papanicolaou and endocervical brush smears. J Reprod Med 1991;36:267–269.

23. Grossman MB, Clofine R. The efficacy of an endocervical brush in obtaining adequate Papanicolaou smears. J Am Osteopath Assoc 1991;91:875–879.

24. Lai-Goldman M, Nieberg RK, Mulcahy D, Wiesmeier E. The Cytobrush for evaluating routine cervicovaginal-endocervical smears. J Reprod Med 1990;35:959–963.

25. Koonings PP, Dickinson K, d'Ablaing G III, Schlaerth JB. A randomized clinical trial comparing the Cytobrush and cotton swab for Papanicolaou smears. Obstet Gynecol 1992;80:241–245.

26. Ruffin MT IV, Van Noord GR. Improving the yield of endocervical elements in a Pap smear with the use of the cytology brush. Fam Med 1991;23:365–369.

27. Davey-Sullivan B, Gearhart J, Evers CG, Cason Z, Replogle WH. The Cytobrush effect on Pap smear adequacy. Fam Pract Res J 1991;11:57–64.

28. Buntinx F, Boon ME, Beck S, Knottnerus JA, Essed GGM. Comparison of Cytobrush sampling, spatula sampling, and combined Cytobrush-spatula sampling of the uterine cervix. Acta Cytol 1991;35:64–68.

29. Fokke HE, Salvatore CM, Schipper MEI, Bleker OP. The quality of the Pap smear. Eur J Gynaecol Oncol 1992;13:445–448.

30. McCord ML, Stovall TG, Meric JL, Summitt RL Jr, Coleman SA. Cervical cytology: a randomized comparison of four sampling methods. Am J Obstet Gynecol 1992;166:1772–1779.

31. Cauthen DB, Cullison M, Symm B, Peterson RF. Use effectiveness of the Cytobrush in the primary care setting. J Am Board Fam Pract 1991;5:365–368.

32. Szarewski A, Curran G, Edwards R, Cuzick J, Kocjan G, Bounds W, Guillebaud J. Comparison of four cytologic sampling techniques in a large family planning center. Acta Cytol 1993;37:457–460.

33. Alons-van Kordelaar JJM, Boon ME. Diagnostic accuracy of squamous cervical lesions studied in spatula-cytobrush smears. Acta Cytol 1988;32:801–804.

34. Elias A, Linthorst G, Bekker B, Vooijs PG. The significance of endocervical cells in the diagnosis of cervical epithelial changes. Acta Cytol 1983;27:225–229.

35. Mauney M, Eide D, Sotham J. Rates of condyloma and dysplasia in Papanicolaou smears with and without endocervical cells. Diagn Cytopathol 1990;6:18–21.

36. Kivlahan C, Ingram E. Papanicolaou smears without endocervical cells: are they inadequate? Acta Cytol 1986; 30:258–260.

37. Mitchell H, Medley G. Longitudinal study of women with negative cervical smears according to endocervical status. Lancet 1991;337:741–742.

38. Harrison DD, Hernandez E, Dunton CJ. Endocervical brush versus cotton swab for obtaining cervical smears at a clinic: a cost comparison. J Reprod Med 1993;38:285–288.

39. Slawson DC, Bennett JH, Herman JM. Are Papanicolaou smears enough? Acetic acid washes of the cervix as adjunctive therapy: a HARNET study. J Fam Pract 1992;35:271–277.

40. Van Le L, Broekhuizen FF, Janzer-Steele R, Behar M, Samter T. Acetic acid visualization of the cervix to detect cervical dysplasia. Obstet Gynecol 1993;81:293–295.

41. Lerman C, Miller SM, Scarborough R, Hanjani P, Nolte S, Smith D. Adverse psychologic consequences of positive cytologic cervical screening. Am J Obstet Gynecol 1991;165:658–662.

42. Lauver D, Rubin M. Women's concerns about abnormal Papanicolaou test results. J Obstet Gynecol Neonatal Nurs 1991;20:154–159.

43. Wolfe C, Doherty I, Raju KS, Holtom R, Richardson P. First steps in the development of an information and counselling service for women with an abnormal smear result. Eur J Obstet Gynecol Reprod Biol 1992;45:201–206.

44. Wilkinson C, Jones JM, McBride J. Anxiety caused by abnormal result of cervical smear test: a controlled trial. BMJ 1990;300:440.

45. Stewart DA, Lickrish GM, Sierra S, Parkin H. The effect of educational brochures on knowledge and emotional distress in women with abnormal Papanicolaou smears. Obstet Gynecol 1993;81:280–282.

46. Hocutt JE Jr, Clark RC, Pfenninger JL. Papanicolaou testing and colposcopic screening. J Fam Pract 1992; 34:38–40.

47. Cecchini S, Bonardi R, Mazzotta A, Grazzini G, Iossa A, Ciatto S. Testing cervicography and cervicoscopy as screening tests for cervical cancer. Tumori 1993;79:22–25.

48. Ferris DG, Payne P, Frisch LE, Milner FH, diPaola FM, Petry LJ. Cervicography: adjunctive cervical cancer screening by primary care clinicians. J Fam Pract 1993;37:158–164.

49. Szarewski A, Cuzick J, Edwards R, Butler B, Singer A. The use of cervicography in a primary screening service. Br J Obstet Gynaecol 1991;98:313–317.

50. Blythe JG. Cervicography: a preliminary report. Am J Obstet Gynecol 1985;152:192–197.

51. Tawa K, Forsythe A, Cove JK, et al. A comparison of the Papanicolaou smear and the cervigram: sensitivity, specificity, and cost analysis. Obstet Gynecol 1988;71:229–235.

52. Hockstad RL. A comparison of simultaneous cervical cytology, HPV testing, and colposcopy. Fam Pract Res J 1992;12:53–60.

53. Nathan PM, Moss TR. Screening colposcopy in genitourinary medicine. Int J STD AIDS 1991;2:342–345.

54. Olatunbosun OA, Okonofua FE, Ayangade SO. Screening for cervical neoplasia in an African population: simultaneous use of cytology and colposcopy. Int J Gynecol Obstet 1991;36:39–42.

55. Rodney WM, Huff M, Euans D, Hutchins C, Clement K, McCall JW III. Colposcopy in family practice: pilot studies of pain prophylaxis and patient volume. Fam Pract Res J 1992;12:91–98.

56. Richart RM, Wright TC Jr. Controversies in the management of low-grade cervical intraepithelial neoplasia. Cancer 1993;71:1413–1421.

57. Kataja V, Syrjanen S, Jarvi RM, Yliskoski M, Saarikoski A, Syrjanen K. Prognostic factors in cervical human papillomavirus infections. Sex Trans Dis 1992;19:154–160.

58. Bauer HM, Greer CE, Chambers JC, Tashiro CJ, Chimera J, Reingold A, Manos MM. Genital human papillomavirus infection in female university students as determined by a PCR-based method. JAMA 1991;265:472–477.

59. Zazove P, Reed BD, Gregoire L, Gorenflo DW, Lancaster WD, Ruffin MT IV, Hruszcyzk J. Presence of human papillomavirus infection of the uterine cervix as determined by different detection methods in a low-risk community-based population. Arch Fam Med 1993;2:1250–1257.

60. Sedlacek TV, Sedlacek AE, Neff DK, Rando RF. The clinical role of human papilloma virus typing. Gyn Oncol 1991;42:222–226.

61. American College of Obstetricians and Gynecologists. Cervical cytology: evaluation and management of abnormalities. Technical Bulletin no. 183. Washington, DC: American College of Obstetricians and Gynecologists, 1993.

62. Cramer DW. The role of cervical cytology in the declining morbidity and mortality of cervical cancer. Cancer 1974;34:2018–2027.

63. Miller AB, Lindsay J, Hill GB. Mortality from cancer of the uterus in Canada and its relationship to screening for cancer of the cervix. Int J Cancer 1976;17:602–612.

64. Anderson GH, Boyes DA, Benedet JL, et al. Organisation and results of the cervical cytology screening programme in British Columbia, 1955–85. BMJ 1988;296:975–978.

65. Johanneson G, Geirsson G, Day N. The effect of mass screening in Iceland, 1965–1974, on the incidence and mortality of cervical carcinoma. Int J Cancer 1978;21:418–425.

66. Laara E, Day NE, Hakama M. Trends in mortality from cervical cancer in the Nordic countries: association with organized screening programmes. Lancet 1987;1:1247–1249.

67. Boon ME, de Graaf Guilloud JC, Rietveld WJ, Wijsman-Grootendorst A. Effect of regular 3-yearly screening on the incidence of cervical smears: the Leiden experience. Cytopathology 1990;1:201–210.

68. Costa MJ, Grimes C, Tackett E, Naib ZM. Cervicovaginal cytology in an indigent population: comparison of results for 1964, 1981 and 1989. Acta Cytol 1991;35:51–56.

69. Benedet JL, Anderson GH, Matisic JP. A comprehensive program for cervical cancer detection and management. Am J Obstet Gynecol 1992;166:1254–1259.

70. Sigurdsson K. Effect of organized screening on the risk of cervical cancer: evaluation of screening activity in Iceland, 1964–1991. Int J Cancer 1993;54:563–570.

71. La Vecchia C, Decarli A, Gentile A, et al. Pap smear and the risk of cervical neoplasia: quantitative estimates from a case-control study. Lancet 1984;2:779–782.

72. Clarke EA, Anderson TW. Does screening by Pap smears help prevent cervical cancer? A case-control study. Lancet 1979;2:1–4.

73. Aristizabal N, Cuello C, Correa P, et al. The impact of vaginal cytology on cervical cancer risks in Cali, Colombia. Int J Cancer 1984;34:5–9.

74. Berrino F, Gatta G, d'Alto M, et al. Efficacy of screening in preventing invasive cervical cancer: a case-control study in Milan, Italy. IARC Sci Publ 1986;76:111–123.

75. Herrero R, Brinton LA, Reeves WC, Brenes MM, De Britton RC, Gaitan E, Tenorio F. Screening for cervical cancer in Latin America: a case-control study. Int J Epidemiol 1992;21:1050–1056.

76. Skrabanek P. Cervical cancer screening. Lancet 1987;1:1432–1433.

77. Miller AB, Visentin T, Howe GR. The effect of hysterectomies and screening on mortality from cancer of the uterus in Canada. Int J Cancer 1981;27:651–657.
78. Yu S, Miller AB, Sherman GJ. Optimising the age, number of tests, and test interval for cervical screening in Canada. J Epidemiol Community Health 1982;36:1–10.
79. Brinton LA, Tashima KT, Lehman HF, et al. Epidemiology of cervical cancer by cell type. Cancer Res 1987; 47:1706–1711.
80. Eddy DM. Screening for cervical cancer. Ann Intern Med 1990;113:214–226.
81. International Agency for Research on Cancer Working Group on Evaluation of Cervical Cancer Screening Programmes. Screening for squamous cervical cancer: duration of low risk after negative results of cervical cytology and its implication for screening policies. BMJ 1986;293:659–664.
82. American Cancer Society. Guidelines for the cancer-related checkup: an update. Atlanta: American Cancer Society, 1993.
83. American College of Obstetricians and Gynecologists. Recommendations on frequency of Pap test screening. Committee Opinion no. 152. Washington, DC: American College of Obstetricians and Gynecologists, 1995.
84. American Academy of Family Physicians. Age charts for periodic health examination. Kansas City, MO: American Academy of Family Physicians, 1994. (Reprint no. 510.)
85. American College of Physicians. Screening for cervical cancer. In: Eddy DM, ed. Common screening tests. Philadelphia: American College of Physicians, 1991:413–414.
86. Canadian Task Force on the Periodic Health Examination. Canadian guide to clinical preventive health care. Ottawa: Canada Communication Group, 1994:884–889.
87. American Medical Association. AMA guidelines for adolescent preventive services (GAPS): recommendations and rationale. Chicago: American Medical Association, 1994.
88. Green M, ed. Bright Futures: guidelines for health supervision of infants, children and adolescents. Arlington, VA: National Center for Education in Maternal and Child Health, 1994.
89. American Academy of Pediatrics. Guidelines for health supervision II. Elk Grove Village, IL: American Academy of Pediatrics, 1988.
90. U.S. Bureau of the Census. Statistical abstract of the United States, 1993. 113th ed. Washington, DC: Bureau of the Census, 1993.
91. Weisman CS, Celentano DD, Hill MN, et al. Pap testing: opinion and practice among young obstetricians-gynecologists. Prev Med 1986;15:342–351.
92. Cervical cancer screening: summary of an NIH consensus statement. BMJ 1980;281:1264–1266.
93. Wright VC, Riopelle MA. Age at time of intercourse v. chronological age as a basis for Pap smear screening. Can Med Assoc J 1982;127:127–131.
94. Canadian Task Force on Cervical Cancer Screening Programs. Cervical cancer screening programs: summary of the 1982 Canadian task force report. Can Med Assoc J 1982;127:581–589.
95. Webb MJ, Sheehan TM. Invasive carcinoma of the cervix in young women. Aust NZ Obstet Gynaecol 1989; 29:47–51.
96. Miller BE, Flax SD, Arheart K, Photopulos G. The presentation of adenocarcinoma of the uterine cervix. Cancer 1993;72:1281–1285.
97. Van Wijngaarden WJ, Duncan ID. Rationale for stopping cervical screening in women over 50. BMJ 1993; 306:967–971.
98. Calle EE, Flanders WD, Thun MJ, Martin LM. Demographic predictors of mammography and Pap smear screening in US women. Am J Public Health 1993;83:53–60.
99. Mandelblatt J, Traxler M, Lakin P, Kanetsky P, Kao R. Mammography and Papanicolaou smear use by elderly poor black women. Harlem Study Team. J Am Geriatr Soc 1992;40:1001–1007.
100. Mandelblatt J, Gopaul I, Wistreich M. Gynecologic care of elderly women: another look at Papanicolaou smear testing. JAMA 1986;256:367–371.
101. Mandelblatt JS, Fahs MC. The cost-effectiveness of cervical cancer screening for low-income elderly women. JAMA 1988;259:2409–2413.
102. Kleinman JC, Kopstein A. Who is being screened for cervical cancer? Am J Public Health 1981;71:73–75.
103. Hayward RA, Shapiro MF, Freeman HE, et al. Who gets screened for cervical and breast cancer? Results from a new national survey. Arch Intern Med 1988;148:1177–1181.
104. Nasca PC, Ellish N, Caputo TA, Saboda K, Metzger B. An epidemiologic study of Pap screening histories in women with invasive carcinomas of the uterine cervix. NY State J Med 1991;91:152–156.
105. Mayer JA, Slymen DJ, Drew JA, Wright BL, Elder JP, Williams SJ. Breast and cervical cancer screening in older women: the San Diego Medicare Preventive Health Project. Prev Med 1992;21:395–404.

106. Harlan LC, Bernstein AB, Kessler LG. Cervical cancer screening: who is not screened and why? Am J Public Health 1991;81:885–891.

107. Koss LG. The Papanicolaou test for cervical cancer detection: a triumph and a tragedy. JAMA 1989;261:737–743.

108. Mandelblatt J, Traxler M, Lakin P, Kanetsky P, Thomas L, Chauhan P, Matseoane S, Ramsey E, and the Harlem Study Group. Breast and cervical cancer screening of poor, elderly, black women: clinical results and implications. Am J Prev Med 1993;9:133–138.

109. Marcus AC, Crane LA, Kaplan CP, et al. Improving adherence to screening follow-up among women with abnormal Pap smears: results from a large clinic-based trial of three intervention strategies. Med Care 1992;30:216–230.

110. Curtis P, Skinner B, Varenholt JJ, Addison L, Resnick J, Kebede M. Papanicolaou smear quality assurance: providing feedback to physicians. J Fam Pract 1993;36:309–312.

111. Paskett ED, White E, Carter WB, Chu J. Improving follow-up after an abnormal Pap smear: a randomized controlled trial. Prev Med 1990;19:630–641.

112. Pachiarz JA, Abbott MI, Gorman B, Henneman CE, Kuhl M. Continuous quality improvement of Pap smears in an ambulatory care facility. QRB Qual Rev Bull 1992;18:229–235.

113. El-Sadr W, Oleske JM, Agins BD, et al. Evaluation and management of early HIV infection. Clinical practice guideline no. 7. Rockville, MD: Agency for Health Care Policy and Research, 1994:60–65. (AHCPR Publication No. 94-0572.)

10. Screening for Prostate Cancer

RECOMMENDATION

Routine screening for prostate cancer with digital rectal examinations, serum tumor markers (e.g., prostate-specific antigen), or transrectal ultrasound is not recommended.

Burden of Suffering

Prostate cancer is the most common noncutaneous cancer in American men.[1] After lung cancer, it accounts for more cancer deaths in men than any other single cancer site. Prostate cancer accounted for an estimated 244,000 new cases and 40,400 deaths in the U.S. in 1995.[1] Risk increases with age, beginning at age 50, and is also higher among African American men. Because it is more common in older men, prostate cancer ranks 21st among cancers in years of potential life lost.[2] The age-adjusted death rate from prostate cancer increased by over 20% between 1973 and 1991.[3] The lifetime risk of dying from prostate cancer is 3.4% for American men.[3] The reported incidence of prostate cancer has increased in recent years by 6% per year, a trend attributed to increased early detection efforts.[4] Because local extension beyond the capsule of the prostate rarely produces symptoms, about one to two thirds of patients already have local extracapsular extension or distant metastases at the time of diagnosis.[5] Ten-year survival rates are 75% when the cancer is confined to the prostate, 55% for those with regional extension, and 15% for those with distant metastases.[6] The potential morbidity associated with progression of prostate cancer is also substantial, including urinary tract obstruction, bone pain, and other sequelae of metastatic disease.

Accuracy of Screening Tests

The principal screening tests for prostate cancer are the digital rectal examination (DRE), serum tumor markers (e.g., prostate-specific antigen [PSA]), and transrectal ultrasound (TRUS). The reference standard for these tests is pathologic confirmation of malignant disease in tissue obtained by biopsy or surgical resection. The sensitivity and specificity of screening tests for prostate cancer cannot be determined with certainty, however, because biopsies are generally not performed on patients with negative screening test results. False-negative results are unrecognized un-

119

less biopsies are performed for other reasons (e.g., abnormal results on another screening test, tissue obtained from transurethral prostatic resection). The resulting incomplete information about the number of true- and false-negative results makes it impossible to properly calculate sensitivity and specificity. Only the positive predictive value (PPV)—the probability of cancer when the test is positive—can be calculated with any confidence.

Even the PPV is subject to uncertainty because of the inaccuracies of the usual reference standard. Needle biopsy, the typical reference standard used for calculating sensitivity and specificity, has limited sensitivity. One study suggested that as many as 19% of patients with an initially negative needle biopsy (but abnormal screening test results) had evidence of cancer on a second biopsy.[7] Moreover, studies vary in the extent to which the gland is sampled during needle biopsy. Recent studies, in which larger numbers of samples are obtained from multiple sections of the gland, provide a different reference standard than the more limited needle biopsies performed in older studies. These methodologic problems account for the large variation in the reported sensitivity, specificity, and PPV of prostate cancer screening tests and the current controversy over their true values.

DRE is the oldest screening test for prostate cancer. Its sensitivity is limited, however, because the examining finger can palpate only the posterior and lateral aspects of the gland. Studies suggest that 25–35% of tumors occur in portions of the prostate not accessible to the examining finger.[8] In addition, Stage A tumors, by definition, are nonpalpable. Most recent studies report that DRE has a sensitivity of 55–68% in detecting prostate cancer in asymptomatic men,[9,10] but values as low as 18–22% have also been reported in studies using different screening protocols.[11,12] The DRE also has limited specificity, producing a large proportion of false-positive results. The reported PPV in asymptomatic men is 6–33%[10,13–15] but appears to be somewhat higher when performed by urologists rather than by general practitioners.[16]

Elevations in certain serum tumor markers (e.g., PSA and prostatic acid phosphatase) provide another means of screening for prostate cancer. In screening studies, a PSA value greater than 4 ng/dL has a reported sensitivity of over 80% in detecting prostate cancer in asymptomatic men,[10] although a sensitivity as low as 29% has also been reported in studies using different screening protocols.[11] Prostatic acid phosphatase has a much lower sensitivity (12–20% for Stage A and B disease) and PPV (below 5%) than PSA,[17] and its role in screening has largely been replaced by PSA. PSA elevations are not specific for prostate cancer. Benign prostatic conditions such as hypertrophy and prostatitis can produce false-positive results; about 25% of men with benign prostatic hypertrophy (BPH) and no malignancy have an elevated PSA level.[18]

In most screening studies involving asymptomatic men, the reported

PPV of PSA in detecting prostate cancer is 28–35%.[10,19–21] In many instances, however, other screening tests (e.g., DRE) are also positive. The PPV of PSA when DRE is negative appears to be about 20%.[22] It is unclear whether the same PPV applies when screening is performed in the general population. Participants in most screening studies are either patients seen in urology clinics or volunteers recruited from the community through advertising. Studies suggest that such volunteers have different characteristics than the general population.[23] For example, in one screening study, 53% of the volunteers had one or more symptoms of prostatism.[10] Since PPV is a function of the prevalence of disease, routine PSA testing of the general population, if it had a lower prevalence of prostate cancer than volunteers, would generate a higher proportion of false-positive results than has been reported in the literature. A significant difference in prevalence in the two populations has not, however, been demonstrated.

Several techniques have been proposed to enhance the specificity and PPV of the PSA test. The serum concentration of PSA appears to be influenced by tumor volume, and some investigators have suggested that PSA density (the PSA concentration divided by the gland volume as measured by TRUS) may help differentiate benign from malignant disease.[24–26] According to these studies, a PSA density greater than 0.15 ng/mL may be more predictive of cancer. Other studies suggest that the rate of change (PSA velocity), rather than the actual PSA level, is a better predictor of the presence of prostate cancer. An increase of 0.75 ng/mL or higher per year has a reported specificity of 90% and 100% in distinguishing prostate cancer from BPH and normal glands, respectively.[27] PSA values tend to increase with age, and investigators have therefore proposed age-adjusted PSA reference ranges.[28,29] Current evidence is inadequate to determine the relative superiority of any of these measures or to prove conclusively that any is superior to absolute values of PSA.[30] The most effective method to increase the PPV of PSA screening is to combine it with other screening tests. In a large screening study, the combination of an elevated PSA and abnormal DRE achieved a PPV of 49%. Even with this improved accuracy, however, combined DRE and PSA screening led to the performance of needle biopsies on 18% of the screened population,[10] raising important public policy issues (see below).

A large proportion of cancers detected by PSA screening may be latent cancers, indolent tumors that are unlikely to produce clinical symptoms or affect survival. Autopsy studies indicate that histologic evidence of prostate cancer is present in about 30% of men over age 50. The reported prevalence of prostate cancer in men without previously known prostate cancer during their lifetimes is 10–42% at age 50–59, 17–38% at age 60–69, 25–66% at age 70–79, and 18–100% at age 80 and older.[31–37] Recent autopsy studies have even found evidence of carcinoma in 30% of men aged 30–49.[38] Although patients who undergo autopsy may not be entirely representative of the general population, these prevalence rates, combined with census data,[39] suggest that millions of American men have prostate cancer. Fewer than 40,000 men in the U.S. die each year from prostate cancer, however, suggesting that only a subset of cancers in the population are clinically significant. Natural history studies indicate that most prostate cancers grow slowly over a period of many years.[40] Thus, many men with early prostate cancer (especially older men) will die of other causes (e.g., coronary artery disease) before their cancer becomes clinically apparent. Because a means of distinguishing definitively between indolent and progressive cancers is not yet available, widespread screening is likely to detect a large proportion of cancers whose effect on future morbidity and mortality is uncertain.

Recent screening studies have suggested, however, that cancers detected by PSA screening may be of greater clinical importance than latent cancers found on autopsy. Studies of asymptomatic patients with nonpalpable cancers detected through PSA screening have reported extracapsular extension, poorly differentiated cell types, tumor volumes exceeding 3 mL, and metastases in 31–38% of cancers that were pathologically staged.[20,41–43] In a retrospective review of radical prostatectomies performed on patients with nonpalpable prostate cancer detected by PSA screening, 65% had a volume greater than 1 mL, and surgical margins were positive in 26% of cases.[44] In a similar series, the mean tumor volume was 7.4 mL and 30% of the tumors had penetrated the capsule.[45]

The sensitivity of PSA for clinically important cancers was examined in a recent nested case-control study among 22,000 healthy physicians participating in a long-term clinical trial.[46] Archived blood samples collected at enrollment were compared for 366 men who were diagnosed clinically with prostate cancer during a 10-year follow-up period and 1,098 matched controls without cancer. PSA was elevated (>4 ng/mL) in 46% of the men who subsequently developed prostate cancer and 9% of the control group (i.e., sensitivity 46%, specificity of 91%). For cancers diagnosed within the first 4 years of follow-up, the sensitivity of PSA was 87% for aggressive cancers but only 53% for nonaggressive cancers (i.e., small, well-differentiated tumors), suggesting that PSA is more sensitive for clinically important disease. Given the low incidence of aggressive prostate cancer in this study (1% over 10 years), the reported specificity of 91% would generate a PPV (10–15%) that is lower than that reported from studies using routine biopsies (28–35%).[10] Furthermore, this study could not address the central question of whether PSA would have identified aggressive cancers at a potentially curable stage.

TRUS is a third means of screening for prostate cancer, but its performance characteristics limit its usefulness as a screening test. In most studies, TRUS has a reported sensitivity of 57–68% in detecting prostate cancer in asymptomatic men.[9,10] Because TRUS cannot distinguish between benign and malignant nodules, its PPV is lower than PSA. Although a PPV as high as 31% has been reported for TRUS,[47] its reported PPV when other screening tests are normal is only 5–9%.[15,19] Even when cancers are detected, the size of tumors is often underestimated by TRUS. The discomfort and cost of the procedure further limit its role in screening.

Effectiveness of Early Detection

There is currently no evidence that screening for prostate cancer results in reduced morbidity or mortality, in part because few studies have prospectively examined the health outcomes of screening. A case-control study found little evidence that DRE screening prevents metastatic disease; the relative risk of metastatic prostate cancer for men with one or more screening DREs compared with men with none was 0.9 (95% confidence interval, 0.5–1.7).[48] A cohort study also reported little benefit from DRE screening,[49] but its methodologic design has been criticized. Randomized controlled trials of DRE and PSA screening, which are expected to provide more meaningful evidence than is currently available, are currently under way in the U.S. and Europe.[50] The results of these studies, however, will not be available for over a decade. Therefore, recommendations for the next 10 years will depend on indirect evidence for or against effectiveness.

Indirect evidence that early detection of prostate cancer improves outcome is limited. Survival appears to be longer for persons with early-stage disease; 5-year survival is 87% for Stage A (nonpalpable) tumors, 81% for Stage B (palpable, organ-confined cancer), 64% for Stage C (local extracapsular penetration), and 30% for Stage D (metastatic).[5] Due to recent screening efforts, prostate cancer is now increasingly diagnosed at a less advanced stage. As with survival advantages observed with other cancers, however, it is not known to what extent lead-time and length biases account for differences in observed survival rates (see Chapter ii). The frequently indolent nature of prostate cancer makes length bias a particular problem in interpreting stage-specific survival data. Successful treatment of indolent tumors may give a false impression that "cure" was due to treatment. Prostate cancers detected through screening are more likely to be organ-confined than cancers detected by other means.[20] Proponents of radical prostatectomy often argue that such cancers are potentially curable by removing the gland. As already noted, however, current evidence is inadequate to determine with certainty whether these organ-confined tumors are destined to progress or affect longevity; thus the need for treatment is often unclear.

Even if the need for treatment is accepted, the effectiveness of available treatments is unproven. Stage C and Stage D disease are often incurable, and the efficacy of treatment for Stage B prostate cancer is uncertain. Currently available evidence about the effectiveness of radical prostatectomy, radiation therapy, and hormonal treatment derives largely from case-series reports without internal controls, usually involving carefully selected patients and surrogate outcome measures for monitoring progression (e.g., PSA levels).[51-55] Although men treated for organ-confined prostate cancer have a normal life expectancy, it is not clear how much their prognosis owes to treatment. The only randomized controlled trial of prostate cancer treatment, which compared radical prostatectomy with expectant management, reported no difference in cumulative survival rates over 15 years, but the study was conducted in the 1970s and suffered from several design flaws.[56,57] Randomized controlled trials to evaluate the effectiveness of current therapies for early disease are being launched in the U.S. and Europe, but results are not expected for 10–15 years.[58,59]

Some observational studies suggest that survival for early-stage prostate cancer may be good even without treatment. A Swedish population-based cohort study of men with early-stage, initially untreated prostate cancer found that, after 12.5 years, 10% had died of prostate cancer and 56% had died of other causes. The 10-year disease-specific survival rate (adjusted for deaths from other causes) for the study population was 85%. Cancer-related morbidity was significant, however. Over one third of the cancers progressed through regional extension, and 17% metastasized. The patient's age and the tumor stage did not significantly influence survival rates, but tumor grade (degree of differentiation) did affect survival; the 5-year survival rate was only 29% for poorly differentiated tumors.[59-61] Critics of the study have argued that the high survival rates were due to the relatively large proportion of older men and of tumors detected incidentally during transurethral prostatic resection, and that Swedish data are not generalizable to the U.S.[22,62] Other studies have reported similar results; in one series of selected men with well- and moderately differentiated cancer and extracapsular (nonmetastatic) extension, 5- and 9-year survival rates were 88% and 70%, respectively, without treatment.[63] Reported 10-year disease-specific survival for expectant management of palpable but clinically localized prostate cancer is 84–96%.[64-66] Finally, it is unclear whether reported survival rates in these studies, in which many cancers were detected without screening, are generalizable to screen-detected cancers.

Reviewers have attempted to compare the efficacy of treatment and watchful waiting by pooling the results of uncontrolled studies. An analysis of six studies concluded that conservative management of clinically localized prostate cancer (delayed hormone therapy but no surgical or radiation therapy) was associated with a 10-year disease-specific survival rate of 87% for men with well- or moderately differentiated tumors and 34% for poorly differentiated tumors.[67] The assumptions used in the model are not universally accepted, however.[68,69] A structured literature review concluded that the median annual rates of metastatic disease and prostate cancer mortality were 1.7% and 0.9%, respectively, without treatment.[70] This study was criticized for including a large proportion of patients with well-differentiated tumors and those receiving early androgen deprivation therapy.[71] Another review concluded that the annual rates for metastasis and mortality were higher (2.5% and 1.7%, respectively), but the review was limited to patients with palpable clinically localized cancers and excluded studies of cancers found incidentally at prostatectomy. In this population, disease-specific survival was estimated to be 83% for deferred treatment, 93% for radical prostatectomy, and 74% for external radiation therapy.[72] Thus, the effectiveness of treatment when compared with watchful waiting remains uncertain.

Uncertainties about the effectiveness of treatment are important because of its potentially serious complications. Needle biopsy, the diagnostic procedure performed on about 20% of men screened with DRE and PSA,[10] is generally safe but results in infection in 0.3–5% of patients, septicemia in 0.6% of patients, and significant bleeding in 0.1% of patients.[19,73–75] The potential adverse effects of radical prostatectomy are more substantial. Although urologists at specialized centers report operative mortality rates of 0.2–0.3%,[55,76] published rates in clinical studies and national databases range between 0.7% and 2%.[6,70,77–79] An examination of Medicare claims files estimated that the 30-day mortality rate was 0.5%.[80] The reported incidence of impotence varies between 20% and 85%,[11,51,70,79,81,82] depending on definitions for impotence and whether bilateral nerve-sparing techniques are used. Other complications of prostatectomy include incontinence (2–27%), urethral stricture (10–18%), thromboembolism (10%), and permanent rectal injuries (3%).[11,51,70,77,83–87] A study of Medicare patients who underwent radical prostatectomy in the late 1980s reported a 30-day operative mortality rate of 1% and a 4–5% incidence of perioperative cardiopulmonary complications. Over 30% wore pads to control wetting, 6% underwent corrective surgery for incontinence, and 2% required the use of an indwelling catheter. Over 60% reported partial erections and 15% underwent treatment for sexual dysfunction; 20% had dilatations or surgical procedure for strictures.[88] Studies of generally healthy and younger patients who have undergone radical prostatectomy in recent years have noted considerably fewer complications.[55]

Complications of radiation therapy include death (about 0.2–0.5%), acute gastrointestinal and genitourinary complications (8–43%), chronic complications requiring surgery or prolonged hospitalization (2%), impotence (40–67%), urethral stricture (3–8%), and incontinence (1–2%).[89] Three-dimensional conformal radiotherapy, a recently introduced technique for more precise, high-dose treatment, is reported to produce acute and chronic gastrointestinal or genitourinary complications in 55–76%

and 11–12% of patients, respectively.[90] Complication rates in studies of radiation therapy cannot be compared with confidence to reported complication rates for surgery because of differences in study designs and patient populations.

Recent decision analyses have combined current estimates of the benefits and harms to predict whether early treatment improves survival. A frequently cited decision analysis for men aged 60–75 concluded that, in most cases of clinically localized prostate cancer, neither surgery nor radiation therapy significantly improved life expectancy.[91] According to the model, treatment generally results in less than 1 year of improvement in quality-adjusted survival. In men over age 70, the analysis suggested that treatment was more harmful than watchful waiting. The study has been criticized because the subjects consisted largely of older men with low-volume, low-grade tumors and because the probability estimates used in the model may be incorrect.[71,92] Defenders of the study note that the data were adjusted for age and tumor grade (but not stage). Retrospective quality-of-life analyses have reported similar findings, noting that men who have undergone radical prostatectomy or radiation therapy for localized prostate cancer generally report lower quality of life due to impaired sexual, urinary, and bowel function than untreated men, even after controlling for the sexual and urinary dysfunction that is common in this age group.[93]

Other decision analyses have examined whether screening itself improves survival. Although older analyses suggested a modest benefit from screening,[94,95] more recent models have reached more pessimistic conclusions when quality-of-life adjustments are incorporated. One analysis concluded that screening and treatment result in an average loss of 3.5 quality-adjusted months of life.[96] Another decision analysis concluded that one-time screening of men aged 50–70 with either DRE or PSA would increase life expectancy by 0–0.2 days and 0.6–1.6 days, respectively, but quality-adjusted life would be decreased by 1.8–7.1 days and 2.1–9.5 days, respectively, per patient screened.[97] The assumptions and calculations used in this model have also been criticized.[98] A recent analysis of annual screening after age 50 concluded that screening would result in an average loss of 0.7 quality-adjusted life-years per patient screened.[98a]

Recommendations of Other Groups

The American Cancer Society[99] recommends an annual DRE for both prostate and colorectal cancer, beginning at age 40. It recommends that the annual examination of men age 50 and older should include a serum PSA measurement and that PSA screening should begin at age 40 for African American men and those with a family history of prostate cancer.[100] Similar recommendations have been issued by the American Urological Association[101] and the American College of Radiology.[102] In 1994, the Food and Drug Administration expanded the licensure for the PSA test to include screening.[103] The Canadian Task Force on the Periodic Health Examination (CTF) recommended against the routine use of PSA or TRUS as part of the periodic health examination; while recognizing the limitations of DRE, they concluded that the evidence was not sufficient to recommend that physicians discontinue use of DRE in men aged 50–70.[104] A 1995 report by the Office of Technology Assessment concluded that research to date had not determined whether or not systematic early screening for prostate cancer with PSA or DRE would save lives, and that the choice to have screening or forego it would depend on patient values.[105] The recommendations of the American College of Physicians and American Academy of Family Physicians are currently under review. In 1992, the American Urological Association concluded that the value of TRUS as an independent screening procedure has not been established and should be reserved for patients with an abnormal DRE or PSA.[106]

Discussion

In summary, prostate cancer is a serious public health problem in the United States, accounting for 35,000–40,000 deaths each year and substantial morbidity from disease progression and metastatic complications. Autopsy studies indicate, however, that these cases arise from a much larger population of latent prostate cancers that are present in over nine million American men. Although screening tests such as PSA have adequate sensitivity to detect clinically important cancers at an early stage, they are also likely to detect a large number of cancers of uncertain clinical significance. The natural history of prostate cancer is currently too poorly understood to determine with certainty which cancers are destined to produce clinical symptoms or affect survival, which cancers will grow aggressively, and which will remain latent. Prostate cancer has a complex biology with many unanswered questions about heterogeneity, tumor-host interactions, and prognostic stratification.

More fundamentally, there is no evidence to determine whether or not early detection and treatment improve survival. For men with well- and moderately differentiated disease, treatment appears to offer little benefit over expectant management, whereas the most aggressive tumors may have spread beyond the prostate by the time they are detected by screening. Observed survival advantages for men with early-stage disease may be due to length bias and other statistical artifacts rather than an actual improvement in clinical outcome. Although it is possible that treatment is beneficial for an unknown proportion of men with early prostate cancer, definitive evidence regarding effectiveness will not be available for over a decade, when ongoing randomized controlled trials are completed. In the interim years, during which thousands of deaths from prostate cancer are predicted, screening might be justified for its potential benefit were it not for its potential harms. Widespread screening will subject many men to anxiety from abnormal test results and the discomfort of prostate biopsies; aggressive treatment for screen-detected cancers will expose thousands of men to the risks of incontinence, impotence, death, and other sequelae without clear evidence of benefit. Decision-analysis models suggest that the negative impact of these complications on quality of life may outweigh the potential benefits of treatment, but the designs and assumptions of these models are controversial. The absence of proof that screening can reduce mortality from prostate cancer, together with the clear potential that screening will increase treatment-related morbidity, argues against a policy of routine screening in asymptomatic men.

The economic implications of widespread prostate screening, although not a principal argument against its appropriateness, also warrant attention. A full discussion of the cost effectiveness of prostate screening is beyond the scope of this chapter. Moreover, cost effectiveness cannot be properly determined without evidence of clinical effectiveness. Nonetheless, it is clear that routine screening of the 28 million American men over age 50,[39] as recommended by some groups, would be costly. Researchers have predicted that the first year of mass screening would cost the country $12–28 billion.[6,11] This investment might be worthwhile if the morbidity and mortality of prostate cancer could be reduced through early detection—given certain assumptions, prostate cancer screening might even achieve cost-benefit ratios comparable to breast cancer screening[107]— but there is currently little evidence to support these assumptions. The costs of this form of screening, with its emphasis on older men, is likely to increase in the future with the advancing age of the United States population; the number of American men over age 55 is expected to nearly double in the next 30 years, from 23 million men in 1994 to 44 million by 2020.[39]

There is some evidence that the recent increase in prostate screening may be generating a poorly controlled expansion in the performance of radical prostatectomies, creating an unnecessary iatrogenic morbidity in a growing population of surgical patients. The rising incidence of prostate cancer due to increased screening has been accompanied by a tripling in rates for radical prostatectomy in the U.S.[4] If early detection and treatment are effective, they are most likely to benefit men under age 70 rather than older men. As already noted, 10-year survival for early-stage prostate cancer approaches 90%. Thus, most men over age 70, who face a life expectancy of just over 10 years, are more likely to die of other causes than of prostate cancer. Subjecting these men to the risks of biopsy and treatment is often unwarranted, and many proponents of prostate screening therefore recommend against screening after age 70. Nonetheless, studies indicate that radical prostatectomy rates for men aged 70–79 increased 4-fold in 1984–1990, and the trend appears to be continuing in this decade. Population-based rates for prostatectomy in men aged 70–79, many of whom are unlikely to benefit from the procedure, appear to be the same as in men aged 60–69.[78] According to an American College of Surgeons survey, one out of three men undergoing radical prostatectomy in 1990 was age 70 or older.[79]

The lack of evidence regarding the benefits of prostate screening and the considerable risks of adverse effects make it important for clinicians to inform patients who express an interest in screening about the consequences of testing before they consent to screening. Although such counseling is proper for all forms of screening, the need for informed consent is especially important for prostate cancer screening because of current uncertainty about its effectiveness and because the proper choice for an individual is highly dependent on personal preferences. Screening is more likely to be chosen by men with strong fears of prostate cancer and by those who can accept the risks of incontinence, impotence, and other treatment complications. Screening is less likely to be chosen by men who are skeptical of the risks of cancer and the effectiveness of treatment and who have strong fears that treatment complications will jeopardize their quality of life.

CLINICAL INTERVENTION

Routine screening for prostate cancer with DRE, serum tumor markers (e.g., PSA), or TRUS is not recommended ("D" recommendation). Patients who request screening should be given objective information about the potential benefits and harms of early detection and treatment. Patient education materials that review this information are available.[108] If screening is to be performed, the best-evaluated approach is to screen with DRE and PSA and to limit screening to men with a life expectancy greater than 10 years. There is currently insufficient evidence to determine the need and optimal interval for repeat screening or whether PSA thresholds must be adjusted for density, velocity, or age.

The draft update of this chapter was prepared for the U.S. Preventive Services Task Force by Steven H. Woolf, MD, MPH. See also the relevant background paper: U.S. Preventive Services Task Force. Screening for prostate cancer: commentary on the recommendations of the Canadian Task Force on the Periodic Health Examination. Am J Prev Med 1994;10:187–193.

REFERENCES

1. Wingo PA, Tong T, Bolden S. Cancer statistics, 1995. CA Cancer J Clin 1995;45:8–30.
2. Ries LAG, Hankey BF, Miller BA, et al. Cancer statistics review 1973–88. Bethesda: National Cancer Institute, 1991. (NIH Publication no. 91-2789.)
3. Ries LAG, Miller BA, Hankey BF, Kosary CL, Harras A, Edwards BK, eds. SEER Cancer statistics review, 1973–1991: Tables and graphs. Bethesda: National Cancer Institute, 1994:371. (NIH Publication no. 94-2789.)
4. Lu-Yao GL, Greenberg ER. Changes in prostate cancer incidence and treatment in USA. Lancet 1994;343:251–254.
5. Mettlin C, Jones GW, Murphy GP. Trends in prostate cancer care in the United States, 1974–1990: observations from the patient care evaluation studies of the American College of Surgeons Commission on Cancer. CA Cancer J Clin 1993;43:83–91.
6. Kramer BS, Brown ML, Prorok PC, Potosky AL, Gohagan JK. Prostate cancer screening: what we know and what we need to know. Ann Intern Med 1993;119:914–923.
7. Keetch DW, Catalona WJ, Smith DS. Serial prostatic biopsies in men with persistently elevated serum prostate specific antigen values. J Urol 1994;151:1571–1574.
8. McNeal JE, Bostwick DG, Kindrachuk RA, et al. Patterns of progression in prostate cancer. Lancet 1986;1:60–63.
9. Catalona WJ, Smith DS, Ratliff TL, et al. Measurement of prostate-specific antigen in serum as a screening test for prostate cancer. N Engl J Med 1991;324:1156–1161.
10. Catalona WJ, Richie JP, Ahmann FR, et al. Comparison of digital rectal examination and serum prostate specific antigen in the early detection of prostate cancer: results of a multicenter clinical trial of 6,630 men. J Urol 1994;151:1283–1290.
11. Optenberg SA, Thompson IM. Economics of screening for carcinoma of the prostate. Urol Clin North Am 1990; 17:719–737.
12. Vihko P, Kontturi O, Ervast J, et al. Screening for carcinoma of the prostate: rectal examination and enzymatic radioimmunologic measurements of serum acid phosphatase compared. Cancer 1985;56:173–177.
13. Chodak GW, Keller P, Schoenberg HW. Assessment of screening for prostate cancer using the digital rectal examination. J Urol 1989;141:1136–1138.
14. Varenhorst E, Berglund K, Lofman O, Pedersen K. Inter-observer variation in assessment of the prostate by digital rectal examination. Br J Urol 1993;72:173–176.
15. Babaian R, Mettlin C, Kane R, et al. The relationship of prostate-specific antigen to digital rectal examination and transrectal ultrasonography. Cancer 1992;69:1195–1200.
16. Pedersen KV, Carlsson P, Varenhorst E, et al. Screening for carcinoma of the prostate by digital rectal examination in a randomly selected population. BMJ 1990;300:1041–1044.
17. Lowe FC, Trauzzi SJ. Prostatic acid phosphatase in 1993: its limited clinical utility. Urol Clin North Am 1993; 20:589–595.
18. Oesterling JE. Prostate-specific antigen: a critical assessment of the most useful tumor marker for adenocarcinoma of the prostate. J Urol 1991;145:907–923.
19. Cooner WH, Mosley BR, Rutherford CL Jr, et al. Prostate cancer detection in a clinical urological practice by ultrasonography, digital rectal examination and prostate specific antigen. J Urol 1990;143:1146–1152.
20. Catalona WJ, Smith DS, Ratliff TL, Basler JW. Detection of organ-confined prostate cancer is increased through prostate-specific antigen-based screening. JAMA 1993;270:948–954.
21. Bretton PR. Prostate-specific antigen and digital rectal examination in screening for prostate cancer: a community-based study. South Med J 1994;87:720–723.
22. Andriole GL, Catalona WJ. Using PSA to screen for prostate cancer: the Washington University experience. Urol Clin North Am 1993;20:647–651.
23. Demark-Wahnefried W, Catoe KE, Paskett E, Robertson CN, Rimer BK. Characteristics of men reporting for prostate cancer screening. Urology 1993;42:269–275.
24. Benson MC, Whang IS, Pantuck A, et al. Prostate-specific antigen density: a means of distinguishing benign prostatic hypertrophy and prostate cancer. J Urol 1992;147:815–816.
25. Bazinet M, Meshref AW, Trudel C, et al. Prospective evaluation of prostate-specific antigen density and systematic biopsies for early detection of prostatic carcinoma. Urology 1994;43:44–52.

26. Semjonow A, Hamm M, Rathert P, Hertle L. Prostate-specific antigen corrected for prostate volume improves differentiation of benign prostatic hyperplasia and organ-confined prostatic cancer. Br J Urol 1994;73:538–543.
27. Carter HB, Pearson JD, Metter EJ, et al. Longitudinal evaluation of prostate-specific antigen levels in men with and without prostate disease. JAMA 1992;267:2215–2220.
28. Oesterling JE, Jacobsen SJ, Chute CG, et al. Serum prostate-specific antigen in a community-based population of healthy men: establishment of age-specific reference ranges. JAMA 1993;270:860–864.
29. Dalkin BL, Ahmann FR, Kopp JB. Prostate specific antigen levels in men older than 50 years without clinical evidence of prostatic carcinoma. J Urol 1993;150:1837–1839.
30. Shinohara K, Wolf JS Jr, Narayan P, Carroll PR. Comparison of prostate specific antigen with prostate specific antigen density for 3 clinical applications. J Urol 1994;152:120–123.
31. Franks LM. Latent carcinoma of the prostate. J Pathol Bacteriol 1954;68:603–616.
32. Bostwick DG, Cooner WH, Denis L, et al. The association of benign prostatic hyperplasia and cancer of the prostate. Cancer 1992;70:291–301.
33. Breslow N, Chan CW, Dhom G, et al. Latent carcinoma of prostate at autopsy in seven areas. Int J Cancer 1977;20:680–688.
34. Baron E, Angrist A. Incidence of occult adenocarcinoma of the prostate after fifty years of age. Arch Pathol 1941;32:787–793.
35. Edwards CN, Steinthorsson E, Nicholson D. An autopsy study of latent prostatic cancer. Cancer 1953;6:531–554.
36. Halpert B, Schmalhorst WR. Carcinoma of the prostate in patients 70 to 79 years old. Cancer 1966;19:695–698.
37. Scott R Jr, Mutchnik DL, Laskowski TZ, Schmalhorst WR. Carcinoma of the prostate in elderly men: incidence, growth characteristics and clinical significance. J Urol 1969;101:602–607.
38. Sakr WA, Haas GP, Cassin BF, Pontes JE, Crissman JD. The frequency of carcinoma of the prostate in young male patients. J Urol 1993;150:379–385.
39. U.S. Bureau of the Census. Statistical Abstract of the United States, 1993. 113th ed. Washington, DC: U.S. Bureau of the Census, 1993.
40. Scardino PT. Early detection of prostate cancer. Urol Clin North Am 1989;16:635–655.
41. Epstein JI, Walsh PC, Carmichael M, Brendler CB. Pathologic and clinical findings to predict tumor extent of nonpalpable (stage T1c) prostate cancer. JAMA 1994;271:368–374.
42. Smith DS, Catalona WJ. The nature of prostate cancer detected through prostate specific antigen based screening. J Urol 1994;152:1732–1736.
43. Mettlin C, Murphy GP, Lee F, Littrup PJ, Chesley A, Babaian R, et al. Characteristics of prostate cancer detected in the American Cancer Society National Prostate Cancer Detection Project. J Urol 1994;152:1737–1740.
44. Scaletscky R, Koch MO, Eckstein CW, Bicknell SL, et al. Tumor volume and stage in carcinoma of the prostate detected by elevations in prostate specific antigen. J Urol 1994;152:129–131.
45. Stormont TJ, Farrow GM, Myers RP, et al. Clinical stage B0 or T1c prostate cancer: nonpalpable disease identified by elevated serum prostate-specific antigen concentration. Urology 1993;41:3–8.
46. Gann PH, Hennekens CH, Stampfer MJ. A prospective evaluation of plasma prostate-specific antigen for detection of prostatic cancer. JAMA 1995;273:289–294.
47. Lee F, Littrup PJ, Torp-Pedersen ST, et al. Prostate cancer: comparison of transrectal US and digital rectal examination for screening. Radiology 1988;168:389–394.
48. Friedman GD, Hiatt RA, Quesenberry CP Jr, et al. Case-control study of screening for prostatic cancer by digital rectal examinations. Lancet 1991;337:1526–1529.
49. Gerber GS, Thompson IM, Thistad R, et al. Disease-specific survival following routine prostate cancer screening by digital rectal examination. JAMA 1993;269:61–64.
50. Gohagan JK, Prorok PC, Kramer BS, Cornett JE. Prostate cancer screening in the Prostate, Lung, Colorectal and Ovarian Cancer Screening Trial of the National Cancer Institute. J Urol 1994;152:1905–1909.
51. Walsh PC, Partin AW, Epstein JI. Cancer control and quality of life following anatomical radical retropubic prostatectomy: results at 10 years. J Urol 1994;152:1831–1836.
52. Catalona WJ, Smith DS. 5-year tumor recurrence rates after anatomical radical retropubic prostatectomy for prostate cancer. J Urol 1994;152:1837–1842.
53. Hanks GE, Hanlon A, Schultheiss T, Corn B, Shipley WU, Lee WR. Early prostate cancer: the national results of radiation treatment from the Patterns of Care and Radiation Therapy Oncology Group stud-

ies with prospects for improvement with conformal radiation and adjuvant androgen deprivation. J Urol 1994;152:1775–1780.

54. Bagshaw MA, Cox RS, Hancock SL. Control of prostate cancer with radiotherapy: long-term results. J Urol 1994;152:1781–1785.

55. Zincke H, Oesterling JE, Blute ML, Bergstralh EJ, Myers RP, Barrett DM. Long-term (15 years) results after radical prostatectomy for clinically localized (Stage T2c or lower) prostate cancer. J Urol 1994;152:1850–1857.

56. Byar DK, Corle DK. VACURG randomized trial of radical prostatectomy for Stages I and II prostate cancer. Veterans Administration Cooperative Urological Research Group. Urology 1981;17(suppl): 7–11.

57. Graversen PH, Nielsen KT, Gasser TC, et al. Radical prostatectomy versus expectant primary treatment in stages I and II prostatic cancer: a 15-year follow-up. Urology 1990;36:493–498.

58. Wilt TJ, Brawer MK. The Prostate Cancer Intervention Versus Observational Trial: a randomized trial comparing radical prostatectomy versus expectant management for the treatment of clinically localized prostate cancer. J Urol 1994;152:1910–1914.

59. Johansson JE. Expectant management of early stage prostatic cancer: Swedish experience. J Urol 1994; 152:1753–1756.

60. Johansson JE, Adami HO, Andersson SO, et al. High 10-year survival rate in patients with early, untreated prostatic cancer. JAMA 1992;267:2191–2196.

61. Johansson JE. Watchful waiting for early stage prostate cancer. Urology 1994;43:138–142.

62. Walsh PC. Using prostate-specific antigen to diagnose prostate cancer: sailing in uncharted waters. Ann Intern Med 1993;119:948–949.

63. Adolfsson J. Deferred treatment of low grade stage T3 prostate cancer without distant metastases. J Urol 1993;149:326–329.

64. Adolfsson J, Carstensen J, Lowhagen T. Deferred treatment in clinically localised prostatic carcinoma. Br J Urol 1992;69:183–187.

65. Adolfsson J, Ronstrom L, Lowhagen T, Carstensen J, Hedlund PO. Deferred treatment of clinically localized low grade prostate cancer: the experience from a prospective series at the Karolinska Hospital. J Urol 1994;152:1757–1760.

66. Warner J, Whitmore WF Jr. Expectant management of clinically localized prostatic cancer. J Urol 1994;152:1761–1765.

67. Chodak GW, Thisted RA, Gerber GS, et al. Results of conservative management of clinically localized prostate cancer. N Engl J Med 1994;330:242–248.

68. Catalona WJ. Conservative management of prostate cancer [letter]. N Engl J Med 1994;330:1830–1831.

69. Scardino PT, Beck JR, Miles BJ. Conservative management of prostate cancer [letter]. N Engl J Med 1994; 330:1831.

70. Wasson JH, Cushman CC, Bruskewitz RC, Littenberg B, Mulley AG Jr, Wennberg JE, and the Prostate Disease Patient Outcome Research Team. A structured literature review of treatment for localized prostate cancer. Arch Fam Med 1993;2:487–493.

71. Walsh PC. Editorial comments on: A decision analysis of alternative treatment for clinically localized prostate cancer. J Urol 1993;150:1330–1331.

72. Adolfsson J, Steineck G, Whitmore W. Recent results of management of palpable clinically localized prostate cancer. Cancer 1993;72:310–322.

73. Desmond PM, Clark J, Thompson IM, et al. Morbidity with contemporary prostate biopsy. J Urol 1993;150:1425–1426.

74. Aus G, Hermansson CG, Hugosson J, et al. Transrectal ultrasound examination of the prostate: complications and acceptance by patients. Br J Urol 1993;71:457–459.

75. Hammerer P. Huland H. Systematic sextant biopsies in 651 patients referred for prostate evaluation. J Urol 1994;151:99–102.

76. Andriole GL, Smith DS, Ganeesh R, Goodnough L, Catalona WJ. Early complications of contemporary anatomical radical retropubic prostatectomy. J Urol 1994;152:1858–1860.

77. Catalona WJ, Avioli LV. Diagnosis, staging, and surgical treatment of prostatic carcinoma. Arch Intern Med 1987;147:361–363.

78. Lu-Yao GL, McLerran D, Wasson J, Wennberg JE. An assessment of radical prostatectomy: time trends, geographic variation, and outcomes. JAMA 1993;269:2633–2636.

79. Murphy GP, Mettlin C, Menck H, Winchester DP, Davidson AM. National patterns of prostate cancer treatment by radical prostatectomy: results of a survey by the American College of Surgeons Commission on Cancer. J Urol 1994;152:1817–1819.

80. Mark DH. Mortality of patients after radical prostatectomy: analysis of recent Medicare claims. J Urol 1994; 152:896–898.

81. Catalona WJ, Bigg SW. Nerve-sparing radical prostatectomy: evaluation of results after 250 patients. J Urol 1990;143:538–544.

82. Walsh PC. Radical prostatectomy, preservation of sexual function, cancer control. Urol Clin North Am 1987;14:663–666.

83. Andriole GL, Catalona WJ. Prostate carcinoma. Annu Rev Med 1994;45:351–359.

84. Narayan P, Jajodia P. Prostatic oncology. Clin Geriatr Med 1990;6:131–161.

85. Gibbons RP, Correa RJ, Brannen GE, et al. Total prostatectomy for localized prostatic cancer. J Urol 1984;131:73–77.

86. Ahmann FR. Dilemmas in managing prostate carcinoma (Pt 1): localized disease. Geriatrics 1985;40:34–42.

87. Middleton RG, Smith JA, Melzer RB, et al. Patient survival and local recurrence rate following radical prostatectomy for prostatic carcinoma. J Urol 1986;136:422–431.

88. Fowler FJ, Barry MJ, Roman A, et al. Patient-reported complications and follow-up treatment following radical prostatectomy: the national Medicare experience: 1988–1990. Urology 1993;42:622–629.

89. Shipley WU, Zietman AL, Hanks GE, et al. Treatment related sequelae following external beam radiation for prostate cancer: a review with an update in patients with stages T1 and T2 tumor. J Urol 1994;152:1799–1805.

90. Leibel SA, Zelefsky MJ, Kutcher GJ, Burman CM, Kelson S, Fuks Z. Three-dimensional conformal radiation therapy in localized carcinoma of the prostate: interim report of a phase 1 dose-escalation study. J Urol 1994; 152:1792–1798.

91. Fleming C, Wasson JH, Albertsen PC, Barry MJ, Wennberg JE, et al. A decision analysis of alternative treatment strategies for clinically localized prostate cancer. JAMA 1993;269:2650–2658.

92. Beck JR, Kattan MW, Miles BJ. A critique of the decision analysis for clinically localized prostate cancer. J Urol 1994;152:1894–1899.

93. Litwin MS, Hays RD, Fink A, Ganz PA, Leake B, Leach GE, Brook RH. Quality-of-life outcomes in men treated for localized prostate cancer. JAMA 1995;273:129–135.

94. Thompson IM, Rounder JB, Teague JL, et al. Impact of routine screening for adenocarcinoma of the prostate on stage distribution. J Urol 1987;137:424–426.

95. Love RR, Fryback DG, Kimbrough SR. A cost-effectiveness analysis of screening for carcinoma of the prostate by digital examination. Med Decis Making 1985;5:263–278.

96. Mold JW, Holtgrave DR, Bisonni RS, et al. The evaluation and treatment of men with asymptomatic prostate nodules in primary care: a decision analysis. J Fam Pract 1992;34:561–568.

97. Krahn MD, Mahoney JE, Eckman MH, Trachtenberg J, Pauker SG, Detsky AS. Screening for prostate cancer: a decision analytic view. JAMA 1994;272:773–780.

98. Miles BJ, Kattan MW, Giesler RB, et al. Screening for prostate cancer [letter]. JAMA 1995;273:1173–1174.

98a. Cantor SB, Spann SJ, Volk RJ, Cardenas MP, Warren MM. Prostate cancer screening: a decision analysis. J Fam Pract 1995;41:33–41.

99. American Cancer Society. Guidelines for the cancer-related checkup: an update. Atlanta: American Cancer Society, 1993.

100. Mettlin C, Jones G, Averette H, et al. Defining and updating the American Cancer Society guidelines for the cancer-related checkup: prostate and endometrial cancers. CA Cancer J Clin 1993;43:42–46.

101. American Urological Association, Executive committee report. Baltimore: American Urological Association, January 1992.

102. American College of Radiology, Resolution #36, approved October 1991.

103. Prostate specific antigen test approved. FDA Medical Bulletin, vol 25 no 1, February 1995:4.

104. Canadian Task Force on the Periodic Health Examination. Canadian guide to clinical preventive health care. Ottawa: Canada Communication Group, 1994:812–823.

105. Office of Technology Assessment. Costs and effectiveness of prostate cancer screening in elderly men. Washington, DC: Government Printing Office, 1995. (Publication no. OTA-BP-H-145.)

106. American Urological Association. Early detection of prostate cancer and use of transrectal ultrasound.

In: American Urological Association 1992 Policy Statement Book. Baltimore: American Urological Association, 1992.

107. Littrup PJ, Goodman AC, Mettlin CJ, et al. The benefit and cost of prostate cancer early detection. CA Cancer J Clin 1993;43:134–149.

108. Hahn DL, Roberts RG. PSA screening for asymptomatic prostate cancer: truth in advertising. J Fam Pract 1993; 37:432–436.

11. Screening for Lung Cancer

RECOMMENDATION

Routine screening for lung cancer with chest radiography or sputum cytology in asymptomatic persons is not recommended. All patients should be counseled against tobacco use (see Chapter 54).

Burden of Suffering

Cancer of the lung is the leading cause of death from cancer in both men and women in the U.S. An estimated 172,000 new cases will be diagnosed in 1995, with an estimated 153,000 deaths.[1] Lung cancer has one of the poorest prognoses of all cancers, with a 5-year survival rate of less than 13%.[1] Important risk factors for lung cancer include tobacco use and certain environmental carcinogen exposures. Tobacco is associated with 87% of all cases of cancer of the lung, trachea, and bronchus.[2]

Accuracy of Screening Tests

The chest radiograph (x-ray) and sputum cytomorphologic examination (cytology) lack sufficient accuracy to be used in routine screening of asymptomatic persons. The accuracy of the chest x-ray is limited by the capabilities of the technology and observer variation among radiologists. Suboptimal technique, insufficient exposure, and poor positioning and cooperation of the patient can obscure pulmonary nodules or introduce artifacts.[3] Radiologists frequently disagree on the interpretation of chest x-rays (interobserver variability). In one study, over 40% of these disagreements were considered potentially significant.[4] Most errors are false-negative interpretations, and pulmonary and hilar masses are among the most commonly missed diagnoses. From 10% to 20% of the incorrect radiologic diagnoses or indeterminate results require follow-up testing for clarification.[4] Interpretation of chest x-rays by primary care physicians is less accurate than interpretation by radiologists. Discrepancies were identified in 58% of chest x-rays read by both family physicians and radiologists.[5] Current radiographic technologies require greater than 20 doublings of tumor size to reach the 1 cm^3 needed for the lower limit of chest imaging sensitivity. By the time lung cancer is suspected on chest x-ray, micrometastatic dissemination has often occurred, limiting the effectiveness of early detection.[6]

Furthermore, the yield of screening chest radiography is low, largely due to the low prevalence of lung cancer in asymptomatic individuals, even those at high risk. Of the initial 31,360 screening x-rays of asymptomatic smokers in the National Cancer Institute (NCI) Cooperative Early Lung Cancer Detection Program, 256 (0.82%) were interpreted as "suspicious for cancer," and only 121 (0.39% of those screened) were diagnosed with lung cancer.[7] Other studies have confirmed a low yield of performing chest x-rays on asymptomatic persons.[8,9]

Sputum cytology is an even less effective screening test, largely due to its low sensitivity compared to chest x-ray.[6] Of the 160 lung cancers detected by dual screening in the NCI study, 123 (77%) would have been detected by chest x-ray alone and 67 (42%) would have been detected by cytologic examination alone.[7] The majority of incident cases detected in subsequent screenings were detected by chest x-ray.[10] In other trials using dual screening, sensitivity of chest x-ray ranges from 40% to 50%, versus 10% to 20% for sputum cytology.[11] Mass screening to detect lung cancer with tests that lack a high sensitivity will be inefficient.[12]

Effectiveness of Early Detection

Lung cancer is usually asymptomatic until it has reached an advanced stage, when the treatment outcome is poor. Five-year survival for all stages is 11–14%; for Stage I it is 42–47%.[1] Under optimal conditions, survival can be higher.[10,12,13] Early detection of Stage I cases through screening might be expected to improve survival, but the small amount of available evidence does not show that screening reduces lung cancer mortality.

The efficacy of chest radiographic screening for lung cancer was first investigated in the 1960s. A controlled prospective study involving over 55,000 persons found that those receiving chest x-rays every 6 months had a larger proportion of resectable tumors, but mortality for lung cancer remained the same when compared with controls who received examinations only at the beginning and end of the trial.[14] Similar findings were reported in the Philadelphia Pulmonary Neoplasm Research Project[15] and, more recently, in a case-control study.[16] In addition, the results of one of the three centers participating in the NCI Cooperative Early Lung Cancer Detection Program provide indirect evidence of the limited efficacy of radiographic screening. In this study, persons receiving chest x-rays and sputum cytology every 4 months had the same lung cancer mortality as persons advised to obtain annual testing.[17]

No prospective randomized study with adequate follow-up time has compared radiographic screening with no screening. A case-control study in Japan compared the screening histories of 273 fatal cases of lung cancer to 1,269 controls, and although the data suggest a trend toward a decreased risk of lung cancer mortality in those screened with chest x-rays (with or without sputum cytologic tests), the difference was not statistically significant.[18]

Three large clinical trials published by the NCI Cooperative Early Lung Cancer Detection Program examined the efficacy of dual screening (chest x-ray and sputum cytology) in over 30,000 male smokers aged 45 or older.[7,10,19–23] Two trials comparing annual dual screening with annual radiographic screening tested the incremental benefit of adding sputum cytology to radiographic screening.[20,21] The third trial, which compared dual screening every 4 months with advice to receive the same tests annually, examined the benefit of frequent dual screening compared to usual medical care.[22] In each study, lung cancer mortality did not differ between experimental and control groups. Although early-stage, resectable tumors were more common and 5-year survival significantly higher in groups receiving regular dual screening, lead-time and length biases may have been responsible for these findings. A randomized prospective trial of dual screening in Czechoslovakia produced similar results.[24] The investigators found no substantial difference in the number or causes of death between study groups.

The NCI is currently conducting the multicenter PLCO (prostate, lung, colorectal, and ovarian cancers) Trial, which will compare annual chest radiographic testing with usual care in both men and women.[25]

Recommendations of Other Groups

No organizations currently recommend routine screening of either the general population or of smokers for lung cancer with either chest x-rays or sputum cytology.[26–31]

Discussion

Lung cancer is the leading cause of cancer mortality. Although screening may increase early detection of resectable early cancers, controlled trials provide no significant evidence that lung cancer screening reduces mortality from this disease. To the weakness of the evidence for screening must be added the substantial costs of routine testing,[9] including false-positive results that lead to unnecessary expense and morbidity from follow-up procedures.[32] Current research and clinical trials of chemoprevention,[33] as well as research in early detection markers such as monoclonal antibodies,[6,34] may improve efficacy in prevention or early identification of lung cancer. Primary prevention—mainly through discouraging tobacco use—is a more effective strategy than screening to reduce lung cancer morbidity and mortality.[11] Unless ongoing trials find a benefit of periodic chest x-rays, the cost, inconvenience, and potential harms of screening cannot be justified.

CLINICAL INTERVENTION

Routine screening of asymptomatic persons for lung cancer with chest radiography or sputum cytology is not recommended ("D" recommendation). All patients should be counseled against tobacco use (see Chapter 54).

The draft update of this chapter was prepared for the U.S. Preventive Services Task Force by Kathlyne Anderson, MD, MOH, and Donald M. Berwick, MD, MPP.

REFERENCES

1. Wingo PA, Tong T, Bolden S. Cancer statistics, 1995. CA Cancer J Clin 1995;45:8–30.
2. Department of Health and Human Services. Reducing the health consequences of smoking: 25 years of progress. A report of the Surgeon General. Rockville, MD: DHHS, 1989. (Publication no. DHHS (PHS) 89-8411.)
3. Tape TG, Mushlin AL. The utility of routine chest radiographs. Ann Intern Med 1986;104:663–670.
4. Herman PG, Gerson DE, Hessel SJ, et al. Disagreements in chest roentgenogram interpretation. Chest 1975; 68:278–282.
5. Kuritzky L, Haddy RI, Curry RW Sr. Interpretation of chest roentgenograms by primary care physicians. South Med J 1987;80:1347–1351.
6. Mulshine JL, Tockman MS, Smart CR. Considerations in the development of lung cancer screening tools. J Natl Cancer Inst 1989;81:900–906.
7. The National Cancer Institute Cooperative Early Lung Cancer Detection Program. Summary and conclusions. Am Rev Respir Dis 1984;130:565–567.
8. Rucker L, Frye EB, Staten MA. Usefulness of screening chest roentgenograms in preoperative patients. JAMA 1983;250:3209–3211.
9. Hubbel FA, Greenfield S, Tyler JL, et al. The impact of routine admission chest x-ray films on patient care. N Engl J Med 1985;312:209–213.
10. Melamed MR, Flehinger BJ, Zamen MB, et al. Screening for early lung cancer: results of the Memorial Sloan-Kettering study in New York. Chest 1984;86:44–53.
11. Marfin AA, Schenker MB. Screening for lung cancer: effective tests awaiting effective treatment. In: Harber P, Balmes JR, eds. Occupational medicine state of the art review: prevention of pulmonary disease. Philadelphia: Hanley & Belfus, 1991:111–131.
12. Wright JL, Coppin C, Mullen BJ, et al. Surgical treatment of lung cancer: promise and problems of early diagnosis. Can J Surg 1986;29:205–208.
13. Moores DW, McKneally MF. Treatment of Stage 1 lung cancer (T1N0M0, T2N0M0). Surg Clin North Am 1987;67: 937–943.
14. Brett GZ. The value of lung cancer detection by six-monthly chest radiographs. Thorax 1968;23:414–420.
15. Weiss W. Survivorship among men with bronchogenic carcinoma: three studies in populations screened every six months. Arch Environ Health 1971;22:168–173.
16. Ebeling K, Nischan P. Screening for lung cancer: results from a case-control study. Int J Cancer 1987;40:141–144.
17. Sanderson DR. Lung cancer screening: the Mayo study. Chest 1986;89(suppl):324S.
18. Sobue T, Suzuki T, Naruke T, and the Japanese Lung-Cancer-Screening Research Group. A case-control study for evaluating lung-cancer screening in Japan. Int J Cancer 1992;50:230–237.
19. Berlin NI, Buncher CR, Fontana RS, et al. The National Cancer Institute Cooperative Early Lung Cancer Detection Program: results of the initial screen (prevalence): introduction. Am Rev Respir Dis 1984;130:545–549.
20. Flehinger BJ, Melamed MR, Zaman MB, et al. Early lung cancer detection: results of the initial (prevalence) radiologic and cytologic screening in the Memorial Sloan-Kettering study. Am Rev Respir Dis 1984;130:555–560.
21. Frost JK, Ball WC Jr, Levin ML, et al. Early lung cancer detection: results of the initial (prevalence) radiologic and cytologic screening in the John Hopkins study. Am Rev Respir Dis 1984;130:549–554.

22. Fontana RS, Sanderson DR, Taylor WF, et al. Early lung cancer detection: results of the initial (prevalence) radiologic and cytologic screening in the Mayo Clinic study. Am Rev Respir Dis 1984;130:561–565.

23. Tockman MS, Frost JK, Stitik FP, et al. Screening and detection of lung cancer. In: Aisner J, ed. Lung cancer. New York: Churchill Livingstone, 1985:25–40.

24. Kubik A, Parkin DM, Khlat M, et al. Lack of benefit from semi-annual screening for cancer of the lung: follow-up report of a randomized controlled trial on a population of high-risk males in Czechoslovakia. Int J Cancer 1990;45:26–33.

25. Kramer BS, Gohagan J, Prorok PC, Smart C. A National Cancer Institute sponsored screening trial for prostatic, lung, colorectal, and ovarian cancers. Cancer 1993;71:589–593.

26. American Cancer Society. Guidelines for the cancer-related checkup: an update. Atlanta: American Cancer Society, 1993.

27. American Academy of Family Physicians. Age charts for periodic health examination. Kansas City, MO: American Academy of Family Physicians, 1994. (Reprint no. 510.)

28. American College of Radiology. ACR standard for adult chest radiography, 2d ed. Reston, VA: American College of Radiology, 1993.

29. Tockman MS, Becklake MR, Clausen JL, et al. American Thoracic Society. Screening for adult respiratory disease. Am Rev Respir Dis 1983;128:768–774.

30. Eddy DM, ed. Screening for lung cancer. In: Common screening tests. Philadelphia: American College of Physicians, 1991:312–325.

31. Canadian Task Force on the Periodic Health Examination. Canadian guide to clinical preventive health care. Ottawa: Canada Communication Group, 1994:780–787.

32. Bailar JC 3d. Screening for lung cancer: where are we now? Am Rev Respir Dis 1984;130:541–542.

33. Benner SE, Lippman SM, Hong WK. Chemoprevention strategies for lung and upper aerodigestive tract cancer. Cancer Res 1992;52(suppl):2758S–2763S.

34. Tockman MS, Gupta PK, Myers JD, et al. Sensitive and specific monoclonal antibody recognition of human lung cancer antigen on preserved sputum cells: a new approach to early lung cancer detection. J Clin Oncol 1988;6:1685–1693.

12. Screening for Skin Cancer—
Including Counseling to Prevent Skin Cancer

RECOMMENDATION

There is insufficient evidence to recommend for or against either routine screening for skin cancer by primary care providers or counseling patients to perform periodic skin self-examinations. A recommendation to consider referring patients at substantially increased risk of malignant melanoma to skin cancer specialists for evaluation and surveillance may be made on other grounds (see *Clinical Intervention*). Counseling patients at increased risk of skin cancer to avoid excess sun exposure is recommended, based on the proven efficacy of risk reduction, although the effectiveness of counseling has not been well established. There is insufficient evidence to recommend for or against sunscreen use for the primary prevention of skin cancer.

Burden of Suffering

Over 800,000 new cases of skin cancer are diagnosed each year.[1] More than 95% of these are basal cell (BCC) and squamous cell (SCC) carcinomas, also referred to as nonmelanomatous skin cancers (NMSC). These are highly treatable and rarely metastasize, but local tissue destruction may cause disfigurement or functional impairment if these tumors are not detected early.[2] They account for approximately 2,100 deaths each year.[1] The risk of NMSC is increased by a personal history of NMSC; older age; light eyes, skin, or hair; poor ability to tan; and substantial cumulative lifetime sun exposure.[3-5]

Malignant melanoma (MM) is less common than NMSC but is far deadlier. An estimated 34,100 new cases and 7,200 deaths (2.2/100,000 population) from MM occurred in the U.S. in 1995.[1,6] The incidence rate varies by race: 9.2/100,000 in whites, 1.9/100,000 in Hispanics, and 0.7–1.2/100,000 in blacks and Asians.[7] In the past two decades, increases of 4%/year in MM incidence and nearly 2%/year in mortality have been reported.[6,8] With a median age at diagnosis of 53 years,[9] MM ranks second among adult-onset cancers in years of potential life lost per death.[10] Significant risk factors for MM besides white race include melanocytic pre-

141

cursor or marker lesions (e.g., atypical moles, certain congenital moles), increased numbers of common moles, immunosuppression, and a family or personal history of skin cancer, especially MM.[11-23] Fewer than 5% of the population have melanocytic precursor lesions, which have a high malignant potential and may account for as many as 40% of melanomas.[24] For persons with the rare familial atypical mole and melanoma (FAM-M) syndrome, the MM risk is increased 100-fold or more,[11-13] and the cumulative lifetime risk may approach 100%.[11] Persons with intermittent intense sun exposure or severe sunburns in childhood also appear to have an increased risk that varies by MM subtype.[17,19,20,25-27] Persons with poor tanning ability, freckles, or light skin, hair, and eye color may have a small increased risk of MM.[17-20,28]

Accuracy of Screening Tests

The principal screening test for skin cancer is physical examination of the skin by a clinician. Detection of a suspicious lesion constitutes a positive screening test, which then should be confirmed by skin biopsy. The true sensitivity and specificity of the skin examination are unknown.[29] In virtually all studies evaluating the accuracy of the skin examination, only clinically suspicious lesions were biopsied and only screen-positive persons were followed; therefore, sensitivity and specificity cannot be determined accurately. One study of persons presenting to free skin cancer screening clinics for screening by dermatologists estimated sensitivity of the examination using population incidence rates to estimate false-negative rates; sensitivities were 97% for MM, 94% for BCC, and 89% for SCC.[30] Two or more risk factors for skin cancer were present in 78% of those screened, however, so sensitivities may have been overestimated.[31] Among persons with positive screening clinic examinations, the likelihood of histologic confirmation has been reported to be 40% for MM, 43% and 57% for BCC, and 14% and 75% for SCC.[30,32] For persons presenting for skin examination to skin clinics, the likelihood of histologic confirmation given a clinical diagnosis of MM is 38–64% for dermatologists and 72–84% for skin cancer specialists.[33-35] Among patients biopsied by dermatologists who had histologically confirmed MM, the diagnosis was suspected in 62–85% of cases.[34,36] In a randomized community study evaluating screening by expert dermatologists, histologic examination confirmed the clinical diagnosis of SCC in 38% of cases and of BCC in 59%.[37] In vivo epiluminescence microscopy appears to improve dermatologists' diagnostic accuracy for skin lesions,[38,39] but it is not a practical screening tool for primary care physicians.

Primary care physicians and others lacking specialized training in dermatology would be expected to have greater difficulty in evaluating skin lesions. Several studies have reported that, compared to dermatologists, nondermatologists make significantly fewer correct diagnoses of skin lesions (including MM and BCC) from color photographs.[40–42] In one such study, at least five of six photographs of MM were correctly identified by 69% of the dermatologists but by only 12% of the nondermatologists; at least one of two atypical moles was recognized by 96% of the dermatologists but by only 42% of the nondermatologists.[40]

One factor affecting the yield of screening for skin cancer is the proportion of the body surface examined. Only 20% of MM occur on normally exposed body surfaces, in contrast to 85–90% of NMSC.[9,27] Dermatologists estimate that detection of MM is 2–6 times more likely with a total-body skin examination (TSE).[43,44] A second factor that affects yield is the frequency of examination. If the interval between examinations is too long, new cancers may not be detected before they have progressed to an advanced stage. There are no published data available, however, with which to determine the optimal frequency of examination in the general population; annual or biennial intervals have been recommended on the basis of clinical judgment. Poor patient compliance with recommendations for yearly total skin examinations may reduce the effectiveness of this intervention; in one study, only 22/524 (4.2%) patients returned for the yearly TSE that was recommended on the first visit.[45]

In terms of risk to the patient, no serious adverse effects associated with TSE and follow-up biopsy have been reported, and experts view it as acceptable and safe.[33] Embarrassment may be an adverse effect,[46] because modesty is one of the main reasons given for refusing a TSE.[44] Medical expenses may also be increased because office visits must be lengthened to accommodate complete undressing, "chaperoning," examination, and redressing,[46] and because more frequent referrals and biopsies are likely to result. There are no controlled studies evaluating any adverse effects of TSE.

Patient self-examination would be expected to be less accurate than physician examination in evaluating skin lesions. One study evaluated patients' ability to apply a seven-point checklist to the skin lesion that prompted their referral to a dermatologist.[35] The patient checklist had a sensitivity of 71%, specificity of 99%, and positive predictive value of 7% for MM diagnosis, using the dermatologist's clinical diagnosis as the "gold standard." The sensitivity and specificity using histologic diagnosis as the reference standard would likely be lower. No data were found evaluating the ability of patients to detect suspicious lesions, the accuracy of periodic skin self-examination, or the efficacy of self-examination instructions in reducing errors.

Effectiveness of Early Detection

Early treatment might reduce morbidity and disfigurement for patients with BCC and SCC,[2] but no studies were found that have evaluated whether such cancers discovered by screening have a better outcome than those which present clinically.

For MM, there have also been no controlled trials evaluating the impact of screening on morbidity or mortality. A time-series study of an educational campaign to encourage MM screening by primary providers in Scotland found a trend toward a reduction in both thick tumors ($p < 0.05$) and mortality (not statistically tested) in women (but not men) after the campaign.[47] Women were overrepresented in the screened population, which may explain the difference in mortality by sex. No control group was included, so differences due to historical trends or other factors cannot be excluded. The authors noted that in Denmark, which has comparable incidence rates, the MM mortality in women rose during this period.

More data are available on the effect of screening by dermatologists on MM thickness. In two large case series of persons with atypical moles who were screened regularly by dermatologists, all MM detected were either thin (< 0.89 mm) or in situ.[13,15] Time series in the general population, and cohort studies in FAM-M syndrome kindreds and in persons with a prior MM, have reported that screening by dermatologists detected significantly thinner tumors when compared to historical population, kindred, or personal index cases.[47-51] Several countries have reported a consistent decline over the past 3–4 decades in median thickness of MM, although this decline has not been directly linked to screening programs.[52,53] None of these studies used concurrent unscreened controls to differentiate the effects of screening programs from historical trends or lead-time and length biases.

If clinician screening does in fact result in detection of significantly thinner MM, mortality might be reduced. Case series and a prediction model (validated on subsequent incident cases) have reported that survival is directly related to lesion thickness at the time of resection.[9,39,54-56] For example, 5-year survival is 95–99% for persons with lesions ≤ 0.75 mm, 66–77% for 1.51–4.0 mm, 41–51% for 4.76–9.75 mm, and 5% for those with disseminated MM. The likelihood of recurrence after resection also correlates with lesion thickness. A MM < 1 mm thick is associated with an 8-year disease-free survival rate of 90%, compared with 74% for lesions 1–2 mm thick.[57] Although it is possible that lead-time and length biases account for some of these differences, these data suggest that persons in whom thinner MM are detected experience a better outcome than those detected with more advanced disease.

Data on the effectiveness of early detection by skin self-examination are limited. Preliminary analyses from a population-based case-control study retrospectively evaluating the efficacy of skin self-examination in patients with MM suggest a protective effect of skin awareness and self-examination,[58,59] but final results from this study have not yet been published.

Primary Prevention

Primary prevention of skin cancer may involve limiting exposure to solar radiation (by limiting sun exposure, avoiding tanning facilities, and wearing protective clothing) or applying sunscreen preparations. Although the effectiveness of these maneuvers has not been evaluated in clinical trials, avoiding sun exposure or using protective clothing is likely to decrease the risk of MM and NMSC, since both types of cancer have been associated with sun exposure in numerous cohort and case-control studies.[3,4,17,19,20,25–27] Use of tanning facilities has not been directly linked to cancer risk, but skin damage after use is common.[60,61] Many adolescents report using such facilities,[61] and severe sunburns occurring at a young age may increase the risk of subsequent melanoma.[17,19,20,26,27] The principal adverse effect associated with avoiding exposure to ultraviolet and other solar radiation is failure to acquire a suntan, which may be perceived as undesirable by some.[48,62,63]

The evidence that sunscreens prevent skin cancer is less clear. Sunscreen agents are formulated and tested for their ability to prevent the acute effects of solar ultraviolet radiation (i.e., sunburn).[64] Most currently available sunscreens block ultraviolet B (UVB) wavelengths, and a few block ultraviolet A (UVA) rays.[65] Only the physical sunblocks (e.g., zinc oxide, talc, etc.) block all solar rays. A randomized controlled trial evaluated the regular use of UVA- and UVB-blocking sunscreens by persons ≥40 years of age with previous solar keratoses (which are precursors of SCC, although their risk of malignant transformation is low).[66] The development of solar keratoses over a 6-month period was significantly reduced, implying that the risk of SCC may also be reduced. The generalizability of the results achieved by these highly motivated volunteers is unknown, and the study did not adequately describe investigator blinding, lesion classification, or the adequacy of randomization. Studies in albino laboratory rodents have also reported that sunscreens can reduce the incidence of tumors resembling human SCC after UV radiation.[64,67–69] Animal data are more limited for MM, but a recent study in mice reported that sunscreen failed to protect against UV radiation-induced increases in melanoma incidence, although it did prevent sunburn.[70] In a fish model, both UVA and visible light, which are not blocked by many currently available sunscreens, were highly effective in inducing melanomas.[71] Several case-control and cohort studies found either no effect or a significantly increased risk of BCC[72] and MM[73,74] in sunscreen users, after adjusting their risk estimates for phenotype (e.g., hair color, tendency to sunburn). The increased risk found in several of these studies may be due to residual confounding, since in all studies adjustment for phenotype reduced the crude risk estimates. It is also possible that sunscreens may increase skin cancer risk by encouraging susceptible persons to prolong exposure of greater skin surface areas to solar rays that are not blocked by most currently used sunscreens. There is as yet no direct evidence that sunscreens prevent skin cancer in humans, but clinical trials of sunscreen in humans are unlikely to be conducted due to cost and time constraints. Sunscreens are associated with mild to moderate side effects in 1–2% of users, including contact and photocontact dermatitis, contact urticaria, and comedogenicity, although these are readily reversible when use is discontinued.[65,75,76]

There are few data examining the effectiveness of counseling patients to protect themselves from sunlight. A case series evaluating counseling given at the time of removal of a skin cancer, and on a yearly basis thereafter, reported increased use of protective clothing and sunscreen and reduced deliberate tanning at 2–6-year follow-up.[77] This study included only the two-thirds of patients who complied with follow-up and was not able to determine how much of the effect seen was due to the surgery alone. There is also evidence from case series that public education can increase knowledge and beliefs about the health risks of sun exposure,[48,78] but cross-sectional surveys give conflicting results about whether knowledgeable persons act on this information.[62,63,79] Community and worksite educational interventions to reduce the risk of skin cancer, including one with a concurrent control group, have demonstrated significantly increased use of sun protection measures, such as hats, shirts, and staying in the shade, after the intervention.[80,81] Whether the results of such educational interventions can be generalized to clinician counseling is not known. No studies on the effectiveness of counseling in reducing skin cancer incidence or mortality were found.

Recommendations of Other Groups

The American Cancer Society recommends monthly skin self-examination for all adults[8] and physician skin examination every 3 years in persons 20–39 years old and annually in persons $\geq$ 40 years old.[82] The American Academy of Dermatology,[2,83] and a National Institutes of Health (NIH) Consensus Panel[84] recommend regular screening visits for skin cancer and patient education concerning periodic skin self-examinations. The NIH Consensus Panel also recommended that some family members of patients with MM be enrolled in surveillance programs.[84] The Canadian Task Force on the Periodic Health Examination does not recommend for or against routine screening for skin cancer or periodic skin self-examination, but suggests that TSE for a very select subgroup of individuals at high risk (e.g., those with familial atypical mole and melanoma syndrome) may be prudent.[85] The American Academy of Family Physicians recommends complete skin examination for adolescents and adults with increased recreational or occupational exposure to sunlight, a family or personal history of skin cancer, or evidence of precursor lesions; these recommendations are under review.[86] The American Cancer Society,[8] the American Academy of Dermatology,[2,83] the American Medical Association,[87] and the NIH Consensus Panel[84] all recommend patient education concerning sun avoidance and sunscreen use. The American Academy of Family Physicians recommends skin protection from ultraviolet light for all persons with increased exposure to sunlight.[86] The Canadian Task Force recommends avoidance of sun exposure and use of protective clothing, but it does not recommend either for or against sunscreen use for the prevention of skin cancer.[85] The American Academy of Dermatology,[88] the American Medical Association,[87] the American Cancer Society,[89] and the NIH Consensus Panel[84] have recommended avoiding artificial tanning devices.

Discussion

Basal cell and squamous cell skin carcinomas are very common but are slow-growing and rarely metastasize. It is unlikely that population screening would substantially improve the already excellent outcome of persons with these tumors. The principal potential benefit of periodic skin examination lies in discovering early MM. The sensitivity and specificity of skin examination by primary physicians, and the optimal frequency of such examinations, is unknown, however. MM is, in addition, uncommon in the general population (lifetime risk of about 1.0%).[90] Since 99% of patients who would be examined annually under a policy of routine screening would never have MM, it is also important to consider the potential adverse effects as well as the cost/benefit ratio of skin cancer screening. Neither of these has been adequately evaluated.[33,39] No controlled studies have demonstrated that screening for MM by primary providers improves outcome, although a time series study suggests a possible mortality benefit. There is thus weak evidence that screening by primary clinicians is effective in improving clinical outcome. In persons at very high risk for MM (i.e., those with melanocytic precursor or marker lesions), referral to skin cancer specialists for evaluation may be justified based on high burden of suffering, minimal adverse effects of TSE, and greater accuracy of the TSE by such specialists; however, there is no direct evidence that screening this population reduces mortality. There is currently only limited evidence of the efficacy of skin self-examination in reducing melanoma mortality, but preliminary results from a population-based case-control study appear promising.

There is fair evidence of the efficacy and safety of sun avoidance and use of protective clothing for the prevention of skin cancer, and weaker evidence to support avoiding artificial tanning devices. There is also fair evidence from one randomized controlled trial, supported by animal data, that sunscreens that block UVA and UVB rays are efficacious in preventing squamous cell cancer precursors, but data are limited on the efficacy of sunscreens in preventing skin cancer. There is also good evidence of mild, reversible adverse effects of sunscreens. Community or worksite educational interventions may increase the use of these sun protection measures, but the effectiveness of clinician counseling in modifying such behaviors is not established.

CLINICAL INTERVENTION

There is insufficient evidence to recommend for or against routine screening for skin cancer by primary care providers using total-body skin examination ("C" recommendation). Clinicians should remain alert for skin lesions with malignant features (i.e., asymmetry, border irregularity, color variability, diameter > 6 mm, or rapidly changing lesions)[84] when examining patients for other reasons, particularly patients with established risk factors. Such risk factors include clinical evidence of melanocytic precursor or marker lesions (e.g., atypical moles, certain congenital moles), large numbers of common moles, immunosuppression, a family or personal history of skin cancer, substantial cumulative lifetime sun exposure, intermittent intense sun exposure or severe sunburns in childhood, freckles, poor tanning ability, and light skin, hair, and eye color. Appropriate biopsy specimens should be taken of suspicious lesions.

Persons with melanocytic precursor or marker lesions (e.g., atypical moles [also called dysplastic nevi], certain congenital nevi, familial atypical mole and melanoma syndrome) are at substantially increased risk for MM. A recommendation to consider referring these patients to skin cancer specialists for evaluation and surveillance may be made on the grounds of patient preference or anxiety due to high burden of suffering, the greater accuracy of TSE when performed by such specialists, and the relatively limited adverse effects from TSE and follow-up skin biopsy, although evidence of benefit from such referral is lacking.

There is also insufficient evidence to recommend for or against counseling patients to perform periodic self-examination of the skin ("C" recommendation). Clinicians may wish to educate patients with established risk factors for skin cancer (see above) concerning signs and symptoms suggesting cutaneous malignancy and the possible benefits of periodic self-examination.

Avoidance of sun exposure, especially between the hours of 10:00 AM and 3:00 PM,[65] and the use of protective clothing such as shirts and hats when outdoors are recommended for adults and children at increased risk of skin cancer (see above) ("B" recommendation). Counseling such patients to avoid excess sun exposure and use protective clothing is recommended, based on the established efficacy of risk reduction from sun avoidance, the potential for large health benefits, low cost, and low risk of

adverse effects from such counseling, even though the effectiveness of such counseling is less well established ("C" recommendation).

There is insufficient evidence to recommend for or against counseling patients to use sunscreens to prevent skin cancer ("C" recommendation). The routine use of sunscreens that block both UVA and UVB radiation may be appropriate for persons who have previously had solar keratosis and who cannot avoid sun exposure, in order to prevent additional solar keratoses, which have a small malignant potential.

The draft update of this chapter was prepared for the U.S. Preventive Services Task Force by Carolyn DiGuiseppi, MD, MPH.

REFERENCES

1. Wingo PA, Tong T, Bolden S, et al. Cancer statistics, 1995. CA Cancer J Clin 1995;45:8–30.
2. Committee on Guidelines of Care, American Academy of Dermatology. Guidelines of care for basal cell carcinoma. J Am Acad Dermatol 1992;26:117–120.
3. Glass AG, Hoover RN. The emerging epidemic of melanoma and squamous cell skin cancer. JAMA 1989; 262:2097–2100.
4. Urback R. Incidence of nonmelanoma skin cancer. Dermatol Clin 1991;9:751–755.
5. Karagas MR, Stukel TA, Greenberg ER, et al. Risk of subsequent basal cell carcinoma and squamous cell carcinoma of the skin among patients with prior skin cancer. JAMA 1992;267;3305–3310.
6. Centers for Disease Control and Prevention. Deaths from melanoma—United States, 1973–1992. MMWR 1995;44:337, 343–347.
7. American Cancer Society. Cancer facts and figures for minority Americans—1991. Atlanta: American Cancer Society, 1991:5.
8. American Cancer Society. Cancer facts and figures—1995. Atlanta: American Cancer Society, 1995.
9. Koh HK. Cutaneous melanoma. N Engl J Med 1991;325:171–182.
10. Albert VA, Koh HK, Geller AC, et al. Years of potential life lost: another indicator of the impact of cutaneous malignant melanoma on society. J Am Acad Dermatol 1990;23:308–310.
11. Greene MH, Clark WH, Tucker MA, et al. High risk of malignant melanoma in melanoma-prone families with dysplastic nevi. Ann Intern Med 1985;102:458–465.
12. MacKie RM, McHenry P, Hole D. Accelerated detection with prospective surveillance for cutaneous malignant melanoma in high-risk groups. Lancet 1993;341:1618–1620.
13. Rigel DS, Rivers JK, Kopf AW, et al. Dysplastic nevi. Markers for increased risk for melanoma. Cancer 1989; 63:386–389.
14. Halpern AC, Guerry D IV, Elder DE, et al. Dysplastic nevi as risk markers of sporadic (nonfamilial) melanoma. Arch Dermatol 1991;127:995–999.
15. Tiersten AD, Grin CM, Kopf AW, et al. Prospective follow-up for malignant melanoma in patients with atypical-mole (dysplastic-nevus) syndrome. J Dermatol Surg Oncol 1991;17:44–48.
16. Lorentzen M, Pers M, Bretteville-Jensen G. The incidence of malignant transformation in giant pigmented nevi. Scand J Plast Reconstr Surg 1977;11:163–167.
17. Holman CDJ, Armstrong BK, Heenan PJ, et al. The causes of malignant melanoma: results from the West Australian Lions Melanoma Research Project. Recent Results Cancer Res 1986;102:18–37.
18. Reynolds P, Austin DF. Epidemiologic-based screening strategies for malignant melanoma of the skin. Prog Clin Biol Res 1984;156:245–254.
19. Evans RD, Kopf AW, Lew RA, et al. Risk factors for the development of malignant melanoma—I: review of case-control studies. J Dermatol Surg Oncol 1988;14:393–408.
20. Dubin N, Moseson M, Pasternack BS. Sun exposure and malignant melanoma among susceptible individuals. Environ Health Perspect 1989;81:139–151.
21. Tucker MA, Misfeldt D, Coleman CN, et al. Cutaneous malignant melanoma after Hodgkins's disease. Ann Intern Med 1985;102:37–41.

22. Greene MH, Young TI, Clark WH Jr. Malignant melanoma in renal-transplant recipients. Lancet 1981;1:1196–1199.
23. Tucker MA, Boice JK Jr, Hoffman DA. Second cancer following cutaneous melanoma and cancers of the brain, thyroid, connective tissue, bone, and eye in Connecticut, 1935–82. Natl Cancer Inst Monogr 1985;68:161–189.
24. Rhodes AR. Melanocytic precursors of cutaneous melanoma. Estimated risks and guidelines for management. Med Clin North Am 1986;70:3–37.
25. Nelemans PJ, Groenendal H, Kiemeney LALM, et al. Effect of intermittent exposure to sunlight on melanoma risk among indoor workers and sun-sensitive individuals. Environ Health Perspect 1993;101:252–255.
26. Cascinelli N, Marchesini R. Increasing incidence of cutaneous melanoma, ultraviolet radiation and the clinician. Photochem Photobiol 1989;50:497–505.
27. Koh HK, Kligler BE, Lew RA. Sunlight and cutaneous malignant melanoma: evidence for and against causation. Photochem Photobiol 1990;51:765–779.
28. Weinstock MA, Colditz GA, Willett WC, et al. Melanoma and the sun: the effect of swimsuits and a "healthy" tan on the risk of nonfamilial malignant melanoma in women. Am J Epidemiol 1991;134:462–470.
29. Miller AB, Chamberlain J, Day NE, et al. Report on a workshop of the UICC project on evaluation of screening for cancer. Int J Cancer 1990;46:761–769.
30. Koh HK, Caruso A, Gage I, et al. Evaluation of melanoma/skin cancer screening in Massachusetts. Cancer 1990;65:375–379.
31. Koh HK, Geller AC, Miller DR, et al. Who is being screened for melanoma/skin cancer? Characteristics of persons screened in Massachusetts. J Am Acad Dermatol 1991;24:271–277.
32. Bolognia JL, Berwick M, Fine JA. Complete follow-up and evaluation of a skin cancer screening in Connecticut. J Am Acad Dermatol 1990;23:1098–1106.
33. Koh HK, Lew RA, Prout MN. Screening for melanoma/skin cancer: theoretic and practical considerations. J Am Acad Dermatol 1989;20:159–172.
34. Grin CM, Kopf AW, Welkovich B, et al. Accuracy in the clinical diagnosis of malignant melanoma. Arch Dermatol 1990;126:763–766.
35. Keefe M, Dick DC, Wakeel RA. A study of the value of the seven-point checklist in distinguishing benign pigmented lesions from melanoma. Clin Exp Dermatol 1990;15:167–171.
36. Rampen FHJ, Rumke P. Referral pattern and accuracy of clinical diagnosis of cutaneous melanoma. Acta Dermato-Venereol (Stockh) 1988;68:61–64.
37. Green A, Leslie D, Weedon D. Diagnosis of skin cancer in the general population: clinical accuracy in the Nambour survey. Med J Aust 1988;148:447–450.
38. Steiner A, Pehamberger H, Wolff K. In vivo epiluminescence microscopy of pigmented skin lesions. II. Diagnosis of small pigmented skin lesions and early detection of malignant melanoma. J Am Acad Dermatol 1987;17:584–591.
39. Friedman RJ, Rigel DS, Silverman MK, et al. Malignant melanoma in the 1990s: the continued importance of early detection and the role of physician examination and self-examination of the skin. CA Cancer J Clin 1991;41:201–226.
40. Cassileth BR, Clark WH, Lusk EJ. How well do physicians recognize melanoma and other problem lesions? J Am Acad Dermatol 1986;14:555–560.
41. Ramsey DL, Fox AB. The ability of primary care physicians to recognize the common dermatoses. Arch Dermatol 1981;117:620–622.
42. Wagner RF, Wagner D, Tomich JM, et al. Diagnoses of skin diseases: dermatologists vs. nondermatologists. J Dermatol Surg Oncol 1985;11:476–479.
43. Rigel DS, Friedman RJ, Kopf AW, et al. Importance of complete cutaneous examination for the detection of malignant melanoma. J Am Acad Dermatol 1986;14:857–860.
44. Lookingbill DP. Yield from a complete skin examination: findings in 1157 new dermatology patients. J Am Acad Dermatol 1988;18:31–37.
45. Lee G, Massa MC, Welykyj S, et al. Yield from total skin examination and effectiveness of skin cancer awareness program: findings in 874 new dermatology patients. Cancer 1991;67:202–205.
46. Epstein E. Crucial importance of the complete skin examination [letter]. J Am Acad Dermatol 1985;13:151–153.
47. MacKie RM, Hole D. Audit of public education campaign to encourage earlier detection of malignant melanoma. BMJ 1992;304:1012–1015.

48. Theobald T, Marks R, Hill D, et al. "Goodbye Sunshine": effects of a television program about melanoma on beliefs, behavior, and melanoma thickness. J Am Acad Dermatol 1991;25:717–723.

49. Masri GD, Clark WH Jr, Guerry D VI, et al. Screening and surveillance of patients at high risk for malignant melanoma result in detection of earlier disease. J Am Acad Dermatol 1990;22:1042–1048.

50. Vasen HFA, Bergman W, Van Haeringen A, et al. The familial dysplastic nevus syndrome. Natural history and the impact of screening on prognosis. A study of nine families in the Netherlands. Eur J Cancer Clin Oncol 1989;25:337–341.

51. Titus-Ernstoff L, Barnhill RL, Ernstoff MS, et al. Usefulness of frequent skin examination for the early detection of second primary cutaneous melanoma. Cancer Detect Prev 1989;13:317–321.

52. Sober AJ, Lew RA, Koh HK, et al. Epidemiology of cutaneous melanoma: an update. Dermatol Clin 1991;9:617–629.

53. Drzewiecki KT, Frydman H, Andersen PK, et al. Malignant melanoma: changing trends in factors influencing metastasis-free survival from 1964 to 1982. Cancer 1990;65:362–366.

54. Clark WH Jr, Elder DE, Guerry D IV, et al. Model predicting survival in stage I melanoma based on tumor progression. J Natl Cancer Inst 1989;81:1893–1904.

55. Keefe M, MacKie RM. The relationship between risk of death from clinical stage 1 cutaneous melanoma and thickness of primary tumour: no evidence for steps in risk. Br J Cancer 1991;64:598–602.

56. Ho VC, Sober AJ. Therapy for cutaneous melanoma: an update. J Am Acad Dermatol 1990;22:159–176.

57. Veronesi U, Cascinelli N. Narrow excision (1-cm margin): a safe procedure for thin cutaneous melanoma. Arch Surg 1991;126:438–441.

58. Berwick M, Roush G, Thompson WD. Evaluating the efficacy of skin self-exam and other surveillance measures in persons at various levels of risk for cutaneous malignant melanoma: an ongoing case-control study. Prog Clin Biol Res 1989;293:297–305.

59. Berwick M, Dubin N, Roush G, et al. Early detection and lethal melanoma in Connecticut: a preliminary analysis. In: Gallagher RP, Elwood JM, eds. Epidemiological aspects of cutaneous malignant melanoma. Boston: Kluwer Academic Publishers, 1994:265–271.

60. The darker side of indoor tanning: skin cancer, eye damage, skin aging, allergic reactions. Rockville, MD: U.S. Public Health Service, 1987. (DHHS Publication no. FDA-87-8270.)

61. Oliphant JA, Forster JL, McBride CM. The use of commercial tanning facilities by suburban Minnesota adolescents. Am J Public Health 1994;84:476–478.

62. Cockburn J, Hennrikus D, Scott R, et al. Adolescent use of sun-protection measures. Med J Aust 1989;151:136–140.

63. Keesling B, Friedman HS. Psychosocial factors in sunbathing and sunscreen use. Health Psychol 1987;6:477–493.

64. Young AR. Senescence and sunscreens. Br J Dermatol 1990;122:S111–S114.

65. O'Donoghue MN. Sunscreen: one weapon against melanoma. Dermatol Clin 1991;9:789–793.

66. Thompson SC, Jolley D, Marks R. Reduction of solar keratoses by regular sunscreen use. N Engl J Med 1993;329:1147–1151.

67. Gurish MF, Robert LK, Krueger GG, et al. The effect of various sunscreen agents on skin damage and the introduction of tumor susceptibility in mice subjected to ultraviolet irradiation. J Invest Dermatol 1981;76:246–251.

68. Kligman LH, Akin FJ, Kligman AM. Sunscreens prevent ultraviolet photocarcinogenesis. J Am Acad Dermatol 1980;3:30–35.

69. Snyder DS, May M. Ability of PABA to protect mammalian skin from ultraviolet light-induced skin tumors and actinic damage. J Invest Dermatol 1975;65:543–546.

70. Wolf P, Donawho CK, Kripke ML. Effect of sunscreens on UV radiation-induced enhancement of melanoma growth in mice. J Natl Cancer Inst 1994;86:99–105.

71. Setlow RB, Grist E, Thompson K, et al. Wavelengths effective in induction of malignant melanoma. Proc Natl Acad Sci USA 1991;90:6666–6670.

72. Hunter DJ, Colditz GA, Stampfer MJ, et al. Risk factors for basal cell carcinoma in a prospective cohort of women. Ann Epidemiol 1990;1:13–23.

73. Beitner H, Norell SE, Ringborg U, et al. Malignant melanoma: aetiological importance of individual pigmentation and sun exposure. Br J Dermatol 1990;122:43–51.

74. Holman CDJ, Armstrong BK, Heenan PJ. Relationship of cutaneous malignant melanoma to individual sunlight-exposure habits. J Natl Cancer Inst 1986;76:403–414.

75. Dromgoole SH, Maibach HI. Sunscreening agent intolerance: contact and photocontact sensitization and contact urticaria. J Am Acad Dermatol 1990;22:1068–1078.

76. Farr PM, Diffey BL. Adverse effects of sunscreens in photosensitive patients. Lancet 1989;1:429–430.

77. Robinson JK. Compensation strategies in sun protection behaviors by a population with nonmelanoma skin cancer. Prev Med 1992;21:754–765.

78. Putnam GL, Yanagisako KL. Skin cancer comic book: evaluation of a public educational vehicle. Cancer Detect Prev 1982;5:349–356.

79. Public awareness of the effects of sun on skin. A survey conducted for the American Academy of Dermatology. Princeton, NJ: Opinion Research Corporation, 1987.

80. Borland RM, Hocking B, Godkin GA, et al. The impact of a skin cancer control education package for outdoor workers. Med J Aust 1991;154:686–688.

81. Lombard D, Neubauer TE, Canfield D, et al. Behavioral community intervention to reduce the risk of skin cancer. J Appl Behav Anal 1991;24:677–686.

82. American Cancer Society. Guidelines for the cancer-related checkup: an update. Atlanta: American Cancer Society, 1993.

83. Committee on Guidelines of Care, American Academy of Dermatology. Guidelines of care for nevi I (nevocellular nevi and seborrheic keratoses). J Am Acad Dermatol 1992;26:629–631.

84. NIH Consensus Development Panel on Early Melanoma. Diagnosis and treatment of early melanoma. JAMA 1992;268:1314–1319.

85. Canadian Task Force on the Periodic Health Examination. Canadian guide to clinical preventive health care. Ottawa: Canada Communication Group, 1994:850–861.

86. American Academy of Family Physicians. Age charts for periodic health examination. Kansas City, MO: American Academy of Family Physicians, 1994. (Reprint no. 510.)

87. Council on Scientific Affairs. Harmful effects of ultraviolet radiation. JAMA 1989;262:380–384.

88. Bickers DR, Epstein JH, Fitzpatrick TB, et al. Risks and benefits from high-intensity ultraviolet A sources used for cosmetic purposes. J Am Acad Dermatol 1985;12:380–381.

89. Fry now. Pay later. Atlanta: American Cancer Society, 1986. (Publication no. 2611-LE.)

90. Ries LAG, Miller BA, Hankey BF, et al, eds. SEER cancer statistics review, 1973–1991: tables and graphs. Bethesda: National Cancer Institute, 1994. (NIH Publication no. 94-2789.)

13. Screening for Testicular Cancer

RECOMMENDATION

There is insufficient evidence to recommend for or against routine screening of asymptomatic men in the general population for testicular cancer by physician examination or patient self-examination. Recommendations to discuss screening options with selected high-risk patients may be made on other grounds (see *Clinical Intervention*).

Burden of Suffering

Testicular cancer is a relatively uncommon disease, with an overall annual incidence of about 4/100,000 men.[1] It is, however, the most common form of cancer in young men between ages 20 and 35,[2] accounting for an estimated 7,100 new cases and 370 deaths in the U.S. in 1995.[3] The peak annual incidence ranges from 8 to 14/100,000 men between 20 and 35 years of age, with a smaller peak in early childhood.[4] The incidence in black men is less than one fifth that of white men.[4] The major predisposing risk factor is cryptorchidism.[1] In men with a history of cryptorchidism, 80–85% of testicular tumors occur in the cryptorchid testicle, while 15–20% occur in the contralateral testicle. Other risk factors include previous cancer in the other testicle, a history of mumps orchitis, inguinal hernia, or hydrocele in childhood, and high socioeconomic status.[1]

Ninety-six percent of testicular cancers are of germ cell origin, of which seminoma is the most common type. Prognosis and treatment depend on the cell type and stage of disease; however, recent advances in treatment have resulted in a 92% overall 5-year survival.[3] Even among the small proportion of patients (12%) with advanced disease at diagnosis, 5-year survival is close to 70%.[4]

Accuracy of Screening Tests

The two screening tests proposed for testicular cancer are physician palpation of the testes and self-examination of the testes by the patient. Detection of a suspicious testicular mass constitutes a positive test, and the diagnosis is confirmed by biopsy and histologic examination of tissue. There is no information on the sensitivity, specificity, or positive predictive value of testicular examination in asymptomatic persons whether done by providers or by patients. Even if they were known, measures of sensitivity and specificity for palpation of the testes might not be very meaningful because of the low incidence of testicular cancer and the high cure rate. If sensitivity is defined as the probability that disease, when present, is detected at a curable stage, then sensitivity is probably high because the overall cure rate (in the absence of systematic screening) is 92%. The negative predictive value is probably also quite good due to the low incidence of the disease. The positive predictive value, however, of palpation of the testes is probably very low due to the low incidence of disease and large number of other causes of scrotal masses.

There is evidence from older literature that between 26% and 56% of patients presenting initially to their physician with testicular cancer are first diagnosed as having epididymitis, testicular trauma, hydrocele, or other benign disorders,[6–8] and these patients often receive treatment for these conditions before the cancer is diagnosed.[7,9,10]

There have been few studies of whether counseling men to perform self-examination motivates them to adopt this practice or to perform it correctly. Research to date has demonstrated only that education about testicular cancer and self-examination may enhance knowledge and self-reported claims of performing testicular examination.[11,12] One study found that men who reviewed an educational checklist on how to perform self-examination were able to demonstrate greater skill when self-examination was performed moments later; they were also able to recall the contents of the checklist in a telephone survey months later.[13] Few studies, however, have examined whether education or self-examination instructions actually increase the performance of self-examination. It is also unclear whether persons who detect testicular abnormalities seek medical attention promptly. Patients with testicular symptoms may wait as long as several months before contacting a physician.[6]

Finally, no studies have been conducted to test whether persons who perform testicular self-examination are more likely to detect early-stage tumors or have better survival than those who do not practice self-examination.[5] Published evidence that self-examination can detect testicular cancer in asymptomatic persons is limited to a small number of case reports.[14]

Tumor markers, including α-fetoprotein and human chorionic gonadotropin are useful in following nonseminomatous testicular cancers but are not useful for early detection or screening.[1,15]

Effectiveness of Early Detection

The prognosis for advanced stages of testicular cancer has improved dramatically in the past decade with the introduction of better chemotherapy. Current cure rates are greater than 80%.[5,16] Survival, however, is still better for patients with Stage I cancer than in those with more advanced disease, and the treatment of early cancer has less cost and morbidity. Treatment for all types and stages of testicular cancer includes removal of the involved testicle. The current 5-year survival for Stage I seminoma treated with radiotherapy is 97%.[3] Stage I nonseminomatous cancers (e.g., teratoma, embryonal carcinoma, choriocarcinoma) treated with radical retroperitoneal lymph node dissection have a reported 3–5-year survival approaching 90%.[17] With the advent of cisplatin-based chemotherapeutic regimens, a 3-year survival of 90–100% has been reported. Reported survival in patients with disseminated testicular cancer, however, is lower (about 67–80%), and these persons require intensive treatment with chemotherapeutic agents that produce a variety of systemic side effects.[3,5,16]

Although lead-time and length biases may account for part of the improved survival observed for persons with early-stage testicular cancer, it is likely that the prognosis is better for persons with less advanced disease. No studies have been done to determine whether screening increases the proportion of cancers diagnosed at early stages, or improves outcomes. Even without screening, 60–80% of seminomas are Stage I at diagnosis.[17] There is evidence that once testicular symptoms have appeared, diagnostic delays are associated with more advanced disease and lower survival.[6,7,18]

The appropriate management and follow-up of patients with a history of an undescended testicle is controversial.[19,20] It is known that orchiopexy at puberty does not reduce malignant transformation. It is uncertain whether earlier orchiopexy prior to school age, which is now common practice, will prevent development of testicular cancer.[19] Giwercman et al. found carcinoma in situ in 2% of men with a history of cryptorchidism who had testicular biopsies.[20] They predicted 50% of these lesions would progress to invasive cancer and recommended that testicular biopsy be offered to all men with a history of cryptorchidism. Many experts recommend that intraabdominal testes should be removed.[1] The survival for patients with a history of cryptorchidism who develop testicular cancer is excellent, as it is in noncryptorchid patients. No studies have been done to evaluate benefits of formal screening of men with a history of cryptorchidism.

Recommendations of Other Groups

The American Cancer Society recommends a cancer checkup that includes testicular examination every 3 years for men over 20 and annually for those over 40.[21] No recommendation is given for testicular self-examination. The American Academy of Family Physicians recommends a clinical testicular examination for men aged 13–39 years who have a history of cryptorchidism, orchiopexy, or testicular atrophy; this policy is currently under review.[22] The American Academy of Pediatrics recommends testes self-examination beginning at age 18 years.[23] The Canadian Task Force on the Periodic Health Examination concluded that there is insufficient evidence to include or exclude routine screening for testicular cancer by palpation in the periodic health examination.[24]

Discussion

There is no direct experimental evidence on which to base a recommendation for or against screening for testicular cancer by either physician examination or patient self-examination, since no studies of screening have been done. It seems unlikely that screening would substantially improve the already favorable outcome in this uncommon disease. If a population of 100,000 men aged 15–35 years were screened with a 100% sensitive test, at most 10 cancers would be detected. At least nine of these would be expected to be cured in the absence of a formal screening program. It is unknown whether the tenth patient would also be cured as a result of the cancer being detected by screening. A primary care physician with 1,500 males in his/her practice could expect to detect one testicular cancer every 15–20 years. The vast majority of men screened by either physician or self-palpation would have normal examinations; of those with suspicious masses, most would have benign disease (false positives). Many of these cases, however, would require referral to urologists, radiographic studies, or invasive procedures (e.g., biopsy or inguinal exploration) before malignancy could be ruled out.[17] These interventions would incur considerable costs and possible morbidity.

Men with a history of undescended testes or testicular atrophy have a much greater incidence of testicular cancer. Although screening in this population has also not been shown to improve outcome, it would be expected to have a much higher yield than screening in the general population.

CLINICAL INTERVENTION

There is insufficient evidence to recommend for or against routine screening of asymptomatic men for testicular cancer by physician examination or patient self-examination ("C" recommendation). Patients with an increased risk of testicular cancer (those with a history of cryptorchidism or atrophic testes) should be informed of their increased risk of testicular cancer and counseled about the options for screening. Such patients may then elect to be screened or to perform testicular self-examination. Adolescent and young adult males should be advised to seek prompt medical attention if they notice a scrotal abnormality.

The draft update of this chapter was prepared for the U.S. Preventive Services Task Force by Paul S. Frame, MD.

REFERENCES

1. Vogt HB, McHale MS. Testicular cancer: role of primary care physicians in screening and education. Postgrad Med 1992;92:93–101.
2. Schottenfeld D, Warshauer ME. Testis. In: Schottenfeld D, Fraumeni JF, eds. Cancer epidemiology and prevention. Philadelphia: WB Saunders, 1982:947–957.
3. Wingo PA, Tong T, Bolden S. Cancer statistics, 1995. CA Cancer J Clin 1995;45:8–30.
4. Ries LAG, Miller BA, Hankey BF, et al, eds. SEER cancer statistics review, 1973–1991: tables and graphs. Bethesda: National Cancer Institute, 1994. (NIH Publication no. 94-2789.)
5. Westlake SJ, Frank JW. Testicular self-examination: an argument against routine teaching. Fam Pract 1987;4:143–148.
6. Bosl GJ, Vogelzang NJ, Goldman A, et al. Impact of delay in diagnosis on clinical stage of testicular cancer. Lancet 1981;2:970–972.
7. Field TE. Common errors occurring in the diagnosis of testicular neoplasms and the effect of these errors on prognosis. J Roy Army Med Corps 1964;110:152–155.
8. Patton JF, Hewitt CB, Mallis N. Diagnosis and treatment of tumors of the testis. JAMA 1959;171:2194–2198.
9. Prout GR, Griffin PP. Testicular tumors: delay in diagnosis and influence on survival. Am Fam Phys 1984;29:205–209.
10. Earlier diagnosis of testicular tumors [editorial]. BMJ 1980;280:961.
11. Marty PJ, McDermott RJ. Three strategies for encouraging testicular self-examination among college-aged males. J Am Coll Health 1986;34:253–258.
12. Ostwald SK, Rothenberger J. Development of a testicular self-examination program for college men. J Am Coll Health 1985;33:234–239.
13. Friman PC, Finney JW, Glasscock SG, et al. Testicular self-examination: validation of a training strategy for early cancer detection. J Appl Behav Anal 1986;19:87–92.
14. Garnick MB, Mayer RJ, Richie JP. Testicular self-examination [letter]. N Engl J Med 1980;302:297.
15. Rowland RG. Serum markers in testicular germ-cell neoplasms. Hematol Oncol Clin North Am 1988;2:485–489.
16. Williams SD, Birch R, Einhorn LH, et al. Treatment of disseminated germ-cell tumors with cisplatin, bleomycin, and either vinblastine or etoposide. N Engl J Med 1987;316:1435–1440.
17. Fung CY, Garnick MB. Clinical stage I carcinoma of the testis: a review. J Clin Oncol 1988;6:734–750.
18. Post GJ, Belis JA. Delayed presentation of testicular tumors. South Med J 1980;73:33–35.
19. Hawtrey CE. Undescended testis and orchiopexy: recent observations. Pediatr Rev 1990;11:305–308.
20. Giwercman A, Bruun E, Frimodt-Möller C, Skakkebaek NE. Prevalence of carcinoma in situ and other histopathological abnormalities in testes of men with a history of cryptorchidism. J Urol 1989;142:998–1002.
21. American Cancer Society. Guidelines for the cancer-related checkup: an update. Atlanta: American Cancer Society, 1993.
22. American Academy of Family Physicians. Age charts for the periodic health examination. Kansas City, MO: American Academy of Family Physicians, 1994. (Reprint no. 510.)
23. American Academy of Pediatrics. Guidelines for health supervision II. Elk Grove Village, IL: American Academy of Pediatrics, 1988.
24. Canadian Task Force on the Periodic Health Examination. Canadian guide to clinical preventive health care. Ottawa: Canada Communication Group, 1994:892–898.

14. Screening for Ovarian Cancer

RECOMMENDATION

Routine screening for ovarian cancer by ultrasound, the measurement of serum tumor markers, or pelvic examination is not recommended. There is insufficient evidence to recommend for or against the screening of asymptomatic women at increased risk of developing ovarian cancer.

Burden of Suffering

Ovarian cancer is the fifth leading cause of cancer deaths among U.S. women and has the highest mortality of any of the gynecologic cancers.[1] It accounted for an estimated 26,600 new cases and 14,500 deaths in 1995.[1] The lifetime risk of dying from ovarian cancer is 1.1%.[1a] The overall 5-year survival rate is at least 75% if the cancer is confined to the ovaries and decreases to 17% in women diagnosed with distant metastases.[2,3] Symptoms usually do not become apparent until the tumor compresses or invades adjacent structures, ascites develops, or metastases become clinically evident.[4] As a result, two thirds of women with ovarian cancer have advanced (Stage III or IV) disease at the time of diagnosis.[2,5,6] Carcinoma of the ovary is most common in women over age 60.[7] Other important risk factors include low parity and a family history of ovarian cancer.[8-10] Less than 0.1% of women are affected by hereditary ovarian cancer syndrome, but these women may face a 40% lifetime risk of developing ovarian cancer.[11]

Accuracy of Screening Tests

Potential screening tests for ovarian cancer include the bimanual pelvic examination, the Papanicolaou (Pap) smear, tumor markers, and ultrasound imaging. The pelvic examination, which can detect a variety of gynecologic disorders, is of unknown sensitivity in detecting ovarian cancer. Although pelvic examinations can occasionally detect ovarian cancer,[12,13] small, early-stage ovarian tumors are often not detected by palpation,[14,15] due to the deep anatomic location of the ovary. Thus, ovarian cancers detected by pelvic examination are generally advanced[7,16-18] and associated with poor survival.[16] The pelvic examination may also produce false positives when benign adnexal masses (e.g., functional cysts) are found.[16,19] The Pap smear may occasionally reveal malignant ovarian cells,[20] but it is not considered a valid screening test for ovarian carcinoma.[16–18,21] Studies indicate that the Pap smear has a sensitivity for ovarian cancer of only 10–30%.[16]

Serum tumor markers are often elevated in women with ovarian cancer. Examples of these markers include carcinoembryonic antigen, ovarian cystadenocarcinoma antigen, lipid-associated sialic acid, NB/70K, TAG 72.3, CA15-3, and CA-125. CA-125 is elevated in 82% of women with advanced (Stage III or IV) ovarian cancer,[22] and it is also elevated, although less frequently, in women with earlier stage disease.[23] In studies of women with known or suspected ovarian cancer, the reported sensitivities of CA-125 in detecting Stage I and Stage II cancers are 29–75% and 67–100%, respectively.[24–30] These cases may not be representative of asymptomatic women in the general population, however. In screening studies, including a recent study of more than 22,000 women, the reported sensitivity was 53–85%.[13,31] Evidence is limited on whether tumor markers become elevated early enough in the natural history of occult ovarian cancer to provide adequate sensitivity for screening. Studies of stored sera have found that about one half of women who developed ovarian cancer had elevated CA-125 levels (>35 U/mL) 18 months[23] to 3 years[32] before their diagnosis. Further research is needed, however, to provide more reliable data on the sensitivity of this and other tumor markers in detecting early-stage ovarian cancer in asymptomatic women.

Tumor markers may have limited specificity. It has been reported that CA-125 is elevated in 1% of healthy women, 6–40% of women with benign masses (e.g., uterine fibroids, endometriosis, pancreatic pseudocyst, pulmonary hamartoma), and 29% of women with nongynecologic cancers (e.g., pancreas, stomach, colon, breast).[22,33] Reported specificity in screening studies is about 99%.[13,31] It may be possible to improve the specificity of CA-125 measurement by selective screening of postmenopausal women,[34] modifying the assay technique,[35] adding other tumor markers to CA-125,[36] requiring a higher concentration or persistent elevation of CA-125 levels over time, or combining CA-125 measurement with ultrasound (see below). Prospective studies involving asymptomatic women are needed, however, to provide definitive data on the performance characteristics of these techniques when used as screening tests.

Ultrasound imaging has also been evaluated as a screening test for ovarian cancer, since it is able to estimate ovarian size, detect masses as small as 1 cm, and distinguish solid lesions from cysts.[17,37] Transvaginal color-flow Doppler ultrasound can also identify vascular patterns associated with tumors.[38,39] In screening studies, the reported sensitivity and specificity of transabdominal or transvaginal ultrasound are 50–100% and 76–97%, respectively,[3,14,15,40–43] but small sample sizes, limited follow-up, and outdated techniques may limit the validity of the data. Studies have shown that routine ultrasound testing of asymptomatic women has a low yield in detecting ovarian cancer and generates a large proportion of false-positive re-sults that often require diagnostic laparotomy or laparoscopy. In one study, ultrasound screening of 805 high-risk women led to 39 laparotomies, which revealed one ovarian carcinoma, two borderline tumors, one cancer of the cecum, and five cystadenomas.[40] A transvaginal ultrasound study of 600 pa-tients with previous breast cancer revealed 18 patients with complex cysts or enlarged ovaries. Laparotomy was performed on 21 patients, four of whom had ovarian cancer (positive predictive value of 22%); the use of color-flow imaging appeared to increase the positive predictive value.[44]

In a larger study, ultrasound was performed routinely on 5,678 asymp-tomatic female volunteers over age 45 or with a history of previous breast or gynecologic cancer.[44a] Two Stage I ovarian cancers were detected in a total of 6,920 scans performed over 2 years. Another report from the same center indicated that 14,356 ultrasound examinations performed over 3 years on 5,489 asymptomatic women over age 45 detected five ovarian can-cers.[45] Although the sensitivity and specificity of the test were excellent (100% and 94.6%, respectively), the positive predictive value in this low-risk study population was only 2.6% and follow-up was of short duration. It has been calculated from these results and other data that ultrasound screening of 100,000 women over age 45 would detect 40 cases of ovarian cancer, but at a cost of 5,398 false positives and over 160 complications from diagnostic laparoscopy.[46]

It may be possible to improve accuracy by combining ultrasound with other screening tests, such as the measurement of CA-125. This approach has been examined as a method of discriminating between benign and ma-lignant adnexal masses in preoperative patients.[47] Further research is needed, however, to determine the sensitivity, specificity, and positive pre-dictive value of performing these tests in combination to screen asympto-matic women. One prospective study[12] screened 1,010 asymptomatic postmenopausal women over age 45 with pelvic examination and CA-125 measurement; those with abnormal results received an ultrasound exami-nation. Although one ovarian cancer was detected (all three screening tests were positive in this woman), the study demonstrated poor positive predictive value with each of the three screening tests. No abnormality was discovered in 28 of the 31 women with elevated CA-125. Fibroids and be-nign cysts were responsible for over half of the 28 abnormal pelvic exami-nations. There were 13 abnormal ultrasound examinations; 12 of these women consented to laparotomy, which revealed six benign ovarian cysts, two fimbrial cysts, two women with no surgical findings, one woman with adhesions, and the ovarian cancer. A more recent report from the same center found that the combination of abdominal ultrasound and sequen-tial CA-125 measurements had a sensitivity of 58–79%, a specificity of about 100%, and a positive predictive value of 27%.[31] Another program that screened 597 women with transvaginal color-flow Doppler ultrasound and CA-125 measurements detected abnormalities in 115 patients, only one of whom had ovarian cancer.[48]

Effectiveness of Early Detection

There is no direct evidence from prospective studies that women with early-stage ovarian cancer detected through screening have lower mortality from ovarian cancer than do women with more advanced disease. A large body of indirect evidence, however, suggests that this is the case. Although lead-time and length biases may be responsible, it is known that survival from ovarian cancer is related to stage at diagnosis. The 5-year survival rate is 89% for localized disease, 36% for women with regional metastases, and 17% for women with distant metastases.[1] Studies have shown that the most important prognostic factor in patients with advanced ovarian cancer is the size of residual tumor after treatment.[4,7] Surgical debulking and chemotherapy for ovarian cancer appear to be more effective in reducing the size of residual tumor when ovarian cancer is detected early.[4] Although these observations provide suggestive evidence that early detection may be beneficial, conclusive proof will require properly conducted prospective studies comparing long-term mortality from ovarian cancer between screened and nonscreened cohorts. A large clinical trial to obtain this evidence has recently been launched by the National Cancer Institute.[49] Under the most optimistic assumptions (100% sensitivity, 30% reduction in 5-year mortality with screening, no lead-time bias), annual pelvic examinations of 40-year-old women would reduce 5-year mortality from ovarian cancer in the population by less than 0.0001%.[50] Modeling studies that have examined annual CA-125 testing or a single screening with transvaginal ultrasound and CA-125 measurement have found that either approach would increase life expectancy by an average of less than 1 day per woman screened.[51,52]

Recommendations of Other Groups

There are no official recommendations to screen routinely for ovarian cancer in asymptomatic women by performing ultrasound or serum tumor marker measurements. The American College of Physicians (ACP),[53] the Canadian Task Force on the Periodic Health Examination,[54] and the American College of Obstetricians and Gynecologists[55] recommend against such screening. A National Institutes of Health Consensus Conference on Ovarian Cancer recommended taking a careful family history and performing an annual pelvic examination on all women.[56] The pelvic examination, including palpation of the adnexae, is mentioned in a recommendation on Pap testing issued by the American Cancer Society, National Cancer Institute, American College of Obstetricians and Gynecologists,

American Medical Association, American Nurses Association, American Academy of Family Physicians, and the American Medical Women's Association.[57] Specifically, the pelvic examination (and Pap smear) is recommended annually for all women who are or have been sexually active or have reached age 18. Although Pap testing may be performed less frequently once three annual smears have been normal, the American Cancer Society specifies that the pelvic examination be performed with the Pap test every 1–3 years in women aged 18–40 years and annually thereafter.[58]

The NIH Consensus Conference concluded that women with presumed hereditary cancer syndrome should undergo annual pelvic examinations, CA-125 measurements, and transvaginal ultrasound until childbearing is completed or at age 35, at which time prophylactic bilateral oopherectomy was recommended.[56] The ACP recommends counseling high-risk women about the potential benefits and harms of screening.[53] The Canadian Task Force on the Periodic Health Examination found insufficient evidence to recommend for or against screening for ovarian cancer in high-risk women.[54]

Discussion

The sensitivity and specificity of available screening tests for ovarian cancer in asymptomatic women are uncertain and require further study. Although various tests can detect occasional asymptomatic tumors, there is currently no evidence that routine screening will improve overall health outcomes. The large majority of women with abnormal screening test results do not have cancer, yet will require invasive procedures (laparoscopy or laparotomy) to rule out malignancy. Given the risks, inconvenience, and substantial costs of follow-up testing, and the current lack of evidence that screening reduces morbidity or mortality from ovarian cancer, routine screening cannot be recommended. Trials to determine the benefits and risks of ovarian cancer screening are under way. There is also no evidence to support routine screening in women with a history of ovarian cancer in a first-degree relative. Although such women are at increased risk and stand to benefit more from interventions that reduce ovarian cancer mortality, the effectiveness of screening has yet to be determined for any group of women. Referral to a specialist may be appropriate for women whose family history suggests hereditary ovarian cancer syndrome, due to the very high risk of cancer in this disorder.

CLINICAL INTERVENTION

Screening asymptomatic women for ovarian cancer with ultrasound, the measurement of serum tumor markers, or pelvic examination is not recommended ("D" recommendation). There is insufficient evidence to rec-

ommend for or against the screening of asymptomatic women at increased risk of ovarian cancer ("C" recommendation).

The draft update of this chapter was prepared for the U.S. Preventive Services Task Force by Steven H. Woolf, MD, MPH, based in part on a paper prepared for the Clinical Efficacy Assessment Panel of the American College of Physicians by Karen J. Carlson, MD, et al. See relevant background paper: Carlson KJ, Skates SJ, Singer DE. Screening for ovarian cancer. Ann Intern Med 1994;121:124–132.

REFERENCES

1. Wingo PA, Tong T, Bolden S. Cancer statistics, 1995. CA Cancer J Clin 1995;45:8–30.
1a. Ries LAG, Miller BA, Hankey BF, et al, eds. SEER cancer statistics review, 1973–1991: tables and graphs. Bethesda: National Cancer Institute, 1994. (NIH Publication no. 94-2789.)
2. Pettersson F, ed. Annual report on the results of treatment of gynecologic cancer. Int J Gynecol Obstet 1991;36(suppl):238–277.
3. Goswamy RK, Campbell S, Whitehead MI. Screening for ovarian cancer. Clin Obstet Gynecol 1983;10:621–643.
4. Slotman BJ, Rao BR. Ovarian cancer: etiology, diagnosis, prognosis, surgery, radiotherapy, chemotherapy and endocrine therapy. Anticancer Res 1988;8:417–434.
5. Richardson GS, Scully RE, Nikrui N, et al. Common epithelial cancer of the ovary. N Engl J Med 1985;312:415–424.
6. Young RC. Ovarian cancer treatment: progress or paralysis. Semin Oncol 1984;11:327–329.
7. Young JL, Percy CL, Asire AJ, eds. SEER Program: incidence and mortality, 1973–1977. National Cancer Institute, Monograph 57. Washington, DC: Government Printing Office, 1981:75.
8. Whittemore AS, Harris R, Itnyre J, et al. Characteristics relating to ovarian cancer risk: collaborative analysis of 12 US case-control studies. II. Invasive epithelial ovarian cancers in white women. Am J Epidemiol 1992;136:1184–1203.
9. Kerlikowske K, Brown JS, Grady DG. Should women with familial ovarian cancer undergo prophylactic oopherectomy? Obstet Gynecol 1992;80:700–707.
10. Amos CI, Struewing JP. Genetic epidemiology of epithelial ovarian cancer. Cancer 1993;71:566–572.
11. Biesecker B, Boehnke M, Calzone K. Genetic counseling for families with inherited susceptibility to breast and ovarian cancer. JAMA 1993;269:1970–1974.
12. Jacobs I, Stabile I, Bridges J, et al. Multimodal approach to screening for ovarian cancer. Lancet 1988;1:268–271.
13. Einhorn N, Sjovall K, Knapp RC, Hall P, Scully RE, Bast RC, Zurawski VR. Prospective evaluation of serum CA 125 levels for the early detection of ovarian cancer. Obstet Gynecol 1992;80:14–18.
14. Van Nagell JR, DePriest PD, Puls NE, Donaldson ES, Gallion HH, Pavlik EJ, et al. Ovarian cancer screening in asymptomatic postmenopausal women by transvaginal sonography. Cancer 1991;68:458–462.
15. Andolf E, Jorgensen C, Astedt B. Ultrasound examination for detection of ovarian carcinoma in risk groups. Obstet Gynecol 1990;75:106–109.
16. Smith LH, Oi RH. Detection of malignant ovarian neoplasm: a review of the literature. 1. Detection of the patient at risk; clinical, radiological and cytological detection. Obstet Gynecol Surv 1984;39:313–328.
17. Lynch HT, Albano WA, Lynch JF, et al. Surveillance and management of patients at high genetic risk for ovarian carcinoma. Obstet Gynecol 1982;59:589–596.
18. Hall DJ, Hurt WG. The adnexal mass. J Fam Pract 1982;14:135–140.
19. Griffiths CT. Carcinoma of the ovary and fallopian tube. In: Holland JF, Frei E, eds. Cancer medicine. Philadelphia: Lea & Febiger, 1982:1958–1969.
20. Graham JB, Graham RM, Schueller EF. Preclinical detection of ovarian cancer. Cancer 1964;17:1414.
21. Rubin P, Bennett JM. Ovarian cancer. In: Bakeman RP, ed. Clinical oncology for medical students and physicians: a multidisciplinary approach. 5th ed. New York: American Cancer Society, 1978:114–120.
22. Bast RC, Klug TL, St John E, et al. A radioimmunoassay using a monoclonal antibody to monitor the course of epithelial ovarian carcinoma. N Engl J Med 1983;309:883–887.

23. Zurawski VR Jr, Orjaseter H, Andersen A, et al. Elevated serum CA 125 levels prior to diagnosis of ovarian cancer neoplasia: relevance for early detection of ovarian cancer. Int J Cancer 1988;42:677–680.

24. Zurawski VR Jr, Knapp RC, Einhorn N, et al. An initial analysis of preoperative serum CA 125 levels in patients with early stage ovarian carcinoma. Gynecol Oncol 1988;30:7–14.

25. Patsner B, Mann WJ. The value of preoperative serum CA 125 levels in patients with a pelvic mass. Am J Obstet Gynecol 1988;159:873–876.

26. Mogensen O, Mogensen B, Jakobsen A. CA 125 in the diagnosis of pelvic masses. Eur J Cancer Clin Oncol 1989;25:1187–1190.

27. Cruickshank DJ, Fullerton WT, Klopper A. The clinical significance of pre-operative serum CA 125 in ovarian cancer. Br J Obstet Gynaecol 1987;94:692–695.

28. Zanaboni F, Vergadoro F, Presti M, Gallotti P, Lombardi F, Bolis G. Tumor antigen CA 125 as a marker of ovarian epithelial carcinoma. Gynecol Oncol 1987;28:61–67.

29. Brioschi PA, Irion O, Bischof P, Bader M, Forni M, Krauer F. Serum CA 125 in epithelial ovarian cancer: a longitudinal study. Br J Obstet Gynaecol 1987;94:196–201.

30. Schilthuis MS, Aalders JG, Bouma J, et al. Serum CA 125 levels in epithelial ovarian cancer: relation with findings at second-look operations and their role in the detection of tumour recurrence. Br J Obstet Gynaecol 1987;94:202–207.

31. Jacobs I, Davies AP, Bridges J, et al. Prevalence screening for ovarian cancer in postmenopausal women by CA 125 measurement and ultrasonography. BMJ 1993;306:1030–1034.

32. Helzllsouer KJ, Bush TL, Alberg AJ, Bass KM, Zacer H, Comstock GW. Prospective study of serum CA125 levels as markers of ovarian cancer. JAMA 1993;269:1123–1126.

33. Di-Xia C, Schwartz P, Xinguo L, et al. Evaluation of CA 125 levels in differentiating malignant from benign tumors in patients with pelvic masses. Obstet Gynecol 1988;72:23–27.

34. Zurawski VR Jr, Broderick SF, Pickens P, et al. Serum CA 125 levels in a group of nonhospitalized women: relevance for the early detection of ovarian cancer. Obstet Gynecol 1987;69:606–611.

35. Klug TL, Green PJ, Zurawski VR Jr, et al. Confirmation of a false-positive result in CA 125 immunoradiometric assay caused by human anti-idiotypic immunoglobulin. Clin Chem 1988;34:1071–1076.

36. Jacobs IJ, Oram DH, Bast RC. Strategies for improving the specificity of screening for ovarian cancer with tumor-associated antigens CA125, CA15-3, and TAG 72.3. Obstet Gynecol 1992;80:396–399.

37. Campbell S, Goessens L, Goswamy R, et al. Real-time ultrasound for determination of ovarian morphology and volume: a possible early screening test for ovarian cancer? Lancet 1982;1:425–426.

38. Bourne T, Campbell S, Steer C, Whitehead MI, Collins WP. Transvaginal colour flow imaging: a possible new screening technique for ovarian cancer. BMJ 1989;299:1367–1370.

39. Kurjak A, Zalud I, Alfirevic Z. Evaluation of adnexal masses with transvaginal color ultrasound. J Ultrasound Med 1991;10:295–297.

40. Andolf E, Svalenius E, Astedt B. Ultrasonography for early detection of ovarian carcinoma. Br J Obstet Gynaecol 1986;93:1286–1289.

41. Campbell S, Royston P, Bhan V, Whitehead MI, Collins WP. Novel screening strategies for early ovarian cancer by transabdominal ultrasonography. Br J Obstet Gynaecol 1990;97:304–311.

42. Rodriguez MH, Platt LD, Medearis AL, Lacarra M, Lobo RA. The use of transvaginal ultrasonography for evaluation of postmenopausal size and morphology. Am J Obstet Gynecol 1988;159:810–814.

43. Bourne TH, Campbell S, Reynolds KM, et al. Screening for early familial ovarian cancer with transvaginal ultrasonography and colour flow imaging. BMJ 1993;306:1025–1029.

44. Weiner Z, Beck D, Shteiner M, et al. Screening for ovarian cancer in women with breast cancer with transvaginal sonography and color flow imaging. J Ultrasound Med 1993;12:387–393.

44a. Goswamy RK, Campbell S. Screening for ovarian cancer. IARC Sci Publ 1986;76:305–309.

45. Campbell S, Bhan V, Royston J, et al. Screening for early ovarian cancer. Lancet 1988;1:710–711.

46. Jacobs I. Screening for early ovarian cancer. Lancet 1988;2:171–172.

47. Finkler NJ, Benacerraf B, Lavin PT, et al. Comparison of serum CA 125, clinical impression, and ultrasound in the preoperative evaluation of ovarian masses. Obstet Gynecol 1988;72:659–664.

48. Karlan BY, Raffel LJ, Crvenkovic G, et al. A multidisciplinary approach to the early detection of ovarian carcinoma: rationale, protocol design, and early results. Am J Obstet Gynecol 1993;169:494–501.

49. Kramer BS, Gohagan J, Prorok PC, Smart C. A National Cancer Institute sponsored screening trial for prostatic, lung, colorectal, and ovarian cancers. Cancer 1993;71:589–593.

50. Eddy DM. Annual pelvic examination. Ann Intern Med 1990;113:803.

51. Skates SJ, Singer DE. Quantifying the potential benefit of CA125 screening for ovarian cancer. J Clin Epidemiol 1991;44:365–380.

52. Schapira MM, Matchar DB, Young MJ. The effectiveness of ovarian cancer screening: a decision-analysis model. Ann Intern Med 1993;118:838–843.
53. American College of Physicians. Screening for ovarian cancer. Ann Intern Med 1994;121:141–142.
54. Canadian Task Force on the Periodic Health Examination. Canadian guide to clinical preventive health care. Ottawa: Canada Communication Group, 1994:869–881.
55. American College of Obstetricians and Gynecologists. Routine cancer screening. Committee Opinion no. 128. Washington, DC: American College of Obstetricians and Gynecologists, 1993.
56. National Institutes of Health. Ovarian cancer: screening, treatment, and follow-up. National Institutes of Health Consensus Conference Statement, April 5–7, 1994.
57. Fink DJ. Change in American Cancer Society checkup guidelines for detection of cervical cancer. CA Cancer J Clin 1988;38:127–128.
58. American Cancer Society. Guidelines for the cancer-related checkup: an update. Atlanta: American Cancer Society, 1993.

15. Screening for Pancreatic Cancer

RECOMMENDATION

Routine screening for pancreatic cancer in asymptomatic persons, using abdominal palpation, ultrasonography, or serologic markers, is not recommended.

Burden of Suffering

Cancer of the pancreas is the fifth leading cause of cancer deaths in the U.S., accounting for an estimated 27,000 deaths in 1995 (8.4 deaths/100,000 persons).[1,1a] Worldwide, the age-adjusted incidence and mortality of pancreatic cancer have been increasing since the 1930s,[2,3] although in the U.S. these rates have declined since the early 1970s.[1,1a] Incidence rates may be overestimated, because an important proportion of pancreatic cancer diagnoses (as many as half in some studies) are not histologically confirmed.[4] Pancreatic cancer is more common in men, blacks, cigarette smokers, and older persons (the majority of cases being diagnosed between ages 65 and 79).[1,2,3,5] The risk of pancreatic cancer is increased in patients with diabetes, including those with long-standing (≥ 5 years) diabetes.[5a] Familial aggregations of pancreatic cancer are rare but have been described.[2,6]

Since initial symptoms are usually nonspecific (e.g., abdominal pain and weight loss) and are frequently disregarded, some 80–90% of patients have regional and distant metastases by the time they are diagnosed.[5,7] Only 3% of the 24,000 patients annually diagnosed with pancreatic cancer live more than 5 years after diagnosis.[1,1a] Of pancreatic adenocarcinomas, which account for more than 90% of all pancreatic neoplasms,[5] only about 4–16% are resectable at diagnosis,[4,8–12] and the 5-year survival rate is less than 1%.[7] In addition, 5-year survival does not indicate cure, since further decrements in survival occur after 5 years.[13,14]

Accuracy of Screening Tests

Adenocarcinoma is the principal form of pancreatic neoplasm for which screening has been considered; in this chapter, "pancreatic cancer" refers to adenocarcinoma. There are no reliable screening tests for detecting pancreatic cancer in asymptomatic persons. The deep anatomic location of the pancreas makes detection of small localized tumors unlikely during the routine abdominal examination. Even in patients with confirmed pancreatic cancer, an abdominal mass is palpable in only 15–25% of cases.[4,5,15,16]

Imaging procedures such as magnetic resonance imaging and computed tomography are too costly to use as routine screening tests, while more accurate tests such as endoscopic retrograde cholangiopancreatography and endoscopic ultrasound are inappropriate for screening asymptomatic patients due to their invasiveness.[17,18] Abdominal ultrasonography is a noninvasive screening test, but there is little information on the efficacy of abdominal ultrasound as a screening test for pancreatic cancer in asymptomatic persons. In symptomatic patients with suspected disease it has a reported sensitivity of 40–98% and a specificity as high as 90–94%.[15,19,20] Conventional ultrasonography is limited by visualization difficulties in the presence of bowel gas or obesity and by its range of resolution (2–3 cm).[7,18,20] Even tumors <2 cm in diameter are frequently associated with metastatic disease,[8,11,21] thus limiting the ability of ultrasound to detect early disease.

Most persons with pancreatic malignancy have elevated levels of certain serologic markers such as CA19-9, peanut agglutinin, pancreatic oncofetal antigen, DU-PAN-2, carcinoembryonic antigen, α-fetoprotein, CA-50, SPan-1, and tissue polypeptide antigen.[22–25] None of these markers is, however, tumor specific or organ specific;[25] elevations of various serologic markers also occur in significant proportions of persons with benign gastrointestinal diseases or malignancies other than pancreatic cancer.[17,22,24,25] Most of these markers have been studied exclusively in high-risk populations, such as symptomatic patients with suspected pancreatic cancer. CA19-9 has probably achieved the widest acceptance as a serodiagnostic test for pancreatic carcinoma in symptomatic patients, with an overall sensitivity of approximately 80% (68–93%) and specificity of 90% (73–100%); sensitivity was highest in patients with more advanced disease.[23,24] Among healthy subjects, CA19-9 has good specificity (94–99%)[26–28] but nevertheless generates a large proportion of false-positive results due to the very low prevalence of pancreatic cancer in the general population.[29] A study of a mass screening of more than 10,000 asymptomatic persons for pancreatic cancer in Japan,[30] using either ultrasonography alone or CA19-9 plus elastase-1, found the likelihood of pancreatic cancer given a positive screening test to be 0.5%; only one of the four cancers discovered could be curably resected.

The predictive value of a positive test could be improved if a population at substantially higher risk could be identified. Diabetes mellitus in older adult patients might be useful as a marker for a population at high risk of having pancreatic cancer.[3,31,32] Cohort studies have reported incidences of pancreatic cancer among diabetic patients ranging from 51 to

166/100,000 person-years.[5a] Studies evaluating screening efficacy might therefore be warranted in this population.

Effectiveness of Early Detection

Evidence that early detection can lower morbidity or mortality from pancreatic cancer is not conclusive. The reported 5-year survival for localized disease based on 1983–1990 national data is only 9%, not substantially higher than the 5-year survival with regional (4%) and distant (2%) metastases.[1a] A comprehensive review of published reports on surgical resection of pancreatic cancer estimated an overall 5-year survival rate of 8% for small tumors without evidence of local or distant spread.[8] In part, this low rate may reflect the fact that a proportion of patients with localized disease cannot be operated on because of concomitant medical problems, advanced age, or other reasons.[10,11,13] Patients who have small localized tumors that are resected for attempted cure, which account for only 4–16% of the total, may have better 5-year survival rates (as high as 37–48% in the most experienced centers),[8–13,21,33] although the designs of most studies of surgical outcome suffer from lead-time, length, and selection biases. The morbidity associated with surgical resection is high (15–53%), but perioperative mortality is now less than 7% in the hands of experienced surgeons.[8,9,13,33,34]

Reports on the effectiveness of adjuvant external beam and/or intraoperative radiotherapy in improving survival among curatively resected patients, using historical controls, have yielded inconsistent results.[35–37] In one small randomized controlled trial,[38] corroborated by a subsequent case series by the same authors,[39] an adjuvant treatment program using combined radiation and chemotherapy following curative resection was associated with a significant median survival advantage of 9 months and a 5-year survival advantage of 14.5% in treated versus control cases; however, the study was closed early due to poor subject accrual and it did not control for the substantially greater frequency of clinic visits by cases. Adverse effects of combined radiation and chemotherapy include leukopenia and gastrointestinal toxicity.[38,40] Intraoperative radiotherapy frequently causes gastrointestinal bleeding, which may be life-threatening.[37] Additional randomized controlled trials of adjuvant therapy are needed to confirm its effectiveness in improving survival in patients with early pancreatic carcinoma. New modalities being explored include immunotherapy[41] and hormonal therapy.[42]

Primary Prevention

Cigarette smoking has been consistently associated with a modestly increased risk of pancreatic cancer in numerous cohort and case-control studies of populations in the U.S., Canada, Europe, and Japan.[3,43–46] A clear dose-response relationship has not been demonstrated, however, nor have the biologic mechanisms underlying this association been adequately delineated. Cohort and case-control studies suggest that former smokers have a decreased risk of pancreatic cancer compared with current smokers,[43,44,47–49] but estimates of the duration of abstinence required to show a reduction in risk have varied from as few as 1–3 years to as many as 10–20 years, and some studies have found no risk reduction at all associated with smoking cessation.[43,45] In addition, a number of these studies suffer from selection, misclassification, and other biases. Although the causal relationship between smoking and pancreatic cancer requires further study, counseling patients to discontinue smoking (see Chapter 54) is easily justified by its established efficacy in preventing other malignancies (e.g., lung cancer), coronary artery disease, and other serious disorders.

Several cohort studies and many population-based case-control studies have reported positive associations between pancreatic cancer and dietary factors such as meat, eggs, carbohydrates, refined sugar, cholesterol, fat, and total calorie intake, as well as negative (protective) associations with intake of vegetables and fruits.[3,46,48,50–56] However, study results are inconsistent; many studies suffer from selection, misclassification, and other biases; and large numbers of comparisons make significance testing problematic. Further research to define nutritional risk factors for pancreatic cancer is therefore needed. Studies of the relationship between increased alcohol consumption and pancreatic cancer have yielded inconsistent results;[3,45–48,57,58] few have adequately assessed level and duration of intake, or evaluated the possibility of a link between alcohol, pancreatitis, and pancreatic cancer. Current epidemiologic evidence does not support an association between pancreatic cancer and coffee consumption.[3,58,59]

Recommendations of Other Groups

No groups recommend routine screening for pancreatic cancer in asymptomatic persons. The Canadian Task Force on the Periodic Health Examination recommends against such screening.[60]

Discussion

Given the lack of evidence for improved outcome with early detection of pancreatic cancer, the invasive nature of diagnostic tests likely to follow a positive screening test (e.g., endoscopic ultrasound, laparotomy), and the fact that most positive screening tests would be false positives, screening for pancreatic cancer cannot be recommended at this time. Primary prevention of pancreatic cancer may be possible through clinical efforts directed at the use of tobacco products.

CLINICAL INTERVENTION

Routine screening for pancreatic cancer in asymptomatic persons, using abdominal palpation, ultrasonography, or serologic markers, is not recommended ("D" recommendation). All patients should be counseled regarding use of tobacco products (see Chapter 54). Counseling to reduce fat and cholesterol intake and to increase intake of fruits and vegetables may be recommended on other grounds (see Chapter 56).

The draft update of this chapter was prepared for the U.S. Preventive Services Task Force by Carolyn DiGuiseppi, MD, MPH.

REFERENCES

1. Wingo PA, Tong T, Bolden S. Cancer statistics, 1995. CA Cancer J Clin 1995;45:8–30.
1a. Ries LAG, Miller BA, Hankey BF, et al, eds. SEER cancer statistics review, 1973–1991: tables and graphs. Bethesda: National Cancer Institute, 1994. (NIH Publication no. 94-2789.)
2. Gordis L, Gold EB. Epidemiology of pancreatic cancer. World J Surg 1984;8:808–821.
3. Boyle P, Hsieh C-C, Maisonneuve P, et al. Epidemiology of pancreas cancer (1988). Int J Pancreatol 1989;5:327–346.
4. Gudjonsson B. Cancer of the pancreas—50 years of surgery. Cancer 1987;60:2284–2303.
5. Arnar D, Theodors A, Isaksson HJ, et al. Cancer of the pancreas in Iceland. An epidemiologic and clinical study, 1974–85. Scand J Gastroenterol 1991;26:724–730.
5a. Everhart J, Wright D. Diabetes mellitus as a risk factor for pancreatic cancer: a meta-analysis. JAMA 1995; 273:1605–1609.
6. Lynch HT, Fitzsimmons ML, Smyrk TC, et al. Familial pancreatic cancer: clinicopathologic study of 18 nuclear families. Am J Gastroenterol 1990;85:54–60.
7. Poston G, Williamson R. Causes, diagnosis, and management of exocrine pancreatic cancer. Compr Ther 1990;16:36–42.
8. Russell RCG. Surgical resection for cancer of the pancreas. Baillieres Clin Gastroenterol 1990;4:889–916.
9. Michelassi F, Erroi F, Dawson PJ, et al. Experience with 647 consecutive tumors of the duodenum, ampulla, head of the pancreas, and distal common bile duct. Ann Surg 1989;210:544–556.
10. Gall FP, Kessler H, Hermanek P. Surgical treatment of ductal pancreatic carcinoma. Eur J Surg Oncol 1991;17:173–181.
11. Nix GAJJ, Dubbelman C, Wilson JHP, et al. Prognostic implications of tumor diameter in carcinoma of the head of the pancreas. Cancer 1991;67:529–535.
12. Bottger T, Zech J, Weber W, et al. Relevant factors in the prognosis of ductal pancreatic carcinoma. Acta Chir Scand 1990;156:781–788.
13. Tsuchiya R, Tsunoda T, Ishida T, et al. Resection for cancer of the pancreas—the Japanese experience. Baillieres Clin Gastroenterol 1990;4:931–939.
14. Livingston EH, Welton ML, Reber HA. Surgical treatment of pancreatic cancer. The United States experience. Int J Pancreatol 1991;9:153–157.
15. Nordback I, Hyoty M, Auvinen O. Improved detection of cancer of the body or tail of the pancreas. Eur J Surg 1991;157:33–37.
16. Ceuterick M, Gelin M, Rickaerr F, et al. Pancreaticoduodenal resection for pancreatic or periampullary tumors—a ten-year experience. Hepatogastroenterology 1989;36:467–473.
17. Carter DC. Cancer of the pancreas. Gut 1990;31:494–496.
18. Grimm H, Maydeo A, Soehendra N. Endoluminal ultrasound for the diagnosis and staging of pancreatic cancer. Baillieres Clin Gastroenterol 1990;4:869–888.
19. Wang TH, Lin JT, Chen DS, et al. Noninvasive diagnosis of advanced pancreatic cancer by real-time ultrasonography, carcinoembryonic antigen, and carbohydrate antigen 19-9. Pancreas 1986;1:219–223.
20. DelMaschio A, Vanzulli A, Sironi S, et al. Pancreatic cancer versus chronic pancreatitis: diagnosis with CA 19-9 assessment, US, CT, and CT-guided fine-needle biopsy. Radiology 1991;178:95–99.

21. Tsuchiya R, Tomioka T, Izawa K, et al. Collective review of small carcinomas of the pancreas. Ann Surg 1986;203:77–81.
22. Rhodes JM, Ching CK. Serum diagnostic tests for pancreatic cancer. Baillieres Clin Gastroenterol 1990;4:833–853.
23. Steinberg W. The clinical utility of the CA 19-9 tumor-associated antigen. Am J Gastroenterol 1990;85:350–355.
24. Satake K, Chung Y-S, Yokomatsu H, et al. A clinical evaluation of various tumor markers for the diagnosis of pancreatic cancer. Int J Pancreatol 1990;7:25–36.
25. Satake K. Diagnosis of pancreatic cancer. Serological markers. Int J Pancreatol 1991;9:93–98.
26. Del Villano BC, Brennan S, Brock P, et al. Radioimmunometric assay for a monoclonal antibody defined tumor marker, CA 19-9. Clin Chem 1983;29:549–552.
27. Ritts RE Jr, Del Villano BC, Go VLW, et al. Initial clinical evaluation of an immunoradiometric assay for CA 19-9 using the NCI serum bank. Int J Cancer 1984;33:339–445.
28. Fabris C, Del Favero G, Basso D, et al. Serum markers and clinical data in diagnosing pancreatic cancer: a contrastive approach. Am J Gastroenterol 1988;83:549–553.
29. Frebourg T, Bercoff E, Manchon N, et al. The evaluation of CA 19-9 antigen level in the early detection of pancreatic cancer. A prospective study of 866 patients. Cancer 1988;62:2287–2290.
30. Homma T, Tsuchiya R. The study of the mass screening of persons without symptoms and of the screening of outpatients with gastrointestinal complaints or icterus for pancreatic cancer in Japan, using CA19-9 and elastase-1 or ultrasonography. Int J Pancreatol 1991;9:119–124.
31. Rosa JA, Van Linda BM, Abourizk NN. New-onset diabetes mellitus as a harbinger of pancreatic carcinoma. A case report and literature review. J Clin Gastroenterol 1989;11:211–215.
32. Ishikawa O, Ohhigashi H, Wada A, et al. Morphologic characteristics of pancreatic carcinoma with diabetes mellitus. Cancer 1989;64:1107–1112.
33. Crist DW, Sitzmann JV, Cameron JL. Improved hospital morbidity, mortality, and survival after the Whipple procedure. Ann Surg 1987;206:358–365.
34. Trede M, Schwall G. The complications of pancreatectomy. Ann Surg 1988;207:39–47.
35. Hiraoka T. Extended radical resection of cancer of the pancreas with intraoperative radiotherapy. Baillieres Clin Gastroenterol 1990;4:985–993.
36. Shibamoto Y, Manabe T, Baba N, et al. High dose, external beam and intraoperative radiotherapy in the treatment of resectable and unresectable pancreatic cancer. Int J Radiol Oncol Biol Phys 1990;19:605–611.
37. Heijmans JH, Hoekstra HJ, Mehta DM. Is adjuvant intra-operative radiotherapy (IORT) for resectable and unresectable pancreatic carcinoma worthwhile? Hepatogastroenterology 1986;36:474–477.
38. Kalser MH, Ellenberg SS. Pancreatic cancer: adjuvant combined radiation and chemotherapy following curative resection. Arch Surg 1985;120:899–903.
39. Gastrointestinal Tumor Study Group. Further evidence of effective adjuvant combined radiation and chemotherapy following curative resection of pancreatic cancer. Cancer 1987;59:2006–2010.
40. Arbuck SG. Chemotherapy for pancreatic cancer. Baillieres Clin Gastroenterol 1990;4:953–968.
41. Buchler M, Friess H, Malfertheiner P, et al. Studies of pancreatic cancer utilizing monoclonal antibodies. Int J Pancreatol 1990;7:151–156.
42. Andren-Sandberg A, Johansson J. Influence of sex hormones on pancreatic cancer. Int J Pancreatol 1990;7: 167–176.
43. Office on Smoking and Health, Centers for Disease Control and Prevention. The health benefits of smoking cessation. Atlanta: Department of Health and Human Services, 1990:155–159. (Publication no. CDC-90-8416.)
44. Howe GR, Jain M, Burch JD, Miller AB. Cigarette smoking and cancer of the pancreas: evidence from a population-based case-control study in Toronto, Canada. Int J Cancer 1991;47:323–323.
45. Ghadirian P, Simard A, Baillargeon J. Tobacco, alcohol, and coffee and cancer of the pancreas. A population-based, case-control study in Quebec, Canada. Cancer 1991;67:2664–2670.
46. Hirayama T. Epidemiology of pancreatic cancer in Japan. Jpn J Clin Oncol 1989;19:208–215.
47. Farrow DC, Davis S. Risk of pancreatic cancer in relation to medical history and the use of tobacco, alcohol and coffee. Int J Cancer 1990;45:816–820.
48. Olsen GW, Mandel JS, Gibson RW, et al. A case-control study of pancreatic cancer and cigarettes, alcohol, coffee and diet. Am J Public Health 1989;79:1016–1019.

49. Bueno de Mesquita HB, Maisonneuve P, Moerman CJ, et al. Life-time history of smoking and exocrine carcinoma of the pancreas: a population-based case-control study in the Netherlands. Int J Cancer 1991;49:816–822.

50. Bueno de Mesquita HB, Moerman CJ, Runia S, Maisonneuve P. Are energy and energy-providing nutrients related to exocrine carcinoma of the pancreas? Int J Cancer 1990;46:435–444.

51. Farrow DC, Davis S. Diet and the risk of pancreatic cancer in men. Am J Epidemiol 1990;132:423–431.

52. Baghurst PA, McMichael AJ, Slavotinek AH, et al. A case-control study of diet and cancer of the pancreas. Am J Epidemiol 1991;134:167–179.

53. Bueno de Mesquita HB, Maisonneuve P, Runia S, Moerman CJ. Intake of foods and nutrients and cancer of the exocrine pancreas: a population-based case-control study in the Netherlands. Int J Cancer 1991;48:540–549.

54. Ghadirian P, Simard A, Baillargeon, et al. Nutritional factors and pancreatic cancer in the francophone community in Montreal, Canada. Int J Cancer 1991;47:1–6.

55. Zatonski W, Przewozniak K, Howe GR, et al. Nutritional factors and pancreatic cancer: a case-control study from south-west Poland. Int J Cancer 1991;48:390–394.

56. Howe GR, Jain M, Miller AB. Dietary factors and risk of pancreatic cancer: results of a Canadian population-based case-control study. Int J Cancer 1990;45:604–608.

57. Cuzick J, Babiker AG. Pancreatic cancer, alcohol, diabetes mellitus and gall-bladder disease. Int J Cancer 1989; 43:415–421.

58. Jain M, Howe GR, St. Louis P, et al. Coffee and alcohol as determinants of risk of pancreas cancer: a case-control study from Toronto. Int J Cancer 1991;47:384–389.

59. Gordis L. Consumption of methylxanthine-containing beverages and risk of pancreatic cancer. Cancer Lett 1990;52:1–12.

60. Canadian Task Force on the Periodic Health Examination. Canadian guide to clinical preventive health care. Ottawa: Canada Communication Group, 1994:862–869.

16. Screening for Oral Cancer

RECOMMENDATION

There is insufficient evidence to recommend for or against routine screening of asymptomatic persons for oral cancer by primary care clinicians. All patients should be counseled to discontinue the use of all forms of tobacco (see Chapter 54) and to limit consumption of alcohol (see Chapter 52). Clinicians should remain alert to signs and symptoms of oral cancer and premalignancy in persons who use tobacco or regularly use alcohol.

Burden of Suffering

The term "oral cancer" includes a diverse group of tumors arising from the oral cavity. Usually included are cancers of the lip, tongue, pharynx, and oral cavity. The annual incidence of oral cancer in the U.S. is about 11/100,000 population, with a male/female ratio greater than 2:1.[1] Oral cancer is responsible for 2% of all cancer deaths in the U.S., and it is projected to account for over 28,000 new cases and about 8,400 deaths in 1995.[2]

Fifty-three percent of oral cancers have spread to regional or distant structures at the time of diagnosis.[1] Overall 5-year survival is 52%, but it ranges from 79% for localized disease to 19% if distant metastases are present.[1] The natural history of each type of cancer can be quite different. Cancer of the lip accounts for 11% of new cases of oral cancer but only 1% of deaths. In contrast, cancer of the pharynx accounts for 31% of new cases of oral cancer but 50% of deaths.[1] The median age at diagnosis of oral cancers is 64 years, and 95% occur in persons over age 40. About half of all oropharyngeal cancers and the majority of deaths from this disease occur in persons over age 65.[1]

Use of tobacco in all forms and, to a lesser extent, alcohol abuse are the major risk factors for the development of oral cancer.[3] The risk of oral cancer is increased 6–28 times in current smokers,[4] and the effects of tobacco and alcohol account for 90% of oral cancer in the U.S.[5] In parts of India and Asia where chewing tobacco or betel nut is very common, the incidence of oral cancer is 3 times higher than in the U.S.[5] In several areas of India, oral cancer accounts for 40% of all female cancer deaths.[5] Other risk factors for oral cancer include occupational exposures, solar radiation (for cancer of the lip), and the presence of premalignant lesions such as

Alternative screening tests for oral cancer have been p
tolonium chloride rinses to stain suspicious lesions,[13,14] but further research is needed to evaluate the accuracy and acceptability of these techniques before routine use in the general population can be considered.

Effectiveness of Early Detection

No controlled trials of screening for oral cancer that include data on clinical outcomes have been reported. There is consistent evidence that persons with early-stage oral cancer have a better prognosis than those

diagnosed with more advanced disease.[1,2] Because of the possible effects of lead-time and length bias, however, these observational data are not sufficient to prove that screening and earlier detection improve the prognosis in patients with oral cancer. Some authors have questioned the effectiveness of early detection in improving prognosis.[15] Prospective trials of screening for oral cancer, although difficult and expensive to conduct in the general population, might be feasible in high-risk populations in which the incidence of oral cancer is substantially greater.

Several studies have examined treatment of oral leukoplakia, a form of premalignancy, as a means of preventing oral cancer. Primary treatment of oral leukoplakia and prevention of second primary lesions in patients with treated oral cancer have been studied in several randomized, placebo-controlled chemoprevention trials of high-dose isotretinoin (13-cis-retinoic acid).[16–18] These studies demonstrated that isotretinoin was effective in promoting remission of leukoplakia and preventing the occurrence of second primary oral cancers.[17] Leukoplakia relapsed in a majority of cases within 3–6 months after discontinuation of therapy, however, and the rate of toxicity of treatment was high (mild to moderate side effects in up to 79% of patients). A trial of alternate maintenance therapies after isotretinoin induction for leukoplakia suggested that low-dose isotretinoin was more effective in maintaining remissions than β-carotene and caused fewer side effects than high-dose therapy: 12% of participants experienced severe toxicity and 42% had moderate toxicity from low-dose isotretinoin, including dry skin, cheilitis, and conjunctivitis.[18]

Uncontrolled trials using β-carotene demonstrated variable reductions (up to 71%) in the occurrence of oral leukoplakia and mucosal dysplasia.[19–21] In a randomized trial, however, the majority of patients with leukoplakia progressed during β-carotene treatment.[18] Although side effects of β-carotene are minimal, older male smokers who took β-carotene for 5–8 years experienced slightly higher rates of lung cancer and overall mortality in a recently completed trial in Finland.[22] Research is currently in progress on alternative agents (e.g., vitamin E) and combinations of therapies.[23]

Recommendations of Other Groups

The American Cancer Society recommends a cancer checkup that includes oral examination every 3 years for persons over age 20 and annually for those over age 40.[24] The Canadian Task Force on the Periodic Health Examination concluded that there was insufficient evidence to include or exclude screening for oral cancer in the periodic health examination of persons in the general population, but suggested that annual oral examination by a physician or dentist should be considered for persons over 60 with risk factors for oral cancer (e.g., smokers and regular drinkers).[25] Although the National Institutes of Health no longer issue specific clinical guidelines regarding screening for oral cancer, both the National Cancer Institute and the National Institute of Dental Research support efforts to promote the early detection of oral cancers during routine dental examinations.[8,26]

Discussion

Primary prevention strategies, such as counseling patients regarding the use of tobacco and alcohol, may have a greater impact on the morbidity and mortality associated with oral cancer than measures aimed at early detection. There is good evidence that tobacco use and excessive consumption of alcohol are both independent and synergistic risk factors for oral cancer.[3] Over 90% of oropharyngeal cancer deaths are associated with smoking.[5] In addition to smoking and alcohol, oral cancer is also associated with the use of snuff and chewing tobacco.[27]

Oral cancer is a relatively uncommon cancer in the United States. Even among high-risk groups such as smokers, oral cancer accounts for a relatively small proportion (<2%) of all deaths.[4] Available screening tests for oral cancer are limited to the physical examination of the mouth, a test of undetermined sensitivity, specificity, and positive predictive value. Despite the strong association between stage at diagnosis and survival, there are few controlled data to determine whether routine screening in the primary care setting leads to earlier diagnosis or reduced mortality from oral cancer. Given the significant morbidity and mortality associated with advanced oral cancer and its treatment, clinicians may wish to include careful examinations for oral cancer in asymptomatic persons at significantly increased risk for the disease (see Clinical Intervention); direct evidence of a benefit of screening in any group, however, is lacking. It is also appropriate to refer patients for regular visits to a dentist, for whom complete examination of the oral cavity is often more feasible (see Chapter 61).

CLINICAL INTERVENTION

There is insufficient evidence to recommend for or against routine screening of asymptomatic persons for oral cancer by primary care clinicians ("C" recommendation). Although direct evidence of a benefit is lacking, clinicians may wish to include an examination for cancerous and precancerous lesions of the oral cavity in the periodic health examination of persons who chew or smoke tobacco (or did so previously), older persons who drink regularly, and anyone with suspicious symptoms or lesions detected through self-examination. All patients, especially those at increased risk, should be advised to receive a complete dental examination on a regular basis (see Chapter 61). All adolescent and adult patients should be asked to describe their use of tobacco (Chapter 54) and alcohol (Chapter 52). Appropriate counseling should be offered to those persons who smoke cigarettes, pipes, or cigars, those who use chewing tobacco or snuff, and those who have evidence of alcohol abuse. Persons with increased exposure to sunlight should be advised to take protective measures when outdoors to protect their lips and skin from the harmful effects of ultraviolet rays (see Chapter 12).

The draft update of this chapter was prepared for the U.S. Preventive Services Task Force by Paul S. Frame, MD, based on materials prepared for the Canadian Task Force on the Periodic Health Examination by Carl Rosati, MD, FRCSC.

REFERENCES

1. Ries LAG, Miller BA, Hankey BF, et al, eds. SEER cancer statistics review, 1973–1991: tables and graphs. Bethesda: National Cancer Institute, 1994. (NIH Publication no. 94-2789.)
2. Wingo PA, Tong T, Bolden S. Cancer statistics, 1995. CA Cancer J Clin 1995;45:8–30.
3. Vokes EE, Weichselbaum RR, Lippman SM, et al. Head and neck cancer. N Engl J Med 1993;328:184–194.
4. Centers for Disease Control and Prevention. Cigarette smoking—attributable mortality and years of potential life lost—United States, 1990. MMWR 1993;42:645–649.
5. Silverman S Jr. Oral cancer. Atlanta: American Cancer Society, 1990.
6. Epstein JB, Silverman S. Head and neck malignancies associated with HIV infection. Oral Surg Oral Med Oral Pathol 1992;73:193–200.
7. Mashberg A, Meyers H. Anatomical site and size of 222 early asymptomatic oral squamous carcinomas. Cancer 1976;37:2149–2157.
8. Department of Health and Human Services, National Cancer Institute. Tobacco effects in the mouth. Bethesda: Public Health Service, 1992. (DHHS Publication no. (NCI) 92-3330.)
9. Mehta FS, Bhonsle RB, Daftary DK, et al. Detection of oral cancer using basic health workers in an area of high oral cancer incidence in India. Cancer Detect Prev 1986;9:219–225.
10. Warnakulasuriya KAAS, Nanayakkara BG. Reproducibility of an oral cancer and precancer detection program using a primary health care model in Sri Lanka. Cancer Detect Prev 1991;15:331–334.
11. Elwood JM, Gallagher RP. Factors influencing early diagnosis of cancer of the oral cavity. Can Med Assoc J 1985;133:651–656.
12. Fedele DJ, Jones JA, Niessen LC. Oral cancer screening in the elderly. J Am Geriatr Soc 1991;39:920–925.
13. Mashberg A. Final evaluation of tolonium chloride rinse for screening of high-risk patients with asymptomatic squamous carcinoma. J Am Dent Assoc 1983;106:319–323.
14. Rosenberg D, Cretin S. Use of meta-analysis to evaluate tolonium chloride in oral cancer screening. Oral Surg Oral Med Oral Pathol 1989;67:621–627.
15. Williams RG. The early diagnosis of carcinoma of the mouth. Ann R Coll Surg Engl 1981;63:423–425.
16. Hong WK, Endicott J, Itri LM, et al. 13-cis-retinoic acid in the treatment of oral leukoplakia. N Engl J Med 1986;315:1501–1505.
17. Hong WK, Lippman SM, Itri LM, et al. Prevention of second primary tumors with isotretinoin in squamous cell carcinoma of the head and neck. N Engl J Med 1990;323:795–801.
18. Lippman SM, Batsakis JG, Toth BB, et al. Comparison of low dose isotretinoin with beta carotene to prevent oral carcinogenesis. N Engl J Med 1993;328:15–20.
19. Malaker K, Anderson BJ, Beecroft WA, et al. Management of oral mucosal dysplasia with β-carotene retinoic acid: a pilot crossover study. Cancer Detect Prev 1991;15:335–340.
20. Garewal HS. Potential role of β-carotene in prevention of oral cancer. Am J Clin Nutr 1991;53:294S–297S.
21. Stich HF, Mathew B, Sankaranarayanan R, et al. Remission of precancerous lesions in the oral cavity of tobacco chewers and maintenance of the protective effect of β-carotene or vitamin A. Am J Clin Nutr 1991;53:298S–304S.

22. The Alpha-tocopherol, Beta Carotene Cancer Prevention Study Group. The effect of vitamin E and beta carotene on the incidence of lung cancer and other cancers in male smokers. N Engl J Med 1994;330:1029–1035.

23. Benner SE, Winn RJ, Lippman SM, et al. Regression of oral leukoplakia with alpha-tocopherol: a Community Clinical Oncology Program chemoprevention study. J Natl Cancer Inst 1993;85:44–47.

24. American Cancer Society. Guidelines for the cancer-related checkup: an update. Atlanta: American Cancer Society, 1993.

25. Canadian Task Force on the Periodic Health Examination. Canadian guide to clinical preventive health care. Ottawa: Canada Communication Group, 1994:838–847.

26. National Institute of Dental Research. Detecting oral cancer: a guide for dentists. Bethesda: National Institute of Dental Research, 1994.

27. Connoly GN, Winn DM, Hecht SS, et al. The reemergence of smokeless tobacco. N Engl J Med 1986;314:1020–1027.

17. Screening for Bladder Cancer

RECOMMENDATION

Routine screening for bladder cancer with urine dipstick, microscopic urinalysis, or urine cytology is not recommended in asymptomatic persons. All patients who smoke tobacco should be routinely counseled to quit smoking (see Chapter 54).

Burden of Suffering

Bladder cancer is an important cause of morbidity and mortality in the U.S., primarily in older men. Over 50,000 new cases and over 11,000 deaths due to bladder cancer are predicted to occur in 1995 in the U.S.[1] Risk rises steeply with age; over half of all deaths from bladder cancer occur after age 70. The incidence of bladder cancer is 3–4 times higher in men than women, and roughly twice as high in white men compared to black men.[2,3] Among white men, the annual incidence of bladder cancer after age 65 is approximately 2/1,000 persons (vs. 0.1/1,000 under 65), and the lifetime probability of developing cancer is over 3%.[3] The probability of dying from bladder cancer is much smaller, however—less than 1%. Cigarette smoking markedly increases the risk for bladder cancer (relative risk among smokers vs. nonsmokers = 1.5–7);[4,5] nearly half of all new cases of bladder cancer occur in current or former smokers.[2] Occupational exposure to chemicals used in dye, leather, and tire and rubber industries has also been associated with increased risks of bladder cancer.[4] Despite initial reports, positive associations between bladder cancer and consumption of coffee or artificial sweeteners have not been confirmed.[2,6,7]

Accuracy of Screening Tests

Early asymptomatic bladder cancer may be associated with occult bleeding (microscopic hematuria) or the presence of dysplastic cells in the urine. The definition of significant hematuria varies, but more than 3–5 red blood cells (RBCs) per high-powered field in microscopic analysis of the urine sediment is usually considered abnormal.[8] Urine dipsticks, which detect peroxidase activity of hemoglobin, provide a quick, inexpensive, and sensitive test for hematuria, and have largely supplanted microscopic urinalysis for screening in asymptomatic patients. Depending on the reference standard used (>2 or >5 RBCs per high-powered field on microscopy), dipstick urinalysis has a sensitivity of 91–100% and a specificity of 65–99% for detecting microscopic hematuria.[9-16] Dipsticks facilitate testing of serial urine specimens at home, which increases the detection of intermittent hematuria. False-positive dipstick results may be produced by myoglobin in the urine, and false-negative results may result from high concentrations of ascorbic acid, or from prolonged exposure of dipsticks to air.[8]

Although dipsticks are reasonably accurate for detecting hematuria, microscopic hematuria is not specific for bladder cancer or other urologic cancers. Of the various other causes of microscopic hematuria in asymptomatic patients, most are either benign (e.g., benign prostatic hypertrophy (BPH), exercise, renal cysts, urethral trauma, menstrual bleeding) or of questionable importance (bladder stones, dysplasia, asymptomatic infection). In three separate studies, 46–55% of men with asymptomatic hematuria had no identifiable source of bleeding.[17-19]

Two large outpatient studies have used urine dipsticks to screen for hematuria in asymptomatic populations at increased risk of bladder cancer. In a study by Messing, older men (mean age 65) screened their urine daily for 14 days. Of 1,340 men completing screening, 21% had at least one positive screen and 16 (1.2%) had urologic cancers (9 bladder, 1 renal, and 6 prostate).[18] Britton recruited 3,152 male outpatients over 60 years old to test their urine 10 times (daily or weekly). At least one screen was positive in 20% of men (12% on initial screen), and 22 (0.5%) had cancer (17 bladder and 5 prostate).[19] Among men undergoing full evaluation for hematuria, the positive predictive values (PPV) of serial dipstick screening for malignancy in these two studies were 8% and 6%, respectively; one third of men with hematuria refused or had an incomplete workup in each study. Similar results have been reported in other populations: among 272 Japanese men with 5 or more RBCs on urinalysis, 6% had urologic cancers.[17] Hematuria has a higher PPV (26–33%) if other urologic disorders are included as useful outcomes of screening,[18,20] but the benefit of early detection of many of these conditions (bladder stones, mild obstruction, urinary tract infection) remains unproven in asymptomatic individuals (also see Chapter 31).

The yield of onetime screening for bladder cancer in the general outpatient population appears to be much lower. In a retrospective review of over 20,000 men over 35 and women over 55 receiving a personal health appraisal, dipstick screening detected only three cases of cancer (one bladder, two prostate).[21] Prevalence of positive dipstick results ranged from 3–9% over a 7-year period. In a second study of almost 2,700 outpatients, 13% of screened men and women had hematuria (at least one RBC on urine sediment), but only 2% of those with microscopic hematuria had serious urologic disease.[22,23] In each of these studies, only 0.5% of all patients (3–4% of men over age 55) with asymptomatic hematuria were diagnosed with urologic cancers within 3 years of a positive screen.

Urine cytology is more specific but less sensitive than microscopic hematuria as a screen for early bladder cancer. Because cytology is technically difficult and significantly more expensive than dipstick urinalysis, its use as an initial screening test has been limited to high-risk occupational screening programs. Specificity for cytology has been estimated to be as high as 95%,[24] and sequential screening combining urine dipstick and urine cytology may be able to reduce the false-positive rate of screening while maintaining sensitivity for clinically important cancers. Among men with dipstick hematuria in one screening study, urine cytology detected 10 of 17 patients with bladder cancer with a specificity of 96%; 6 of the 7 cases missed were well-differentiated, superficial lesions with a good prognosis.[19] Rapid tests based on other tumor markers are under investigation.[25]

Effectiveness of Early Detection

Survival in patients with bladder cancer is strongly associated with stage at diagnosis. Although most cancers are superficial at time of diagnosis, currently 10–20% of all cases of bladder cancer have invaded the muscular wall of the bladder when first diagnosed, with a much worse prognosis. Five-year survival for patients with superficial disease is over 90%, but falls to less than 50% with invasive disease.[1] The rationale for screening is that detecting and treating early asymptomatic bladder cancers may prevent progression to invasive disease, or allow for more effective treatment of noninvasive tumors, which have a high rate of recurrence. Many cases detected on screening, however, are low-grade transitional cell cancers with low propensity for invasion; in contrast, since aggressive cancers may invade early, periodic screening may have a limited potential for detecting lethal bladder cancers at an early, treatable stage.[26]

In the prospective screening studies cited above, all 26 cases of bladder cancer detected by screening were early tumors confined to superficial areas of the bladder (Stage T0 or T1).[18,19] Compared to outcomes of cancers developing in the general population, cases detected by screening appeared to be less likely to progress over 3 years[27] or lead to death within 2 years.[28] Because of lead-time and length biases (see Chapter ii, Methodology), however, comparing case-survival is not sufficient to establish a benefit of screening, without information on rates of cancer and death in a comparable unscreened population. The incidence of invasive and fatal bladder cancer among screened men is very low, and it is also quite low in the general population of older men (<1/1,000 per year). Larger studies, with a comparable unscreened group and longer follow-up, are needed to determine whether screening improves the outcome of bladder cancer in high-risk populations. Despite early detection and treatment, 10 of 16 cancers detected by screening recurred within 3 years in one study.[27]

Recommendations of Other Groups

No major organization recommends screening for bladder cancer in asymptomatic adults. The Canadian Task Force on the Periodic Health Examination recommends against routine screening in asymptomatic individuals and concludes that there is insufficient evidence for or against screening in specific high risk groups.[29] The American Cancer Society has not issued any specific guidelines on screening for bladder cancer.

Discussion

Dipstick and microscopic urinalysis are simple and sensitive tests for detecting hematuria from early tumors, but they are not sufficiently specific to be practical for screening for bladder cancer in the general population. Even among older high-risk populations, the predictive value of a positive screening test is low (5–8%). As a result, many persons without cancer will require diagnostic workups for false-positive test results and will be subjected to the costs, discomforts, and risks of cystoscopy and intravenous pyelography. More important, there is no proof that early detection significantly improves the prognosis for the small minority of patients found to have urologic malignancies. Most of the bladder cancers detected have a good prognosis in the absence of screening: 5-year survival for all bladder cancer is currently close to 80%.[1] Due to the frequent multifocal nature of bladder cancer, recurrences are common despite early detection and treatment. Conversely, the most lethal tumors become invasive early in the course of disease, and the potential to detect them at an earlier stage may be limited. Only a prospective study that includes an unscreened comparison group can determine whether screening is effective in reducing morbidity or mortality from bladder cancer (or other urologic cancers), and whether the benefits are sufficient to justify the costs and risks of screening and early treatment. In the absence of such evidence, routine screening cannot be recommended, due to the high rate of false-positive results, and the possibility of harm to asymptomatic patients, few of whom have cancer. Primary prevention may offer a safer and more effective strategy than screening for reducing mortality from urologic cancer, since smoking accounts for nearly half of all deaths from cancers of the bladder and kidney.[2]

CLINICAL INTERVENTION

Routine screening for bladder cancer with microscopic urinalysis, urine dipstick, or urine cytology is not recommended in asymptomatic persons ("D" recommendation). Persons working in high-risk professions (e.g., dye or rubber industries) may be eligible for screening at the worksite, although the benefit of this has not been determined. Men and women who smoke cigarettes should be advised that smoking significantly increases the

risk for bladder cancer, and all smokers should be routinely counseled to quit smoking (see Chapter 54).

The draft update for this chapter was prepared for the U.S. Preventive Services Task Force by David Atkins, MD, MPH, with contributions from materials prepared by Sarvesh Logsetty, MD, for the Canadian Task Force on the Periodic Health Examination.

REFERENCES

1. Wingo PA, Tong T, Bolden S. Cancer statistics, 1995. CA Cancer J Clin 1995;45:8–30.
2. National Cancer Institute. Cancer of the bladder. Bethesda: National Cancer Institute, 1990. (NIH Publication no. 90-722.)
3. Ries LAG, Miller BA, Hankey BF, et al, eds. SEER cancer statistics review 1973–1991: tables and graphs. Bethesda: National Cancer Institute, 1994. (NIH Publication no. 94-2789.)
4. Anton-Culver H, Lee-Felstein A, Taylor TH. Occupation and bladder cancer risk. Am J Epidemiol 1992;136:89–94.
5. Slattery ML, Schumacher MC, West DW, et al. Smoking and bladder cancer. The modifying effect of cigarettes on other factors. Cancer 1988;61:402–408.
6. Viscoli CM, Lachs MS, Horwitz RI. Bladder cancer and coffee drinking: a summary of case-control research. Lancet 1993;341:1432–1437.
7. Chappel CI. A review and biological risk assessment of sodium saccharin. Regul Toxicol Pharmacol 1992;15:253–270.
8. Woolhandler S, Pels RJ, Bor DH, et al. Dipstick urinalysis screening of asymptomatic adults for urinary tract disorders: I. hematuria and proteinuria. JAMA 1989;262:1214–1219.
9. Loo SY, Scottolini AG, Luangphinith S, et al. Urine screening strategy employing dipstick analysis and selective culture: an evaluation. Am J Clin Pathol 1984;81:634–642.
10. Sewell DL, Burt SP, Gabbert NJ, et al. Evaluation of the Chemstrip 9 as a screening test for urinalysis and urine culture in men. Am J Clin Pathol 1985;83:740–743.
11. Mariani AJ, Luangphinith S, Loo S, et al. Dipstick chemical urinalysis: an accurate cost-effective screening test. J Urol 1984;132:64–66.
12. Hearne CR, Donnell MG, Fraser CG. Assessment of new urinalysis dipstick. Clin Chem 1980;26:170–171.
13. Shaw ST, Poon SY, Wong ET. Routine urinalysis: is the dipstick enough? JAMA 1985;253:1596–1600.
14. Szwed JJ, Schaust C. The importance of microscopic examination of the urinary sediment. Am J Med Technol 1982;48:141–143.
15. Smalley DL, Bryan JA. Comparative evaluation of biochemical and microscopic urinalysis. Am J Med Technol 1983;49:237–239.
16. Schumann GB, Greenberg NF. Usefulness of microscopic urinalysis as a screening procedure. Am J Clin Pathol 1979;71:452–456.
17. Muramaki S, Igarashi T, Hara S, Shimazaki J. Strategies for asymptomatic microscopic hematuria: a prospective study of 1,034 patients. J Urol 1990;144:99–101.
18. Messing EM, Young TB, Hunt VB, et al. Home screening for hematuria: results of a multi-clinic study. J Urol 1992;148:289–292.
19. Britton JP, Dowell AC, Whelan P, Harris CM. A community study of bladder cancer screening by the detection of occult urinary bleeding. J Urol 1992;148:788–790.
20. Messing EM, Young TB, Hunt VB, et al. The significance of asymptomatic microhematuria in men 50 or more years old: findings of a home screening study using urinary dipsticks. J Urol 1987;137:919–922.
21. Hiatt RA, Ordonez JD. Dipstick urinalysis screening, asymptomatic microhematuria, and subsequent urological cancers in a population-based sample. Cancer Epidemiol Biomarkers Prev 1994;3:1–5.
22. Mohr DN, Offord KP, Owen RA, et al. Asymptomatic microhematuria and urologic disease. JAMA 1986;256:224–229.
23. Mohr DN, Offord KP, Melton LJ. Isolated asymptomatic microhematuria: a cross sectional analysis of test-positive and test-negative patients. J Gen Intern Med 1987;2:318–324.
24. Farrow GM. Pathologist's role in bladder cancer. Semin Oncol 1979;6:198–206.
25. Attallah AM, Helmi H, El-Helali E, et al. A dipstick, dot-ELISA assay for the rapid detection of bladder cancer. Cancer Detect Prev 1991;15:495–499.

26. Farrow GM. Pathology of carcinoma in situ of the urinary bladder and related lesions. J Cell Biochem 1992;16(Suppl I):39–43.
27. Whelan P, Britton JP, Dowell AC. Three-year follow-up of bladder tumors found on screening. Br J Urol 1993;72:893–896.
28. Messing EM, Young TB, Hunt VB, et al. Comparison of bladder cancer outcome in men undergoing hematuria home screening versus those with standard clinical presentations. Urology 1995;45:387–397.
29. Canadian Task Force on the Periodic Health Examination. Canadian guide to clinical preventive health care. Ottawa: Canada Communication Group, 1994:826–836.

18. Screening for Thyroid Cancer

RECOMMENDATION

Routine screening for thyroid cancer using neck palpation or ultrasonography is not recommended for asymptomatic children or adults. There is insufficient evidence to recommend for or against screening persons with a history of external head and neck irradiation in infancy or childhood, but recommendations for such screening may be made on other grounds (see *Clinical Intervention*).

Burden of Suffering

Thyroid cancer accounts for an estimated 14,000 new cancer cases and more than 1,000 deaths in the U.S. each year.[1] The annual incidence is about 4/100,000 population.[2] Women account for 77% of new cases and 61% of deaths.[1] Current overall 5-year survival with treatment is 95% in whites and 90% in blacks,[1] but is much lower with some histologic types (e.g., medullary, anaplastic).[3–5] Among those at substantially increased risk for thyroid cancer are persons exposed to external upper body (especially head and neck) irradiation during infancy or childhood, and individuals with a family history of thyroid cancer or multiple endocrine neoplasia type 2 (MEN 2) syndrome.[6–10] The risk of radiation-induced thyroid nodularity and cancer increases with radiation dose and decreases with increasing age at which irradiation occurred.[7–12] In several large cohort studies, the absolute excess risk of thyroid cancer associated with low-dose irradiation given before 18 years of age ranged from 0.3 to 12.5/10,000 person-years per Gy (Gy = radiation dose).[8–10] Medullary thyroid cancer, which comprises about 10% of all thyroid malignancies, is inherited in one fourth of cases as part of the autosomal dominant MEN 2 syndrome.[6,13]

Accuracy of Screening Tests

Common screening tests for thyroid cancer include neck palpation and ultrasonography to detect nodules. Screening for medullary thyroid cancer as part of the autosomal dominant syndrome MEN 2 is performed at specialized centers[13a] rather than by primary care providers and will not be considered further in this chapter. Diagnostic procedures such as scintigraphy and fine-needle aspiration with cytology are generally reserved for persons with evidence of nodular disease or goiter.

The accuracy of neck palpation as a screening test varies with the examiner's technical skill and the size of the mass.[14] Among asymptomatic persons, palpation had a reported sensitivity of 38% for any thyroid disease (compared to examination at surgery for hyperparathyroidism), and 4 of 6 thyroid tumors were missed by palpation.[15] Compared to ultrasonographic examination, the sensitivity of neck palpation for detection of solitary thyroid nodules was only 15%, although no nodules were malignant.[16] Of 821 patients with no history of thyroid abnormalities and without clinically palpable nodules at autopsy, 100 had solitary nodules on macroscopic inspection of serially sectioned glands, and 17 had primary thyroid cancer.[17] Direct palpation of the excised thyroid gland at autopsy had a sensitivity for solitary nodules of only 24% compared to macroscopic inspection. These studies suggest a negative examination does not appreciably decrease the probability of thyroid nodules or cancer.

Neck palpation for thyroid nodularity has a high specificity in asymptomatic persons (93–100%), but routine palpation for thyroid nodules as a screening test to detect thyroid cancer generates many false-positive results because only a small proportion of nodular thyroid glands are neoplastic.[14,17,18] Periodic screening by palpation of almost 77,000 Japanese women detected thyroid cancer in 0.14%; the likelihood of thyroid cancer in the presence of a palpable thyroid abnormality was 6%.[18] A similarly high false-positive rate has been reported when ultrasonography is used as a screening test for thyroid abnormalities. In Finnish studies, ultrasound screening of 354 asymptomatic persons detected 56 solitary nodules, but none was malignant on biopsy.[16,19] Those falsely identified as positive by screening tests must undergo the inconvenience, expense, and anxiety of needless additional testing, including invasive tests such as biopsy, to rule out cancer.

Persons exposed to upper body irradiation in childhood have a higher prevalence of thyroid cancer, but also have a higher prevalence of thyroid nodularity.[8–11] It is unclear what effect a history of irradiation has on the likelihood of thyroid cancer in the presence of palpable thyroid nodularity. Periodic screening by neck palpation of 1,500 patients with a history of thyroid irradiation detected carcinoma in 1%.[20] The likelihood of thyroid cancer given detection of any nodular disease was only 3%, but the likelihood of malignancy among patients with nodular disease that was suspicious for cancer (e.g., solitary nodules) was not reported. Only 17% of the patients with nodularity actually underwent surgery, of whom 20% had thyroid cancer.

Effectiveness of Early Detection

The benefits of early detection of thyroid cancer in the general population are not well defined. For all histologic types, 5-year survival is significantly better with earlier stage at diagnosis.[3] A cohort study of mass screening found a significantly higher 7-year cumulative survival rate in patients whose cancer was detected by screening (98%) when compared with those presenting with symptoms (90%).[18] Cancers detected by screening were significantly more likely to have a favorable histology, however, and both lead-time and length biases are likely in this study. There have been no controlled trials demonstrating that asymptomatic persons detected by screening have a better outcome than those who present with clinical symptoms or signs. In addition, not all cancers detected through screening are likely to present clinically during the patient's lifetime. In autopsy studies in the U.S., the prevalence of occult thyroid carcinoma in adults ranges from 2–13%;[17,21,22] in contrast, the annual incidence of thyroid carcinoma is only about 4/100,000 population.[2]

Recommendations of Other Groups

The American Cancer Society recommends screening for thyroid cancer by palpation every 3 years in persons aged 21–40 years and annually in those more than 40 years old.[23] The American Academy of Family Physicians recommends palpation for thyroid nodules in adults with a history of upper body irradiation;[24] this recommendation is currently under review. The Canadian Task Force on the Periodic Health Examination concluded that there was poor evidence for either inclusion or exclusion of screening for thyroid cancer in the periodic health examination.[25]

Discussion

Given the lack of evidence that early detection of thyroid cancer by screening improves outcome, the high prevalence and uncertain clinical significance of occult throid carcinoma, the poor sensitivity of neck palpation in the detection of thyroid nodules, the fact that most positive screening tests would be false-positives, and the invasive nature of diagnostic tests (e.g., biopsy) likely to follow a positive screening test, routine screening for thyroid cancer cannot be recommended at this time. For persons irradiated in childhood, the greater likelihood of having both thyroid nodules and malignancy means that the yield from screening is likely to be higher. The clinical benefits of such screening have not been established, however.

CLINICAL INTERVENTION

Screening asymptomatic adults or children for thyroid cancer using either neck palpation or ultrasonography is not recommended ("D" recommendation). Although there is insufficient evidence to recommend for or against such screening in asymptomatic persons with a history of external

upper body (primarily head and neck) irradiation in infancy or childhood, recommendations for periodic palpation of the thyroid gland in such persons may be made on other grounds, including patient preference or anxiety regarding their increased risk of cancer ("C" recommendation).

The draft update of this chapter was prepared for the U.S. Preventive Services Task Force by Carolyn DiGuiseppi, MD, MPH.

REFERENCES

1. Wingo PA, Tong T, Bolden S. Cancer statistics, 1995. CA Cancer J Clin 1995;45:8–30.
2. Clark OH, Quan-Yang D. Thyroid cancer. Med Clin North Am 1991;75:211–234.
3. Akslen LA, Haldorsen T, Thoresen SO, et al. Survival and causes of death in thyroid cancer: a population-based study of 2479 cases from Norway. Cancer Res 1991;51:1234–1241.
4. Demeter JG, De Jong SA, Lawrence AM, et al. Anaplastic thyroid carcinoma: risk factors and outcome. Surgery 1991;110:956–963.
5. Flynn MB, Tarter J, Lyons K, et al. Frequency and experience with carcinoma of the thyroid at a private, a Veterans Administration, and a university hospital. J Surg Oncol 1991;48:164–170.
6. Grauer A, Raue F, Gagel RF. Changing concepts in the management of hereditary and sporadic medullary thyroid carcinoma. Endocrinol Metab Clin North Am 1990;19:613–635.
7. Kaplan MM. Progress in thyroid cancer. Endocrinol Metab Clin North Am 1990;19:469–478.
8. Ron E, Modan B, Preston D, et al. Thyroid neoplasia following low-dose radiation in childhood. Radiat Res 1989;120:516–531.
9. Shore RE, Hildreth N, Dvoretsky P, et al. Thyroid cancer among persons given x-ray treatment in infancy for an enlarged thymus gland. Am J Epidemiol 1993;137:1068–1080.
10. Tucker MA, Morris Jones PH, Boice JD Jr, et al. Therapeutic radiation at a young age is linked to secondary thyroid cancer. Cancer Res 1991;51:2885–2888.
11. Pottern LM, Kaplan MM, Larsen PR, et al. Thyroid nodularity after childhood irradiation for lymphoid hyperplasia: a comparison of questionnaire and clinical findings. J Clin Epidemiol 1990;43:449–460.
12. Nagataki S, Shibata Y, Inoue S, et al. Thyroid diseases among atomic bomb survivors in Nagasaki. JAMA 1994;272:364–370.
13. Bergholm U, Adami H-O, Bergstrom R, et al. Clinical characteristics in sporadic and familial medullary thyroid carcinoma. A nationwide study of 249 patients in Sweden from 1959 through 1981. Cancer 1989;63:1196–1204.
13a. Lips CJM, Landsvoter RM, Hoppener JWM, et al. Clinical screening as compared with DNA analysis in families with multiple endocrine neoplasia type 2A. N Engl J Med 1994;331:828–835.
14. Brander A, Viikinkoski P, Tuuhea J, et al. Clinical versus ultrasound examination of the thyroid gland in common clinical practice. J Clin Ultrasound 1992;20:37–42.
15. Christensen SB, Tibblin S. The reliability of the clinical examination of the thyroid gland: a prospective study of 100 consecutive patients surgically treated for hyperparathyroidism. Ann Chir Gynaecol 1985;74:151–154.
16. Brander A, Viikinkoski P, Nickels J, et al. Thyroid gland: US screening in a random adult population. Radiology 1991;181:683–687.
17. Mortensen JB, Woolner LB, Bennett WA. Gross and microscopic findings in clinically normal thyroid glands. J Clin Endocrinol Metab 1955;15:1270–1280.
18. Ishida T, Izuo M, Ogawa T, et al. Evaluation of mass screening for thyroid cancer. Jpn J Clin Oncol 1988;18:289–295.
19. Brander A, Viikinkoski P, Nickels J, et al. Thyroid gland: US screening in middle-aged women with no previous thyroid disease. Radiology 1989;173:507–510.
20. Shimaoka K, Bakri K, Sciascia M, et al. Thyroid screening program: follow-up evaluation. NY State J Med 1982; 1184–1187.
21. Sampson RJ, Woolner LB, Bahn RC, et al. Occult thyroid carcinoma in Olmsted County, Minnesota: prevalence at autopsy compared with that in Hiroshima and Nagasaki, Japan. Cancer 1974;34:2072–2076.

22. Nishiyama RH, Ludwig GK, Thompson NW. The prevalence of small papillary thyroid carcinomas in 100 consecutive necropsies in an American population. In: DeGroot LJ, ed. Radiation-associated thyroid carcinoma. New York: Grune & Stratton, 1977:123–125.

23. American Cancer Society. Guidelines for the cancer-related checkup: an update. Atlanta: American Cancer Society, 1993.

24. American Academy of Family Physicians. Age charts for periodic health examination. Kansas City, MO: American Academy of Family Physicians, 1994. (Reprint no. 510.)

25. Canadian Task Force on the Periodic Health Examination. Canadian guide to clinical preventive health care. Ottawa: Canada Communication Group, 1994:611–618.

19. Screening for Diabetes Mellitus

RECOMMENDATION

There is insufficient evidence to recommend for or against routine screening for diabetes mellitus in asymptomatic adults. There is also insufficient evidence to recommend for or against universal screening for gestational diabetes. Although the benefit of early detection has not been established for any group, clinicians may decide to screen selected persons at high risk of diabetes on other grounds (see *Clinical Intervention*). Screening with immune markers to identify persons at risk for developing insulin-dependent diabetes is not recommended in the general population.

Burden of Suffering

Approximately 14 million persons in the U.S. have diabetes mellitus.[1] Non-insulin-dependent diabetes mellitus (NIDDM) or Type II diabetes accounts for 90–95% of all cases of diabetes in the U.S., while insulin-dependent diabetes mellitus (IDDM) or Type I diabetes accounts for the remaining 5–10%.[1–4] An estimated half of all persons with diabetes (primarily patients with NIDDM) are currently unaware of their diagnosis.[2] Diabetes may cause life-threatening metabolic complications, and is the seventh leading cause of death in the U.S., contributing to roughly 160,000 deaths each year.[1,3] It is also an important risk factor for other leading causes of death such as coronary heart disease and cerebrovascular disease.[4] Diabetes is the most common cause of polyneuropathy, with approximately 50% of diabetics affected within 25 years of diagnosis,[5] and is responsible for over 50% of the 120,000 annual nontraumatic amputations in the U.S.[6] Diabetic nephropathy is now the leading cause of end-stage renal disease in the U.S.[7] and, if current trends continue, will soon account for 50% of all patients with renal failure.[8] Diabetes is the leading cause of blindness in adults ages 20–74 and accounts for over 8,000 new cases of blindness each year.[9] Infants born of diabetic women are at increased risk of fetal malformation, prematurity, spontaneous abortion, macrosomia, and metabolic derangements.[10,11] Compared to persons without diabetes, diabetic patients have a higher hospitalization rate, longer hospital stays, and increased ambulatory care visits.[3,12] The total annual economic burden of diabetes is believed to approach $100 billion in the U.S.[13]

The onset of NIDDM is usually after age 30, and the prevalence steadily increases with advancing age. It is estimated that nearly 20% of the U.S. population aged 65–74 has diabetes.[2] The prevalence of NIDDM is markedly increased in Native Americans and is also higher among black and Hispanic populations.[3] The prevalence of NIDDM is greater than 70% in Pima Indians 55 years of age and older.[14] Other risk factors for diabetes include family history, obesity, and a previous history of gestational diabetes or impaired glucose tolerance. IDDM has an earlier onset (usually before age 30), a much shorter asymptomatic period, and a more severe clinical course than NIDDM.

Gestational diabetes mellitus (GDM), the development of glucose intolerance during pregnancy, occurs in 3–5% of all pregnancies and is the most common medical problem of pregnancy.[3,15] Risk factors for GDM include obesity, increased maternal age, hypertension, glucosuria, a family history of diabetes, and a history of a macrosomic, stillborn, or congenitally malformed infant. GDM is a risk factor for fetal macrosomia and is associated with other neonatal complications, such as hyperbilirubinemia and hypoglycemia. Macrosomia—most commonly defined as birth weight above 4,000 or 4,500 g—is not itself a morbid condition but is associated with increased risk of operative delivery (cesarean section or vacuum or forceps delivery) and birth trauma (e.g., clavicular fracture, shoulder dystocia, and peripheral nerve injury).[16–19] In some series, the incidence of shoulder dystocia in infants over 4,000 g is close to 2%.[20] Women with a history of GDM are also at increased risk for developing NIDDM later in life.[21]

Accuracy of Screening Tests

The diagnosis of diabetes in many nonpregnant patients is based on typical symptoms (polyuria, polydypsia) in association with clear elevation of glucose (fasting plasma glucose > 140 mg/dL [7.8 mM]). Many asymptomatic persons, however, may have abnormal glucose metabolism and be at increased risk for complications of diabetes.

Diagnosis of Diabetes in Asymptomatic Persons. The National Diabetes Data Group (NDDG)[22] and World Health Organization (WHO)[23] have issued similar criteria for diagnosing diabetes in asymptomatic persons, based on elevated fasting plasma glucose (>140 mg/dL) or an abnormal plasma or serum glucose using a 2-hour 75 g oral glucose tolerance test (OGTT). NDDG criteria for a positive OGTT (> 200 mg/dL at 2 hours and before 2 hours) differ slightly from WHO criteria (glucose > 200 mg/dL at 2 hours alone). Abnormal glucose measurements on more than one occasion are required for a diagnosis of diabetes.[22,23] The complex diagnostic criteria reflect both the difficulty in distinguishing diabetic from nondiabetic patients on the basis of a single measurement, and the substantial test-retest variability of the OGTT. The coefficient of variation for OGTT ranges from 20% to 35%.[24,25] To improve reliability of the OGTT in nonpregnant adults, the American Diabetes Association (ADA) recommends that patients eat an unrestricted diet for 3 days preceding the test and fast overnight before the test.[26]

Both the NDDG and WHO recognize an intermediate form of disordered glucose metabolism, impaired glucose tolerance (IGT), based on intermediate results of the OGTT (140–200 mg/dL).[22,23] Patients with IGT are at increased risk of developing frank diabetes, but rates of progression are highly variable. IGT is also a risk factor for cardiovascular disease.[25] A significant number of individuals diagnosed with IGT revert to normal on repeat testing,[25] and the treatment implications of IGT alone are uncertain.

Diagnosis of Gestational Diabetes. The diagnosis of GDM is traditionally based on two or more abnormal values during a 3-hour glucose tolerance test using 100 g glucose.[22,27] NDDG diagnostic criteria are based on extrapolations from standards for whole blood glucose originally derived by O'Sullivan[28] to identify mothers at risk of developing diabetes in long-term follow-up. The conversion factor used to develop criteria for plasma glucose measurements may have been incorrect, however,[29] and others have proposed modified criteria with lower thresholds as more sensitive predictors of adverse pregnancy outcomes.[30] Outside of North America, the diagnosis of GDM is usually based on WHO criteria using a 2-hour 75 g glucose tolerance test.[23] The prevalence of GDM varies considerably depending on whether WHO, NDDG, or modified criteria of Carpenter and Coustan[30] are used.[15,31] In addition to poorly standardized criteria for a positive OGTT in pregnancy, the lack of studies on the reproducibility of the 100 g glucose tolerance test contributes to ongoing controversy over the diagnosis of GDM.[32–34]

Because diagnostic glucose tolerance testing is too time-consuming and expensive for routine screening, various blood or urine tests have been examined for their ability to identify three distinct at-risk populations among asymptomatic persons: persons with undiagnosed NIDDM, pregnant women with GDM, and individuals at high risk of developing IDDM.

Screening for Non-Insulin-Dependent Diabetes. The most commonly used screening tests for NIDDM include measurement of serum or plasma glucose in fasting or postprandial specimens, measurement of glycosylated proteins in blood, and detection of glucose in urine. The sensitivity and specificity of the fasting plasma glucose (compared to diagnostic oral glucose tolerance testing) depends on the threshold set to define an abnormal screening result. A single fasting glucose above 140 mg/dL is specific for diabetes (>99%) but sensitivity varies widely among different populations (21–75%).[35–40] Using a lower threshold (>123 mg/dL) improves sensitivity (40–88%), while maintaining reasonably high specificity (97–99%).[35–40] A random (i.e., nonfasting) plasma glucose greater than 140 mg/dL has a sensitivity of 45% and a specificity of 86%.[41] The ADA recommends that a fasting plasma glucose greater than 115 mg/dL, or a random glucose greater than 160 mg/dL, be considered a positive screen to be confirmed with OGTT.[26]

The nonenzymatic attachment of glucose to circulating proteins, primarily hemoglobin and albumin, reflects overall metabolic control in diabetic populations. A number of studies have evaluated hemoglobin A1c (HbA1c) and serum fructosamine as screening tests for diabetes.[40,42–45] Test characteristics are more variable than fasting plasma glucose, with sensitivity ranging from 15% to 93% and specificity from 84% to 99%.

Presence of glucose in the urine is fairly specific but less sensitive than most blood tests for NIDDM. In population-based screening using semiquantitative urine dipstick, a "trace positive" dipstick result or greater has a reported sensitivity of 23–64% and specificity of 98–99%.[40,46] In a high-risk population, quantitative assays of urine glucose achieved high sensitivity (81%) with high specificity (98%), comparable to both fasting plasma glucose and glycosylated protein assays.[40]

Sensitivity of all screening tests increases with the severity of hyperglycemia among the diabetic population.[40] Both the sensitivity and positive predictive value of screening tests will be highest in high-risk populations such as Native Americans and African Americans, where undiagnosed diabetes and severe hyperglycemia are more prevalent.[40] In the asymptomatic general population, where the prevalence of undiagnosed diabetes is only 1–3%, a greater proportion of diabetic patients may be missed by screening, and many persons with a positive screening test will not have diabetes. Screening asymptomatic persons may have some harmful effects, including an increase in false-positive diagnoses; in a review of 112 patients being treated for diabetes in a general practice, nine (8%) patients, all without classic symptoms, were found not to have diabetes on further evaluation.[47] Even a true-positive diagnosis could have adverse consequences for an asymptomatic person if it causes "labeling" effects[48] or difficulty obtaining insurance.

Screening for GDM. The Third International Workshop Conference on Gestational Diabetes has recommended screening pregnant women at 24–28 weeks of gestation with a 50 g 1-hour oral glucose challenge test, performed in fasting or nonfasting state.[27] Patients with plasma glucose of

140 mg/dL (7.8 mM) or greater at 1 hour should undergo a diagnostic 3-hour OGTT. There is no single threshold that accurately separates normal from abnormal results on the glucose challenge test, however.[27] Estimates of sensitivity of screening under this protocol range from 71% to 83% with a specificity of 78%–87%.[30,49,50] Sensitivity is increased by using a lower threshold for a positive screen[30,51] and by testing in the fasting state.[49] A large prospective study of nearly 4,300 pregnant women reported that using higher cutpoints (142–149 mg/dL) and adjusting for time since last meal could reduce the misclassification of patients based on initial screening tests.[52] Reproducibility of the 1 hour glucose challenge test is only fair,[53] but it improves with advancing gestational age.[54] In an unselected pregnant population (prevalence of GDM approximately 3%), fewer than one in five women with a positive glucose challenge test will meet criteria for gestational diabetes on a full OGTT.[52]

The elevations in plasma glucose in GDM are less pronounced than in IDDM or NIDDM. As a result, neither serum glycosylated proteins[51,55–58] nor urine glucose[34] are sufficiently sensitive for detecting GDM. In addition, glucosuria is common among nondiabetic pregnant women. Random blood glucose has been advocated as a simpler and less costly screening test for GDM[59,60] but its test performance has not been fully evaluated. A large prospective study is comparing fasting and random plasma glucose to oral glucose challenge for detecting GDM and for predicting adverse perinatal outcomes.[52]

Screening for Patients at Risk for IDDM. A growing body of evidence indicates that IDDM is a genetically linked autoimmune disorder, in which progressive destruction of insulin-producing pancreatic islet cells eventually leads to complete dependence on exogenous insulin.[61] Islet cell autoantibodies and insulin autoantibodies are present in the majority of patients with newly diagnosed IDDM,[62] and may precede the onset of clinical symptoms by months to years. Immunoassays for islet cell antibodies remain difficult to standardize,[63] however, and appear to be of limited value for screening in the general population. In individuals without a family history of IDDM, the prevalence of islet cell autoantibodies ranges from 0.3% to 4.0% and the chance of developing IDDM in antibody-positive individuals is estimated to be less than 10%.[64] The potential value of immune markers is greater in high-risk individuals (i.e., first-degree relatives of affected patients). Several studies report that a combination of immune markers and measures of insulin responsiveness can identify a population at very high risk (up to 70%) of developing IDDM.[62,63,65] This high risk may make such persons appropriate candidates for experimental interventions to reduce the risk of progression to IDDM. Only 10% of all cases of IDDM, however, occur in persons with a positive family history.

Effectiveness of Early Detection

Asymptomatic NIDDM. Up to 20% of patients with newly diagnosed NIDDM already have early retinopathy, suggesting that the onset of diabetes may be many years (estimated 9–12 years) before clinical diagnosis, and that the microvascular changes may precede overt symptoms in many patients.[66] Earlier detection through screening might provide an opportunity to reduce the progression of microvascular or macrovascular disease due to asymptomatic hyperglycemia. Animal models of diabetes suggest that hyperglycemia is the underlying cause of microvascular complications,[67] and numerous epidemiologic studies confirm that the degree of hyperglycemia and duration of disease are associated with microvascular complications such as nephropathy, retinopathy, and neuropathy.[5,68–72] Direct evidence that improving glucose control reduces the incidence of these complications has only recently become available, and only for patients with IDDM. In the Diabetes Control and Complications Trial (DCCT), over 1,400 subjects with IDDM were randomized to intensive insulin therapy versus conventional treatment. Intensive insulin therapy improved average blood glucose, significantly reduced progression of existing retinopathy, and significantly lowered the incidence of retinopathy, neuropathy, and nephropathy in all patients.[73,74]

The DCCT study is generally regarded as providing strong evidence of the role of hyperglycemia in diabetic microvascular disease, but questions remain about extrapolating its results to the management of patients with NIDDM.[75] The incidence of microvascular complications is lower in NIDDM than IDDM, and the largest controlled trial to date of treatment of NIDDM (the University Group Diabetes Program study) found no effect of improved glucose control with insulin or drug therapy on retinopathy.[76] More definitive results may come from the U.K. Prospective Diabetes Study (UKPDS), which randomized 2,520 patients with newly diagnosed NIDDM controlled with diet to diet alone, or additional therapy with chlorpropamide, glibenclamide, metformin, or insulin.[77] Three-year results indicated that patients receiving drug or insulin therapy had significantly better glucose control but greater weight gain and more frequent episodes of hypoglycemia.[78] Data on other clinical outcomes are not yet available.

Patients with diabetes are at significantly increased risk for coronary heart disease, stroke, and peripheral vascular disease; cardiovascular diseases combined account for the majority of deaths in diabetic patients. The risk of cardiovascular disease, however, is not clearly associated with either disease duration or degree of glycemic control. The rate of increase in coronary heart disease risk over time is similar in patients with NIDDM and in nondiabetic patients.[79,80] In 8-year follow-up of almost 500 diabetic men and women, disease duration was associated with risk of ischemic heart disease in patients with IDDM but not in those with NIDDM,[81] and there was no correlation between cerebrovascular and peripheral vascular events and diabetes duration. Detecting such an association may be complicated by difficulty in accurately ascertaining the onset of diabetes in patients with NIDDM. Insulin resistance and hyperinsulinemia may be more important determinants of macrovascular complications than degree of glucose control.[79,82] In the UGDP study, neither cardiovascular disease nor mortality was reduced by improved glucose control in the intervention groups,[76] but the interpretation of these findings has been criticized.[83] Drug therapy for NIDDM carries the risk of hypoglycemia. In the UKPDS study, the annual incidence of hypoglycemia was 28% for patients on glibenclamide, and 33% for those on insulin; episodes requiring medical therapy occurred in 1.4% of subjects each year.[78]

The majority of individuals in the U.S. who have disordered glucose metabolism have IGT.[84] Untreated, most persons with IGT do not develop diabetes, but the reported cumulative incidence of diabetes at 10 years has varied from 15% to 61%.[25] Progression to diabetes is highest in some Native American populations.[85] There is little direct evidence of a benefit of detecting and treating IGT.[86,87] Prospective studies of interventions to prevent progression to frank diabetes in patients with IGT have produced conflicting results. One trial of dietary and pharmacologic treatment[88] and a nonrandomized trial of diet and physical activity training[89] each reported a reduced incidence of diabetes, whereas other prospective studies have reported no effect on the rate of progression to diabetes.[90–92]

Gestational Diabetes. GDM is associated with increased risk of fetal macrosomia, birth trauma, neonatal hypoglycemia, and perinatal mortality.[93–96] No properly controlled trial has examined the benefit of universal or selective screening compared to routine care without screening. In two retrospective analyses, no significant difference in macrosomia or in birth trauma was found in women screened for GDM compared to unscreened control populations.[97,98] Because women screened for GDM are more likely to be at high risk, such studies cannot reliably exclude a benefit of screening.[98]

The clearest benefit of screening is the potential for treatment to reduce the incidence of fetal macrosomia in women with GDM. Although modified diet can reduce hyperglycemia in GDM, only one controlled trial has examined the effect of dietary therapy on clinical outcomes in GDM.[99] A total of 158 women with mild GDM (positive by NDDG criteria but not WHO criteria) were randomized to diet treatment or no therapy; there were no significant differences in perinatal outcomes, although slightly fewer infants over 4,000 g were born to diet-treated mothers (3 vs. 5).[100] Several randomized controlled trials have demonstrated that diet and insulin (compared to diet alone) results in improved glucose control and reduced incidence of macrosomia in women with GDM.[94,101,102] Macrosomia was not significantly reduced in a fourth trial, but 15% of the women assigned to diet therapy received insulin because glucose control was inadequate.[103] An overview of four randomized trials estimated that treatment of GDM with diet and insulin, compared to diet alone, reduced the incidence of macrosomia by two thirds (6% vs. 17%).[104] Despite a reduction in macrosomia, there were no significant differences in rates of cesarean section, forceps delivery, or birth trauma between treated and control groups in any of the prospective trials, however. There was only one reported instance of shoulder dystocia among 140 births in the two trials reporting this outcome.[101,104] In a retrospective analysis of 445 gestational diabetics, women who received both insulin and dietary treatment had significantly lower rates of birth trauma and operative delivery than women who received dietary treatment alone or no intervention.[96] Since treatment was not randomly assigned, factors other than treatment may have contributed to the differences in outcomes.

The benefit of improved glucose control on other outcomes in GDM, including perinatal mortality, remains uncertain. Although several case series have reported marked improvements in perinatal death rates with treatment of GDM,[95,97,105-107] none of these studies employed an appropriate control group. The use of historical controls (i.e., outcomes of prior pregnancies) or general population controls is likely to exaggerate the apparent benefits of treatment. In an overview of five randomized trials, there was no significant difference in perinatal mortality among women treated with diet and insulin (2.7%) and those treated with diet alone (3.2%).[104] Moreover, in trials conducted after 1975, there were no perinatal deaths in treated or control groups.[100,104] In one trial, insulin treatment was associated with lower rates of neonatal jaundice and nonsignificant reductions in admissions to the neonatal ICU.[108] At the same time, treatment of GDM may have adverse effects for some women. In one retrospective analysis, women with GDM who maintained tight glucose control (mean glucose < 87 mg/dL) had a higher incidence of small-for-gestational age infants than nondiabetic controls.[109]

Degrees of hyperglycemia more subtle than in GDM may result in increased maternal and neonatal complication rates.[110-112] The incidence of macrosomia and preeclampsia/eclampsia is higher in women who demonstrate at least one abnormal result among the four measurements in a glucose tolerance test. The prevalence of mildly hyperglycemic pregnant women who do not meet the criteria for GDM but are at increased risk during pregnancy is unknown.

Although treatment of GDM can reduce macrosomia, the impact of widespread screening and treatment on the overall incidence of macrosomia and dystocia may be quite small. The reported incidence of macrosomia in the general population varies from 1% to 8%,[93,113] and most macrosomic infants are born to women without GDM.[114] Gestational diabetes was responsible for only 5% of infants over 4,500 g in one study,[115] and it is estimated to account for only 5% of shoulder dystocia cases in this country.[116] Other factors such as maternal obesity, gestational weight gain, and maternal age may be more important determinants of macrosomia and adverse outcomes.[117] In a prospective study of GDM controlled with diet, the only significant predictor of birth weight was maternal weight at delivery; plasma glucose levels were poor predictors of birth weight.[118]

Persons at Risk for IDDM. Earlier diagnosis of IDDM could be of considerable benefit if treatment could arrest the disease process before severe insulinopenia and hyperglycemia had developed. A number of recent trials have examined whether immunosuppressive agents can delay disease progression in patients with new-onset IDDM.[61] Although some patients have experienced prolonged remissions, the benefit has not been sustained in most patients, and the serious adverse effects of immunosuppressive agents are likely to preclude their use in completely asymptomatic persons. There have been several promising small trials of other interventions to prevent IDDM in high-risk asymptomatic persons, enrolling individuals identified by autoantibodies levels and other physiologic measures.[63,119,120] Multicenter randomized clinical trials are currently underway to determine whether prophylactic regimens of insulin or nicotinamide can prevent progression to IDDM in such high-risk subjects.[61]

Recommendations of Other Groups

The Canadian Task Force on the Periodic Health Examination (CTF),[121] the American College of Physicians (ACP),[122] and the American Academy of Family Physicians[123] recommend against routine screening for diabetes among asymptomatic nonpregnant adults; each of these organizations concluded that selective screening may be reasonable among individuals at high risk of developing diabetes (e.g., older obese persons, those with a strong family history). AAFP policy is currently under review. The ADA recommends screening all individuals with a careful history and measuring fasting glucose on those with identified risk factors for developing diabetes, including obesity, family history, history of GDM, selected medical conditions, or selected ethnic background.[124] A 1994 report of the WHO concluded that population screening for NIDDM was not justified, but that opportunistic screening of high-risk persons may be useful to permit earlier intervention.[125]

The ACP,[122] the ADA,[124] and the Third International Workshop Conference on Gestational Diabetes[27] recommend universal screening for GDM in pregnant women between weeks 24 and 28 using a 1-hour glucose tolerance test. The American College of Obstetricians and Gynecologists and the American Academy of Pediatrics do not recommend universal screening in pregnancy but strongly recommend screening pregnant women in certain high-prevalence populations (e.g., Native Americans) and those with specific risk factors (age over 30, family history of diabetes, previous macrosomia, malformed or stillborn infants, hypertension, or glucosuria).[126,127] The CTF concluded that there was insufficient evidence to recommend for or against universal screening for GDM, but suggested close monitoring of women with risk factors for GDM.[121]

Discussion

Screening for diabetes in asymptomatic adults suffers from two important limitations: the lack of a practical screening test that is both sensitive and specific, and insufficient evidence that detection of diabetes in the asymptomatic period significantly improves long-term outcomes. Even if improving glucose control can reduce long-term complications of NIDDM, many other factors must be considered in determining the likely benefits and risks of screening in asymptomatic persons: efficacy of diet or medications in reducing glucose levels; compliance of asymptomatic persons with lifestyle advice; possible risks of drug or insulin therapy; inconvenience and costs of screening, follow-up, and treatment; and the potential adverse effects of screening (false-positive diagnoses, "labeling" of asymptomatic persons). Targeting screening to high-risk groups (certain ethnic populations, older overweight subjects) and emphasizing interventions that are inexpensive and safe (exercise, prudent diet, and weight loss) are likely to minimize the potential adverse effects of screening. Since most of these interventions are recommended for all adults, the additional benefit of screening to promote lifestyle interventions remains uncertain. If the ongoing UKPDS trial demonstrates important clinical benefits from more intensive interventions (i.e., drug or insulin therapy) in patients with minimally symptomatic NIDDM, this would provide stronger support for screening for diabetes among asymptomatic adults.

The value of widespread screening for GDM is also unproven. Important questions remain about the diagnostic gold standard, the optimal screening test, and the appropriate management of GDM. Although there is good evidence that insulin treatment can reduce the incidence of macrosomia in GDM, evidence of an effect on clinically important perinatal outcomes (birth trauma, operative delivery, neonatal metabolic derangements, or perinatal mortality) is much weaker. The high risk associated with GDM in earlier cohorts primarily reflects adverse outcomes in women who were older, overweight, or otherwise at increased risk. Universal screening is likely to have only a small impact on the overall incidence of macrosomia and birth trauma and may subject many low-risk women to the inconvenience, costs and possible risks of follow-up testing, dietary restriction, or insulin management. A 1988 study estimated that universal screening would cost $8,000 per case of macrosomia prevented.[122] By one estimate, however, up to 10,000 women would need to be screened to prevent 50 cases of macrosomia, 6 cases of shoulder dystocia, and 1 case of shoulder girdle injury (few of which cause lasting problems).[128] Targeting screening to women with risk factors for GDM (including older age), with emphasis on dietary management of GDM, is likely to minimize the adverse effects and costs of screening. Direct evidence of a benefit of screening on important clinical outcomes is not available for any group, however.

Immune markers are not sufficiently specific to recommend their use in the general population at this time. Screening persons with a family history of IDDM using immune markers and physiologic measurements can identify a small number of persons at very high risk of developing IDDM. Patients with a family history account for only 10% of all cases of IDDM, however, and trials of interventions to prevent IDDM in high-risk patients have not yet been completed.

Primary prevention may be a more effective means to reduce diabetes-associated morbidity than widespread screening. Diet, exercise, and weight reduction can safely improve glucose tolerance and are likely to have independent benefits on other important chronic diseases (see Chapters 55 and 56). Whether diabetes screening improves compliance with generally recommended lifestyle interventions has not been determined.

CLINICAL INTERVENTION

There is insufficient evidence to recommend for or against routine screening for NIDDM in nonpregnant adults ("C" recommendation). Although evidence of a benefit of early detection is not available for any group, clinicians may decide to screen selected persons at high risk of NIDDM on other grounds, including the increased predictive value of a positive test in individuals with risk factors and the potential (although unproven) benefits of reducing asymptomatic hyperglycemia through diet and exercise. Individuals at higher risk of diabetes include obese men and women over 40, patients with a strong family history of diabetes, and members of certain ethnic groups (Native Americans, Hispanics, African Americans). In persons without risk factors, screening for asymptomatic disease is much less likely to be of benefit, due to the low burden of disease and the poor predictive value of screening tests in low-risk persons. Measurement of fasting plasma glucose is recommended by experts as the screening test of choice; the frequency of screening is left to clinical discretion.

There is also insufficient evidence to recommend for or against routine screening for GDM ("C" recommendation). Although a beneficial effect of screening on perinatal morbidity has not been clearly demonstrated for any group, clinicians may decide to screen high-risk pregnant women on other grounds, including the higher burden of disease, and the potential clinical benefits from reducing macrosomia due to GDM. Risk factors for GDM include obesity, older maternal age, a family history of diabetes, and a history of macrosomia, fetal malformation, or fetal death. The 1-hour 50 g glucose challenge test, with confirmation of abnormal results with a 3-hour 100 g oral glucose tolerance test, is the screening test recommended by expert panels in the U.S.

Screening with immune markers to identify asymptomatic individuals at risk for developing IDDM is not recommended in the general population ("D" recommendation).

The draft update of this chapter was prepared for the U.S. Preventive Services Task Force by M. Carrington Reid, MD, PhD, Harold C. Sox, Jr., MD, Richard Comi, MD, and David Atkins, MD, MPH.

REFERENCES

1. National Diabetes Information Clearinghouse. Diabetes statistics. Bethesda: National Institute of Diabetes and Digestive and Kidney Diseases, 1994. (NIH Publication no. 94-3822.)
2. Harris MI. Undiagnosed NIDDM: clinical and public health issues. Diabetes Care 1993;16:642–652.
3. American Diabetes Association. Diabetes—1996 vital statistics. Alexandria, VA: American Diabetes Association, 1995.
4. Alberti KGMM, DeFronzo RA, Zimmet P, eds. International textbook of diabetes mellitus. New York: John Wiley and Sons, 1995.
5. Harati Y. Diabetic peripheral neuropathies. Ann Intern Med 1987;107:546–559.
6. Centers for Disease Control. Lower extremity amputations among persons with diabetes mellitus—Washington, 1988. MMWR 1991;40:737–741.
7. Viberti GC, Yip-Messent J, Morocutti A. Diabetic nephropathy: future avenue. Diabetes Care 1992; 15:1216–1225.
8. Breyer JA. Diabetic nephropathy in insulin-dependent patients. Am J Kidney Dis 1992;20:533–547.
9. Centers for Disease Control and Prevention. Public health focus: prevention of blindness associated with diabetic retinopathy. MMWR 1993;42:191–195.
10. Garner P. Type I diabetes mellitus and pregnancy. Lancet 1995;346:157–161.
11. Miodonovik M, Mimouni F, Dignan PSJ, et al. Major malformations in infants of IDDM women: vasculopathy and early-trimester poor glycemic control. Diabetes Care 1988;11:713–718.
12. Centers for Disease Control and Prevention. Surveillance for diabetes mellitus—United States, 1980–1989. MMWR 1993;42(SS-2):1–20.
13. American Diabetes Association. Direct and indirect costs of diabetes in the United States in 1992. Alexandria, VA: American Diabetes Association, 1993.
14. Knowler WC, Saad MS, Pettitt DJ, et al. Determinants of diabetes mellitus in the Pima Indians. Diabetes Care 1993;16(Suppl 1):216–226.
15. Magee MS, Walden CE, Benedetti TJ, et al. Influence of diagnostic criteria on the incidence of gestational diabetes and perinatal morbidity. JAMA 1993;269:609–615.
16. Gross TL, Sokol RJ, Williams T, et al. Shoulder dystocia: a fetal-physician risk. Am J Obstet Gynecol 1987;156:1408–1418.
17. McFarland LV, Raskin M, Daling JR, et al. Erb/Duchenne's palsy: a consequence of fetal macrosomia and method of delivery. Obstet Gynecol 1986;68:784–788.
18. Modanlou HD, Dorchester WL, Thorosian A, et al. Macrosomia—maternal, fetal, and neonatal implications. Obstet Gynecol 1980;55:420–424.
19. Sandmire HF, O'Halloin TJ. Shoulder dystocia: its incidence and associated risk factors. Int J Gynaecol Obstet 1988;26:65–73.

20. Cunningham FG, ed. Williams obstetrics. 19th ed. Norwalk, CT: Appleton & Lange, 1993.

21. Harris MI. Gestational diabetes may represent discovery of preexisting glucose intolerance. Diabetes Care 1988;11:402–411.

22. National Diabetes Data Group. Classification and diagnosis of diabetes mellitus and other categories of glucose tolerance. Diabetes 1979;28:1039–1057.

23. Expert Committee on Diabetes Mellitus—World Health Organization. Technical Report Series no. 646. Geneva: World Health Organization, 1980.

24. Home P. The OGTT: gold that does not shine. Diabetes Med 1988;5:313–314.

25. Yudkin JS, Alberti KG, McLarty DG, et al. Impaired glucose tolerance. Is it a risk factor for diabetes or a diagnostic ragbag? BMJ 1990;301:397–402.

26. American Diabetes Association. Office guide to diagnosis and classification of diabetes mellitus and other categories of glucose intolerance. Diabetes Care 1993;16(Suppl 2):4–6.

27. Metzger BE. Summary and recommendations of the Third International Workshop Conference on Gestational Diabetes Mellitus. Diabetes 1991;40(Suppl 2):197–201.

28. O'Sullivan JB, Gellis SS, Dandrow RV, et al. The potential diabetic and her treatment in pregnancy. Obstet Gynecol 1966;27:683–689.

29. Sacks DA, Salim AF, Greenspoon JS, et al. Do the current standards for glucose tolerance testing in pregnancy represent a valid conversion of O'Sullivan's original criteria? Am J Obstet Gynecol 1989;161:638–641.

30. Carpenter MW, Coustan DR. Criteria for screening tests for gestational diabetes. Am J Obstet Gynecol 1982; 144:768–773.

31. Li DFH, Wong VCW, O'Hoy KM, et al. Evaluation of the WHO criteria for 75 g oral glucose tolerance test in pregnancy. Br J Obstet Gynaecol 1987;94:847–850.

32. Canadian Task Force on the Periodic Health Examination. Periodic health examination, 1992 update: 1. Screening for gestational diabetes mellitus. Can Med Assoc J 1992;147:435–443.

33. Naylor CD. Diagnosing gestational diabetes: is the gold standard valid? Diabetes Care 1989;12:565–572.

34. Singer DE, Coley CM, Samet JH, et al. Tests of glycemia in diabetes mellitus. Ann Intern Med 1989; 110:125–137.

35. Cockram CS, Lau JT, Chan AY, et al. Assessment of glucose tolerance test criteria for diagnosis of diabetes in Chinese subjects. Diabetes Care 1992;15:988–990.

36. Blunt BA, Barrett-Connor E, Wingard DL. Evaluation of fasting plasma glucose as screening test for NIDDM in older adults. Diabetes Care 1991;14:989–993.

37. Seikikawa A, Tominaga M, Takahashi K, et al. Is examination of fructosamine levels valuable as a diagnostic test for diabetes mellitus. Diabet Res Clin Pract 1990;8:187–192.

38. Swai ABM, Harrison K, Chuwa LM, et al. Screening for diabetes: does measurement of serum fructosamine help? Diabet Med 1988;5:648–652.

39. Hanson RI, Nelson RG, McCance DR, et al. Comparison of screening tests for non-insulin dependent diabetes mellitus. Arch Intern Med 1993;153:2133–2140.

40. Modan M, Harris MI. Fasting plasma glucose in screening for NIDDM in the U.S. and Israel. Diabetes Care 1994;17:436–439.

41. Bourn D, Mann J. Screening for noninsulin dependent diabetes mellitus and impaired glucose tolerance in a Dunedin general practice—is it worth it? NZ Med J 1992;105:208–210.

42. Croxson SC, Absalom S, Burden AC. Fructosamine in diabetes screening of the elderly. Ann Clin Biochem 1991;28:279–282.

43. Guillausseau PJ, Charles MA, Paolaggi F, et al. Comparison of HbA1 and fructosamine in diagnosis of glucose-tolerance abnormalities. Diabetes Care 1990;13:898–900.

44. Forrest RD, Jackson CA, Gould BJ, et al. Four assay methods for glycated hemoglobin compared as screening tests for diabetes mellitus: the Islington diabetes survey. Clin Chem 1988;34:145–148.

45. Little RR, England JD, Wiedmeyer H, et al. Relationship of glycosylated hemoglobin to oral glucose tolerance. Diabetes 1988;37:60–64.

46. Anderson DKG, Lundblad E, Svardsudd K. A model for early diagnosis of type II diabetes mellitus in primary health care. Diabetes Med 1993;10:167–173.

47. Patchett P, Roberts D. Diabetic patients who do not have diabetes: investigation of register of diabetic patients in general practice. BMJ 1994;308:1225–1226.

48. Haynes RB, Sackett DL, Taylor DW, et al. Increased absenteeism after detection and labelling of hypertensive patients. N Engl J Med 1978;299:741–744.

49. Coustan DR, Widness JA, Carpenter MW, et al. Should the fifty-gram, one-hour plasma glucose screening test for gestational diabetes be administered in the fasting or fed state? Am J Obstet Gynecol 1986;154:1031–1035.

50. O'Sullivan JB, Mahan CM. Criteria for the oral glucose tolerance test in pregnancy. Diabetes 1964;13:278–285.

51. Roberts AB, Baker JR, Metcalf P, et al. Fructosamine compared with a glucose load as a screening test for gestational diabetes. Obstet Gynecol 1990;76:773–775.

52. Sermer M, Naylor CD, Gare DJ, et al. Impact of time since last meal on the gestational glucose challenge test. The Toronto Tri-Hospital Gestational Diabetes Project. Am J Obstet Gynecol 1994;171: 607–616.

53. Sacks DA, Abu-Fadil S, Greenspoon JS, et al. How reliable is the fifty-gram one-hour glucose screening test? Am J Obstet Gynecol 1989;161:642–645.

54. Espinosa de los Monteros A, Carino N, Ramirez A. The reproducibility of the 50-gram, 1-hour glucose screen for diabetes in pregnancy. Obstet Gynecol 1993;82:515–518.

55. Menon U, Ranjan M, Jasper P, et al. Evaluation of plasma fructosamine as a screening test for gestational diabetes. Aust NZ J Obstet Gynaecol 1991;31:25–26.

56. Corcoy R, Cerqueira MJ, Pedreno J, et al. Serum fructosamine is not a useful screening test for gestational diabetes. Eur J Obstet Gynecol Reprod Biol 1990;38:217–220.

57. Comtois R, Desjarlais F, Nguyen M, et al. Clinical usefulness of estimation of serum fructosamine concentration as screening test for gestational diabetes. Am J Obstet Gynecol 1989;160:651–654.

58. Cefalu WT, Prather KL, Chester DL, et al. Total serum glycosylated proteins in detection and monitoring of gestational diabetes. Diabetes Care 1990;13:872–875.

59. Lind T. Antenatal screening using random blood glucose values. Diabetes 1985;34(Suppl 2):17–20.

60. Hatem M, Dennis KJ. A random plasma glucose method for screening abnormal glucose tolerance in pregnancy. Br J Obstet Gynaecol 1987;94:213–216.

61. Atkinson MA, Maclaren NK. The pathogenesis of insulin-dependent diabetes mellitus. N Engl J Med 1994;331:1428–1444.

62. Riley WJ, Maclaren NK, Krischer J, et al. A prospective study of the development of diabetes in relatives of patients with insulin-dependent diabetes. N Engl J Med 1990;323:1167–1172.

63. Eisenbarth GS, Verge CF, Allen H, et al. The design of trials for prevention of IDDM. Diabetes 1993;42:941–946.

64. Bingley PJ, Bonifacio E, Shattock M, et al. Can islet cell antibodies predict IDDM in the general population? Diabetes Care 1993;16:45–50.

65. Bonifacio E, Bingley PJ, Shattock M, et al. Quantification of islet-cell antibodies and prediction of insulin-dependent diabetes. Lancet 1990;335:147–149.

66. Harris MI, Klein R, Welbourn TA, et al. Onset of NIDDM occurs at least 4–7 years before clinical diagnosis. Diabetes Care 1992;15:815–819.

67. Brownlee M. Glycation and diabetic complications. Diabetes 1994;43:836–841.

68. Takazakura E, Nakamoto Y, Hayakawa H, et al. Onset and progression of diabetic glomerulosclerosis: a prospective study based on serial renal biopsies. Diabetes 1975;24:1–9.

69. Miki E, Fukuda M, Kuzuya T, et al. Relation of the course of retinopathy to control of diabetes, age, and therapeutic agents in diabetic Japanese patients. Diabetes 1969;18:773–780.

70. Chase HP, Jackson WE, Hoops SL, et al. Glucose control and the renal and retinal complications of insulin-dependent diabetes mellitus. JAMA 1989;261:1155–1160.

71. Reichard P, Berglund B, Britz A, et al. Intensified conventional insulin treatment retards the microvascular complications of insulin-dependent diabetes mellitus (IDDM): the Stockholm Diabetes Intervention Study (SDIS) after 5 years. J Intern Med 1991;230:101–108.

72. Dahl-Jorgensen K, Bjoro T, Kierulf P, et al. Long term glycemic control and kidney function in insulin-dependent diabetes mellitus. Kidney Int 1992;41:920–923.

73. Diabetes Control and Complications Trial Research Group. The effect of intensive treatment of diabetes on the development and progression of long-term complications in insulin-dependent diabetes mellitus. N Engl J Med 1993;329:977–986.

74. The Diabetes Control and Complications Trial. The effect of intensive diabetes therapy on the development and progression of neuropathy. Ann Intern Med 1995;122:561–568.

75. Lasker RD. The Diabetes Control and Complications Trial. Implications for policy and practice. N Engl J Med 1993;329:1035–1036.

76. University Group Diabetes Program. Effects of hypoglycemic agents on vascular complications in patients with adult-onset diabetes. VIII. Evaluation of insulin therapy: final report. Diabetes 1982; 31(Suppl 5):1–81.

77. U.K. Prospective Diabetes Study Group. UK Prospective Diabetes Study (UKPDS) VIII. Study design, progress and performance. Diabetologia 1991;34:877–890.

78. United Kingdom Prospective Diabetes Study Group. United Kingdom Prospective Diabetes Study (UKPDS) 13: relative efficacy of randomly allocated diet, sulphonylurea, insulin or metformin in patients with newly diagnosed non-insulin dependent diabetes followed for three years. BMJ 1995; 310:83–88.

79. Donahue RP, Orchard TJ. Diabetes mellitus and macrovascular complications. Diabetes Care 1992;15:1141–1155.

80. Jarrett RJ, Shipley MJ. Type 2 (non-insulin-dependent) diabetes mellitus and cardiovascular disease— putative association versus common antecedents; further evidence from the Whitehall Study. Diabetologia 1988;31:737–740.

81. Morrish NJ, Stevens LK, Jarrett RJ, et al. Risk factors for macrovascular disease in diabetes mellitus: the London follow-up to the WHO multinational study of vascular disease in diabetics. Diabetologia 1991;34:590–594.

82. Welborn TA, Wearne K. Coronary heart disease incidence and cardiovascular mortality in Busselton with reference to glucose and insulin concentrations. Diabetes Care 1979;2:154–160.

83. Kilo C, Miller JP, Williamson JR. The Achilles heel of the University Group Diabetes Program. JAMA 1980;243:450–457.

84. Harris MI. Impaired glucose tolerance in the U.S. population. Diabetes Care 1989;12:464–474.

85. Saad MF, Knowler WC, Pettitt DJ, et al. Transient impaired glucose tolerance in Pima indians: is it important? BMJ 1988;297:1438–1441.

86. Genuth SM, Houser HB, Carter JR, et al. Observations on the value of mass indiscriminate screening for diabetes mellitus based on a five-year follow-up. Diabetes 1978;27:377–383.

87. Bennett PH, Knowler WC. Early detection and intervention in diabetes mellitus: is it effective? J Chronic Dis 1984;37:653–656.

88. Sartor G, Schersten B, Carlstrom S, et al. Ten-year follow-up of subjects with impaired glucose tolerance: prevention of diabetes by tolbutamide and diet regulation. Diabetes 1980;29:41–49.

89. Eriksson KF, Lindgarde F. Prevention of type 2 (non-insulin-dependent) diabetes mellitus by diet and physical exercise. The 6-year Malmo feasibility study. Diabetologia 1991;34:891–898.

90. Keen H, Jarrett RJ, McCartney P. The ten-year follow-up of the Bedford survey (1962–1972) glucose tolerance and diabetes. Diabetologia 1982;22:73–78.

91. Jarrett RJ, Keen H, Fuller JH, et al. Treatment of borderline diabetes: controlled trial using carbohydrate restriction and phenformin. BMJ 1977;2:861–865.

92. Jarrett RJ, Keen H, McCartney P. The Whitehall Study: ten year follow-up report on men with impaired glucose tolerance with reference to worsening of diabetes and predictors of death. Diabetic Med 1984;1:279–283.

93. Langer O, Berkus MD, Huff RW, et al. Shoulder dystocia: Should the fetus weighing > 4000 grams be delivered by cesarean section? Am J Obstet Gynecol 1991;165:831–837.

94. O'Sullivan JB, Charles D, Mahan CM, et al. Gestational diabetes and perinatal mortality rate. Am J Obstet Gynecol 1973;116:901–904.

95. Hod M, Merlob P, Friedman S, et al. Gestational diabetes mellitus—a survey of perinatal complications in the 1980's. Diabetes 1991;40(Suppl 2):74–78.

96. Coustan DR, Imarah J. Prophylactic insulin treatment of gestational diabetes reduces the incidence of macrosomia, operative delivery, and birth trauma. Am J Obstet Gynecol 1984;150:836–842.

97. Gabbe SG, Mestman JH, Freeman RK, et al. Management and outcome of Class A diabetes mellitus. Am J Obstet Gynecol 1977;127:465–469.

98. Santini DL, Ales KL. The impact of universal screening for gestational glucose intolerance on outcome of pregnancy. Surg Gynecol Obstet 1990;170:427–436.

99. Hunter DJS, Keirse MJNC. Gestational diabetes. In: Chalmers I, Enkin MW, Keirse MJNC, eds. Effective care in pregnancy and childbirth. Oxford: Oxford University Press, 1989:403–410.

100. Li DFH, Wong VCW, O'Hoy KMKY, et al. Is treatment needed for mild impairment of glucose in pregnancy? A randomized controlled trial. Br J Obstet Gynaecol 1987;94:851–854.

101. Coustan DR, Lewis SB. Insulin therapy for gestational diabetes. Obstet Gynecol 1978;51:306–310.

102. Thompson DJ, Porter KB, Gunnells DJ, et al. Prophylactic insulin in the management of gestational diabetes. Obstet Gynecol 1990;75:960–964.

103. Persson B, Strangenberg M, Hansson U, et al. Gestational diabetes mellitus (GDM) comparative evaluation of two treatment regimens, diet versus insulin and diet. Diabetes 1985;11(Suppl 2):101–105.

104. Walkinshaw SA. Diet + insulin vs diet alone for 'gestational diabetes.' In: Enkin MW, Keirse MJNC, Renfrew MJ, Neilson JP, eds. Pregnancy and childbirth module. Cochrane Database of Systematic Reviews: Review No. 06650, 20 April 1993, "Cochrane Updates on Disk," Oxford: Update Software, 1994, Disk Issue 1.

105. Adashi EY, Pinto H, Tyson JE. Impact of maternal euglycemia on fetal outcome in diabetic pregnancy. Am J Obstet Gynecol 1979;133:268–274.

106. Roversi GD, Gargiulo M, Nicolini U, et al. A new approach to the treatment of diabetic women: report of 479 cases seen from 1963 to 1975. Am J Obstet Gynecol 1979;135:567–576.

107. Gyves MT, Rodman HM, Little AB, et al. A modern approach to management of pregnant diabetics: a two-year analysis of perinatal outcomes. Am J Obstet Gynecol 1977;128:606–616.

108. Langer O, Anyaegbunam A, Brustman L, et al. Management of women with one abnormal oral glucose tolerance test value reduces adverse outcome in pregnancy. Am J Obstet Gynecol 1989;161: 593–599.

109. Langer O, Levy J, Brustman L, et al. Glycemic control in gestational diabetes mellitus—how tight is tight enough: small for gestational age vs. large for gestational age? Am J Obstet Gynecol 1989;161: 646–653.

110. Berkus MD, Langer O. Glucose tolerance test: degree of glucose abnormality correlates with neonatal outcome. Obstet Gynecol 1993;81:345–348.

111. Langer O, Brustman L, Anyaegbunam A, et al. The significance of one abnormal glucose tolerance test value on adverse outcome in pregnancy. Am J Obstet Gynecol 1987;157:758–763.

112. Lindsay MK, Graves W, Klein L. The relationship of one abnormal glucose tolerance test value and pregnancy outcome. Obstet Gynecol 1989;73:103–106.

113. Shelley-Jones DC, Beischer NA, Sheedy MT, et al. Excessive birth weight and maternal glucose tolerance—a 19-year review. Aust NZ J Obstet Gynaecol 1992;32:318–324.

114. Braveman P, Showstack J, Browner W, et al. Evaluating outcomes of pregnancy in diabetic women: epidemiologic considerations and recommended indicators. Diabetes Care 1988;11:281–287.

115. Spellacy WN, Miller S, Winegar A, et al. Macrosomia: maternal characteristics and infant complications. Obstet Gynecol 1985;66:158–161.

116. Hopwood HG. Shoulder dystocia: fifteen years' experience in a community hospital. Am J Obstet Gynecol 1982;144:162–166.

117. Johnson JW, Longmate JA, Frentzen B. Excessive maternal weight and pregnancy outcome. Am J Obstet Gynecol 1992;167:353–370.

118. Jacobson JD, Cousins L. A population-based study of maternal and perinatal outcome to patients with gestational diabetes. Am J Obstet Gynecol 1989;161:981–986.

119. Keller RJ, Eisenbarth GS, Jackson RA. Insulin prophylaxis in individuals at high risk of type I diabetes. Lancet 1993;341:927–928.

120. Elliot RB, Chase HP. Prevention or delay of type I (insulin-dependent) diabetes: progression to overt IDDM despite oral nicotinamide. Diabetologia 1991;34:362–365.

121. Canadian Task Force on the Periodic Health Examination. Canadian guide to clinical preventive health care. Ottawa: Canada Communication Group, 1994:16–23, 601–609.

122. Singer DE, Samet JH, Coley CM, Nathan DM. Screening for diabetes mellitus. In: Eddy DM, ed. Common screening tests. Philadelphia: American College of Physicians, 1991:154–178, 404–405.

123. American Academy of Family Physicians. Age charts for periodic health examination. Kansas City, MO: American Academy of Family Physicians, 1994. (Reprint no. 510.)

124. American Diabetes Association. Position Statement, screening for diabetes. Diabetes Care 1993;16 (Suppl 2):7–9.

125. World Health Organization. Prevention of diabetes mellitus: report of a WHO study group. Technical Report Series no. 844. Geneva: World Health Organization, 1994.

126. American College of Obstetricians and Gynecologists. Diabetes and pregnancy. Technical Bulletin no. 200. Washington DC: American College of Obstetricians and Gynecologists, 1994.

127. American Academy of Pediatrics and American College of Obstetricians and Gynecologists. Guidelines for perinatal care, 3rd ed. Elk Grove Village, IL: American Academy of Pediatrics, 1992.

128. Blank A, Metzger BE, Grave GD. Effects of gestational diabetes on perinatal morbidity reassessed. Diabetes Care 1995;18:127–129.

20. Screening for Thyroid Disease

RECOMMENDATION

Routine screening for thyroid disease with thyroid function tests is not recommended for asymptomatic children or adults. There is insufficient evidence to recommend for or against screening for thyroid disease with thyroid function tests in high-risk patients, but recommendations may be made on other grounds (see *Clinical Intervention*). Clinicians should remain alert to subtle symptoms and signs of thyroid dysfunction when examining such patients. Screening for congenital hypothyroidism is discussed in Chapter 45.

Burden of Suffering

Hyperthyroidism and hypothyroidism together account for considerable morbidity in the U.S. The total prevalence of these two disorders in adolescents and adults is estimated to be 1–4%; prevalence is higher in women and persons with Down syndrome, and increases with increasing age.[1–10] The annual incidence in adults has been estimated to be 0.05–0.1% for hyperthyroidism and 0.08–0.2% for hypothyroidism, with the higher incidences cited occurring in elderly women.[2,11] In adolescents, an incidence of 0.06%/year for these two disorders has been reported.[5] Symptoms of thyroid dysfunction, involving the nervous, cardiovascular, and gastrointestinal systems, may have an important impact on health and behavior.[12] Rarely, fatalities may occur due to thyroid storm in hyperthyroidism and myxedema coma in hypothyroidism.[13] Thyroid dysfunction during pregnancy is associated with an increased risk of adverse maternal and fetal outcomes.[14–18] Most patients with thyroid dysfunction will present with typical clinical symptoms and signs within a few months of disease onset, although overt disease may occasionally be overlooked. Studies in which asymptomatic adults of all ages were screened in the clinical setting, often using older, less sensitive tests, detected previously unsuspected thyroid disease in 0.6–0.9% of persons screened.[2,3,19,20]

The clinical diagnosis of thyroid dysfunction can be more difficult in certain high-prevalence populations, including the elderly, those with Down syndrome, and postpartum women, possibly delaying treatment and risking complications.[13] Older persons may experience apathetic hyperthyroidism, without the goiter, ophthalmopathy, and signs of sympathetic nervous system hyperactivity typically seen in younger persons.[21] Typical symptoms and signs of hypothyroidism, like fatigue, constipation, dry skin, and poor concentration, may be confused with symptoms of aging,[22] and may also occur less frequently in elderly hypothyroid patients.[23] Screening persons 60 years or older in the clinical setting detects previously unsuspected hyperthyroidism in 0.1–0.9% and hypothyroidism in 0.7–2.1%.[2,19,24–27] The clinical diagnosis of hypothyroidism may also be overlooked in patients with Down syndrome because some symptoms and signs, such as slow speech, thick tongue, and slow mentation, are typical findings of both conditions.[6,7] Screening persons with Down syndrome has detected previously unrecognized thyroid disease, primarily hypothyroidism, in 2.9% (range 0–6.5%).[6,7,28] Screening reveals thyroid dysfunction, primarily thyroiditis, in 4–6% of postpartum women.[29–32] This dysfunction is sometimes accompanied by nonspecific symptoms, such as fatigue, palpitations, impaired concentration, or depression,[31,33,34] that may be mistakenly attributed to the postpartum condition. Women with a personal or family history of thyroid or autoimmune disease, or with thyroid antibodies, are at increased risk for postpartum thyroid dysfunction.[16,30,35–37] Postpartum thyroid dysfunction is usually transient, but it may require short-term treatment to control symptoms.

Subclinical thyroid dysfunction as typically defined in the literature is a biochemical abnormality,[38] characterized by an abnormal level of thyroid-stimulating hormone (TSH) with otherwise normal thyroid tests and no clinical symptoms. Subclinical hypothyroidism, recognized by an elevated TSH level, is seen in 6–8% of adult women and 3% of adult men.[1] As with overt disease, the prevalence is higher in the elderly and in persons with Down syndrome.[6,7,24,25,27,28,39–41] Progression to overt hypothyroidism occurred in ≤ 2% of patients who had subclinical hypothyroidism without evidence of thyroid autoimmunity or prior thyroid-related disorders and who were followed for 2–15 years; in those with thyroid antibodies, however, progression occurs in about 5–7%/year, and in as many as 20–24%/year in elderly patients with antibodies.[25,28,39,42–45] Other than the risk of developing overt hypothyroidism, the importance of subclinical hypothyroidism is unknown. Case series have suggested adverse effects of an isolated elevated TSH level on blood lipid profile, myocardial function, and neuropsychiatric function,[22,46–48] but controlled observational studies have reported conflicting evidence regarding an association between subclinical hypothyroidism and any of these adverse effects.[49–54]

Subclinical hyperthyroidism, recognized by a subnormal TSH level, is seen in 0.2–5% of the elderly population; ≤ 1%/year progress to overt disease.[11,40,55,56] Subnormal levels of TSH are often transient, returning to normal without intervention.[3,25,57] There is limited evidence of risk from subclinical hyperthyroidism except when it is due to excessive thyroxine replacement. Case series have reported subclinical hyperthyroidism in a number of patients with atrial fibrillation.[58–61] Older controlled observational studies found no association between subclinical hyperthyroidism and atrial fibrillation,[62,63] but a significant association was reported in one carefully controlled cohort study that used a sensitive TSH assay.[57] One controlled study reported a significantly lower total cholesterol level in patients with a subnormal TSH level,[51] suggesting a possible benefit of this condition.

Accuracy of Screening Tests

Thyroid function tests to detect thyroid disease, including total thyroxine (TT_4), free thyroxine (FT_4), and TSH, are influenced by a variety of diagnostic and biologic factors that may affect their accuracy. For example, while TT_4 is usually elevated in hyperthyroidism, it misses 5% of cases that are due to triiodothyronine (T_3) toxicosis.[64] TT_4 concentration is strongly influenced by the concentrations and binding affinities of thyroxine-binding globulin and other thyroid-binding proteins.[38] Falsely abnormal TT_4 results often occur with conditions that affect these proteins, such as pregnancy, use of certain drugs, and nonthyroidal illness.[38,64] FT_4 has the advantage over TT_4 of being independent of thyroid-binding protein concentrations. Equilibrium dialysis (ED), regarded as the reference method for FT_4, is not suitable for routine screening due to its high cost.[38,65] Immunoassay or index (FTI) methods to estimate FT_4 are simpler, less expensive than ED, and have specificities of 93–99% compared to ED;[20,66–68] these methods are not always independent of thyroid-binding protein concentrations, however,[38,69] and they may show substantial interlaboratory variation.[65] TT_4 and FT_4 cannot be reliably measured in ill patients, because a substantial proportion will have abnormal thyroid function in the absence of true thyroid disease, due to "sick euthyroid syndrome."[69–71] Screening with TT_4 or FT_4 will generate many false-positive results in healthy populations.[2,19,20,71] With test specificities in the mid-90% range or lower, the low prevalence of previously unsuspected thyroid disease means that the likelihood of disease given an abnormal test will be quite low. In one study, thyroid disease requiring treatment was found in only 13% of those with abnormal FTI results.[20] Because TT_4 and FT_4 are normal by definition in subclinical thyroid dysfunction, they are not useful as screening tests for this condition.

The immunometric ("sensitive") TSH (sTSH) assays detect low as well as high serum TSH levels, and have become the standard for detecting hyperthyroidism and hypothyroidism. They therefore offer promise as first-line thyroid screening tests. In unselected populations, sTSH has a sensitivity of 89–95% and specificity of 90–96% for overt thyroid dysfunction, as compared to reference standards incorporating clinical history, examination, repeat measurement, and/or additional testing including thyrotropin-releasing hormone tests.[3,40,68] In an asymptomatic older population, the likelihood of thyroid disease given an abnormal sTSH was only 7%, however, reflecting the low prevalence of disease in healthy people.[40] Acutely ill patients, pregnant women, and persons using certain drugs such as glucocorticoids may have false-positive sTSH results,[38,72,73] although specificity is better than for TT_4 and FT_4 when the three tests have been directly compared.[38,74] Newer sTSH assays reduce but do not eliminate false-positive diagnoses in such patients.[75–77] sTSH may respond slowly to abrupt changes in thyroid function,[38] such as those that occur after treatment for hyperthyroidism, but such changes are not generally relevant to the screening of asymptomatic patients.

Effectiveness of Early Detection

Screening for occult thyroid dysfunction in adults would be valuable if there were clinical benefits of early treatment, including relief of previously unrecognized symptoms. We found no studies evaluating the treatment of hyperthyroidism detected by screening in asymptomatic persons, or of subclinical hyperthyroidism in persons with atrial fibrillation. Uncertainties about the benefits of treating hyperthyroidism detected by screening are particularly important because of the costs and potential adverse effects (e.g., agranulocytosis, induced hypothyroidism, surgical complications) of treatment with antithyroid medications, radioactive iodine ablation, or subtotal thyroidectomy.[78,79]

Several studies have evaluated the effectiveness of treating patients with subclinical hypothyroidism. Most of the subjects had previously identified thyroid disease, however, and the results may not apply to asymptomatic patients identified only by screening. In a randomized placebo-controlled trial of 33 women with subclinical hypothyroidism, all with a past history of treated hyperthyroidism, there were significant improvements in myocardial contractility and in previously unrecognized symptoms, but no significant changes in basal metabolic rate, pulse, body weight, skin texture, or serum lipid levels.[80] The long-term clinical importance of subtle changes in myocardial contractility is unknown. An uncontrolled experiment in 17 women identified by screening found a significantly improved mean clinical symptom score after treatment, mixed effects on myocardial function, and no effect on cholesterol, resting heart rate, body mass, or blood pressure.[81] Methodologic flaws make it difficult to interpret the results of this study. Uncontrolled experiments in adult patients, mostly women, with subclinical hypothyroidism due to previously identified thyroid disease have reported variable improvement in myocardial function but little effect on lipoproteins with thyroxine treatment.[82–89] A randomized controlled trial measuring the effects of thyroid replacement on quality of life, lipids, neuropsychological function, bone mineral density, and myocardial function in elderly patients with subclinical hypothyroidism is ongoing (personal communication, Dr. R. Jaeshke, St. Joseph's Hospital, Hamilton, Ontario, August 4, 1995).

In children and adults with Down syndrome and subclinical hypothyroidism, a double-blind crossover placebo-controlled trial failed to document any cognitive, social, or physical changes attributable to 8–14 weeks of thyroxine treatment,[41] although treatment duration may have been inadequate to effect change. There is otherwise little evidence regarding the benefits of early intervention in these individuals.

Thyroxine replacement therapy can have adverse effects with even moderate degrees of overtreatment (as detected by low TSH or high TT_4 levels), including decreased bone density compared to matched controls.[90–93] Reduced bone density could increase the risk of fractures in the elderly, but one large series found no significant difference in risk for fractures (or for ischemic heart disease) in treated patients with normal TSH levels compared to those with suppressed TSH due to overtreatment.[94] The fracture rate in the two groups was the same as in the general population, while the risk of ischemic heart disease was higher in treated patients irrespective of TSH levels. The study was not designed to determine whether the latter finding was due to treatment or to the underlying disease, however. A small randomized controlled trial in postmenopausal women with subclinical hypothyroidism found no bone density reduction after 14 months of appropriate thyroxine treatment.[95] Evidence therefore suggests against an adverse impact of appropriate thyroxine treatment.

Recommendations of Other Groups

No organizations recommend routine screening for thyroid disease in the general population, except screening newborns for congenital hypothyroidism (see Chapter 45). The American Academy of Family Physicians (AAFP)[96] and the American Association of Clinical Endocrinologists[97] recommend measuring thyroid function periodically in all older women. The policy of the AAFP is currently under review. The Canadian Task Force on the Periodic Health Examination recommends maintaining a high index of clinical suspicion for nonspecific symptoms consistent with hypothyroidism when examining perimenopausal and postmenopausal women.[98] The American College of Physicians recommends screening women over age 50 with one or more general symptoms that could be caused by thyroid disease.[99] The American College of Obstetricians and Gynecologists recommends that physicians and patients be aware of the symptoms and risk factors for postpartum thyroid dysfunction, and evaluate patients when indicated.[100] The American Academy of Pediatrics recommends that children with Down syndrome have thyroid screening tests at 4–6 and 12 months of age, and annually thereafter.[101] The American Thyroid Association recommends screening thyroid function in elderly patients, postpartum women, and all patients with autoimmune disease or with a strong family history of thyroid disease, using serum TSH measurement.[64,102]

Discussion

The prevalence of unsuspected thyroid disease in healthy people in the general population is very low. Despite the high specificity of thyroid function tests such as the newer TSH assays, their routine use in the asymptomatic general population results in many false-positive results. Because of the low prevalence of unsuspected disease, only 1 in 5–10 persons with abnormal screening tests will prove to have thyroid disease. Given the low risk, the lack of evidence that treatment of subclinical thyroid disease identified by screening results in important health benefits, and the potential adverse effects of treatment, screening the asymptomatic general population is not recommended.

The prevalence of thyroid disease is higher in certain populations, including elderly persons (particularly women), persons with Down syndrome, and postpartum women, and these patients might be candidates for thyroid function testing if the results could provide an explanation for nonspecific and insidious symptoms, such as fatigue, memory impairment, or depression, that might be attributed mistakenly to other medical or psychiatric causes. Clinicians should therefore maintain a high index of suspicion for such nonspecific symptoms, and for thyroid disease when these types of symptoms are found, when examining high-risk patients. There is, however, little evidence that routinely screening high-risk patients results in important clinical benefits.

CLINICAL INTERVENTION

Routine screening for thyroid disease with thyroid function tests is not recommended for asymptomatic children or adults ("D" recommendation). This recommendation does not mean that clinicians should not monitor thyroid function in patients with a previous history of thyroid disease. There is insufficient evidence to recommend for or against screening for thyroid disease with thyroid function tests in high-risk patients, including elderly persons, postpartum women, and persons with Down syndrome, but recommendations may be made on other grounds, such as the higher prevalence of disease and the increased likelihood that symptoms of thyroid disease will be overlooked in these patients ("C" recommendation).

Clinicians should remain alert for subtle or nonspecific symptoms of thyroid dysfunction when examining such patients, and maintain a low threshold for diagnostic evaluation of thyroid function. Examples of such symptoms include easy fatiguability, weight gain, dry skin or hair, cold intolerance, difficulty concentrating, depression, nervousness, and palpitations. If screening is performed, the preferred test is measurement of thyroid-stimulating hormone (TSH) using a sensitive immunometric or similar assay, because of its superior sensitivity and specificity. Screening for congenital hypothyroidism is discussed in Chapter 45.

The draft update of this chapter was prepared for the U.S. Preventive Services Task Force by Carolyn DiGuiseppi, MD, MPH.

REFERENCES

1. Tunbridge WMG, Evered DC, Hall R, et al. The spectrum of thyroid disease in a community: the Whickham survey. Clin Endocrinol (Oxf) 1977;7:481–493.
2. dos Remedios LV, Weber PM, Feldman R, et al. Detecting unsuspected thyroid dysfunction by the free thyroxine index. Arch Intern Med 1980;140:1045–1049.
3. Eggertsen R, Petersen K, Lundberg P-A, et al. Screening for thyroid disease in a primary care unit with a thyroid stimulating hormone assay with a low detection limit. BMJ 1988;297:1586–1592.
4. Baldwin DB, Rowett D. Incidence of thyroid disorders in Connecticut. JAMA 1978;239:742–744.
5. Rallison ML, Dobyns BM, Meikle AW, et al. Natural history of thyroid abnormalities: prevalence, incidence, and regression of thyroid diseases in adolescents and young adults. Am J Med 1991;91:363–370.
6. Dinani S, Carpenter S. Down's syndrome and thyroid disorder. J Mental Deficiency Res 1990;34: 187–193.
7. Pozzan GB, Rigon F, Girelli ME, et al. Thyroid function in patients with Down syndrome: preliminary results from non-institutionalized patients in the Veneto region. Am J Med Genet Suppl 1990;7:57–58.
8. Falkenberg M, Kagedal B, Norr A. Screening of an elderly female population for hypo- and hyperthyroidism by use of a thyroid hormone panel. Acta Med Scand 1983;214:361–365.
9. Sawin CT, Castelli WP, Hershman JM, et al. The aging thyroid: thyroid deficiency in the Framingham Study. Arch Intern Med 1985;145:1386–1388.
10. Petersen K, Lindstedt G, Lundberg P-A, et al. Thyroid disease in middle-aged and elderly Swedish women: thyroid-related hormones, thyroid dysfunction and goitre in relation to age and smoking. J Intern Med 1991;229:407–414.
11. Sundbeck G, Lundberg P-A, Lindstedt G, et al. Incidence and prevalence of thyroid disease in elderly women: results from the longitudinal population study of elderly people in Gothenburg, Sweden. Age Ageing 1991; 20: 291–298.
12. Gavin LA. The diagnostic dilemmas of hyperthyroxinemia and hypothyroxinemia. Adv Intern Med 1988;33:185–204.
13. Gavin LA. Thyroid crises. Med Clin North Am 1991;75:179–193.
14. Leung AS, Millar LK, Koonings PP, et al. Perinatal outcome in hypothyroid pregnancies. Obstet Gynecol 1993; 81:349–353.
15. Glinoer D, Fernandez Soto M, Bourdoux P, et al. Pregnancy in patients with mild thyroid abnormalities: maternal and neonatal repercussions. J Clin Endocrinol Metab 1991;73:421–427.
16. Glinoer D, Riahi M, Grun J-P, et al. Risk of subclinical hypothyroidism in pregnant women with asymptomatic autoimmune thyroid disorders. J Clin Endocrinol Metab 1994;79:197–204.
17. Davis LE, Lucas MJ, Hankins GDV, et al. Thyrotoxicosis complicating pregnancy. Am J Obstet Gynecol 1989; 160:63–70.
18. Davis LE, Leveno KJ, Cunningham FG. Hypothyroidism complicating pregnancy. Obstet Gynecol 1988;72:108–112.
19. Nolan JP, Tarsa NJ, DiBenedetto G. Case-finding for unsuspected thyroid disease: costs and health benefits. Am J Clin Pathol 1985;83:346–355.

20. Fukazawa H, Sakurada T, Yoshida K, et al. Free thyroxine estimation for the screening of hyper- and hypothyroidism in an adult population. Tohoku J Exp Med 1986;148:411–420.
21. Sawin CT. Thyroid dysfunction in older persons. Adv Intern Med 1991;37:223–248.
22. Levy EG. Thyroid disease in the elderly. Med Clin North Am 1991;75:151–167.
23. Doucet J, Trivalle C, Chassagne P, et al. Does age play a role in clinical presentation of hypothyroidism. J Am Geriatr Soc 1994;42:984–986.
24. Bemben DA, Winn P, Hamm RM, et al. Thyroid disease in the elderly. Part 1. Prevalence of undiagnosed hypothyroidism. J Fam Pract 1994;38:577–582.
25. Parle JV, Franklyn JA, Cross KW, et al. Prevalence and follow-up of abnormal thyrotrophin (TSH) concentrations in the elderly in the United Kingdom. Clin Endocrinol (Oxf) 1991;34:77–83.
26. Bahemuka M, Hodkinson HM. Screening for hypothyroidism in elderly inpatients. BMJ 1975;2:601–603.
27. Drinka PJ, Nolten WE. Prevalence of previously undiagnosed hypothyroidism in residents of a midwestern nursing home. South Med J 1990;83:1259–1261.
28. Selikowitz M. A five-year longitudinal study of thyroid function in children with Down syndrome. Dev Med Child Neurol 1993;35:396–401.
29. Gerstein HC. How common is postpartum thyroiditis? Arch Intern Med 1990;150:1397–1400.
30. Walfish PG, Meyerson J, Provias JP, et al. Prevalence and characteristics of post-partum thyroid dysfunction: results of a survey from Toronto, Canada. J Endocrinol Invest 1992;15:265–272.
31. Amino N, Mori H, Iwatani Y, et al. High prevalence of transient post-partum thyrotoxicosis and hypothyroidism. N Engl J Med 1982;306:849–852.
32. Jansson R, Bernander S, Karlsson A, et al. Autoimmune thyroid dysfunction in the postpartum period. J Clin Endocrinol Metab 1984;58:681–687.
33. Hayslip CC, Fein HG, O'Donnell VM, et al. The value of serum antimicrosomal antibody testing in screening for symptomatic postpartum thyroid dysfunction. Am J Obstet Gynecol 1988;159:203–209.
34. Roti E, Emerson CH. Clinical review 29: postpartum thyroiditis. J Clin Endocrinol Metab 1992;74:3–5.
35. Hidaka Y, Tamaki H, Iwatani Y, et al. Prediction of post-partum Graves' thyrotoxicosis by measurement of thyroid stimulating antibody in early pregnancy. Clin Endocrinol (Oxf) 1994;41:15–20.
36. Solomon BL, Fein HG, Smallridge RC. Usefulness of antimicrosomal antibody titers in the diagnosis and treatment of postpartum thyroiditis. J Fam Pract 1993;36:177–182.
37. Fung HYM, Kologlu M, Collison K, et al. Postpartum thyroid dysfunction in Mid Glamorgan. BMJ 1988;296:241–244.
38. Bayer MF. Effective laboratory evaluation of thyroid status. Med Clin North Am 1991;75:1–26.
39. Rosenthal MJ, Hunt WC, Garry PJ, et al. Thyroid failure in the elderly. JAMA 1987;258:209–213.
40. Okamura K, Ueda K, Sone H, et al. A sensitive thyroid stimulating hormone assay for screening of thyroid functional disorder in elderly Japanese. J Am Geriatr Soc 1989;37:317–322.
41. Tirosh E, Taub Y, Scher A, et al. Short-term efficacy of thyroid hormone supplementation for patients with Down syndrome and low-borderline thyroid function. Am J Ment Retard 1989;93:652–656.
42. Tunbridge WMG, Brewis M, French JM, et al. Natural history of autoimmune thyroiditis. BMJ (Clin Res) 1981;282: 258–262.
43. Helfand M, Crapo LM. Screening for thyroid disease. Ann Intern Med 1990;112:840–849.
44. Gordin A, Lamberg BA. Spontaneous hypothyroidism in symptomless autoimmune thyroiditis. A long-term follow-up study. Clin Endocrinol (Oxf) 1981;15:537–543.
45. Drinka PJ, Nolten WE, Voeks SK, et al. Follow-up of mild hypothyroidism in a nursing home. J Am Geriatr Soc 1991;39:264–266.
46. Pallas D, Koutras DA, Adamopoulos P, et al. Increased mean serum thyrotropin in apparently euthyroid hypercholesterolemic patients: does it mean occult hypothyroidism? J Endocrinol Invest 1991;14:743–746.
47. Haggerty JJ Jr, Garbutt JC, Evans DL, et al. Subclinical hypothyroidism: a review of neuropsychiatric aspects. Int J Psychiatr Med 1990;20:193–208.
48. Glueck CJ, Lang J, Tracy T, et al. The common finding of covert hypothyroidism at initial clinical evaluation for hyperlipoproteinemia. Clin Chim Acta 1991;201:113–122.
49. Althaus BU, Staub JJ, Ryff-De Leche A, et al. LDL/HDL changes in subclinical hypothyroidism: possible risk factors for coronary heart disease. Clin Endocrinol (Oxf) 1988;28:157–163.
50. Staub J-J, Althaus BU, Engler H, et al. Spectrum of subclinical and overt hypothyroidism: effect on thyrotropin, prolactin, and thyroid reserve, and metabolic impact on peripheral target tissues. Am J Med 1992;92:631–642.

51. Parle JV, Franklyn JA, Cross KW, et al. Circulating lipids and minor abnormalities of thyroid function. Clin Endocrinol (Oxf) 1992;37:411–414.

52. Tunbridge WMG, Evered DC, Hall R, et al. Lipid profiles and cardiovascular disease in the Whickham area with particular reference to thyroid failure. Clin Endocrinol (Oxf) 1977;7:495–508.

53. Osterweil D, Syndulko K, Cohen SN, et al. Cognitive function in non-demented older adults with hypothyroidism. J Am Geriatr Soc 1992;40:325–335.

54. Kutty KM, Bryant DG, Farid NR. Serum lipids in hypothyroidism—a reevaluation. J Clin Endocrinol Metab 1978;46: 55–56.

55. Sawin CT, Geller A, Kaplan MM, et al. Low serum thyrotropin (thyroid-stimulating hormone) in older persons without hyperthyroidism. Arch Intern Med 1991;151:165–168.

56. Sundbeck G, Jagenburg R, Johansson P-M, et al. Clinical significance of low serum thyrotropin concentration by chemiluminometric assay in 85-year-old women and men. Arch Intern Med 1991;151: 549–556.

57. Sawin CT, Geller A, Wolf PA, et al. Low serum thyrotropin concentrations as a risk factor for atrial fibrillation in older persons. N Engl J Med 1994;331:1249–1252.

58. Forfar JC, Feek CM, Miller HC, et al. Atrial fibrillation and isolated suppression of the pituitary-thyroid axis: response to specific antithyroid therapy. Int J Cardiol 1981;1:43–48.

59. Forfar JC, Miller HC, Toft AD. Occult thyrotoxicosis: a correctable cause of "idiopathic" atrial fibrillation. Am J Cardiol 1979;44:9–12.

60. Ciaccheri M, Cecchi F, Arcangeli C, et al. Occult thyrotoxicosis in patients with chronic and paroxysmal isolated atrial fibrillation. Clin Cardiol 1984;7:413–416.

61. Bruce SA, Rangedara DC, Lewis RR, et al. Hyperthyroidism in elderly patients with atrial fibrillation and normal thyroid hormone measurements. J Roy Soc Med 1987;80:74–76.

62. Tajiri J, Hamasaki S, Shimada T, et al. Masked thyroid dysfunction among elderly patients with atrial fibrillation. Jpn Heart J 1986;27:183–190.

63. Davies AB, Williams I, John R, et al. Diagnostic value of thyrotrophin releasing hormone tests in elderly patients with atrial fibrillation. BMJ 1985;291:773–776.

64. Surks MI, Chopra IJ, Mariash CN, et al. American Thyroid Association guidelines for use of laboratory tests in thyroid disorders. JAMA 1990;263:1529–1532.

65. Hay ID, Bayer MF, Kaplan MM, et al. American Thyroid Association assessment of current free thyroid hormone and thyrotropin measurements and guidelines for future clinical assays. Clin Chem 1991;37: 2002–2008.

66. Ericsson U-B, Thorell JI. A prospective critical evaluation of in vitro thyroid function tests. Acta Med Scand 1986; 220:47–56.

67. Wilke TJ, Eastment HT. Discriminative ability of tests for free and total thyroid hormones in diagnosing thyroid disease. Clin Chem 1986;32:1746–1750.

68. de los Santos ET, Starich GH, Mazzaferri EL. Sensitivity, specificity, and cost-effectiveness of the sensitive thyrotropin assay in the diagnosis of thyroid disease in ambulatory patients. Arch Intern Med 1989;149;526–532.

69. Cavalieri RR. The effects of nonthyroid disease and drugs on thyroid function tests. Med Clin North Am 1991;75: 27–39.

70. Small M, Buchanan L, Evans R. Value of screening thyroid function in acute medical admissions to hospital. Clin Endocrinol (Oxf) 1990;32:185–191.

71. Drinka PJ, Nolten WE, Voeks S, et al. Misleading elevation of the free thyroxine index in nursing home residents. Arch Pathol Lab Med 1991;115:1208–1211.

72. Finucane P, Rudra T, Church H, et al. Thyroid function tests in elderly patients with and without an acute illness. Age Ageing 1989;18:398–402.

73. Ehrmann DA, Weinberg M, Sarne DH. Limitations to the use of a sensitive assay for serum thyrotropin in the assessment of thyroid status. Arch Intern Med 1989;149:369–372.

74. Klee GG, Hay ID. Sensitive thyrotropin assays: analytic and clinical performance criteria. Mayo Clin Proc 1988;63: 1123–1132.

75. Franklyn JA, Black EG, Betteridge J, et al. Comparison of second and third generation methods for measurement of serum thyrotropin in patients with overt hyperthyroidism, patients receiving thyroxine therapy, and those with nonthyroidal illness. J Clin Endocrinol Metab 1994;78:1368–1371.

76. Spencer CA, LoPresti JS, Guttler RB, et al. Applications of a new chemiluminometric thyrotropin assay to subnormal measurement. J Clin Endocrinol Metab 1990;70:453–460.

77. Wilkinson E, Rae PWH, Thomson KJT, et al. Chemiluminescent third-generation assay (Amerlite TSH-30) of thyroid-stimulation hormone in serum or plasma assessed. Clin Chem 1993;39:2166–2173.
78. Baker B, Shapiro B, Fig LM, et al. Unusual complications of antithyroid drug therapy: four case reports and review of literature. Thyroidology 1989;1:17–26.
79. Franklyn JA. The management of hyperthyroidism. N Engl J Med 1994;330:1731–1738.
80. Cooper DS, Halpern R, Wood LC, et al. L-thyroxine therapy in subclinical hypothyroidism: a double-blind, placebo-controlled trial. Ann Intern Med 1984;101:18–24.
81. Nystrom E, Caidahl K, Fager G, et al. A double-blind cross-over 12-month study of L-thyroxine treatment of women with "subclinical" hypothyroidism. Clin Endocrinol 1988;29:63–76.
82. Caron P, Calazel C, Parra HJ, et al. Decreased HDL cholesterol in subclinical hypothyroidism: the effect of L-thyroxine therapy. Clin Endocrinol (Oxf) 1990;33:519–523.
83. Bell GM, Todd WT, Forfar JC, et al. End-organ responses to thyroxine therapy in subclinical hypothyroidism. Clin Endocrinol 1985;22:83–89.
84. Arem R, Patsch W. Lipoprotein and apolipoprotein levels in subclinical hypothyroidism. Effect of levothyroxine therapy. Arch Intern Med 1990;150:2097–2100.
85. Forfar JC, Wathen CG, Todd WTA, et al. Left ventricular performance in subclinical hypothyroidism. Q J Med 1985;57:857–865.
86. Franklyn JA, Daykin J, Betteridge J, et al. Thyroxine replacement therapy and circulating lipid concentrations. Clin Endocrinol (Oxf) 1993;38:453–459.
87. Ridgway EC, Cooper DS, Walker H, et al. Peripheral responses to thyroid hormone before and after L-thyroxine therapy in patients with subclinical hypothyroidism. J Clin Endocrinol Metab 1981;53:1238–1242.
88. Nilsson G, Nordlander S, Levin K. Studies on subclinical hypothyroidism with special reference to the serum lipid pattern. Acta Med Scand 1976;200:63–67.
89. Lithell H, Boberg J, Hellsing K, et al. Serum lipoprotein and apolipoprotein concentrations and tissue lipoprotein-lipase activity in overt and subclinical hypothyroidism: the effect of substitution therapy. Eur J Clin Invest 1981;11: 3–10.
90. Paul TL, Kerrigan J, Kelly AM, et al. Long-term L-thyroxine therapy is associated with decreased hip bone density in premenopausal women. JAMA 1988;259:3137–3141.
91. Stall GM, Harris S, Sokoll LJ, et al. Accelerated bone loss in hypothyroid patients overtreated with L-thyroxine. Ann Intern Med 1990;113:265–269.
92. Ross DS. Subclinical hyperthyroidism: possible danger of overzealous thyroxine replacement therapy. Mayo Clin Proc 1988;63:1223–1239.
93. Schneider DL, Barrett-Connor EL, Morton DJ. Thyroid hormone use and bone mineral density in elderly women: effects of estrogen. JAMA 1994;271:1245–1249.
94. Leese GP, Jung RT, Guthrie C, et al. Morbidity in patients on L-thyroxine: a comparison of those with a normal TSH to those with a suppressed TSH. Clin Endocrinol (Oxf) 1992;37:500–503.
95. Ross DS. Bone density is not reduced during the short-term administration of levothyroxine to postmenopausal women with subclinical hypothyroidism: a randomized, prospective study. Am J Med 1993;95:385–388.
96. American Academy of Family Physicians. Age charts for periodic health examination. Kansas City, MO: American Academy of Family Physicians, 1994. (Reprint no. 510.)
97. American Association of Clinical Endocrinologists. Clinical practice guidelines for the evaluation of hyperthyroidism and hypothyroidism. Jacksonville, FL: American Association of Clinical Endocrinologists and American College of Endocrinology, 1995.
98. Canadian Task Force on the Periodic Health Examination. Canadian guide to clinical preventive health care. Ottawa: Canada Communication Group, 1994:611–618.
99. Eddy DM. Common screening tests. Philadelphia: American College of Physicians, 1991;406–408.
100. American College of Obstetricians and Gynecologists. Thyroid disease in pregnancy. Technical Bulletin no. 181. Washington, DC: American College of Obstetricians and Gynecologists, 1993.
101. American Academy of Pediatrics Committee on Genetics. Health supervision for children with Down syndrome. Pediatrics 1994;93:855–859.
102. Becker DV, Bigos ST, Gaitan E, et al. Optimal use of blood tests for assessment of thyroid function [letter]. JAMA 1993;269:2736.

21. Screening for Obesity

RECOMMENDATION

Periodic height and weight measurements are recommended for all patients (see *Clinical Intervention*).

Burden of Suffering

Obesity is an excess of body fat.[1] Most epidemiologic studies rely on indices of relative weight, such as body mass index (BMI), an index of body weight that is normalized for height, to estimate the prevalence of obesity.[a] For example, the National Center for Health Statistics currently uses the 85th percentile sex-specific values of BMI for persons aged 20–29 (≥ 27.8 kg/m^2 for men and ≥ 27.3 kg/m^2 for women) from the second U.S. National Health and Nutrition Examination Survey (NHANES II) as a cutoff to define overweight in adults.[2]

Approximately one third of adult Americans aged 20 and older are estimated to be overweight, based on data from NHANES III.[3] Using 1990 census figures, this corresponds to 58 million people. The prevalence of overweight in the United States has increased dramatically during the past 15 years in men and women of all age and ethnic groups, and remains disproportionately high among black and Hispanic women.[3] Other groups that have a high prevalence of obesity include Asian and Pacific Islanders, Native Americans and Alaska Natives, and Native Hawaiians.[4] The prevalence of overweight among adolescents has also increased.[5] Based on NHANES III data, about one fifth of adolescents aged 12–19 are overweight.[5] The prevalence of obesity among younger children is uncertain, but is estimated to be between 5% and 25%,[6] and may also be increasing.[7]

Increased mortality in adults has been clearly documented as a result of morbid obesity, weight that is at least twice the desirable weight.[8,9] Less severe obesity (e.g., as low as 26.4–28.5 kg/m^2) has also been associated with increased mortality in large prospective cohort studies.[10–13] Although some studies have reported greater mortality among the thinnest individuals,[14] a 1993 prospective cohort study that carefully controlled for smoking and illness-related weight loss found a linear relationship between BMI

---

[a] *Overweight* refers to an excess of body weight relative to height that includes all tissues and therefore may reflect varying degrees of adiposity. Despite the distinction between *obesity* and *overweight*, the majority of overweight persons are also obese, and these terms tend to be used interchangeably in the medical literature.

and mortality.[15] Two cohort studies suggest that overweight children and adolescents may have increased mortality as adults.[16,17] Childhood obesity may be a significant risk factor for adult obesity, with adolescent obesity being a better predictor than obesity at younger ages.[8,18,19]

Persons who are overweight are more likely to have adult-onset diabetes, hypertension, and risk factors for other diseases.[8,20] The prevalence of diabetes and hypertension is 3 times higher in overweight adults than in those of normal weight.[21] Observational studies have established a clear association between overweight and hypercholesterolemia and suggest an independent relationship between overweight and coronary artery disease.[8,10,11,20–23] Being overweight has also been associated with several cardiovascular risk factors in children and adolescents, including hypercholesterolemia and hypertension.[24–26] An elevated waist/hip circumference ratio (WHR), which may indicate central adiposity, has been shown to correlate with the presence of these conditions independent of BMI,[27–35] and may predict the complications of obesity in adults better than BMI does.[35,36] Obesity has also been associated with an increased risk of certain cancers (including those of the colon, rectum, prostate, gallbladder, biliary tract, breast, cervix, endometrium, and ovary), and with other disorders such as cholelithiasis, obstructive sleep apnea, venous thromboembolism, and osteoarthritis.[8,20,37] Finally, obesity can affect the quality of life by limiting mobility, physical endurance, and other functional measures,[8] as well as through social, academic, and job discrimination.[38–40]

Accuracy of Screening Tests

Extremely overweight individuals can be identified easily in the clinical setting by their physical appearance. More precise methods may be necessary, however, to evaluate persons who are mildly or moderately overweight. The complications of obesity occur among those with elevated body fat composition, which is most accurately measured by underwater (hydrostatic) weighing, isotopic dilution measures, and other sophisticated techniques that are not suited to clinical practice.[41] Bioelectric impedance, which provides an estimate of total body water from which the percentage of body fat can be calculated, is not widely available in clinical practice. This method has been reviewed elsewhere.[42]

The most common clinical method for detecting obesity is the evaluation of body weight and height based on a table of suggested or "desirable" weights.[e.g.,43–45] These tables generally reflect the weight at which mortality is minimized, and they only approximate the extent of fatness. The criteria for healthy body weight are a matter of controversy among experts and vary considerably as presented in different weight-for-height tables.[46,47] Weights for children and adolescents are typically evaluated in relation to average weight for age, height, and gender. This information can be obtained from growth charts that are based on percentile distributions of body size attained at specific ages.[2] An alternative measure to using weight-for-height tables or growth charts is the BMI, a weight-height index that is calculated by dividing the body weight in kilograms by the square of the height in meters (kg/m^2). The BMI is easily performed, is highly reliable,[48] and has a correlation of 0.7–0.8 with body fat content in adults.[49–52] BMI also correlates with body fat content in children and adolescents.[50,51,53] In adults, overweight has been defined by the National Center for Health Statistics as a BMI $\geq$ 27.8 for men and $\geq$ 27.3 for women (the 85th percentile values for persons aged 20–29 in NHANES II);[2] a BMI at this level has been associated with increased risk of morbidity and mortality.[8] In adolescents, a BMI exceeding the 85th percentile for age and gender has been suggested as one definition for overweight[2] or for those at risk of overweight.[54]

Other anthropometric methods that may be useful in the clinical setting include the measurement of skinfold thickness and the indirect assessment of body fat distribution. Skinfold thickness is a more direct measure of adiposity than BMI and correlates well with body fat content in both adults and children, but this technique requires training and has lower intra- and interobserver reliability than height and weight measurements used to calculate BMI.[55,56] The WHR, the circumference of the waist divided by the circumference of the hips, which may be a better predictor of the sequelae associated with adult obesity than BMI, can also be measured in the clinical setting. The reliability of the WHR is comparable to that of BMI.[57] A WHR greater than 1.0 in men and 0.8 in women has been shown to predict complications from obesity, independent of BMI,[36] although the WHR has not been evaluated in all ethnic groups.

Effectiveness of Early Detection

The purpose of screening for obesity is to assist the obese individual to lose or at least maintain weight and thereby prevent the complications of obesity. Such screening may also assist with counseling other patients regarding maintaining a healthy weight. Most studies of interventions for obesity involve subjects who are overweight; we found no studies evaluating interventions for persons identified solely on the basis of an elevated WHR. Although there is little evidence from prospective studies that weight loss by obese individuals improves their longevity, there is evidence that obesity is associated with increased mortality[8–13] and that weight loss in obese persons reduces important risk factors for disease and mortality.[8,58] Prospective cohort studies[59,60] and randomized clinical trials[61–64,66] have demonstrated that caloric restriction or weight loss reduces systolic and diastolic blood pressures as well as the requirements for antihypertensive medication in obese adults with hypertension. These effects were independent of sodium restriction. In controlled[67] and uncontrolled trials[68,69] of low-calorie diets in obese diabetic patients, weight reduction was associated with improved glycemic control and reduced need for oral hypoglycemic agents and insulin. Weight loss generally improves the blood lipid profile[70–72] and can reduce symptoms related to obstructive sleep apnea.[73,74] To benefit from the detection of obesity, however, patients must be motivated to lose weight, must have access to an efficacious method of reducing body weight, and must maintain the resulting weight loss.

Various weight-reducing regimens are available, but many have only short-term efficacy and fail to achieve long-term weight loss.[6,9,75,76] Research to explain the difficulty in achieving long-term weight loss is ongoing. One theory is that obesity is related to an internal "set-point" that maintains excess body fat in certain individuals.[77] Some evidence suggests that energy expenditure decreases to compensate for reduced body weight,[78] which would tend to return body weight to the usual weight. Such a decrease in energy expenditure could contribute to the failure of most weight-reducing regimens to achieve long-term benefits.

Dietary modification is the most commonly used weight-loss strategy, and can achieve weight reduction over the short-term in both adults and children.[6,76,79] Very-low-calorie diets (< 800 kcal/day), which have been used for moderately to severely obese adults who have failed more conservative approaches,[80] produce greater short-term weight loss than standard low-calorie diets of 1,000–1,500 kcal/day.[76,79,80] Long-term results, however, are similar with both types of programs: the majority of participants eventually return to their pre-treatment weight within 5 years,[76,79] although sustained weight loss may be achieved by some patients.[81–85] Cohort studies and randomized controlled trials of behavioral modification, often combined with dietary therapy, have shown modest long-term benefits in adults[86–88] and children.[89,90] The results of the intensive dietary and behavioral interventions evaluated in these studies may not necessarily be applicable to the type of counseling likely to be given in a busy clinical primary care practice, and referral to other qualified providers or to qualified weight-management programs[1] may be necessary to achieve similar results. The amount of weight loss that can be achieved with exercise, either alone or in combination with other methods, is relatively limited in adults[76,91–93] and children,[94–96] but physical activity may be beneficial in maintaining weight loss[76,92,97,98] and reducing the WHR[92,99] in adults. Numerous randomized clinical trials have shown that various appetite-suppressant drugs can be effective in producing short-term weight loss in adults.[100–109] The effects, however, are limited to periods when the drug is taken, and some studies have shown a plateauing or gradual regain of weight with prolonged use.[76,100,101,104,105,107,110,111] Surgical techniques such as vertical band gastroplasty and gastric bypass may benefit selected adults who are morbidly obese,[112–114] but other procedures such as intragastric balloon insertion have not been shown to be effective.[115–118]

Certain weight reduction methods may cause important adverse effects. Very-low-calorie diets can cause fatigue, hair loss, dizziness, and symptomatic cholelithiasis.[76,119] Pharmacologic agents may cause palpitations, dizziness, insomnia, headache, and gastrointestinal discomfort.[120] Surgical therapies such as gastroplasty and balloon insertion can lead to gastric ulceration, perforation, and bowel obstruction.[121] Some cohort studies have reported that weight change or fluctuation in weight (weight cycling) among adults is associated with increased cardiovascular morbidity and mortality, but a review by the National Task Force on the Prevention and Treatment of Obesity concluded there is insufficient evidence that weight cycling is associated with adverse effects.[122] There is conflicting evidence regarding the potential adverse effects of caloric restriction and weight loss on growth velocity and development in obese children and adolescents.[123–127]

Recommendations of Other Groups

The American Academy of Family Physicians,[128] the American Heart Association,[129] the Institute of Medicine,[130] the American Academy of Pediatrics,[131] the Bright Futures guidelines,[132] and the American Medical Association guidelines for adolescent preventive services (GAPS)[133] all recommend measurement of height and weight as part of a periodic health examination for patients. Bright Futures and GAPS also recommend the determination of BMI for all adolescents.[132,133] The Canadian Task Force on the Periodic Health Examination concluded that there is insufficient evidence to recommend the inclusion or exclusion of height, weight, BMI, or skinfold measurement to screen for obesity in a routine health examination of either children or adults.[134] The Canadian Task Force does, however, recommend measuring and plotting the height and weight of infants and children in order to identify those who are failing to thrive.

Discussion

Evidence is limited that screening for obesity and implementing weight-reducing or weight maintenance strategies are effective in decreasing long-term morbidity and mortality. This is unlikely to improve in the near future due to the difficulty and cost of conducting controlled trials of weight loss with these outcome measures and of separating the effect of obesity from that of other risk factors. An additional obstacle is the low rate of long-term success in maintaining weight loss. Obesity is a chronic disorder that requires continuing treatment, which could explain the failure of short-term interventions in achieving long-term success. Although losing weight has not been proven to reduce morbidity and mortality, it is clear that weight loss reduces an individual's risk for major chronic diseases such as hypertension and coronary artery disease, and it also improves the management of both hypertension and diabetes. Periodic height and weight measurements are inexpensive, rapid, reliable, and require minimal training to perform. They may also be useful for the detection of medical conditions causing unintended weight loss or weight gain, such as cancer or thyroid disorders, and the detection of growth abnormalities in childhood. Once height and weight have been determined, the BMI or standard height and weight tables may be used as a means of evaluating adolescents and adults for obesity. In addition, determination of the WHR may be useful for assessing some adults, particularly those whose weight or BMI is borderline for classification as overweight and who have personal or family medical histories placing them at increased health risk. There are inadequate data to determine the optimal frequency of obesity screening, and this is best left to clinical discretion.

CLINICAL INTERVENTION

Periodic height and weight measurements are recommended for all patients ("B" recommendation). In adults, BMI (body weight in kilograms divided by the square of height in meters) or a table of suggested weights[e.g.,43–45] may be used, along with the assessment of other factors such as medical conditions or WHR, as a basis for further evaluation, intervention, or referral to specialists. In adolescents, a BMI exceeding the 85th percentile for age and gender may be used as a basis for further assessment, treatment, or referral.[54] The height (or length if appropriate) and weight of infants and children may be plotted on a growth chart[e.g.,2] or compared to tables of average weight for height, age, and gender to determine the need for further evaluation, treatment, or referral. The optimal frequency for measuring height and weight in the clinical setting has not been evaluated and is a matter of clinical discretion. There is insufficient evidence to recommend for or against determination of the WHR as a routine screening test for obesity ("C" recommendation).

All patients should receive appropriate counseling to promote physical activity (see Chapter 55) and a healthy diet (see Chapter 56).

The draft update of this chapter was prepared for the U.S. Preventive Services Task Force by Barbara Albert, MD, MS, and Carolyn DiGuiseppi, MD, MPH, based in part on background papers written for the Canadian Task Force on the Periodic Health Examination by James Douketis, MD, William Feldman, MD, FRCPC, and Brenda Beagen, MA.

REFERENCES

1. Institute of Medicine. Weighing the options: criteria for evaluating weight-management programs. Washington, DC: National Academy Press, 1995.

2. Najjar MF, Rowland M. Anthropometric reference data and prevalence of overweight, United States, 1976–80. Vital and health statistics; series 11, no 238. Washington, DC: Government Printing Office, 1987. (DHHS Publication no. (PHS) 87-1688.)

3. Kuczmarski RJ, Flegal KM, Campbell SM, et al. Increasing prevalence of overweight among US adults. JAMA 1994;272:205–211.

4. Kumanyika SK. Special issues regarding obesity in minority populations. Ann Intern Med 1993; 119:650–654.

5. Centers for Disease Control and Prevention. Prevalence of overweight among adolescents—United States, 1988–91. MMWR 1994;43:818–821.

6. Dietz WH. Childhood obesity: susceptibility, cause, and management. J Pediatr 1983;103:676–686.

7. Gortmaker SL, Dietz WH, Sobol AM, et al. Increasing pediatric obesity in the United States. Am J Dis Child 1987;141:535–540.

8. Foster WR, Burton BT, eds. National Institutes of Health consensus conference: health implications of obesity. Ann Intern Med 1985;103:977–1077.

9. Van Itallie TB, Kral JG. The dilemma of morbid obesity. JAMA 1981;246:999–1003.

10. Hubert HB, Feinleib M, McNamara PM, et al. Obesity as an independent risk factor for cardiovascular disease: a 26-year follow-up of participants in the Framingham Heart Study. Circulation 1983;67:968–977.

11. Rhoads GG, Kagan A. The relation of coronary disease, stroke, and mortality to weight in youth and middle age. Lancet 1983;1:492–495.

12. Wilcosky T, Hyde J, Anderson JJ, et al. Obesity and mortality in the Lipid Research Clinics Program Follow-up Study. J Clin Epidemiol 1990;43:743–752.

13. Harris T, Cook EF, Garrison R, et al. Body mass index and mortality among nonsmoking older persons: the Framingham Heart Study. JAMA 1988;259:1520–1524.

14. Manson JE, Stampfer MJ, Hennekens CH, et al. Body weight and longevity: a reassessment. JAMA 1987;257: 353–358.

15. Lee IM, Manson JE, Hennekens CH, et al. Body weight and mortality: a 27-year follow-up of middle-aged men. JAMA 1993;270:2823–2828.

16. Javier Nieto F, Szklo M, Comstock GW. Childhood weight and growth rate as predictors of adult mortality. Am J Epidemiol 1992;136:201–213.

17. Must A, Jacques PF, Dallal GE, et al. Long-term morbidity and mortality of overweight adolescents: a follow-up of the Harvard Growth Study of 1922 to 1935. N Engl J Med 1992;327:1350–1355.

18. Epstein LH, Wing RR, Valoski A, et al. Childhood obesity. Pediatr Clin North Am 1985;32:363–379.

19. Guo SS, Roche AF, Chumlea WC, et al. The predictive value of childhood body mass index values for overweight at age 35 years. Am J Clin Nutr 1994;59:810–819.

20. Pi-Sunyer FX. Medical hazards of obesity. Ann Intern Med 1993;119:655–660.

21. Van Itallie TB. Health implications of overweight and obesity in the United States. Ann Intern Med 1985;103:983–988.

22. Manson JE, Colditz GA, Stampfer MJ, et al. A prospective study of obesity and risk of coronary heart disease in women. N Engl J Med 1990;322:882–889.

23. Willett WC, Manson JE, Stampfer MJ, et al. Weight, weight change, and coronary heart disease in women: risk within the "normal" weight range. JAMA 1995;273:461–465.

24. Smoak CG, Burke GL, Webber LS, et al. Relation of obesity to clustering of cardiovascular disease risk factors in children and young adults. Am J Epidemiol 1987;125:364–372.

25. Aristimuno GG, Foster TA, Voors AW, et al. Influence of persistent obesity in children on cardiovascular risk factors: the Bogalusa Heart Study. Circulation 1984;69:895–904.

26. Burns TL, Moll PP, Lauer RM. The relation between ponderosity and coronary risk factors in children and their relatives: the Muscatine Ponderosity Family Study. Am J Epidemiol 1989;129:973–987.

27. Ohlson LO, Larsson B, Svardsudd K, et al. The influence of body fat distribution on the incidence of diabetes mellitus: 13.5 years of follow-up of the participants in the study of men born in 1913. Diabetes 1985;34:1055–1058.

28. Kaye SA, Folsum AR, Sprafka JM, et al. Increased incidence of diabetes mellitus in relation to abdominal adiposity in older women. J Clin Epidemiol 1991;44:329–334.

29. Freedman DS, Jacobsen SJ, Barboriak JJ, et al. Body fat distribution and male/female differences in lipids and lipoproteins. Circulation 1990;81:1498–1506.
30. Larsson B, Svarsudd K, Welin L, et al. Abdominal adipose tissue distribution, obesity, and risk of cardiovascular disease and death: 13 year follow-up of participants in the study of men born in 1913. BMJ 1984;288:1401–1404.
31. Lapidus L, Bengtsson C, Larsson B, et al. Distribution of adipose tissue and risk of cardiovascular disease and death: a 12 year follow-up of participants in the population study of women in Gothenberg, Sweden. BMJ 1984;289:1257–1261.
32. Ducimetiere P, Richard J, Cambien F. The pattern of subcutaneous fat distribution on middle-aged men and the risk of coronary heart disease: the Paris prospective study. Int J Obesity 1986;10:229–240.
33. Kannel WB, Cupples LA, Ramaswami R, et al. Regional obesity and risk of cardiovascular disease: the Framingham study. J Clin Epidemiol 1991;44:183–190.
34. Folsum AR, Prineas RJ, Kaye SA, et al. Incidence of hypertension and stroke in relation to body fat distribution and other risk factors in older women. Stroke 1990;21:701–706.
35. Folsum AR, Kaye SA, Sellers TA, et al. Body fat distribution and 5-year risk of death in older women. JAMA 1993;269:483–487.
36. Bjorntorp P. Regional patterns of fat distribution. Ann Intern Med 1985;103:994–995.
37. Bray GA. Obesity: basic considerations and clinical approaches. Dis Month 1989;35:449–537.
38. Wadden TA, Stunkard AJ. Social and psychological consequences of obesity. Ann Intern Med 1985;103:1062–1067.
39. Klesges RC, Klem ML, Hanson CL, et al. The effects of applicant's health status and qualifications on simulated hiring decisions. Int J Obesity 1990;14:527–535.
40. Gortmaker SL, Must A, Perrin JM, et al. Social and economic consequences of overweight in adolescence and young adulthood. N Engl J Med 1993;329:1008–1012.
41. Lukaski HC. Methods for the assessment of human body composition: traditional and new. Am J Clin Nutr 1987;46:537–556.
42. National Institute of Diabetes and Digestive and Kidney Disease and the NIH Office of Medical Applications of Research. Bioelectrical impedance analysis in body composition measurement. Technology assessment conference statement, 1994 Dec 12–14. Bethesda: National Institutes of Health, 1994.
43. U.S. Department of Agriculture and U.S. Department of Health and Human Services. Dietary guidelines for Americans. 4th ed. Washington, DC: Department of Agriculture and Department of Health and Human Services, 1996.
44. Metropolitan Life Insurance Company. New weight standards for men and women. Stat Bull Metropol Life Insur Co 1959;40:1–4.
45. Metropolitan Life Insurance Company. Metropolitan height and weight tables. Stat Bull Metropol Life Insur Co 1983;64:2–9.
46. Schulz LO. Obese, overweight, desirable, ideal: where to draw the line in 1986? J Am Diet Assoc 1986;86:1702–1704.
47. Willett WC, Stampfer M, Manson J, et al. New guidelines for Americans: justified or injudicious? Am J Clin Nutr 1991;53:1102–1103.
48. Stewart AW, Jackson RT, Ford MA, et al. Underestimation of relative weight by the self-reported height and weight. Am J Epidemiol 1987;125:122–126.
49. Keys A, Fidanza F, Karvonen MJ, et al. Indices of relative weight and obesity. J Chronic Dis 1972;25:329–343.
50. Deurenberg P, Westrate JA, Seidel JC. Body mass index as a measure of body fatness: age- and sex-specific prediction formulas. Br J Nutr 1991;65:105–114.
51. Roche AF, Siervogel RM, Chumlea WM, et al. Grading body fatness from limited anthropometric data. Am J Clin Nutr 1981;34:2831–2838.
52. Gray DS, Fujioka K. Use of relative weight and body mass index for the determination of adiposity. J Clin Epidemiol 1991;44:545–550.
53. Schey HM, Michieluttie R, Corbett WT, et al. Weight-for-height indices as measures of adiposity in children. J Chronic Dis 1984;37:397–400.
54. Himes JH, Dietz WH. Guidelines for overweight in adolescent preventive services: recommendations from an expert committee. Am J Clin Nutr 1994;59:307–316.
55. Bray GA, Greenway FL, Molitch ME, et al. Use of anthropometric measures to assess weight loss. Am J Clin Nutr 1978;31:769–773.

56. Kispert CP, Merrifield HH. Interrater reliability of skinfold fat measurements. Phys Ther 1987;67: 917–920.

57. Kushi LH, Kaye SA, Folsum AR, et al. Accuracy and reliability of self-measurement of body girth. Am J Epidemiol 1988;128:740–748.

58. Pi-Sunyer FX. Short-term medical benefits and adverse effects of weight loss. Ann Intern Med 1993;119:722–726.

59. Tuck ML, Sowers J, Dornfeld L, et al. The effect of weight reduction on blood pressure, plasma renin activity, and plasma aldosterone levels in obese patients. N Engl J Med 1981;304:930–933.

60. Kannel WB, Brand N, Skinner JJ, et al. The relation of adiposity to blood pressure and the development of hypertension. Ann Intern Med 1967;67:48–59.

61. Fagerberg B, Berglund A, Andersson OK, et al. Weight reduction versus antihypertensive drug therapy in obese men with high blood pressure: effects upon plasma insulin levels and association with changes in blood pressure and serum lipids. J Hypertens 1992;10:1053–1061.

62. Weinsier RL, James LD, Darnell BE, et al. Obesity-related hypertension: evaluation of the separate effects of energy restriction and weight reduction on hemodynamic and neuroendocrine status. Am J Med 1991;90:460–468.

63. Hypertension Prevention Trial Research Group. The Hypertension Prevention Trial: three-year effects of dietary changes on blood pressure. Arch Intern Med 1990;150:153–162.

64. Davis BR, Blaufox MD, Oberman A, et al. Reduction in long-term antihypertensive medication requirements: effects of weight reduction by dietary intervention in overweight persons with mild hypertension. Arch Intern Med 1993;153:1773–1782.

65. *Deleted in proof.*

66. Stevens VJ, Corrigan SA, Obarzanek E, et al. Weight loss intervention in phase 1 of the Trials of Hypertension Prevention. The TOHP Collaborative Research Group. Arch Intern Med 1993;153:849–858.

67. Wing RR, Marcus MD, Salata R, et al. Effects of a very-low-calorie diet on long-term glycemic control in obese type 2 diabetic subjects. Arch Intern Med 1991;151:1334–1340.

68. Kirschner MA, Schneider G, Ertel NH, et al. An eight-year experience with a very-low-calorie formula diet for control of major obesity. Int J Obesity 1988;12:69–80.

69. Fitz JD, Sperling EM, Fein HG. A hypocaloric high-protein diet as primary therapy for adults with obesity-related diabetes: effective long-term use in a community hospital. Diabetes Care 1983;6:328–333.

70. Jalkanen L. The effect of a weight reduction program on cardiovascular risk factors among overweight hypertensives in primary health care. Scand J Soc Med 1991;19:66–71.

71. Dattilo AM, Kris-Etherton PM. Effects of weight reduction on blood lipids and lipoproteins: a meta-analysis. Am J Clin Nutr 1992;56:320–328.

72. Wolf RN, Grundy SM. Influence of weight reduction on plasma lipoproteins in obese patients. Arteriosclerosis 1983;3:160–169.

73. Smith PL, Gold AR, Meyers DA, et al. Weight loss in mildly to moderately obese patients with obstructive sleep apnea. Ann Intern Med 1985;103:850–855.

74. Wittels EH, Thompson S. Obstructive sleep apnea and obesity. Otolaryngol Clin North Am 1990;23: 751–760.

75. Stunkard AJ. Conservative treatments for obesity. Am J Clin Nutr 1987;45:1142–1154.

76. NIH Technology Assessment Conference Panel. Methods for voluntary weight loss and control: Technology Assessment Conference Statement. Ann Intern Med 1993;119:764–770.

77. Bennett WI. Beyond overeating. N Engl J Med 1995;332:673–674.

78. Leibel RL, Rosenbaum M, Hirsch J. Changes in energy expenditure resulting from altered body weight. N Engl J Med 1995;332:621–628.

79. Wadden TA. Treatment of obesity by moderate and severe caloric restriction: results of clinical research trials. Ann Intern Med 1993;119:688–693.

80. National Task Force on the Prevention and Treatment of Obesity. Very low-calorie diets. JAMA 1993;270:967–974.

81. Wadden TA, Syernberg JA, Letizia KA, et al. Treatment of obesity by very low calorie diet, behavior therapy, and their combination: a five-year perspective. Int J Obesity 1989;13(Suppl 2):39–46.

82. Karvetti RL, Hakala P. A seven year follow up of a weight reduction programme in Finnish primary health care. Eur J Clin Nutr 1992;46:743–752.

83. Perri MG, McAllister DA, Gange JJ, et al. Effects of four maintenance programs on the long-term management of obesity. J Consult Clin Psychol 1988;56:529–534.

84. Ginsberg-Fellner F, Knittle JL. Weight-reduction in young obese children. I. Effects on adipose tissue cellularity and metabolism. Pediatr Res 1981;15:1381–1389.
85. Nuutinen O, Knip M. Long-term weight control in obese children: persistence of treatment outcome and metabolic changes. Int J Obesity 1992;16:279–287.
86. Holden J, Darga LL, Olson SM, et al. Long-term follow-up of patients attending a combination very-low calorie diet and behavior therapy weight loss programme. Int J Obesity 1992;16:605–613.
87. Hakala P, Karvetti RL, Ronnemaa T. Group vs. individual weight reduction programmes in the treatment of severe obesity—a five year follow-up study. Int J Obesity 1993;17:97–102.
88. Wing RR. Behavioral treatment of severe obesity. Am J Clin Nutr 1992;55(Suppl 2):545s–551s.
89. Epstein LH, McCurley J, Wing RR, et al. Five year follow-up of family-based behavioral treatments for childhood obesity. J Clin Consult Psychol 1990;58:661–664.
90. Epstein LH, Valoski A, Wing RR, et al. Ten-year follow-up of behavioral, family-based, treatment for obese children. JAMA 1990;264:2519–2523.
91. King AC, Tribble DL. The role of exercise in weight regulation in nonathletes. Sports Med 1991;11: 331–349.
92. Blair SN. Evidence for success of exercise in weight loss and control. Ann Intern Med 1993;119:702–706.
93. Sweeney ME, Hill JO, Heller PA, et al. Severe vs moderate energy restriction with and without exercise in the treatment of obesity: efficiency of weight loss. Am J Clin Nutr 1993;57:127–134.
94. Epstein LH, Wing RR, Koeske R, et al. The effects of diet plus exercise on weight change in parents and children. J Consult Clin Psychol 1984;52:429–437.
95. Epstein LH, Wing RR, Penner BC, et al. Effect of diet and controlled exercise on weight loss in obese children. J Pediatr 1985;107:358–361.
96. Reybrouck T, Vinckx J, Van den Berghe G, et al. Exercise therapy and hypocaloric diet in the treatment of obese children and adolescents. Acta Paediatr Scand 1990;79:84–89.
97. Pavlou KN, Krey S, Steffee WP. Exercise as an adjunct to weight loss and maintenance in moderately obese subjects. Am J Clin Nutr 1989;49:1115–1123.
98. Sikand G, Kondo A, Foreyt JP, et al. Two year follow-up of patients treated with a very low calorie diet and exercise training. J Am Diet Assoc 1988;88:487–488.
99. Wood PD, Stefanick ML, Williams PT, et al. The effects on plasma lipoproteins of a prudent weight-reducing diet, with or without exercise, in overweight men and women. N Engl J Med 1991;325: 461–469.
100. Bray GA. Use and abuse of appetite-suppressant drugs in the treatment of obesity. Ann Intern Med 1993;119: 707–713.
101. Goldstein DJ, Rampey AH, Enas GG, et al. Fluoxetine: a randomized clinical trial in the treatment of obesity. Int J Obesity 1994;18:129–135.
102. Toubro S, Astrup AV, Breum L, et al. Safety and efficacy of long-term treatment with ephedrine, caffeine and an ephedrine/caffeine mixture. Int J Obesity 1993;17(Suppl 1):S69–S72.
103. Weintraub M, Sundaresan PR, Schuster B, et al. Long-term weight control study: I–VII. Clin Pharmacol Ther 1992;51:581–646.
104. Gray DS, Fujioka K, Devine W, et al. Fluoxetine treatment of the obese diabetic. Int J Obesity 1992;16:193–198.
105. Darga LL, Carroll-Michals L, Botsford SJ, et al. Fluoxetine's effect on weight loss in obese subjects. Am J Clin Nutr 1991;54:321–325.
106. Levine LR, Enas GG, Thompson WL, et al. Use of fluoxetine, a selective serotonin-uptake inhibitor, in the treatment of obesity: a dose-response study. Int J Obesity 1989;13:635–645.
107. Guy-Grand B, Crepaldi G, Lefebre P, et al. International trial of long-term dexfenfluramine in obesity. Lancet 1989;2:1142–1145.
108. Enzi G, Crepaldi G, Inelman EM, et al. Efficacy and safety of dexfenfluramine in obese patients: multi-centre study. Clin Neuropharmacol 1988;11(Suppl 1):S173–S178.
109. Weintraub M, Hasday JD, Mushlin AI, et al. A double-blind clinical trial in weight control: use of fenfluramine and phentermine alone and in combination. Arch Intern Med 1984;144:1143–1148.
110. Mathus-Vliegen EM, Van De Voore K, Kok AM, et al. Dexfenfluramine in the treatment of severe obesity: a placebo-controlled investigation of the effects on weight loss, cardiovascular risk factors, food intake and eating behavior. J Intern Med 1992;232:119–127.
111. Andersen T, Astrup A, Quaade F. Dexfenfluramine as adjuvant to a low-calorie formula diet in the treatment of obesity: a randomized clinical trial. Int J Obesity 1992;16:35–40.

112. MacLean LD, Rhode BM, Sampalis J, et al. Results of the surgical treatment of obesity. Am J Surg 1993;165:155–162.
113. MacGregor AM, Rand CS. Gastric surgery in morbid obesity: outcome in patients aged 55 years and older. Arch Surg 1993;128:1153–1157.
114. Mason EE, et al. Impact of vertical banded gastroplasty on mortality from obesity [abstract]. Obes Surg 1991;1:115.
115. Kramer FM, Stunkard AJ, Spiegel TA, et al. Limited weight losses with a gastric balloon. Arch Intern Med 1989;149:411–413.
116. Meshkinpour H, Hsu D, Farivar S. Effects of gastric bubble as a weight reduction device: a controlled, cross-over study. Gastroenterology 1988;95:589–592.
117. Benjamin SB, Maher KA, Cattau EL, et al. Double-blind controlled trial of the Garren-Edwards gastric bubble: an adjunctive treatment for exogenous obesity. Gastroenterology 1988;95:581–588.
118. Lindor KD, Hughes RW, Ilstrup DM, et al. Intragastric balloons in comparison with standard therapy for obesity: a randomised, double-blind trial. Mayo Clin Proc 1987;62:992-996.
119. Everhart JE. Contribution of obesity and weight loss to gallstone disease. Ann Intern Med 1993;119:1029–1035.
120. Physicians' desk reference. 48th ed. Montvale, NJ: Medical Economics Data, 1994.
121. Kral JG. Overview of surgical techniques for treating obesity. Am J Clin Nutr 1992;55:552S–555S.
122. National Task Force on the Prevention and Treatment of Obesity. Weight cycling. JAMA 1994;272:1196–1202.
123. Mallick MJ. Health hazards of obesity and weight control in children: a review of the literature. Am J Public Health 1983;73:78–82.
124. Dietz WH, Hartung R. Changes in height velocity of obese preadolescents during weight reduction. Am J Dis Child 1985;139:705–707.
125. Paige DM. Obesity in childhood and adolescence: special problems in diagnosis and treatment. Postgrad Med 1986;79:233–245.
126. Epstein LH, McCurley J, Valoski A, et al. Growth in obese children treated for obesity. Am J Dis Child 1990;144:1360–1364.
127. Epstein LH, Valoski A, McCurley J. Effect of weight loss by obese children on long-term growth. Am J Dis Child 1993;147:1076–1080.
128. American Academy of Family Physicians. Age charts for periodic health examination. Kansas City, MO: American Academy of Family Physicians, 1994. (Reprint no. 510.)
129. Grundy SM, Greenland P, Herd A, et al. Cardiovascular and risk factor evaluation of healthy American adults. A statement for physicians by an ad hoc committee appointed by the Steering Committee, American Heart Association. Circulation 1987;75:1340A–1362A.
130. National Academy of Sciences, Institute of Medicine. Preventive services for the well population. Washington, DC: National Academy of Sciences, 1978.
131. American Academy of Pediatrics, Committee on Practice and Ambulatory Medicine. Recommendations for preventive pediatric health care. Pediatrics 1995;96:373–374.
132. Green M, ed. Bright Futures: national guidelines for health supervision of infants, children, and adolescents. Arlington, VA: National Center for Education in Maternal and Child Health, 1994.
133. American Medical Association. Guidelines for adolescent preventive services (GAPS): recommendations and rationale. Chicago: American Medical Association, 1994.
134. Canadian Task Force on the Periodic Health Examination. Canadian guide to clinical preventive health care. Ottawa: Canada Communication Group, 1994:334–344, 574–584.

22. Screening for Iron Deficiency Anemia—*Including Iron Prophylaxis*

RECOMMENDATION

Screening for iron deficiency anemia using hemoglobin or hematocrit is recommended for pregnant women and for high-risk infants. There is insufficient evidence to recommend for or against routine screening for iron deficiency anemia in other asymptomatic persons, but recommendations against screening may be made on other grounds (see *Clinical Intervention*). Encouraging parents to breastfeed their infants and to include iron-enriched foods in the diet of infants and young children is recommended (see also Chapter 56). There is currently insufficient evidence to recommend for or against the routine use of iron supplements for healthy infants or pregnant women.

Burden of Suffering

Anemia is defined by the presence of a hemoglobin level that is below the normal range of values for the population (see *Accuracy of Screening Tests*).[1-4] U.S. populations with a high prevalence of anemia include blacks, Alaska Natives and Native Americans, immigrants from developing countries, and individuals of low socioeconomic status.[5-7] Anemia may be due to a variety of underlying conditions. Iron deficiency is an important cause among young children and women of reproductive age in the U.S.[8-10] The prevalence of iron deficiency anemia in U.S. children has declined in recent years[6,11-14] and in 1993 was estimated to be at or below 3% for children aged 1–5.[15] In low-income populations and certain ethnic groups, such as Alaska Natives, the prevalence of iron deficiency anemia in children <5 years of age may be substantially higher, ranging from 10–30% (unpublished data, Centers for Disease Control and Prevention, 1993).[6] Among middle-class children, on the other hand, anemia is uncommon and tends to be mild (i.e., within 1% of the hematocrit level defining anemia).[13,14] The exact prevalence of iron deficiency anemia among pregnant women is uncertain, but national data suggest that <2% of nonpregnant women aged 20–44 years have iron deficiency anemia.[5] Among low-income, pregnant U.S. populations, a low hemoglobin level and/or low hematocrit is present in 6% of white women and 17% of black women during the first trimester and in 25% of white women and 46% of black women during the third trimester.[7] The high rates of anemia in pregnant women may not be attributable to iron deficiency, however. In a large cohort of urban, low-income, mostly minority pregnant women, only 12.5% of anemic women were iron deficient.[16]

As early as the 1960s, researchers demonstrated that, in general, decreased hemoglobin alone does not have readily apparent adverse effects unless it is below 10 g/dL (100 g/L).[17–19] Clearly, persons with markedly reduced hemoglobin levels are at risk for cardiopulmonary and other complications. Reduced work productivity, endurance, and exercise capacity have been associated with anemia or iron deficiency anemia in adults, most of whom were from developing countries.[20–26] Iron deficiency and iron deficiency anemia during infancy and early childhood have been associated with abnormal infant behavior, growth, and development, although it is unclear how much of this association is actually attributable to other factors often associated with iron deficiency (e.g., poor nutrition, low socioeconomic status).[27–35] Hemoglobin levels well below what is considered normal for pregnancy have been associated with increased risk of low birth weight, preterm delivery, and perinatal mortality.[16,36–42]

Accuracy of Screening Tests

The hemoglobin concentration and hematocrit are the principal screening tests for detecting anemia. The World Health Organization hemoglobin cut-points for diagnosing anemia in adults have been widely adopted: men, <13 g/dL; menstruating women, <12 g/dL; pregnant women, <11 g/dL.[1] The Centers for Disease Control and Prevention (CDC) has also produced criteria for anemia: in infancy and childhood, <11 g/dL for 0.5–4.9 years and <11.5 mg/dL for 5.0–11.9 years; in pregnancy, <11 g/dL during the first and third trimesters and <10.5 g/dL in the second trimester.[2] Studies have shown that automated electronic cell counters and chemical analyzers provide accurate and reliable data on red blood cell number and size and on the concentration of hemoglobin.[43,44] Although sampling of capillary blood is more convenient in ambulatory practice and is especially useful for infant testing, results obtained from capillary blood specimens are less reliable than those from venous blood.[45,46] One study found the capillary microhematocrit to have a sensitivity of 90% and a specificity of 44% when compared with values obtained from venous blood with an automated cell counter.[46]

While sensitive for iron deficiency anemia, hemoglobin is not sensitive for iron deficiency because mild deficiency states may not affect hemoglobin levels.[47] Hemoglobin is also nonspecific, since many cases of anemia are due to causes other than iron deficiency.[9,10,16] Reported sensitivity of low hemoglobin for detecting iron deficiency ranges from 8–90% and specificity from 65–99% depending on the population, reference standard and cut-point used.[47–50] In a national sample, detection of a hemoglobin <12 g/dL had a sensitivity of 90% and specificity of 78% for iron deficiency in black women, whereas sensitivity and specificity were 36% and 95% in white women.[50] Other tests (i.e., total iron binding capacity, serum iron, transferrin saturation, erythrocyte protoporphyrin, mean cell volume, red blood cell distribution width, and serum ferritin) may be more accurate for the detection of iron deficiency, but they are poor screening tests for iron deficiency anemia.[48,51–59] Among these tests, serum ferritin has the best sensitivity and specificity for diagnosing iron deficiency in anemic patients.[60]

Effectiveness of Early Detection

Evidence is limited that in the asymptomatic general **adolescent or adult** U.S. population, early detection and treatment significantly reduces morbidity from anemia, iron deficiency, or the conditions that cause them.[17–19,61] This evidence is further limited by the fact that studies often use inconsistent or vague definitions of anemia and iron deficiency. Observational studies in developing countries have reported decreased physical endurance and maximal exercise capacity in association with iron deficiency anemia.[21–24,26] The extent to which this might affect daily activities that do not involve maximal exercise capacity is unknown. Clinical trials and case series from developing countries have reported conflicting results regarding a benefit of iron supplementation on work productivity in anemic or iron-deficient workers.[22,25,62–64] There is little evidence evaluating adverse effects from the mild degree of anemia that is most often detected by screening asymptomatic persons in developed countries. In a Swedish cohort, anemic women (Hgb <12 g/dL) reported no increase in reported infections, fatigue, or other symptoms, but they were significantly more likely to report low work productivity compared to nonanemic women.[20] In a small, randomized placebo-controlled trial of Welsh women with anemia (hemoglobin <10.5 g/dL) detected by population-based screening, iron therapy did not result in clinically or statistically significant improvements in psychomotor function tests, symptoms, or subjective well-being, despite increased hemoglobin concentrations.[65] Trials evaluating the effects of iron supplementation on physiologic outcomes such as running speed and maximum running time in nonanemic, iron-depleted runners have been inconclusive.[66,67] Although the evaluation of anemia may disclose underlying diseases (e.g., occult malignancies) that benefit from early detection,[68] there are no data to suggest that testing for anemia is an effective means of screening for these conditions.

A number of trials have evaluated whether **infants** with iron deficiency anemia benefit from early treatment. Randomized controlled trials have demonstrated the efficacy of iron supplementation in correcting iron deficiency anemia in infants and children, but its effect on clinical outcomes is less clear.[27,28,69,70] Four relatively large, generally well-conducted, randomized controlled trials in developing countries have evaluated the effects of iron supplementation on the behavior and development of anemic infants.[27,28,31,70] Three trials failed to show a significant effect of treatment on standardized developmental test scores after short-term (6–10 days) iron therapy.[27,28,31] In one trial,[31] an additional 3 months of iron therapy for all infants corrected their anemia but did not significantly improve developmental test scores. Another of the trials[27] reported that after 3 months of iron therapy infants whose iron deficiency was completely corrected (36%) had developmental scores similar to iron sufficient subjects, mainly because the scores of the latter group declined. In the remaining 64%, treatment corrected anemia but not iron deficiency, and test scores remained lower in this group. This trial did not have a true placebo group, and other causes of anemia (such as vitamin A deficiency) were not adequately excluded. There was no delayed benefit of iron therapy in this trial; children with hemoglobin ≤10 g/dL as infants still had lower developmental scores at school entry 5 years later.[33] The largest and most recent trial, which enrolled 12–18-month-old infants with hemoglobins ≤ 10.5 g/dL, reported sizable, statistically significant improvements in both mental and motor development after 4 months of oral therapy.[70] A small randomized double-blind placebo-controlled trial[71] in the United Kingdom evaluated 2 months of iron supplementation in urban, underprivileged toddlers (aged 17–19 months) with mild to moderate anemia, using the Denver developmental screening test to assess outcome, which is not as well standardized or validated as the test used in the other trials. Effects on developmental outcomes were inconsistent, but iron supplements significantly increased rate of weight gain. Long-term results were not evaluated. It is unclear why the results of these trials differ, although adequacy and duration of therapy may account for some of the differences.

Clinical trials and a cohort study in **older children** have also demonstrated improved iron and hemoglobin status with therapy,[35,69,72] but evidence for a clinical benefit from treatment of iron deficiency anemia is limited. A double-blind randomized controlled trial in 1,358 9–11-year-old Thai children failed to show any effect of iron treatment on intelligence test scores in anemic children, despite the large sample size.[73] A series of small randomized controlled trials conducted in India did report small improvements in IQ with iron treatment,[74,75] however, and two small randomized, controlled trials suggested a benefit of oral iron on some tests of learning in anemic school-aged Indonesian children.[76,77] All of these studies suffered from important design limitations, such as use of unvalidated tests, multiple significance testing, high dropout rates, and addition of folic acid to the treatment regimen. Conflicting results have been reported concerning the effect of iron supplementation on infection rates in children.[35,78–80] On the other hand, improved growth and weight gain with 3–6 months of iron supplementation have been reported consistently in placebo-controlled trials of anemic, malnourished children in developing countries.[34,35,81,82] Another controlled trial reported a significant benefit from iron treatment on physical performance and submaximal work capacity in anemic Indian boys.[83] It is unclear whether the results of these studies are generalizable to U.S. children, who are likely to be healthy and otherwise adequately nourished.

Early detection and treatment of iron deficiency anemia in **pregnancy** has been assumed to be beneficial because moderate to severe anemia (i.e., <9.0–10.0 g/dL) has been associated with a 2–3-fold increased risk of low birth weight, preterm delivery, and perinatal mortality in numerous cross-sectional and longitudinal observational studies in industrialized countries.[16,36–42,84] The consistency of these results across different study designs and population samples is noteworthy, although such studies do not conclusively prove that anemia directly influences pregnancy outcomes. Many of the studies did not control for other factors that may have had adverse effects (e.g., smoking, maternal malnutrition), or for increases in hemoglobin and hematocrit that occur as gestation approaches term; most did not differentiate iron deficiency anemia from anemia due to other causes. A large body of data suggests that iron supplements are effective in improving the hematologic indices of pregnant women,[85–91] but there is limited evidence that improving hematologic indices in anemic women results in improved clinical outcomes for the mother, fetus, or newborn. Most published trials evaluating the effects of iron supplementation on pregnancy outcomes systematically excluded anemic women (i.e., those with hemoglobins <10 g/dL or hematocrits ≤0.3) and are therefore not necessarily relevant to pregnant women with iron deficiency anemia. They are described later in the chapter (see *Primary Prevention*). One controlled trial enrolled Indian women with hemoglobins as low as 7.0 g/dL who attended rural health centers, randomizing the women by health center to receive either iron and folic acid supplements for 100 days or no supplements.[92] The trial reported a significantly higher mean birth weight and lower rate of low birth weight infants in women who completed 100 days of supplements compared to controls. Among those receiving supplementation, the increase in birth weight was significantly related to rise in hemoglobin. A large (n = 601), retrospective cohort study from Kenya compared women with severe anemia (hemoglobin ≤8.8 g/dL) who were or were not treated with ferrous sulfate.[93] Treatment was associated with markedly reduced preterm delivery and stillbirth rates, and increased mean birth weight, but there was no change in neonatal death rates. Women with "mild anemia" (hemoglobin ≥8.9 g/dL) who received iron therapy before 30 weeks also had lower preterm delivery and perinatal mortality rates compared to those receiving no iron or iron after 30 weeks. Neither significance testing nor adjustment for covariates was performed, limiting the conclusions that can be drawn from these data. The detection of anemia and the determination of its etiology may also lead to the discovery of other correctable obstetrical risks (e.g., poor nutritional status, medical illness) that might otherwise escape detection, but the effectiveness of anemia screening in improving outcomes related to these risks has not specifically been evaluated in developed countries.

Adverse effects of iron therapy include unpleasant gastrointestinal symptoms (e.g., nausea and constipation) that are dose-related and, at normal doses, reversible.[94–97] Iron therapy can cause complications of excessive iron storage in patients with an underlying iron storage disorder (e.g., idiopathic hemochromatosis).[98,99] A potential hazard of iron supplements is unintentional overdosage by children in the home; 20,330 cases of ingestion of iron or iron-containing vitamins by children under 6 years, including 3 fatalities, were reported to poison control centers in 1993.[100] Iron supplements accounted for 30% of fatal pediatric pharmaceutical overdoses occurring between 1983 and 1990.[101] Other potential adverse effects of iron mentioned in the literature (e.g., birth defects, cancer, heart disease, infection, metabolic imbalances of other minerals, and harmfully high hemoglobin levels)[109] have not been proven.

Primary Prevention (Iron Prophylaxis)

Studies of the effects of iron fortification of formula and cereal on healthy, nonanemic infants have focused primarily on laboratory rather than clinical outcomes. Randomized and nonrandomized controlled trials, observational studies, and time series studies have demonstrated substantial reductions in the incidence of iron deficiency and iron deficiency anemia in healthy infants fed iron-fortified formula, iron-fortified cereal, or breast milk (with iron-fortified cereal added at 4–6 months), compared to infants fed cow's milk or unfortified formula.[12,102–107] Evidence is more limited regarding clinical benefits from iron fortification of infant diets. A cohort study reported that infants fed iron-fortified formula beginning at age 6 months had significantly fewer diarrheal episodes compared to infants fed whole cow's milk (0.16 vs. 0.30 per child in the second 6 months of life);

the incidence of other medical conditions (e.g., otitis media, dermatitis, wheezing) did not differ.[106] This study did not have standardized criteria for diagnosing medical conditions and had limited control for potentially confounding variables, however. A controlled trial randomized healthy infants at a mean age of 1.3 months to either iron-fortified or nonfortified milk-based formula.[108] Infants in the fortified group had a significantly greater height (by 0.9 cm) and growth rate at 12 months, but this group was also significantly taller at birth. At 12 months, there were no other statistically significant differences in clinical outcomes, such as weight, number of acute illnesses, or psychomotor development. Intake of the iron-fortified formula may have been insufficient to produce a clinical effect, however; by 8 months of age, 92% of study infants and 85% of controls were drinking cow's milk rather than study formula. In another randomized controlled trial in healthy infants from very low income families, infants randomized to nonfortified formula had significantly worse psychomotor development (Bayley Scales) at 9 and 12 months of age compared to those given iron-fortified formula.[108a] Differences were no longer significant at 15 months, although sample size may have been inadequate: only half the sample was assessed at 15 months. There were no differences at any age in standardized tests of cognitive development or behavior. These results suggest a clinical benefit from iron-fortified formula, but further trials are needed to confirm these results and determine their long-term impact.

Evidence is limited that iron supplementation in healthy pregnant women with mild or no anemia results in important clinical benefits.[109] Clinical trials have reported that iron supplements in healthy pregnant women with initial hemoglobins ≥ 10 g/dL are efficacious in correcting red cell indices and iron stores, but they do not improve birth weight, length of gestation, or other outcome measures when compared to placebo or to no supplements.[110–116] Few of these trials had sufficient statistical power to detect small positive effects of iron supplementation, however. One small randomized controlled trial in young pregnant women suggested a modest beneficial effect of routine iron supplementation on some tests of psychomotor function, but it had important discrepancies in reported data and analyses.[118] In a large randomized controlled trial of healthy, nonanemic pregnant women, routine iron therapy was compared to selective iron therapy given only when a confirmed hemoglobin level below 10 g/dL was detected after 14 weeks.[119] Women in the selective group had poorer self-reported overall health and increased rates of transfusion and operative delivery, although differences were small and may have been due to nonblinding. The routine supplementation group had more subjective side effects attributable to iron, more postdate gestations, and higher perinatal mortality; the latter difference was probably attributable to chance, given small numbers and multiple comparisons. Evidence thus does not confirm important clinical benefits from routine iron supplementation in nonanemic pregnant women.

Cohort studies have reported no important adverse effects with iron-fortified formula,[120,121] nor were serious side effects reported in the clinical trials of iron-fortified food or formula previously cited. Routine iron supplementation may produce mild, reversible gastrointestinal symptoms similar to those seen with iron therapy (see above). In one small, randomized controlled trial, oral iron supplements in iron-sufficient children resulted in significantly less weight gained after 4 months of treatment,[122] but additional studies are needed to confirm these results. Trials of routine iron supplementation in pregnancy have not reported adverse effects on pregnancy outcome. The doses of oral iron typically offered for routine iron supplementation (e.g., in pregnancy) are unlikely to cause complications of excessive iron storage.[98,99] As with iron therapy, an important hazard of iron prophylaxis is unintentional overdosage by children in the home; many reported cases of iron ingestion involve iron-containing prenatal vitamins.[100]

Recommendations of Other Groups

A number of organizations recommend some form of anemia screening during infancy and pregnancy. The Institute of Medicine (IOM), the Canadian Task Force on the Periodic Health Examination, and the Bright Futures report recommend screening high-risk infants (e.g., preterm or low birth weight, low socioeconomic status, those fed with cow's milk or nonfortified formula before 12 months of age) between 6 or 9 and 12 months of age; IOM recommends screening before 3 months in preterm infants.[15,123,124] The American Academy of Pediatrics (AAP) and the American Academy of Family Physicians (AAFP) recommend that all infants receive a hemoglobin or hematocrit measurement once during infancy; the AAP recommends that it be done at or before 9 months of age.[125,126] The recommendations of the AAFP are currently under review. Prenatal screening for anemia is recommended by the Canadian Task Force,[127] the American College of Obstetricians and Gynecologists (ACOG),[128] and the IOM.[15] ACOG recommends measuring a hemoglobin or hematocrit at the earliest prenatal visit and again early in the third trimester;[128] IOM recommends measuring hemoglobin once in each trimester.[15]

Routine screening of older children or nonpregnant adolescents and adults is not advocated by most organizations.[15,124,126,128,129] Some organizations recommend screening selectively in specific high-risk populations: adolescents at increased risk due to heavy menses, chronic weight loss, nutritional deficit, or athletic activity;[124] recent immigrants from undeveloped countries;[129] the institutionalized elderly;[129] and nonpregnant women aged 15–25 or otherwise at increased risk (e.g., with large menstrual blood loss, high parity, poverty, recent immigration).[15] The AAP recommends at least one measurement of hemoglobin or hematocrit for all menstruating adolescents, preferably at age 15 years.[125]

Primary prevention of iron deficiency anemia in infancy by breastfeeding, feeding iron-fortified formula if not breastfeeding, and feeding iron-fortified cereal after 4–6 months of age, is recommended by the Canadian Task Force,[123] IOM,[15] AAP,[130,131] and Bright Futures.[124] The AAFP recommends counseling parents of children under 6 years of age and women of childbearing age on the benefits of iron-enriched food and iron intake.[126] The AAP recommends iron supplements in breastfed term infants who do not receive iron-fortified cereal beginning at 4 months of age.[131] The Canadian Task Force found insufficient evidence to recommend for or against the routine use of iron supplements in pregnant women.[123] The IOM does not recommend routine iron supplements in nonanemic pregnant women.[15] ACOG and AAP recommend dietary supplements including iron during pregnancy if dietary intake is inadequate to meet need, or if there are other risk factors for iron deficiency.[128]

Discussion

The burden of suffering from iron deficiency anemia in the general child, adolescent, and adult populations in the U.S. is low. Although it is prevalent in certain high-risk groups, mild iron deficiency anemia in the absence of symptoms appears to have only subtle health consequences in these individuals. Trials of iron therapy in school children, adolescents, and adults have not proven important clinical benefits in well-nourished populations in developed countries. Thus, there is little evidence to suggest that early detection of iron deficiency anemia in these groups is beneficial. Treatment of some forms of anemia not caused by iron deficiency (e.g., vitamin B_{12} or folate deficiency), and some medical disorders that cause anemia, which would also be detected if hemoglobin measurement was performed routinely, can produce dramatic results. These disorders are too rare in most subgroups of the population to justify mass screening, however. There is therefore little basis for large-scale efforts to screen for anemia in the general population.

There is fair evidence to support screening for anemia in pregnant women, based on numerous observational studies reporting an association between severe to moderate anemia (hemoglobin <9–10 g/dL) and poor pregnancy outcome, and weak evidence from a nonrandomized controlled trial and a cohort study that iron treatment of anemic women improves obstetric outcomes. Women of low socioeconomic status and immigrants from developing countries, among whom iron deficiency anemia is more common, are most likely to benefit from such screening. Because hemoglobin measurement is a nonspecific test for iron deficiency, further evaluation should be performed to identify the etiology of anemia detected by screening. Serum ferritin appears to have the best sensitivity and specificity for diagnosing iron deficiency in anemic patients. Although routine iron supplementation improves hematologic indices and iron status, there is at present insufficient evidence from published clinical research to suggest that routine iron supplementation of healthy pregnant women with hemoglobins ≥10 g/dL is beneficial in improving clinical outcomes for the mother, fetus, or newborn.[109]

The prevalence of iron deficiency anemia in the general infant population is low, and when it occurs in low-risk populations, it tends to be mild. In healthy, low-risk populations, there are few observational data showing adverse effects of iron deficiency anemia, nor have there been trials of early detection and correction of iron deficiency anemia. There is therefore little evidence to support routine hemoglobin measurement in infancy for the detection of iron deficiency anemia. On the other hand, multiple observational studies in high-risk populations (i.e., low socioeconomic status or developing countries) have found an association between iron deficiency anemia in childhood and abnormal growth and development. The largest and most recent trial[70] of iron therapy in a high-risk population showed an important effect of iron therapy on development, while several trials in high-risk, often malnourished, infants and children have found beneficial effects of iron on growth and growth rates. In the U.S., certain infants (e.g., recent immigrants from developing countries, those of low socioeconomic status, members of certain minority and ethnic groups, preterm infants, those who begin cow's milk before 12 months) have a substantially higher prevalence of iron deficiency anemia and may also be more likely to suffer from general malnutrition. There is therefore fair evidence to support screening high-risk infants and toddlers for iron deficiency anemia, using hemoglobin (or hematocrit). As for pregnant women, evaluation to determine the etiology of anemia is appropriate. Both breastfeeding and eating iron-fortified formula and cereal are effective in the primary prevention of iron deficiency anemia. Given the absence of known adverse effects from such dietary interventions, and the other important benefits of breastfeeding (see Chapter 56), evidence supports encouraging mothers to breastfeed and to include iron-enriched foods in the diet of infants and young children.

CLINICAL INTERVENTION

A hemoglobin analysis or hematocrit is recommended for pregnant women at their first prenatal visit ("B" recommendation). There is insufficient evidence to recommend for or against repeated prenatal testing for anemia in asymptomatic pregnant women lacking evidence of medical or obstetrical complications ("C" recommendation). Screening for anemia with hemoglobin or hematocrit in high-risk infants, preferably at 6–12 months of age, is also recommended ("B" recommendation). Examples of high-risk infants include infants living in poverty, blacks, Native Americans and Alaska Natives, immigrants from developing countries, preterm and low birth weight infants, and infants whose principal dietary intake is unfortified cow's milk. Although capillary blood specimens are easier to obtain in infants, a venous blood count provides more accurate and reliable data. Serum ferritin testing may be useful as an additional screening test in selected high-risk infants. There is currently insufficient evidence to recommend for or against periodic screening for high-risk infants not found to be anemic at initial screening ("C" recommendation). There is also insufficient evidence to recommend for or against routine testing for anemia in other asymptomatic persons, but recommendations against such screening may be made on the grounds of low prevalence, cost, and potential adverse effects of iron therapy ("C" recommendation).

Guidelines for normal hemoglobin ranges for infants and pregnant women have been published.[1–4] Appropriate hematological studies and nutrition counseling should be provided for patients found to have anemia. Compared to other diagnostic tests, serum ferritin has the best sensitivity and specificity for detecting iron deficiency in patients found to be anemic. Screening for hemoglobinopathies is discussed in Chapter 43.

Encouraging mothers to breastfeed their infants and advising parents to include iron-enriched foods in the diet of infants and young children is recommended for the primary prevention of iron deficiency anemia ("B" recommendation). There is also good evidence to recommend breastfeeding based on proven benefits unrelated to iron deficiency (see Chapter 56). Pregnant women should receive specific nutritional guidance to enhance fetal and maternal health (see Chapter 56). There is currently insufficient evidence to recommend for or against the routine use of iron supplements for healthy infants or pregnant women who are not anemic ("C" recommendation).

See the relevant background paper: U.S. Preventive Services Task Force. Routine iron supplementation during pregnancy. JAMA 1993;270:2846–2854.

The draft update of this chapter was prepared for the U.S. Preventive Services Task Force by Carolyn DiGuiseppi, MD, MPH, and was based in part on a previously published background paper by the U.S. Preventive Services Task Force (review article by Steven H. Woolf, MD, MPH) and on materials prepared for the Canadian Task Force on the Periodic Health Examination by John W. Feightner, MD, MSc, FCFP.

REFERENCES

1. Cook JD. Clinical evaluation of iron deficiency. Semin Hematol 1982;19:6–18.
2. Centers for Disease Control. CDC criteria for anemia in children and childbearing-aged women. MMWR 1989;38: 400–404.
3. Lockitch G, ed. Handbook of diagnostic biochemistry and hematology in normal pregnancy. Boca Raton, FL: CRC Press, 1993.
4. Gibson RS. Nutritional assessment: a laboratory manual. New York: Oxford University Press, 1993.
5. Pilch SM, Senti FR, eds. Assessment of the iron nutritional status of the US population based on data collected in the second National Health and Nutrition Examination Survey, 1976–1980. Rockville, MD: Life Sciences Research Office, Federation of American Societies for Experimental Biology, 1984.
6. Centers for Disease Control. Pediatric nutrition surveillance system—United States, 1980–1991. MMWR 1992; 41(SS-7):1–24.
7. Kim I, Hungerford DW, Yip R, et al. Pregnancy nutrition surveillance system—United States, 1979–1990. MMWR 1992;41(SS-7):25–41.
8. Dallman PR, Siimes MA, Stekel A. Iron deficiency in infancy and childhood. Am J Clin Nutr 1980;33:86–118.
9. Dallman PR, Yip R, Johnson C. Prevalence and causes of anemia in the United States, 1976 to 1980. Am J Clin Nutr 1984;39:437–445.
10. Yip R, Dallman PR. The roles of inflammation and iron deficiency as causes of anemia. Am J Clin Nutr 1988;48:1295–1300.
11. Expert Scientific Working Group. Summary of a report on assessment of the iron nutritional status of the United States population. Am J Clin Nutr 1985;42:1318–1330.
12. Vazquez-Seoane P, Windom R, Pearson HA. Disappearance of iron-deficiency anemia in a high-risk infant population given supplemental iron. N Engl J Med 1985;313:1239–1240.
13. Yip R, Binkin NJ, Fleshood L, et al. Declining prevalence of anemia among low-income children in the United States. JAMA 1987;258:1619–1623.
14. Yip R, Walsh KM, Goldfarb MG, et al. Declining prevalence of anemia in childhood in a middle-class setting: a pediatric success story? Pediatrics 1987;80:330–334.
15. Institute of Medicine. Iron deficiency anemia: recommended guidelines for the prevention, detection, and management among U.S. children and women of childbearing age. Washington, DC: National Academy Press, 1993.
16. Scholl TO, Hediger ML, Fischer RL, et al. Anemia vs iron deficiency: increased risk of preterm delivery in a prospective study. Am J Clin Nutr 1992;55:985–988.
17. Elwood PC, Waters WE, Greene WJ, et al. Symptoms and circulating hemoglobin level. J Chronic Dis 1969;21: 615–628.
18. Elwood PC. Evaluation of the clinical importance of anemia. Am J Clin Nutr 1973;26:958–964.
19. Elwood PC, Waters WE, Benjamin IT, et al. Mortality and anemia in women. Lancet 1974;1:891–894.
20. Lennartsson J, Bengtsson C, Hallberg L, et al. Characteristics of anaemic women: the population study of women in Goteborg, 1968–1969. Scand J Haematol 1979;22:17–24.
21. Davies CTM, Chukweumeka AC, van Haaren JPM. Iron-deficiency anaemia: its effect on maximum aerobic power and responses to exercise in African males aged 17–40 years. Clin Sci 1973;44:555–562.
22. Basta SS, Soekirman MS, Karyadi D, et al. Iron deficiency anemia and the productivity of adult males in Indonesia. Am J Clin Nutr 1979;32:916-925.
23. Viteri FE, Torun B. Anaemia and physical work capacity. Clin Haematol 1974;3:609–626.
24. Gardner GW, Edgerton VR, Senewiratne B, et al. Physical work capacity and metabolic stress in subjects with iron deficiency anemia. Am J Clin Nutr 1977;30:910–917.
25. Edgerton VR, Gardner GW, Ohira Y, et al. Iron-deficiency anaemia and its effect on worker productivity and activity patterns. BMJ 1979;2:1546–1549.
26. Ohira Y, Edgerton VR, Gardner GW, et al. Work capacity, heart rate and blood lactate responses to iron treatment. Br J Haematol 1979;41:365–372.

27. Lozoff B, Brittenham GM, Wolf AW, et al. Iron deficiency anemia and iron therapy effects on infant developmental test performance. Pediatrics 1987;79:981–995.
28. Lozoff B, Brittenham GM, Viteri FE, et al. The effects of short-term oral iron therapy on developmental deficits in iron-deficient anemic infants. J Pediatr 1982;100:351–357.
29. Walter T, Kovalskys J, Stekel A. Effect of mild iron deficiency on infant mental development scores. J Pediatr 1983;102:519–522.
30. Frindulis H, Scott PH, Belton NR, et al. Combined deficiency of iron and vitamin D in Asian toddlers. Arch Dis Child 1986;61:843–848.
31. Walter T, De Andraca I, Chadud P, et al. Iron deficiency anemia: adverse effects on infant psychomotor development. Pediatrics 1989;84:7–17.
32. Oski FA, Honig AS. The effects of therapy on the development scores of iron-deficient infants. J Pediatr 1978;92:21–25.
33. Lozoff B, Jimenez E, Wolf AW. Long-term developmental outcome of infants with iron deficiency. N Engl J Med 1991;325:687–694.
34. Bhatia D, Seshadri S. Growth performance in anemia and following iron supplementation. Indian Pediatr 1993;30:195–200.
35. Chwang LC, Soemantri AG, Pollitt E. Iron supplementation and physical growth of rural Indonesian children. Am J Clin Nutr 1988;47:496–501.
36. Harrison KA. Anaemia, malaria and sickle cell disease. Clin Obstet Gynecol 1982;9:445–477.
37. Kuizon MD, Cheong RL, Ancheta LP, et al. Effect of anaemia and other maternal characteristics on birthweight. Hum Nutr Clin Nutr 1985;39:419–426.
38. Murphy JF, O'Riordan J, Newcombe RG, et al. Relation of haemoglobin levels in first and second trimester to outcome of pregnancy. Lancet 1986;1:992–994.
39. Klein L. Premature birth and maternal prenatal anemia. Am J Obstet Gynecol 1962;83:588–590.
40. Garn SM, Ridela SA, Petzoid AS, et al. Maternal hematologic levels and pregnancy outcomes. Semin Perinatol 1981;5:155–162.
41. Lieberman E, Ryan KJ, Monson RR, et al. Association of maternal hematocrit with premature labor. Am J Obstet Gynecol 1988;159:107–114.
42. Klebanoff MA, Shiono PH, Selby JV, et al. Anemia and spontaneous preterm birth. Am J Obstet Gynecol 1991;164:59–63.
43. Mayer K, Chin B, Baisley A. Evaluation of the S-plus IV. Am J Clin Pathol 1985;83:40–46.
44. Cox CJ, Habermann TM, Payne BA, et al. Evaluation of the Coulter counter model S-Plus IV. Am J Clin Pathol 1985;84:297–306.
45. Thomas WJ, Collins TM. Comparison of venipuncture blood counts with microcapillary measurements in screening for anemia in one-year-old infants. J Pediatr 1982;101:32–35.
46. Young PC, Hamill B, Wasserman RC, et al. Evaluation of the capillary microhematocrit as a screening test for anemia in pediatric office practice. Pediatrics 1986;78:206–209.
47. Binkin NJ, Yip R. When is anemia screening of value in detecting iron deficiency? In: Hercberg S, Galan P, Dupin H, eds. Recent knowledge on iron and folate deficiencies in the world. Colloq INSERM 1990;197:137–146.
48. Rybo E. Diagnosis of iron deficiency. Scand J Haematol 1985;43(suppl):5–39.
49. Friere WB. Hemoglobin as a predictor of response to iron therapy and its use in screening and prevalence estimates. Am J Clin Nutr 1989;50:1442–1449.
50. Johnson-Spear MA, Yip R. Hemoglobin difference between black and white women with comparable iron status: justification for race-specific anemia criteria. Am J Clin Nutr 1994;60:117–21.
51. Madan N, Rusia U, Manocha A, et al. Detection of iron deficiency in pregnancy by haemoglobin, serum ferritin and protoporphyrin/haem ratio. Indian J Med Res 1988;87:245–251.
52. Lewis GJ, Rowe DF. Can a serum ferritin estimation predict which pregnant women need iron? Br J Clin Pract 1986;40:15–16.
53. Schifman RB, Thomasson JE, Evers JM. Red blood cell zinc protoporphyrin testing for iron deficiency anemia in pregnancy. Am J Obstet Gynecol 1987;157:304–307.
54. Markus HS. Diagnostic investigations in the elderly: the clinical usefulness of serum iron and transferrin measurements in the diagnosis of iron deficiency anemia. An audit. Br J Clin Pract 1989;43:451–453.
55. Yip R, Schwartz S, Deinard AS. Screening for iron deficiency with the erythrocyte protoporphyrin test. Pediatrics 1983;72:214–219.

56. Cook JD, Skikne BS. Iron deficiency: definition and diagnosis. J Intern Med 1989;226:349–355.

57. Diaz-Tejeiro R, Maduell F, Diez J, et al. Red cell distribution width: a method that improves detection of iron deficiency in chronic hemodialysis patients. Nephron 1989;53:379–380.

58. McClure S, Custer E, Bessman D. Improved detection of early iron deficiency in nonanemic subjects. JAMA 1985;253:1021–1023.

59. Jensen BM, Sando SH, Grandjean P, et al. Screening with zinc protoporphyrin for iron deficiency in non-anemic female blood donors. Clin Chem 1990;36:846–848.

60. Guyatt GH, Oxman AD, Ali M, et al. Laboratory diagnosis of iron-deficiency anemia: an overview [published erratum appears in J Gen Intern Med 1992;7:423]. J Gen Intern Med 1992;7:145–153.

61. Shapiro MF, Greenfield S. The complete blood count and leukocyte differential count: an approach to their rational application. Ann Intern Med 1987;106:65–74.

62. Davies CTM, van Haaren JPM. Effect of treatment on physiological responses to exercise in East African industrial workers with iron deficiency anaemia. Br J Ind Med 1973;30:335–340.

63. Gardner GW, Edgerton VR, Barnard RJ, et al. Cardiorespiratory, hematological and physical performance responses of anemic subjects to iron treatment. Am J Clin Nutr 1975;28:982–988.

64. Li R, Chen X, Yan H, et al. Functional consequences of iron supplementation in iron-deficient female cotton mill workers in Beijing, China. Am J Clin Nutr 1994;59:908–913.

65. Elwood PC, Hughes D. Clinical trial of iron therapy on psychomotor function in anaemic women. BMJ 1970;3:254–255.

66. Matter M, Stittfall T, Graves J, et al. The effect of iron and folate therapy on maximal exercise performance in female marathon runners with iron and folate deficiency. Clin Sci 1987;72:415–422.

67. Rowland TW, Deisroth MB, Green GM, et al. The effect of iron therapy on the exercise capacity of nonanemic iron-deficient adolescent runners. Am J Dis Child 1988;142:165–169.

68. Ward MC, Gundroo D, Bailey RJ, et al. Effect of investigation on the management of elderly patients with iron deficiency anaemia. Age Ageing 1990;19:204–206.

69. Smith AW, Hendrickse RG, Harrison C, et al. Iron deficiency anemia and its response to oral iron: report of a study in rural Gambian children treated at home by their mothers. Ann Trop Paediatr 1989;9:6–16.

70. Idjradinata P, Pollitt E. Reversal of developmental delays in iron-deficient anemic infants treated with iron. Lancet 1993;341:1–4.

71. Aukett MA, Parks YA, Scott PH, et al. Treatment with iron increases weight gain and psychomotor development. Arch Dis Child 1986;61:849–857.

72. Bhandari B, Mandowara SL, Bothra K, et al. Effectivity of colloidal ferric salt in childhood iron-deficiency anemia. Indian J Pediatr 1989;56:105–107.

73. Pollitt E, Hathirat P, Kotchabhakdi NJ, et al. Iron deficiency and educational achievement in Thailand. Am J Clin Nutr 1989;50:687–697.

74. Seshadri S, Gopaldas T. Impact of iron supplementation on cognitive functions in preschool and school-aged children: the Indian experience. Am J Clin Nutr 1989;50:675–686.

75. Gopaldas T, Kale M, Bhardwaj P. Prophylactic iron supplementation for underprivileged school boys. II. Impact on selected tests of cognitive function. Indian Pediatr 1985;22:737–743.

76. Soemantri AG. Preliminary findings on iron supplementation and learning achievement of rural Indonesian children. Am J Clin Nutr 1989;50:698–702.

77. Soewondo S, Husaini M, Pollitt E. Effects of iron deficiency on attention and learning processes in preschool children: Bandung, Indonesia. Am J Clin Nutr 1989;50:667–674.

78. Dallman PR. Iron deficiency and the immune response. Am J Clin Nutr 1987;46:329–334.

79. Andelman MB, Sered SR. Utilization of dietary iron by term infants. Am J Dis Child 1966;111:45–55.

80. Damsdaran M, Naidu AN, Sarma KVR. Anemia and morbidity in rural preschool children. Indian J Med Res 1979;69:448–456.

81. Latham MC, Stephenson LS, Kinoti SN, et al. Improvements in growth following iron supplementation in young Kenyan school children. Nutrition 1990;6:159–165.

82. Lawless JW, Latham MC, Stephenson LS, et al. Iron supplementation improves appetite and growth in anemic Kenyan primary school children. J Nutr 1994;124:645–654.

83. Gopaldas T, Kale M, Bhardwaj P. Prophylactic iron supplementation for underprivileged school boys. III. Impact on submaximal work capacity. Indian Pediatr 1985;22:745–751.

84. Scholl TO, Hediger ML. Anemia and iron-deficiency anemia: compilation of data on pregnancy outcome. Am J Clin Nutr 1994;59:492S–501S.

85. Chanarin I, Rothman D. Further observations on the relation between iron and folate status in pregnancy. BMJ 1971;2:81–84.

86. Svanberg B, Arvidsson O, Norrby A, et al. Absorption of supplemental iron during pregnancy: a longitudinal study with repeated bone marrow studies and absorption measurements. Acta Obstet Gynecol Scand Suppl 1976;48: 87–100.

87. Puolakka J, Janne O, Pakarinen A, et al. Serum ferritin in the diagnosis of anemia during pregnancy. Acta Obstet Gynecol Scand Suppl 1980;95:57–63.

88. Taylor DJ, Mallen C, McDougall N, et al. Effect of iron supplementation on serum ferritin levels during and after pregnancy. Br J Obstet Gynaecol 1982;89:1011–1017.

89. Romslo I, Haram K, Sagen N, et al. Iron requirement in normal pregnancy as assessed by serum ferritin, serum transferrin saturation, and erythroprotoporphyrin determinations. Br J Obstet Gynaecol 1983;90:101–107.

90. Dawson EO, McGanity WJ. Protection of maternal iron stores in pregnancy. J Reprod Med 1987;32: 478–487.

91. Suharno D, West CE, Muhilal, et al. Supplementation with vitamin A and iron for nutritional anaemia in pregnant women in West Java, Indonesia. Lancet 1993;342:1325–1328.

92. Agarwal KN, Agarwal DK, Mishra KP. Impact of anaemia prophylaxis in pregnancy on maternal haemoglobin, serum ferritin, and birth weight. Indian J Med Res 1991;94:277–280.

93. Macgregor MW. Maternal anemia as a factor in prematurity and perinatal mortality. Scot Med J 1963;8:134–140.

94. Gilman AG, Rall TW, Nies AS, et al, eds. The pharmacological basis of therapeutics. 8th ed. Elmsford, NY: Pergamon Press, 1990:1282–1292.

95. Careddu P, Scotti A. Controlled, double-blind, multicenter clinical trial of iron protein succinylate in the treatment of iron deficiency in children. Int J Clin Pharmacol Ther Toxicol 1993;31:157–169.

96. Gordeuk VR, Brittenham GM, McLaren CE, et al. Carbonyl iron therapy for iron deficiency anemia. Blood 1986;67:745–752.

97. Cook JD, Carrgaga M, Kahn SG, et al. Gastric delivery system for iron supplementation. Lancet 1990;335:1136–1139.

98. American Medical Association. Drug evaluations. 6th ed. Philadelphia: WB Saunders, 1989:591.

99. Reynolds JEF, ed. Martindale: the extra pharmacopoeia. 29th ed. London, England: The Pharmaceutical Press, 1989:1189–1190.

100. Litovitz TL, Clark LR, Soloway RA. 1993 annual report of the American Association of Poison Control Centers Toxic Exposure Surveillance System. Am J Emerg Med 1994;12:546–584.

101. Litovitz T, Manoguerra A. Comparison of pediatric poisoning hazards: an analysis of 3.8 million exposure incidents. A report from the American Association of Poison Control Centers. Pediatrics 1992;89:999–1006.

102. Miller V, Swaney S, Deinard A. Impact of the WIC program on the iron status of infants. Pediatrics 1985;75:100–105.

103. Walter T, Dallman PR, Pizarro F, et al. Effectiveness of iron-fortified infant cereal in prevention of iron deficiency anemia. Pediatrics 1993;91:976–982.

104. Zlotkin SH, Beaton GH, Tanaka P, et al. Double-blind trial of iron fortification of infant cereals: effect on growth and hematologic status (abstr). Pediatr Res 1993;33:113a.

105. Pizarro F, Yip R, Dallman PR, et al. Iron status with different infant feeding regimens: relevance to screening and prevention of iron deficiency. J Pediatr 1991;118:687–692.

106. Tunnessen WW Jr, Oski FA. Consequences of starting whole cow milk at 6 months of age. J Pediatr 1987;111: 813–816.

107. Greene-Finestone L, Feldman W, Heick H, et al. Prevalence and risk factors of iron depletion and iron deficiency anemia among infants in Ottawa-Carlton. Can Diet Assoc J 1991;52:20–23.

108. Hemminki E, Nemet K, Horvath M, et al. Impact of iron fortification of milk formulas on infant's growth and health. Nutr Res 1995;15:491–503.

108a. Moffatt ME, Longstaffe S, Besant J, et al. Prevention of iron deficiency and psychomotor decline in high-risk infants through use of iron-fortified infant formula: a randomized clinical trial. J Pediatr 1994;125:527–534.

109. U.S. Preventive Services Task Force. Routine iron supplementation during pregnancy. JAMA 1993;270:2846–2854.

110. Hemminki E, Starfield B. Routine administration of iron and vitamins during pregnancy: review of controlled clinical trials. Br J Obstet Gynaecol 1978;85:404–410.

111. Paintin DB, Thomson AM, Hytten FE. Iron and the haemoglobin level in pregnancy. Br J Obstet Gynaecol 1966;73:181–190.

112. Willoughby MLN. An investigation of folic acid requirements in pregnancy, II. Br J Haematol 1967;13:503–509.

113. Primbs K. Eisenbehandlung wahrend der Schwangerschaft—eine Vergleichsstudie [English abstract: iron treatment during pregnancy—a comparative study]. Geburtsh Frauenheilkd 1973;33:552–559.

114. Fleming AF, Martin JD, Hahnel R, et al. Effects of iron and folic acid antenatal supplements on maternal haematology and fetal well-being. Med J Aust 1974;2:429–436.

115. Guldholt IS, Trolle BG, Hvidman LE. Iron supplementation during pregnancy. Acta Obstet Gynecol Scand 1991;70:9–12.

116. Milman N, Agger AO, Nielsen OJ. Iron status markers and serum erythropoietin in 120 mothers and newborn infants. Effect of iron supplementation in normal pregnancy. Acta Obstet Gynecol Scand 1994;73:200–204.

117. *Deleted in proof.*

118. Groner JA, Holtzman NA, Charney E, et al. A randomized trial of oral iron on tests of short-term memory and attention span in young pregnant women. J Adolesc Health Care 1986;7:44–48.

119. Hemminki E, Rimpela U. A randomized comparison of routine versus selective iron supplementation during pregnancy. J Am Coll Nutr 1991;10:3–10.

120. Nelson SE, Zeigler EE, Copeland AM, et al. Lack of adverse reactions to iron-fortified formula. Pediatrics 1988;81:360–364.

121. Oski FA. Iron-fortified formulas and gastrointestinal symptoms in infants: a controlled study. Pediatrics 1980;66:168–170.

122. Idjradinata P, Watkins WE, Pollitt E. Adverse effect of iron supplementation on weight gain of iron-replete young children. Lancet 1994;343:1252–1254.

123. Canadian Task Force on the Periodic Health Examination. Canadian guide to clinical preventive health care. Ottawa: Canada Communication Group, 1994:244–255.

124. Green M, ed. Bright Futures: national guidelines for health supervision of infants, children, and adolescents. Arlington, VA: National Center for Education in Maternal and Child Health, 1994.

125. American Academy of Pediatrics, Committee on Practice and Ambulatory Medicine. Recommendations for preventive pediatric health care. Pediatrics 1995;96:373–374.

126. American Academy of Family Physicians. Age charts for periodic health examination. Kansas City, MO: American Academy of Family Physicians, 1994. (Reprint no. 510.)

127. Canadian Task Force on the Periodic Health Examination. The periodic health examination. Can Med Assoc J 1979;121:1194–1254.

128. American Academy of Pediatrics and American College of Obstetricians and Gynecologists. Guidelines for perinatal care. 3d ed. Washington, DC: American College of Obstetricians and Gynecologists, 1992.

129. Eddy DM, ed. Common screening tests. Philadelphia: American College of Physicians, 1991.

130. American Academy of Pediatrics Committee on Nutrition. Iron-fortified infant formulas. Pediatrics 1989;84:1114–1115.

131. American Academy of Pediatrics, Committee on Nutrition. Iron supplementation for infants. Pediatrics 1976; 58:765–768. (Reaffirmed June 1992. American Academy of Pediatrics. Policy reference guide of the American Academy of Pediatrics. 7th ed. A comprehensive guide to AAP policy statements issued through December 1993. Elk Grove Village, IL: American Academy of Pediatrics, 1994.)

23. Screening for Elevated Lead Levels in Childhood and Pregnancy

RECOMMENDATION

Screening for elevated lead levels by measuring blood lead at least once at age 12 months is recommended for all children at increased risk of lead exposure. All children with identifiable risk factors should be screened, as should all children living in communities in which the prevalence of blood lead levels requiring individual intervention, including residential lead hazard control or chelation therapy, is high or is undefined (see *Clinical Intervention*). Evidence is currently insufficient to recommend an exact community prevalence below which targeted screening can be substituted for universal screening. Clinicians can seek guidance from their local or state health department. There is insufficient evidence to recommend for or against routine screening for lead exposure in asymptomatic pregnant women, but recommendations against such screening may be made on other grounds. There is also insufficient evidence to recommend for or against counseling families about the primary prevention of lead exposure, but recommendations may be made on other grounds. Recommendations regarding the primary prevention of lead poisoning by population-wide environmental interventions are beyond the scope of this chapter.

Burden of Suffering

Prevalence. The prevalence of elevated blood lead levels in the U.S. population has declined 78% in the past decade,[1] due primarily to marked declines in lead in gasoline, soldered cans, and air.[1-6] In a 1988–1991 national survey of children aged 1–5 years, 9% and 0.5% had blood lead levels ≥10 μg/dL and ≥25 μg/dL, respectively, down from 88% and 9% a decade before.[7] (The units μg/dL will be used throughout this chapter; to convert to μmol/L, divide by 20.72.) Prevalence varies widely among different communities and populations, however, with studies reporting 2–41% of children having blood lead levels ≥10 μg/dL, 0–3% ≥25 μg/dL, and 0–0.5% ≥40 μg/dL.[8-19] Current national data for pregnant women have not been published, but only 0.5% of U.S. women aged 12–49 years of age have blood lead levels ≥10 μg/dL.[7] Two large surveys of low-income pregnant women found 0%[20] and 6%[21] with blood lead levels >15 μg/dL.

Risk Factors for Elevated Lead Levels. The highest mean blood lead levels in the U.S. occur in children aged 1–2 years (mean 4.1 μg/dL) and in adults ≥50 years of age (4.0 μg/dL), with the lowest in adolescents (1.6 μg/dL).[7] Among adults, geometric mean levels are significantly higher in males than in females. Correlates of higher blood lead levels at all ages include minority race/ethnicity, central city residence, low income, low educational attainment, and residence in the Northeast region of the U.S.[7,22] These factors are associated with increased exposure to important lead sources, including dilapidated, pre-1950 housing with lead-based paint, lead-soldered pipes and household lead dust; and lead in dust and soil from heavy traffic and industry.[22–27] Other potential sources of household lead exposure include clothing or waste material brought home by workers in lead-based industries or hobbies, lead-based paint and dust contamination in pre-1950 housing that is undergoing remodeling or renovation, dietary intake from lead-soldered cans and lead-based pottery, and traditional ethnic remedies.[23,24,28]

Neurotoxic Effects of Lead Exposure in Children. Very high levels of inorganic lead exposure can produce serious neurologic complications, which may result in death or long-term sequelae.[23] A growing number of studies have reported associations between neurotoxic effects and blood lead levels once thought to be harmless. Adequately designed and conducted prospective cohort studies from a broad range of child populations have reported that a rise in blood lead from 10 to 20 μg/dL is associated with a likely decrement of about 2 points (reported range –6 to +1) in intelligence test scores (IQ).[29–35] In these studies, the mean blood lead levels at age 1–2 years (7.7–35.4 μg/dL) were higher than the current U.S. mean for this age group (4 μg/dL), but most levels were below 35 μg/dL. A meta-analysis[36] that included the five oldest of these cohort studies concluded that a doubling of blood lead levels from 10 to 20 μg/dL measured at age 2 years was associated with a statistically significant mean reduction of 1–2 IQ points; evidence was inconclusive regarding an association of IQ with mean postnatal blood lead levels. Although most cross-sectional studies evaluating the association of tooth and blood lead with IQ suffer from methodologic problems such as selection bias and limited adjustment for covariates, they have been generally consistent in reporting small negative effects of elevated lead levels on IQ.[e.g., in 36,37] A meta-analysis that included studies of whole tooth lead published since 1979 reported a statistically significant 1 point reduction in IQ associated with a doubling of tooth lead from 5 to 10 μg/g.[36] Evidence is not sufficient to quantify the exact nature of the relationship between IQ and higher blood lead levels (i.e., 40–100 μg/dL). Cross-sectional studies[38–42] have consistently reported small, inverse associations between blood or tooth lead and reaction (attentional) performance, but studies evaluating the effect of mildly elevated lead levels on other measures of neurodevelopmental function (e.g., behavior, learning disorders, auditory function) have produced inconclusive results. These have been less thoroughly evaluated than IQ, however.

In most studies, the size of the estimates of lead effects on IQ are reduced when adjusted for potentially confounding variables,[36] suggesting that some of the observed association may be due to imperfectly measured or unmeasured covariates. Studies in rodents and primates, however, which can avoid most of the methodologic weaknesses of observational studies in humans, report cognitive, attentional, and behavioral deficits, as well as auditory and visual dysfunction, with mildly elevated blood lead levels,[43–45] supporting a causal relationship between low-level lead exposure and neurotoxic effects in children. Studies demonstrating laboratory abnormalities (e.g., impaired vitamin D metabolism) in persons with blood lead levels as low as 10–15 μg/dL[23,46–48] also support a causal relationship.

Adverse Effects of Lead Exposure on Pregnancy Outcomes. The effects of very high blood lead levels during pregnancy on reproductive outcomes such as abortion and stillbirth have been recognized for many years.[23] Observational studies in pregnant women with blood lead levels <30 μg/dL have reported associations between elevated levels and birth weight, length of gestation (including preterm delivery), and neonatal head circumference.[49–56] The associations have been small, variable in direction of effect, and not statistically significant in most studies. These studies failed to detect important effects on other reproductive outcomes. Inconsistent results may be due in part to imprecise measures of fetal lead exposure.[55–59] All but one[34] of six previously cited cohort studies,[29–34] as well as the meta-analysis described above,[36] reported no association between antenatal or perinatal maternal blood lead levels and full-scale IQ measured at preschool or school age. Although very high lead levels in pregnancy are clearly hazardous, the adverse effects on the fetus of antepartum lead levels in the range typically found in the U.S. are not established.

Other Adverse Effects of Lead Exposure. Lead exposure affects many organ systems, including cardiovascular, renal, and hepatic, but most clinically apparent (i.e., symptomatic) effects occur with blood lead levels ≥50 μg/dL.[23,60–63] Small increases in systolic blood pressure have been associated with mildly elevated blood lead levels (i.e., 1–3 mm Hg for a rise in blood lead from 10 to 20 μg/dL) in most large, population-based, cross-sectional studies evaluating nonpregnant adults and pregnant women.[64–70] In children, evidence of blood pressure effects is more limited: one cross-sectional study found no association between elevated blood lead levels (range 7–70 μg/dL) and elevated blood pressure.[71] Adverse effects on height from lead levels well below 40 μg/dL have been suggested by analyses of national cross-sectional data,[72,73] but cohort studies with more extensive covariate adjustment report either transient or no effect of elevated lead levels (peak sample means 11–17 μg/dL) on growth.[35,74,75]

Accuracy of Screening Tests

Screening tests considered for detecting lead exposure include blood lead and free erythrocyte (or zinc) protoporphyrin levels. Blood lead concentration is the more sensitive of the two for detecting modest lead exposure, but its accuracy, precision and reliability can be affected by environmental lead contamination during blood collection, day-to-day biologic variability, and laboratory analytic variation. Lead contamination of collecting equipment, and skin contamination during capillary sampling, may each positively bias blood lead levels by up to 1.0 μg/dL, on average, although individual effects of skin contamination may be much greater.[76–80] Studies defining abnormal results as blood lead levels above 10 or 20 μg/dL have reported false-positive rates of 3–9% for capillary sampling compared to simultaneously collected venous blood lead.[77–78] Day-to-day biologic variability and trends over time contribute to higher false-positive rates for initial capillary samples when compared to results from venous testing done at a later date.[77,81] False-negative rates with capillary sampling appear to be lower, reported in one study as 1–8% compared to venous blood.[78] In published surveys,[76,82] 80–90% of clinical laboratories participating in proficiency testing programs met performance criteria for blood lead (within ±4 μg/dL of target values, for values <40 μg/dL[82]); unpublished national data show >95% of participating laboratories meeting these criteria and >80% achieving accuracy to within ±2 μg/dL of target values (unpublished data, Centers for Disease Control and Prevention, November 1993). Nonparticipating laboratories are likely to be less proficient. Reported blood lead values may differ by as much as 5 μg/dL from true values due to these sources of variability and bias, which may affect the predictive value of a positive test. Results from capillary samples may vary even more, although recent studies suggest the positive bias can be reduced with increased attention to reducing skin lead contamination.[77,78]

The erythrocyte protoporphyrin (EP) test, an indirect measure of lead exposure based on lead's effects on the hematopoietic system, is unaffected by contamination with environmental lead and is easily performed on capillary blood specimens, making it more acceptable for use with young patients. Erythrocyte (or zinc) protoporphyrin is insensitive, however, to modest elevations in blood lead levels.[21,83–89] The test also lacks specificity,[21,83,84,86,87,90] thus limiting its predictive value. In one study, EP measurements were taken on 47,230 suburban and rural children; although 4.7% of the children had an elevated erythrocyte protoporphyrin level, only 0.6% had elevated blood lead levels.[91]

In communities where there is a low prevalence of lead levels requiring individual intervention with chelation or residential lead hazard control, blood lead screening will have a low yield, and many unaffected children will be tested at potentially high cost and inconvenience. A questionnaire that can predict those at high risk for elevated lead levels would allow targeted screening in low prevalence areas, increasing the yield of blood testing by increasing the pretest probability of elevated lead levels in those who are tested. Cross-sectional studies[13–15,92–93a] in urban and suburban, mostly midwestern, populations have shown that one or more positive responses to five questions (about exposures to deteriorated paint from older or renovated housing, to other lead-poisoned children, or to lead-related hobbies or industry)[128] detects 64–87% of children with blood lead levels ≥10 μg/dL. Three studies reported higher sensitivities (81–100%) for blood lead levels ≥15–20 μg/dL.[15,92,93a] None of these studies evaluated the ability of questionnaires to detect levels above 20 μg/dL, in part because so few patients had levels so high. Specificity among the studies ranged from 32% to 75%. In the samples with a lower prevalence (2–7%) of levels ≥10 μg/dL, the proportion of those with a negative questionnaire who had elevated blood lead levels was predictably low (0.2–3.5%), but increased to 19% when the population prevalence of elevated lead levels was higher (17–28%).

Effectiveness of Early Detection

Detection of lead exposure before the development of potentially irreversible complications permits the clinician to recommend environmental interventions to limit further exposure and, when necessary, to begin medical treatment with chelating agents. Early detection may also result in interventions that prevent exposure of other children to lead (the child with elevated blood lead level acting as a sentinel for a hazardous environment). There is relatively little convincing evidence that these interventions improve health, however. One issue is that most available studies in asymptomatic children evaluate the effects of various interventions on blood lead levels rather than on clinical outcomes. Second, blood lead levels typically decline with the passage of time. On average, blood lead levels in childhood decrease with age after peaking at about 2 years of age, even without intervention.[7] Longitudinal studies of asymptomatic children with elevated lead levels have shown reductions in blood lead levels after short- and long-term follow-up in the absence of any intervention,[94,95] a result attributable at least in part to regression to the mean, random variation, and laboratory error. To evaluate adequately the effects of interventions on blood lead levels, studies must take into account these changes over time, preferably by the use of controls who do not receive the intervention.

Effect of Screening on Clinical Outcomes. Evidence is not available to demonstrate that universal screening for blood lead results in better clinical outcomes than either screening targeted to high-risk persons or individualized testing in response to clinical suspicion. Several older studies reported that, compared to historical results from individualized testing, intensive screening programs targeted to children in high-risk neighborhoods reduced case fatality rates, mortality rates, and proportions of children detected with very high blood lead levels or who developed symptomatic lead poisoning.[96–98] In the absence of concurrent controls, it is not clear whether the reported reductions in mortality and case fatality rates were due to screening, or to improvements in medical care over time. Reductions in mean lead levels may also have been due to secular trends, changes in screening tests, and to screening greater numbers of children, including many at low risk for severe lead poisoning. Thus, the available evidence regarding the efficacy of screening programs is weak.

Effect of Interventions to Lower Blood Lead Levels on Clinical Outcomes. In contrast to substantial evidence that chelating agents benefit children with symptomatic lead poisoning, few studies have compared potential clinical benefits of chelation therapy with its adverse effects in asymptomatic children. Ethical considerations preclude such trials for children with blood lead levels above 45 μg/dL. A large randomized controlled trial assessing the effect of chelation therapy on IQ in young children with venous blood lead concentrations of 20–45 μg/dL is currently under way (G. Rhoads, personal communication, Environmental and Occupational Health Sciences Institute, Piscataway, NJ, January 1994). An observational study[99,100] compared children with blood lead levels between 13 and 46 μg/dL (median 30 μg/dL), who did and did not receive EDTA chelation therapy depending on the results of a lead mobilization test. There was no effect of chelation on IQ at either 7 weeks or 6 months follow-up after controlling for age and initial IQ. Changes in concentrations of blood lead, bone lead, and EP also did not differ significantly between chelated and unchelated children. The greatest reductions in blood lead were associated with the highest initial lead levels, independent of chelation. The method of treatment assignment (i.e., based on a positive mobilization test) was most likely to have biased the study toward finding an effect of chelation, yet no effect was observed. There is thus little evidence presently available to confirm a clinical benefit from chelation therapy for children with lead levels <45 μg/dL. A comprehensive literature review found no studies evaluating clinical effects of residential lead hazard control. Their effects on blood lead levels are reviewed below.

Effects of Chelation Therapy on Blood Lead Levels. In uncontrolled experiments and case series in asymptomatic children with initial blood lead levels ranging from 40 to 471 μg/dL, chelating agents reduced blood lead levels substantially, to levels <40–70 μg/dL (varying with initial levels); these reductions were maintained for weeks to years after therapy was discontinued.[101–105] Most of these children were also returned to homes that had undergone lead hazard reduction, and the effect of this additional intervention was not specifically evaluated. Chelating agents have caused short-term reductions in blood lead levels in children whose pretreatment values ranged from 20 to 49 μg/dL in nonrandomized comparative trials, cohort studies, and uncontrolled experiments; these reductions have not been sustained over longer periods in the absence of repeated or continuing chelation therapy or environmental interventions.[104,106–109] Most of these studies did not report whether chelation therapy was combined with environmental interventions. With such weak evidence, including the previously cited cohort study reporting no effects of chelation on IQ,[99] it is difficult to make a convincing argument that chelation therapy to lower moderately elevated blood lead levels has a long-term benefit.

Effect of Residential Lead Hazard Control on Blood Lead Levels. For most asymptomatic children with elevated lead levels, the primary goal of intervention is to reduce exposure to lead-contaminated paint, dust, and soil in the child's home environment, since these sources account for most excessive lead exposure. Residential lead-based paint hazard control methods have become increasingly effective for reducing exposure to lead paint and lead-contaminated dust.[25,110,111] These new techniques are now replacing the older strategies, which often created lead dust during the intervention process, but there are currently few published studies of their effect on blood lead levels.

Because most published studies used older, less effective techniques, the effects of residential interventions on blood lead reported in the literature, and outlined below, probably indicate the minimum possible benefit of residential lead-paint and lead-contaminated dust hazard control. In an early cohort study[112] of 184 children with initial blood lead levels ≥50 μg/dL, children discharged after chelation therapy to lead-free (i.e., new or completely gutted and renovated) housing had significantly lower mean blood lead levels when compared to children exposed to "legally abated" or to inadequately abated housing (28.8 μg/dL vs. 38.5 and 57 μg/dL, respectively). Children in lead-free housing also had fewer recurrences of levels ≥50 μg/dL at 12 and 24–30 months follow-up. A nonrandomized trial[113] of households with children having initial blood lead levels >29 μg/dL compared more intensive experimental lead-reduction procedures with the lead-reduction procedures commonly in use in the study community. Neither intervention had any effect on mean dust or blood lead levels as tested 6 months after abatement, but an untreated control group was not included. Published[114] and unpublished[115] retrospective cohort studies suggest that residential lead paint hazard control is associated with modest declines (4–10 μg/dL) in mean blood lead levels in children with initial blood lead levels ≥ 25 μg/dL, although in one study[114] those with initial blood lead levels <35 μg/dL benefitted little from intervention. Case series and uncontrolled experiments, both weak study designs, have also evaluated lead-paint hazard control efforts in children with initial blood lead levels of 25–55 μg/dL;[100,116–119] several were published only as abstracts or summaries.[115,120] These studies reported statistically significant declines in mean blood lead levels, ranging from 2.5 to 10.2 μg/dL, 6–12 months after residential lead-based paint hazard control. All of the studies cited suffer from important design flaws, such as substantial drop-out rates and inadequate control for confounding variables such as season and age. Despite their flaws, the consistency of the results from these studies suggests a small, beneficial effect of lead-based paint hazard control on blood lead levels. As noted, there are as yet no published studies evaluating the effects on blood lead levels of newer residential lead hazard control techniques.

There are important problems with using one-time residential lead-paint hazard control as the sole method to reduce lead exposure in children.[121] Poor, inner-city families tend to move frequently, so that treating the current residence may have limited long-term benefit to the child, although benefit may accrue to other children moving in to that residence (see below). Residential lead-paint hazard control is costly and labor-intensive, resulting in low rates of intervention, especially in poor communities.[24,122] Lead dust is ubiquitous and highly mobile, so that recontamination by nearby lead sources, including soil lead, may occur after lead-paint hazard control efforts take place in a dwelling.[110,123,124] These problems indicate a need for additional individual interventions, as well as more comprehensive community-based interventions, to reduce household lead exposure.

The small effect noted in studies evaluating lead-paint hazard control methods may be attributable in part to recontamination of the dwelling by nearby lead sources and from subsequent deterioration of painted surfaces.[110,123,124] Several studies have evaluated measures designed to reduce ongoing lead-dust contamination from lead-contaminated paint and soil. In a nonrandomized controlled trial among children with blood lead levels of 30–49 μg/dL, having a research team wet-mop all lead-contaminated interior surfaces twice a month with a high-phosphate detergent cleanser resulted in significantly greater adjusted declines in mean blood lead levels of children in intervention households compared to children in control households (6.9 vs. 0.7 μg/dL) at 1-year follow-up.[125] There have been no controlled studies to evaluate whether counseling families to perform similar cleaning would be equally effective in reducing blood lead levels. In one uncontrolled experiment, the families of 78 children with blood lead levels of 10–35 μg/dL, who were living in the vicinity of a defunct lead smelter, received intensive (30–45 minutes) in-home education and literature on prevention of lead exposure.[126] The mean blood lead levels in the 51 (65%) children who had follow-up blood lead levels at 4 months declined from 15.0 to 7.8 μg/dL (and maximum levels from 35.0 to 12.7 μg/dL). Without concurrent controls, it is not possible to determine how much regression to the mean and seasonal and age variations contributed to these reductions in blood lead levels. There is also evidence that clinician counseling at the worksite to reduce lead dust ingestion by workers (e.g., through personal hygiene practices) can significantly reduce mean blood lead levels at 1-year follow-up,[127] but this study also lacked controls and may not be generalizable to the residential setting.

A third focus of residential lead hazard control is exposure to soil lead. In a randomized controlled trial[123] of young children with initial blood lead levels of 7–24 μg/dL, extensive soil abatement, one-time dust abatement, and removal of loose interior paint resulted in a statistically significant reduction in mean blood lead levels of 1.2–1.3 μg/dL compared to loose paint removal alone. This clinically insignificant decline was associated with a substantial reduction in soil lead from a median 2,000 to 105 ppm. Preliminary results of the U.S. Environmental Protection Agency's Three City Urban Soil Lead Abatement Demonstration Project similarly suggest that substantial declines in soil lead cause only modest reductions in mildly elevated blood lead concentrations.[124] The small effect was due at least in part to rapid recontamination with dust lead in households undergoing soil abatement. Among children living near a closed lead smelter, only 3% of the variance in blood lead levels was attributable to soil lead.[127a]

An important potential benefit of residential lead hazard control is its effect on the lead levels or clinical outcomes of other children who live in the same household as a child identified with elevated lead levels, or who subsequently move into the remediated residence. The literature review revealed no published evidence evaluating the effect of residential lead hazard control measures on such children. Based on the biokinetics of lead,[23] it is reasonable to believe that environmental interventions conducted before children are exposed are likely to prevent increases in blood lead levels more effectively than the same interventions in children who have already been exposed.

Effect of Nutritional Interventions on Blood Lead Levels. In most settings, neither residential lead-based paint or dust hazard control nor chelation therapy is routinely offered to children with blood lead levels <20 μg/dL, but some experts have recommended offering these children dietary counseling to reduce their blood lead levels.[128] Diets deficient in calories, calcium, and zinc have been associated with increased gastrointestinal absorption of lead,[129,130] but there is only limited evidence that counseling to correct such nutritional inadequacies will reduce blood lead levels or prevent further increases. Results of experimental studies of the effects of iron deficiency on lead absorption and retention in adult humans have been equivocal.[129,131] In a cohort study of children with initial blood lead levels of 13–46 μg/dL,[99] all children who were iron deficient or depleted were prescribed iron supplementation. Although most children were still iron deficient at the end of the study, there were improvements in ferritin level that were not associated with either declines in blood lead or improvements in cognitive function. Cross-sectional and cohort studies have failed to establish a clear association between mean blood lead levels and measures of iron status in women at midpregnancy or delivery, in newborns (cord blood), or in children.[57,99,131–134]

Adverse Effects of Screening and Intervention. The most common adverse effects of screening for elevated lead levels are false-positive fingerstick results, and the anxiety, inconvenience, work or school absenteeism, and financial costs associated with return visits and repeat tests. An EDTA lead mobilization test, used for some children with blood lead levels of 30–44 μg/dL,[135] requires intramuscular or intravenous infusion, a stay at the clinical center for at least 8 hours, and for young children, application of urine collection bags.[136] Residential lead-based paint and dust hazard control, when improperly done,[25] may produce acute increases in blood lead levels in resident children and abatement workers, occasionally necessitating hospitalization and chelation therapy.[113,116,137–139] Currently recommended techniques for lead hazard reduction are likely to reduce these adverse effects.[25] Chelating agents for asymptomatic lead poisoning have also been associated with important adverse effects. EDTA and dimercaprol (BAL) have transient renal, hepatic, and other toxicity, require intravenous or intramuscular injection, and generally require hospitalization for administration.[128,140,141] Common adverse effects of d-penicillamine are penicillin-like sensitivity reactions and transient nephrotoxicity; there are rare life-threatening reactions.[96,105,107,128] Succimer (meso-2,3-dimercaptosuccinic acid, or DMSA) causes mild gastrointestinal and systemic symptoms, rashes, and transient elevations in liver function tests, in up to 10% of cases.[104,106,108,142]

Recommendations of Other Groups

Several states mandate either universal screening for lead exposure or selective screening of populations at high risk for lead exposure.[143] Periodic screening of children with blood lead measurement is also required for Medicaid's Early and Periodic Screening, Diagnostic, and Treatment Program.[144] The American Academy of Pediatrics[145] and the Bright Futures guidelines[146] recommend: *(a)* screen all children for lead exposure at about 12 months of age, and possibly again at about 24 months of age; *(b)* take a history of lead exposure (using questionnaires provided with the guidelines) between the ages of 6 months and 6 years to identify high-risk children who should be screened earlier or more frequently; and *(c)* provide education to parents on safe environmental, occupational, nutritional and hygiene practices to protect their children from lead exposure. Follow-up screening intervals should be based on risk assessment and previous blood lead levels. The Centers for Disease Control and Prevention (CDC) recommends screening all children at 12 months of age using a blood lead test, except in communities where no childhood lead poisoning problem exists; high-risk children require earlier and more frequent screening.[128] The American Academy of Family Physicians (AAFP)[147] and the Canadian Task Force on the Periodic Health Examination[148] recommend screening all children who are at high risk of lead exposure (e.g., due to exposure to heavy traffic and industry, or to dilapidated older housing). The recommendations of the AAFP are currently under review. The American Medical Association recommends regularly screening all children under the age of 6 years for lead exposure through history-taking and, when appropriate, blood lead testing.[149] They recommend that the decision to employ universal or targeted screening be made based on prevalence studies of blood lead levels in the local pediatric population.

No major organizations currently recommend screening pregnant women for elevated lead levels.

Discussion

There is fair evidence that screening for elevated lead levels in asymptomatic children at increased risk for lead exposure will improve clinical outcomes. Because there have been no controlled trials directly evaluating screening for elevated lead levels, this conclusion is based on a chain of evidence constructed from studies of weaker design. First, in young asymptomatic children, blood lead levels as low as 10 μg/dL are associated with measurable neurodevelopmental dysfunction. Second, although the national prevalence of elevated lead levels has declined substantially in the past decade, a high prevalence persists in some communities, particularly poor urban communities in the northeastern U.S. Third, measurement of venous blood lead concentration is a convenient, reliable, precise and reasonably valid screening test for assessing lead exposure. Fourth, current interventions, including residential lead hazard control and chelation therapy, can reduce blood lead levels in children identified with levels ≥25 μg/dL, although the quality of evidence supporting their effectiveness is weak and a beneficial effect on IQ or other clinical outcomes has not yet been demonstrated. There is also weak evidence that screening high-risk children for elevated lead levels results in improved clinical outcome compared to historical controls identified by case-finding. Based on this evidence of the current burden of suffering and the effectiveness of early detection, the Task Force recommends screening children at increased risk for lead exposure.

While no studies have evaluated a specific age at which to screen, the natural history of blood lead levels in children, which increase most rapidly between 6 and 12 months and peak at age 18–24 months, suggests that screening at about 12 months of age is likely to be most effective for the early detection of elevated lead levels.

For those children who are screened and found to have initial blood lead levels <25 μg/dL, there is as yet little evidence regarding the effectiveness of early detection and intervention, or of repeated screening to detect further increases in blood lead. Longitudinal and cross-sectional studies suggest that in children ≥2 years, most such levels will decline naturally with time, but elevated levels may persist in children who are chronically exposed.[101]

There is no direct evidence comparing the outcomes of universal screening with the outcomes from targeted screening for elevated lead levels. Recent studies indicate that the prevalence of elevated blood levels in the U.S. has declined dramatically in the past decade, but that local prevalence is highly variable, with more than 10-fold differences between communities. In a community with a low prevalence of elevated blood lead levels, universal screening may result in disproportionate risks and costs relative to benefits. The prevalence level at which targeted screening can replace universal screening is a public health policy decision requiring consideration of factors in addition to the scientific evidence for effectiveness of early detection, such as available resources, competing public health needs, and costs and availability of alternative approaches to reducing lead exposure. Good quality analyses are needed to determine the population prevalence below which universal lead screening is not cost-effective. Clinicians can consult with their local or state health department regarding appropriate screening policy for the local child population.

In communities where data suggest that universal screening is not indicated, there may nevertheless be some children who are at increased risk of blood lead levels in the range for which individual intervention by chelation therapy or residential lead hazard control has been demonstrated to be effective. These children may have had exposure to lead sources such as lead-based hobbies or industries, traditional ethnic remedies, or lead-based pottery. Selective blood lead screening of such high-risk children is appropriate even in low prevalence communities. There is fair evidence that a validated questionnaire of known and acceptable sensitivity and specificity can identify those at high risk. In several studies, the CDC[128] and similar questionnaires correctly identified 64% to 87% of urban and sub-urban children who had blood lead levels ≥10 µg/dL. These questionnaires have not been adequately evaluated as a screening tool to detect higher blood lead levels (e.g., ≥20–25 µg/dL), or to detect exposure in other populations (e.g., migrant workers, rural communities). Locale-specific questionnaires that inquire about likely local sources of lead exposure may lead to improved prediction.

As is the case in children, there are no controlled trials evaluating screening for elevated lead levels in pregnant women, nor are there sufficient data to construct an adequate chain of evidence demonstrating benefit. The prevalence of levels >15 µg/dL appears to be quite low in pregnant women. There is fair evidence that mildly elevated lead levels during pregnancy are associated with small increases in antepartum blood pressure, but limited evidence that these levels have important adverse effects on reproductive or other outcomes, including intelligence of offspring. An extensive literature search failed to identify studies evaluating screening or intervention for lead exposure in pregnant women. There are potentially important adverse effects of chelation therapy on the fetus, and of residential lead hazard control on both the pregnant woman and fetus if they are not performed according to established standards. Removal to a lead-free environment would theoretically be effective in reducing lead exposure but has not been specifically evaluated in pregnancy. There is thus insufficient evidence to recommend for or against screening pregnant women for the detection of elevated lead levels.

Population-based interventions for the primary prevention of lead exposure are likely to be more effective, and may be more cost-effective, than office-based screening, treatment and counseling. Community, regional, and national environmental lead hazard reduction efforts, such as reducing lead in industrial emissions, gasoline, and cans, have proven highly effective in reducing population blood lead levels.[1–6,150,151] Remaining important sources of lead (e.g., lead paint and pipes in older homes, lead-contaminated soil) are, however, more difficult to address on a population-wide basis. Studies of community-based efforts to reduce lead exposure from these and other sources in order to prevent the occurrence of elevated lead levels are ongoing.[25,110,152] Evaluation of the effectiveness of community-based interventions, and recommendations regarding their use, are beyond the scope of this document.

CLINICAL INTERVENTION

Screening for elevated lead levels by measuring blood lead at least once at age 12 months is recommended for all children at increased risk of lead exposure ("B" recommendation). All children with identifiable risk factors should be screened, as should children living in communities in which the prevalence of blood lead levels requiring individual intervention, including chelation therapy or residential lead hazard control, is high or is undefined. If capillary blood is used, elevated lead levels should be confirmed by measurement of venous blood lead. The optimal frequency of screening for lead exposure in children, or for repeated testing of children previously found to have elevated blood lead levels, is unknown and is left to clinical discretion; consideration should be given to the degree of elevation, the interventions provided, and the natural history of lead exposure, including the typical peak in lead levels at 18–24 months of age.

In communities where the prevalence of blood lead levels requiring individual intervention is low, a strategy of targeted screening, possibly using locale-specific questionnaires of known and acceptable sensitivity and specificity, can be used to identify high-risk children who should have blood lead testing. Examples of individual risk factors include: *(a)* living in or frequently visiting an older home (built before 1950) with dilapidated paint or with recent or ongoing renovation or remodeling, *(b)* having close contact with a person who has an elevated lead level, *(c)* living near lead industry or heavy traffic, *(d)* living with someone whose job or hobby involves lead exposure, *(e)* using lead-based pottery, or *(f)* taking traditional ethnic remedies that contain lead.[128] There is currently insufficient evidence to recommend an exact population prevalence below which targeted screening can be substituted for universal screening. The results of cost-benefit analyses, available resources and public health priorities are among the determinants of the prevalence below which targeted screening is recommended for a community. Clinicians can seek guidance from their local or state health department.

There is insufficient evidence to recommend for or against routine screening for lead exposure in asymptomatic pregnant women ("C" recommendation). Recommendations against such screening may be made on the grounds of limited and conflicting evidence regarding the current burden of suffering, high costs, and the potential for adverse effects from intervention.

There is insufficient evidence to recommend for or against trying to prevent lead exposure by counseling families to control lead dust by repeated household cleaning, or to optimize caloric, iron, and calcium intake specifically to reduce lead absorption ("C" recommendation). For high-risk individuals or those living in high-prevalence communities, such recommendations may be made on other grounds, including minimal risk of adverse effects from the cleaning or the dietary advice, and the additional, unrelated benefits from optimizing nutrition (see Chapter 22, Screening for Iron Deficiency Anemia, and Chapter 56, Counseling to Promote a Healthy Diet).

Recommendations regarding community- or population-based interventions for the primary prevention of lead poisoning, assessment of community lead contamination, or the setting of community priorities for lead hazard reduction, are beyond the scope of this document.

The draft update of this chapter was prepared for the U.S. Preventive Services Task Force by Carolyn DiGuiseppi, MD, MPH.

REFERENCES

1. Pirkle JL, Brody DJ, Gunter EW, et al. The decline in blood lead levels in the United States. The National Health and Nutrition Examination Surveys (NHANES). JAMA 1994;272:284–291.
2. Annest JL, Pirkle JL, Makuc D, et al. Chronological trend in blood lead levels between 1976 and 1980. N Engl J Med 1983;308:1373–1377.
3. Centers for Disease Control and Prevention. Blood lead levels—United States, 1988–1991. MMWR 1994;43:545–548.
4. Hayes EB, McElvaine MD, Orbach HG, et al. Long-term trends in blood lead levels among children in Chicago: relationship to air lead levels. Pediatrics 1994;93:195–200.
5. Davis JM, Elias RW, Grant LD. Current issues in human lead exposure and regulation of lead. Neurotoxicology 1993;14:15–28.
6. Galal-Gorchev H. Dietary intake, levels in food and estimated intake of lead, cadmium, and mercury. Food Addit Contam 1993;10:115–128.
7. Brody DJ, Pirkle JL, Kramer RA, et al. Blood lead levels in the US population. Phase 1 of the third National Health and Nutrition Examination Survey (NHANES III, 1988–1991). JAMA 1994;272:277–284.
8. Gellert GA, Wagner GA, Maxwell RM, et al. Lead poisoning among low-income children in Orange County, California. A need for regionally differentiated policy. JAMA 1993;270:69–71.
9. Blumenthal HT, Mayfield R. An update on blood lead levels in pediatric patients of a neighborhood health center and an analysis of sources of exposure. J Natl Med Assoc 1995;87:99–104.
10. Rifai N, Cohen G, Wolf M, et al. Incidence of lead poisoning in young children from inner-city, suburban, and rural communities. Ther Drug Monit 1993;15:71–74.
11. Gottlieb K, Koehler JR. Blood lead levels in children from lower socioeconomic communities in Denver, Colorado. Arch Environ Health 1994;49:260–266.
12. Norman EH, Bordley WC, Hertz-Picciotto I, et al. Rural-urban blood lead differences in North Carolina children. Pediatrics 1994;94:59–64.
13. Tejeda D, Wyatt D, Rostek B, et al. Do questions about lead exposure predict elevated lead levels? Pediatrics 1994;93:192–194.
14. Binns HJ, LeBailly SA, Poncher J, et al. Is there lead in the suburbs? Risk assessment in Chicago suburban pediatric practices. Pediatrics 1994;93:164–171.
15. Nordin JD, Rolnick SJ, Griffin JM. Prevalence of excess lead absorption and associated risk factors in children enrolled in a midwestern health maintenance organization. Pediatrics 1994;93:172–177.
16. Taubman B, Wiley C, Henretig F. Prevalence of elevated blood lead levels in a suburban middle class private practice. Arch Pediatr Adolesc Med 1994;148:757–760.
17. Maskarinec G. Blood lead levels among children in Hawaii. Hawaii Med J 1993;52:242–250.

18. Cook M, Chappell WR, Hoffman RE, et al. Assessment of blood lead levels in children living in a historic mining and smelting community. Am J Epidemiol 1993;137:447–455.

19. Kimbrough R, LeVois M, Webb D. Survey of lead exposure around a closed lead smelter. Pediatrics 1995;95:550–554.

20. Fredeen DJ, Ehlinger EP, Cruikshank SH, et al. Lead levels among pregnant women in Hennepin County. Minn Med 1992;75:29–32.

21. Flanigan GD Jr, Mayfield R, Blumenthal HT. Studies on lead exposure in patients of a neighborhood health center: Part II. A comparison of women of childbearing age and children. J Natl Med Assoc 1992;84:23–27.

22. Sargent JD, Brown MJ, Freeman JL, et al. Childhood lead poisoning in Massachusetts communities: its association with sociodemographic and housing characteristics. Am J Public Health 1995;85:528–534.

23. Committee on Measuring Lead in Critical Populations, National Research Council. Measuring lead exposure in infants, children, and other sensitive populations. Washington, DC: National Academy Press, 1993.

24. Agency for Toxic Substances and Disease Registry. The nature and extent of lead poisoning in children in the United States: a report to Congress. Atlanta: Department of Health and Human Services, Public Health Service, 1988. (Publication no. DHHS-99-2966.)

25. Department of Housing and Urban Development. Comprehensive and workable plan for the abatement of lead-based paint in privately owned housing. Report to Congress. Washington, DC: Department of Housing and Urban Development, 1990. (Publication no. HUD-PDR-1295.)

26. Environmental Protection Agency. Reducing lead in drinking water: a benefit analysis. Washington, DC: Environmental Protection Agency, Office of Policy Planning and Evaluation, 1986.

27. Arnetz BB, Nicolich MJ. Modelling of environmental lead contributors to blood lead in humans. Int Arch Occup Environ Health 1990;62:397–402.

28. Centers for Disease Control and Prevention. Lead poisoning associated with use of traditional ethnic remedies—California, 1991–1992. MMWR 1993;42:521–524.

29. Baghurst PA, McMichael AJ, Wigg NR, et al. Environmental exposure to lead and children's intelligence at the age of seven years. The Port Pirie Cohort Study. N Engl J Med 1992;327:1279–1284.

30. Cooney G, Bell A, Stravou C. Low level exposure to lead and neurobehavioural development: the Sydney Study at seven years. In: Farmer JG, ed. Proceedings of Heavy Metals in the Environment Conference, Edinburgh, September 1991;1:16–19.

31. Bellinger DC, Stiles KM, Needleman HL. Low-level lead exposure, intelligence and academic achievement: a long-term follow-up study. Pediatrics 1992;90:855–861.

32. Dietrich KN, Berger OG, Succop PA, et al. The developmental consequences of low to moderate prenatal and postnatal lead exposure: intellectual attainment in the Cincinnati Lead Study Cohort following school entry. Neurotoxicol Teratol 1993;15:37–44.

33. Ernhart CB, Morrow-Tlucak M, Wolf AW, et al. Low-level lead exposure in the prenatal and early preschool periods: intelligence prior to school entry. Neurotoxicol Teratol 1989;11:161–170.

34. Wasserman GA, Graziano JH, Factor-Litvak P, et al. Consequences of lead exposure and iron supplementation on childhood development at age 4 years. Neurotoxicol Teratol 1994;16:233–240.

35. Wolf AW, Jimenez E, Lozoff B. No evidence of developmental ill effects of low-level lead exposure in a developing country. J Dev Behav Pediatr 1994;15:224–231.

36. Pocock SJ, Smith M, Baghurst P. Environmental lead and children's intelligence: a systematic review of the epidemiological evidence. BMJ 1994;309:1189–1197.

37. Needleman HL, Gatsonis CA. Low-level lead exposure and the IQ of children. A meta-analysis of modern studies. JAMA 1990;263:673–678.

38. Winneke G, Brockhaus A, Ewers U, et al. Results from the European multicenter study on lead neurotoxicity in children: implications for risk assessment. Neurotoxicol Teratol 1990;12:553–559.

39. Winneke G, Beginn U, Ewert T, et al. Comparing the effects of perinatal and later childhood lead exposure on neuropsychological outcome. Environ Res 1985;38:155–167.

40. Winneke G, Kramer U, Brockhaus A, et al. Neuropsychological studies in children with elevated tooth-lead concentrations. Int Arch Occup Environ Health 1983;51:231–252.

41. Winneke G, Brockhaus A, Collet W, et al. Modulation of lead-induced performance deficit in children by varying signal rate in a serial choice reaction task. Neurotoxicol Teratol 1989;11:587–592.

42. Hatzakis A, Kokkevi A, Katsouyanni K, et al. Psychometric intelligence and attentional performance deficits in lead-exposed children. In: Proceedings of the International Conference: heavy metals in the environment. 1987;1:204–209.

43. Otto DA, Fox DA. Auditory and visual dysfunction following lead exposure. Neurotoxicology 1993;14:191–208.

44. Cory-Slechta DA. The behavioral toxicity of lead: problems and perspectives. Adv Behav Pharmacol 1984;4: 211–255.

45. Rice DC. Lead-induced changes in learning: evidence for behavioral mechanisms from experimental animal studies. Neurotoxicol 1993;14:167–178.

46. Staessen JA, Lauwerys RR, Buchet J-P, et al. Impairment of renal function with increasing blood lead concentrations in the general population. N Engl J Med 1992;327:151–156.

47. Factor-Litvak P, Stein Z, Graziano J. Increased risk of proteinuria among a cohort of lead-exposed pregnant women. Environ Health Perspect 1993;101:418–421.

48. Graziano JH, Slavkovic V, Factor-Litvak P, et al. Depressed serum erythropoietin in pregnant women with elevated blood lead. Arch Environ Health 1991;46:347–350.

49. Ernhart CB, Wolf AW, Kennard MJ, et al. Intrauterine exposure to low levels of lead: the status of the neonate. Arch Environ Health 1986;41:287–291.

50. McMichael AJ, Vimpani GV, Robertson EF, et al. The Port Pirie cohort study: maternal blood lead and pregnancy outcome. J Epidemiol Community Health 1986;40:18–25.

51. Bellinger D, Leviton A, Rabinowitz M, et al. Weight gain and maturity in fetuses exposed to low levels of lead. Environ Res 1991;54:151–158.

52. Murphy MJ, Graziano JH, Popovac D, et al. Past pregnancy outcomes among women living in the vicinity of a lead smelter in Kosovo, Yugoslavia. Am J Public Health 1990;80:33–35.

53. Lindbohm M-L, Sallmen M, Anttila A, et al. Paternal occupational lead exposure and spontaneous abortion. Scand J Work Environ Health 1991;17:95–103.

54. Laudanski T, Sipowicz M, Modzelewski P, et al. Influence of high lead and cadmium soil content on human reproductive outcome. Int J Gynecol Obstet 1991;36:309–315.

55. Dietrich KN, Krafft KM, Bornschein RL, et al. Low-level fetal lead exposure effect on neurobehavioral development in early infancy. Pediatrics 1987;80:721–730.

56. Factor-Litvak P, Graziano JH, Kline JK, et al. A prospective study of birthweight and length of gestation in a population surrounding a lead smelter in Kosovo, Yugoslavia. Int J Epidemiol 1991;20:722–728.

57. Milman N, Christensen JM, Ibsen KK. Blood lead and erythrocyte zinc protoporphyrin in mothers and newborn infants. Eur J Pediatr 1988;147:71–73.

58. Ernhart CB. A critical review of low-level prenatal lead exposure in the human: I. Effects on the fetus and newborn. Reprod Toxicol 1992;6:9–19.

59. Baghurst PA, Robertson EF, Oldfield RK, et al. Lead in the placenta, membranes, and umbilical cord in relation to pregnancy outcome in a lead-smelter community. Environ Health Perspect 1991;90: 315–320.

60. Chisolm JJ Jr. The use of chelating agents in the treatment of acute and chronic lead intoxication in childhood. J Pediatr 1968;73:1–38.

61. Pueschel SM, Kopito L, Schwachman H. Children with an increased lead burden: a screening and follow-up study. JAMA 1972;222:462–466.

62. Nuyts GD, Daelemans RA, Jorens PG, et al. Does lead play a role in the development of chronic renal disease? Nephrol Dial Transplant 1991;6:307–315.

63. Hu H. A 50-year follow-up of childhood plumbism. Hypertension, renal function, and hemoglobin levels among survivors. Am J Dis Child 1991;145:681–687.

64. Grandjean P, Hollnagel H, Hedegaard L, et al. Blood lead-blood pressure relations: alcohol intake and hemoglobin as confounders. Am J Epidemiol 1989;129:732–739.

65. Elwood PC, Yarnell JWG, Oldham PD, et al. Blood pressure and blood lead in surveys in Wales. Am J Epidemiol 1988;127:942–945.

66. Schwartz J. Lead, blood pressure, and cardiovascular disease in men and women. Environ Health Perspect 1991;91:71–75.

67. Moller L, Kristensen TS. Blood lead as a cardiovascular risk factor. Am J Epidemiol 1992;136:1091–1100.

68. Dolenc P, Staessen JA, Lauwerys RR, et al. Short report: low-level lead exposure does not increase the blood pressure in the general population. J Hypertens 1993;11:589–593.

69. Hense HW, Filipiak B, Keil U. The association of blood lead and blood pressure in population surveys. Epidemiology 1993;4:173–179.

70. Rabinowitz M, Bellinger D, Leviton A, et al. Pregnancy hypertension, blood pressure during labor, and blood lead levels. Hypertension 1986;10:447–451.

71. Selbst SM, Sokas RK, Henretig FM, et al. The effect of blood lead on blood pressure in children. J Environ Pathol Toxicol Oncol 1993;12:213–218.

72. Schwartz J, Angle C, Pitcher H. Relationship between childhood blood lead levels and stature. Pediatrics 1986;77:281–288.

73. Frisancho AR, Ryan AS. Decreased stature associated with moderate blood lead concentrations in Mexican-American children. Am J Clin Nutr 1991;54:516–519.

74. Shukla R, Dietrich KN, Bornschein RL, et al. Lead exposure and growth in the early preschool child: a follow-up report from the Cincinnati Lead Study. Pediatrics 1991;88:886–892.

75. Greene T, Ernhart CB. Prenatal and preschool age lead exposure: relationship with size. Neurotoxicol Teratol 1991;13:417–427.

76. Jacobson BE, Lockitch G, Quigley G. Improved sample preparation for accurate determination of low concentrations of lead in whole blood by graphite furnace analysis. Clin Chem 1991;37:515–519.

77. Parsons PJ, Raciti KA, Esernio-Jenssen D. Evaluation and improvement of sample collection procedures for the determination of blood lead. Third semi-annual report to the Center for Environmental Health and Injury Control, Centers for Disease Control and Prevention. Atlanta: Centers for Disease Control and Prevention, 1993.

78. Schlenker TL, Fritz CJ, Mark D, et al. Screening for pediatric lead poisoning: comparability of simultaneously drawn capillary and venous blood samples. JAMA 1994;271:1346–1348.

79. Schonfeld DJ, Cullen MR, Rainey PM, et al. Screening for lead poisoning in an urban pediatric clinic using samples obtained by fingerstick. Pediatrics 1994;94:174–179.

80. Lyngbye T, Jorgensen PJ, Grandjean P, et al. Validity and interpretation of blood lead levels: a study of Danish school children. Scand J Clin Lab Invest 1990;50:441–449.

81. Schonfeld DJ, Rainey PM, Cullen MR, et al. Screening for lead poisoning by fingerstick in suburban pediatric practices. Arch Pediatr Adolesc Med 1995;149:447–450.

82. Parsons PJ. Monitoring human exposure to lead: an assessment of current laboratory performance for the determination of blood lead. Environ Res 1992;57:149–162.

83. Blumenthal HT, Flanigan GD, Mayfield R. Studies on lead exposure in patients of a neighborhood health center: Part I. Pediatric patients. J Natl Med Assoc 1991;83:1065–1072.

84. Mahaffey KR, Annest JL. Association of erythrocyte protoporphyrin with blood lead level and iron status in the second National Health and Nutrition Examination Survey, 1979–1980. Environ Res 1986;41:328–338.

85. Debaun MR, Sox HC. Setting the optimal erythrocyte protoporphyrin screening decision threshold for lead poisoning: a decision analytic approach. Pediatrics 1991;88:121–131.

86. Parsons PJ, Reilly AA, Hussain A. Observational study of erythrocyte protoporphyrin screening test for detecting low lead exposure in children: impact of lowering the blood lead action threshold. Clin Chem 1991;37:216–225.

87. McElvaine MD, Orbach HG, Binder S, et al. Evaluation of the erythrocyte protoporphyrin test as a screen for elevated blood lead levels. J Pediatr 1991;119:548–550.

88. Leung FY, Bradley C, Pellar TG. Reference intervals for blood lead and evaluation of zinc protoporphyrin as a screening test for lead toxicity. Clin Biochem 1993;26:491–496.

89. Rolfe PB, Marcinak JF, Nice AJ, et al. Use of zinc protoporphyrin measured by the Protofluor-Z hematofluorometer in screening children for elevated blood lead level. Am J Dis Child 1993;147:66–68.

90. Marcus AH, Schwartz J. Dose-response curves for erythrocyte protoporphyrin vs blood lead: effects of iron status. Environ Res 1987;44:221–227.

91. Guthrie R, Orfanos A, Widger K, et al. Screening suburban/rural children for lead exposure, iron deficiency. Am J Public Health 1988;78:856–857.

92. Schaffer SJ, Szilagyi PG, Weitzman M. Lead poisoning risk determination in an urban population through the use of a standardized questionnaire. Pediatrics 1994;93:159–163.

93. Rooney BL, Hayes EB, Allen BK, et al. Development of a screening tool for prediction of children at risk for lead exposure in a midwestern clinical setting. Pediatrics 1994;93:183–187.

93a. Striph KB. Prevalence of lead poisoning in a suburban practice. J Fam Pract 1995;41:65–71.

94. McCusker J. Longitudinal changes in blood lead level in children and their relationship to season, age, and exposure to paint or plaster. Am J Public Health 1979;69:348–352.

95. Reigart JR, Whitlock NH. Longitudinal observations of the relationship between free erythrocyte porphyrins and whole blood lead. Pediatrics 1976;57:54–59.

96. Sachs HK, Blanksma LA, Murray EF, et al. Ambulatory treatment of lead poisoning: report of 1,155 cases. Pediatrics 1970;46:389–396.

97. Sachs HK. Effect of a screening program on changing patterns of lead poisoning. Environ Health Perspect 1974;7:41–45.

98. Browder A, Joselow M, Louria DB, et al. Evaluation of screening programs for childhood lead poisoning by analysis of hospital admissions. Am J Public Health 1974;64:914–915.

99. Ruff HA, Bijur PE, Markowitz M, et al. Declining blood lead levels and cognitive changes in moderately lead-poisoned children [comments in JAMA 1993;270:827–829]. JAMA 1993;269:1641–1646.

100. Markowitz ME, Bijur PE, Ruff H, et al. Effects of calcium disodium versenate (CaNa$_2$EDTA) chelation in moderate childhood lead poisoning. Pediatrics 1993;92:265–271.

101. Moel DI, Sachs HK, Drayton MA. Slow, natural reduction in blood lead level after chelation therapy for lead poisoning in childhood. Am J Dis Child 1986;140:905–908.

102. Chisolm JJ Jr. Chelation therapy in children with subclinical plumbism. Pediatrics 1974;53:441–443.

103. Vitale LF, Rosalinas-Bailon A, Folland D, et al. Oral penicillamine therapy for chronic lead poisoning in children. J Pediatr 1973;83:1041–1045.

104. Graziano JH, LoIacono NJ, Moulton T, et al. Controlled study of meso-2,3-dimercaptosuccinic acid for the management of childhood lead intoxication. J Pediatr 1992;120:133–139.

105. Marcus SM. Experience with D-penicillamine in treating lead poisoning. Vet Hum Toxicol 1982;24:18–20.

106. Graziano JH, LoIacono NJ, Meyer P. Dose-response study of oral 2,3-dimercaptosuccinic acid in children with elevated blood lead concentrations. J Pediatr 1988;113:751–757.

107. Shannon M, Graef J, Lovejoy FH Jr. Efficacy and toxicity of D-penicillamine in low-level lead poisoning. J Pediatr 1988;112:799–804.

108. Liebelt EL, Shannon M, Graef JW. Efficacy of oral meso-2,3-dimercaptosuccinic acid therapy for low-level childhood plumbism. J Pediatr 1994;124:313–317.

109. Shannon M, Grace A, Graef JW. Use of penicillamine in children with small lead burdens [letter]. N Engl J Med 1989;321:979–980.

110. Office of Policy Development and Research, Department of Housing and Urban Development. Lead-based paint abatement demonstration (FHA). Washington, DC: Department of Housing and Urban Development, 1991. (Publication no. HUD-1316-PDR.)

111. Farfel MR, Chisolm JJ Jr, Rohde CA. The longer-term effectiveness of residential lead paint abatement. Environ Res 1994;66:217–221.

112. Chisolm JJ Jr, Millits ED, Quaskey SA. The relationship between the level of lead absorption in children and the age, type and condition of housing. Environ Res 1985;38:31–45.

113. Farfel MR, Chisolm JJ Jr. Health and environmental outcomes of traditional and modified practices for abatement of residential lead-based paint. Am J Public Health 1990;80:1240–1245.

114. Staes C, Matte T, Copley CG, et al. Retrospective study of the impact of lead-based paint hazard remediation on children's blood lead levels in St. Louis, Missouri. Am J Epidemiol 1994;139: 1016–1026.

115. Rust SW, Burgoon DA, Pierce BK, et al. Draft report on a summary of studies addressing the efficacy of lead abatement. Columbus, OH: Battelle, 1993.

116. Amitai Y, Brown MJ, Graef JW, et al. Residential deleading: effects on the blood lead levels of lead-poisoned children. Pediatrics 1991;88:893–897.

117. Rosen JF, Markowitz ME, Bijur PE, et al. L-line x-ray fluorescence of cortical bone lead compared with the CaNa$_2$EDTA test in lead-toxic children [Correction published in Proc Natl Acad Sci USA 1989;86:7595]. Proc Natl Acad Sci USA 1989;86:685–689.

118. Rosen JF, Markowitz ME, Bijur PE, et al. Sequential measurements of bone lead content by L x-ray fluorescence in CaNa$_2$EDTA-treated lead-toxic children. Environ Health Perspect 1991;93:271–277.

119. Rosen JF, Markowitz ME. Trends in the management of childhood lead poisonings. Neurotoxicology 1993;14: 211–218.

120. Swindell S, Charney E. Does home abatement lower blood lead levels in children with Class II lead poisoning [abstr]? Am J Dis Child 1992;146:478.

121. Mushak P, Crocetti AF. Methods for reducing lead exposure in young children and other risk groups: an integrated summary of a report to the U.S. Congress on childhood lead poisoning. Environ Health Perspect 1990;89:125–135.

122. Foster JD, Louria DB, Stinson L. Influence of documented lead poisoning on environmental modification programs in Newark, New Jersey. Arch Environ Health 1979;34:368–371.

123. Weitzman M, Aschengrau A, Bellinger D, et al. Lead-contaminated soil abatement and urban children's blood lead levels [comments in JAMA 1993;270:829–830]. JAMA 1993;269:1647–1654.

124. Environmental Protection Agency. Three city urban soil lead abatement demonstration project (fact sheet). Washington, DC: Environmental Protection Agency, 1992. (Publication no. 9355.4-10FSa.)

125. Charney E, Kessler B, Farfel M, et al. Childhood lead poisoning. A controlled trial of the effect of dust-control measures on blood lead levels. N Engl J Med 1983;309:1089–1093.

126. Kimbrough RD, LeVois M, Webb DR. Management of children with slightly elevated blood lead levels. Pediatrics 1994;93:188–191.

127. Porru S, Donato F, Apostoli P, et al. The utility of health education among lead workers: the experience of one program. Am J Ind Med 1993;22:473–481.

127a. Kimbrough R, LeVois M, Webb D. Survey of lead exposure around a closed lead smelter. Pediatrics 1995;95:550–554.

128. Centers for Disease Control and Prevention. Preventing lead poisoning in young children. A statement by the Centers for Disease Control—October 1991. Atlanta: Department of Health and Human Services, 1991.

129. Mahaffey KR. Nutritional factors in lead poisoning. Nutr Rev 1981;39:353–362.

130. Ziegler EE, Edwards BB, Jensen RL, et al. Absorption and retention of lead by infants. Pediatr Res 1978;12:29–34.

131. Markowitz ME, Rosen JF, Bijur PE. Effects of iron deficiency on lead excretion in children with moderate lead intoxication. J Pediatr 1990;116:360–364.

132. Ernhart CB, Wolf AW, Sokol RJ, et al. Fetal lead exposure: antenatal factors. Environ Res 1985; 38:54–66.

133. Carraccio CL, Bergman GE, Daley BP. Combined iron deficiency and lead poisoning in children. Clin Pediatr 1987;26:644–647.

134. Graziano JH, Popovac D, Factor-Litvak, et al. Determinants of elevated blood lead during pregnancy in a population surrounding a lead smelter in Kosovo, Yugoslavia. Environ Health Perspect 1990;89: 95–100.

135. Glotzer DE, Bauchner H. Management of childhood lead poisoning: a survey. Pediatrics 1992;89:614–618.

136. Markowitz ME, Rosen JF. Need for the lead mobilization test in children with lead poisoning. J Pediatr 1991;119:305–310.

137. Amitai Y, Graef JW, Brown MJ, et al. Hazards of "deleading" homes of children with lead poisoning. Am J Dis Child 1987;141:758–760.

138. Rey-Alvarez S, Menke-Hargrave T. Deleading dilemma: pitfall in the management of childhood lead poisoning. Pediatrics 1987;79:214–217.

139. Feldman RG. Urban lead mining: lead intoxication among deleaders. N Engl J Med 1978;298: 1143–1145.

140. Chisolm JJ Jr. Treatment of acute lead intoxication—choice of chelating agents and supportive therapeutic measures. Clin Toxicol 1970;3:527–540.

141. Moel DI, Kumar K. Reversible nephrotoxic reactions to a combined 2,3-dimercapto-1-propanol and calcium disodium ethylenediaminetetraacetic acid regimen in asymptomatic children with elevated blood lead levels. Pediatrics 1982;70:259–262.

142. Mann KV, Travers JD. Succimer, an oral lead chelator. Clin Pharmacol 1991;10:914–922.

143. Alliance to End Childhood Lead Poisoning. Guide to state lead screening laws. Washington, DC: Alliance to End Childhood Lead Poisoning, 1991.

144. Medicaid Bureau, Health Care Financing Administration, Department of Health and Human Services. EPSDT: a guide for educational programs. Baltimore: Department of Health and Human Services, 1992:12.

145. American Academy of Pediatrics, Committee on Environmental Health. Lead poisoning: from screening to primary prevention. Pediatrics 1993;92:176–183.

146. Green M, ed. Bright Futures: guidelines for health supervision of infants, children and adolescents. Arlington, VA: National Center for Education in Maternal and Child Health, 1994.

147. American Academy of Family Physicians. Age charts for periodic health examination. Kansas City, MO: American Academy of Family Physicians, 1994. (Reprint no. 510.)

148. Canadian Task Force on the Periodic Health Examination. Canadian guide to clinical preventive health care. Ottawa: Canada Communication Group, 1994:268–288.

149. American Medical Association Council on Scientific Affairs. Report 6: lead poisoning among children. Chicago: American Medical Association, December 1994.

150. Prpic-Majic D, Pongracic J, Hrsak J, et al. A follow-up study in a lead smelter community following the introduction of an effective pollution control system. Isr J Med Sci 1992;28:548–556.

151. Yankel AJ, von Lindern IH, Walter SD. The Silver Valley Study: the relationship between childhood blood lead levels and environmental exposure. J Air Pollut Control Assoc 1977;27:763–767.
152. Department of Health and Human Services, Department of Housing and Urban Development, and Environmental Protection Agency. Report of the Interagency Task Force on the Prevention of Lead Poisoning: a report to Congress. Washington, DC: Department of Health and Human Services, December 1993.

24. Screening for Hepatitis B Virus Infection

RECOMMENDATION

Screening with hepatitis B surface antigen (HBsAg) to detect active (acute or chronic) hepatitis B virus (HBV) infection is recommended for all pregnant women at their first prenatal visit. The test may be repeated in the third trimester in women who are initially HbsAg negative and who are at increased risk of HBV infection during pregnancy. Routine screening for HBV infection in the general population is not recommended. Certain persons at high risk may be screened to assess eligibility for vaccination (see *Clinical Intervention*).

Burden of Suffering

Each year in the U.S., an estimated 200,000–300,000 persons become infected with HBV, more than 10,000 require hospitalization, and 250 die of fulminant disease.[1,2] The greatest reported incidence occurs in adults aged 20–39.[3,4] Of note, the number of reported cases peaked in 1985 and has shown a continuous gradual decline since that time.[4] While most infections resolve with time, it is estimated that 1.0–1.25 million individuals have chronic, asymptomatic HBV infection (i.e., chronic carriers).[5] This places them at risk for developing chronic active hepatitis, cirrhosis, and primary hepatocellular carcinoma (PHC). In the population as a whole, 50–67% of acute HBV infections are asymptomatic, whereas over 90% of early childhood infections are asymptomatic.[3,6] Individuals with asymptomatic infections are still at risk for the development of chronic HBV infection and its sequelae. An estimated 22,000 births occur to HBV-infected women each year in the U.S.[6] Infants whose mothers are positive for hepatitis B e antigen (HBeAg) have a 70–90% chance of becoming infected perinatally.[6-8] Infections during infancy, while estimated to represent only 1–3% of cases, account for 20–30% of chronic infections.[6] The risk of developing a chronic HBV infection (i.e., carrier state) is inversely related to age at the time of infection.[6,9,10] This risk is 85–90% for infected infants and rapidly decreases to a steady risk of 6–10% in older children and adults. The risk of developing PHC or cirrhosis depends on the length of time that an individual has been chronically infected. It is estimated that infants who become chronically infected have a 25% lifetime risk and adults have a 15% lifetime risk of PHC or cirrhosis.[3] An estimated 5,000 hepatitis B-related deaths occur each year as a result of cirrhosis and PHC, with the median age of death occurring in the fifth decade of life.[1,11–13]

The principal risk factors for HBV infection in the U.S. are injecting illicit drugs; heterosexual contact with HBV-infected persons or with persons at high risk for HBV infection (e.g., injection drug users); sexual contact with multiple sex partners; and male homosexual activity.[14–17] In 1990, heterosexual activity accounted for 27% of cases, homosexual activity for 11%, and injection drug use for 14%.[15] No associated risk factor can be identified in over 30% of patients with HBV infection.[6] In recent years, a growing number of injection drug users have become infected; currently, between 60% and 80% of persons who use illicit drugs parenterally have serologic evidence of HBV infection.[1] In a study of inner-city pregnant women, those who presented for delivery without prenatal care, with a positive drug screen, or with a past history of any illicit drug use were at increased risk for HbsAg positivity.[18] For example, those with no prenatal care and positive urine drug screens were 29 times more likely to be seropositive than those without these risk factors. Alaska Natives, Pacific Islanders, immigrants and refugees from HBV endemic areas (including Asia, Africa, and Eastern Europe), hemodialysis patients and staff, and residents and staff in institutions for the developmentally disabled, are also at increased risk.[1,19]

Accuracy of Screening Tests

The principal screening test for detecting current (acute or chronic) HBV infection is the identification of HBsAg. Immunoassays for detecting HBsAg have a reported sensitivity and specificity of greater than 98%.[20–20d] Spontaneous clearance of HBsAg occurs each year in 1% of persons with chronic HBV infection.[21]

Effectiveness of Early Detection

There is good evidence that early detection of HBsAg in pregnant women can prevent infection in the newborn. Controlled trials,[22–30a] a cohort study,[31] and multiple time series[8,32,33] have shown that hepatitis B vaccine alone and in combination with hepatitis B immune globulin (HBIG) is effective in preventing the development of chronic HBV infection in infants born to HBsAg-positive mothers. Vaccine, in combination with a single dose of HBIG given within 12 hours of birth, is 75–95% efficacious in preventing chronic HBV infection,[22,25–27,30–31] whereas vaccine alone has an efficacy of 65–96%.[22,26,27,29,30a] Although the ranges of efficacy overlap, the efficacy of hepatitis B vaccine in combination with HBIG was generally greater than that of vaccine alone in studies that directly compared the two strategies, with the difference reaching statistical significance in two studies.[24,31]

In the past, prenatal testing for HBsAg was recommended only for pregnant women at high risk of having acquired HBV infection.[34] Recent studies in urban and minority populations have shown that only 35–65% of HBsAg-positive mothers are identified when testing is restricted to high-risk groups.[35–39] It is thought that many women at risk are not tested because their sexual and drug-related histories are not discussed with clinicians or because their clinicians are unfamiliar with perinatal transmission of HBV and recommended preventive measures.[40] In addition, many women who have asymptomatic chronic HBV infection may not acknowledge having risk factors even when a careful history is taken.

Detecting acute or chronic HBV infection may also be important in preventing virus transmission to others besides newborns. Screening tests coupled with counseling have the potential to influence certain behaviors (e.g., having sex with multiple partners, sharing needles among injection drug users, donating blood products) in infected persons, and thereby prevent transmission. Sexual contacts and persons with possible percutaneous exposure may also be identified in the process and offered vaccination (see Chapter 67). The effectiveness of routine screening of asymptomatic persons in the clinical setting as a means of reducing HBV transmission needs further study, however. Routine counseling on preventive behaviors to reduce the risk of infection and transmission, and appropriate vaccination, may be more effective strategies (see Chapters 62, 65, and 66).

There is little evidence that early detection of asymptomatic HBV infection reduces the risk of developing chronic liver disease or its complications. Interferon eliminates HBsAg positivity in some individuals with a diagnosis of chronic hepatitis B,[41–45] but whether this results in a reduction in long-term morbidity and mortality has not been adequately evaluated.

A strategy of targeting high-risk populations for screening and immunizing those found to be seronegative has been ineffective in reducing the population incidence of HBV infection.[5,16] This approach has failed as a public health strategy because a high percentage (>30%) of patients have no identifiable risk factors[6] and because high-risk individuals (e.g., injection drug users) may not have access to screening and vaccination services. Nevertheless, individuals known to be at high risk who are found to be seronegative on screening can be immunized and thus protected from HBV infection (see Chapters 65 and 66).

Recommendations of Other Groups

The Advisory Committee on Immunization Practices (ACIP),[5] the American College of Obstetricians and Gynecologists,[46,47] the American Academy of Pediatrics,[47,48] and the American College of Physicians (ACP)[49] recommend that all pregnant women be tested for HBsAg during an early prenatal visit. The test may be repeated in the third trimester if acute hepatitis is suspected, an exposure to hepatitis has occurred, or the woman practices a high-risk behavior such as injection drug use. No major organizations recommend universal screening of nonpregnant individuals for HBV infection. ACIP and ACP recommend making decisions to test potential vaccine recipients for prior infection on the basis of cost-effectiveness, and state that testing in groups with the highest risk of HBV infections (i.e., HBV marker prevalence >20%)[1] is usually cost-effective.[1,49]

Discussion

Because many HBsAg-positive women are not detected during pregnancy when only high-risk women are screened, routine HBsAg testing of all pregnant women is a more effective strategy for the prevention of perinatal HBV transmission. It has been calculated that screening all of the more than four million pregnant women each year in the U.S. would detect about 22,000 HBsAg-positive mothers, and treatment of their newborns would prevent the development of chronic HBV infection in an estimated 6,000 neonates each year.[50] Several studies have demonstrated that the long-term benefits of preventing chronic liver disease make routine prenatal HBsAg testing as cost-effective as other widely implemented prenatal and blood donor screening practices.[39,51-53] Despite current recommendations for universal vaccination of newborns against HBV (see Chapter 65), screening all pregnant women for HBV infection is recommended as an effective intervention because the vaccine alone appears to be less efficacious than the combination of vaccine and HBIG in preventing HBV infection of infants exposed to HBsAg-positive mothers.

A recommendation for universal screening of the general population would require proof that intervention reduces the morbidity and mortality associated with asymptomatic chronic HBV infection, or that it reduces or prevents HBV transmission. While interferon therapy appears promising as an intervention, current data are insufficient to recommend its use in asymptomatic HBV-infected persons in order to improve clinical outcome. Similarly, there is little evidence to support screening and counseling seropositive persons as an effective intervention to prevent HBV transmission. Given the low burden of suffering, lack of evidence of benefit, and the costs and inconvenience associated with testing, universal screening in the nonpregnant population cannot be recommended at this time.

Routine vaccination with hepatitis B vaccine is discussed in Chapters 65 and 66. Prevaccination screening is likely to be cost-effective and should be considered in high-risk groups where the rate of previous infection is high (e.g., >20–40%), in order to avoid vaccinating immune individuals or persons with chronic HBV infections.[54-56] In these populations, screening with antibody to hepatitis B core antigen (anti-HBc), which identifies all previously infected individuals, including those with chronic HBV infection, may be preferable.[5] In other high-risk adolescents and adults, routine vaccination without screening may be more cost-effective (see Chapters 65 and 66).

CLINICAL INTERVENTION

Screening with hepatitis B surface antigen (HBsAg) to detect active (acute or chronic) HBV infection is recommended for all pregnant women at their first prenatal visit ("A" recommendation). The test may be repeated in the third trimester if the woman is initially HBsAg-negative and engages in high-risk behavior such as injection drug use or if exposure to hepatitis B virus during pregnancy is suspected. Infants born to HBsAg-positive mothers should receive hepatitis B immune globulin (HBIG) (0.5 mL) intramuscularly within 12 hours of birth. Hepatitis B vaccine, at the appropriate dosage, should be administered intramuscularly concurrently with HBIG (at a different injection site). The second and third doses of vaccine should be given 1 and 6 months after the first dose. Depending on the brand of vaccine utilized, the dosage of vaccine given to an infant born to a HBsAg-positive mother may differ from that given routinely to infants born to HBsAg-negative mothers. For neonates born to women whose HBsAg-status is unknown at the time of delivery, administering vaccine within 12 hours of birth, using the same dosage as that for infants whose mothers are HbsAg-positive, is recommended. Maternal testing for HBsAg-should be performed at the same time. If the mother is found to be HBsAg-positive, HBIG should be administered to her infant as soon as possible and within 7 days of birth. Contacts (sexual or household) of HBsAg-positive pregnant women should be either vaccinated or tested to determine susceptibility to HBV and vaccinated if susceptible (see also Chapter 67). The decision to do prevaccination testing may be made based on cost-effectiveness analysis.

Routine screening for HBV infection in the general population is not recommended ("D" recommendation). There is insufficient evidence to recommend for or against routinely screening asymptomatic high-risk individuals for HBV infection in order to determine eligibility for vaccination, but recommendations for screening may be made based on cost-effectiveness analyses ("C" recommendation). Such analyses suggest that screening is usually cost-effective in groups with an HBV marker prevalence >20%.[1,49] See Chapters 65 and 66 for further recommendations on hepatitis B vaccination and Chapter 67 for information about passive and ac-

tive immunization of persons with possible exposure to HBV-infected individuals or blood products. Counseling on preventive behaviors to reduce the risk of HBV infection and transmission is discussed in Chapter 62.

The draft update of this chapter was prepared for the U.S. Preventive Services Task Force by Peter W. Pendergrass, MD, MPH, and Carolyn DiGuiseppi, MD, MPH.

REFERENCES

1. Centers for Disease Control. Protection against viral hepatitis: recommendations of the Immunization Practices Advisory Committee. MMWR 1990;39:1–26.
2. Centers for Disease Control. Update on hepatitis B prevention: recommendations of the Immunization Practices Advisory Committee. MMWR 1987;36:353–360,366.
3. Shapiro CN. Epidemiology of hepatitis B. Pediatr Infect Dis J 1993;12:433–437.
4. Centers for Disease Control and Prevention. Summary of notifiable diseases, United States, 1993. MMWR 1994;42(53):1–74.
5. Centers for Disease Control. Hepatitis B virus: a comprehensive strategy for eliminating transmission in the United States through universal childhood vaccination. Recommendations of the Immunization Practices Advisory Committee (ACIP). MMWR 1991;40(RR-13):1–25.
6. Margolis HS, Alter MJ, Hadler SC. Hepatitis B: evolving epidemiology and implications for control. Semin Liver Dis 1991;11:84–92.
7. Stevens CE, Beasley RP, Tsui J, et al. Vertical transmission of hepatitis B antigen in Taiwan. N Engl J Med 1975;292:771–774.
8. Stevens CE, Toy PT, Tong MJ, et al. Perinatal hepatitis B virus transmission in the United States: prevention by passive-active immunization. JAMA 1985;253:1740–1745.
9. McMahon BJ, Alward WL, Hall DB, et al. Acute hepatitis B virus infection: relation of age to the clinical expression of disease and subsequent development of the carrier state. J Infect Dis 1985;151: 599–603.
10. Edmunds WJ, Medley GF, Nokes DJ, et al. The influence of age on the development of the hepatitis B carrier state. Proc R Soc Lond B Biol Sci 1993;253:197–201.
11. Beasley RP, Hwang LY. Epidemiology of hepatocellular carcinoma. In: Vyas GN, Dienstag JL, Hoofnagle JH, eds. Viral hepatitis and liver disease. Orlando, FL: Grune & Stratton, 1984:209–224.
12. Beasley RP. Hepatitis B virus as the etiologic agent in hepatocellular carcinoma: epidemiologic considerations. Hepatology 1982;2:21S–26S.
13. Beasley RP, Hwang LY, Lin CC, et al. Hepatocellular carcinoma and HBV: a prospective study of 22,707 men in Taiwan. Lancet 1981;2:1129–1133.
14. Centers for Disease Control. Changing patterns of groups at high risk for hepatitis B in the United States. MMWR 1988;37:429–432,437.
15. Alter MJ. Community acquired viral hepatitis B and C in the United States. Gut 1992;34(2 Suppl):S17–S19.
16. Alter MJ, Hadler SC, Margolis HS, et al. The changing epidemiology of hepatitis B in the United States: need for alternative vaccination strategies. JAMA 1990;263:1218–1222.
17. Centers for Disease Control. Hepatitis Surveillance Report no. 54. Atlanta: Centers for Disease Control, 1992.
18. Silverman NS, Darby MJ, Ronkin SL, et al. Hepatitis B prevalence in an unregistered prenatal population. JAMA 1991;266:2852–2855.
19. Centers for Disease Control. Screening for hepatitis B virus infection among refugees arriving in the United States, 1979–1991. MMWR 1991;40:784–786.
20. Centers for Disease Control and Prevention. Sensitivity of the test for antibody to hepatitis B surface antigen, United States. MMWR 1993;42:707–710.
20a. Ferguson M, Pipkin PA, Heath AB, et al. Working standards for hepatitis B surface antigen for use in the UK Blood Transfusion Service: results of a collaborative study. Vox Sang 1993;65:303–308.
20b. Toplikar E, Carlomagno A, Rojkin LF, et al. Development of an enzyme immunoassay for the detection of hepatitis B surface antigen employing monoclonal antibodies. J Clin Lab Anal 1993;7: 324–328.
20c. Jakob R. A multiple center clinical study of third-generation enzyme immunoassays for hepatitis B surface antigen and hepatitis B core IgM class antibody. Eur J Clin Chem Clin Biochem 1993;31:259–266.

20d. McCready JA, Morens D, Fields HA, et al. Evaluation of enzyme immunoassay (EIA) as a screening method for hepatitis B markers in an open population. Epidemiol Infect 1991;107:673–684.

21. Beasley RP. Hepatitis B virus: the major etiology of hepatocellular carcinoma. Cancer 1988;61: 1942–1956.

22. Lo K-J, Tsai Y-T, Lee S-D, et al. Immunoprophylaxis of infection with hepatitis B virus in infants born to hepatitis B surface antigen-positive carrier mothers. J Infect Dis 1985;152:817–822.

23. Halliday ML, Kang L-Y, Rankin JG, et al. An efficacy trial of a mammalian cell-derived recombinant DNA hepatitis B vaccine in infants born to mothers positive for HBsAg, in Shanghai, China. Int J Epidemiol 1992;21:564–573.

24. Sehgal A, Gupta I, Sehgal R, et al. Hepatitis B vaccine alone or in combination with anti-HBS immunoglobulin in the perinatal prophylaxis of babies born to HBsAg carrier mothers. Acta Virol 1992; 36:359–366.

25. Beasley RP, Hwang LY, Lee GCY, et al. Prevention of perinatally transmitted hepatitis B virus infections with hepatitis B immune globulin and hepatitis B vaccine. Lancet 1983;2:1099–1102.

26. Wong VCW, Ip HMH, Reesink HW, et al. Prevention of the HBsAg carrier state in newborn infants of mothers who are chronic carriers of HBsAg and HBeAg by administration of hepatitis B vaccine and hepatitis B immunoglobulin: double-blind randomized placebo controlled study. Lancet 1984;1: 921–926.

27. Ip HMH, Lelie PN, Wong VCW, et al. Prevention of hepatitis B virus carrier state in infants according to maternal serum levels of HBV DNA. Lancet 1989;1:406–410.

28. Poovorawan Y, Sanpavat S, Pongpunlert W, et al. Comparison of a recombinant DNA hepatitis B vaccine alone or in combination with hepatitis B immune globulin for the prevention of perinatal acquisition of hepatitis B carriage. Vaccine 1990;8S:S56–S62.

29. Xu Z-Y, Liu C-B, Francis D, et al. Prevention of perinatal acquisition of hepatitis B virus carriage using vaccine: preliminary report of a randomized, double-blind placebo controlled and comparative trial. Pediatrics 1985;76:713–718.

30. Assateerawatt A, Tanphaichitr VS, Suvatte V, et al. Immunogenicity and efficacy of a recombinant DNA hepatitis B vaccine, GenHevac B Pasteur in high risk neonates, school children and healthy adults. Asian Pac J Allergy Immunol 1993;11:85–91.

30a. Xu Z-Y, Duan S-C, Margolis HS, et al. Long-term efficacy of active postexposure immunization of infants for prevention of hepatitis B virus infection. J Infect Dis 1995;171:54–60.

31. Hsu H-M, Chen D-S, Chuang C-H, et al. Efficacy of a mass hepatitis B vaccination program in Taiwan. Studies on 3464 infants of hepatitis B surface antigen-carrier mothers. JAMA 1988;260:2231–2235.

32. Poovorawan Y, Sanpavat S, Pongpunlert W, et al. Protective efficacy of a recombinant DNA hepatitis B vaccine in neonates of HBe antigen-positive mothers. JAMA 1989;261:3278–3281.

33. Stevens CE, Taylor PE, Tong MJ, et al. Yeast-recombinant hepatitis B vaccine: efficacy with hepatitis B immune globulin in prevention of perinatal hepatitis B virus transmission. JAMA 1987;257:2612–2616.

34. Immunization Practices Advisory Committee. Postexposure prophylaxis of hepatitis B. MMWR 1984; 33:285–290.

35. Kumar ML, Dawson NV, McCullough AJ, et al. Should all pregnant women be screened for hepatitis B? Ann Intern Med 1987;107:273–277.

36. Jonas MM, Schiff ER, O'Sullivan MJ, et al. Failure of Centers for Disease Control criteria to identify hepatitis B infection in a large municipal obstetrical population. Ann Intern Med 1987;107:335–337.

37. Summers PR, Biswas MK, Pastorek JG II, et al. The pregnant hepatitis B carrier: evidence favoring comprehensive antepartum screening. Obstet Gynecol 1987;69:701–704.

38. Wetzel AM, Kirz DS. Routine hepatitis screening in adolescent pregnancies: is it cost effective? Am J Obstet Gynecol 1987;156:166–169.

39. Delage G, Montplaisir S, Remy-Prince S, et al. Hepatitis B Virus Transmission Study Group. Prevalence of hepatitis B virus infection in pregnant women in the Montreal area. Can Med Assoc J 1986;134: 897–901.

40. Immunization Practices Advisory Committee. Prevention of perinatal transmission of hepatitis B virus: prenatal screening of all pregnant women for hepatitis B surface antigen. MMWR 1988;37:341–346,351.

41. Hoofnagle JH, Peters M, Mullen KD, et al. Randomized, controlled trial of recombinant human alpha-interferon in patients with chronic hepatitis B. Gastroenterology 1988;95:1318–1325.

42. Brook MG, Chan G, Yap I, et al. Randomized controlled trial of lymphoblastoid interferon alfa in European men with chronic hepatitis B virus infection. BMJ 1989;299:652–656.

43. Saracco G, Mazzella G, Rosina F, et al. A controlled trial of human lymphoblastoid interferon in chronic hepatitis B in Italy. Hepatology 1989;10:336–341.

44. Korenman J, Baker B, Waggoner J, et al. Long-term remission of chronic hepatitis B after alpha-interferon therapy. Ann Intern Med 1991;114:629–634.

45. Perrollo RP, Schiff ER, Davis GL, et al. A randomized controlled trial of interferon alfa-2b alone and after prednisone withdrawal for the treatment of chronic hepatitis B. N Engl J Med 1990;323:295–301.

46. Committee on Obstetrics: Maternal and Fetal Medicine, American College of Obstetricians and Gynecologists. Guidelines for hepatitis B virus screening and vaccination during pregnancy. Int J Gynaecol Obstet 1993;40: 172–174.

47. American Academy of Pediatrics and American College of Obstetricians and Gynecologists. Guidelines for perinatal care. 3rd ed. Washington, DC: American College of Obstetricians and Gynecologists, 1992.

48. American Academy of Pediatrics. Hepatitis B. In: Peter G, ed. 1994 Red Book: report of the Committee on Infectious Diseases. 23rd ed. Elk Grove Village, IL: American Academy of Pediatrics, 1994:224–238.

49. American College of Physicians Task Force on Adult Immunization and Infectious Diseases Society of America. Guide for adult immunization. 3rd ed. Philadelphia: American College of Physicians, 1994.

50. West DJ, Margolis HS. Prevention of hepatitis B virus infection in the United States: a pediatric perspective. Pediatr Infect Dis J 1992;11:866–874.

51. Arevalo JA, Washington AE. Cost-effectiveness of prenatal screening and immunization for hepatitis B virus [erratum appears in JAMA 1988;260:478]. JAMA 1988;259:365–369.

52. Kane MA, Hadler SC, Margolis HS, et al. Routine prenatal screening for hepatitis B surface antigen. JAMA 1988; 259:408–409.

53. Krahn M, Detsky AS. Should Canada and the United States universally vaccinate infants against hepatitis B? Med Decision Making 1993;13:4–20.

54. Holliday SM, Faulds D. Hepatitis B vaccine: a pharmacoeconomic evaluation of its use in the prevention of hepatitis B virus infection. Pharmacoeconomics 1994;5:141–171.

55. Bloom BS, Hillman AL, Fendrick AM, et al. A reappraisal of hepatitis B virus vaccination strategies using cost-effectiveness analysis. Ann Intern Med 1993;118:298–306.

56. Kwan-Gett TS, Whitaker RC, Kemper KJ. A cost-effectiveness analysis of prevaccination testing for hepatitis B in adolescents and preadolescents. Arch Pediatr Adolesc Med 1994;148:915–920.

25. Screening for Tuberculous Infection—*Including Bacille Calmette-Guérin Immunization*

RECOMMENDATION

Screening for tuberculous infection with tuberculin skin testing is recommended for asymptomatic high-risk persons. Bacille Calmette-Guérin (BCG) vaccination should be considered only for selected high-risk individuals (see *Clinical Intervention*).

Burden of Suffering

About 10–15 million persons in the United States are infected with *Mycobacterium tuberculosis*.[1] More than 24,000 reported cases of tuberculosis (TB) occurred in the U.S. in 1994.[1a,2] This disease is associated with considerable morbidity from pulmonary and extrapulmonary pathology. Pulmonary symptoms are progressive and include cough, hemoptysis, dyspnea, and pleuritis. Extrapulmonary TB can involve the bones, joints, pericardium, and lymphatics, and it can cause spinal cord compression from Pott's disease. Death is more common in older patients and infants, with estimated case-fatality rates ranging from 0.3% in adolescents to 18.5% in the elderly.[3] Newborns and infants also experience significant morbidity from this disease.

The incidence of TB is greatest in Asians, Pacific Islanders, blacks, American Indians, Alaska Natives, and Hispanics. About one third of all reported cases in the U.S. occur in blacks, 20% occur in Hispanics, 14% occur in Asians and Pacific Islanders, and 1% occur in American Indians and Alaska Natives.[2] About 30% of new cases occur in foreign-born immigrants.[2] The prevalence in homeless persons is 1–7% for clinically active TB and 18–51% for asymptomatic *M. tuberculosis* infection.[4]

After experiencing a steady decline from 1963 to 1984, reported TB cases increased by 20% from 1985 to 1992.[2] A disproportionately large number of new cases are occurring among black and Hispanic persons, among whom there was a 41% increase in reported TB cases between 1985 and 1992.[2] Infection with human immunodeficiency virus (HIV) is a major contributor to the recent increase in TB cases. Persons infected with HIV are more than 100 times more likely to develop active TB than are persons with competent immune systems, and the onset of the disease is often more rapid.[5] Reports of multidrug-resistant TB have also increased in recent years. Nationally, the proportion of new cases resistant to both isoniazid (INH) and rifampin increased from 0.5% in 1982 to 3.3% in the first quarter of 1991.[6] In New York City, as many as 33% of cases are resistant to INH or rifampin.[7] Reported case-fatality rates in patients with multidrug-resistant TB, most of whom are infected with HIV, have been as high as 72–89% (the rate is about 30–40% for immunocompetent individuals).[5] The latest data indicate a 9% decrease in annually reported TB cases from 1992 to 1994, in part reflecting intensified federal, state, and local TB control efforts.[1a]

Accuracy of Screening Tests

Tuberculin skin testing is the principal means of detecting *M. tuberculosis* infection in asymptomatic persons. Although some authors recommend chest radiography as a first-line test in high-risk populations,[8] roentgenography is generally considered to be inappropriate as the initial screening test for detecting tuberculous infection in asymptomatic persons. It is important, however, as a follow-up test to identify active pulmonary TB in infected persons identified through tuberculin testing. The most accurate tuberculin skin test is the Mantoux test, in which 5 units (5 TU) of tuberculin purified protein derivative (PPD) are injected intradermally to detect delayed hypersensitivity reactions within 48–72 hours.

The frequency of false-positive and false-negative tuberculin skin tests depends on a number of variables, including immunologic status, the size of the hypersensitivity reaction, and the prevalence of atypical mycobacteria. In certain geographic areas, cross-reacting atypical mycobacteria (as well as previous BCG vaccination) can produce intermediate size reactions, thereby limiting the specificity of the test.[9–11] False-positive results can also be produced by improper technique (e.g., measuring erythema rather than induration), hypersensitivity to PPD constituents, an Arthus reaction, and cellulitis. Prior BCG vaccination may produce false-positive indurations, but these are generally less than 10 mm in diameter. Moreover, because many BCG vaccinees either lose their immunity over time or do not convert, large indurations cannot be confidently attributed to prior BCG vaccination.[12,13] False-negative reactions, which are estimated to occur in about 5–10% of patients, can be observed early in infection before hypersensitivity develops, in anergic individuals and those with severe illnesses (including active TB), in newborns and infants less than 3 months of age, and as a result of improper technique in handling the PPD solution, administering the intradermal injection, and interpreting the results.[11] Other limitations of the Mantoux test include the time and skill required for proper administration and variability among clinicians in interpreting results.[14]

Multiple puncture tests (e.g., tine, Mono-Vacc) are less expensive and easier to administer than the Mantoux test. Studies evaluating the accuracy of these devices, however, have produced inconsistent results. In general, the evidence suggests that multiple puncture tests have poor specificity and may have inadequate sensitivity when compared with the Mantoux test.[15–17] Some of this inaccuracy is due to inconsistencies in the dose of injected tuberculin delivered by multiple puncture tests. Patient compliance can also affect the effectiveness of tuberculin skin testing because patients must return to the clinician 48–72 hours after the injection to have the test interpreted. Studies in pediatric patients report noncompliance rates of 28–82%.[18–20]

Persons who are tuberculin test negative may need repeat testing, but there are inadequate data from which to determine the optimal frequency of PPD screening. In the absence of such data, clinical decisions regarding the need for repeat testing and its frequency should be based on the likelihood of further exposure to TB and the clinician's level of confidence in the accuracy of the test results. Some negative reactions to tuberculin skin tests require immediate retesting (two-step testing) to help determine whether future positive reactions are due to the booster phenomenon or to new conversion. A positive result on the second test, typically performed 1–3 weeks later, suggests that the patient has been previously infected (boosted reaction), whereas a negative result on the second test followed by a positive result on subsequent testing suggests recent conversion. Two-step testing has become more common in screening health care workers[21] and other population groups (e.g., elderly nursing home residents) for tuberculous infection.

Effectiveness of Early Detection

The early detection of tuberculin reactivity is of potential benefit because chemoprophylaxis with INH is an effective means of preventing the subsequent development of active TB.[22] A review of 14 controlled trials found that efficacy in preventing clinical disease ranges between 25% and 88% among persons assigned to a 1-year course of INH.[22] Among individuals who complete the course of chemoprophylaxis, efficacy is greater than 90%.[23,24] Some studies suggest that 6 months of INH therapy in adults are nearly as effective as 12 months of treatment.[23,26] Preventive INH therapy is also of potential public health value in preventing future disease activity and transmission of the organism to household members and other close contacts.

A number of factors, however, limit the effectiveness of INH chemoprophylaxis. Some organisms are resistant to INH and other agents.[5] Patient compliance with a 6–12-month regimen is often difficult. The most important limitation of INH is its potential hepatotoxicity. INH-induced hepatitis occurs in about 0.3–2.3% of patients,[27] the frequency increasing with age and other factors (e.g., alcohol use). The condition can be fatal, but the exact frequency of fatal INH-induced hepatitis is uncertain. Mortality rates for persons with INH-related hepatitis were reported to be as high as 4–7% in one major study, with risk increasing directly with age (zero for persons less than 20 years of age, 0.3% for persons 20–34 years of age, 1.2% for persons 35–49 years of age, 2.3% for persons 50–64 years of age).[28] These data may overestimate the actual mortality from INH-induced hepatitis because the local incidence of cirrhosis-related deaths was increased in one of the communities participating in the study.[29] More recent analyses of published and unpublished data have estimated that the incidence of fatal INH-induced hepatitis is about 1–14/100,000 persons started on preventive therapy.[30,31] The risk may be lowered by performing periodic liver function tests while patients take INH. In persons who develop complications from INH, the resulting interruption of INH therapy before completion of the 1-year course may also lower the effectiveness of TB prevention.[24]

Although the benefits of INH probably outweigh its side effects in persons at high risk for developing active TB (see *Clinical Intervention* for description of high-risk groups), it is uncertain from available data whether low-risk, asymptomatic persons with a reactive tuberculin skin test are at sufficient risk of developing TB to justify the risks of INH-induced hepatitis. Epidemiologic calculations suggest that the annual incidence of TB in a low-risk population is less than 0.1%,[32,33] and that the lifetime probability of developing active TB ranges from 1.2% at age 20 to 0.37% at age 80.[34] Depending on the risk of INH-induced hepatitis, it is possible for complications from INH treatment to be more likely than the development of TB. In the absence of definitive clinical studies to clarify this issue, investigators have used decision analysis techniques to compare the benefits and risks of INH in tuberculin skin reactors of different ages. The results of these analyses have been inconsistent. One group concluded that benefits outweigh risks until the patient exceeds age 45;[35] another found that treatment was beneficial at all ages;[27] and another analysis concluded that INH should be withheld at all ages in the absence of other risk factors.[34] A decision analysis in young adults concluded that treatment was not beneficial in this age group.[32] An analysis for elderly tuberculin skin reactors concluded that INH would neither improve nor worsen 5-year survival but would decrease the risk of developing active disease.[33] An analysis for HIV-infected injection drug users concluded that, with the exception of black women, such patients would benefit from INH therapy even in the absence of tuberculin skin testing.[36]

Bacille Calmette-Guérin (BCG) Vaccination

Primary prevention through vaccination represents an alternative approach to the prevention of TB. BCG, a live vaccine derived from attenuated *Mycobacterium bovis,* has been used worldwide for more than 50 years to prevent TB. Clinical trials of the efficacy of BCG have yielded inconsistent results since the early 1930s, however, with reported levels of protection ranging from –56% to 80%.[37,38] Observational studies have shown that the incidence of the disease is lower in vaccinated children than in unvaccinated controls.[39–43] Factors contributing to the wide variation in results in BCG vaccine efficacy include genetic changes in the bacterial strains as well as differences in production techniques, methods of administration, and the populations and environments in which the vaccine has been studied.[44] A meta-analysis of 14 trials and 12 case-control studies concluded that BCG offered 50% protection against TB overall and 64–71% protection against TB meningitis and TB-related death.[45]

The potential adverse effects of BCG vaccination include prolonged ulceration and local adenitis, which occur in about 1–10% of vaccinees. The risk varies with the type of vaccine used, the population, and the methods used to measure complications. Osteomyelitis and death from disseminated BCG infection are estimated to occur in one case per million doses administered.[44]

In the U.S., where the risk of becoming infected with *M. tuberculosis* is relatively low, the disease can currently be controlled most successfully by screening and early treatment of infected persons. However, BCG vaccination may have a role in the U.S. for persons with special exposures to individuals with active TB, such as uninfected children who are at high risk for continuous or repeated exposure to infectious persons who are undetected or untreated,[44] or a future role in light of escalating multidrug resistance.

Recommendations of Other Groups

The Centers for Disease Control and Prevention (CDC), American Thoracic Society (ATS), and other members of the Advisory Committee for Elimination of Tuberculosis recommend screening the following groups for tuberculous infection: persons infected with HIV; close contacts of persons with TB; persons with medical risk factors associated with TB; immigrants from countries with high TB prevalence; medically underserved low-income populations; injection drug users; and residents and employees of high risk facilities.[46] Similar recommendations have been issued by the American Academy of Family Physicians.[55] Although the Canadian

Task Force on the Periodic Health Examination recommends screening high-risk groups, it gave an "E" recommendation (good evidence against performing the maneuver in the periodic health examination) to screening low-risk persons.[46a] The American Academy of Pediatrics (AAP) recommends against routine annual skin testing of children who lack risk factors and live in low-prevalence communities. The AAP does recommend annual Mantoux testing of high-risk children, as well as consideration of less frequent periodic testing (e.g., at ages 1, 4–6, and 11–16 years) of low-risk children who live in high-prevalence communities or have unreliable histories.[47] The Bright Futures guidelines recommend annual testing for persons of low socioeconomic status, those in high prevalence areas, those exposed to TB, and immigrants.[48] The American Medical Association's Guidelines for Adolescent Preventive Services (GAPS) recommend annual testing for adolescents in high-risk settings including those in homeless shelters, correctional institutions, and health care facilities.[49]

Recommendations on how to perform tuberculin skin testing have been issued by the CDC and ATS.[11] The CDC has recently issued guidelines on preventing transmission in health care facilities, which include specific recommendations on the categories of health care workers to include in skin-testing programs and the frequency with which they should be tested.[50] Guidelines for the treatment of converters have been issued in a joint statement by the ATS, AAP, CDC, and Infectious Disease Society of America.[51,52] The CDC has also issued recommendations on multidrug preventive therapy for converters with suspected contact with drug-resistant TB.[5] Screening certain populations for tuberculous infection is required by law in 44 states.[7]

Recommendations on BCG vaccination have been issued in a joint statement by the Immunization Practices Advisory Committee and the Advisory Committee for Elimination of Tuberculosis.[44] They recommended limiting BCG vaccination in the U.S. to tuberculin-negative infants and children who cannot be placed on INH and who have continuous exposure to persons with active disease, those with continuous exposure to patients with organisms resistant to INH or rifampin, and those belonging to groups with a rate of new infections greater than 1% per year and for whom the usual surveillance and treatment programs may not be operationally feasible.

CLINICAL INTERVENTION

Screening for tuberculous infection by tuberculin skin testing is recommended for all persons at increased risk of developing tuberculosis (TB) ("A" recommendation). Asymptomatic persons at increased risk include persons infected with HIV, close contacts of persons with known or sus-

pected TB (including health care workers), persons with medical risk factors associated with TB, immigrants from countries with high TB prevalence (e.g., most countries in Africa, Asia, and Latin America), medically underserved low-income populations (including high-risk racial or ethnic minority populations), alcoholics, injection drug users, and residents of long-term care facilities (e.g., correctional institutions, mental institutions, nursing homes). The Mantoux test involves the intradermal injection of 5 units of tuberculin PPD and the subsequent examination of the injection site 48–72 hours later. Current minimum criteria for a positive skin test, based on observational data and expert opinion, are 15-mm diameter for low-risk individuals, 10-mm diameter for high-risk individuals (e.g., immigrants, medically underserved low-income populations, injection drug users, residents of long-term care facilities, persons with conditions that increase TB risk, infants, and children less than 4 years of age), and 5-mm diameter for persons at very high risk (e.g., persons infected with HIV, persons with abnormal chest radiographs, recent contacts of infected persons). Prior BCG vaccination is not currently considered a valid basis for dismissing positive results. Persons with negative reactions who are at increased risk of anergy (e.g., HIV-infected individuals) can be skin-tested for anergy,[53] but this procedure is now considered optional in current CDC guidelines.[46] Treatment decisions in HIV-infected anergic patients should be made on an individual basis.[54] The frequency of tuberculin skin testing is a matter of clinical discretion.

Persons with a positive PPD test should receive a chest x-ray and clinical evaluation for TB. Those lacking evidence of active infection should receive INH prophylaxis if they meet criteria defined in recent guidelines.[52] Briefly, these criteria recommend INH prophylaxis in persons under 35 years of age who are from high-prevalence countries; medically underserved, low-income, high-prevalence populations; or long-term care facilities. It is also recommended in persons of any age with HIV infection or increased risk of HIV infection, other medical conditions that increase the risk of TB, or close contact with patients with newly diagnosed TB or skin test conversion. Screening for HIV infection may be indicated in recent converters (see Chapter 28). Patients with possible exposure to drug-resistant TB should be treated according to current recommendations for multidrug preventive therapy.[5] Directly observed therapy—observation of the patient by a health care worker as the medication is taken—may be indicated in patients who are unlikely to be compliant.

BCG vaccination against TB should be considered only for tuberculin-negative infants and children who cannot be placed on INH and who have continuous exposure to persons with active disease, those with continuous exposure to patients with organisms resistant to INH or rifampin, and those belonging to groups with a rate of new infections greater than 1%

per year and for whom the usual surveillance and treatment programs may not be operationally feasible ("B" recommendation). These groups may also include persons with limited access to or willingness to use health care services.

The draft update of this chapter was prepared for the U.S. Preventive Services Task Force by Steven H. Woolf, MD, MPH.

REFERENCES

1. Centers for Disease Control. National action plan to combat multidrug-resistant tuberculosis. MMWR 1992;41(RR-11):5–48.
1a. Centers for Disease Control and Prevention. Tuberculosis morbidity—United States, 1994. MMWR 1995;44:387–389, 395.
2. Centers for Disease Control and Prevention. Tuberculosis morbidity—United States, 1993. MMWR 1994;43:361–366.
3. Centers for Disease Control and Prevention. Tuberculosis statistics in the United States, 1990. Atlanta: Centers for Disease Control and Prevention, 1992.
4. Centers for Disease Control. Prevention and control of tuberculosis among homeless persons: recommendations of the Advisory Council for the Elimination of Tuberculosis. MMWR 1992;41(RR-5): 13–23.
5. Centers for Disease Control. Management of persons exposed to multidrug-resistant tuberculosis. MMWR 1992;41(RR-11):61–71.
6. Bloch AB, Cauthen GM, Onorato IM, et al. Nationwide survey of drug-resistant tuberculosis in the United States. JAMA 1994;271:665–671.
7. Centers for Disease Control and Prevention. Tuberculosis control laws—United States, 1993. MMWR 1993;42(RR-15):1–28.
8. Davidson PT. Routine screening for tuberculosis on hospital admission. Chest 1988;94:228–230.
9. Tuberculin, PPD: generic statement. Fed Reg 1977;42:52709–52712.
10. Mellor J. False-positive results of Mantoux tests. Can Med Assoc J 1985;132:1403.
11. American Thoracic Society. Diagnostic standards and classification of tuberculosis. Am Rev Respir Dis 1990;142:725–735.
12. Snider DE Jr. Bacille Calmette-Guerin vaccinations and tuberculin skin tests. JAMA 1985;253: 3438–3439.
13. Skotniski EM. Post-BCG tuberculin testing: interpreting results and establishing essential baseline data. Can J Public Health 1993;84:307–308.
14. Bearman JE, Kleinman H, Glyer VV, et al. A study of variability in tuberculin test reading. Am Rev Respir Dis 1964;90:913–919.
15. Rudd RM, Gellert AR, Venning M. Comparison of Mantoux, tine, and "Imotest" tuberculin tests. Lancet 1982;2:515–518.
16. Catanzaro A. Multiple puncture skin test and Mantoux test in Southeast Asian refugees. Chest 1985; 87:346–350.
17. Hansen JP, Falconer JA, Gallis HA, et al. Inadequate sensitivity of tuberculin tine test for screening employee populations. J Occup Med 1982;24:602–604.
18. Maqbool S, Asnes RS, Grebin B. Tine test compliance in a clinic setting. Pediatrics 1975;55:388–391.
19. Weinberger HL, Terry C. Tuberculin testing in a pediatric outpatient clinic. J Pediatr 1969;75:111–115.
20. Asnes RS, Maqbool S. Parent reading and reporting of children's tuberculin skin test results. Chest 1975;68 (Suppl 3):459–462.
21. Snider DE Jr, Cauthen GM. Tuberculin skin testing of hospital employees: infection, "boosting," and two-step testing. Am J Infect Control 1984;12:305–311.
22. Comstock GW, Woolpert SF. Preventive therapy. In: Kubica GP, Wayne LG, eds. The mycobacteria: a source book. New York: Marcel Dekker, 1984:1071–1081.
23. International Union Against Tuberculosis, Committee on Prophylaxis. Efficacy of various durations of isoniazid preventive therapy for tuberculosis: five years of follow-up in the IUAT trial. Bull WHO 1982; 60:555–564.

24. Stead WW, Teresa T, Harrison RW, et al. Benefit-risk considerations in preventive treatment for tuberculosis in elderly persons. Ann Intern Med 1987;107:843–845.

25. Deleted in proof.

26. Snider DE Jr, Caras GJ, Koplan JP. Preventive therapy with isoniazid: cost-effectiveness of different durations of therapy. JAMA 1986;255:1579–1583.

27. Rose DN, Schechter CB, Silver AL. The age threshold for isoniazid chemoprophylaxis: a decision analysis for low-risk tuberculin reactors. JAMA 1986;256:2709–2713.

28. Kopanoff DE, Snider DE Jr, Caras GJ. Isoniazid-related hepatitis: a U.S. Public Health Service cooperative surveillance study. Am Rev Respir Dis 1978;117:991–1001.

29. Comstock GW. Prevention of tuberculosis among tuberculin reactors: maximizing benefits, minimizing risks. JAMA 1986;256:2729–2730.

30. Snider DE Jr, Caras GJ. Isoniazid-associated hepatitis deaths: a review of available information. Am Rev Respir Dis 1992;145:494–497.

31. Salpeter SR. Fatal isoniazid-induced hepatitis: its risk during chemoprophylaxis. West J Med 1993;159:560–564.

32. Taylor WC, Aronson MD, Delbanco TL. Should young adults with a positive tuberculin test take isoniazid? Ann Intern Med 1981;94:808–813.

33. Cooper JK. Decision analysis for tuberculosis preventive treatment in nursing homes. J Am Geriatr Soc 1986;34:814–817.

34. Tsevat J, Taylor WC, Wong JB, et al. Isoniazid for the tuberculin reactor: take it or leave it. Am Rev Respir Dis 1988;137:215–220.

35. Comstock GW, Edwards PQ. The competing risks of tuberculosis and hepatitis for adult tuberculin reactors. Am Rev Respir Dis 1975;111:573–577.

36. Jordan TJ, Lewit EM, Montgomery RL, Reichman LB. Isoniazid as preventive therapy in HIV-infected intravenous drug abusers: a decision analysis. JAMA 1991;265:2987–2991.

37. Clemens JD, Chuong JJH, Feinstein AR. The BCG controversy: a methodological and statistical reappraisal. JAMA 1983;249:2362–2369.

38. Tripathy SP. Fifteen-year follow-up of the Indian BCG prevention trial. In: International Union Against Tuberculosis. Proceedings of the XXVIth IUAT World Conference on Tuberculosis and Respiratory Diseases. Singapore: Professional Postgraduate Services International, 1987:69–72.

39. Romanus V. Tuberculosis in Bacillus Calmette-Guerin-immunized children in Sweden: a ten-year evaluation following the cessation of general Bacillus Calmette-Guerin immunization of the newborn in 1975. Pediatr Infect Dis 1987;6:272–280.

40. Smith PG. Case-control studies of the efficacy of BCG against tuberculosis. In: International Union Against Tuberculosis. Proceedings of the XXVIth IUAT World Conference on Tuberculosis and Respiratory Diseases. Singapore: Professional Postgraduate Services International, 1987:73–79.

41. Padungchan S, Konjanart S, Kasiratta S, et al. The effectiveness of BCG vaccination of the newborn against childhood tuberculosis in Bangkok. Bull WHO 1986;64:247–258.

42. Tidjani O, Amedome A, ten Dam HG. The protective effect of BCG vaccination of the newborn against childhood tuberculosis in an African community. Tubercle 1986;67:269–281.

43. Slutkin G. Management of tuberculosis in urban homeless indigents. Public Health Rep 1986;101:481–485.

44. Immunization Practices Advisory Committee. Use of BCG vaccines in the control of tuberculosis: a joint statement by the ACIP and the Advisory Committee for Elimination of Tuberculosis. MMWR 1988;37:663–664, 669–675.

45. Colditz GA, Brewer TF, Berkey CS, et al. Efficacy of BCG vaccine in the prevention of tuberculosis: meta-analysis of the published literature. JAMA 1994;271:698–702.

46. Centers for Disease Control and Prevention. Screening for tuberculosis and tuberculosis infection in high-risk populations: recommendations of the Advisory Committee for Elimination of Tuberculosis. MMWR 1995;44(RR-11):19–34.

46a. Canadian Task Force on the Periodic Health Examination. Canadian guide to clinical preventive health care. Ottawa: Canada Communication Group, 1994:754–765.

47. American Academy of Pediatrics, Committee on Infectious Diseases. Screening for tuberculosis in infants and children. Pediatrics 1994;93:131–134.

48. Green M, ed. Bright Futures: guidelines for health supervision of infants, children and adolescents. Arlington, VA: National Center for Education in Maternal and Child Health, 1994.

49. American Medical Association. AMA guidelines for adolescent preventive services (GAPS): recommendations and rationale. Chicago: American Medical Association, 1994.
50. Centers for Disease Control and Prevention. Guidelines for preventing the transmission of Mycobacterium tuberculosis in health-care facilities, 1994. MMWR 1994;43(RR-13):1–132.
51. American Thoracic Society. Control of tuberculosis in the United States. Am Rev Respir Dis 1992;146:1623–1633.
52. American Thoracic Society. Treatment of tuberculosis and tuberculosis infection in adults and children. Am J Respir Crit Care Med 1994;149:1359–1374.
53. Centers for Disease Control. Purified protein derivative (PPD)-tuberculin anergy and HIV infection: guidelines for anergy testing and management of anergic persons at risk of tuberculosis. MMWR 1991;40(RR-5):1–5.
54. Centers for Disease Control and Prevention. USPHS/IDSA guidelines for the prevention of opportunistic infections in persons with human immunodeficiency virus: a summary. MMWR 1995;44(RR-8):1–34.
55. American Academy of Family Physicians. Age charts for periodic health examination. Kansas City, MO: American Academy of Family Physicians, 1994. (Reprint no. 510.)

26. Screening for Syphilis

RECOMMENDATION

Routine serologic screening for syphilis is recommended for all pregnant women and for persons at increased risk of infection (see *Clinical Intervention*). See Chapter 62 for recommendations on counseling to prevent sexually transmitted diseases.

Burden of Suffering

Syphilis is caused by infection with the bacterium *Treponema pallidum* which can be transmitted congenitally or by sexual contact. In 1994, 20,627 cases of primary and secondary syphilis were reported in the United States.[1] Primary syphilis produces ulcers of the genitalia, pharynx, or rectum, and secondary syphilis is characterized by contagious skin lesions, lymphadenopathy, and condylomata lata.[2] Systemic spread, including invasion of the central nervous system, can occur early in infection and may be symptomatic during early or late stages of syphilis. The disease then evolves into a latent phase in which syphilis is clinically inapparent. If left untreated, as many as one third of patients progress to have potentially severe late gummatous, cardiovascular, and neurologic complications.[3] Cardiovascular syphilis produces aortic disease (insufficiency, aneurysms, aortitis), and neurosyphilis can result in meningitis, peripheral neuropathy (e.g., tabes dorsalis), meningovascular brain lesions, and psychiatric illness. Persons with tertiary syphilis may have decreased life expectancy, and they often experience significant disability and diminished productivity as a result of their symptoms. Long-term hospitalization is often necessary for patients with severe neurologic deficits or psychiatric illness. Syphilis has been associated epidemiologically with acquisition and transmission of infection with human immunodeficiency virus (HIV).[4,5]

The incidence of syphilis has decreased by 50% since 1990, but it is still high and now approximates 1970 rates.[1] A growing proportion of cases is being reported among commercial sex workers and persons who use illicit drugs, especially those using crack cocaine and those who exchange sex for drugs.[6,7] There are pronounced geographic differences in the incidence of syphilis in different communities. In recent data, nearly all counties with a high incidence of reported syphilis cases (more than 10/100,000 persons) were in large metropolitan areas or in southern states; nearly two thirds of all counties in the U.S. reported no cases of primary or secondary syphilis in the most recent year.[1] The incidence of reported infections among Hispanics and blacks is 5–60 times higher than that in non-Hispanic whites.[1] Individual communities may experience substantial fluctuations in incidence rates independent of national trends.

The incidence of congenital syphilis had increased sharply in the last 15 years, but it has fallen since 1991.[1] Congenital syphilis results in fetal or perinatal death in 40% of affected pregnancies, as well as in an increased risk of medical complications in surviving newborns.[8] The incidence of congenital syphilis increased steadily in the United States from 1978 to 1991,[9] reaching 108 cases per 100,000 live births in 1991.[1] (The reporting definition changed in 1989 to reflect both confirmed cases and infants at high risk of infection.) The rate dropped from 1991 to 1994, to 56 cases per 100,000 live births.[1]

Accuracy of Screening Tests

Serologic tests are currently the mainstay for syphilis diagnosis and management. Nontreponemal tests are used to screen patients for the presence of nonspecific reagin antibodies that appear and rise in titer following infection. Although VDRL (Venereal Disease Research Laboratory) and RPR (rapid plasma reagin) are the most commonly used nontreponemal tests, others are available. The sensitivity of nontreponemal tests varies with the levels of antibodies present during the stages of disease. In early primary syphilis, when antibody levels may be too low to detect, results may be nonreactive, and the sensitivity of nontreponemal tests is 62–76%.[10] Antibody levels rise as disease progresses; titers usually peak during secondary syphilis, when the sensitivity of nontreponemal tests approaches 100%. In late syphilis, titers decline, and previously reactive results revert to nonreactive in 25% of patients; in untreated late syphilis, test sensitivity averages only 70%.[10] Nontreponemal test titers decline or revert to normal after successful treatment.

Nontreponemal tests can produce sustained or transient false-positive reactions due to preexisting conditions (e.g., collagen vascular diseases, injection drug use, advanced malignancy, pregnancy) or infections (e.g., malaria, tuberculosis, viral and rickettsial diseases), or due to laboratory-associated errors.[10–12] The specificity of nontreponemal tests is 75–85% in persons with preexisting diseases or conditions, and it approaches 100% in persons without them.[10,13] Because nontreponemal serodiagnostic tests may be falsely positive, all reactive results in asymptomatic patients should be confirmed with a more specific treponemal test such as fluorescent treponemal antibody absorption (FTA-ABS), which has a sensitivity of 84% in primary syphilis and almost 100% for other stages, and a specificity of 96%.[14] Two less expensive and easier to perform confirmatory tests are the

MHA-TP (microhemagglutination assay for antibodies to *Treponema pallidum*) and HATTS (hemagglutination treponemal test for syphilis).[13]

Treponemal tests should not be used as initial screening tests in asymptomatic patients, as they are considerably more expensive and remain reactive in patients with previous, treated infection. Used in concert with nontreponemal tests, however, the positive predictive value of treponemal tests is high, and reactive results are likely to represent true infection with syphilis. Treponemal tests may also be useful in patients with suspected late syphilis and nonreactive nontreponemal tests, since declining antibody titers may produce false-negative nontreponemal tests. All test results should be evaluated in concert with a clinical diagnosis and history.

Infection with HIV may alter the clinical presentation and performance of serologic tests for syphilis. Co-infection with HIV and syphilis does not generally impair the sensitivity of syphilis testing, although there are sporadic reports of absent or delayed response to nontreponemal tests. [14,15] In contrast, HIV infection may reduce the specificity of syphilis testing; several studies have noted increased reactivity to nontreponemal tests among HIV-infected persons without syphilis.[15,16] Persistence of elevated nontreponemal titers after treatment for syphilis has also been reported in some HIV-infected persons, making it difficult to confirm the adequacy of treatment.[17,18] At the same time, treponema-specific tests may become nonreactive after treatment of syphilis in HIV-infected persons, limiting the ability to document past infection.[14,19,20]

Effectiveness of Early Detection

Early detection of syphilis in asymptomatic persons permits the initiation of antibiotic therapy to eradicate the infection, thereby preventing both clinical disease and transmission to sexual contacts. Antibiotic therapy with penicillin G benzathine (or tetracycline hydrochloride if neurosyphilis has been excluded) has been shown to be highly effective in eliminating *T. pallidum*. Early detection and penicillin treatment during pregnancy have the added benefit of reducing the risk to the fetus of acquiring congenital syphilis.[9] Prenatal antibiotic therapy is effective in preventing congenital syphilis when the mother is treated with penicillin early in pregnancy (desensitization for penicillin allergy may be required).[21] Failures can occur, however, if women are treated with erythromycin, an antibiotic with limited efficacy in preventing congenital syphilis, or if antibiotic therapy is not started until the third trimester.[21]

Recommendations of Other Groups

The American College of Obstetricians and Gynecologists and the American Academy of Pediatrics recommend routine prenatal screening for syphilis at the first prenatal visit, after exposure to an infected partner, and in the third trimester for patients at high risk.[22,23] In the event of incomplete or equivocal data on maternal serology or treatment, neonatal testing is recommended. The American Academy of Family Physicians[24] and the American College of Physicians[25] recommend serologic screening for syphilis in high-risk adults (prostitutes, persons who engage in sex with multiple partners in areas in which syphilis is prevalent, contacts of persons with active syphilis). The American Academy of Family Physicians,[24] American Academy of Pediatrics,[22,26] American Medical Association,[27] and Bright Futures[28] all recommend routine syphilis screening for sexually active adolescents at increased risk. The Centers for Disease Control and Prevention recommends obtaining serology for syphilis from all women at the first prenatal visit.[21] In communities and populations with high syphilis prevalence or for patients at high risk, serologic testing should be repeated during the third trimester and again at delivery.[21] The Canadian Task Force on the Periodic Health Examination recommends testing for syphilis in pregnant women and sexually active persons in high-risk groups.[29]

Discussion

Since the annual incidence of syphilis is less than 10 cases per 100,000 persons,[1] routine screening of the general population is likely to have low yield. Populations at increased risk due to high-risk sexual activities include commercial sex workers, persons who exchange sex for drugs, persons with other sexually transmitted diseases (STDs) including HIV, and contacts of persons with active syphilis. The value of screening for asymptomatic infection in other persons will depend on both individual risk factors (e.g., the number and nature of sex partners) and on local epidemiology. Experience with HIV and other STDs demonstrates that sexual history is not sufficiently sensitive to identify infected persons in high-risk communities; some persons may not report risk factors, and even monogamous patients may be at risk from an infected partner. Conversely, in communities where syphilis is uncommon, screening asymptomatic persons is likely to detect few cases of syphilis, even when patients have high-risk behaviors.

Routine screening in both high- and low-risk areas is justified among pregnant women, because of the severe neonatal morbidity and mortality associated with congenital syphilis, as well as its potential preventability. Determination of sexual risk factors is often insensitive in pregnant women, who may be reluctant to admit some behaviors or unaware of risk factors in their partners.[10] Several studies have demonstrated that prenatal screening for syphilis is cost-effective, even when the prevalence of the disease among pregnant women is as low as 0.005%.[30,31] Currently, congenital syphilis occurs in 0.05% of all live births.[1]

CLINICAL INTERVENTION

Routine serologic testing for syphilis is recommended for all pregnant women and for persons at increased risk for infection, including commercial sex workers, persons who exchange sex for money or drugs, persons with other STDs (including HIV), and sexual contacts of persons with active syphilis ("A" recommendation). The local incidence of syphilis in the community and the number of sex partners reported by an individual should also be considered in identifying persons at high risk of infection. The optimal frequency for such testing has not been determined and is left to clinical discretion.

All pregnant women should be tested at their first prenatal visit. For women at high risk of acquiring syphilis during pregnancy (e.g., women in the high-risk groups listed above), repeat serologic testing is recommended in the third trimester and at delivery. Follow-up serologic tests should be obtained to document decline in titers after treatment. They should be performed using the same test initially used to document infection (e.g., VDRL or RPR) to ensure comparability.

See Chapter 62 for recommendations on counseling to prevent sexually transmitted diseases.

The draft update of this chapter was prepared for the U.S. Preventive Services Task Force by James G. Kahn, MD, MPH, and A. Eugene Washington, MD, MSc.

REFERENCES

1. Division of STD/HIV Prevention. Sexually Transmitted Disease Surveillance, 1994. U.S. Department of Health and Human Services, Public Health Service. Atlanta: Centers for Disease Control and Prevention, 1995.
2. Hook EW, Marra CM. Acquired syphilis in adults. N Engl J Med 1992;326:1060–1069.
3. Clark EG, Danbolt N. The Oslo study of the natural course of untreated syphilis: an epidemiologic investigation based on a restudy of the Boeck-Bruusgaard material. Med Clin North Am 1964;48:613–623.
4. Stamm WE, Handsfield HH, Rompalo AM, et al. The association between genital ulcer disease and acquisition of HIV infection in homosexual men. JAMA 1988;260:1429–1433.
5. Wasserheit JN. Epidemiological synergy: Interrelationships between human immunodeficiency virus infection and other sexually transmitted diseases. Sex Transm Dis 1992;19:61–77.
6. Centers for Disease Control. Relationship of syphilis to drug use and prostitution—Connecticut and Philadelphia, Pennsylvania. MMWR 1988;37:755–758, 764.
7. Marx R, Aral SG, Rolfs RT, Sterk CE, Kahn JG. Crack, sex and STD. Sex Transm Dis 1991;18:92–101.
8. Marx R, Aral SG, Rolfs RT, Sterk CE, Kahn JG. Guidelines for the prevention and control of congenital syphilis. MMWR 1988;(Suppl 1):37.
9. Marx R, Aral SG, Rolfs RT, Sterk CE, Kahn JG. Congenital syphilis, United States, 1983–1985. MMWR 1986;35: 625–628.
10. Hart G. Syphilis tests in diagnostic and therapeutic decision making. Ann Intern Med 1986;104: 368–376.
11. Hart G. Screening to control infectious diseases. Rev Infect Dis 1980;2:701–712.
12. Feder HM, Manthous C. The asymptomatic patient with a positive VDRL test. Am Fam Phys 1988;37: 185–190.
13. Wentworth BB, Thompson MA, Peter CR, et al. Comparison of a hemagglutination treponemal test for syphilis (HATTS) with other serologic methods for the diagnosis of syphilis. Sex Transm Dis 1978;5: 103–111.

14. Larsen SA, Kraus SJ, Whittington WL. Diagnostic tests. In: Larsen SA, Hunter EF, Kraus SJ, eds. A manual of tests for syphilis. Washington, DC: American Public Health Association, 1990.
15. Young H. Syphilis: new diagnostic directions [editorial review]. Int J STD AIDS 1992;3:391–413.
16. Rompalo AM, Cannon RO, Quinn TC, Hook EW. Association of biologic false-positive reactions for syphilis with human immunodeficiency virus infection. J Infect Dis 1992;165:1124–1126.
17. Telzak EF, Greenberg MS, Harrison J, Stoneburner RL, Schultz S. Syphilis treatment response in HIV-infected individuals. AIDS 1991;5:591–595.
18. Chirgwin K, Augenbraun MH, Bazile JB, Marcel A. Serologic response to treatment of late syphilis in HIV infected patients: correlation with CD4 count. International Conference on AIDS. July 19–24, 1992, vol 8, p B148 [abstr. POB 3370].
19. Notenboom R, MacFadden DK. Reliability of syphilis tests in patients with HIV. International Conference on AIDS. July 19–24, 1992, vol 8, p B94 [abstr. POB 3044].
20. Johnson PD, Graves SR, Stewart L, Warren R, Dwyer B, Lucas CR. Specific syphilis serological tests may become negative in HIV infection. AIDS 1991;5:419–423.
21. Centers for Disease Control and Prevention. Sexually transmitted diseases treatment guidelines. MMWR 1993; 42(RR-14):1–102.
22. American Academy of Pediatrics and American College of Obstetricians and Gynecologists. Guidelines for perinatal care. 3rd ed. Washington, DC: AAP and ACOG, 1992:133–135.
23. American Academy of Pediatrics. 1994 Red Book: report of the Committee on Infectious Diseases. 23rd ed. Elk Grove Village, IL: American Academy of Pediatrics, 1994:445–455.
24. American Academy of Family Physicians. Age charts for periodic health examination. Kansas City, MO: American Academy of Family Physicians, 1994. (Reprint no. 510.)
25. Hart G. Syphilis tests in diagnostic and therapeutic decision making. In: Sox HC Jr, ed. Common diagnostic tests: use and interpretation. 2nd ed. Philadelphia: Lea & Febiger, 1986.
26. American Academy of Pediatrics. Role of the pediatrician in management of sexually transmitted diseases in children and adolescents. Pediatrics 1987;79:454–456.
27. American Medical Association. Guidelines for adolescent preventive services (GAPS): recommendations and rationale. Chicago: American Medical Association, 1994:xxxv.
28. Green M, ed. Bright Futures: guidelines for health supervision of infants, children, and adolescents. Arlington, VA: National Center for Education in Maternal and Child Health, 1994.
29. Canadian Task Force on the Periodic Health Examination. Canadian guide to clinical preventive health care. Ottawa: Canada Communication Group, 1994:982.
30. Stray-Pedersen B. Economic evaluation of maternal screening to prevent congenital syphilis. Sex Transm Dis 1983;10:167–172.
31. Williams K. Screening for syphilis in pregnancy: an assessment of the costs and benefits. Commun Med 1985;7:37–42.

27. Screening for Gonorrhea—
Including Ocular Prophylaxis in Newborns

RECOMMENDATION

Routine screening for Neisseria gonorrhoeae is recommended for asymptomatic women at high risk of infection (see *Clinical Intervention*). All high-risk women should be screened during pregnancy. There is insufficient evidence to recommend for or against screening all pregnant women or screening asymptomatic men. Recommendations to screen selected high-risk young men may be made on other grounds (see *Clinical Intervention*). Routine screening is not recommended for the general adult population. Ocular antibiotic prophylaxis of all newborn infants is recommended to prevent gonococcal ophthalmia neonatorum.

Burden of Suffering

Nearly 420,000 *N. gonorrhoeae* infections were reported in the U.S. in 1994;[1] the actual number of new infections is estimated to be closer to 800,000 per year, due to incomplete reporting.[2] Between 10% and 20% of untreated gonococcal infections in women lead to pelvic inflammatory disease (PID), which may require hospitalization or surgery.[3] PID is an important cause of chronic pelvic pain, ectopic pregnancy, and infertility; approximately one out of four women with a prior history of PID is unable to conceive.[4] Pregnant women with gonococcal infections are at increased risk for obstetric complications (e.g., stillbirth, low birth weight).[5,6] Infected women can give birth to infants with gonococcal conjunctivitis (ophthalmia neonatorum), a condition that often produces blindness if not treated.[5] Gonococcal infections produce urethritis, epididymitis, and proctitis in men, but few long-term complications. Disseminated gonococcal infection can cause tenosynovitis, septic arthritis, endocarditis, and meningitis, especially in persons with complement disorders.

The overall incidence of gonorrhea has steadily declined in the U.S. since 1975,[1,7] but rates of infection have remained very high in some groups of young men and women.[8] Over 60% of gonococcal infections occur in persons under age 25;[7] adolescents (ages 15–19) have rates of infection comparable to young adults (ages 20–24). A number of demographic and behavioral characteristics are associated with higher reported rates of gonorrhea: being unmarried, urban residence, low socioeconomic status, early sexual activity, multiple sex contacts, and a prior history of gonorrhea.[10,11] Rates of gonorrhea are highest in poor, minority communities in large cities and in the rural Southeast. Black male and female adolescents have a 10–20-fold higher rate of infection than their Hispanic or white counterparts.[7,8,11] Geographic variation is substantial, with the highest rates of infection in the Southeastern states.[1,7] Since most data come from public health clinics, the demographics of reported disease may not be entirely representative of the true distribution of infection.

Up to 80% of women infected with gonorrhea are asymptomatic,[12] and asymptomatic men and women comprise an important reservoir for new infection. Nearly half of all male partners of infected women, and over three quarters of female partners of infected men, are infected.[13,14] While the majority of infected men eventually develop symptoms, initial asymptomatic periods may last up to 45 days.[15] The prevalence of asymptomatic gonorrhea in high-risk communities is generally higher in women (4–5%)[16,17] than in men (1.5–2.5%).[15,18,19] Asymptomatic gonorrhea was uncommon, however, among women at a university health clinic (0.4%),[17] private practice patients in Montreal (0.4%),[20] and non-Medicaid patients in Boston (<1%).[21] Among asymptomatic male adolescents screened at urban teen clinics or detention centers, up to 5% are infected with *N. gonorrhoeae*.[22–25]

The majority of pharyngeal infections are asymptomatic, but infection may be transmitted to genital sites through oral sex[26] or progress to disseminated gonococcal infection.[27] Pharyngeal gonorrhea, however, usually occurs in association with anogenital infection, and it responds to usual treatment regimens for anogenital gonorrhea (i.e., broad-spectrum cephalosporins and fluoroquinolones).[9] Persons with gonorrhea may be infected with other sexually transmitted diseases (chlamydia, syphilis, HIV); up to 50% of persons with gonorrhea have a coexistent chlamydial infection.[12]

The frequency of antibiotic-resistant *N. gonorrhoeae* has steadily increased in the U.S. Recent surveillance data estimate that 32% of gonorrhea isolates nationwide are resistant to penicillin or tetracycline.[28] These organisms are currently sensitive to broad-spectrum cephalosporins such as ceftriaxone and several other antibiotics, but the emergence of new resistance remains a concern.[9]

Accuracy of Screening Tests

The most sensitive and specific test for detecting gonococcal infection in asymptomatic persons is direct culture from sites of exposure (urethra, endocervix, throat, rectum). Under quality-controlled conditions, the sensitivity of culture is high for both male and female anogenital gonorrhea, and for pharyngeal gonococcal infections. In women, a single endocervical culture is estimated to have a sensitivity of 80–95%.[29,30] Sensitivity of cultures may be limited by inadequate clinical specimens, improper storage, transport or processing, and inhibition of growth by antibiotics in selective culture mediums.[31]

Microscopic examination of Gram-stained urethral or cervical specimens can detect infection with *N. gonorrhoeae*. The sensitivity of Gram-stained urethral specimens is higher in symptomatic men (90–95%) than in asymptomatic men (70%).[31] The Gram stain is less sensitive for cervical infections in women (30–65%), and it is not useful for diagnosing pharyngeal or rectal infections. The specificity of stained smears is high in men (97–99%), but lower in women (90–97%), due to presence of vaginal flora.[31]

In clinical settings where handling and storage of culture medium is difficult, other methods of testing have become increasingly popular. DNA probes and enzyme immunoassays (EIA) are currently the most widely used nonculture diagnostic tests. Compared to culture, the sensitivity, specificity, and positive predictive value (PPV) of EIA are generally high using urethral specimens from symptomatic men (>95%).[32,33] Accuracy of EIA is significantly lower in endocervical specimens, however: sensitivity 60–100%, specificity 70–98%, and PPV 78–85%.[32–35] Among patients in sexually transmitted disease (STD) clinics (prevalence of gonorrhea 9–10%), a DNA probe had a very high sensitivity and specificity (97–99%) and high PPV (>90%) and was more sensitive than a single culture.[36,37] The accuracy of nonculture tests has not been adequately studied in an asymptomatic, primary care population, however. Among asymptomatic persons, in whom the prevalence of gonorrhea is often very low, a substantial proportion of positive EIA or DNA probe results may be false positives.[32,34] Serology is neither sufficiently sensitive nor specific for use in screening. None of the nonculture tests provides information on antibiotic susceptibility.

Screening for gonorrhea in asymptomatic men has been limited by the discomfort and inconvenience of obtaining urethral specimens.[24] EIA using urine specimens produces accurate results in symptomatic men,[38] but when used to screen a low-prevalence population, the majority of positive EIA results have been false positives.[39] Urine dipstick for leukocyte esterase (LE) is an inexpensive, rapid, and noninvasive test for urethritis in men. Among asymptomatic high-risk young men (ages 15–25, prevalence of infection 3%), urinary LE had a sensitivity of 46–60% and a specificity of 93–96% for gonorrhea.[24,25] The PPV of LE in an asymptomatic population is low (30–43%), although some false-positive results may be due to other infections that require treatment (e.g., chlamydia).

Information from the sexual history and clinical examination have been used to improve screening strategies. In one study of 1,441 women in Boston undergoing routine pelvic examinations, five factors were independently associated with gonococcal infection: partners with gonorrhea or urethral discharge, endocervical bleeding induced by swab, age at first intercourse less than 16, payment by Medicaid (a proxy measure for low socioeconomic status), and low abdominal or pelvic pain.[21] The prevalence of infection among women with one or more risk factors was 2.5%, compared to 0.2% for women with no risk factors. In a second study, young age (under 20), vaginal discharge, or a sex partner suspected of having gonorrhea identified all infected women in a low-income, urban population (prevalence of gonorrhea 3%).[17]

Effectiveness of Early Detection

Early detection and treatment of gonococcal infection in asymptomatic persons offers the potential benefits of preventing future complications of infection, reducing transmission to uninfected partners, and identifying sexual contacts who are likely to be infected. Due to ethical considerations that preclude placebo-controlled trials of treatment, the benefits of early detection are based largely on indirect evidence: the effectiveness of antibiotic treatment and the high morbidity of untreated gonorrhea. The decline in the reported incidence of gonorrhea over the last two decades and decline in hospitalizations for PID may also indicate a benefit of current screening strategies, but other factors (increased use of condoms) have presumably had an impact as well.[7] Due to high rates of reinfection among those at greatest risk, screening may be of little benefit to some individuals unless it is accompanied by measures to prevent future infections. Early detection and treatment of gonorrhea during pregnancy has the potential to decrease morbidity from the obstetric complications of gonococcal infections, although this benefit has never been tested in a controlled trial.

Ocular Prophylaxis of Newborn Infants

Between 30% and 50% of infants exposed to gonococci will develop ophthalmia in the absence of treatment.[40] Gonococcal ophthalmia can cause severe conjunctivitis and lead to corneal scarring, abscess, eye perforation, and permanent blindness.[41] Blindness due to ophthalmia neonatorum declined dramatically with the institution of widespread prophylaxis of infants with silver nitrate. Studies of ocular prophylaxis in developing countries, using historical controls, report reductions of 80–90% in the transmission of gonococcal ophthalmia neonatorum with prophylaxis with silver nitrate, tetracycline or erythromycin.[42,43] In a U.S. study, failure rates were similar after prophylaxis with silver nitrate, erythromycin, or tetracycline (0.03–0.1%).[44] A recent controlled trial in Kenya reported that povidone-iodine, erythromycin, and silver nitrate were each effective in preventing conjunctivitis due to *N. gonorrhoeae*.[45] Tetracycline-resistant strains of gonorrhea have been reported in the U.S. and other countries.[45] The optimal prophylactic agent against penicillinase-producing strains of *N. gonorrhoeae* (PPNG) has not been determined.

Recommendations of Other Groups

The Canadian Task Force on the Periodic Health Examination advises against routine screening for gonorrhea in the general population but recommends screening of high-risk patients: individuals under 30 years, particularly adolescents, with at least two sex partners in the previous year; prostitutes; sexual contacts of individuals known to have an STD; and persons under age 16 years at first intercourse.[46] The Centers for Disease Control and Prevention (CDC) recommends screening asymptomatic women in the following priority groups: all pregnant women, sexually active adolescents, and women with multiple sex partners.[9,12] The American Academy of Family Physicians recommends screening prostitutes, persons with multiple sex partners or whose sex partner has multiple sex contacts, sexual contacts of persons with culture-proven gonorrhea, or persons with a history of repeated episodes of gonorrhea.[47] These recommendations are under review. Bright Futures,[48] the American Medical Association Guidelines for Adolescent Preventive Services (GAPS),[49] and the American Academy of Pediatrics (AAP)[50] recommend annual screening of sexually active adolescents. The AAP recommends dipstick urinalysis for leukocytes in all adolescents.[51] An expert panel convened in 1994 by the Institute of Medicine, National Academy of Sciences, is developing recommendations for public health strategies to control STDs, including gonorrhea.

The American College of Obstetricians and Gynecologists (ACOG) recommends obtaining endocervical cultures in pregnant women during their first prenatal visit only if they are in one of the high-risk categories for gonorrhea.[10] ACOG and CDC recommend repeating culture late in the third trimester for high-risk women.[10,12] ACOG recommends that all cases of gonorrhea should be diagnosed or confirmed by culture to facilitate antimicrobial susceptibility testing.[10] The American Academy of Pediatrics,[52] American Academy of Family Physicians,[47] and CDC[2] recommend administering ointment or drops containing tetracycline, erythromycin, or 1% silver nitrate solution to the eyes of all infants shortly after birth (within 1 hour). In the absence of universal prenatal screening for gonorrhea, the Canadian Task Force also recommends universal ocular prophylaxis with any of these antibiotic agents.[46]

Discussion

Gonorrhea remains an important public health problem and a major source of morbidity for women. Although definitive proof (e.g., controlled trials) that screening reduces future morbidity is not available, selective screening of high-risk women can be justified by the substantial prevalence of asymptomatic infection, the availability of accurate screening tests and effective treatments, and the high morbidity of untreated gonorrhea in women. Early identification and treatment of asymptomatic individuals is also likely to reduce transmission of gonorrhea. The benefits of early detection may be reduced by the high likelihood of reinfection unless effective measures are taken to identify and treat sex partners.

Performing routine cultures for gonorrhea on all sexually active adults would be inefficient due to the low prevalence of infection in the general population and the wide variation in the rates of gonorrhea in different communities. Clinicians must base their decision to screen for gonorrhea on both individual risk factors and the local epidemiology of disease, realizing that sexual history is often an unreliable indicator of actual risk of infection. Therefore, routine screening of all sexually active young women may be more effective in communities where gonorrhea is prevalent, while more selective screening is appropriate when the rate of infection is known to be low.

In men, the prevalence of asymptomatic infection and the morbidity from gonorrhea is much lower than in women. Asymptomatic men, however, represent an important reservoir for transmitting infection, and opportunities to identify and treat infected men are often limited. Screening asymptomatic men with currently available urine tests may generate a large proportion of false-positive results. As more reliable, noninvasive methods for testing men become available (e.g., polymerase or ligase chain reaction assays of urine), screening young men may help reduce the incidence of gonorrhea in high-risk communities. The effectiveness of such a strategy, however, deserves to be tested in a prospective study.

The primary rationale for screening all pregnant women has been the prevention of ophthalmia neonatorum. Due to the low prevalence of gonorrhea in average-risk pregnant women, and the efficacy of universal ocular prophylaxis with antibiotic ointment, the benefits of screening for gonorrhea in all pregnant women are uncertain. Screening pregnant women at high risk for gonorrhea, however, may also help prevent other complications associated with gonococcal infection during pregnancy.

CLINICAL INTERVENTION

Routine screening for gonorrhea is recommended for asymptomatic women at high risk of infection ("B" recommendation). High-risk groups include commercial sex workers (prostitutes), persons with a history of re-peated episodes of gonorrhea, and young women (under age 25) with two or more sex partners in the last year. Actual risk, however, will depend on the local epidemiology of disease. Clinicians may wish to consult local health authorities for guidance in identifying high-risk populations in their community. In communities with high prevalence of gonorrhea, broader screening of sexually active young women may be warranted. Clinicians should remain alert for findings suggestive of cervical infection (e.g., mu-copurulent discharge, cervical erythema or friability) during routine pelvic examinations.

Screening is recommended at the first prenatal visit for pregnant women who fall into one of the high-risk categories ("B" recommenda-tion). An additional test in the third trimester is recommended for those at continued risk of acquiring gonorrhea. There is insufficient evidence to recommend for or against universal screening of pregnant women ("C" recommendation). Erythromycin 0.5% ophthalmic ointment, tetracycline 1% ophthalmic ointment, or 1% silver nitrate solution should be applied topically to the eyes of all newborns as soon as possible after birth and no later than 1 hour after birth ("A" recommendation).

There is insufficient evidence to recommend for or against screening high-risk men for gonorrhea ("C" recommendation). In selected clinical settings where asymptomatic infection is highly prevalent in men (e.g., adolescent clinics serving high-risk populations), screening sexually active young men may be recommended on other grounds, including the poten-tial benefits of early treatment for preventing transmission to uninfected sex partners. Screening men with urine LE dipstick is convenient and in-expensive, but requires confirmation of positive results. Routine screen-ing of men or women is not recommended in the general population of low-risk adults ("D" recommendation). The optimal frequency of screen-ing has not been determined and is left to clinical discretion.

Culture of endocervical specimens is the preferred method for screen-ing asymptomatic women. When EIA or DNA probe tests are used for ini-tial screening, verification of positive results may be necessary, depending on the underlying risk in the patient and potential adverse consequences of a false-positive result. Treatment should employ regimens effective against penicillin- and tetracycline-resistant organisms and should include treatment for co-infection with chlamydia and treatment of sex partners.[9] All sexually active individuals should be counseled about effective means of preventing STDs (see Chapter 62). Clinicians should follow local gonorrhea disease-reporting requirements.

The draft update of this chapter was prepared for the U.S. Preventive Services Task Force by Mark S. Smolinski, MD, MPH, and David Atkins, MD, MPH, based in part on materials prepared for the Canadian Task Force on the Periodic Health Examination by Brenda Beagan, MSc, Elaine E. L. Wang, MD, CM, FRCPC, and Richard B. Goldbloom, MD, FRCPC.

REFERENCES

1. Centers for Disease Control and Prevention. Summary of notifiable diseases, United States, 1994. MMWR 1995; 43(53):1–80.
2. Centers for Disease Control and Prevention, Division of STD/HIV Prevention. 1993 annual report. Atlanta: Centers for Disease Control and Prevention, 1993.
3. Hook EW III, Handsfield HH. Gonococcal infections in the adult. In: Holmes KK, Mardh P-A, Sparling PF, Wiesner PJ, eds. Sexually transmitted diseases. 2nd ed. New York: McGraw-Hill, 1990:149–165.
4. Westrom L. Effect of acute pelvic inflammatory disease on fertility. Am J Obstet Gynecol 1975;121:707–713.
5. Brunham RC, Holmes KK, Embree JE. Sexually transmitted diseases in pregnancy. In: Holmes KK, Mardh P-A, Sparling PF, Wiesner PJ, eds. Sexually transmitted diseases. 2nd ed. New York: McGraw-Hill, 1990:771–801.
6. Elliot B, Brunham RC, Laga M, et al. Maternal gonococcal infection as a preventable risk factor for low birth weight. J Infect Dis 1990;161:531–536.
7. Centers for Disease Control and Prevention, Division of STD/HIV Prevention. Sexually transmitted disease surveillance, 1994. Atlanta: Centers for Disease Control and Prevention, 1995.
8. Webster LA, Berman SM, Greenspan JR. Surveillance for gonorrhea and primary and secondary syphilis among adolescents, United States—1981–1991. In: CDC Surveillance Summaries, August 13, 1993. MMWR 1993;42(SS-3):1–11.
9. Centers for Disease Control and Prevention. 1993 sexually transmitted diseases treatment guidelines. MMWR 1993;42(RR-14):56–67.
10. American College of Obstetricians and Gynecologists. Gonorrhea and chlamydial infections. ACOG Technical Bulletin no. 190. Washington, DC: American College of Obstetricians and Gynecologists, 1994.
11. Rice RJ, Roberts PL, Handsfield HH, Holmes KK. Sociodemographic distribution of gonorrhea incidence: implications for prevention and behavioral research. Am J Public Health 1991;81:1252–1258.
12. Centers for Disease Control. Sexually transmitted diseases. Clinical practice guidelines. Atlanta: Centers for Disease Control, 1991.
13. Potterat JJ, Dukes RL, Rothenberg RB. Disease transmission by heterosexual men with gonorrhea: an empirical estimate. Sex Transm Dis 1987;14:107–110.
14. Kamwendo F, Johansson E, Moi H, et al. Gonorrhea, genital chlamydia infection, and nonspecific urethritis in male partners of women hospitalized and treated for acute pelvic inflammatory disease. Sex Transm Dis 1993;20:143–146.
15. Handsfield HH, Lipman TO, Harnish JP, et al. Asymptomatic gonorrhea in men. N Engl J Med 1974;290:117–123.
16. Allard R, Robert J, Turgeon P, Lepage Y. Predictors of asymptomatic gonorrhea among patients seen by private practitioners. Can Med Assoc J 1985;133:1135–1139, 1146.
17. Rosenthal GE, Mettler G, Pare S, et al. A new diagnostic index for predicting cervical infection with either *Chlamydia trachomatis* or *Neisseria gonorrhoeae.* J Gen Intern Med 1990;5:319–326.
18. Alexander-Rodriquez T, Vermund SH. Gonorrhea and syphilis in incarcerated urban adolescents: prevalence and physical signs. Pediatrics 1987;80:561–564.
19. McNagny SE, Parker RM, Zenilman JM, Lewis JS. Urinary leukocyte esterase test: a screening method

for the detection of asymptomatic chlamydial and gonococcal infections in men. J Infect Dis 1992;165: 573–576.

20. Vincelette J, Baril JG, Allard R. Predictors of chlamydial infection and gonorrhea among patients seen by private practitioners. Can Med Assoc J 1991;144:713–721.

21. Phillips RS, Hanff PA, Wertheimer A, Aronson MD. Gonorrhea in women seen for routine gynecologic care: criteria for testing. Am J Med 1988;85:177–182.

22. Demetriou E, Sackett R, Welch DF, et al. Evaluation of an enzyme immunoassay for detection of *Neisseria gonorrhoeae* in an adolescent population. JAMA 1984;252:247–250.

23. O'Brien SF, Bell TA, Farrow JA. Use of a leukocyte esterase dipstick to detect *Chlamydia trachomatis* and *Neisseria gonorrhoeae* urethritis in asymptomatic adolescent male detainees. Am J Public Health 1988;78:1583–1584.

24. Shafer MA, Schachter J, Moscicki AB, et al. Urinary leukocyte esterase screening test for asymptomatic chlamydial and gonococcal infections in males. JAMA 1989;262:2562–2565.

25. Johnson J, Neas B, Parker DE, et al. Screening for urethral infection in adolescent and young adult males. J Adolesc Health 1993;14:356–361.

26. Hutt DM, Judson FN. Epidemiology and treatment of oropharyngeal gonorrhea. Ann Intern Med 1986;104:655–658.

27. Roochvarg LB, Lovchik JC. Screening for pharyngeal gonorrhea in adolescents. J Adolesc Health 1991; 12:269–272.

28. Gorwitz RJ, Nakashima AK, Moran JS. Sentinel surveillance for antimicrobial resistance in Neisseria gonorrhoeae—United States, 1988–1991. In: CDC surveillance summaries, August 13, 1993. MMWR 1993;42:29–39.

29. Goh BT, Varia KB, Ayliffe PF, Lim FKS. Diagnosis of gonorrhea by gram-stained smears and cultures in men and women: role of the urethral smear. Sex Transm Dis 1985;12:135–139.

30. Romanowski B, Harris JRW, Wood H, Kessock-Philip S: Improved diagnosis of gonorrhea in women. Sex Transm Dis 1986;13:93–96.

31. Centers for Disease Control. Guide for the diagnosis of gonorrhea using culture and gram-stained smear. Atlanta: Centers for Disease Control, 1991.

32. Stamm WE, Cole B, Fennell C, et al. Antigen detection for the diagnosis of gonorrhea. J Clin Microbiol 1984; 19:399–403.

33. D'Angelo L, Mohla C, Sneed J, Woodward K. Diagnosing gonorrhea: a comparison of rapid and standard techniques. J Adolesc Health Care 1987;8:344–348.

34. Lieberman RW, Wheelock JB. The diagnosis of gonorrhea in a low-prevalence female population: enzyme immunoassay versus culture. Obstet Gynecol 1987;69:743–746.

35. Thomason HJL, Gelbart SM, Sobieski VJ, et al. Effectiveness of Gonozyme for detection of gonorrhea in low-risk pregnant and gynecologic populations. Sex Transm Dis 1989;16:28–31.

36. Stary A, Kopp W, Zahel B, et al. Comparison of DNA-probe test and culture for the detection of *Neisseria gonorrhoeae* in genital samples. Sex Transm Dis 1993;20:243–247.

37. Vlaspolder F, Mutsaers JA, Blog F, et al. Value of DNA probe assay (Gen-Probe) compared with that of culture for diagnosis of gonococcal infection. J Clin Microbiol 1993;31:107–110.

38. Roongpisuthipong A, Lewis JS, Kraus SJ, et al. Gonococcal urethritis diagnosed from enzyme immunoassay of urine sediment. Sex Transm Dis 1988;15:192–195.

39. Papapetropoulou M, Detorakis J, Arkoulis A, Vervitas J. Screening for asymptomatic gonorrhea in males: a comparison of four techniques. J Chemother 1990;2:37–39.

40. Foster A, Klauss V. Ophthalmia neonatorum in developing countries. N Engl J Med 1995;332:600–601.

41. O'Hara MA. Ophthalmia neonatorum. Pediatr Clin North Am 1993;40:715–725.

42. Laga M, Plummer FA, Piot P, et al. Prophylaxis of gonococcal and chlamydial ophthalmia neonatorum. A comparison of silver nitrate and tetracycline. N Engl J Med 1988;318:653–657.

43. Lund RJ, Kibel MA, Knight GL, et al. Prophylaxis against gonococcal ophthalmia neonatorum. A prospective study. S Afr Med J 1987;72:620–622.

44. Hammerschlag MR, Cummings C, Roblin P, et al. Efficacy of neonatal ocular prophylaxis for the prevention of chlamydial and gonococcal conjunctivitis. N Engl J Med 1989;320:769–772.

45. Isenberg SJ, Apt L, Wood M. A controlled trial of povidone-iodine as prophylaxis against ophthalmia neonatorum. N Engl J Med 1995;332:562–566.

46. Canadian Task Force on the Periodic Health Examination. Canadian guide to clinical preventive health care. Ottawa: Canada Communication Group, 1994:168–175, 720–729.

47. American Academy of Family Physicians. Age charts for periodic health examination. Kansas City, MO: American Academy of Family Physicians, 1994. (Reprint no. 510.)
48. Green M, ed. Bright Futures: national guidelines for health supervision of infants, children, and adolescents. Arlington, VA: National Center for Education in Maternal and Child Health, 1994.
49. American Medical Association. Guidelines for adolescent preventive services (GAPS): recommendations and rationale. Chicago: American Medical Association, 1994.
50. American Academy of Pediatrics. Gonococcal infections. In: Peter G, ed. 1994 Red Book: report of the Committee on Infectious Diseases. 23rd ed. Elk Grove Village, IL: American Academy of Pediatrics, 1994:195–202.
51. American Academy of Pediatrics, Committee on Practice and Ambulatory Medicine. Recommendations for preventive pediatric health care. Pediatrics 1995;96:373–374.
52. American Academy of Pediatrics. Prophylaxis and treatment of neonatal gonococcal infections. Pediatrics 1980;65:1047–1048.

28. Screening for Human Immunodeficiency Virus Infection

RECOMMENDATION

Clinicians should assess risk factors for human immunodeficiency virus (HIV) infection by obtaining a careful sexual history and inquiring about injection drug use in all patients. Periodic screening for infection with HIV is recommended for all persons at increased risk of infection (see *Clinical Intervention*). Screening is recommended for all pregnant women at risk for HIV infection, including all women who live in states, counties, or cities with an increased prevalence of HIV infection. There is insufficient evidence to recommend for or against universal screening among low-risk pregnant women in low-prevalence areas, but recommendations to counsel and offer screening to all pregnant women may be made on other grounds (see Clinical Intervention). Screening infants born to high-risk mothers is recommended if the mother's antibody status is not known. All patients should be counseled about effective means to avoid HIV infection (see Chapter 62).

Burden of Suffering

It is estimated that 0.8–1.2 million persons in the U.S. are infected with the human immunodeficiency virus (HIV-1) and that 40,000–80,000 new infections occur each year.[1,2] Most people infected with HIV eventually develop the acquired immunodeficiency syndrome (AIDS), defined by opportunistic infections or severe immune dysfunction.[3] Within 10 years of infection with HIV, about 50% of persons develop clinical AIDS, and another 40% or more develop other illnesses associated with HIV infection.[4] A small proportion (5–10%) of persons remain well 10–15 years after HIV infection,[5] but there is currently no available curative treatment for AIDS. Of the 476,899 cases of AIDS reported to the Centers for Disease Control and Prevention (CDC) through June 1995, 62% had died, including over 90% of those diagnosed before 1988.[6] HIV infection is now the leading cause of death among men ages 25–44, and the fifth leading cause of years of potential life lost before age 65.[7,8] By the end of 1995, it is projected that there will be 130,000–205,000 persons living with AIDS in the U.S., at an annual cost of treatment in excess of $15 billion.[9]

High-Risk Groups. Men who have sex with men and injection drug users (IDUs) together accounted for over 80% of AIDS cases reported in 1994.[6] HIV infection is widely prevalent in these groups.[10] In seroprevalence surveys conducted in 1991–1992 at STD clinics and drug treatment facilities, the median prevalence of HIV infection among men having sex with men was 26% (range 4–47%)[a] and ranged from 2–7% among IDUs in Western cities to 12–40% among IDUs on the East Coast.[10] HIV infection is also prevalent among heterosexual persons with other STDs (median 0.6%), prisoners (range 1–15%), and residents of homeless shelters (range 1–21%).[10] Very high rates of HIV infection (up to 30%) have been detected among inner-city young adults who smoke crack, especially among women who exchange sex for drugs.[11] More than 10,000 cases of AIDS have been attributed to transfusion of infected blood or blood components (i.e., clotting factor) between 1977 and 1985, but the current risk of becoming infected from blood or tissue products is extremely low.[12]

Pregnant Women. By July 1995, over 5,900 cases of AIDS had been attributed to perinatal infection.[6] An estimated 0.17% of all childbearing women in the U.S. were infected with HIV in 1991–1992, but prevalence varied from 0–0.05% in 16 states to 0.6% in New York State. Of 144 urban family planning clinics conducting blinded surveillance, 13 reported a prevalence of HIV infection over 1%.[10] Of the estimated 7,000 infants born to infected mothers each year, 80% are born in 20 states where prevalence of antibody-positive newborns was 0.1% or greater.[13] The probability of vertical transmission from mother to infant is between 13% and 35%,[14–16] increasing with severity of disease in the mother.[17]

General Population. The distribution of new AIDS cases may not reflect the changing pattern of the HIV epidemic due to the long delay between infection and clinical AIDS. Heterosexual transmission is the most rapidly growing source of new AIDS cases, accounting for 10% of new AIDS cases in 1994 (up from 2% in 1985).[6] It is the leading cause of new HIV infections in American women.[6,18] Young black and Hispanic women in large East Coast cities are at greatest risk (due to the higher prevalence of HIV in their male partners and the more efficient transmission of virus from men to women during intercourse),[19] but women of all races experienced comparable increases in heterosexually acquired AIDS cases between 1992 and 1994.[18] Large surveys in 1991–1992 of Job Corps applicants ages 16–21 (seroprevalence 0.27%), military recruits (seroprevalence 0.06%), and pa-

---

[a]Data from patients at STD clinics, by selecting for high-risk sexual practices, will overstate the rate of infection in the general population of homosexual and bisexual men.

tients at urban hospitals (range 0.1–5.8%) indicate that the prevalence of HIV infection varies markedly among different demographic groups and geographic areas.[10] The rate of AIDS and the prevalence of HIV are substantially higher in Atlantic Coast states than in Midwest and Mountain states, in large metropolitan areas (population 500,000 or greater) than in smaller cities or rural areas, and in black and Hispanic young persons than in whites, Native Americans, or Asians/Pacific Islanders.[6,10,20] Blinded screening of over 20,000 primary care patients in smaller cities and rural areas detected HIV in 0.15% of all patients without known disease, however.[10] The regional variations in HIV prevalence generally mirror the local prevalence of infection among drug users. IDUs account for a large proportion of new HIV infections[21] and are a leading source of heterosexual and perinatal transmission of HIV.[6]

Accuracy of Screening Tests

The initial screening test to detect antibodies to HIV is the enzyme immunoassay (EIA). Commercially available EIAs use antigens from whole disrupted virus (first generation), recombinant viral proteins (second generation), or chemically synthesized peptides (third generation).[22] EIA results are considered "reactive" only when a positive result has been confirmed in a second test of the original sample. In subjects with clinical AIDS, the sensitivity of EIA is close to 100%, but newly infected individuals may not develop detectable antibodies for periods of weeks to months after infection.[23] The median interval between infection and seropositivity has been estimated at 3 months with earlier EIAs, with 95% seroconverting within 6 months.[24] Estimates based on more sensitive third-generation EIAs, which may be positive within 1 week of peak antigen levels, suggest that the "window" period with current tests is substantially shorter (3–4 weeks).[25,25a] Specificity of EIA is above 99.5% with most tests. Third-generation EIAs had specificities of 99.7–99.9% when tested against uninfected controls.[25–27] False-positive results can be caused by nonspecific reactions in persons with immunologic disturbances (e.g., systemic lupus erythematosus or rheumatoid arthritis), multiple transfusions, or recent influenza or rabies vaccination.[28,29] Food and Drug Administration (FDA) approval has been granted to rapid tests (<15 minutes) using colorimetric assays,[30] and to an EIA-based test using oral fluid samples collected with a cotton pad.[31,32] Although these tests are sensitive and specific (>99%), neither method is recommended for the definitive diagnosis of HIV infection.[33]

To prevent the serious consequences of a false-positive diagnosis of HIV infection, confirmation of positive EIA results is necessary, using an independent test with high specificity. The Western blot (WB) is the most commonly used confirmatory test in the U.S. Indirect immunofluorescence assay (IFA), which is less expensive and less time-consuming, is also approved for confirmatory testing.[34] The specificity of WB is close to 100% under controlled settings,[35] but it is dependent on the skill and experience of the laboratory and on criteria used to determine positive WB results.[33,35] The sensitivity of WB was 98.5% and specificity 92.5% in a 1989 CDC quality control survey of 140 laboratories;[26] most errors involved misclassification of positive or negative samples as "indeterminate." Criteria for interpreting WB have been developed to improve accuracy in clinical testing.[35] Many laboratories doing a large volume of HIV testing achieved sensitivities and specificities of 100%.[36]

The precise false-positive rate of current HIV testing is not known. A false-positive rate of less than 1 in 100,000 was reported in experienced, centralized laboratories using careful quality control procedures.[37,38] In practice, false-positive diagnoses can result from contaminated or mislabeled specimens,[39] cross-reacting antibodies,[33] failure to perform confirmatory tests,[40] misinterpretation of WB patterns, or misunderstanding of reported results by clinicians or patients.[41] In one study, 8 of 900 women referred for treatment of HIV were not infected on repeat testing.[40] To prevent errors due to mistakes in specimen handling or WB interpretation, a consensus laboratory panel recommended confirming all new diagnoses of HIV with tests on a freshly obtained specimen.[42]

Indeterminate Western Blot Results. Indeterminate WB results, due to antibody patterns that do not meet full criteria for positive test, occur in 3–8% of EIA-positive specimens.[33,43] In a survey of over 1 million newborn specimens for maternal HIV antibody, <1 in 4,000 screened samples produced an indeterminate WB result.[43a] An indeterminate WB result may indicate evolving antibody response in recently infected subjects, but in low-risk persons it usually represents the presence of nonspecific antibodies. Follow-up of nearly 700 EIA positive/WB indeterminate blood donors documented seroconversion in only eight subjects, all but one of whom reported a high-risk behavior.[43-45] An indeterminate WB is more significant in high-risk subjects, but the risk of seroconversion is variable (13–28%).[44,46] Antibodies to p24 antigen were present in 29 of 30 subjects who subsequently converted.[43,44] A new indeterminate WB in subjects who were previously seronegative is more likely to represent recent infection.[47] Seroconversion usually occurs within 2–3 months (range 2–16 weeks in one study).[44] A stable indeterminate WB after 6 months can be assumed to be due to nonspecific antibody reaction rather than HIV infection.[33,48]

Viral Culture and Polymerase Chain Reaction Assays. Viral culture is the most specific test for HIV infection, but it is time-consuming, expensive, technically difficult, and insufficiently sensitive for use as a screening test.[22] Polymerase chain reaction (PCR) can detect viral genetic material in subjects who have not yet developed antibodies, but trace levels of contamination can produce false-positive results.[22] In proficiency testing of five experienced laboratories, sensitivity of PCR was 98–100% and specificity was 96–100%.[49] With newer, more sensitive EIAs, the additional value of screening with PCR is small in adults. In over 250 high-risk persons with nonreactive EIAs, PCR detected only two confirmed cases of HIV.[50–53] Since PCR is not 100% specific, a large proportion of positive PCR results in seronegative patients may be false positives. Despite their limitations as screening tests, viral culture, PCR, and viral antigen assays are useful for evaluating patients with symptoms of acute HIV infection.

Diagnosis of HIV in Infants. Diagnosing infection in infants born to HIV-infected mothers is difficult, since maternal antibodies to HIV are present in both infected and uninfected infants. Uninfected infants serorevert an average of 10 months after birth, but maternal antibody may persist up to 18 months.[54] Viral culture and PCR are highly specific for infection in infants, although PCR is occasionally positive in infants who eventually serorevert and are presumed not to be infected.[55] Reported sensitivity for culture is 60–90%[22,56] and 84–98% for PCR, increasing after 3 months.[57,58] Using culture and/or PCR, an estimated 50% of infected infants can be identified at birth, and up to 90% by 3 months.[59] Other tests for perinatal infection include assays for viral antigen (sensitivity 30–60%)[56,59] and IgA (sensitivity 50–80%).[59,60]

Screening by Risk Factor Assessment. Patient history is an important but imperfect way to assess risk for HIV infection. Patients may conceal high-risk behaviors, and others (especially women in high-risk areas) may be unknowingly at risk from an infected sex partner. In high-prevalence family planning clinics, testing women who reported drug use or an IDU partner detected only 41–57% of all cases.[61,62] Offering testing routinely to all women resulted in greater acceptance (up to 96%),[61] and detected 87% of all HIV infections.[62] Even in low-prevalence areas such as Sweden, 37% of infected pregnant women did not report clear risk factors for HIV.[63] There are few data comparing the sensitivity of targeted versus routine screening in male patients. In a seroprevalence study in primary care practices, physicians were not aware of HIV risk factors in roughly one third of infected patients.[10]

Consent, Confidential Versus Anonymous Testing, and Partner Notification. There is general consensus that informed consent should be obtained prior to HIV testing.[14,64] The diagnosis of HIV has serious consequences, and compulsory testing may discourage persons from seeking care. Alternate forms of consent—right of refusal (i.e., passive consent) versus explicit consent, active recommendation versus nondirective counseling—have been considered to facilitate screening during pregnancy.[13,65] Universal newborn screening without consent of the mother was considered but rejected by the New York State legislature.[66]

Half of all states require confidential reporting of HIV-infected persons by name to state or local health departments, and all require reporting of AIDS patients.[6,67] Partner notification (contact tracing) can alert exposed persons to the need to be tested. Between 50% and 90% of sex partners can be identified through organized partner notification programs,[68] and costs per case identified compare favorably to screening high-risk groups.[69]

In one trial, offering the option of anonymous testing resulted in higher rates of testing.[70] Two thirds of all patients at a public clinic (and a majority of seropositive patients) chose anonymous testing over confidential testing.[71] Test kits that would allow individuals to submit specimens (blood or saliva) collected at home for anonymous testing, using coded identifiers, are being considered by the FDA.[71a]

Frequency of Testing. The appropriate frequency of HIV screening is not known, but it depends in part on the incidence of new infections. Rates are highest among IDUs in Northeastern cities (3–6 infections/100 patient-years [py]),[21] compared to less than 1/100 py in homosexual men in most cities,[72] and 0.04/100 py among military personnel aged 25–29.[73] Due to the low incidence of new infection and increased sensitivity of new tests, repeat testing simply to confirm an initial negative EIA is rarely indicated.

Effectiveness of Early Detection

Detection of asymptomatic HIV infection permits early treatment to slow disease progression, interventions to reduce perinatal transmission, and counseling to prevent transmission of virus to uninfected sex partners or persons sharing injection needles.

Effectiveness of Early Therapy in Asymptomatic Adults. Antiretroviral medications (e.g., zidovudine [ZDV or AZT], didanosine, zalcitabine) reduce mortality in AIDS patients and delay progression to AIDS in symptomatic HIV infection.[74,75] Due to eventual resistance developed by the HIV virus,[76] however, there is no clear benefit of initiating antiretroviral therapy (with current drugs as monotherapies) before patients become symptomatic.[74,77,78] In an overview of six randomized, controlled trials (RCTs) of ZDV for asymptomatic HIV infection, there was no long-term benefit of early treatment versus deferred treatment (begun at onset of symptoms) on survival or progression to AIDS.[79] For asymptomatic patients with more advanced immunodeficiency (CD4 200–500/µL), early ZDV delayed progression to AIDS or AIDS-related complex over the short-term but did not improve outcomes beyond the first 1–2 years.[74,79,80] In Concorde, the largest and longest trial—over 1,700 men and women with asymptomatic HIV infection followed over 3 years—there was no significant difference between patients receiving early versus deferred treatment in the combined incidence of AIDS or death (18% in each group), or in total mortality (8% and 6%, respectively).[81] The early benefits from delaying disease progression are offset by the adverse effects of ZDV (e.g., nausea, headache, and fatigue).[82] Early combination antiretroviral therapy, by reducing drug resistance, may be more effective than monotherapy in reducing viral burden and delaying immunodeficiency, but long-term clinical trials of these approaches have not yet been completed.[83,84]

Chemoprophylaxis can reduce the risk of *Pneumocystis carinii* pneumonia (PCP) in patients with more advanced immunodeficiency. The annual incidence of PCP rises to 18–25% in persons with CD4 < $200/\mu L$,[85,86] and half of all HIV-infected persons are still asymptomatic at this stage of disease.[85,87,88] In retrospective analyses, prophylaxis with trimethoprim-sulfamethoxazole (TMP-SMX) or inhaled pentamidine reduced the incidence of primary PCP by 67–83%,[86,89–91] delayed onset of AIDS by 6–12 months, and prolonged survival in those with low CD4 count by almost 1 year.[92–94] In a recent 3-year trial, TMP-SMX, dapsone, and inhaled pentamidine were equally effective as initial therapy for primary prophylaxis against PCP.[95] TMP-SMX was more effective in shorter studies[89,90,96] and for patients with CD4 < 100,[95] and it is recommended as the preferred prophylactic agent;[97] long-term therapy is limited by the high incidence of side effects (e.g., leukopenia, fever, rash, or gastrointestinal side effects). TMP-SMX and dapsone also provide protection against toxoplasmosis,[98,99] an uncommon complication of asymptomatic HIV infection in the U.S.[95] Long-term benefits of chemoprophylaxis are limited by the continuing decline in immune function.[92]

HIV-infected persons infected with *Mycobacterium tuberculosis* are at increased risk of developing active tuberculosis, primarily at CD4 counts below $500/\mu L$. In a randomized trial among asymptomatic HIV-infected persons in Haiti, an endemic tuberculosis area, chemoprophylaxis with isoniazid reduced the incidence of tuberculosis nearly 75% and delayed progression to AIDS.[100] In a U.S. cohort study, isoniazid prophylaxis reduced tuberculosis among HIV-positive, PPD-positive drug users.[101,102] Decision analyses suggest that the benefits of prophylaxis may outweigh risks in both PPD-positive and anergic patients with HIV when exposure to tuberculosis is prevalent (e.g., in IDUs, homeless persons, and immigrants from endemic areas; see Chapter 25).[103] Chemoprophylaxis with rifabutin is also effective against *Mycobacterium avium* complex (MAC), but few asymptomatic patients have sufficiently advanced disease (CD4 < $75/\mu L$) to warrant MAC prophylaxis.[97]

Effectiveness of Early Therapy in Asymptomatic Children. There are few randomized trials of interventions in asymptomatic HIV-infected children, but TMP-SMX is safe and effective for PCP prophylaxis in other immunocompromised children.[104] PCP may be the first indication that infants are infected with HIV: 44% of the children who developed PCP in one study had never been evaluated for HIV.[105] Between 7% and 20% of children with HIV develop PCP within the first year of life (peak incidence between 3 and 9 months),[105,106] and mortality is high (up to 30%).[107] Adverse reactions (rash, cytopenia) from TMP-SMX occur in up to 15% of HIV-infected children. New CDC guidelines for PCP prophylaxis in infants recommend prophylaxis for all HIV- infected or possibly infected infants during the first year of life.[107] Studies are currently under way to evaluate the benefit of different antiretroviral therapies in asymptomatic children.

A variety of precautions are routinely recommended for HIV-infected children and adults, due to the increased susceptibility to viral and bacterial infections:[108–110] vaccination against influenza, pneumococcus, hepatitis B, and *Haemophilus influenzae;*[111] avoidance of oral (live virus) polio vaccine in children;[112] attention to nutrition;[113] avoiding uncooked foods and high-risk sexual practices; and more frequent Papanicolaou (Pap) screening for women (due to an increased risk of invasive cervical cancer).[67,114] The benefit of these interventions in persons with asymptomatic HIV infection has not been determined.

Effectiveness of Early Intervention in Asymptomatic Pregnant Women. A randomized placebo-controlled trial (ACTG 076) demonstrated that a regimen of ZDV begun between weeks 14 and 34 of pregnancy and continued through delivery and for 6 weeks in newborn infants significantly reduced perinatal HIV infection (8.3% vs. 25.5%) among infants born to seropositive mothers with mildly symptomatic HIV infection (CD4 > $200/\mu L$).[16] ZDV is associated with a low incidence of severe side effects in mothers or infants, but the long-term effects on the health of infants, and on the course of HIV disease in mothers, are not known. Cesarean delivery is also associated with lower rates of vertical transmission; a trial of operative versus vaginal delivery in HIV-infected pregnancies is under way in Italy.[115]

Identifying seropositive women during pregnancy may have other important benefits: some women may be candidates for PCP prophylaxis; male partners can be advised to be tested and to use condoms; infants can be monitored for evidence of HIV infection and started on appropriate therapy; and early involvement of social services may facilitate care for infected mothers and infants. Infected mothers are advised to avoid breast-feeding: a meta-analysis of cohort studies estimated that breastfeeding increases vertical transmission by 14%.[116] The extent to which early detection actually leads to these benefits is difficult to estimate. There is no clear effect of testing and counseling on fertility decisions: in two U.S. studies, pregnancy rates were similar for HIV-positive and HIV-negative women.[117] Infected women were more likely to choose abortion than uninfected women in one study,[118] but the large majority of women with HIV chose to continue the pregnancy.[63]

Effectiveness of Testing and Counseling to Prevent Transmission of HIV. Determining whether HIV testing and counseling reduces HIV transmission is complicated by many factors:[119] a paucity of well-controlled trials; variable quality of counseling interventions; reliance on intermediate endpoints, such as self-reported changes in behavior; differences between screened and unscreened patients in observational studies; population-wide changes in high-risk behavior; and the uncertain importance of testing versus counseling. The effect of testing and counseling varies with the specific behavior and population being targeted.[117] Programs that targeted couples in which one member was infected provide the strongest evidence of the benefits of testing and counseling: compared with historical controls, counseled couples increased regular condom use and significantly reduced the rate of seroconversion in partners.[120-123]

Among homosexual men, high-risk sexual practices and new HIV infections have declined substantially since the development of HIV tests. Community-wide changes may have been more important than identification of seropositive persons, however, and there are worrisome signs of persisting unsafe practices among younger gay men.[124] Condom use is generally higher among seropositive men than seronegative or untested men, but longitudinal studies suggest increasing use of condoms across all groups.[125-127] Unprotected anal intercourse and number of sex partners have declined over time in both tested and untested men. The absolute change in risk may be greater in seropositive men, who engage in higher-risk behavior at baseline.[128] A substantial proportion of seropositive men continue to have sex with multiple partners and engage in oral intercourse; 5–15% continue unprotected anal intercourse.[128]

The effects of screening in injection drug users are less consistent. Among drug users in treatment, drug use and needle sharing decline after HIV counseling and testing but also declined among unscreened patients.[117,129] In a community survey, IDUs who had received testing and counseling were half as likely to share needles as untested subjects.[130] Testing has inconsistent effects on high-risk sexual behavior among drug users. Seropositive IDUs are more likely to report condom use in some cross-sectional studies, but 30–70% use condoms only occasionally or not at all.[117,131]

Counseling and testing patients at STD clinics has had variable results. Rate of recurrent STDs was unchanged 1 year after testing in one study,[132] was lower among HIV-positive than HIV-negative subjects in another (15% vs. 23%),[133] and declined among seropositive patients while rising among seronegative patients in a third.[134] In one randomized trial, testing and counseling reduced unprotected intercourse more than counseling alone.[135] Other longitudinal studies suggest little change in sexual behavior in seronegative subjects after testing and counseling. Routine testing and counseling among students at a college health clinic did not improve low rates of condom use.[136] Among women tested in community health clinics, seronegative women did not reduce sexual risk factors after testing and counseling, compared with untested controls.[137]

Efforts to modify high-risk behaviors in infected and high-risk persons are often hindered by substance abuse, poverty, limited education, denial, or economic necessity (i.e., prostitutes). A minority of seropositive persons abstain completely from sex or drug use after diagnosis. Those who do not may have trouble obtaining condoms or clean needles but may not inform sex partners that they are infected.[138] Female partners of infected men may minimize risk or be unable to get their male partner to consistently use a condom.[139]

Adverse Effects of Testing and Counseling. The diagnosis of HIV infection can have significant adverse effects, among them intense anxiety, depression, somatization, or anger.[140,141] Among 1,718 newly diagnosed patients with HIV, 21% met criteria for depression at first visit, but psychological distress was related more to symptoms than diagnosis and diminished with time.[142] Testing reduces anxiety in high-risk persons who are seronegative. Despite recent efforts to improve public perceptions and attitudes, the stigma associated with the diagnosis of HIV/AIDS is still significant.[143] Disclosure of test results can result in disrupted personal relationships, domestic violence, social ostracism, and discriminatory action, such as loss of employment, housing, health insurance, and educational opportunities.[144] Recent legislation and the expanded case definitions for AIDS may help prevent some forms of discrimination and help ensure medical care for those with more advanced infection. Information on the frequency or consequences of false-positive diagnoses are largely anecdotal. Although retesting and follow-up can resolve most errors, misdiagnosis may cause irreparable harm (divorce, abortion, etc.). Finally, negative test results may provide false reassurance unless patients are counseled about their continuing risk of infection from drug use and high-risk sexual activity.

Recommendations of Other Groups

Counseling and HIV testing of high-risk individuals are recommended by the CDC[14] and numerous medical organizations: the Canadian Task Force on the Periodic Health Examination (CTF),[145] the American Academy of Family Physicians,[146] the American Medical Association (AMA),[147] the

American College of Obstetricians and Gynecologists (ACOG),[114] the American College of Physicians, and the Infectious Disease Society of America.[148] High-risk individuals include men who have sex with men; persons seeking treatment for STDs; injection drug users and their sex partners; recipients of transfusion between 1978 and 1985; and persons who have had multiple sex partners or exchanged sex for money or drugs. Bright Futures[149] and the AMA Guidelines for Adolescent Preventive Services (GAPS)[150] recommend offering HIV testing to all at-risk adolescents, including those with more than one sex partner in the last 6 months.

The CDC recommends that health care facilities where the prevalence of infection exceeds 1%, or the AIDS diagnosis rate is greater than 1/1,000 hospital discharges, consider routine, voluntary screening among patients aged 15–54 years.[151] The AMA approves of routine HIV testing in the clinical setting, based on local considerations such as planned medical procedures and local seroprevalence.[147] GAPS[150] and AAFP[146] recommend offering screening to sexually active adolescents and adults from high-prevalence communities.

The U.S. Public Health Service (PHS) released new guidelines in 1995, recommending that all pregnant women be routinely counseled and encouraged to have HIV testing.[152] Similar policies have been approved by American Academy of Pediatrics (AAP)[65] and ACOG.[153] Pregnant women should be screened as soon as the woman is known to be pregnant; repeat testing may be indicated near delivery for women at high risk of infection. The CTF (prior to ACTG 076) concluded there was insufficient evidence to recommend for or against routine screening in pregnancy, due to the low rate of infection in Canada.[145] In cases where the HIV serostatus of the mother is not known, PHS and AAP guidelines suggest that health care providers educate the mother about benefits to her infant and encourage her to allow testing for the newborn.[65,152] A 1991 Institute of Medicine task force (before ACTG 076) recommended voluntary screening of all pregnant women in high-prevalence areas and of high-risk women in other areas, but it found insufficient evidence to recommend routine newborn screening.[64]

Both the AMA and the AAP have endorsed alternate procedures for pretest counseling and consent, including right of refusal, to facilitate routine testing in specific situations. Mandatory testing for HIV is currently required on entrance to the military, and for donors of blood, organs, and tissue; federal prisoners; and persons seeking to immigrate to the U.S. Individual state laws vary regarding mandatory testing, confidentiality of results, informed consent, and reporting of seropositive persons to public health officials.[67] The CDC recommends that seropositive persons be instructed how to notify their partners, but suggests that physicians or health department personnel should use confidential procedures to ensure that partners are notified.[14]

Discussion

Early detection of asymptomatic HIV infection can reduce morbidity and mortality in infected persons, but the long-term benefits are currently limited by the relentless course of disease in most patients. The most compelling argument for early detection is the potential to prevent transmission of HIV, which may occur over many years before infected persons develop symptoms of HIV infection. Although there is only indirect evidence that screening reduces the incidence of new HIV infections, even small changes in transmission will have important public health benefits.

Screening is most important in the high-risk groups that currently account for the large majority of AIDS cases and new HIV infections.[154] The ability of ZDV to reduce perinatal transmission of HIV provides strong evidence of the benefit of screening during pregnancy. In high-risk communities, offering HIV testing to all pregnant women is more acceptable to patients, easier to implement, and more sensitive than screening on the basis of self-reported risk factors. In areas where HIV infection is uncommon, however, the choice between targeted screening and universal screening is a policy decision. Universal screening may detect occasional cases of HIV infection among women without reported risk factors, but it will subject many women at negligible risk to the potential harms from a false-positive or indeterminate test result. If specificity of testing is 99.98%, routine screening in low-risk populations (e.g., pregnant women in low-prevalence states) will generate one false-positive and many additional indeterminate results for every true-positive. Although indeterminate and false-positive results can generally be resolved with follow-up testing, some women may decide to terminate the pregnancy before infection status can be definitively determined. Counseling and testing many thousands of low-risk women to detect a single case of HIV may also divert resources from more important issues. If routine testing can be provided with the combination of accuracy and low costs achieved by large, centralized screening programs,[37,63,155] the justification for universal screening would be stronger.

A growing number of HIV infections occur in persons who are infected through heterosexual contact. The risk of heterosexual transmission varies widely among different communities, with the highest risk among poor minority women in large cities and the rural South. In high-risk communities or clinics, routine screening of sexually active young women and men may be appropriate. In populations where prevalence of infection is low, more selective screening is likely to be more efficient: 5% of women and 12% of men report multiple sex partners within the last 12 months without consistent condom use.[156] Deciding what constitutes a "high-risk" community is a policy decision,[64] depending in part on available data and resources for testing. A prevalence of 1/1,000 among newborns,[157] or an AIDS diagnosis rate of more than 1/1,000 hospital discharges,[151] has been used to justify routine screening in other settings. Community prevalence provides only a crude measure of individual risk, however, and should not replace careful assessment of high-risk behaviors in each patient.

Screening for HIV in high-risk groups is cost-effective under a wide range of assumptions. In an analysis of federally funded programs (where HIV prevalence was 2.6%) testing and counseling activities saved money even if only one new infection is avoided for every 100 seropositive subjects identified.[158] In Sweden, where prevalence of infection is only 0.01% in pregnant women, routine prenatal HIV testing costs approximately $10 per patient and $100,000 per case identified.[63] Screening is less cost-effective in asymptomatic adults if only the benefits from early treatment are considered.[154] Revised cost-effectiveness analyses of alternate screening strategies for asymptomatic persons are needed, incorporating new data on antiretroviral therapy in pregnant and nonpregnant adults, regional variations in prevalence, targeted versus universal screening, and the costs of testing and counseling in the primary care setting.

CLINICAL INTERVENTION

Clinicians should assess risk factors for HIV infection in all patients by obtaining a careful sexual history and inquiring about drug use. Counseling and testing for HIV should be offered to all persons at increased risk for infection: those seeking treatment for sexually transmitted diseases; men who have had sex with men after 1975; past or present injection drug users; persons who exchange sex for money or drugs, and their sex partners; women and men whose past or present sex partners were HIV-infected, bisexual, or injection drug users; and persons with a history of transfusion between 1978 and 1985 ("A" recommendation).

Pregnant women in these categories, and those from communities (e.g., states, counties, or cities) where the prevalence of seropositive newborns is increased (e.g., ≥0.1%) should be counseled about the potential benefit to their infant of early intervention for HIV, and offered testing as soon as the woman is known to be pregnant ("A" recommendation). Repeat testing may be indicated in the third trimester of pregnancy for women at high risk of recent exposure to HIV. There is insufficient evidence to recommend for or against universal prenatal screening for HIV in low-prevalence communities ("C" recommendation). A policy of offering screening to all pregnant women may be recommended on other grounds, including patient preference, easier implementation, and increased sensitivity compared to screening based on community prevalence and reported risk factors. Careful quality control measures and patient counseling are essential to limit the potential adverse effects from indeterminate and false-positive test results during pregnancy. Testing infants born to high-risk mothers, with permission of mother, is recommended when antibody status of mother is unknown. ("B" recommendation).

There is insufficient evidence to recommend for or against routine HIV screening in persons without identified risk factors ("C" recommendation). Recommendations to screen sexually active young women and men in high-risk communities can be made on other grounds, based on the increasing burden of heterosexual transmission and the insensitivity of screening based on self-reported risk factors. Similarly, routine HIV screening may be reasonable in groups such as prisoners, runaway youth, or homeless persons, where the prevalence of high-risk behaviors and HIV is generally high. The definition of high-risk community is imprecise. Clinicians should consult local public health authorities for advice and information on the epidemiology of HIV infection in their communities. More selective screening may be appropriate in low-risk areas. Testing should not be performed in the absence of informed consent and pretest counseling, which should includes the purpose of the test, the meaning of reactive and nonreactive results, measures to protect confidentiality, and the need to notify persons at risk. Patients who wish to be tested anonymously should be advised of appropriate testing facilities.

A positive test requires at least two reactive EIAs and confirmation with WB or IFA, performed by experienced laboratories that receive regular external proficiency testing. A separate sample should be submitted for persons found to be seropositive for the first time, to rule out possible error in specimen handling. Patients with indeterminate WB results should be evaluated individually to determine whether findings are likely to represent recent seroconversion. Repeat testing should be performed 3–6 months after indeterminate test results, or sooner if recent seroconversion is suspected. A stable indeterminate WB pattern is not indicative of HIV infection.

Seropositive patients should receive information regarding the meaning of the results, the distinctions between casual nonsexual contact and proven modes of HIV transmission, measures to reduce risk to themselves and others, symptoms requiring medical attention, and available community resources for HIV-infected persons. Clinicians should explore potential barriers to changing high-risk behavior in seropositive and seronegative individuals. Guidelines for HIV counseling have been published by the PHS.[159] Seropositive persons should be evaluated for severity of immune dysfunction and screened for other infectious diseases such as tuberculosis (see Chapter 25). Guidelines for the management of early HIV infection and prevention of opportunistic infections have been published by the Agency for Health Care Policy and Research[67] and the CDC.[97,107,111] Arrangements for follow-up medical care are especially important for drug users, who may require assistance in gaining entrance to a drug treatment program (see Chapter 53). All seropositive individuals should be encouraged to notify sex partners, persons with whom injection needles have been shared, and others at risk of exposure. Seropositive cases should be reported confidentially or anonymously to public health officials in accordance with local regulations.

Persons with nonreactive test results should be informed that the risk of acquiring subsequent HIV infection can be prevented by maintaining monogamous sexual relationships with uninfected partners. Other measures to reduce the risk of infection (consistent use of condoms, etc.) should be specifically mentioned (see Chapter 62). The frequency of repeat testing of seronegative individuals is a matter of clinical discretion. Periodic testing is most important in patients who continue high-risk activities. In patients with recent high-risk exposure (e.g., sex with HIV-infected partner), repeat testing at 3 months may be useful to rule out initial false-negative tests.

The draft update of this chapter was prepared for the U.S. Preventive Services Task Force by David Atkins MD, MPH.

REFERENCES

1. Centers for Disease Control and Prevention. Projections of the numbers of persons diagnosed with AIDS and the number of immunosuppressed HIV-infected persons—United States, 1992–1994. MMWR 1992;41(RR-18):1–29.
2. Centers for Disease Control. Update: public health surveillance for HIV infection—United States, 1989 and 1990. MMWR 1990;39:853, 859–861.
3. Centers for Disease Control and Prevention. 1993 revised classification system for HIV infection and expanded surveillance case definition for AIDS among adolescents and adults. MMWR 1992;41(RR-17):1–19.
4. Alcabes P, Munoz A, Vlahov D, et al. Incubation period of human immunodeficiency virus. Epidemiol Rev 1993;15:303–318.
5. Buchbinder SP, Katz MH, Hessol NA, et al. Long-term HIV infection without immunologic progression. AIDS 1994;8:1123–1128.
6. Centers for Disease Control and Prevention. HIV/AIDS surveillance report, 1995;7(1):1–34.
7. National Center for Health Statistics. Annual summary of births, marriages, divorces, and deaths: United States, 1993. Monthly vital statistics report; vol 42 no 13. Hyattsville, MD: Public Health Service, 1994:18–19.
8. Centers for Disease Control and Prevention. Years of potential life lost before age 65—United States, 1990 and 1991. MMWR 1993;42:251–253.
9. Hellinger FJ. Forecasts of the costs of medical care for persons with HIV: 1992–1995. Inquiry 1992;29: 356–365.
10. National Center for Infectious Diseases, Division of HIV/AIDS. National HIV serosurveillance summary—results through 1992. Vol 3. Atlanta: Centers for Disease Control and Prevention, 1993. (Publication no. HIV/NCID/11-93/036.)
11. Edlin BR, Irwin KL, Faruque S, et al. Intersecting epidemics—crack cocaine use and HIV infection among inner-city young adults. Multicenter Crack Cocaine and HIV Infection Team. N Engl J Med 1994;331:1422–1427.
12. Busch MP. HIV and blood transfusion: focus on seroconversion. Vox Sang 1994;67 (Suppl 3):13–18.

13. U.S. Public Health Service. Use of AZT to prevent perinatal transmission (ACTG 076): workshop on implications for treatment, counseling, and HIV testing. June 6–7, 1994. Bethesda: Public Health Service, 1994.

14. Centers for Disease Control. Public Health Service guidelines for counseling and antibody testing to prevent HIV infection and AIDS. MMWR 1987;36:509–515.

15. European Collaborative Study. Children born to women with HIV-1 infection: natural history and risk of transmission. Lancet 1991;337:253–260.

16. Connor EM, Sperling RS, Gelber R, et al. Reduction of maternal-infant transmission of HIV-1 with zidovudine treatment. N Engl J Med 1994;331:1173–1180.

17. Peckham C, Gibb C. Mother-to-child transmission of the human immunodeficiency virus. N Engl J Med 1995;333:298–302.

18. Centers for Disease Control and Prevention. Heterosexually acquired AIDS—United States, 1993. MMWR 1994;43:155–160.

19. Padian NS, Shiboski SC, Jewell NP. Female-to-male transmission of human immunodeficiency virus. JAMA 1991;266:1664–1667.

20. Centers for Disease Control and Prevention. AIDS among racial/ethnic minorities—United States, 1993. MMWR 1994;43:644–647, 653–655.

21. Holmberg SD. Emerging epidemiologic patterns of HIV in the United States. AIDS Res Hum Retrovir 1994;10(Suppl 2):81.

22. Schochetman G. Diagnosis of HIV infection. Clin Chim Acta 1992;211:1–26.

23. Imagawa DT, Lee MH, Wolinsky SM, et al. Human immunodeficiency virus type 1 infection in homosexual men who remain seronegative for prolonged periods. N Engl J Med 1989;320:1458–1462.

24. Horsburgh CR Jr, Ou CY, Jason J, et al. Duration of human immunodeficiency virus infection before detection of antibody. Lancet 1989;2:637–640.

25. Zaaijer HL, Exel-Oehlers PV, Kraaijeveld T, et al. Early detection of antibodies to HIV-1 by third-generation assays. Lancet 1992;340:770–772.

25a. Brown A, and the Planning Committee, Conference on Human Retrovirus Testing, Association of State and Territorial Public Health Laboratory Directors. 10th annual ASTPHLD Conference on HIV Testing summary report. CDC/NCID Focus, vol 5 no 6. Atlanta: Centers for Disease Control and Prevention, 1995:7–8.

26. Centers for Disease Control. Update: serologic testing for HIV-1 antibody—United States, 1988 and 1989. MMWR 1990;39:380–383.

27. Ascher DP, Roberts C. Determination of the etiology of seroreversals in HIV testing by antibody fingerprinting. J Acquired Immune Defic Syndr 1993;6:241–244.

28. Esteva MH, Blasini AM, Ogly D, Rodriquez MA. False positive results to antibody to HIV in two men with systemic lupus erythematosus. Ann Rheum Dis 1992;51:1071–1073.

29. MacKenzie WR, Davis JP, Peterson DE, et al. Multiple false-positive serologic tests for HIV, HTLV-1, and hepatitis C following influenza vaccination, 1991. JAMA 1992;268:1015–1017.

30. Malone JD, Smith ES, Sheffield J, et al. Comparative evaluation of six rapid serologic tests for HIV-1 antibody. J Acquired Immune Defic Syndr 1993;6:115–119.

31. Tamashiro H, Constantine NT. Serologic diagnosis of HIV infection using oral fluid samples. Bull WHO 1994;72:135–143.

32. Food and Drug Administration. Oral fluid specimen test for HIV-1 approved. JAMA 1995;273:613.

33. Report of the Ninth Annual Conference on Human Retrovirus Testing. Washington, DC: Association of State and Territorial Public Health Laboratory Directors, 1994.

34. Sullivan MT, Mucke H, Kadey SD, et al. Evaluation of an indirect immunofluorescence assay for confirmation of human immunodeficiency virus type 1 antibody in U.S. blood donor sera. J Clin Microbiol 1992;30:2509–2510.

35. Centers for Disease Control. Interpretation and use of the Western blot assay for serodiagnosis of human immunodeficiency virus type 1 infections. MMWR 1989;38(Suppl 7):1–7.

36. Gerber AR, Valdiserri RO, Johnson CA, et al. Quality of laboratory performance in testing for human immunodeficiency virus type 1 antibody. Arch Pathol Lab Med 1991;115:1091–1096.

37. Burke DS, Brundage JF, Redfield RR, et al. Measurement of the false-positive rate in a screening program for human immunodeficiency virus infections. N Engl J Med 1988;319:961–964.

38. MacDonald KL, Jackson B, Bowman RJ, et al. Performance characteristics of serologic tests for human immunodeficiency virus type 1 (HIV-1) antibody among Minnesota blood donors. Ann Intern Med 1989;110:617–621.

39. Mahoney A, Parry JV, Mortimer PP. Cross-contamination and "confirmed" positive anti-HIV results [letter]. Lancet 1991;338:953–954.

40. Sheon AR, Fox, HE, Alexander G, et al. Misdiagnosed HIV infection in pregnant women: implications for clinical care. Public Health Rep 1994;109:694–699.

41. Craven DE, Steger KA, LaChapelle R, et al. Factitious HIV infection: the importance of documenting infection. Ann Intern Med 1994;121:763–766.

42. Report of the Eighth Annual Conference on Human Retrovirus Testing. Washington, DC: Association of State and Territorial Public Health Laboratory Directors, 1993.

43. Kleinman S. The significance of HIV-1 indeterminate Western blot results in blood donor populations. Arch Pathol Lab Med 1990;114:298–303.

43a. Gwinn M, Redus MA, Granade TC. HIV-1 serologic test results for one million newborn dried-blood specimens: assay performance and implications for screening. J Acquired Immune Defic Syndr 1992; 5:505–512.

44. Healey DS, Maskill WJ, Howard TS, et al. HIV-1 Western blot: development and assessment of testing to resolve indeterminate reactivity. AIDS 1992;6:629–633.

45. Dock NL, Kleinman SH, Rayfield MA, et al. Human immunodeficiency virus infection and indeterminate Western blot patterns. Arch Intern Med 1991;151:525–530.

46. Celum CL, Coombs RW, Lafferty W, et al. Indeterminate human immunodeficiency virus type 1 western blots: seroconversion risk, specificity of supplemental tests, and an algorithm for evaluation. J Infect Dis 1991;164:657–664.

47. Phair J, Hoover D, Huprika J, et al. The significance of Western blot assays indeterminate for antibody to HIV in a cohort of homosexual/bisexual men. J Acquired Immune Defic Syndr 1992;5:988–992.

48. Jackson JB, MacDonald KL, Cadwell J, et al. Absence of HIV infection in blood donors with indeterminate Western blot tests for antibody to HIV-1. N Engl J Med 1990;322:217–222.

49. Sheppard HW, Ascher MS, Busch MP, et al. A multicenter proficiency trial of gene amplification (PCR) for the detection of HIV-1. J Acquired Immune Defic Syndr 1991;4:277–283.

50. Kelen GD, Chanmugam A, Meyer WA, et al. Detection of HIV-1 by polymerase chain reaction and culture in seronegative intravenous drug users in an inner-city emergency department. Ann Emerg Med 1993;22:769–775.

51. Yerly S, Chamot E, Déglon JJ, et al. Absence of chronic human immunodeficiency virus infection without seroconversion in intravenous drug users: a prospective and retrospective study. J Infect Dis 1991;164:965–968.

52. Brettler DB, Somasundaran M, Forsberg AF, et al. Silent human immunodeficiency virus type 1 infection: a rare occurrence in a high-risk heterosexual population. Blood 1993;80:2396–2400.

53. Eble BE, Busch MP, Khayam-Bashi H, et al. Resolution of infection status of human immunodeficiency virus (HIV)-seroindeterminate donors and high-risk seronegative individuals with polymerase chain reaction and virus culture: absence of persistent silent HIV type 1 infection in a high-prevalence area. Transfusion 1992;32:503–508.

54. Centers for Disease Control and Prevention. 1994 revised classification system for human immunodeficiency virus in children less than 13 years of age. MMWR 1994;43(RR-12):1–10.

55. De Rossi AD, Ades AE, Mammano F, et al. Antigen detection, virus culture, polymerase chain reaction, and in vitro antibody production in the diagnosis of vertically transmitted HIV-1 infection. AIDS 1991; 5:15–20.

56. Burgard M, Mayaux MJ, Blanche S, et al. The use of viral culture and p24 antigen testing to diagnose human immunodeficiency virus infection in neonates. N Engl J Med 1992;327:1192–1197.

57. Comeau AM, Harris JA, McIntosh K, et al. Polymerase chain reaction in detecting HIV infection among seropositive infants: relation to clinical status and age to results of other assays. J Acquired Immune Defic Syndr 1992;5:271–278.

58. Scarlatti G, Lombardi V, Plebani A, et al. Polymerase chain reaction, virus isolation and antigen assay in HIV-1 antibody-positive mothers and their children. AIDS 1991;5:1173–1178.

59. Report of a consensus workshop. Early diagnosis of HIV infection in infants. J Acquired Immune Defic Syndr 1992;5:1169–1178.

60. Quinn TC, Kline RL, Halsey N, et al. Early diagnosis of perinatal HIV infection by detection of viral-specific IgA antibodies. JAMA 1991;266:3439–3442.

61. Lindsay MK, Johnson N, Peterson HB, et al. Human immunodeficiency virus infection among inner-city adolescent parturients undergoing routine voluntary screening. Am J Obstet Gynecol 1992;167: 1096–1099.

62. Barbacci M, Repke JT, Chaisson RE. Routine prenatal screening for HIV infection. Lancet 1991;337: 709–711.

63. Lindgren S, Bohlin AB, Forsgren M, et al. Screening for HIV-1 antibodies in pregnancy: results from the Swedish national programme. BMJ 1993;307:1447–1451.

64. Hardy LM, ed. HIV screening of pregnant women and newborns. Committee on Prenatal and Newborn Screening for HIV Infection, Institute of Medicine. Washington, DC: National Academy Press, 1991.

65. American Academy of Pediatrics, Provisional Committee on Pediatric AIDS. Perinatal human immunodeficiency virus testing. Pediatrics 1995;95:303–307.

66. Bayer R. Ethical challenges posed by zidovudine treatment to reduce vertical transmission of HIV. N Engl J Med 1994;331:1223–1225.

67. El-Sadr W, Oleske JM, Agins BD, et al. Evaluation and management of early HIV infection. Clinical Practice Guideline no. 7. Rockville, MD: Agency for Health Care Policy and Research, 1994. (AHCPR Publication no. 94-0572.)

68. Washington AE, Kahn JG, Showstack JA, et al. Updated estimates of the impact and cost of HIV prevention in injection drug users. Final report from the Institute of Health Policy Studies, University of California, San Francisco to Centers for Disease Control and Prevention, Division of STD/HIV Prevention. San Francisco: Institute of Health Policy Studies, University of California, San Francisco, 1992.

69. Giesecke J, Ramstedt K, Granath F, et al. Efficacy of partner notification for HIV infection. Lancet 1991;338:1096–1100.

70. Fehrs LJ, Fleming D, Foster LR, et al. Trial of anonymous vs. confidential human immunodeficiency virus testing. Lancet 1988;2:379–382.

71. Centers for Disease Control and Prevention. Differences between anonymous and confidential registrants for HIV testing—Seattle, 1986–1992. MMWR 1993;42:53–56.

71a. Bayer R, Stryker J, Smith MD. Testing for HIV infection at home. N Engl J Med 1995;332:1296–1299.

72. Sheppard HW, Busch MP, Louie PH, et al. HIV-1 PCR and isolation in seroconverting and seronegative homosexual men: absence of long-term immunosilent infection. J Acquired Immune Defic Syndr 1993;6:1339–1346.

73. Withers BG, Kelley PW, McNeil JG. A brief review of the epidemiology of HIV in the US Army. Mil Med 1992;157:80–84.

74. Sande MA, Carpenter CCJ, Cobbs CG, et al. Antiretroviral therapy for adult HIV-infected patients. JAMA 1993;270:2583–2589.

75. Lundgren JD, Phillips AN, Pedersen C, et al. Comparison of long-term prognosis of patients with AIDS treated and not treated with zidovudine. JAMA 1994;271:1088–1092.

76. Erice A, Balfour HH. Resistance of human immunodeficiency virus type 1 to antiretroviral agents: a review. Clin Infect Dis 1994;18:149–156.

77. Bartlett JG. Zidovudine now or later? N Engl J Med 1993;329:351–352.

78. Gazzard BG. After Concorde: suggests no place for zidovudine as sole treatment for asymptomatic HIV positive patients. BMJ 1992;306:1016–1017.

79. Ioannidis JPA, Cappelleri JC, Lau J, et al. Early or deferred zidovudine therapy in HIV-infected patients without an AIDS-defining illness. Ann Intern Med 1995;122:856–866.

80. Volberding PA, Lagakos SW, Grimes JM, et al. The duration of zidovudine benefit in persons with asymptomatic HIV infection. JAMA 1994;272:437–442.

81. Concorde Coordinating Committee. Concorde: MRC/ANRS randomized double-blind controlled trial of immediate and deferred zidovudine in symptom-free HIV infection. Lancet 1994;343:871–881.

82. Lenderking WR, Gelber RD, Cotton DJ, et al. Evaluation of the quality of life associated with zidovudine treatment in asymptomatic human immunodeficiency virus infection. N Engl J Med 1994;330: 738–743.

83. Collier AC, Coombs RW, Fischl MA, et al. Combination therapy with zidovudine and didanosine compared with zidovudine alone in HIV-1 infection. Ann Intern Med 1993;119:786–793.

84. Johnson VA. Combination therapy: more effective control of HIV type 1? AIDS Res Hum Retroviruses 1994;10:907–912.

85. Phair J, Munoz A, Detels R, et al. The risk of Pneumocystis carinii pneumonia among men infected with human immunodeficiency virus type 1. N Engl J Med 1990;322:161–165.

86. Hirschel B, Lazzarin A, Chopard P, et al. A controlled study of inhaled pentamidine for primary prevention of Pneumocystis carinii pneumonia. N Engl J Med 1991;324:1079–1083.

87. Hutchinson CM, Wilson C, Reichart CA, et al. CD4 lymphocyte concentrations in patients with newly

identified HIV infection attending STD clinics. Potential impact on publicly funded health care resources. JAMA 1991;266:253–256.

88. Centers for Disease Control and Prevention. Recommendations for prophylaxis against Pneumocystis carinii pneumonia for adults and adolescents infected with human immunodeficiency virus. MMWR 1992;41(RR-4):1–11.

89. Wormser GP, Horowitz HW, Duncanson FP, et al. Low-dose intermittent trimethoprim-sulfamethoxazole for prevention of Pneumocystis carinii pneumonia in patients with human immunodeficiency virus infection. Arch Intern Med 1991;151:688–692.

90. Ruskin J, LaRiviere M. Low-dose co-trimoxazole for prevention of Pneumocystis carinii pneumonia in human immunodeficiency virus disease. Lancet 1991;337:468–471.

91. Graham NMH, Zeger SL, Park LP, et al. Effect of zidovudine and Pneumocystis carinii pneumonia prophylaxis on progression of HIV-1 infection to AIDS. Lancet 1991;338:266–269.

92. Hoover DR, Saah AJ, Bacellar H, et al. Clinical manifestations of AIDS in the era of Pneumocystis prophylaxis. N Engl J Med 1993;329:1922–1926.

93. Graham NMH, Zeger SL, Park LP, et al. The effects on survival of early treatment of human immunodeficiency virus infection. N Engl J Med 1992;326:1037–1042.

94. Osmond D, Charlebois E, Lang W, et al. Changes in AIDS survival time in two San Francisco cohorts of homosexual men, 1983 to 1993. JAMA 1994;271:1083–1087.

95. Bozzette SA, Finkelstein DM, Spector SA, et al. for the NIAID AIDS Clinical Trials Group. A randomized trial of three antipneumocystis agents in patients with advanced immunodeficiency virus infection. N Engl J Med 1995;332: 693–699.

96. Schneider MME, Hopelman AIM, Schattenkerk JK, et al. A controlled trial of aerosolized pentamidine or trimethoprim-sulfamethoxazole as primary prophylaxis against Pneumocystis carinii pneumonia in patients with human immunodeficiency virus infection. N Engl J Med 1992;327:1836–1841.

97. Centers for Disease Control and Prevention. USPHS/IDSA guidelines for the prevention of opportunistic infections in persons with human immunodeficiency virus: a summary. MMWR 1995;44(RR-8):1–34.

98. Girard PM, Landman R, Gaudebout C, et al. Dapsone-pyrimethamine compared with aerosolized pentamidine as primary prophylaxis against Pneumocystis carinii pneumonia and toxoplasmosis in HIV infection. N Engl J Med 1993;328:1514–1520.

99. Carr A, Tindall B, Brew BJ. Low-dose trimethoprim-sulfamethoxazole prophylaxis for toxoplasmic encephalitis in patients with AIDS. Ann Intern Med 1992;117:106–111.

100. Pape JW, Jean SS, Ho JL, et al. Effect of isoniazid prophylaxis on incidence of active tuberculosis and progression of HIV infection. Lancet 1993;342:268–272.

101. Selwyn PA, Sckell BM, Alcabes P, et al. High risk of active tuberculosis in HIV-infected drug users with cutaneous anergy. JAMA 1992;268:504–509.

102. Centers for Disease Control. Tuberculosis and human immunodeficiency virus infection; recommendations of the Advisory Committee for the Elimination of Tuberculosis (ACET). MMWR 1989;38:236–238, 243–250.

103. Centers for Disease Control. Purified protein derivative (PPD)-tuberculin anergy and HIV infection: guidelines for management of anergic persons at risk of tuberculosis. MMWR 1991;40(RR-5):1–5.

104. Hughes WT, Kuhn S, Chaudhary S, et al. Successful chemoprophylaxis for Pneumocystis carinii pneumonitis. N Engl J Med 1977;297:1419–1426.

105. Simonds RJ, Oxtoby MJ, Caldwell MB, et al. Pneumocystis carinii pneumonia among US children with perinatally acquired HIV infection. JAMA 1993;270:470–478.

106. European Collaborative Study. CD4 T cell count as predictor of Pneumocystis carinii pneumonia in children born to mothers infected with HIV. BMJ 1994;308:437–440.

107. Centers for Disease Control and Prevention. 1995 revised guidelines for prophylaxis against Pneumocystis carinii pneumonia for children infected or perinatally exposed to human immunodeficiency virus. MMWR 1995;44(RR-4):1–11.

108. Jewett JF, Hecht FM. Preventive health care for adults with HIV infection. JAMA 1993;269:1144–1153.

109. Gerber AR, Valdiseri RO, Holtgrave DR, et al. Preventive services guidelines for primary care clinicians caring for adults and adolescents infected with the human immunodeficiency virus. Arch Fam Med 1993;2:969–979.

110. O'Connor PG, Selwyn PA, Schottenfeld RS. Medical care for injection-drug users with human immunodeficiency virus infection. N Engl J Med 1994;331:450–459.

111. Centers for Disease Control and Prevention. Recommendations of the Advisory Committee on Im-

munization Practices (ACIP): use of vaccines and immunoglobulins for persons with altered immunocompetence. MMWR 1993; 42(RR-4):1–18.

112. Onorato IM, Markowitz LE, Oxtoby MJ. Childhood immunizations, vaccine-preventable diseases and infection with immunodeficiency virus. Pediatr Infect Dis J 1988;6:588–595.

113. Raiten DJ. Nutrition and HIV infection: a review and evaluation of the extant knowledge of the relationship between nutrition and HIV infection. Bethesda: Life Science Research Office of the Federation of American Societies for Experimental Biology, 1990.

114. American College of Obstetricians and Gynecologists. Human immunodeficiency virus infection. Technical Bulletin no. 169. Washington, DC: American College of Obstetricians and Gynecologists, 1992.

115. The European Collaborative Study. Caesarean section and risk of vertical transmission of HIV-1 infection. Lancet 1994;343:1464–1467.

116. Dunn DT, Newell ML, Ades ED, Peckham CS. Risk of human immunodeficiency virus type 1 transmission through breastfeeding. Lancet 1992;340:585–588.

117. Higgins DL, Galavotti C, O'Reilly KR, et al. Evidence for the effects of HIV antibody counseling and testing on risk behaviors. JAMA 1991;266:2419–2429.

118. Selwyn PA, Carter RJ, Schoenbaum EE, et al. Knowledge of antibody status and decisions to continue or terminate pregnancy among intravenous drug users, JAMA 1989;261:3567–3571.

119. Auerbach JD, Wypijewska C, Brodie HKH, eds. AIDS and behavior: an integrated approach. Committee on Substance Abuse and Mental Health Issues in AIDS Research, Division of Biobehavioral Sciences and Mental Disorders, Institute of Medicine. Washington, DC: National Academy Press, 1994.

120. Kamenga M, Ryder RW, Jingu M, et al. Evidence of marked sexual behavior change associated with low HIV-1 seroconversion in 149 married couples with discordant HIV-1 serostatus: experience at an HIV counseling center in Zaire. AIDS 1991;5:61–67.

121. Padian NS, O'Brien TR, Chang YC, et al. Prevention of heterosexual transmission of human immunodeficiency virus through couple counseling. J Acquired Immune Defic Syndr 1993;6:1043–1048.

122. Allen S, Tice J, Van de Perre P, et al. Effect of serotesting with counselling on condom use and seroconversion among HIV discordant couples in Africa. BMJ 1992;304:1605–1609.

123. Allen S, Serufilira A, Bogaerts J, et al. Confidential HIV testing and condom promotion in Africa. JAMA 1992;268:3338–3343.

124. Stall R. How to lose the fight against AIDS among gay men. BMJ 1994;309:685–686.

125. Fox R, Odaka NJ, Brookmeyer R, et al. Effect of HIV antibody disclosure on subsequent sexual activity in homosexual men. AIDS 1987;1:241–246.

126. van Griensven GJP, de Vroome EMM, Tielman RAP, et al. Impact of HIV antibody testing on changes in sexual behavior among homosexual men in the Netherlands. Am J Public Health 1988;78: 1575–1577.

127. McCusker J, Stoddard AM, Mayer KH, et al. Effects of HIV antibody test knowledge on subsequent sexual behaviors in a cohort of homosexually active men. Am J Public Health 1988;78:462–467.

128. Calzavara LM, Coates R, Johnson K, et al. Sexual behavior in a cohort of male sexual contacts of men with HIV disease: a three year overview. Can J Public Health 1991;82:151–156.

129. Calsyn DA, Saxon AJ, Freeman G, Whittaker S. Ineffectiveness of AIDS antibody testing in reducing high-risk behaviors among injection drug users. Am J Public Health 1992;82:573–575.

130. Watters JK, Estilo MJ, Clark GL, Lorvick J. Syringe and needle exchange as HIV/AIDS prevention for injection drug users. JAMA 1994;271:115–120.

131. Vanichseni S, Choopanya K, Des Jarlais DC, et al. HIV testing and sexual behavior among intravenous drug users in Bangkok, Thailand. J Acquired Immune Defic Syndr 1992;5:1119–1123.

132. Landis SE, Earp JL, Koch GG. Impact of HIV testing and counseling on subsequent sexual behavior. AIDS Educ Prev 1992;4:61–70.

133. Zenilman JM, Erickson B, Fox R, et al. Effect of HIV post-test counseling on STD incidence. JAMA 1992;267:843–845.

134. Otten MW, Zaidi AA, Wroten JE, et al. Changes in sexually transmitted disease rates after HIV testing and posttest counseling, Miami, 1988 to 1989. Am J Public Health 1993;83:529–533.

135. Wenger NS, Linn LS, Epstein M. Reduction of high-risk sexual behavior among heterosexuals undergoing HIV antibody testing: a randomized clinical trial. Am J Public Health 1991;81:1580–1584.

136. Wenger NS, Greenberg JM, Hilborne LH, et al. Effect of HIV antibody testing and AIDS education on communication about HIV risk and sexual behavior. Ann Intern Med 1992;117:905–911.

137. Ickovics JR, Morrill AC, Beren SE, et al. Limited effects of HIV counseling and testing for women. JAMA 1994;272:443–448.

138. Marks G, Richardson JL, Maldonado N, et al. Self-disclosure of HIV infection to sexual partners. Am J Public Health 1991;81:1321–1322.

139. Centers for Disease Control. Drug use and sexual behaviors among sex partners of injecting drug users—United States 1988–1990. MMWR 1991;40:855–860.

140. National Institute of Mental Health. Coping with AIDS: psychological and social considerations in helping people with HTLV-III infection. Rockville, MD: Alcohol, Drug Abuse, and Mental Health Administration, 1986. (Publication no. DHHS (ADM) 85-1432.)

141. Cleary PD, Van Decanter N, Rogers TF, et al. Depressive symptoms in blood donors notified of HIV infection. Am J Public Health 1993;83:534–539.

142. Lyketsos CG, Hoover DR, Guccione M, et al. Depressive symptoms as predictors of medical outcomes in HIV infection. JAMA 1993;270:2563–2567.

143. Herek GM, Capitano JP. Public reactions to AIDS in the United States: a second decade of stigma. Am J Public Health 1993;83:574–577.

144. Department of Health and Human Services. AIDS: A public health challenge. State issues, policies, and programs. Vol 1. Assessing the problem. Washington, DC: Intergovernmental Health Policy Project, 1987.

145. Canadian Task Force on the Periodic Health Examination. Canadian guide to clinical preventive health care. Ottawa: Canada Communication Group, 1994:708–718.

146. American Academy of Family Physicians. Age charts for periodic health examination. Kansas City, MO: American Academy of Family Physicians, 1994. (Reprint no. 510.)

147. American Medical Association. HIV blood test counseling. Physician guidelines. 2nd ed. Chicago: American Medical Association, 1993.

148. American College of Physicians and Infectious Disease Society of America. Human immunodeficiency virus (HIV) infection. Ann Intern Med 1994;120:310–319.

149. American Medical Association. Guidelines for adolescent preventive services (GAPS): recommendations and rationale. Chicago: American Medical Association, 1994.

150. Green M, ed. Bright Futures: national guidelines for health supervision of infants, children, and adolescents. Arlington, VA: National Center for Education in Maternal and Child Health, 1994.

151. Centers for Disease Control and Prevention. Recommendations for HIV testing services in inpatients and outpatients in acute-care hospital settings. MMWR 1993;42(RR-2):1–6.

152. Centers for Disease Control and Prevention. U.S. Public Health Service recommendations for human immunodeficiency virus counseling and voluntary testing for pregnant women. MMWR 1995;44(RR-7):1–15.

153. American College of Obstetricians and Gynecologists, Committee on Obstetric Practice. Zidovudine for the prevention of vertical transmission of human immunodeficiency virus. Committee Opinion no. 148. Washington, DC: American College of Obstetricians and Gynecologists, 1994.

154. McCarthy BD, Wong JB, Munoz A. Who should be screened for HIV infection? Arch Intern Med 1993;153:1107–1116.

155. Brown AE, Burke DS. Cost of HIV testing in the U.S. Army [letter]. N Engl J Med 1995;332:963.

156. Berrios DC, Hearst N, Coates TJ, et al. HIV antibody testing among those at risk for infection. The National AIDS Behavioral Surveys. JAMA 1993;270:1576–1580.

157. Task Force on Pediatric AIDS. Perinatal human immunodeficiency virus (HIV) testing. Pediatrics 1992;89:791–794.

158. Holtgrave DR, Valdiserri RO, Gerber AR, et al. Human immunodeficiency virus counseling, testing, referral, and partner notification services. Arch Intern Med 1993;153:1225–1230.

159. Centers for Disease Control and Prevention. Technical guidance on HIV counseling. MMWR 1993;42(RR-2):8–17.

29. Screening for Chlamydial Infection—*Including Ocular Prophylaxis in Newborns*

RECOMMENDATION

Routine screening for Chlamydia trachomatis infection is recommended for all sexually active female adolescents, high-risk pregnant women, and other asymptomatic women at high risk of infection (see *Clinical Intervention*). There is insufficient evidence to recommend for or against routine screening in asymptomatic men. Recommendations to screen selected high-risk male adolescents may be made on other grounds (see *Clinical Intervention*). Routine screening is not recommended for the general adult population. See Chapter 27 for recommendations regarding ocular prophylaxis to prevent ophthalmia neonatorum.

Burden of Suffering

Infection with *C. trachomatis* is the most common bacterial sexually transmitted disease (STD) in the U.S., affecting an estimated 4 million persons at a cost of $2.4 billion each year.[1,2] The medical consequences and costs of infection are greatest in women, who may develop urethritis, cervicitis, or pelvic inflammatory disease (PID; i.e., salpingitis or endometritis). Chlamydial infections are responsible for 25–50% of the 2.5 million cases of PID that are reported annually in the U.S.[3] PID is an important cause of infertility and ectopic pregnancy in American women and may lead to chronic pelvic pain. Data from other countries suggest that infection with chlamydia may be a cofactor in heterosexual transmission of HIV infection.[4] In men, chlamydia is responsible for 30–40% of the 4–6 million visits each year for nongonococcal urethritis and half of over 150,000 cases of acute epididymitis.[1]

Up to 25% of men and 70% of women with chlamydial infection are asymptomatic.[5] Immunologic surveys suggest that chlamydial infection increases the risk of infertility and ectopic pregnancy even in women who never develop clinical PID, most likely because the symptoms of salpingitis may be mild or nonspecific.[1] Asymptomatic infections in men and women also serve as an important reservoir for new infections.

Age is the strongest demographic predictor of chlamydial infection. Men and women under 25 account for the large majority of cases,[6] and prevalence of infection is highest among young women age 15–19. Although risk factors for chlamydia are similar to those for other STDs, chlamydia is distinct in that the prevalence of infection is substantial (>5%) among sexually active female adolescents in general, regardless of race, place of residence, or socioeconomic status.[1,7] For example, infection was present in 5–8% of North American female college students at student health clinics[8,9] and 8–26% of teenage girls attending adolescent clinics.[10,11] The high risk in young women probably reflects both behavioral and physiologic factors (increased exposure of cervical columnar epithelium in young women).[12] Other important risk factors for chlamydial infection include having multiple sex partners, a new sex partner, or an infected sex partner; inconsistent use of barrier contraceptives; and cervical ectopy on examination.[1,7,13–18] Among 1,800 women ages 15–34 screened in a health maintenance organization, marital status was the single strongest predictor of infection: prevalence was less than 1% among married women, 7% among single women, and 3–4% among those divorced or living as married.[15] Chlamydial infection is more prevalent among blacks than among whites or Hispanics.[15,19] In routine screening, women with vaginal discharge, cervicitis, or cervical friability (i.e., bleeding induced by swab) were more likely to be infected.[7,15] Chlamydial infection is common among women with other STDs, incarcerated women,[20] and women seeking abortions.[21] In high-risk urban communities, chlamydia was detected in 6–11% of asymptomatic, sexually active male adolescents.[22,23]

The overall prevalence of chlamydial infection among pregnant women in the U.S. is estimated to be about 5%, but it varies widely (0–37%), depending on age and other risk factors.[24] Many sites serving younger women and high-risk urban communities have reported a substantially higher prevalence of infection (10–25%).[25,26] Infection during pregnancy increases the risk of endometritis, both after delivery and after elective abortion.[1,27] Each year more than 155,000 infants are born to chlamydia-infected mothers, and the organism is transmitted to the fetus in over half of deliveries.[24] Neonatal infection can result in ophthalmia neonatorum and pneumonia.

Accuracy of Screening Tests

The most specific test for chlamydial infection in asymptomatic persons is culture. Urethral and endocervical cultures have been estimated to have a sensitivity of about 70–90% and a specificity of 100%.[1,22] In addition to its variable sensitivity, culture is expensive, not uniformly available, requires careful handling of specimens, and takes 3–7 days for results. In one study, one fourth of women with positive cultures did not return for therapy.[28] In men, screening with culture requires obtaining specimens with urethral swabs, which is unacceptable to many asymptomatic men.[22]

A variety of nonculture tests are now available, offering the advantages of easier handling and processing, lower costs, wider availability, and more timely results. Commercially available tests employ enzyme immunoassay (EIA), direct fluorescent antibody (DFA), DNA probe, polymerase chain reaction (PCR), or solid-phase colorimetric assays[28] to detect chlamydia in urethral or cervical specimens. Tests using ligase chain reaction (LCR) are awaiting Food and Drug Administration (FDA) approval.[29] Of these tests, EIA and DFA tests have been most widely evaluated, with reported sensitivities of 70–90% and high specificity (97–99%).[1] False-positive EIA results may result from cross-reaction with other vaginal flora or urinary pathogens, but confirmation of positive tests using blocking antibody increases specificity to close to 100%. Studies in STD clinics indicate that DNA probe, PCR, and LCR can each be very sensitive and specific (>95%).[30,31] Sensitivity of commercial PCR and DNA probe kits was significantly lower (60–75%) in some studies,[32,33] however, and the performance of these assays for screening asymptomatic patients needs further evaluation. The arrival of competitively priced, commercial kits is likely to make these increasingly popular alternatives to chlamydia culture.

The ability to detect chlamydial infection in centrifuged, first-void urine specimens may make screening asymptomatic men more feasible.[22–24] Urine dipsticks can detect leukocyte-esterase (LE) activity, an indicator of urethritis or upper urinary infections. However, the sensitivity of LE testing for chlamydial infection is variable (40–100%),[1] and the low predictive value of LE in asymptomatic young men (11% in one study[22]) necessitates use of confirmatory tests. Testing urine specimens with EIA is more sensitive (77–91%) and specific (97–100%), but it substantially increases the cost per confirmed case.[22,34] PCR and LCR assays appear to have the highest sensitivity and specificity (95–99%) for chlamydia using urine specimens.[23,29,35] A recent study reported that LCR assays of urine were also very sensitive and specific for chlamydial infection in women (94% and 99.9%, respectively).[36]

Even with highly specific tests, the likelihood that a positive result indicates true infection varies with the prevalence of infection in the population being screened. Assuming a sensitivity of 80% and specificity of 98%, the positive predictive value of a test will range from 82% when prevalence of chlamydia is high (10%), to only 45% when prevalence is low (2%). As a result, independent confirmation of positive results from some nonculture tests may be necessary to prevent false-positive results in low-risk patients.

In prospective studies of screening in low-risk populations, risk scores based on age, other risk factors, and findings on physical examination successfully identified a subpopulation of high-risk women (prevalence 6% or higher) who accounted for the large majority of all infections.[15,16,37]

Effectiveness of Early Detection

Early detection of chlamydial infections in asymptomatic persons permits initiation of antibiotic therapy to eradicate infection. The benefits of detecting and treating asymptomatic infection in pregnancy have been demonstrated in several large cohort studies of high-risk women screened at the first prenatal visit.[26,38] Infected women who received erythromycin had significantly lower rates of preterm delivery, rupture of membranes, and low birth weight compared to infected women who were untreated or treatment failures. In one study, treatment was associated with lower perinatal mortality among children.[26] Some of the benefit may have been due to effects of erythromycin on pathogens other than *Chlamydia* or underlying differences between treated and untreated women.

Eradication of asymptomatic infection is also likely to reduce the complications of chlamydial infection in nonpregnant women. Proving a benefit on long-term se-quelae of infection (e.g., infertility and ectopic pregnancy) is difficult, but a recent trial in a large health maintenance organization demonstrated that at-risk women randomized to receive routine chlamydia screening were less than half as likely to develop PID over the next year (1% vs. 2.2%).[37] Hospitalizations for PID also declined in Sweden in association with increased chlamydia screening, but other changes in sexual behavior are likely to have contributed to this trend.[39] Treatment effectively eradicates chlamydial infection, but it has traditionally required an extended course of medication. A 7-day course of tetracycline or doxycycline results in a short-term cure in 92–100% of women and 97–100% of men.[1] Single-dose therapy with azithromycin is as effective as doxycycline and may be a suitable alternative when noncompliance is a concern.[40] The benefits of early detection are limited by high rates of reinfection or treatment failure in some populations.[1] In follow-up studies of adolescent women treated for chlamydia, 26–39% are infected 2–5 years later.[41,42] Treatment failures are usually due to failure to treat sex partners, noncompliance with therapy, or reinfection. Referral of sex partners of cases is important, since up to one third of male partners, and a majority of female partners, are infected.[5]

Chlamydia may cause epididymitis, but serious complications of chlamydial infection are uncommon in men. Although screening and treating high-risk young men has the potential to reduce the incidence of chlamydia, the impact of routine screening in men has not been examined prospectively, or compared to the current strategy of screening women and treating male partners. A variety of other factors will influence whether screening men will significantly reduce the incidence of new infections: duration of asymptomatic period, rates of transmission from asymptomatic men to their female partners, compliance with treatment, and rates of re-infection in young men.

Ocular Prophylaxis in Newborns

Between 20% and 50% of all infants born to infected mothers develop chlamydial conjunctivitis, but there is conflicting evidence of the benefit of universal ocular prophylaxis with topical antibiotics (erythromycin, tetracycline, or silver nitrate) after birth to reduce the incidence of chlamydial ophthalmia neonatorum.[43–45] In a recent trial in Kenya, where maternal chlamydial infection is common, povidone-iodine was significantly more effective than erythromycin or silver nitrate for preventing chlamydial conjunctivitis in newborns.[46] The failure rate of ocular prophylaxis for chlamydia has been estimated to be 7–19%, and chlamydial ophthalmia (unlike gonococcal ophthalmia) is rarely associated with serious ocular complications.[45] In a trial among infants born to low-risk American women, prophylaxis with silver nitrate or erythromycin reduced the incidence of conjunctivitis compared to placebo (8–9% vs. 15%); regardless of treatment, however, most cases were mild and due to organisms other than chlamydia.[47]

Recommendations of Other Groups

Screening for chlamydia in asymptomatic sexually active female adolescents (under 20 years old), and in other women with risk factors for infection, is recommended by the Centers for Disease Control and Prevention (CDC),[1] the American College of Obstetricians and Gynecologists (ACOG),[48] the American Academy of Pediatrics (AAP),[49] Bright Futures,[50] the American Medical Association,[51] the American Academy of Family Physicians (AAFP),[52] and the Canadian Task Force for the Periodic Health Examination (CTF);[53] AAFP recommendations are under review. Some of these organizations also make these recommendations for adolescent males and young men at high risk. Risk factors cited by various organizations include age under 25, new or multiple sex partners in the past 3 months, inconsistent use of barrier contraception, the presence of mucopurulent cervicitis or cervical friability, the diagnosis of other STDs, and others. An expert panel convened in 1994 by the Institute of Medicine, National Academy of Sciences, is developing recommendations for public health strategies to control STDs, including chlamydia.

The CTF recommends that all pregnant women be screened for asymptomatic chlamydial infection.[53] Both ACOG and CDC recommend screening with chlamydial culture in high-risk pregnant women (including those under age 25), at the initial prenatal visit and/or in the third trimester.[1,48] No major organization recommends routine screening of the general population. The CDC, CTF, AAP, and AAFP all recommend routine ocular antibiotic prophylaxis for all newborns, primarily to prevent ophthalmia neonatorum due to *Neisseria gonorrhoeae* rather than *Chlamydia* (see Chapter 27).[1,45,49,52] Ocular prophylaxis is required by law in most states in the U.S.

Discussion

The substantial long-term morbidity from chlamydia in women, the high prevalence of asymptomatic infection, and the availability of reliable screening tests and effective treatments all suggest that screening for asymptomatic chlamydial infection may be a useful strategy. There is now preliminary evidence from one trial that screening high-risk asymptomatic, nonpregnant women can reduce the incidence of PID. Screening and treatment of infected women and their partners is also likely to reduce the incidence of new infections, although conclusive proof of this is not available. While high-risk sexual behavior is an important determinant of risk of chlamydial infection, the generally high prevalence of chlamydia among sexually active female adolescents supports routine screening in this population.[7]

The optimal criteria for screening other women depend on the local burden of disease and resources available for screening. Risk of infection depends on both individual sexual behavior and the prevalence of chlamydia in the community. Where the prevalence of infection is documented to be low (<5%), targeting screening to women with multiple risk factors for infection may be most efficient. Because self-reported sexual history is often an unreliable indicator of risk, however, broader screening of young women may be preferable in practices or communities where chlamydia is highly prevalent.

There is fair evidence that treatment of chlamydial infection during pregnancy is associated with improved outcomes for both infants and mothers. Due to the low prevalence of infection in women who are older or married, universal screening is not indicated in pregnancy. Since the primary benefit of treatment in pregnancy is to prevent perinatal and postpartum complications, screening high-risk women in the third trimester is likely to be effective and reduce the opportunity for reinfection prior to delivery. Although ocular prophylaxis appears to reduce the risk of chlamydial ophthalmia neonatorum, screening and treating high-risk mothers may be a more effective means of preventing chlamydial infections in newborn infants.

Screening is less likely to benefit asymptomatic men, but screening young men using urine-based tests (LE, EIA, or PCR) may be a useful strategy to prevent spread of infection in communities where chlamydia is common. Whether routine screening in men is effective in reducing the incidence of chlamydial infection deserves further study, however.

Nonculture methods are appropriate alternatives to cell culture for diagnosis of infection. The choice of optimal testing strategy will depend on available resources, the prevalence of chlamydia, and the potential adverse consequences of false-positive diagnoses. Newer methods such as PCR or LCR are likely to offer advantages due to improved sensitivity and specificity; further evaluations of new commercial test kits are needed in asymptomatic populations before specific recommendations can be made.

Cost-effectiveness analyses have concluded that screening for chlamydia with nonculture tests is cost-effective during routine gynecologic visits[54-56] and during pregnancy[57] when prevalence of infection exceeds 6–8%. Others have suggested that screening is cost-effective at even lower prevalence.[13] Screening asymptomatic adolescent males with urine-based tests was calculated to be cost-saving, primarily by reducing infections in female partners, but has not been compared to the current strategy of screening women.[34]

CLINICAL INTERVENTION

Routine screening for asymptomatic infection with *Chlamydia trachomatis* during pelvic examination is recommended for all sexually active female adolescents and for other women at high risk for chlamydial infection ("B" recommendation). Patient characteristics associated with a higher prevalence of infection include: history of prior STD, new or multiple sex partners, age under 25, inconsistent use of barrier contraceptives, cervical ectopy, and being unmarried. Actual risk will depend on number of risk factors and local epidemiology of chlamydial infection. Clinicians may wish to consult local public health authorities for guidance in identifying high-risk populations within their community. Algorithms to identify high-risk women have been published.[15,16] In clinical settings where the prevalence of infection is known to be high (e.g., some urban family planning clinics), routine screening of all women is appropriate. Clinicians should remain alert for findings suggestive of chlamydial infection (e.g., mucopurulent discharge, cervical erythema, or cervical friability) during pelvic examination of asymptomatic women.

Pregnant women at high risk of infection (including age under 25) should be tested for chlamydia ("B" recommendation). The optimal tim-

ing of screening in pregnancy is uncertain. There is insufficient evidence to recommend for or against screening all women during pregnancy ("C" recommendation).

There is insufficient evidence to recommend for or against routine screening in high-risk men ("C" recommendation). In clinical settings where asymptomatic infection is highly prevalent in men (e.g., urban adolescent clinics), screening sexually active young men may be recommended on other grounds, including the potential to prevent transmission to uninfected sex partners. Routine screening for chlamydia is not recommended in the general population of low-risk adults ("D" recommendation).

In women, endocervical specimens should be obtained for cell culture or nonculture assays. Verification of positive nonculture results may be necessary, depending on the underlying risk in the patient and potential adverse consequences of a false-positive result. The choice of screening test for asymptomatic men is left to clinical discretion. Urine LE dipstick is much less expensive than urine assays using EIA, PCR, or LCR, but it is also less sensitive and specific for asymptomatic chlamydial infection. The optimal frequency of testing has not been determined for women or men and is left to clinical discretion.

Routine ocular antibiotic prophylaxis with silver nitrate, erythromycin, or tetracycline is recommended for all newborn infants to prevent ophthalmia neonatorum due to gonorrhea and is required by law in most states (see Chapter 27). There is insufficient evidence to recommend for or against universal ocular prophylaxis of newborns solely for the prevention of chlamydial conjunctivitis ("C" recommendation).

The draft update of this chapter was prepared for the U.S. Preventive Services Task Force by David Atkins, MD, MPH, based in part on background materials prepared by H. Oladele Davies, MD, MSc, FRCPC, and Richard B. Goldbloom, MD, FRCPC, for the Canadian Task Force on the Periodic Health Examination.

REFERENCES

1. Centers for Disease Control and Prevention. Recommendations for the prevention and management of *Chlamydia trachomatis* infections, 1993. MMWR 1993;42(RR-12):1–39.
2. Washington AE, Katz P. Cost of and payment sources for pelvic inflammatory disease. Trends and projections, 1983 through 2000. JAMA 1991;266:2565–2569.
3. Rolfs RT, Galaid EI, Zaidi AA. Pelvic inflammatory disease: trends in hospitalizations and office visits, 1979 through 1988. Am J Obstet Gynecol 1992;166:983–990.
4. Plummer FA, Simonsen JN, Cameron DW, et al. Cofactors in male-female sexual transmission of human immunodeficiency virus type 1. J Infect Dis 1991;163:233–239.
5. Cates W, Wasserheit JN. Genital chlamydial infections: epidemiology and reproductive sequelae. Am J Obstet Gynecol 1991;164:1771–1781.
6. Zimmerman HL, Potterat JJ, Dukes RL, et al. Epidemiologic differences between chlamydia and gonorrhea. Am J Public Health 1990;80:1338–1342.
7. Vincelette J, Baril JG, Allard R. Predictors of chlamydial infection and gonorrhea among patients seen by private practitioners. Can Med Assoc J 1991;144:713–721.
8. Swinker M, Young S, Cleavenger R, et al. Prevalence of *Chlamydia trachomatis* cervical infection in a col-

lege gynecological clinic: relationship to other infections and clinical features. Sex Transm Dis 1988;15: 133–136.

9. McCormack W, Rosner B, McComb D, et al. Infection with *Chlamydia trachomatis* in female college students. Am J Epidemiol 1985;121:107–115.

10. Fraser J, Rettig P, Kaplan D. Prevalence of cervical *Chlamydia trachomatis* and *Neisseria gonorrhoeae* in female adolescents. Pediatrics 1983;71:333–336.

11. Chacko M, Lovchik J. *Chlamydia trachomatis* infection in sexually active adolescents: prevalence and risk factors. Pediatrics 1984;73:836–840.

12. Stamm WE, Mårdh PA. *Chlamydia trachomatis*. In: Holmes KK, Mårdh PA, Sparling PF, Wiesner PJ, eds. Sexually transmitted diseases. 2nd ed. New York: McGraw-Hill, 1990:917–926.

13. Handsfield HH, Jasman LL, Roberts PL, et al. Criteria for selective screening of *Chlamydia trachomatis* infection in women attending family planning clinics. JAMA 1986;255:1730–1734.

14. Masse R, Lapierre H, Rousseau H, Lefebvre J, Remis R. *Chlamydia trachomatis* cervical infection: prevalence and determinants among women presenting for routine gynecologic examination. Can Med Assoc J 1991;145:953–961.

15. Stergachis A, Scholes D, Heidrich FE, et al. Selective screening for *Chlamydia trachomatis* infection in a primary care population of women. Am J Epidemiol 1993;138:143–153.

16. Rosenthal GE, Mettler G, Pare S, et al. A new diagnostic index for predicting cervical infection with either *Chlamydia trachomatis* or *Neisseria gonorrhoeae*. J Gen Intern Med 1990;5:319–326.

17. Johnson BA, Poses RM, Fortner CA, et al. Derivation and validation of a clinical diagnostic model for chlamydial cervical infection in university women. JAMA 1990;264:3161–3165.

18. Phillips RS, Hanff PA, Holmes MD, et al. *Chlamydia trachomatis* cervical infections in women seeking routine gynecological care: criteria for selective testing. Am J Med 1989;86:515–520.

19. Centers for Disease Control and Prevention. Chlamydial prevalence and screening practices—San Diego County, California, 1993. MMWR 1994;43:366–369, 375.

20. Holmes MD, Sayfer SM, Bickell NA, et al. Chlamydia cervical infection in jailed women. Am J Public Health 1993;83:551–555.

21. Amortegul A, Meyer M, Gnatuk C. Prevalence of *Chlamydia trachomatis* and other microorganisms in women seeking abortions in Pittsburgh, Pennsylvania, United States of America. Genitourin Med 1992; 62:88–92.

22. Shafer M, Schacter J, Moncada J, et al. Evaluation of urine-based screening strategies to detect *Chlamydia trachomatis* among sexually active asymptomatic young males. JAMA 1993;270:2065–2070.

23. Jaschek G, Gaydos CA, Welsh LA, Quinn TC. Direct detection of *Chlamydia trachomatis* in urine specimens from symptomatic and asymptomatic men by using rapid polymerase chain reaction assay. J Clin Microbiol 1993;31:1209–1212.

24. Smith JR, Taylor-Robinson D. Infection due to *Chlamydia trachomatis* in pregnancy and the newborn. Ballieres Clin Obstet Gynaecol 1993;7:237–355.

25. Maguire N, Jordan A, Ehya H. Detection of *Chlamydia trachomatis* in cervical smears from pregnant population. Arch Pathol Lab Med 1990;114:204–207.

26. Ryan GJ, Abdella T, McNeeley G, Baselski V, Drummond D. *Chlamydia trachomatis* infection in pregnancy and effect of treatment on outcome. Am J Obstet Gynecol 1990;162:34–39.

27. Blackwell AL, Thomas PD, Wareham K, Emery SJ. Health gains from screening for infection of the lower genital tract in women attending for termination of pregnancy. Lancet 1993;342:206–210.

28. Hook EW III, Spitters C, Reichart CA, et al. Use of cell culture and a rapid diagnostic assay for *Chlamydia trachomatis* screening. JAMA 1994;272:867–870.

29. Chernesky M, Lee H, Schachter J, et al. Diagnosis of *Chlamydia trachomatis* urethral infection in symptomatic and asymptomatic men by testing first-void urine in a ligase chain reaction assay. J Infect Dis 1994;170:1308–1311.

30. Vogels WH, van Voorst Vader PC, Schroder FP. *Chlamydia trachomatis* infection in a high-risk population: comparison of polymerase chain reaction and cell culture for diagnosis and follow-up. J Clin Microbiol 1993;31:1103–1107.

31. Warren R, Dwyer B, Plackett M, et al. Comparative evaluation of detection assays for *Chlamydia trachomatis*. J Clin Microbiol 1993;31:1663–1666.

32. Bauwens JE, Clark AM, Stamm WE. Diagnosis of *Chlamydia trachomatis* endocervical infections by a commercial polymerase chain reaction assay. J Clin Microbiol 1993;31:3023–3027.

33. Blanding J, Hirsch L, Stranton N, et al. Comparison of the Clearview chlamydia, the PACE 2 assay, and culture for the detection of *Chlamydia trachomatis* from cervical specimens in a low-prevalence population. J Clin Microbiol 1993;31:1622–1625.

34. Genc M, Ruusuvaara L, Mårdh P. An economic evaluation of screening for *Chlamydia trachomatis* in adolescent males. JAMA 1993;270:2057–2064.
35. Bauwens JE, Clark AM, Loeffelholz MJ, et al. Diagnosis of *Chlamydia trachomatis* urethritis in men by polymerase chain reaction assay of first-catch urine. J Clin Microbiol 1993;31:3013–3016.
36. Lee HH, Chernesky MA, Schachter J, et al. Diagnosis of *Chlamydia trachomatis* genitourinary infection in women by ligase chain reaction assay of urine. Lancet 1995;345:213–216.
37. Scholes D, Stergachis A, Heidrich FE, et al. Selective screening for chlamydia reduces the incidence of pelvic inflammatory disease: results from a randomized intervention trial. In: Orfila J, Byrne GI, Chernesky MA, et al, eds. Chlamydia infections: proceedings of the Eighth International Symposium on Human Chlamydia Infections. Bologna: Societa Editrice Esculapio, 1994.
38. Cohen L, Veille J-C, Calkins B. Improved pregnancy outcomes following successful treatment of chlamydial infection. JAMA 1990;263:3160–3163.
39. Westrom L. Decrease in incidence of women treated in hospital for acute salpingitis in Sweden. Genitourin Med 1988;64:59–63.
40. Martin DH, Mroczkowski TF, Dalu ZA, et al. A controlled trial of a single dose of azithromycin for the treatment of chlamydial urethritis and cervicitis. N Engl J Med 1992;327:921–925.
41. Jones RB. Treatment of *Chlamydia trachomatis* infections of the urogenital tract. In: Bowie WR, Caldwell HD, Jones RP, et al, eds. Chlamydia infections: proceedings of the Seventh International Symposium on Human Chlamydial Infections. Cambridge: Cambridge University Press, 1990:509–518.
42. Hillis SD, Nakashima A, Marchbanks PA, et al. Risk factors for recurrent *Chlamydia trachomatis* infections in women. Am J Obstet Gynecol 1994;170:801–806.
43. Hammerschlag MR, Chandler JW, Alexander ER, et al. Erythromycin ointment for ocular prophylaxis of neonatal chlamydial infection. JAMA 1980;244:2291–2293.
44. Hammerschlag MR, Cummings C, Robilin P, et al. Efficacy of neonatal ocular prophylaxis for the prevention of chlamydial and gonorrheal conjunctivitis. N Engl J Med 1989;320:769–772.
45. Canadian Task Force on the Periodic Health Examination. Periodic health examination, 1992 update: 4. Prophylaxis for gonococcal and chlamydial ophthalmia neonatorum. Can Med Assoc J 1992;147:1449–1454.
46. Isenberg SJ, Apt L, Wood M. A controlled trial of povidone-iodine as prophylaxis against ophthalmia neonatorum. N Engl J Med 1995;332:562–566.
47. Bell TA, Grayston JT, Krohn A, et al. Randomized trial of silver nitrate, erythromycin, and no eye prophylaxis for the prevention of conjunctivitis among newborns not at risk for gonococcal ophthalmitis. Pediatrics 1993;92:755–760.
48. American College of Obstetricians and Gynecologists. Gonorrhea and chlamydial infections. Technical Bulletin no. 190. Washington, DC: American College of Obstetricians and Gynecologists, 1994.
49. American Academy of Pediatrics. 1994 Red Book: report of the Committee on Infectious Diseases. 23rd ed. Elk Grove Village, IL: American Academy of Pediatrics, 1994.
50. Green M, ed. Bright Futures: guidelines for health supervision of infants, children and adolescents. Arlington, VA: National Center for Education in Maternal and Child Health, 1994.
51. American Medical Association. AMA guidelines for adolescent preventive services (GAPS): recommendations and rationale. Chicago: American Medical Association, 1994.
52. American Academy of Family Physicians. Age charts for periodic health examination. Kansas City, MO: American Academy of Family Physicians, 1994. (Reprint no. 510.)
53. Canadian Task Force on the Periodic Health Examination. Canadian guide to clinical preventive health care. Ottawa: Canada Communication Group, 1994:168–175, 732–742.
54. Phillips RS, Aronson MD, Taylor WC, et al. Should tests for *Chlamydia trachomatis* cervical infection be done during routine gynecologic visits? An analysis of the costs of alternative strategies. Ann Intern Med 1987;107:188–194.
55. Nettleman MD, Jones RB. Cost-effectiveness of screening women at moderate risk for genital infections caused by *Chlamydia trachomatis*. JAMA 1988;260:207–213.
56. Estany A, Todd M, Vasques M, McLaren R. Early detection of genital chlamydial infection in women: an economic evaluation. Sex Transm Dis 1989;16:21–27.
57. Nettleman M, Bell T. Cost-effectiveness of prenatal screening for *Chlamydia trachomatis*. Am J Obstet Gynecol 1991;164:1289–1294.

30. Screening for Genital Herpes Simplex

RECOMMENDATION

Routine screening for genital herpes simplex virus (HSV) infection by viral culture or other tests is not recommended for asymptomatic persons, including asymptomatic pregnant women. There is insufficient evidence to recommend for or against the examination of pregnant women in labor for signs of active genital HSV lesions, although recommendations to do so may be made on other grounds (see *Clinical Intervention*). See Chapter 62 for recommendations on counseling to prevent sexually transmitted diseases.

Burden of Suffering

Primary genital herpes simplex virus (HSV) infection occurs in approximately 200,000–500,000 Americans each year,[1] mostly in adolescents and young adults. Between 25 and 31 million individuals are chronically infected.[1,2] Both HSV types 1 (HSV-1) and 2 (HSV-2) can infect the genitalia, but HSV-2 causes the majority of primary and recurrent genital herpes infections.[3] Most HSV-2 infections are asymptomatic, detected only by seroconversion;[4,5] 16% of the adult population is HSV-2 seropositive.[2] In symptomatic genital herpes, the chief clinical morbidity is painful, pruritic vesicles that may coalesce into large ulcerative lesions.[3] Systemic symptoms, such as fever, headache, myalgia, and malaise, are reported by two thirds of patients with primary first-episode genital herpes, and serious complications such as meningitis (reported in 8%) may ensue.[3] After initial infection, the virus enters a latent state in spinal cord ganglia. Infected persons may periodically experience viral reactivations that can be asymptomatic, characterized by viral shedding alone, or symptomatic, marked by a recurrence of signs and symptoms that are less severe than those of primary genital herpes.[3] The sexual contacts of individuals with either symptomatic or asymptomatic disease are at risk of becoming infected.[6]

In pregnant women, the rate of genital herpes reported as a maternal risk factor on birth certificates is 8.0/1,000 live births.[7] Pregnant women with genital HSV infection can transmit the virus to their newborns. The majority (82–87%) of neonatal infections occur during delivery, but some also occur in utero or postnatally.[8–10] In 1984 it was estimated that the minimum annual incidence of neonatal HSV infections in the United States, based on voluntary reporting, was 4/100,000 live births;[11] intensive local surveillance in one county in Washington found a rate of 12/100,000 live births.[12] One fourth of HSV-infected neonates develop disseminated disease and one third have encephalitis.[13,14] Even with antiviral treatment, the mortality rate is 57% among infants with disseminated disease and 15% among those with encephalitis.[13] Severe neurologic impairment occurs in about one third of those who survive encephalitis or disseminated disease.[13,14] Among infants with infection apparently limited to mucocutaneous involvement, death or severe impairment is rare but other complications such as visual impairment or seizures occur in about 5%.[13,14]

Accuracy of Screening Tests

History and physical examination are not adequate screening tests for either active (i.e., transmissible) or latent genital HSV infection, because most infected persons are asymptomatic;[4,5,15] their clinical manifestations may resemble a number of other causes of genital ulcerations;[16] and viral shedding in association with recurrent disease may be asymptomatic.[3,17]

The most commonly used test for detecting active genital HSV infection is viral culture. The sensitivity of this test is variable, however, depending upon the viral titer present, ranging in one study from 93% for vesicles to 72% for ulcers and 27% for crusted lesions, and from 82% for ulcerative lesions in first episodes to 43% for ulcerative lesions in recurrent episodes.[16,18] Since the viral titer in asymptomatic shedding is 10–100 times less than that in symptomatic episodes,[17] the sensitivity of viral culture for detecting HSV infection in asymptomatic individuals is likely to be low. In addition, conventional viral culture is time-consuming and technically demanding, and only 40–48% of positive results are available within 24 hours.[19–21] Viral culture techniques may be modified to produce final test results within 16–24 hours, but sensitivity is then reduced by 5–20% compared with final conventional culture results in symptomatic patients;[20–24] sensitivity is likely to be reduced further in asymptomatic patients.

Other rapid screening methods, such as cytology and direct fluorescent antibody staining, are widely available but are substantially less sensitive than is conventional viral culture.[6] Newer methods, not yet licensed for clinical diagnostic testing for HSV, include enzyme immunoassay (EIA), polymerase chain reaction (PCR), and DNA hybridization. EIA and PCR show concordance of >93% with the results of conventional viral culture in symptomatic women.[25–28] In one study in asymptomatic pregnant women, PCR had a reported concordance of 100% with conventional culture.[27] EIA, however, had a concordance of only 59% with conventional viral culture in a large study of samples taken primarily from "presumed asymptomatic" pregnant women.[25] EIA can provide results within several hours, whereas even with automated techniques PCR currently requires more than a day to process and is extremely labor intensive. Both EIA and PCR may react with nonviable virus or viral particles,[25-28] thus overestimating the risk of infectivity. Results from studies of DNA hybridization appear less promising, with a sensitivity of 25% and specificity of 88% compared to conventional culture,[22] and 43% and 71%, respectively, compared to cytology,[29] on samples from symptomatic patients.

An estimated 35–80% of infants with neonatal herpes are born to women with no known history of genital herpes or physical signs of infection at delivery.[10,12,13] Therefore, screening asymptomatic pregnant women has the potential of identifying unrecognized active HSV infections. In order for routine screening at the onset of labor to be useful for clinical decision making regarding surgical or medical intervention to prevent neonatal herpes, rapid and accurate methods of detecting asymptomatic HSV infections likely to be transmitted would be needed. The yield of routine screening by viral culture in asymptomatic pregnant women is quite low; large-scale screening studies have isolated HSV by culture from only 0.20–0.35% at the time of delivery.[30-32] A positive viral culture does not necessarily mean an infant will become infected during delivery. The risk of acquiring neonatal herpes infection from an asymptomatic pregnant woman with active viral shedding from reactivated disease is less than 5%, whereas from a woman with first-episode genital disease the risk is 33%.[31] A negative culture, however, does not eliminate an infant's risk of infection. In one large cohort study, the mothers of 30% (3 of 10) of the infected newborns were culture negative at the time of delivery,[31] and in a case series of infants with neonatal herpes, 61% (54 of 89) of the pregnant women had negative cultures within the 2 weeks before delivery.[33] In asymptomatic women with a history of recurrent herpes, surveillance cultures during the 4 weeks before delivery did not correlate with viral shedding at delivery.[34] Thus, screening near term is not adequate to predict accurately the likelihood of HSV transmission from asymptomatic pregnant women to their offspring.

Antibody testing can accurately distinguish HSV-seropositive from HSV-seronegative persons and therefore may be useful to detect asymptomatic carriers at potential risk for transmitting disease, as well as persons susceptible to primary infection. Commercial assays are insensitive to recent infections, however, and they are unreliable for distinguishing HSV-2 from HSV-1 antibodies.[35,36] Antibody test results do not indicate whether the virus is currently capable of being transmitted.

Effectiveness of Early Detection

The detection of HSV infection in asymptomatic, nonpregnant individuals would be useful if treatment were available to either eradicate latent HSV infection or to prevent transmission to sex partners by eliminating or reducing viral shedding. There is currently no effective treatment for eradicating latent herpes infection. Both episodic and continuous oral acyclovir reduce viral shedding, lesion healing time, and local and systemic symptoms during symptomatic primary first-episode and recurrent genital HSV infections.[37-42] When used continuously for up to 4 years, oral acyclovir produces only minor side effects and minimal emergence of resistant strains in immunologically normal individuals.[41-43] The beneficial effects of acyclovir on lesion healing and viral shedding in symptomatic individuals have not been documented to prevent or reduce transmission to sex partners, however. Based on a single, small before-after study, oral acyclovir does not appear to prevent asymptomatic viral shedding,[44] and no studies have evaluated its ability to decrease infectivity and disease transmission during episodes of asymptomatic shedding.

Routine screening for HSV-2 antibodies may be useful to identify persons with previously unrecognized infection,[4] who could then be instructed in the recognition of recurrent episodes. Such instruction results in recognition of clinically symptomatic genital herpes on follow-up in 50% of seropositive persons with previously unrecognized infection.[45] Counseling seropositive persons to avoid sexual activity or to use condoms during symptomatic episodes may reduce transmission of herpes to their sex partners.[45,46] Among a series of 144 couples with one partner with recurrent herpes and one without antibody, all of whom were advised to abstain from skin-to-skin contact during active episodes and about the risks of transmission during asymptomatic periods, acquisition of genital herpes occurred in 6% who used barrier contraception and 14% who did not (p = 0.19), but only 15% of couples used condoms routinely.[47] Although not specifically designed to evaluate counseling, this study suggests a limited benefit from knowledge of susceptibility. The effectiveness of this strategy in preventing HSV-2 transmission has not been evaluated adequately; it may not provide any incremental benefit over routine counseling of all sexually active adults regarding prevention of sexually transmitted diseases.[48]

The early detection of active HSV infection may be of greater importance during pregnancy because cesarean delivery can be performed. This has the potential to reduce the exposure of the neonate to virus in the birth canal that occurs during vaginal delivery, although the evidence for the effectiveness of this intervention is limited. Small, uncontrolled case series of symptomatic women with positive genital cultures during the 1-2 weeks before delivery[49,50] or with positive cervical cultures at the time of delivery[51] suggest a protective effect of cesarean deliveries; no controlled trials have evaluated this intervention. None of these studies differentiated primary from recurrent infections, which have different rates of HSV transmission. Cesarean delivery is clearly not completely effective, since large case series of newborns infected with HSV reveal that 19–33% of them were delivered by cesarean delivery.[11,33,52] Information concerning the effectiveness of cesarean delivery in preventing neonatal herpes transmission by asymptomatic pregnant women comes from a large cohort study that screened such women by viral culture during early labor.[31] In this study, 8% (1 of 13) of infants delivered by cesarean delivery to culture-positive women became infected, compared to 14% (6 of 43) of infants delivered vaginally to culture-positive women. Drawing conclusions from this study is difficult, however, because sample size was insufficient to establish statistical significance; reasons for selection of vaginal delivery are not given; and differences between the two groups in the proportions of primary versus recurrent infections, site of positive culture (i.e., cervical vs. other), and duration of rupture of membranes are not delineated. Thus, the benefit of cesarean delivery in either symptomatic or asymptomatic culture-positive women is not established.

Even if cesarean delivery does offer some benefit in preventing the transmission of HSV to newborns, more definitive studies would be needed to determine the proper indications for abdominal delivery. For example, it is not clear whether cesarean delivery would be indicated when the risk of herpes transmission is low, e.g., in the setting of asymptomatic viral shedding, recurrent symptomatic disease, or when labial but not cervical cultures are positive.[31,34,51,53] In these relatively low-risk situations, the potential benefit to the fetus of averting HSV infection may not outweigh the known risk of complications in the mother and infant due to cesarean delivery. In cohort studies, cesarean delivery has been associated with increases in both maternal morbidity and mortality compared to vaginal delivery,[54–56] even when stratified by maternal diagnosis. A 1993 decision analysis model calculated that cesarean delivery for herpes lesions at delivery in women with recurrent genital HSV leads to 1,580 excess (i.e., performed solely to prevent HSV transmission) cesarean deliveries for every neonate saved from death or neurologic sequelae, and 0.57 maternal deaths for every neonatal death prevented; total costs were $2.5 million per case of HSV averted, and $203,000 per quality adjusted life-year (QALY) gained.[57] These estimates are sensitive to risk of vertical transmission (estimated to be 1%) and to the efficacy of cesarean delivery (estimated to be 80%); reductions in either of these could result in maternal deaths exceeding neonatal mortality. The decision analysis results change dramatically if only women with primary HSV infections are entered. In women with herpes lesions at delivery but no previous history of genital HSV, nine excess cesarean deliveries would be performed for every neonate saved, with 0.004 maternal deaths per neonatal death prevented, at a total savings of more than $38,000, saving $2600 per QALY gained. Net benefits persisted across all likely ranges of values entered into the model.

Serologic screening may prove useful for the prevention of primary HSV-2 infections in pregnancy. One study screened pregnant women and their partners for type-specific antibodies to herpes, and found that 10% (18 of 190) of the women were seronegative with seropositive partners, and therefore were at risk of contracting a primary HSV-2 infection during pregnancy; 7 of 18 couples continued to have unprotected intercourse after being informed of their serologic status, and 1 of the 7 seroconverted during pregnancy.[5] Studies evaluating the effectiveness of counseling such couples to abstain from sexual intercourse or to use condoms regularly during pregnancy to prevent neonatal herpes transmission have not been performed.

Another potential strategy for preventing the transmission of HSV to newborns is offering prophylactic acyclovir to pregnant women with recurrent herpes. A case series of 15 pregnant women with recurrent genital herpes demonstrated that suppressive treatment with acyclovir after 38 weeks of gestation was well tolerated with no toxicity to the mothers or infants.[58] None of the women experienced new symptomatic recurrences or asymptomatic viral shedding after beginning treatment and none of their infants developed neonatal infection. In a pilot randomized controlled trial, women with recurrent herpes who received acyclovir continuously at least 1 week before expected term had significantly fewer HSV recurrences/positive cultures and a significantly lower rate of cesarean delivery for herpes.[59] Four randomized controlled studies are currently being conducted, in the United States, Norway, and England, to determine the effectiveness and safety of prophylactic acyclovir in reducing the risks of asymptomatic shedding, cesarean delivery, and neonatal transmission when given in late pregnancy to women with histories of recurrent herpes (H. Watts, personal communication, July 1995; L. Scott, personal communication, July 1995).[60,61] Although acyclovir has not been found to be teratogenic in standard animal testing, and no recognizable pattern of birth defects has been detected among 601 reported cases of exposure during pregnancy, current data are only sufficient to exclude a teratogenic risk of at least 2-fold over the 3% baseline risk of birth defects.[62,63]

Recommendations of Other Groups

The American College of Obstetricians and Gynecologists,[64] the American Academy of Pediatrics,[65] the Canadian Task Force on the Periodic Health Examination,[66] and the Infectious Disease Society of America[67] recommend against surveillance cultures for herpes infections in asymptomatic pregnant women. All four groups suggest careful examination of all women at the time of delivery and culture of active lesions, with cesarean delivery for women with positive findings on clinical examination.[64-67] No organizations currently recommend screening for genital herpes simplex virus or antibody in the asymptomatic general population.

Discussion

There are currently no commercially available tests that are adequate to detect latent HSV-2 infections in asymptomatic patients. Even if accurate type-specific serology becomes widely available, there is no proven treatment to eradicate latent infection or to eliminate viral shedding in order to prevent disease transmission. Similarly, there is limited evidence that counseling persons known to have HSV offers any benefit over routine counseling of all sexually active adults to prevent sexually transmitted diseases. Evidence does not therefore support screening the asymptomatic general population for HSV infection.

For pregnant women (and those planning conception), the potential benefit of detecting asymptomatic and unrecognized HSV infection is the prevention of neonatal HSV transmission. The risk of transmitting HSV to their infants is slightly increased in pregnant women with asymptomatic shedding of HSV due to reactivated disease at delivery, and it is substantially increased in women with primary HSV infection at delivery. Culture results at the onset of labor are rarely available in time to affect clinical decision making, and there is good evidence that positive viral cultures in the weeks prior to delivery do not accurately predict the risk of neonatal HSV transmission. More rapid tests that could be performed at the onset of labor are either substantially less sensitive than culture or not yet widely available. Women with primary first-episode HSV infection at delivery are more likely to present with symptoms and signs detectable by physical examination, but such examinations have not been shown to be sensitive or specific. Even if the diagnosis of HSV is made by physical examination during labor, the evidence supporting the effectiveness of cesarean delivery in preventing neonatal HSV transmission is of poor quality, while there is fair evidence that cesarean delivery increases risk to the mother and fetus compared to vaginal delivery. A recent decision analysis predicts that if cesarean delivery prevents 85% of neonatal HSV infections that occur following vaginal delivery, a physical examination at labor for symptoms or signs of genital herpes would minimize the ratio of excess cesarean deliveries to cases of neonatal HSV infection averted, compared to other screening methods or no screening.[68] Another model that evaluated performing a physical examination at delivery, followed by cesarean delivery for women with genital herpes lesions, found clear evidence of benefit only for women with no history of genital herpes.[57] For women with recurrent herpes, the risk to the mother may outweigh that to the neonate, depending on assumptions made about the efficacy of cesarean delivery and the likely HSV transmission rate.

The use of acyclovir in pregnancy to reduce neonatal HSV has not been adequately evaluated, but trials are ongoing.

Although a history of genital herpes does not accurately predict HSV seropositivity, if the pregnant woman who lacks such a history has a partner known to have genital herpes, counseling to prevent HSV transmission to the woman could prevent primary HSV infection, thereby preventing neonatal HSV at little cost or risk to the patient. When commercially available, HSV serotyping at the first prenatal visit with serotesting of the partners of those who are HSV-2 seronegative would allow more accurate detection of pregnant women at risk for primary HSV infection. The effectiveness of counseling such women regarding primary prevention has not been demonstrated, however.

CLINICAL INTERVENTION

Routine screening for genital herpes simplex in asymptomatic persons, using culture, serology, or other tests, is not recommended ("D" recommendation). See Chapter 62 for recommendations on counseling to prevent sexually transmitted diseases.

Routine screening for genital herpes simplex infection in asymptomatic pregnant women, by surveillance cultures or serology, is also not recommended ("D" recommendation). Clinicians should take a complete sexual history on all adolescent and adult patients (see Chapter 62).

As part of the sexual history, clinicians should consider asking all pregnant women at the first prenatal visit whether they or their sex partner(s) have had genital herpetic lesions. There is insufficient evidence to recommend for or against routine counseling of women who have no history of genital herpes, but whose partners do have a positive history, to use condoms or abstain from intercourse during pregnancy ("C" recommendation); such counseling may be recommended, however, on other grounds, such as the lack of health risk and potential benefits of such behavior.

There is also insufficient evidence to recommend for or against the examination of all pregnant women for signs of active genital HSV lesions during labor and the performance of cesarean delivery on those with lesions ("C" recommendation); recommendations to do so may be made on other grounds, such as the results of decision analyses and expert opinion. There is not yet sufficient evidence to recommend for or against routine use of systemic acyclovir in pregnant women with recurrent herpes to prevent reactivations near term ("C" recommendation).

The draft update of this chapter was prepared for the U.S. Preventive Services Task Force by Paul Denning, MD, MPH, and Carolyn DiGuiseppi, MD, MPH.

REFERENCES

1. Centers for Disease Control and Prevention, Division of STD/HIV Prevention. 1993 annual report. Atlanta: Centers for Disease Control and Prevention, 1994.
2. Johnson RE, Nahmias AJ, Magder LS, et al. A seroepidemiologic survey of the prevalence of herpes simplex virus type 2 infection in the United States. N Engl J Med 1989;321:7–12.
3. Corey L, Adams HG, Brown ZA, et al. Genital herpes simplex virus infections: clinical manifestations, course, and complications. Ann Intern Med 1983;98:973–983.
4. Koutsky LA, Stevens CE, Holmes KK, et al. Underdiagnosis of genital herpes by current clinical and viral-isolation procedures. N Engl J Med 1992;326:1533–1539.
5. Kulhanjian JA, Soroush V, Au DS, et al. Identification of women at unsuspected risk of primary infection with herpes simplex virus type 2 during pregnancy. N Engl J Med 1992;326:916–920.
6. Mertz GJ. Genital herpes simplex virus infections. Med Clin North Am 1990;74:1433–1454.
7. Ventura SJ, Martin JA, Taffel SM, et al. Advance report of final natality statistics. Monthly vital statistics report; vol 43 no 5 (suppl). Hyattsville, MD: National Center for Health Statistics, 1994.
8. Baldwin S, Whitley RJ. Teratogen update: intrauterine herpes simplex virus infection. Teratology 1989;39:1–10.
9. Hutto C, Arvin A, Jacobs R, et al. Intrauterine herpes simplex virus infections. J Pediatr 1987;110: 97–101.
10. Yeager AS, Arvin AM. Reasons for the absence of a history of recurrent genital infections in mothers of neonates infected with herpes simplex virus. Pediatrics 1984;73:188–193.
11. Stone KM, Brooks CA, Guinan ME, et al. National surveillance for neonatal herpes simplex virus infections. Sex Transm Dis 1989;16:152–156.
12. Sullivan-Bolyai J, Jull HF, Wilson C, et al. Neonatal herpes simplex virus infection in King County, Washington: increasing incidence and epidemiologic correlates. JAMA 1983;250:3059–3062.
13. Whitley R, Arvin A, Prober C, et al. Predictors of morbidity and mortality in neonates with herpes simplex virus infections. The National Institute of Allergy and Infectious Diseases Collaborative Antiviral Study Group. N Engl J Med 1991;324:450–454.
14. Whitley R, Arvin A, Prober C, et al. A controlled trial comparing vidarabine with acyclovir in neonatal herpes simplex virus infection. N Engl J Med 1991;324:444–449.
15. Koelle DM, Benedetti J, Langenberg A, et al. Asymptomatic reactivation of herpes simplex virus in women after the first episode of genital herpes. Ann Intern Med 1992;116:433–437.
16. Corey L, Holmes KK. Genital herpes simplex virus infections: current concepts in diagnosis, therapy, and prevention. Ann Intern Med 1983;98:973–983.
17. Corey L, Spear PG. Infections with herpes simplex viruses (pt 1 of 2). N Engl J Med 1986;314:686–691.
18. Mosely RC, Corey L, Benjamin D, et al. Comparison of viral isolation, direct immunofluorescence, and indirect immunoperoxidase techniques for detection of genital herpes simplex virus infection. J Clin Microbiol 1981;13:913–918.
19. Zimmerman SJ, Moses E, Sofat N, et al. Evaluation of a visual, rapid, membrane enzyme immunoassay for the detection of herpes simplex virus antigen. J Clin Microbiol 1991;29:842–845.
20. Espy MJ, Wold AD, Jespersen DJ, et al. Comparison of shell vials and conventional tubes seeded with rhabdomyosarcoma and MRC-5 cells for the rapid detection of herpes simplex virus. J Clin Microbiol 1991;29:2701–2703.
21. Johnston SL, Siegel CS. Comparison of enzyme immunoassay, shell vial culture, and conventional cell culture for the rapid detection of herpes simplex virus. Diagn Microbiol Infect Dis 1990;13:241–244.
22. Seal LA, Toyama PS, Fleet KM, et al. Comparison of standard culture methods, a shell vial assay, and a DNA probe for the detection of herpes simplex virus. J Clin Microbiol 1991;29:650–652.
23. Johnson FB, Luker G, Chow C. Comparison of shell vial culture and the suspension-infection method for the rapid detection of herpes simplex viruses. Diagn Microbiol Infect Dis 1993;16:61–66.
24. Johnson FB, Visick EM. A rapid culture alternative to the shell-vial method for the detection of herpes simplex virus. Diagn Microbiol Infect Dis 1992;15:673–678.
25. Verano L, Michalski FJ. Herpes simplex virus antigen direct detection in standard virus transport medium by DuPont Herpchek enzyme-linked immunosorbent assay. J Clin Microbiol 1990;28: 2555–2558.
26. Baker DA, Pavan-Langston D, Gonik B, et al. Multicenter clinical evaluation of the DuPont Herpchek HSV ELISA, a new rapid diagnostic test for the direct detection of herpes simplex virus. Adv Exp Med Biol 1990;263:71–76.

27. Hardy DA, Arvin AM, Yasukawa LL, et al. Use of polymerase chain reaction for successful identification of asymptomatic genital infection with herpes simplex virus in pregnant women at delivery. J Infect Dis 1990;162:1031–1035.

28. Gonik B, Seibel M, Berkowitz A, et al. Comparison of two enzyme-linked immunosorbent assays for detection of herpes simplex virus antigen. J Clin Microbiol 1991;29:436–438.

29. Kobayashi TK. Comparison of immunocytochemistry and in situ hybridization in the cytodiagnosis of genital herpetic infection. Diagn Cytopathol 1992;8:53–60.

30. Simkovich JW, Soper DE. Asymptomatic shedding of herpesvirus during labor. Am J Obstet Gynecol 1988;158: 588–589.

31. Brown ZA, Benedetti J, Ashley R, et al. Neonatal herpes simplex virus infection in relation to asymptomatic maternal infection at the time of labor. N Engl J Med 1991;324:1247–1252.

32. Prober CG, Hensleigh PA, Boucher FD, et al. Use of routine viral cultures at delivery to identify neonates exposed to herpes simplex virus. N Engl J Med 1988;318:887–891.

33. Whitley RJ, Corey L, Arvin A, et al. Changing presentation of herpes simplex virus infection in neonates. J Infect Dis 1988;158:109–116.

34. Arvin AM, Hensleigh PA, Prober CG, et al. Failure of antepartum maternal cultures to predict the infant's risk of exposure to herpes simplex virus at delivery. N Engl J Med 1986;315:796–800.

35. Nahmias AJ, Lee FK, Pereira L, et al. Monoclonal antibody immunoaffinity purified glycoprotein for the detection of herpes simplex virus type 1 and type 2 specific antibodies in serum. In: Lopez C, Roizman B, eds. Human herpesvirus infections: pathogenesis, diagnosis, and treatment. New York: Raven Press, 1986:203–210.

36. Ashley R, Cent A, Maggs V, et al. Inability of enzyme immunoassays to discriminate between infections with herpes simplex virus types 1 and 2. Ann Intern Med 1991;115:520–526.

37. Bryson YJ, Dillon M, Lovett M, et al. Treatment of first episodes of genital herpes simplex virus infection with oral acyclovir. N Engl J Med 1983;308:916–921.

38. Nilsen AE, Aasen T, Halsos AM, et al. Efficacy of oral acyclovir in the treatment of initial and recurrent genital herpes. Lancet 1982;2:571–573.

39. Mertz GJ, Critchlow CW, Benedetti J, et al. Double-blind placebo-controlled trial of oral acyclovir in first-episode genital herpes simplex virus infection. JAMA 1984;252:1147–1151.

40. Reichman RC, Badger GJ, Mertz GJ, et al. Treatment of recurrent genital herpes simplex infections with oral acyclovir: a controlled trial. JAMA 1984;251:2103–2107.

41. Baker DA, Blythe JG, Kaufman R, et al. One-year suppression of frequent recurrences of genital herpes with oral acyclovir. Obstet Gynecol 1989;73:84–87.

42. Kaplowitz LG, Baker D, Gelb L, et al. Prolonged continuous acyclovir treatment of normal adults with frequently recurring genital herpes simplex virus infection. JAMA 1991;265:747–751.

43. Molin L, Ruhnek-Forsbeck M, Svennerholm B. One year acyclovir suppression of frequently recurring genital herpes: a study of efficacy, safety, virus sensitivity and antibody response. Scand J Infect Dis Suppl 1991;80:33–39.

44. Straus SE, Seidlin M, Takiff HE, et al. Effect of oral acyclovir treatment on symptomatic and asymptomatic virus shedding in recurrent genital herpes. Sex Transm Dis 1989;16:107–113.

45. Langenberg A, Benedetti J, Jenkins J, et al. Development of clinically recognizable genital lesions among women previously identified as having "asymptomatic" herpes simplex virus type 2 infection. Ann Intern Med 1989;110: 882–887.

46. Corey L, Koutsky LA. Underdiagnosis of genital herpes [letter]. N Engl J Med 1992;327:1099.

47. Mertz GJ, Benedetti J, Ashley R, et al. Risk factors for the sexual transmission of genital herpes. Ann Intern Med 1992;116:197–202.

48. Kaplan J. Underdiagnosis of genital herpes [letter]. N Engl J Med 1992;327:1098–1099.

49. Grossman JH, Wallen WC, Sever JL. Management of genital herpes simplex virus infection during pregnancy. Obstet Gynecol 1981;58:1–4.

50. Boehm FH, Estes W, Wright PF, et al. Management of genital herpes simplex virus infection occurring during pregnancy. Am J Obstet Gynecol 1981;141:735–740.

51. Nahmias AJ, Josey WE, Naib ZM, et al. Perinatal risk associated with maternal genital herpes simplex virus infection. Am J Obstet Gynecol 1971;110:825–834.

52. Koskiniemi M, Happonen J-M, Jarvenpaa A-L, et al. Neonatal herpes simplex virus infection: a report of 43 patients. Pediatr Infect Dis J 1989;8:30–35.

53. Prober CG, Sullender WM, Yasukawa LL, et al. Low risk of herpes simplex virus infections in neonates exposed to the virus at the time of vaginal delivery to mothers with recurrent genital herpes simplex virus infections. N Engl J Med 1987;316:240–244.

54. Bashore RA, Phillips WH Jr, Brinkman CR 3d. A comparison of the morbidity of midforceps and cesarean delivery. Am J Obstet Gynecol 1990;162:1428–1434.

55. Petitti DB, Cefalo RC, Shapiro S, et al. In-hospital maternal mortality in the United States: time trends and relation to method of delivery. Obstet Gynecol 1982;59:6–12.

56. Lehmann DK, Mabie WC, Miller JM Jr, et al. The epidemiology and pathology of maternal mortality: Charity Hospital of Louisiana in New Orleans, 1965–1984. Obstet Gynecol 1987;69:833–840.

57. Randolph AG, Washington AE, Prober CG. Cesarean delivery for women presenting with genital herpes lesions. Efficacy, risks, and costs. JAMA 1993;270:77–82.

58. Frenkel LM, Brown ZA, Bryson YJ, et al. Pharmacokinetics of acyclovir in the term human pregnancy and neonate. Am J Obstet Gynecol 1991;164:569–576.

59. Stray-Pedersen B. Acyclovir in late pregnancy to prevent neonatal herpes simplex [letter]. Lancet 1990;336:756.

60. Brocklehurst P, Carney O, Helson K, et al. Acyclovir, herpes, and pregnancy [letter]. Lancet 1990;336:1594–1595.

61. Stray-Pedersen B. Acyclovir, herpes, and pregnancy [letter]. Lancet 1990;336:1595.

62. Eldridge R, Andrews E, Tilson H, et al. Pregnancy outcomes following systemic prenatal acyclovir exposure—June 1, 1984–June 30, 1993. MMWR 1993;42:806–809.

63. Centers for Disease Control. Sexually transmitted diseases: treatment guidelines. Atlanta: Centers for Disease Control, 1989:14–16.

64. American College of Obstetricians and Gynecologists. Perinatal herpes simplex virus infections. Technical Bulletin no. 122. Washington, DC: American College of Obstetricians and Gynecologists, 1988:1–5.

65. American Academy of Pediatrics. Herpes simplex. In: Peter G, ed. 1994 Red Book: report of the Committee on Infectious Diseases. 23rd ed. Elk Grove Village, IL: American Academy of Pediatrics, 1994:242–252.

66. Canadian Task Force on the Periodic Health Examination. Canadian guide to clinical preventive health care. Ottawa: Canada Communication Group, 1994:108–115.

67. Prober CG, Corey L, Brown ZA, et al. The management of pregnancies complicated by genital infections with herpes simplex virus. Clin Infect Dis 1992;15:1031–1038.

68. Libman MD, Dascal A, Kramer MS, et al. Strategies for the prevention of neonatal infection with herpes simplex virus: a decision analysis. Rev Infect Dis 1991;13:1093–1104.

31. Screening for Asymptomatic Bacteriuria

RECOMMENDATION

Screening for asymptomatic bacteriuria by urine culture is recommended for all pregnant women (see *Clinical Intervention*). There is insufficient evidence to recommend for or against routine screening for asymptomatic bacteriuria in diabetic or ambulatory elderly women, but recommendations against such screening may be made on other grounds. Routine screening for asymptomatic bacteriuria in other persons is not recommended.

Burden of Suffering

Asymptomatic bacteriuria is defined as a significant bacterial count (usually $\geq 10^5$ or 10^6 organisms/mL) present in the urine of a person without symptoms. Asymptomatic bacteriuria may precede symptomatic urinary tract infection, characterized by dysuria, frequency, pain, fever, etc., which accounts for over 6 million outpatient visits each year.[1] Urinary tract infection may be associated with renal insufficiency and increased mortality in adults, but these complications rarely occur among those without underlying structural and functional diseases of the urinary tract.[2] In both institutionalized and noninstitutionalized elderly, urinary tract infection is the most common cause of bacteremia, which may be associated with a 10–30% case fatality rate.[3,4] Most such bacteremia occurs in residents with indwelling catheters or urinary tract abnormalities, however. Similarly, most of the 300,000 hospitalizations each year for urinary tract infections[1] involve patients with indwelling urethral catheters.

In children, asymptomatic bacteriuria may be a sign of underlying urinary tract abnormalities. About 10–35% of infants and children with asymptomatic bacteriuria have vesicoureteral reflux and 6–37% have renal scarring or other abnormalities (the lower prevalences generally reflecting more stringent definitions of abnormality),[2,5–8] whereas such abnormalities are uncommon in the general population of children.[2,9] Children with major structural abnormalities, chronic pyelonephritis, or severe vesicoureteral reflux are at increased risk of renal scarring, obstructive renal atrophy, hypertension, and renal insufficiency.[2] Pyelonephritis, reflux nephropathy, and urinary tract malformations may cause as much as one

347

fifth of cases of renal failure in children.[10] In pregnancy, 13–27% of untreated women with asymptomatic bacteriuria develop pyelonephritis, usually requiring hospitalization for treatment.[11–14] Bacteriuria in pregnant women increases the risk for preterm delivery and low birth weight about 1.5–2-fold, and may also increase the risk of fetal and perinatal mortality.[15–23]

The risk of acquiring bacteriuria varies with age and sex. Asymptomatic bacteriuria in term infants is more common in males (estimated prevalence of 2.0–2.9% vs. 0.0–1.0% in females), but it is considerably more common in girls after age 1 (0.7–2.7% in girls vs. 0.0–0.4% in boys).[2,5–8,24] Approximately 5–6% of girls have at least one episode of bacteriuria between first grade and their graduation from high school, and as many as 80% of these children experience recurrent infections.[2] Asymptomatic bacteriuria in adulthood is more prevalent in women than men (3–5% vs. <1% in those under 60 years), and its prevalence increases with age.[25–27] Asymptomatic bacteriuria is a common finding in older persons, especially those who are very old (20% of women and 10% of men >80 years old living in the community) or institutionalized (30–50% of women and 20–30% of men).[3,4] Bacteriuria occurs in 2–7% of pregnant women; of those who are not bacteriuric at initial screening, 1–2% will develop bacteriuria later in the pregnancy.[28–30] An increased prevalence of asymptomatic bacteriuria (about 10–20%) has been reported in asymptomatic diabetic women, although several studies have found no increase when compared to matched nondiabetic controls or to expected age- and sex-specific population rates.[2,31–34]

Accuracy of Screening Tests

The most accurate test for bacteriuria is urine culture, but laboratory charges make this test expensive for routine screening in populations that have a low prevalence of asymptomatic bacteriuria. The most commonly used tests for detecting bacteriuria in asymptomatic persons are dipstick urinalysis and direct microscopy. The dipstick test is rapid, inexpensive, and requires little technical expertise. The dipstick leukocyte esterase (LE) test, which detects esterases released from degraded white blood cells, is an indirect test for bacteriuria. When compared with culture (at least 100,000 organisms/mL), it has a sensitivity of 72–97% and a specificity of 64–82%.[35–40] The nitrite reduction test, which detects nitrites produced by urinary bacteria (usually limited to Gram-negative bacteria), has variable sensitivity (35–85%) but good specificity (92–100%).[35–39,41–49] In children, dipstick testing for LE and/or nitrites has been found to have sensitivity and specificity of around 80% compared to quantitative culture.[50–57] Among pregnant women, a sensitivity of only 50% for dipstick testing compared to culture has been reported.[30] False-positive and false-negative urinalysis results are due to a variety of factors, including specimen contamination, certain organisms, and the timing of specimen collection. The sensitivity of this test can be improved by obtaining first-morning specimens, preferably on consecutive days, instead of performing random collection.[41] Many of the studies assessing the accuracy of dipstick testing in children and adults do not describe the patients included. A proportion of these patients were undoubtedly symptomatic, possibly leading to bias in the accuracy estimates. In one study, dipstick sensitivity was significantly lower (56% vs. 92%) and specificity significantly higher (78% vs. 42%) in patients with few symptoms and a low prior probability of bacteriuria, compared to patients with a high prior probability of bacteriuria (i.e., those with dysuria, frequency, etc.).[58]

Examination of the sediment by microscopic urinalysis to detect bacteria and white blood cells has also been evaluated as a screening test for bacteriuria. In children (including symptomatic patients), microscopy performs similarly to dipstick testing for detection of bacteriuria.[50] In pregnant women, microscopic analysis, with either bacteriuria or pyuria indicating a positive test, had a sensitivity of 83% but a specificity of only 59%.[30] In hospitalized adults, only 3% of urine specimens that were macroscopically (including dipstick) negative had clinically significant abnormalities detected by routine microscopic examination.[59,60] Microscopy has limited value as a screening test for asymptomatic persons because of the cost, time, and technique required.[30]

In populations with a low prevalence of urinary tract disorders, most positive screening tests are falsely positive. Thus, in asymptomatic men, and in asymptomatic women under age 60, a dipstick test has a positive predictive value for significant bacteriuria of less than 10% (assuming a sensitivity of 85% and a specificity of 70%).[20,25,43] In children, the likelihood of bacteriuria in the presence of a positive dipstick screening test has been estimated at 0.1% for boys and 4% for girls.[57] In groups at increased risk for urinary tract infection, the positive predictive value of dipstick tests is higher: 13% in pregnant women, 18% in women over age 60, 33% in diabetic women, and 44% in institutionalized older persons.[20,25,29,32,41,43,61-64] The predictive value of bacteriuria found on microscopic urinalysis among pregnant women was 4.2–4.5%.[30]

Urine screening tests are generally performed on a clean-catch specimen. In infants and young children, collection of a "clean" urine specimen is difficult, and as a result few studies of the accuracy of screening tests have included infants. Adhesive polyethylene bag specimens are the most acceptable choice, but these may have a significant contamination rate (false positives). Compared to suprapubic aspiration, positive results on bag specimens indicate true bacteriuria in only 7.5% of specimens.[65] The collection of confirmatory sterile culture specimens by suprapubic aspiration or urethral catheterization is too invasive and costly to be considered in a screening protocol for asymptomatic infants, as is routine screening by urethral catheterization.

Effectiveness of Early Detection

The early detection of asymptomatic bacteriuria may reduce the rate of bacteriuria and prevent symptomatic infection and its complications. Some observational studies suggest that persons with untreated asymptomatic bacteriuria are at increased risk of developing symptomatic urinary tract infection[66,67] and other complications (e.g., structural damage, renal insufficiency, hypertension, or mortality).[41,61–64,68–71] Evidence is not conclusive, however, that these clinical outcomes are caused by bacteriuria (especially in the absence of a structural abnormality), or that early treatment results in important clinical benefits. A randomized placebo-controlled trial of conventional treatment for asymptomatic bacteriuria in both **young and middle-aged women** (ages 20–65) reported no significant differences in the prevalence of bacteriuria or incidence of symptomatic urinary tract infection at 1-year follow-up.[66] Another randomized controlled trial (available only in abstract form) among women ages 16–69 years with asymptomatic bacteriuria reported significant reductions in bacteriuria at 1 and 3 years with vigorous individualized antimicrobial therapy, but did not report on clinical outcomes.[72] Among a cohort of middle-aged women (38–60 years) screened for asymptomatic bacteriuria, the prevalence of asymptomatic bacteriuria at 6-year follow-up in women identified with asymptomatic bacteriuria and appropriately treated remained significantly higher than in the nonbacteriuric group (23% vs. 5%) and 58% of the treated women had recurrent or persistent infection within 2 years of treatment.[25] Studies evaluating the treatment or natural history of asymptomatic bacteriuria are not available for **young or middle-aged men.**

Randomized controlled trials in **institutionalized elderly women**[73] **and men**[74] found no decreases in genitourinary morbidity with treatment of asymptomatic bacteriuria despite a reduced prevalence of bacteriuria. In both studies, life-table analyses suggested a survival advantage for the untreated group, but the differences were not statistically significant. In women, treatment was associated with an increased incidence of adverse antimicrobial drug effects and increased reinfections.[73]

Among noninstitutionalized **ambulatory elderly women**, a randomized controlled trial reported that treatment significantly reduced the prevalence of bacteriuria at 6-month follow-up.[67] Symptomatic urinary tract infection and mortality rates were 16.4% and 4.9%, respectively, without treatment, compared to 7.9% and 3.2%, respectively, with treatment, but these differences were not statistically significant; sample size may have been inadequate to detect a difference, however. In a nonrandomized controlled trial in noninstitutionalized elderly women, treatment of asymptomatic bacteriuria did not significantly reduce mortality (adjusted relative risk 0.92, 95% confidence interval, 0.57 to 1.57), although wide confidence intervals do not exclude the possibility of a substantial benefit.[75] A large cohort study from the same center reported no association between asymptomatic bacteriuria and mortality in ambulatory elderly women after control for confounding, even though the cure rate with treatment was 83% compared to a 16% spontaneous remission rate in untreated patients.[75] It is not clear whether the possible but unproven benefits from treatment of such women justify routine screening or the potential adverse effects of antibiotic therapy, including drug toxicity and the development of resistant organisms while treating recurrent infections. No controlled trials of therapy for asymptomatic bacteriuria in **noninstitutionalized elderly men** have been reported. In a prospective cohort study of 234 elderly men followed for up to 4.5 years, 29 (12%) had asymptomatic bacteriuria at initial screening, and 20 (8%) became positive in follow-up.[76] Of untreated bacteriuric subjects, 76% spontaneously cleared. Only five bacteriuric subjects were treated for symptomatic infection, with prompt recurrence of asymptomatic bacteriuria in three; no adverse outcomes from symptomatic infection were reported. Cohort and cross-sectional studies that have included elderly ambulatory men have reported no differences in mortality, chronic genitourinary symptoms, or systemic symptoms such as anorexia, fatigue, or malaise between those with and without asymptomatic bacteriuria, after adequate adjustment for confounding variables.[77–79]

Although some trials of elderly patients may have included **persons with diabetes,** we found no controlled clinical trials specifically evaluating the effectiveness of early detection of asymptomatic bacteriuria in diabetics for improving clinical outcome. Case series suggest treatment of asymptomatic bacteriuria usually clears bacteriuria and may reduce clinical symptoms, but bacteriuria recurs in more than two thirds of treated patients.[80–83] Continuous suppressive antibiotic therapy in diabetic patients can prevent re-infection but provides no posttreatment benefit.[80,81] The long-term consequences of asymptomatic bacteriuria in this population are undefined, although in one series persistent bacteriuria did not appear to contribute to renal damage.[83]

The early detection of asymptomatic bacteriuria is of greater potential value for **pregnant women,** in whom bacteriuria is an established risk factor for serious complications, including acute pyelonephritis, preterm delivery, and low birth weight. Randomized controlled trials, cohort studies, and a meta-analysis of 8 randomized clinical trials have shown that treatment of asymptomatic bacteriuria during pregnancy can significantly reduce the incidence of symptomatic urinary tract infection, low birth weight, and preterm delivery.[12-14,18,20,28,84] There is little evidence regarding the optimal periodicity of screening in pregnancy. A urine culture obtained at 12–16 weeks of pregnancy will identify 80% of women who will ultimately have asymptomatic bacteriuria in pregnancy,[85] with an additional 1–2% identified by repeated monthly screening.

In **children**, detection of bacteriuria might lead to the identification of correctable abnormalities of the urinary tract and the prevention of renal scarring, obstructive atrophy, hypertension, and renal insufficiency. However, in three randomized controlled trials in girls aged 5–15 years, treatment of asymptomatic bacteriuria did not significantly reduce emergence of symptoms, pyelonephritis, renal scarring, or persistence of vesicoureteral reflux.[86-88] In two of these trials,[86,87] sample sizes may have been too small to detect important differences, but adverse outcomes were rare in both groups. Treated and control subjects had similar growth, blood pressure, renal growth, and concentrating capacity at the end of follow-up, ranging from 12 to 48 months. In longitudinal studies from the Oxford-Cardiff Cohort screening program, girls with asymptomatic bacteriuria in childhood had an increased prevalence of asymptomatic bacteriuria in pregnancy, and among those with asymptomatic bacteriuria and renal scarring, increased preeclampsia, hypertension, and obstetric interventions.[89,90] On the other hand, in pregnant women with a history of symptomatic urinary tract infection in childhood, there were no differences in preeclampsia or operative delivery, although asymptomatic bacteriuria was again more common.[91] All pregnancies in these studies had satisfactory maternal and fetal outcomes.

Most of the complications from urinary tract abnormalities are thought to occur before children reach school age,[2] and therefore screening might be more effective in **younger children**. There have been no studies, however, proving that preschool urinalyses result in lower morbidity from recurrent infection or in less renal damage.[2,92] Several studies have evaluated the natural history of asymptomatic bacteriuria detected in infancy and followed through the preschool years. In a Swedish cohort of 3,581 screened newborns, 50 infants were identified with asymptomatic bacteriuria, of whom 3 (<0.1%) were treated for underlying renal or urologic abnormalities and 2 were treated for pyelonephritis that occurred within 2 weeks of testing.[8,93] All 45 infants with untreated asymptomatic bacteriuria followed for up to 7 years cleared either spontaneously (80%) or after antibiotic treatment for other conditions (20%). Three subsequently developed cystitis and 20% had recurrences of asymptomatic bacteriuria, but none had major renal or urologic abnormalities as measured by concentrating capacity and urography at a median follow-up of 32 months. Forty infants developed symptomatic urinary tract infection in the first year of age, but only 2 (5%) had evidence of bacteriuria on previous screening. In another cohort of 1,617 healthy infants followed for 5 years, screening for asymptomatic bacteriuria detected 5 cases (0.3%) with high-risk lesions (such as obstructive uropathy, vesicoureteral junction ectopia, etc).[94] Whether early detection of bacteriuria improved prognosis was not established by this study. In 113 infants less than 1 year old undergoing urologic evaluation, the proportion of abnormal kidneys on dimercapto-succinic acid (DMSA) scan did not differ between those with and without urinary tract infection (33% vs. 28%), suggesting that renal scarring from reflux may occur independently of bacteriuria.[95] Renal abnormalities detectable by ultrasound are found in 1.4% of infants who are considered normal,[2,96] compared to 6% of infants with asymptomatic bacteriuria.[8] However, these infants might have been detected outside the screening program as their symptoms developed.

The effectiveness of detecting asymptomatic bacteriuria in patients with indwelling or intermittent urethral catheterization, of periodic screening in patients with known urologic structural abnormalities, or of follow-up of symptomatic urinary tract infection with repeat cultures, is not discussed in this report. These forms of testing are considered within the domain of diagnostic studies for patients with existing medical or surgical conditions, rather than a part of routine screening tests for asymptomatic persons.

Recommendations of Other Groups

The American Academy of Family Physicians (AAFP) recommends periodic screening by dipstick combining leukocyte esterase and nitrite tests to detect bacteriuria in preschool children, those who are morbidly obese, persons with diabetes or a history of gestational diabetes, and persons aged 65 years and older.[97] The recommendations of the AAFP are currently under review. The American College of Physicians recommends against routine screening of adults for asymptomatic bacteriuria with urinalysis or urine culture.[98] The Canadian Task Force on the Periodic Health Examination recommends against routinely screening asymptomatic infants, children, elderly men, or institutionalized elderly women for bacteriuria, and found insufficient evidence to recommend for or against screening noninstitutionalized elderly women.[99] Bright Futures does not recommend routine urinalyses in infants, children, or adolescents.[100] The American Academy of Pediatrics (AAP) recommends routine urinalysis at age 5, and dipstick urinalysis for leukocytes for all adolescents, preferably at age 15 years.[102]

The American College of Obstetricians and Gynecologists and the AAP recommend a urinalysis, including microscopic examination and infection screen, at the first prenatal visit, with the need for additional laboratory evaluations including urine culture determined by findings obtained from the history and physical examination.[101] The Canadian Task Force recommends a urine culture at 12–16 weeks of pregnancy.[99]

Discussion

Screening for asymptomatic bacteriuria is important during pregnancy, where there is strong evidence that treatment is efficacious in improving outcome. Given the benefits of detecting asymptomatic bacteriuria in pregnancy, prenatal testing should be carried out by urine culture (rather than by urinalysis) to reduce the risk of false negatives. A specimen obtained at 12–16 weeks will detect most cases of asymptomatic bacteriuria. There are, however, inadequate data to determine the optimal frequency of subsequent urine testing during pregnancy.

Screening for asymptomatic bacteriuria in school-age girls has been shown to produce little clinical benefit in controlled trials. The effectiveness of screening school-age boys for asymptomatic bacteriuria has not been evaluated, but because the prevalence is extremely low in this population and the specificity of screening tests is only about 80% in children, most positive tests will be false positives (estimated at 99.9% in one overview[57]), with the potential for consequent adverse effects including unnecessary antibiotic therapy and invasive testing. Screening in infants, toddlers, and preschool children might be beneficial in preventing renal damage, but its effectiveness has not been established and cohort studies suggest little risk from untreated asymptomatic bacteriuria. In addition, no accurate and noninvasive screening test is available for infants or toddlers in diapers. Given an 80% sensitivity and specificity of current screening methods, and a 1% prevalence of asymptomatic bacteriuria in girls and 0.03% in boys, screening 100,000 children is estimated to result in 19,897 false-positive tests, or nearly 1 in 5 children screened.[57]

Trials of routine screening have shown no benefit for institutionalized elderly persons and suggest the occurrence of adverse consequences such as unintended drug effects and increased reinfection rates. Screening is therefore not justified in this population. Screening urinalysis might be appropriate in certain high-risk groups, such as diabetic and noninstitutionalized elderly women, but firm evidence of benefit is not available. Several trials in ambulatory elderly women have found no clinical benefit from screening for asymptomatic bacteriuria, but sample sizes were small and do not exclude the possibility of important benefits. Potential benefits must be balanced against the high likelihood of reinfection after treatment in these groups and the adverse effects associated with antibiotic use. Screening is not justified in the general adolescent and adult population, or in ambulatory elderly men, because unrecognized, serious urinary tract disorders are uncommon, the positive predictive value of screening urinalysis is low, and the effectiveness of early detection and treatment is unproven.

CLINICAL INTERVENTION

Screening for asymptomatic bacteriuria with urine culture is recommended for pregnant women at 12–16 weeks of gestation ("A" recommendation). The optimal frequency for subsequent periodic urine cultures during pregnancy has not been determined and is left to clinical discretion. The urine specimen should be obtained in a manner that minimizes contamination. Routine screening for asymptomatic bacteriuria with leukocyte esterase or nitrite testing in pregnant women is not recommended because of poor test characteristics compared to urine culture ("D" recommendation).

There is currently insufficient evidence to recommend for or against routine screening for asymptomatic bacteriuria with leukocyte esterase or nitrite testing in ambulatory elderly women or in women with diabetes ("C" recommendation), but recommendations against such screening may be made on other grounds, including a high likelihood of recurrence and the potential adverse effects of antibiotic therapy. Routine screening for bacteriuria with leukocyte esterase or nitrite testing is not recommended for other asymptomatic persons, including school-aged girls ("E" recommendation), institutionalized elderly ("E" recommendation), and other children, adolescents, and adults ("D" recommendation). Screening for asymptomatic bacteriuria with microscopy testing is not recommended ("D" recommendation).

The draft update of this chapter was prepared for the U.S. Preventive Services Task Force by Carolyn DiGuiseppi, MD, MPH, based in part on materials prepared for the Canadian Task Force on the Periodic Health Examination by Michael B.H. Smith, MB, BCh, CCFP, FRCPC, and Lindsay E. Nicolle, MD.

REFERENCES

1. National Center for Health Statistics. Detailed diagnoses and procedures for patients discharged from short-stay hospitals: United States, 1985. Vital and Health Statistics, series 13, no. 90. Washington, DC: Government Printing Office, 1987. (Publication no. DHHS (PHS) 87-1751.)
2. Kunin CM. Detection, prevention and management of urinary tract infections, 4th ed. Philadelphia: Lea & Febiger, 1987.
3. Nicolle LE. Urinary tract infection in the elderly. J Antimicrob Chemother 1994;33(Suppl A):99–109.
4. Nicolle LE. Urinary tract infections in long-term care facilities. Infect Control Hosp Epidemiol 1993; 14:220–225.
5. Asscher AW, McLachlan MSF, Verrier Jones R, et al. Screening for asymptomatic urinary-tract infection in schoolgirls: a two-centre feasibility study. Lancet 1973;2:1–4.
6. Lindberg U, Claesson I, Hanson LA, et al. Asymptomatic bacteriuria in schoolgirls. I. Clinical and laboratory findings. Acta Paediatr Scand 1975;64:425–431.

7. Savage DCL, Wilson MI, McHardy M, et al. Covert bacteriuria of childhood: a clinical and epidemiological study. Arch Dis Child 1973;48:8–20.
8. Wettergren B, Hellstron M, Stokland E, et al. Six year follow-up of infants with bacteriuria on screening. BMJ 1990; 301:845–848.
9. Jones BW, Headstream JW. Vesicoreflux in children. J Urol 1958;80:1067–1069.
10. Gruskin AB, Baluarte HJ, Dabbagh S. Hemodialysis and peritoneal dialysis. In: Edelmann CM Jr, ed. Pediatric kidney disease. Boston: Little, Brown, 1992.
11. Andriole VT. Advances in the treatment of urinary infections. J Antimicrob Chemother [Suppl A] 1982;9:163–172.
12. Little PJ. The incidence of urinary infection in 5,000 pregnant women. Lancet 1966;2:925–928.
13. Kincaid-Smith P, Buller M. Bacteriuria in pregnancy. Lancet 1965;1:395–399.
14. Campbell-Brown M, McFadyen R, Seal DV, Stephenson ML. Is screening for bacteriuria in pregnancy worthwhile? BMJ 1987;294:1579–1582.
15. Gilstrap LC, Levens KJ, Cunningham FG, et al. Renal infection and pregnancy outcome. Am J Obstet Gynecol 1981;141:709–716.
16. McGrady GA, Daling JR, Peterson DR. Maternal urinary tract infection and adverse fetal outcomes. Am J Epidemiol 1985;121:377–381.
17. Naeye RL. Urinary tract infections and the outcome of pregnancy. Adv Nephrol 1986;15:95–102.
18. Romero R, Oyarzun E, Mazor M, et al. Meta-analysis of the relationship between asymptomatic bacteriuria and preterm delivery/low birth weight. Obstet Gynecol 1989;73:576–582.
19. Institute of Medicine, Division of Health Promotion and Disease Prevention. Preventing low birth weight. Washington, DC: National Academy Press, 1985.
20. Kass EH. Pyelonephritis and bacteriuria. Ann Intern Med 1962;56:46–53.
21. Williams JD, Reeves DS, Condie AP, et al. Significance of bacteriuria during pregnancy. In: Kass EH, Brumfitt W, eds. Infections of the urinary tract: proceedings of the third International Symposium on Pyelonephritis. Chicago: University of Chicago Press, 1978:8–18.
22. Zinner SH, Kass EH. Long-term (10 to 14 years) follow-up of bacteriuria of pregnancy. N Engl J Med 1971; 285:820–824.
23. Schieve LA, Handler A, Hershow R, et al. Urinary tract infection during pregnancy: its association with maternal morbidity and perinatal outcome. Am J Public Health 1994;84:405–410.
24. Verrier Jones K, Asscher AW. Urinary tract infection and vesicoureteral reflux. In: Edelmann CM Jr, ed. Pediatric kidney disease. Boston: Little, Brown, 1992.
25. Bengtsson C, Bengtsson U, Lincoln K. Bacteriuria in a population sample of women. Acta Med Scand 1980;208: 417–423.
26. Evans DA, Williams DN, Laughlin LW, et al. Bacteriuria in a population-based cohort of women. J Infect Dis 1978; 138:768–773.
27. Switzer S. Bacteriuria in a healthy population and its relation to hypertension and pyelonephritis. N Engl J Med 1961; 264:7–10.
28. Patterson TF, Andriole VT. Bacteriuria in pregnancy. Infect Dis Clin North Am 1987;1:807–822.
29. Norden CW, Kass EH. Bacteriuria of pregnancy: a critical appraisal. Annu Rev Med 1968;19:431–470.
30. Bachman JW, Heise RH, Naessens JM, et al. A study of various tests to detect asymptomatic urinary tract infections in an obstetric population. JAMA 1993;270:1971–1974.
31. Zhanel GG, Harding GKM, Nicolle LE. Asymptomatic bacteriuria in patients with diabetes mellitus. Rev Infect Dis 1991;13:150–154.
32. National Diabetes Data Group. Diabetes in America: diabetes data compiled 1984. Washington, DC: Government Printing Office, 1985. (Publication no. DHHS (NIH) 85-1468.)
33. Perez-Luque EL, de la Luz Villalpando M, Malacara JM. Association of sexual activity and bacteriuria in women with non-insulin-dependent diabetes mellitus. J Diabetes Comp 1992;6:254–257.
34. Brauner A, Flodin U, Hylander B, et al. Bacteriuria, bacterial virulence and host factors in diabetic patients. Diabetes Med 1993;10:550–554.
35. Loo SY, Scottolini AG, Luangphinith S, et al. Urine screening strategy employing dipstick analysis and selective culture: an evaluation. Am J Clin Pathol 1984;81:634–642.
36. Oneson R, Groschel DH. Leukocyte esterase activity and nitrite test as a rapid screen for significant bacteriuria. Am J Clin Pathol 1985;83:84–87.
37. Pfaller MA, Koontz FP. Laboratory evaluation of leukocyte esterase and nitrite tests for the detection of bacteriuria. J Clin Microbiol 1985;21:840–842.

38. Jones C, MacPherson DW, Stevens DL. Inability of the Chemstrip LN compared with quantitative urine culture to predict significant bacteriuria. J Clin Microbiol 1986;23:160–162.
39. Doern GV, Saubolle MA, Sewell DL. Screening for bacteriuria with the LN strip test. Diagn Microbiol Infect Dis 1986; 4:355–358.
40. Males BM, Bartholomew WR, Amsterdam D. Leukocyte esterase-nitrite and bioluminescence assays as urine screens. J Clin Microbiol 1985;22:531–534.
41. Alwall N, Lohi A. Factors affecting the reliability of screening tests for bacteriuria I. Acta Med Scand 1973;193:499–503.
42. James GP, Paul KL, Fuller JB. Urinary nitrite and urinary tract infection. Am J Clin Pathol 1978;70: 671–678.
43. Kunin CM, DeGroot JE. Self-screening for significant bacteriuria. JAMA 1975;231:1349–1353.
44. Czerwinski AW, Wilkerson RG, Merrill JA, et al. Further evaluation of the Griess test to detect significant bacteriuria. Am J Obstet Gynecol 1971;110:677–681.
45. Finnerty FA, Johnson AC. A simplified accurate method for detecting bacteriuria. Am J Obstet Gynecol 1968;101: 238–243.
46. Kincaid-Smith P, Bullen M, Mills J, et al. The reliability of screening tests for bacteriuria in pregnancy. Lancet 1964; 2:61–62.
47. Takagi LR, Mruz RM, Vanderplow MG. Screening obstetric outpatients for bacteriuria. J Reprod Med 1975;15: 229–231.
48. Archbald FJ, Verma U, Tajani NA. Screening for asymptomatic bacteriuria with Microstix. J Reprod Med 1984;29: 272–274.
49. Sleigh JD. Detection of bacteriuria by a modification of the nitrite test. BMJ 1965;1:765–767.
50. Lohr JA. Use of routine urinalysis in making a presumptive diagnosis of urinary tract infection in children. Pediatr Infect Dis J 1991;10:646–650.
51. Cannon HJ Jr, Goetz ES, Hamoudi AC, et al. Rapid screening and microbiological processing of pediatric urine specimens. Diagn Microbiol Infect Dis 1986;4:11–17.
52. Marsik FJ, Owens D, Lewandowski J. Use of the leukocyte esterase and nitrite tests to determine the need for culturing urine specimens from a pediatric and adolescent population. Diagn Microbiol Infect Dis 1986;4:181–183.
53. Goldsmith BM, Campos JM. Comparison of urine dipstick, microscopy, and culture for the detection of bacteriuria in children. Clin Pediatr 1990;29:214–218.
54. Shaw KN, Hexter D, McGowan KL, et al. Clinical evaluation of a rapid screening test for urinary tract infections in children. J Pediatr 1991;118:733–736.
55. Weinberg AG, Gan VN. Urine screen for bacteriuria in symptomatic pediatric outpatients. Pediatr Infect Dis 1991; 10:651–654.
56. Lohr JA, Portilla MG, Geuder TG, et al. Making a presumptive diagnosis of urinary tract infection by using a urinalysis performed in an on-site laboratory. J Pediatr 1993;122:22–25.
57. Kemper KJ, Avner ED. The case against screening urinalyses for asymptomatic bacteriuria in children. Am J Dis Child 1992;146:343–346.
58. Lachs MS, Nachamkin I, Edelstein PH, et al. Spectrum bias in the evaluation of diagnostic tests: lessons from the rapid dipstick test for urinary tract infection. Ann Intern Med 1992;117:135–140.
59. Schumann GB, Greenberg NF. Usefulness of macroscopic urinalysis as a screening procedure. Am J Clin Pathol 1979;71:452–456.
60. Schumann GB, Greenberg NF, Henry JB. Microscopic look at urine often unnecessary. JAMA 1978;239:13–14.
61. Dontas AS, Papanayiotou P, Marketos S, et al. Bacteriuria in old age. Lancet 1966;2:305–306.
62. Walkey FA, Judge TG, Thompson J, et al. Incidence of urinary tract infection in the elderly. Scott Med J 1967;12: 411–414.
63. Dontas AS, Papanayiotou P, Marketos SG, et al. The effect of bacteriuria on renal function patterns in old age. Clin Sci 1968;34:73–81.
64. Sourander LB, Kasanen A. A 5-year follow-up of bacteriuria in the aged. Gerontol Clin 1972;14: 274–281.
65. Burns MJ, Burns JL, Krieger JN. Pediatric urinary tract infection. Diagnosis, classification, and significance. Pediatr Clin North Am 1987;34:1111–1120.
66. Asscher AW, Sussman M, Waters WE, et al. Asymptomatic significant bacteriuria in the non-pregnant woman. II. Response to treatment and follow-up. BMJ 1969;1:804–806.

67. Boscia JA, Kobasa WD, Knight RA, et al. Therapy vs. no therapy for bacteriuria in elderly ambulatory nonhospitalized women. JAMA 1987;257:1067–1071.

68. Sussman M, Asscher AW, Waters WE, et al. Asymptomatic significant bacteriuria in the non-pregnant woman. I. Description of a population. BMJ 1969;1:799–803.

69. Nordenstam GR, Branberg CA, Oden AS, et al. Bacteriuria and mortality in an elderly population. N Engl J Med 1986;314:1152–1156.

70. Dontas AS, Kasviki-Charvati P, Papanayiotou P, et al. Bacteriuria and survival in old age. N Engl J Med 1981;304:939–943.

71. Evans DA, Kass EH, Hennekens CH, et al. Bacteriuria and subsequent mortality in women. Lancet 1982;1:156–158.

72. Evans DA, Brauner E, Warren JW, et al. Randomized trial of vigorous antimicrobial therapy of bacteriuria in a community population [abstract]. In: Program and Abstracts of the Twenty-Seventh Interscience Conference on Antimicrobial Agents and Chemotherapy. New York: American Society for Microbiology, 1987:148.

73. Nicolle LE, Mayhew WJ, Bryan L. Prospective, randomized comparison of therapy and no therapy for asymptomatic bacteriuria in institutionalized elderly women. Am J Med 1987;83:27–33.

74. Nicolle LE, Bjornson J, Harding GKM, MacDonell JA. Bacteriuria in elderly institutionalized men. N Engl J Med 1983;309:1420–1425.

75. Abrutyn E, Mossey J, Berlin JA, et al. Does asymptomatic bacteriuria predict mortality and does antimicrobial treatment reduce mortality in elderly ambulatory women? Ann Intern Med 1994;120: 827–833.

76. Mims AD, Norman DC, Jamamura RH, et al. Clinically inapparent (asymptomatic) bacteriuria in ambulatory elderly men: epidemiologic, clinical, and microbiological findings. J Am Geriatr Soc 1990;38: 1209–1214.

77. Heinamaki P, Haavisto M, Hakulinen T, et al. Mortality in relation to urinary characteristics in the very aged. Gerontology 1986;32:167–171.

78. Nordenstam GR, Brandberg CA, Oden AS, et al. Bacteriuria and mortality in an elderly population. N Engl J Med 1986;314:1152–1156.

79. Boscia JA, Kobasa WD, Abrutyn E, et al. Lack of association between bacteriuria and symptoms in the elderly. Am J Med 1986;81:979–982.

80. Di Mauro M, Leonardi R, La Bella G, et al. Chronic prophylaxis of urinary tract infections in diabetic patients. A controlled study. Minerva Med 1990;81:69–74.

81. Forland M, Thomas VL. The treatment of urinary tract infections in women with diabetes mellitus. Diabetes Care 1985;8:499–506.

82. Forland M, Thomas V, Shelokov A. Urinary tract infections in patients with diabetes mellitus: studies on antibody coating of bacteria. JAMA 1977;238:1924–1926.

83. Batalla MA, Balodimos MC, Bradley RF. Bacteriuria in diabetes mellitus. Diabetologia 1971;7:297–301.

84. Kass EH. Bacteriuria and pyelonephritis of pregnancy. Trans Assoc Am Phys 1959;72:257–264.

85. Stengvist K, Dahlen-Nelsson I, Lidin-Janson G, et al. Bacteriuria in pregnancy: frequency and risk of acquisition. Am J Epidemiol 1989;129:372–379.

86. Savage DCL, Howie G, Adler K, et al. Controlled trial of therapy in covert bacteriuria in childhood. Lancet 1975; 1:358–361.

87. Lindberg U. Asymptomatic bacteriuria in school girls. V: The clinical course and response to treatment. Acta Paediatr Scand 1975;64:718–724.

88. Cardiff-Oxford Bacteriuria Study Group. Sequelae of covert bacteriuria in schoolgirls. Lancet 1978;1: 889–893.

89. McGladdery SL, Aparicio S, Verrier-Jones K, et al. Outcome of pregnancy in an Oxford-Cardiff cohort of women with previous bacteriuria. Q J Med 1992;83:533–539.

90. Sacks SH, Verrier Jones K, Roberts R, et al. Effect of symptomless bacteriuria in childhood on subsequent pregnancy. Lancet 1987;2:991–994.

91. Martinell J, Jodal U, Lidin-Janson G. Pregnancies in women with and without renal scarring after urinary infections in childhood. BMJ 1990;300:840–844.

92. Schwartz GJ, Edelmann CM. Screening for bacteriuria in children. Kidney 1975;8:11–14.

93. Wettergren B, Jodal U, Jonasson G. Epidemiology of bacteriuria during the first year of life. Acta Paediatr Scand 1985;74:925–933.

94. Siegel SR, Siegel B, Sokoloff BZ, et al. Urinary infection in infants and preschool children. Am J Dis Child 1980;134:369–372.

95. Farnsworth RH, Rossleigh MA, Leighton DM, et al. The detection of reflux nephropathy in infants by 99m-technetium dimercaptosuccinic acid studies. J Urol 1991;145:542–546.

96. Steinhart JM, Kuhn JP, Eisenberg B, et al. Ultrasound screening of healthy infants for urinary tract abnormalities. Pediatr 1988;82:609–614.

97. American Academy of Family Physicians. Age charts for periodic health examination. Kansas City, MO: American Academy of Family Physicians, 1994. (Reprint no. 510.)

98. Komaroff AL. Urinalysis and urine culture in women with dysuria. In: Sox HC Jr, ed. Common diagnostic tests: use and interpretation. 2nd ed. Philadelphia: American College of Physicians, 1990: 286–301.

99. Canadian Task Force on the Periodic Health Examination. Canadian guide to clinical preventive health care. Ottawa: Canada Communication Group, 1994:100–106, 220–230, 966–973.

100. Green M, ed. Bright Futures: guidelines for health supervision of infants, children and adolescents. Arlington VA: National Center for Education in Maternal and Child Health, 1994.

101. American Academy of Pediatrics and American College of Obstetricians and Gynecologists. Guidelines for perinatal care. 3rd ed. Washington, DC: American College of Obstetricians and Gynecologists, 1992.

102. Committee on Practice and Ambulatory Medicine, American Academy of Pediatrics. Recommendations for preventive pediatric health care. Pediatrics 1995;96:373–374.

32. Screening for Rubella—

Including Immunization of Adolescents and Adults

RECOMMENDATION

Routine screening for rubella susceptibility by history of vaccination or by serology is recommended for all women of childbearing age at their first clinical encounter. Susceptible nonpregnant women should be offered rubella vaccination; susceptible pregnant women should be vaccinated immediately after delivery. An equally acceptable alternative for nonpregnant women of childbearing age is to offer vaccination against rubella without screening (see *Clinical Intervention*). There is insufficient evidence to recommend for or against screening or routine vaccination of young men in settings where large numbers of susceptible young adults of both sexes congregate, such as military bases and colleges. Routine screening or vaccination of other young men, of older men, and of postmenopausal women is not recommended.

Burden of Suffering

Rubella is generally a mild illness; when contracted by pregnant women, however, especially those in the first 16 weeks of pregnancy, it frequently causes serious complications including miscarriage, abortion, stillbirth, and congenital rubella syndrome (CRS).[1,2] The 1964 rubella pandemic in the U.S. caused over 12 million infections, 11,000 fetal losses, and 20,000 cases of CRS in infants.[3] The most common manifestations of CRS are hearing loss, developmental delay, growth retardation, and cardiac and ocular defects.[1,2] The lifetime costs of treating a patient with CRS were estimated in 1985 to exceed $220,000.[3]

Since 1969, when rubella vaccine became available in the U.S. and universal childhood immunization was initiated, no major periodic rubella epidemics have occurred. The incidence of reported cases has declined dramatically, to an estimated incidence rate of 0.1/100,000 population (192 cases) and an indigenous CRS incidence rate of 0/100,000 live births (no cases reported) in 1993.[4] Outbreaks of rubella infection have continued to occur, however; in 1991, for example, 1,401 rubella infections were reported (0.6/100,000), one third of which occurred among adolescents and young adults (ages 15–29 years), resulting in 31 cases of CRS (0.8/100,000).[4,5] Most recent outbreaks have occurred in settings where many unvaccinated children and young adults are gathered (e.g., religious communities that refuse vaccination, colleges, prisons, and work places), and among persons in specific racial/ethnic groups (e.g., Asians/Pacific Islanders and Hispanics) who are often unvaccinated.[4,6,7] The highest risk for CRS occurs in Amish women, for whom the rate in one Pennsylvania county was 14/1,000 live births in 1991, compared to 0.006/1,000 for the general U.S. population.[4]

Accuracy of Screening Tests

One way to prevent rubella infection in adults is to screen for susceptibility, by serologic tests for antibodies or by vaccination history, and to administer vaccine to susceptible persons. Vaccine trials and cohort studies have shown that most patients with hemagglutination-inhibition (HI) antibody are protected from clinical disease.[8–10] HI is a labor-intensive test, however, and it can be associated with both false-positive and false-negative results.[1,8,11] Faster, more convenient laboratory methods (e.g., enzyme immunoassay and latex agglutination) have now replaced HI in most laboratories.[1,12] Using HI as the comparison standard, these tests have sensitivities of 92–100% and specificities of 71–100%.[11,13–15] The apparently low specificities of some newer methods are due to their ability to detect low levels of rubella antibody that are undetectable by HI methods and are therefore reported as "false positives."[1,16,17] There have been no controlled trials to determine if these low levels confer immunity against wild virus,[1] but other clinical and in vitro evidence suggests that they are protective.[16,18–22] These newer tests, therefore, appear to be both more accurate and more convenient than HI when performed in laboratories with demonstrated proficiency.

A history of rubella vaccination can identify many who may be protected. Despite a variety of design flaws in some of the available studies (such as selection biases and small sample sizes), most demonstrate that persons with a positive history of having received rubella vaccine are significantly more likely to be seropositive (median 92%, range 82–97%) than those without such a history (median 74%, range 62–83%).[18,23–30] A positive rubella vaccination history documented by vaccination card, school record, or medical record is more likely to be associated with seropositivity than is an undocumented history (although this difference was not statistically significant in some studies),[18,25–27] and it is therefore preferred. A positive history of rubella infection is substantially less likely to correctly predict rubella immunity than is a positive history of vaccination;[18,23-25] therefore, a history of infection is not adequate for determining susceptibility.

Effectiveness of Early Detection

Rubella vaccine, once administered, is efficacious. Efficacy studies in healthy vaccinees show that ≥90% have protection against clinical rubella illness,[31-35] and seropositivity is long-lasting.[36-39] After the initiation of universal child immunization in 1969, the incidence of both rubella and CRS dropped markedly (see above).[1,4] Adverse reactions from the RA27/3 live attenuated rubella vaccine (the only rubella vaccine currently licensed in the U.S.) are generally mild in children.[40,41] Joint symptoms after vaccination are common in adults but rarely persist; the incidence is higher in women than men and increases with increasing age at vaccination.[1,9,42,43] Vaccination of persons who are already immune rarely induces the joint symptoms seen with primary immunization of susceptible adults.[44,45]

Because an estimated 6–12% of the young adult population is seronegative,[30,46] and because CRS continues to occur in the U.S. despite recommendations for universal childhood vaccination (see Chapter 65),[4] it has been recommended by some authorities that clinicians also direct efforts toward vaccinating susceptible adolescents and young adults, particularly women of childbearing age.[1] Several factors may reduce the effectiveness of a strategy to prevent CRS by screening (with history of vaccination or serology) and vaccinating susceptibles. The screening test may falsely identify some susceptible persons as immune; of 21 infants with CRS in 1990, 71% of their mothers had had a positive serologic test and 43% gave a history of vaccination.[47] Persons correctly identified as susceptible may not be offered or accept the vaccine; vaccination rates after serologic screening in different populations have ranged from 37% to 88%.[18,24,26,27,48-56] Seronegative women are more likely than are seronegative men to accept immunization,[55,57] with the highest rates of follow-up vaccination (78–87%) occurring in susceptible postpartum women.[52-54]

The effectiveness of a strategy of screening and follow-up vaccination to prevent CRS may be assessed by its effect on the incidence of CRS and of rubella infection and susceptibility in women of childbearing age. No controlled studies have evaluated the effectiveness of screening and vaccinating susceptible persons in reducing the incidence of CRS. CRS occurrence has decreased over time in some, but not all, countries that have employed selective vaccination of susceptible adolescent and adult females as their sole strategy to reduce CRS.[58-60] Evidence that screening and follow-up vaccination can reduce the likelihood of rubella infection was provided by a severe rubella outbreak in Iceland, where identical rates of protection from infection occurred in screened and immunized (98.5%) and in naturally immune (99%) schoolgirls.[61] Evidence regarding rubella susceptibility is supplied by a cohort study from Scotland. Six to seven years after a screening program for schoolgirls took place, 98.7% of girls who had originally been naturally immune had circulating antibodies, compared to 95.1% of those who had been vaccinated as susceptibles and 42.8% of a small group of susceptibles who had refused vaccination.[62] Case series from Iceland[61,63] and cross-sectional studies from Great Britain[52,64] also show a reduction in susceptibility among women of childbearing age using this strategy. There is thus fair evidence that screening and immunizing susceptible females of childbearing age reduces both rubella susceptibility and infection and, by inference, CRS.

An alternative strategy to prevent rubella infection in women of childbearing age is routine vaccination without screening. In addition to protecting those who have not been previously vaccinated, such a strategy would eliminate most susceptibility due to primary vaccine failure (failure to develop antibodies after initial vaccination). Primary vaccine failure occurs in 2–5% of RA27/3 vaccine recipients,[65–70] and a second rubella vaccination results in seroconversion in most cases.[9,18] Antibodies have been found in 99.2% of schoolchildren after two doses of rubella vaccine, compared to 94.6% after one dose.[28] In Sweden and Finland, vaccine programs in which all adolescent girls are routinely immunized (as well as all children at age 14–18 months) have been associated with substantially reduced occurrence of both seronegativity and of rubella infection in female compared to male adolescents and adults.[71,72] These data provide fair evidence for routine vaccination of all nonpregnant women of childbearing age to reduce rubella susceptibility and infection and, therefore, CRS.

The rubella vaccine is contraindicated during pregnancy because of the theoretical possibility of teratogenicity, although there have been no reported cases of rubella vaccine-related birth defects in the United States after inadvertent vaccination of 321 susceptible pregnant women within 3 months of conception.[1] Similarly reassuring results have been reported from Great Britain and Germany.[73,74] Based on reported data, the true risk for CRS in susceptible women vaccinated during pregnancy using the RA27/3 vaccine may be zero, and the probability is 95% that the true risk is less than 1.7%.[75] Because a measurable iatrogenic risk cannot be excluded, however, vaccination of susceptible women who are known to be pregnant should be postponed until the postpartum period.[75] The virus has been isolated in breast milk and in breast-fed infants after postpartum vaccination,[76] but no adverse consequences from such exposure have been reported.[76,77] A greater disadvantage of postpartum immunization is that it often occurs too late to prevent CRS; 61% of reported cases have occurred with the first live birth.[78]

In settings where large numbers of young adults are gathered (e.g., military bases and colleges), outbreaks of rubella are not uncommon, and males and females are infected at similar rates.[79–82] Rubella screening or routine vaccination of young men in such settings might reduce the risk of spreading rubella to susceptible pregnant women. There is weak evidence from a single before-after study that universal rubella screening and follow-up vaccination of military recruits is effective in preventing rubella infection and eliminating epidemic rubella.[83] A small cohort study using the older Cendehill vaccine found that routine vaccination of young male military recruits reduced rubella susceptibility, clinical disease, and viral shedding.[10] In a before-after study of 256 college athletes (62% male) screened serologically with follow-up vaccination of susceptibles, the proportion with documented immunity by serology increased from 93% to 96%, and 8 of the remaining 9 seronegative students were vaccinated but did not receive follow-up testing.[84] There is, however, no direct evidence that either screening or routine vaccination of males in these settings reduces CRS. For young men not living in such settings, no evidence was found to support either screening or routine vaccination in reducing susceptibility, infection, or CRS.

There are few data concerning rubella screening or vaccination in older men or in women past childbearing age. Because men ages 40 years and older and postmenopausal women account for only a small proportion (<10%) of recent rubella cases,[5,85] have a high rate of natural immunity (85–95%),[59,86] have a greater likelihood of postvaccine joint reactions,[9] and are at little direct risk if they do become infected, routine screening or vaccination of this population does not seem to be justified despite the fact that these persons might, on rare occasions, transmit rubella to susceptible women of childbearing age.

Recommendations of Other Groups

The American Academy of Pediatrics (AAP),[87] American College of Obstetricians and Gynecologists (ACOG),[88] American College of Physicians,[89] and Advisory Committee for Immunization Practices (ACIP)[1] recommend vaccinating all adolescents and adults (particularly women and persons in colleges, health care settings, and military institutions) who have no contraindications and who lack documented evidence of either rubella immunization on or after the first birthday or of serologic evidence of immunity. Routine serologic testing of men and nonpregnant women is not recommended by these organizations. The American Medical Association[90] and Bright Futures[91] recommend rubella vaccination (as measles-mumps-rubella [MMR]) for all adolescents who have not had two previous MMR vaccinations. The American Academy of Family Physicians recommends rubella antibody testing in all women of childbearing age who lack evidence of immunity.[92] AAP,[87] ACOG,[89] and ACIP[1] recommend routine prenatal or antepartum serologic screening of all pregnant women not known to be immune, and postpartum vaccination of those found to be susceptible. The Canadian Task Force on the Periodic Health Examination recommends serologic screening of women of childbearing age, with vaccination of seronegative nonpregnant women immediately and seronegative pregnant women after delivery. They also recommend universal vaccination of women of childbearing age without screening as an acceptable alternative. The Canadian Task Force does not recommend for or against universal vaccination of young men in settings where large numbers of young persons are gathered.[93]

Discussion

When administered to children, the current rubella vaccine is efficacious in the induction of rubella immunity and in the prevention of rubella infection and CRS. Recent cases of rubella and CRS have been associated with outbreaks among groups of unvaccinated persons, leading to infections of unvaccinated pregnant women.[4,7] The added coverage provided by the two MMR vaccinations many will receive during childhood to meet current recommendations for measles immunization (see Chapter 65) should eliminate most primary vaccine failures, and will increase the rate of primary immunization among women of childbearing age. Therefore, the incidence of CRS will probably decline as the current cohort of highly immunized female children and adolescents enters its childbearing years.

In the intervening years, however, many women of childbearing age will remain unimmunized and, therefore, susceptible to rubella infection. Universal screening and follow-up vaccination of susceptible females would reduce rubella susceptibility, infections, and CRS; however, the effectiveness of this strategy in the clinical setting may be limited by incomplete screening, imperfect screening tests, and failure to vaccinate susceptibles. Routine vaccination of all women of childbearing age, without screening, also seems to be effective in reducing rubella infections; it avoids the problem of noncompliance with return visits, and if given as MMR also provides immunity to other infectious diseases, but it results in vaccination of many women who are already immune. Because the adverse effects of vaccinating immune persons appear to be minimal, cost and convenience are likely to be the determining factors in deciding which strategy should be used. In one study, the most cost-effective strategy was record review followed by vaccination, if at least 75% of patients had records available; otherwise, vaccination of all persons without screening was most cost-effective.[23] On the other hand, a study from Iceland found that serologic screening of females ages 12–40 followed by vaccination of seronegatives and follow-up retesting was more cost-effective than routine vaccination.[94] These estimates are sensitive to the prevalence of immunity, compliance with follow-up, and the costs of screening, vaccine, and follow-up.

Whether either strategy (screening for susceptibility or routine vaccination of women of childbearing age) is justified by expected benefits compared to costs is not clear. An analysis of a premarital rubella screening program found that costs did not justify benefits unless at least 85% of seronegatives were vaccinated.[95,96] Variation in the cost of the screening tests and vaccines, the prevalence of immunity, and the likelihood of rubella exposure will influence these results, however. The impact and benefit-cost ratio of strategies to reduce rubella susceptibility are likely to be greatest in settings where many women are unvaccinated (and are therefore at higher risk for acquiring rubella), such as certain religious communities and communities with many unimmunized immigrants from developing countries. Cost-benefit analyses concerning rubella screening and vaccination of women in various settings are needed.

CLINICAL INTERVENTION

All children without contraindications should receive MMR vaccine at age 12–15 months and again at age 4–6 years (see Chapter 65). To reduce further the incidence of CRS, screening for rubella susceptibility by history of vaccination or by serology is recommended for all women of childbearing age at their first clinical encounter ("B" recommendation). A documented history of vaccination is more accurate than an undocumented history in determining rubella immunity and is therefore preferred. All susceptible nonpregnant women of childbearing age should be offered vaccination. Susceptible pregnant women should be vaccinated in the immediate postpartum period. An equally acceptable alternative for nonpregnant women of childbearing age is to offer vaccination against rubella without screening ("B" recommendation). The decision of which strategy to use should be tailored to the individual clinician's practice population, depending on the availability of vaccination records, the reliability of the vaccination history, the rate of immunity, the cost of serologic testing, and the cost and likelihood of follow-up vaccination for susceptible persons identified by serologic testing.

There is insufficient evidence to recommend for or against routine screening or vaccination of young men to prevent CRS in settings where large numbers of susceptible young adults of both sexes congregate, such as military bases and colleges ("C" recommendation). Recommendations to give MMR vaccine in these settings may be made on other grounds, however, such as prevention of measles (see Chapter 66). Routine screening or

vaccination of other young men, of older men, or of postmenopausal women, is not recommended ("D" recommendation).

Guidelines for the administration of MMR vaccine, and its contraindications, have been published by ACIP.[1] The National Childhood Vaccine Injury Act requires that the date of administration, the manufacturer and lot number, and the name, address, and title of the person administering the vaccine be recorded in the patient's permanent medical record (or in a permanent office log or file).[97]

The draft update of this chapter was prepared for the U.S. Preventive Services Task Force by Carolyn DiGuiseppi, MD, MPH.

REFERENCES

1. Centers for Disease Control. Rubella prevention: recommendations of the Advisory Committee for Immunization Practices (ACIP). MMWR 1990;39(RR-15):1–18.
2. Freij BJ, South MA, Sever JL. Maternal rubella and the congenital rubella syndrome. Clin Perinatol 1988;15:247–257.
3. Orenstein WA, Bart KJ, Hinman AR, et al. The opportunity and obligation to eliminate rubella from the United States. JAMA 1984;251:1988–1994.
4. Centers for Disease Control and Prevention. Rubella and congenital rubella syndrome—United States, January 1, 1991–May 7, 1994. MMWR 1994;43:391, 397–401.
5. Centers for Disease Control and Prevention. Summary of notifiable diseases, United States—1991. MMWR 1992;40: 3–12.
6. Centers for Disease Control. Outbreaks of rubella among the Amish—United States, 1991. MMWR 1991;40: 264–265.
7. Centers for Disease Control. Increase in rubella and congenital rubella syndrome—United States, 1988–90. MMWR 1991;40:93–99.
8. Cradock-Watson JE. Laboratory diagnosis of rubella: past, present and future. Epidemiol Infect 1991;107:1–15.
9. Best JM. Rubella vaccines: past, present and future. Epidemiol Infect 1991;107:17–30.
10. Horstmann DM, Liebhaber H, Le Bouvier GL, et al. Rubella: reinfection of vaccinated and naturally immune persons exposed in an epidemic. N Engl J Med 1970;283:771–778.
11. Fayram SL, Akin S, Aarnaes SL, et al. Determination of immune status in patients with low antibody titers for rubella virus. J Clin Microbiol 1987;25:178–180.
12. Skendzel LP, Edson DC. Latex agglutination test for rubella antibodies: report based on data from the College of American Pathologists surveys, 1983–1985. J Clin Microbiol 1986;24:333–335.
13. Field PR, Ho DW, Cunningham AL. Evaluation of rubella immune status by three commercial enzyme-linked immunosorbent assays. J Clin Microbiol 1988;26:990–994.
14. Skendzel LP, Edson DC. Evaluation of enzyme immunosorbent rubella assays. Arch Pathol Lab Med 1985; 109:391–393.
15. Steece RS, Talley MS, Skeels MR, et al. Comparison of enzyme-linked immunosorbent assay, hemagglutination inhibition, and passive latex agglutination for determination of rubella immune status. J Clin Microbiol 1985; 21:140–142.
16. Kleeman KT, Kiefer DJ, Halbert SP. Rubella antibodies detected by several commercial immunoassays in hemagglutination inhibition-negative sera. J Clin Microbiol 1983;18:1131–1137.
17. Morgan-Capner P, Pullen HJM, Pattison JR, et al. A comparison of three tests for rubella antibody screening. J Clin Pathol 1979;32:542–545.
18. Robinson RG, Dudenhoeffer FE, Holroyd HJ, et al. Rubella immunity in older children, teenagers, and young adults: a comparison of immunity in those previously immunized with those unimmunized. J Pediatr 1982;101:188–191.
19. Banatvala JE, Best JM, O'Shea S, Dudgeon JA. Persistence of rubella antibodies after vaccination: detection after experimental challenge. Rev Infect Dis 1985;7:S86–S90.

20. Balfour HH, Groth KE, Edelman CK. Rubella viraemia and antibody responses after rubella vaccination and reimmunisation. Lancet 1981;1:1078–1080.
21. Butler AB, Scott RM, Schydlower M, et al. The immunoglobulin response to reimmunization with rubella vaccine. J Pediatr 1981;99:531–534.
22. Buimovici-Klein E, O'Beirne AJ, Millian SJ, et al. Low level rubella immunity detected by ELISA and specific lymphocyte transformation. Arch Virol 1980;66:321–327.
23. Preblud SR, Gross F, Halsey NA, et al. Assessment of susceptibility to measles and rubella. JAMA 1982; 247:1134–1137.
24. Mills DA, Parker KR, Evans CE. Rubella antibody titres and immunization status in a family practice. Can Med Assoc J 1980;122:549–552.
25. Dales LG, Chin J. Public health implications of rubella antibody levels in California. Am J Public Health 1982;72: 167–172.
26. Nelson DB, Layde MM, Chatton TB. Rubella susceptibility in inner-city adolescents: the effect of a school immunization law. Am J Public Health 1982;72:710–713.
27. Cohen ZB, Rice LI, Felice ME. Rubella seronegativity in a low socioeconomic adolescent female population. Clin Pediatr 1985;24:387–390.
28. Orenstein WA, Herrmann KL, Holmgreen P, et al. Prevalence of rubella antibodies in Massachusetts schoolchildren. Am J Epidemiol 1986;124:290–298.
29. Schum TR, Nelson DB, Duma MA, et al. Increasing rubella seronegativity despite a compulsory school law. Am J Public Health 1990;80:66–69.
30. Murray DL, Lynch MA. Determination of immune status to measles, rubella, and varicella-zoster viruses among medical students: assessment of historical information. Am J Public Health 1988;78:836–838.
31. Chang TW, Desrosiers S, Weinstein L. Clinical and serologic studies of an outbreak of rubella in a vaccinated population. N Engl J Med 1970;283:246–248.
32. Grayston JT, Detels R, Chen KP, et al. Field trial of live attenuated rubella virus vaccine during an epidemic on Taiwan. JAMA 1969;207:1107–1110.
33. Davis WJ, Larson HE, Simsarian JP, et al. A study of rubella immunity and resistance to infection. JAMA 1971; 215:600–608.
34. Baba K, Yabuuchi H, Okuni H, et al. Rubella epidemic in an institution: protective value of live rubella vaccine and serological behavior of vaccinated, revaccinated, and naturally immune groups. Biken J 1978;21:25–31.
35. Greaves WL, Orenstein WA, Hinman AR, et al. Clinical efficacy of rubella vaccine. Pediatr Infect Dis 1983;2:284–286.
36. Horstmann DM, Schluederberg A, Emmons JE, et al. Persistence of vaccine-induced immune responses to rubella: comparison with natural infection. Rev Infect Dis 1985;7(Suppl 1):S80–S85.
37. Hillary IB, Griffith AH. Persistence of rubella antibodies 15 years after subcutaneous administration of Wistar 27/3 strain live attenuated rubella virus vaccine. Vaccine 1988;2:274–276.
38. Enders G, Nickerl U. Rubella vaccination: antibody persistence for 14–17 years and immune status of women without and with a history of vaccination. Immun Infekt 1988;16:58–64.
39. O'Shea S, Woodward S, Best JM, et al. Rubella vaccination: persistence of antibodies for 10–21 years [letter]. Lancet 1988;2:909.
40. Herrmann KL. Rubella in the United States: toward a strategy for disease control and elimination. Epidemiol Infect 1991;107:55–61.
41. Chen RT, Moses JM, Markowitz LE, et al. Adverse events following measles-mumps-rubella and measles vaccinations in college students. Vaccine 1991;9:297–299.
42. Wharton M, Cochi SL, Williams WW. Measles, mumps, and rubella vaccine. Infect Dis Clin North Am 1990;4:47–73.
43. Tingle AJ, Allen M, Petty RE, et al. Rubella-associated arthritis: I. Comparative study of joint manifestations associated with natural rubella infection and RA27/3 rubella immunization. Ann Rheum Dis 1986;45:110–114.
44. Lerman SJ, Nankervis GA, Heggie AD. Immunologic response, virus excretion, and joint reactions with rubella vaccine: a study of adolescent girls and young women given live attenuated virus vaccine (HPV-77:DE-5). Ann Intern Med 1971;74:67–73.
45. Landrigan PJ, Stoffels MA, Anderson E, et al. Epidemic rubella in adolescent boys: clinical features and results of vaccination. JAMA 1974;227:1283–1287.
46. Stehr-Green PA, Cochi SL, Preblud SR, et al. Evidence against increasing rubella seronegativity among adolescent girls [letter]. Am J Public Health 1990;80:88.

47. Lee SH, Ewert DP, Frederick PD, et al. Resurgence of congenital rubella syndrome in the 1990s. Report on missed opportunities and failed prevention policies among women of childbearing age. JAMA 1992; 267:2616–2620.

48. Povar GJ, Maloney M, Watson WN, et al. Rubella screening and follow-up immunization in Vermont. Am J Public Health 1979;69:285–286.

49. Falvo CE, Weiss KE, Liss SM. A rubella screening and immunization program in an adolescent clinic. Am J Public Health 1979;69:283–285.

50. Lieberman E, Faich GA, Simon PR, et al. Premarital rubella screening in Rhode Island. JAMA 1981; 245:1333–1335.

51. Vogt RL, Clark SW. Premarital rubella vaccination program. Am J Public Health 1985;75:1088–1089.

52. Miller CL, Miller E, Sequeira PJL, et al. Effect of selective vaccination on rubella susceptibility and infection in pregnancy. BMJ 1985;291:1398–1401.

53. Edmond E, Zealley H. The impact of a rubella prevention policy on the outcome of rubella in pregnancy. Br J Obstet Gynaecol 1986;93:563–567.

54. Trallero EP, Eguiluz GC, Iraeta MD, et al. Rubella in Guipuzcoa (Basque country, Spain). A four-year serosurvey. Eur J Epidemiol 1991;7:183–187.

55. Hartstein AI, Quan MA, Williams ML, et al. Rubella screening and immunization of health care personnel: critical appraisal of a voluntary program. Am J Infect Control 1983;11:1–9.

56. Weiss KE, Falvo CE, Buimovici-Klein E, et al. Evaluation of an employee health service as a setting for a rubella screening and immunization program. Am J Public Health 1979;69:281–283.

57. Polk BF, White JA, DeGirolami PC, et al. An outbreak of rubella among hospital personnel. N Engl J Med 1980;303:541–545.

58. Swartz TA, Hornstein L, Epstein I. Epidemiology of rubella and congenital rubella infection in Israel, a country with a selective immunization program. Rev Infect Dis 1985;7(suppl):S42–S46.

59. Galazka A. Rubella in Europe. Epidemiol Infect 1991;107:43–54.

60. Tobin JO, Sheppard S, Smithells RW, et al. Rubella in the United Kingdom, 1970–1983. Rev Infect Dis 1985;7(suppl):S47–S52.

61. Rafnar B. Rubella immunization of teenage girls in Iceland and follow-up after a severe rubella epidemic. Bull WHO 1982;60:141–146.

62. Zealley H, Edmond E. Rubella screening and immunisation of schoolgirls: results six to seven years after vaccination. BMJ 1982;284:382–384.

63. Gudmundsdottir S, Antonsdottir A, Gudnadottir S, et al. Prevention of congenital rubella in Iceland by antibody screening and immunization of seronegative females. Bull WHO 1985;63:83–92.

64. Griffiths PD, Baboonian C. Is post partum rubella vaccination worthwhile? J Clin Pathol 1982;35: 1340–1344.

65. Buser F, Nicolas A. Vaccination with RA27/3 rubella vaccine. Am J Dis Child 1971;122:53–56.

66. Schiff GM, Linnemann CC, Shea L, et al. Evaluation of RA27/3 rubella vaccine. J Pediatr 1974;85: 379–381.

67. Balfour HH, Balfour CL, Edelman CK, et al. Evaluation of Wistar RA27/3 rubella virus vaccine in children. Am J Dis Child 1976;130:1089–1091.

68. Weibel RE, Villarejos VM, Klein EB, et al. Clinical and laboratory studies of live attenuated RA27/3 and HPV-77DE rubella virus vaccines. Proc Soc Exp Biol Med 1980;165:44–49.

69. Plotkin SA, Farquhar JD, Katz M, et al. Attenuation of RA27/3 rubella virus in WI-38 human diploid cells. Am J Dis Child 1969;118:178–185.

70. Plotkin SA, Farquhar JD, Ogra PL. Immunologic properties of RA27/3 rubella virus vaccine. JAMA 1973;225:585–590.

71. Bottiger M, Christenson B, Romanus V, et al. Swedish experience of two dose vaccination programme aiming at eliminating measles, mumps, and rubella. BMJ (Clin Res Ed) 1987;295:1264–1267.

72. Ukkonen P, von Bonsdorff C-H. Rubella immunity and morbidity: effects of vaccination in Finland. Scand J Infect Dis 1988;20:255–259.

73. Sheppard S, Smithells RW, Dickson A, et al. Rubella vaccination and pregnancy: preliminary report of a national survey. BMJ 1986;292:727.

74. Enders G. Rubella antibody titers in vaccinated and nonvaccinated women and results of vaccination during pregnancy. Rev Infect Dis 1985;7(Suppl 1):S103–S107.

75. Centers for Disease Control. Rubella vaccination during pregnancy—United States, 1971–1988. MMWR 1989;38: 289–293.

76. Losonsky GA, Fishaut JM, Strussenberg J, et al. Effect of immunization against rubella on lactation products. II. Maternal-neonatal interactions. J Infect Dis 1982;145:661–666.

77. Krogh V, Duffy LC, Wong D, et al. Postpartum immunization with rubella virus vaccine and antibody response in breast-feeding infants. J Lab Clin Med 1989;113:695–699.

78. Kaplan KM, Cochi SL, Edmonds LD, et al. A profile of mothers giving birth to infants with congenital rubella syndrome. Am J Dis Child 1990;144:118–123.

79. Centers for Disease Control. Rubella in universities—Washington, California. MMWR 1982;31: 394–395.

80. Centers for Disease Control. Rubella in hospitals—California. MMWR 1983;32:37–39.

81. Centers for Disease Control. Rubella outbreak among office workers—New York City. MMWR 1985;34: 455–459.

82. Heseltine PNR, Ripper M, Wohlford P. Nosocomial rubella—consequences of an outbreak and efficacy of a mandatory immunization program. Infect Control 1985;6:371–374.

83. Crawford GE, Gremillion DH. Epidemic measles and rubella in Air Force recruits: impact of immunization. J Infect Dis 1981;144:403–410.

84. Cote TR, Sivertson D, Horan JM, et al. Evaluation of a two-dose measles, mumps, and rubella vaccination schedule in a cohort of college athletes. Public Health Rep 1993;108:431–435.

85. Centers for Disease Control and Prevention. Summary of notifiable diseases, United States—1993. MMWR 1994;42 (53):1–73.

86. Bart KJ, Orenstein WA, Preblud SR, et al. Universal immunization to interrupt rubella. Rev Infect Dis 1985; 7(suppl):S177–S184.

87. American Academy of Pediatrics. Rubella. In: Peter G, ed. 1994 Red Book: report of the committee on infectious diseases. 23rd ed. Elk Grove Village, IL: American Academy of Pediatrics, 1994:406–412.

88. American College of Obstetricians and Gynecologists. Rubella and pregnancy. Technical Bulletin no. 171. Washington, DC: American College of Obstetricians and Gynecologists, 1992:1–6.

89. American College of Physicians Task Force on Adult Immunization and Infectious Diseases Society of America. Guide for adult immunization. 3rd ed. Philadelphia: American College of Physicians, 1994: 125–128.

90. American Medical Association. Guidelines for adolescent preventive services (GAPS). Chicago: American Medical Association, 1994:165–167.

91. Green M, ed. Bright Futures: guidelines for health supervision of infants, children, and adolescents. Arlington, VA: National Center for Education in Maternal and Child Health, 1994.

92. American Academy of Family Physicians. Age charts for periodic health examination. Kansas City, MO: American Academy of Family Physicians, 1994. (Reprint no. 510.)

93. Canadian Task Force on the Periodic Health Examination. Canadian guide to clinical preventive health care. Ottawa: Canada Communication Group, 1994:126–135.

94. Gudnadottir M. Cost-effectiveness of different strategies for prevention of congenital rubella infection: a practical example from Iceland. Rev Infect Dis 1985;7:S200–S209.

95. Farber ME, Finkelstein SN. A cost-benefit analysis of a mandatory premarital rubella-antibody screening. N Engl J Med 1979;300:856–859.

96. McCormack WM, Gilfillan RF, Grady GF, et al. Cost-benefit analysis of rubella screening [letter]. N Engl J Med 1979; 301:216–217.

97. Centers for Disease Control. National Childhood Vaccine Injury Act: requirements for permanent vaccination records and for reporting of selected events after vaccination. MMWR 1988;37:197–200.

33. Screening for Visual Impairment

RECOMMENDATION

Vision screening to detect amblyopia and strabismus is recommended once for all children prior to entering school, preferably between ages 3 and 4. Clinicians should be alert for signs of ocular misalignment when examining infants and children. Screening for diminished visual acuity with Snellen visual acuity chart is recommended for elderly persons. There is insufficient evidence to recommend for or against screening for diminished visual acuity among other asymptomatic persons, but recommendations against routine screening may be made on other grounds (see *Clinical Intervention*).

Burden of Suffering

Preschool Children. Undetected vision problems are common in preschool children, with an estimated prevalence of 5–10%.[1] About 2–5% suffer from amblyopia ("lazy eye"; loss of vision due to disuse) and strabismus (ocular misalignment) which, aside from congenital conditions, usually develop between infancy and ages 5–7.[2–4] In the newborn, risk factors for developing strabismus or amblyopia include a family history of ocular malformations, anisometropia (a large difference in refractive power between the two eyes, more than 4 diopters in sphere and/or 2 diopters in astigmatism), congenital cataracts, ocular tumors, premature birth, or birth to a mother who suffered from infection such as rubella, genital herpes, or toxoplasmosis during pregnancy. Since normal vision from birth is necessary for normal binocular development, failure to detect and treat amblyopia, marked anisometropia, or strabismus at an early age may result in irreversible visual deficits. Resulting permanent amblyopia and cosmetic defects may lead to later restrictions in educational and occupational opportunities.[5,6] Patients with amblyopia are at increased risk of blindness from loss of vision in their good eye.[6a]

School-Aged Children. Data are limited regarding the prevalence of uncorrected refractive errors and previously undiagnosed vision problems in elementary school-aged and adolescent children. A community-based examination of all first- to third-grade children in 1984 found visual acuity of 20/30 or better in the better eye in 94–95% of the schoolchildren; 7%, 9%, and 9% of children in first, second, and third grades, respectively, had glasses prescribed. Two percent of children for whom glasses were prescribed were not wearing them.[7] Refractive errors, which often become manifest during school age, rarely carry any serious prognostic implications. Experts disagree on whether an uncorrected refractive error that would be detected by screening has any adverse effects on academic performance in school-aged children.[7,8]

Adolescents and Adults. Refractive errors are the most common visual disorder in the adolescent and adult population. In a study of undetected eye disease in a primary care population (94% African-American), 21% of patients ages 40–59 were diagnosed with an eye disease of which they were not aware.[9] The majority of these cases, however, were not detected by acuity screening (e.g., glaucoma or diabetic retinopathy), most were mild or previously diagnosed, and few required immediate treatment. There are no data to determine the incremental benefit of routine screening of adults to detect early refractive errors compared to waiting for patients to present with complaints of vision problems.

Elders. Visual impairment is a common and potentially serious problem among older people. Personal safety may be compromised; the risk of falling is increased.[10] The rate ratio for fatal car crashes in the elderly is lower in states where vision testing is required for persons over 65 than in states where it is not required.[11] While a reduction in visual acuity may be noticed by an individual, underreporting is common. One small study of patients attending a geriatric day care center showed that one third had unrecognized severe visual loss.[12] Surveys have revealed that up to 25% of older people are wearing inappropriate visual correction.[13] The Baltimore Eye Survey reported that more than half of the 5,300 persons screened had improved vision after refraction and appropriate corrective lenses.[14] In the Beaver Dam Eye Study, visual acuity with current correction was worse than 20/40 in 5% of persons aged 65–74, and was worse than 20/40 in 21% of those 75 years of age or older; the proportion with correctable poor acuity was not reported.[15] A 1995 study found that uncorrected vision problems are common among nursing home residents. Among 499 residents, 17% had bilateral blindness (acuity 20/200) and 19% had impaired vision (<20/40); a substantial proportion of vision problems in this population could have been remedied by adequate refractive correction or treatment of cataracts.[15a]

The most common causes of visual impairment in the elderly include presbyopia, cataract, age-related macular degeneration (ARMD), and glaucoma (see Chapter 34). In persons over age 75 years, 5% have exudative macular degeneration, and 5% have glaucoma.[16–18] The prevalence of cataract increases with age. In persons aged 55–64 years, the Beaver Dam Eye Study found 33% with early cataract and 6% with late cataract; in persons over 75 years these prevalences were 37% and 52%.[17] The frequency of visually significant cataract is higher in women than in men.[17] The causes of blindness vary by race, with whites being more commonly afflicted with macular degeneration and blacks having a higher prevalence of untreated cataract and open-angle glaucoma.[19]

Accuracy of Screening Tests

Preschool Children. Despite the importance of early childhood screening for strabismus and amblyopia, detecting occult visual disorders by screening tests in children under 3 years of age has generally been unsuccessful. Obstacles to screening include the child's inability to cooperate, the time required for testing, and inaccuracy of the tests.[20,21] Some of the techniques for this age group, such as preferential looking, grating acuity cards, refractive screening, and photographic evaluation, have not yet been proven effective.[22,23]

Screening tests for detecting strabismus and amblyopia in the 3–5-year-old child include simple inspection, cover test, visual acuity tests, and stereo vision assessment. Although it is widely recommended,[24] reports are not available of sensitivity or specificity of the cover test performed by primary care providers. Visual acuity tests for children include the Snellen chart, the Landolt C, the tumbling E, the Allen picture cards, grating cards, and others.[25] The specificity of any acuity test for detecting strabismus or amblyopia is imperfect as other conditions may be the cause of the diminished acuity. Snellen letters are estimated to have a sensitivity of only 25%–37%.[26] Refractive screening is not a test for strabismus or amblyopia per se, but may be used to identify amblyogenic risk factors (e.g., anisometropia, or severe hyperopia [farsightedness]).[27]

The Modified Clinical Technique (MCT) includes retinoscopy, cover testing, quantifying ocular misalignment, Snellen acuity, color vision assessment, and external observation.[28] Preferential looking (PL) has been substituted for Snellen acuity in the MCT without loss of predictive power of the MCT but with increase in percentage of young children who were able to complete the test.[23] The MCT, despite a high sensitivity and specificity, cannot be used routinely by primary care physicians for screening because it takes on average about 12 minutes to perform and requires skills and instrumentation not typically found in this setting.

Stereograms such as the Random Dot E (RDE) have been proposed as more effective than visual acuity tests in detecting strabismus and amblyopia.[25,29] The test, in which the child wears Polaroid glasses while viewing the test cards, takes about 1 minute. The RDE has an estimated sensitivity of 54–64%, specificity of 87–90%, positive predictive value of 57%, and negative predictive value of 93%.[30,31]

An evaluation of a preschool vision screening program comprising visual inspection, acuity assessment, and evaluation of stereoacuity, found a combined negative predictive value of 99% for amblyopia, strabismus, and/or high refractive errors.[32] A similar program, evaluated with limited use of definitive examinations, reported a positive predictive value of 72% for screening.[33] A positive screening test does not ensure adequate follow-up. In one practice-based study, nearly half of parents of children who had a positive screen were unaware of that result 2 months later; 15% of children referred to a specialist did not make or keep the subsequent appointment.[34]

School-Aged Children. The public school system in most states has taken on the responsibility of vision screening in school-aged children and making referrals to eye care specialists. In 1992, all but 12 states had mandatory or regulated screening of elementary school-aged children. Screening of visual acuity is generally accomplished with standard Snellen vision charts. Although referral criteria and procedures vary widely, school screening may have a false-positive rate of 30% or more.[35,36]

Elders. Asking screening questions about visual function has yielded mixed results when compared to use of a Snellen acuity chart. The question "Do you have difficulty seeing distant objects?" had sensitivity of 28% in detecting visual acuity worse than 20/40.[37] "(When wearing glasses) Can you see well enough to recognize a friend across the street?" had sensitivity of 48%.[38] A similar question showed lower sensitivity for visual impairment as part of the HANES 1971–72 survey.[39] A brief questionnaire using an additive score formed from three similar questions was found to have sensitivity of 86% and specificity of 90% for visual acuity worse than 20/40 in a combined sample of 248 persons aged 45 years and older selected at random from a community population, and a convenience sample of 118 diabetics from the Wisconsin Epidemiologic Survey of Diabetic Retinopathy.[40]

Impaired visual acuity is readily detected by use of a Snellen chart. Cataracts are detectable by ophthalmoscopy, even by relatively inexperienced health professionals. There are few data on sensitivity and specificity of these examinations in the primary care setting. Funduscopy may reveal characteristic changes of ARMD. While these abnormalities are readily recognized by ophthalmologists and optometrists trained in funduscopy, no studies of the sensitivity of funduscopy by primary care physicians were found in a computerized literature search.[41] Case reports support the usefulness of the Amsler grid to detect early detachment of the retinal pigment epithelium at a point when immediate treatment may be beneficial, but compliance with testing is poor.[42,43]

Effectiveness of Early Detection

Preschool Vision Problems. There is fair evidence based on animal models, and case series and case-control studies in humans, that early detection and treatment of amblyopia and strabismus in infants and young children improves the prognosis for normal eye development.[24,44-49] The success of intervention may be dependent on age, with increased likelihood of attaining normal or near-normal vision with earlier detection and treatment; the older the patient, the longer the duration of treatment needed. In a prospective study of visual acuity screening in matched cohorts of over 700 preschool children, those who were screened had significantly less visual impairment than the controls when reexamined 6–12 months later.[50]

Vision Problems in School-Aged Children, Adolescents, and Nonelderly Adults. There is little evidence that early detection of refractive errors is associated with important clinical benefits, compared with testing based on symptoms. A common justification for regular screening in school-aged children is the concern that undetected vision problems are an important cause of academic difficulty, but there is no evidence that routine screening has important benefits in terms of academic performance.[51,52]

Vision Problems in Elders. Refractive errors are readily correctable with eye glasses or contact lenses. Following refraction and correction, 54% of subjects in the Baltimore Eye Survey improved their visual acuity by at least one line on the Snellen chart and 8% improved by three lines or more. While the impact on physical and social function of these improvements is unknown, it has been demonstrated that restoration of vision following cataract surgery leads to subjective improvements in a variety of vision-related functions, as well as improvements in objective measures of physical and intellectual function.[53]

Although ophthalmologists use differing criteria to determine the optimal time to remove cataracts, a general rule is that surgery should be considered when an otherwise well patient feels that there is a significant impairment to daily life caused by the vision loss. While there are theoretical reasons to believe that earlier referral to an ophthalmologist is desirable for assessment of retinal disease prior to obliteration of the view of the fundus by advancing cataract, in practice most individuals will complain of visual loss and be treated before this occurs.

Randomized clinical trials have shown a beneficial effect of argon laser photocoagulation of choroidal neovascular membranes in selected cases of ARMD.[54] Controlled trials with other wavelengths of light (e.g., krypton) are currently underway. Medical therapy for ARMD, with zinc supplements or interferon, has been reported as case series, but it has not yet been evaluated more rigorously.[55,56]

Recommendations of Other Groups

The Canadian Task Force on the Periodic Health Examination (CTF)[57] concluded that there is fair evidence to recommend visual acuity testing of preschool children. The American Academy of Ophthalmology (AAO),[58] American Optometric Association,[59] American Academy of Pediatrics (AAP),[60] and Bright Futures[61] each recommend examining newborns and infants for ocular problems and screening visual acuity and ocular alignment at age 3 or 4 in children, and every 1–2 years thereafter through adolescence. New guidelines for vision screening in children, outlining which tests to use and criteria for referral, have been developed by the AAP Section on Ophthalmology, in conjunction with the AAO and the American Association for Pediatric Ophthalmology and Strabismus.[62] The American Academy of Family Physicians (AAFP) recommends that all children be screened for eye and vision abnormalities at 3–4 years of age and that clinicians remain alert for vision problems throughout childhood and adolescence.[63]

Periodic comprehensive eye examinations including acuity testing are recommended for all adults by the American Optometric Association and by Prevent Blindness America (formerly National Society to Prevent Blindness)[59] and for adults over age 40 by the American Academy of Ophthalmology.[65] The CTF[41] and the AAFP[63] advise routine screening of visual acuity only for individuals age 65 and over. AAFP recommendations on vision screening are currently under review.

Discussion

No prospective trial has directly assessed the benefits of routine preschool vision screening, but animal models and observational studies provide fair evidence that earlier detection and treatment improves the outcomes in children with strabismus and amblyopia. Screening and early referral is recommended for infants and preschool children in the primary care setting. The optimal age for screening cannot be determined from direct evidence. The recommendation to screen at ages 3–4 years is based primarily on expert opinion, and reflects a compromise between the inability of younger children to cooperate fully with screening and the goal to detect and treat the conditions as early as possible.

Screening older children, adolescents, and adults is less likely to detect vision problems that require early intervention. Although routine screening in asymptomatic persons may detect some persons with early refractive errors, these are readily corrected when patients become symptomatic. It is not certain that the incremental benefit of early detection (compared to evaluation when patients complain of change in vision) is sufficient to justify the costs and inconvenience of routine testing. Any patient with ocular symptoms, however, should be advised to see an eye care specialist.

Vision problems are more prevalent in persons over 65, and they are more likely to lead to serious consequences such as accidental injuries. Questioning elderly patients about vision problems is less sensitive than directly assessing visual acuity. Although the effect on functional outcomes of periodic screening with Snellen chart acuity testing in the elderly has not been directly assessed, there is fair evidence that routine screening leads to improvements in measured acuity, and there is little chance of serious harm from screening. The role of routine screening with funduscopy by the primary care provider is less certain. Funduscopy is likely to be more sensitive than acuity testing for detecting persons with exudative ARMD, especially those with early disease, who may benefit from photocoagulation therapy. The sensitivity and specificity of funduscopy by primary care providers for ARMD is unknown, however.

CLINICAL INTERVENTION

Vision screening for amblyopia and strabismus is recommended for all children once before entering school, preferably between ages 3 and 4 years ("B" recommendation). Clinicians should be alert for signs of ocular misalignment when examining all infants and children. Stereoacuity testing may be more effective than visual acuity testing in detecting these conditions.

There is insufficient evidence to recommend for or against routine screening for diminished visual acuity among asymptomatic schoolchildren and nonelderly adults ("C" recommendation). Recommendations against such screening may be made on other grounds, including the inconvenience and cost of routine screening, and the fact that refractive errors can be readily corrected when they produce symptoms.

Routine vision screening with Snellen acuity testing is recommended for elderly persons ("B" recommendation). The optimal frequency for screening is not known and is left to clinical discretion. Selected questions about vision may also be helpful in detecting vision problems in elderly persons, but they do not appear as sensitive or specific as direct assessment of acuity. There is insufficient evidence to recommend for or against routine screening with ophthalmoscopy by the primary care physician in asymptomatic elderly patients ("C" recommendation).

The draft update of this chapter was prepared for the U.S. Preventive Services Task Force by Joseph N. Blustein, MD, MS, and Dennis Fryback, PhD, based in part on materials prepared for the Canadian Task Force on the Periodic Health Examination by Christopher Patterson, MD, FRCP, and John W. Feightner, MD, MSc, FCFP.

REFERENCES

1. National Center for Health Statistics. Refraction status and motility defects of persons 4–74 years, U.S. 1971–72: Vital health statistics, Series 11, 1978.

2. Ehrlich MI, Reinecke RD, Simons K. Preschool vision screening for amblyopia and strabismus: programs, methods, guidelines. Surv Ophthalmol 1983;28:145–163.

3. Cross AW. Health screening in schools: part I. J Pediatr 1985;107:487–494.

4. Thompson JR, Woodruff G, Hiscox FA, Strong N, Minshull C. The incidence and prevalence of amblyopia detected in childhood. Public Health 1991;105:455–462.

5. Campbell LR, Charney E. Factors associated with delay in diagnosis of childhood amblyopia. Pediatrics 1991;87:178–185.

6. Magramm I. Amblyopia: etiology, detection, and treatment. Pediatr Rev 1992;13:7–14.

6a. Woodruff G. Amblyopia: could we do better? BMJ 1995;310:1153–1154.

7. Helveston EM, Weber JC, Miller K, et al. Visual function and academic performance. Am J Ophthalmol 1985;99:346–355.

8. Rosner J, Rosner J. Comparison of visual characteristics in children with and without learning difficulties. Am J Optom Physiol Optics 1987;84:531–533.

9. Wang F, Ford D, Tielsch JM, et al. Undetected eye disease in a primary care population. Arch Intern Med 1994;154:1821–1828.

10. Hindmarsh JA, Estes EH. Falls in older persons: etiology and interventions. In: Goldbloom RB, Lawrence RS, eds. Preventing disease. Beyond the rhetoric. New York: Springer-Verlag, 1990.

11. Nelson DE, Sacks JJ, Chorba TI. Required vision testing for older drivers. N Engl J Med 1992;326: 1784–1785.

12. McMurdo ME, Baines PS. The detection of visual disability in the elderly. Health Bull 1988;46: 327–329.

13. Stults BM. Preventive health care for the elderly. West J Med 1984;141:832–845.

14. Tielsch JM, Sommer A, Witt K, Katz J, Royall RM. Blindness and visual impairment in an American urban population. The Baltimore Eye Survey. Arch Ophthalmol 1990;108:286–290.

15. Klein R, Klein BE, Linton KL, De MD. The Beaver Dam eye study: visual acuity. Ophthalmology 1991;98:1310–1315.

15a. Tielsch JM, Javitt JC, Coleman A, et al. The prevalence of blindness and visual impairment among nursing home residents in Baltimore. N Engl J Med 1995;332:1205–1209.

16. Klein R, Klein BE, Linton KL. Prevalence of age-related maculopathy. The Beaver Dam eye study. Ophthalmology 1992;99:933–943.

17. Klein BE, Klein R, Linton KL. Prevalence of age-related lens opacities in a population. The Beaver Dam eye study. Ophthalmology 1992;99:546–552.

18. Klein BE, Klein R, Sponsel WE, et al. Prevalence of glaucoma. The Beaver Dam eye study. Ophthalmology 1992;99:1499–1504.

19. Sommer A, Tielsch JM, Katz J, et al. Racial differences in the cause-specific prevalence of blindness in East Baltimore. N Engl J Med 1991;325:1412–1417.

20. Jacobson SG, Mohindra I, Held R. Visual acuity of infants with ocular disease. Am J Ophthalmol 1982;93:198–209.

21. Hall SM, Pugh AG, Hall DMB. Vision screening in the under-5s. BMJ 1982;285:1096–1098.

22. Jarvis SN, Tamhne RC, Thompson L, Francis PM, Anderson J, Colver AF. Preschool vision screening. Arch Dis Child 1991;66:288–294.

23. Schmidt PP. Effectiveness of vision-screening in pre-school populations with preferential-looking cards used for assessment of visual acuity. Optom Vision Sci 1991;68:210–219.

24. Day S, Eggers H, Gammon JA, Spivey BE. Early strabismus/amblyopia screening. Patient Care 1990;24:83–105.

25. Fern KD, Manny RE. Visual acuity of the preschool child: a review. Am J Optom Physiol Optics 1986; 63:319–345.

26. Lieberman S, Cohen AH, Stolzberg M, Ritty JM. Validation study of the New York State Optometric Association (NYSOA) vision screening battery. Am J Optom Physiol Optics 1985;62:165–168.

27. Sjostrand J, Abrahamsson M. Risk factors in amblyopia. Eye 1990;4:787–793.

28. Peters HB. The Orinda study. Am J Optom Physiol Optics 1984;61:361–363.

29. Ruttum MS, Bence SM, Alcorn D. Stereopsis testing in a preschool vision screening program. J Pediatr Ophthalmol Strabismus 1986;23:298–302.

30. Hammond RS, Schmidt PP. A Random Dot E stereogram for the vision screening of children. Arch Ophthalmol 1986;104:54–60.

31. Ruttum MS, Nelson DB. Stereopsis testing to reduce overreferral in preschool vision screening. J Pediatr Ophthalmol Strabismus 1991;28:131–133.

32. De Becker I, MacPherson HJ, LaRoche GR, et al. Negative predictive value of a population-based preschool vision screening program. Ophthalmology 1992;99:998–1003.
33. MacPherson H, Braunstein J, LaRoche GR. Utilizing basic screening principles in the design and evaluation of vision screening programs. Am Orthopt J 1991;41:110–121.
34. Wasserman RC, Croft CA, Brotherton SE. Preschool vision screening in pediatric practice: a study from the Pediatric Research in Office Settings (PROS) Network. American Academy of Pediatrics [published erratum appears in Pediatrics 1992;90:1001]. Pediatrics 1992;89:834–838.
35. Appelboom TM. A history of vision screening. J School Health 1985;55:138–141.
36. Romano PE. Summary and conclusions. Symposium on preschool/school vision and eye screening: current techniques and future trends. Am Orthop J 1988;38:73–80.
37. Stone DH, Shannon DJ. Screening for impaired visual acuity in middle age in general practice. BMJ 1978;2:859–861.
38. Haase KW, Bryant EE. Development of a scale designed to measure functional distance vision loss using an interview technique. Proc Am Stat Assoc 1973;(SS):274–279.
39. Hiller R, Krueger DE. Validity of a survey question as a measure of visual acuity impairment. Am J Public Health 1983;73:93–96.
40. Fryback DG, Martin PA, Klein R, Klein BEK. Short questionnaires about visual function to proxy for measured best-corrected visual acuity. Invest Ophthalmol Visual Sci 1993;34:1422.
41. Canadian Task Force on the Periodic Health Examination. Canadian guide to clinical preventive health care. Ottawa: Canada Communication Group, 1994:932–942.
42. Fine SL. Early detection of extrafoveal neovascular membranes by daily central field evaluation. Ophthalmology 1985;92:603–609.
43. Fine AM, Elman MJ, Ebert JE, Prestia PA, Starr JS, Fine SL. Earliest symptoms caused by neovascular membranes in the macula. Arch Ophthalmol 1986;104:513–514.
44. Epelbaum M, Milleret C, Buisseret P, Dufier JL. The sensitive period for strabismic amblyopia in humans. Ophthalmology 1993;100:323–327.
45. Lithander J, Sjostrand J. Anisometropic and strabismic amblyopia in the age group 2 years and above: a prospective study of the results of treatment. Br J Ophthalmol 1991;75:111–116.
46. Hiscox F, Strong N, Thompson JR, Minshull C, Woodruff G. Occlusion for amblyopia: a comprehensive survey of outcome. Eye 1992;6:300–304.
47. Levartovsky S, Gottesman N, Shimshoni M, Oliver M. Factors affecting long-term results of successfully treated amblyopia: age at beginning of treatment and age at cessation of monitoring. J Pediatr Ophthalmol Strabismus 1992;29:219–223.
48. Rutstein RP, Fuhr PS. Efficacy and stability of amblyopia therapy. Optom Vision Sci 1992;69:747–754.
49. Rubin SE, Nelson LB. Amblyopia. Diagnosis and management. Pediatr Clin North Am 1993;40:727–735.
50. Feldman W, Milner RA, Sackett B, Gilbert S. Effects of preschool screening for vision and hearing on prevalence of vision and hearing problems 6–12 months later. Lancet 1980;2:1014–1016.
51. Hulme C. The implausibility of low-level visual deficits as a cause of children's reading difficulties. Cogn Neuropsychol 1988;5:369–374.
52. Lovegrove W, Martin F, Slaghuis W. A theoretical and experimental case for a visual deficit in specific reading disability. Cogn Neuropsychol 1986;3:225–267.
53. Applegate WB, Miller ST, Elam JT, Freeman JM, Wood TO, Gettlefinger TC. Impact of cataract surgery with lens implantation on vision and physical function in elderly patients. JAMA 1987;257:1064–1066.
54. Argon laser photocoagulation for senile macular degeneration. Results of a randomized clinical trial. Arch Ophthalmol 1982;100:912–918.
55. Newsome DA, Swartz M, Leone NC, Elston RC, Miller E. Oral zinc in macular degeneration. Arch Ophthalmol 1988;106:192–198.
56. Fung WE. Interferon alpha 2a for treatment of age-related macular degeneration [letter]. Am J Ophthalmol 1991; 112:349–350.
57. Canadian Task Force on the Periodic Health Examination. Canadian guide to clinical preventive care. Ottawa: Canada Communication Group, 1994:298–304.
58. American Academy of Ophthalmology. Preferred practice pattern: comprehensive pediatric eye evaluation. San Francisco: American Academy of Ophthalmology, 1992.
59. American Optometric Association. Recommendations for regular optometric care. St. Louis, MO: American Optometric Association, 1994.

60. American Academy of Pediatrics, Committee on Practice and Ambulatory Medicine. Recommendations for preventive pediatric health care. Pediatrics 1995;96:373–374.

61. Green M, ed. Bright Futures: guidelines for health supervision of infants, children and adolescents. Arlington VA: National Center for Education in Maternal and Child Health, 1994.

62. AAP Policy Statement: proposed vision screening guidelines. AAP News, vol 11 no 1. Elk Grove Village, IL: American Academy of Pediatrics, 1995.

63. American Academy of Family Physicians. Age charts for periodic health examination. Kansas City, MO: American Academy of Family Physicians, 1994. (Reprint no. 510.)

34. Screening for Glaucoma

RECOMMENDATION

There is insufficient evidence to recommend for or against routine screening for intraocular hypertension or glaucoma by primary care clinicians. Recommendations to refer high-risk patients for evaluation by an eye specialist may be made on other grounds (see *Clinical Intervention*).

Burden of Suffering

Glaucoma is a disorder defined by slowly progressive loss of vision in association with characteristic signs of damage to the optic nerve. Selective death of retinal ganglion cells leads to the gradual enlargement of the optic cup and loss of vision (beginning with peripheral vision) that are typical of glaucoma.[1] Increased intraocular pressure (IOP) is common in glaucoma and is believed to contribute to the damage to the optic nerve, but it is no longer considered a diagnostic criterion for glaucoma. Glaucoma is the second leading cause of irreversible blindness in the U.S., and the leading cause among African Americans.[2,3] Of the various forms of glaucoma (e.g., congenital, open-angle, closed-angle, secondary), primary open-angle glaucoma (POAG) is the most common in the U.S. (80–90% of cases)[4] and is estimated to be responsible for impaired vision in 1.6 million Americans and blindness in 150,000.[1,4] Annual office visits for glaucoma increased from roughly 2 million in 1975 to almost 9 million in 1992.[4a] POAG is usually asymptomatic until irreversible visual field loss has occurred. One study reported that over the course of 20 years, blindness may develop in up to 75% of persons with glaucoma.[5] There are few data, however, on the natural history of disease in persons with mild visual field defects detected by screening.

The prevalence of glaucoma is 4–6-fold higher in blacks than whites, and it increases steadily with age: among whites, glaucoma is present in 0.5–1.5% of persons under age 65 and 2–4% of those over 75;[6,7] among blacks, 1.2% of 40–49-year-olds and 11.3% of those over 80 have glaucoma.[8] Prevalence of glaucoma is increased in patients with diabetes mellitus, myopia, and a family history of glaucoma.[1] A much larger number of persons have ocular hypertension (usually defined as an IOP > 21 mm Hg), which is a strong risk factor for developing glaucoma. Ocular hypertension is present in 7–13% of the general population, prevalence increasing with age.[3] In the Framingham Study, one fourth of men and women over age 65 had ocular hypertension.[9] The risk of progressing to glaucoma varies directly with level of IOP and duration of follow-up: the proportion of persons developing visual deficits within 5 years was less than 1% for normal IOP (<21 mm Hg), 3–10% for IOP ≥ 21 mm Hg, 6–16% for IOP > 25 mm Hg, and 33% for IOP > 30 mm Hg.[10] Untreated individuals with moderate ocular hypertension (mean IOP 24–26 mm Hg) developed new visual deficits (based on sensitive measures) at a rate of 3–4% per year in recent trials.[11–13] Among patients with untreated ocular hypertension followed for 17–20 years in older series, over 30% developed clinical glaucoma.[14,15]

Accuracy of Screening Tests

There are two potential targets for screening among asymptomatic persons: individuals who have normal vision but are at increased risk for developing glaucoma (i.e., "glaucoma suspects"), and those who have undetected visual field defects (i.e., undiagnosed glaucoma). Up to 50% of persons with glaucomatous visual deficits detected by screening are unaware of their diagnosis.[8]

The three most common screening tests for glaucoma are tonometry, ophthalmoscopy, and perimetry. Tonometers, which include Schiötz, applanation, and noncontact (air puff) devices, are used to measure intraocular pressure. The accuracy and reliability of tonometry is affected by the choice of device, the experience of the examiner, and physiologic variables in the patient.[10,16] The more fundamental problem with tonometry as a screening test is the limited sensitivity and specificity of elevated IOP for current or future cases of glaucoma. Many patients with ocular hypertension (perhaps more than 70%) will never develop vision problems due to glaucoma.[14,15] Isolated measurements of IOP are also insensitive for glaucoma: only half of all patients with documented glaucoma have IOP greater than 21 mm Hg on random measurement, due in part to fluctuations in IOP over time.[4,17] There is no single cutoff value of IOP that provides an acceptable balance of sensitivity and specificity for screening.[1] In the Baltimore Eye Survey, a cutoff of IOP > 18 mm Hg had a sensitivity and specificity of 65% for definite or probable glaucoma; raising the cutoff to 21 mm Hg improved specificity to 92%, but lowered sensitivity to 44%.[4] In population screening, where prevalence of glaucoma is relatively low, less than 5% of those with ocular hypertension will have documented glaucoma.[18]

A second screening test for POAG is direct ophthalmoscopy or slit-lamp examination, which can detect the changes in the optic nerve head (e.g., cupping, pallor, hemorrhage) that often precede the development of visual deficits in glaucoma. Examining the optic disk to screen for glaucoma in the primary care setting is limited by considerable interobserver variation in interpretation of funduscopic findings, even among experts using standardized criteria.[19] Ophthalmologists using direct ophthalmoscopy alone detected fewer than one half of all cases of glaucoma.[20] Primary care clinicians with less skill in ophthalmoscopy and less time to dilate pupils would be expected to have poorer accuracy. Qualitative evaluation of stereoscopic photographs of the optic disk is more sensitive,[21] and disc photography allows for precise measures of disk parameters, which may provide evidence of glaucomatous nerve damage (e.g., vertical and horizontal cup-disk ratios, neuroretinal rim width). No combination of parameters, however, adequately discriminates patients with glaucoma from normal subjects. In the Baltimore survey, various combinations of disk parameters, IOP, and family history had only moderate sensitivity (49–66%) and specificity (79–87%) for glaucoma.[4] Neither slit-lamp examination nor optic disk photography is routinely available in the primary care setting.

The third method of screening for POAG is perimetry, in which patients respond to visual stimuli of varying brightness presented in various locations in their visual field. Reproducible visual field defects currently represent the "gold standard" for diagnosing glaucoma, but diagnostic testing with automated perimetry may take more than 45 minutes and is not feasible for screening.[1] Modified testing strategies can reduce the time needed for screening, but they are less sensitive and specific for glaucoma. Evaluations of these devices report a sensitivity in excess of 90% and a specificity of 70–88%.[17,22,23] False-positive results can be caused by visual disorders other than glaucoma and by unfamiliarity of patients with the testing process. Due to expense and technical difficulties, automated perimetry is not practical for routine use in the primary care setting. Moreover, visual field loss is often a late event in the natural history of glaucoma: by the time visual deficits are evident, up to 50% of nerve fibers may have been lost.[24] Newer techniques (e.g., computer-assisted imaging, specialized photographic methods) for assessing changes in the optic nerve may prove more sensitive for early injury, but they are currently too complicated or expensive to be used for routine screening.[1,17]

Effectiveness of Early Detection

Visual deficits due to glaucoma are not generally reversible, but early treatment is widely believed to prevent or delay the progression to more serious vision problems. The assumption that lowering intraocular pressure improves outcome in patients with glaucoma is based primarily on indirect evidence, however: the strong association between level of intraocular pressure and risk of POAG, the deleterious effects of raised IOP in secondary glaucoma and in animal models, and the progressive nature of untreated glaucoma. Controlled studies of treatment of glaucoma have generally compared different modes of therapy with each other, rather than comparing treatment to no treatment.[25] The majority of patients experience continuing loss of vision despite treatment, however, and change in IOP does not reliably distinguish patients who progress on treatment from those with stable disease.[26,27] A few observational studies have reported a higher incidence of disease progression in those receiving treatment than untreated patients, but these findings are probably biased by more severe disease in treated subjects.[10] Some indirect evidence of treatment effectiveness is provided by a report from Denmark of declining incidence of blindness due to glaucoma over the past 30 years.[28] The disparity in the rates of glaucoma and glaucoma blindness among white and black Americans may also reflect greater access to effective treatment among whites, although the higher prevalence of glaucoma among blacks may have a biologic basis as well.[2,29] Nonetheless, for many patients who would be detected by screening, especially those with mild visual field defects and moderate elevations of intraocular pressure, the natural history of disease and the benefits of early treatment remain uncertain. The Early Manifest Glaucoma Trial, currently under way in Sweden, is randomizing such patients to early treatment with medications and laser therapy or no initial treatment (M.C. Leske, personal communication, Stony Brook, NY, March 1995).

A larger number of controlled studies has been conducted among patients with elevated IOP but no visual deficits. Early trials suffered from various methodologic problems, including small size, insufficient follow-up, or use of less reliable methods for determining visual changes.[30-33] Three recent, well-designed studies have compared ocular timolol treatment to no treatment (or placebo) in patients with normal visual fields and moderate elevations of IOP (<35 mm Hg, mean 24–26 mm Hg). These studies each enrolled larger numbers of patients, followed subjects between 4–8 years, and used automated perimetry to detect or confirm new visual field deficits. A study by Kass et al. randomized one eye to active treatment (and one to placebo) in 62 patients. After 5 years of treatment, new visual deficits developed in 4 timolol-treated eyes and 10 placebo-treated eyes, a result of borderline statistical significance.[11] Systemic effects of timolol on placebo-treated eyes may have diminished the apparent benefit of treatment. A second study by Epstein et al. randomized 107 patients to timolol or placebo: 9 patients on placebo (vs. 4 on active treatment) developed new visual field defects. The benefits of treatment were of borderline significance ($p = 0.07$) using a combined endpoint of visual field changes, increase in cup-disk ratio, or progression to more severe intraocular hypertension (IOP > 32 mm Hg).[12] In contrast, Schulzer et al. found no benefit of timolol treatment, despite enrolling more subjects and more effectively lowering IOP than previous trials (mean 4.5 mm Hg).[13] Over a 6-year study, there were no differences between treated and untreated subjects in the progression to new visual field deficits, disk hemorrhage, or change in photographic appearance of the optic disk. Neither mean IOP nor change in IOP predicted progression of disease in subjects using timolol. The power of each of these trials was reduced by substantial dropout rates among treated subjects (up to 25%).

A meta-analysis of these three trials estimated that treatment reduces the proportion of patients who develop new visual deficits by 25%, but it could not rule out a possible harmful effect of treatment.[25] The difficulty in demonstrating a significant effect in previous clinical studies may be due in part to variations among individuals in their sensitivity to raised IOP, modest effects of treatment on IOP, and poor long-term compliance with therapy. Due to continuing uncertainty about the benefits of treating moderate, isolated intraocular hypertension, a new, large randomized trial is now under way.[34]

The adverse effects of glaucoma treatment are potentially significant. Antiglaucoma medications must be taken for life and are accompanied by a variety of side effects. Eye drops containing cholinergic agonists (e.g., pilocarpine, carbachol, and echothiophate) and adrenergic agonists (epinephrine and dipivefrin) can cause ocular and systemic side effects; topical β blockers (e.g., timolol, levobunolol, metipranol, and betaxolol) can cause bradycardia, bronchospasm, or worsening of congestive heart failure; and oral carbonic anhydrase inhibitors (e.g., acetazolamide, methazolamide) can cause malaise, anorexia, and other adverse systemic effects.[35,36]

Argon laser trabeculoplasty appears to be a relatively safe alternative to medication, but it is expensive and its long-term effectiveness remains uncertain.[1,37] Although laser treatment lowered IOP more effectively than medications in one trial, more than half of laser-treated eyes required medications to control IOP, and no difference in progression to visual deficits was noted in 2-year follow-up.[37] Filtering surgery, which is usually reserved for patients unresponsive to other treatment, achieves greater reductions in IOP but carries a higher risk of serious postoperative ophthalmologic complications, including permanent loss of vision.[1] Trials of surgery as initial treatment for glaucoma are under way.[36]

Recommendations of Other Groups

The American Academy of Ophthalmology recommends a comprehensive eye examination by an ophthalmologist (including examination of the optic disc and tonometry) for all adults beginning around age 40, and periodic reexamination thereafter. Periodic examination every 3–5 years is also recommended for younger black men and women (age 20–39), due to their higher risk of glaucoma.[38] The American Optometric Association recommends regular optometric evaluations (including tonometry) for all adults, and advises primary care clinicians to screen for glaucoma (with ophthalmoscopy and/or tonometry) in high-risk groups, including persons over 50, blacks, diabetics or hypertensives, relatives of glaucoma patients, and others with specific health concerns or medical conditions.[39] Prevent Blindness America (formerly the National Society to Prevent Blindness) recommends that asymptomatic individuals have periodic comprehensive eye examinations beginning at age 20, with increasing frequency for African Americans and others at high risk.[40] A 1988 review by the Office of Technology Assessment of the U.S. Congress concluded that the benefits of screening for glaucoma or ocular hypertension among the elderly were uncertain.[10] The Canadian Task Force on the Periodic Health Examination concluded there was insufficient evidence to recommend for or against screening for glaucoma in the periodic health examination, but stated that referral of high-risk persons to a specialist with access to automated perimetry was "clinically prudent."[41]

Discussion

Glaucoma remains an important cause of blindness and impaired vision in older Americans, especially among blacks. Treatment of glaucoma with medications or surgery to lower intraocular pressure has been the standard of care for many years, and it remains prudent for patients with more severe visual deficits or extreme elevations in intraocular pressure. Definitive evidence to support the benefit of treating persons with early, mild disease is not yet available, however. Controlled treatment trials currently under way may help resolve the questions about early intervention in persons with mild disease and those at increased risk for glaucoma.

Despite a potential benefit of early treatment, the current evidence is not sufficient to recommend for or against routine screening for glaucoma in the primary care setting. There is currently no efficient and reliable method for primary care clinicians to detect patients who have early glaucoma or who are likely to develop glaucoma. While patients with elevated intraocular pressure are at increased risk of developing glaucoma, the majority may never develop significant vision problems, and the benefit of early treatment for such patients remains unproven.

Accurate glaucoma screening is best performed by eye specialists with access to specialized equipment for assessing the appearance and function of the optic nerve (e.g., slit-lamp, automated perimetry). Even experts, however, face limitations in screening patients for early disease. Of the three methods currently available for screening (tonometry, examination of the optic disk, and measurement of visual fields), only the latter is sufficiently sensitive and specific for glaucoma. Perimetry, however, is relatively expensive and time-consuming for use in routine screening, it detects patients relatively late in the disease process, and older patients may have difficulty adequately completing the examination.

Assuming that treatment of early glaucoma is effective, screening will be most useful in populations with an increased prevalence of glaucoma. If newer methods prove able to detect early and specific evidence of glaucoma (e.g., optic nerve damage), routine screening for early disease may become more feasible.

CLINICAL INTERVENTION

There is insufficient evidence to recommend for or against routine screening by primary care clinicians for elevated intraocular pressure or early glaucoma ("C" recommendation). Effective screening for glaucoma is best performed by eye specialists who have access to specialized equipment to evaluate the optic disc and measure visual fields. Recommendations may be made on other grounds to refer high-risk patients for evaluation by eye specialists. This recommendation is based on the substantial prevalence of unrecognized glaucoma in these populations, the progressive nature of untreated disease, and expert consensus that reducing intraocular pressure may slow the rate of visual loss in patients with early glaucoma or severe intraocular hypertension. Populations in whom the prevalence of glaucoma is greater than 1% include blacks over age 40 and whites over age 65. Patients with a family history of glaucoma, patients with diabetes, and patients with severe myopia are also at increased risk and may benefit from screening. The optimal frequency for glaucoma screening has not been determined and is left to clinical discretion.

The draft update of this chapter was prepared for the U.S. Preventive Services Task Force by David Atkins, MD, MPH, with contributions from materials prepared by Christopher Patterson, MD, FRCP, for the Canadian Task Force on the Periodic Health Examination.

REFERENCES

1. Quigley HA. Open-angle glaucoma. N Engl J Med 1993;328:1097–1106.
2. Sommer A, Tielsch JM, Katz J, et al. Racial differences in the cause-specific prevalence of blindness in East Baltimore. N Engl J Med 1991;325:1412–1417.
3. Leske MC. The epidemiology of open-angle glaucoma: a review. Am J Epidemiol 1983;118:166–191.
4. Tielsch JM, Katz J, Singh K, Quigley HA, Gottsch JD, Javitt J,et al. A population-based evaluation of glaucoma screening: the Baltimore Eye Survey. Am J Epidemiol 1991;134:1102–1110.
4a. Schappert SM. Office visits for glaucoma: United States, 1991–92. Advance data from vital and health statistics; no 262. Hyattsville, MD: National Center for Health Statistics, 1995.
5. Grant WM, Burke JF. Why do some people go blind from glaucoma? Ophthalmology 1982;89:991–998.

6. Klein BEK, Klein R, Sponsel WE, et al. Prevalence of glaucoma: the Beaver Dam Eye Study. Ophthalmology 1992;99:1499–1504.

7. Podgor MJ, Leske MC, Ederer F. Incidence estimates for lens changes, macular changes, open-angle glaucoma, and diabetic retinopathy. Am J Epidemiol 1983;118:206–212.

8. Tielsch JM, Sommer A, Katz J, et al. Racial variations in the prevalence of primary open-angle glaucoma. The Baltimore Eye Survey. JAMA 1991;266:369–374.

9. Kahn HA, Leibowitz HM, Ganley JP, et al. The Framingham Eye Study. Am J Epidemiol 1977;106:17–32.

10. Power EJ, Wagner JL, Duffy BM. Screening for open-angle glaucoma in the elderly. Washington, DC: Office of Technology Assessment, Congress of the United States, 1988.

11. Kass MA, Gordon MO, Hoff MR, et al. Topical timolol administration reduces the incidence of glaucomatous damage in ocular hypertensive individuals. Arch Ophthalmol 1989;107:1590–1598.

12. Epstein DL, Krug JH, Hertzmark E, et al. A long-term clinical trial of timolol therapy versus no treatment in the management of glaucoma suspects. Ophthalmology 1989;96:1460–1467.

13. Schulzer M, Drance SM, Douglas GR. A comparison of treated and untreated glaucoma suspects. Ophthalmology 1991;98:301–307.

14. Lundberg L, Wettrell K, Linner E. Ocular hypertension. Acta Ophthalmol 1987;65:705–708.

15. Hovding G, Aasved H. Prognostic factors in the development of manifest open angle glaucoma. Acta Ophthalmol 1986;64:601–608.

16. Thorburn W. The accuracy of clinical applanation tonometry. Acta Ophthalmol 1978;56:1–5.

17. Tielsch JM. Screening for primary open-angle glaucoma: alternative strategies and future directions. J Glaucoma 1992;1:214–218.

18. Sommer AE. Relationship between intraocular pressure and primary open-angle glaucoma among white and black Americans. Arch Ophthalmol 1991;109:1090–1095.

19. Schwartz JT. Methodologic differences and measurement of cup-disc ratio: an epidemiologic assessment. Arch Ophthalmol 1976;94:1101–1105.

20. Wood CM, Bosanquet RC. Limitations of direct ophthalmoscopy in screening for glaucoma. BMJ 1987; 1587–1588.

21. O'Connor DJ, Zeyen T, Caprioli J. Comparison of methods to detect glaucomatous optic nerve damage. Ophthalmology 1993;100:1498–1503.

22. Sommer A, Enger C, Witt K. Screening for glaucomatous visual field loss with automated threshold perimetry. Am J Ophthalmol 1987;103:681–684.

23. Mundorf TK, Zimmerman TJ, Nardin GF, Kendall KS. Automated perimetry, tonometry, and questionnaire in glaucoma screening. Am J Ophthalmol 1989;108:505–508.

24. Quigley HA, Addicks EM, Green R. Optic nerve damage in human glaucoma. III. Quantitative correlation of nerve fiber loss and visual field defect in glaucoma, ischemic neuropathy, papilledema, and toxic neuropathy. Arch Ophthalmol 1982;146:135–146.

25. Rossetti L, Marchetti I, Orzalesi N, et al. Randomized clinical trials on medical treatment of glaucoma: are they appropriate to guide clinical practice? Arch Ophthalmol 1993;111:96–103.

26. Messmer C, Flammer J, Stumpfig D. Influence of betaxolol and timolol on the visual fields of patients with glaucoma. Am J Ophthalmol 1991;112:678–681.

27. O'Brien C, Schwartz B, Takamoto T, Wu DC. Intraocular pressure and the rate of visual field loss in chronic open-angle glaucoma. Am J Ophthalmol 1991;111:491–500.

28. Fuchs J, Nissen KR, Goldschmidt E. Glaucoma blindness in Denmark. Acta Ophthalmol (Copenh) 1992;70:73–78.

29. Javitt JC, McBean AM, Nicholson GA, et al. Undertreatment of glaucoma among black Americans. N Engl J Med 1991;325:1418–1422.

30. Shin DH, Kolker AE, Kass MA, et al. Long-term epinephrine therapy of ocular hypertension. Arch Ophthalmol 1976;94:2059–2060.

31. Becker B, Morton RW. Topical epinephrine in glaucoma suspects. Am J Ophthalmol 1966;62:272–277.

32. Kitazawa Y. Prophylactic therapy of ocular hypertension: a prospective study. Trans Ophthal Soc NZ 1981;33:30–32.

33. Levene RZ. Uniocular miotic therapy. Trans Am Acad Ophthalmol Otol 1975;79:376–380.

34. Rossetti L, Orzalesi N, Liberati A. The medical treatment of open-angle glaucoma [letter; comment]. N Engl J Med 1993;329:735–736.

35. Bartlett JD. Adverse effects of antiglaucoma medications. Optom Clin 1991;1:103–126.

36. American Academy of Ophthalmology. Preferred practice pattern. Primary open-angle glaucoma. San Francisco: American Academy of Ophthalmology, 1992.

37. The Glaucoma Laser Trial Research Group. The Glaucoma Laser Trial (GLT). 2. Results of argon laser trabeculoplasty versus topical medicines. Ophthalmology 1990;97:1403–1413.
38. American Academy of Ophthalmology. Preferred practice pattern. Comprehensive adult eye evaluation. San Francisco: American Academy of Ophthalmology, 1992.
39. American Optometric Association. Recommendations for regular optometric care. St. Louis, MO: American Opto-metric Association, 1994.
40. Prevent Blindness America™. Vision problems in the U.S. Schaumberg, IL: Prevent Blindness America™, 1994.
41. Canadian Task Force on the Periodic Health Examination. Canadian guide to clinical preventive health care. Ottawa: Canada Communication Group, 1994:932–944.

35. Screening for Hearing Impairment

RECOMMENDATION

Screening older adults for hearing impairment by periodically questioning them about their hearing, counseling them about the availability of hearing aid devices, and making referrals for abnormalities when appropriate, is recommended. There is insufficient evidence to recommend for or against routinely screening older adults for hearing impairment using audiometric testing (see _Clinical Intervention_). There is also insufficient evidence to recommend for or against routinely screening asymptomatic adolescents and working-age adults for hearing impairment. Recommendations against such screening, except for those exposed to excessive occupational noise levels, may be made on other grounds (see _Clinical Intervention_). Routine hearing screening of asymptomatic children beyond age 3 years is not recommended. There is insufficient evidence to recommend for or against routine screening of asymptomatic neonates for hearing impairment using evoked otoacoustic emission testing or auditory brainstem response. Recommendations to screen high-risk infants may be made on other grounds (see _Clinical Intervention_). Clinicians examining infants and young children should remain alert for symptoms or signs of hearing impairment.

Burden of Suffering

Prevalence estimates for hearing impairment vary depending on age and the criteria used to define the various causal conditions.[1] For severe congenital and prelingually acquired losses, estimates range from 1 to 3/1,000 live births.[1–5,12,22,30] Moderate and severe hearing losses in early infancy are clearly associated with impaired language development.[6–8] Factors that increase the risk for congenital or delayed-onset sensorineural hearing impairment include family history of hearing impairment, congenital or central nervous system infections, ototoxic drug exposure, prematurity, congenital head and neck deformities, trauma, and several other factors associated with admission to an intensive care nursery.[2,5,9] Chronic and recurrent acute otitis media is commonly associated with temporary hearing loss in infants and school-aged children. Prevalence rates for otitis media are 12% before age 3, 4–18% for ages 4–5, and 3–9% for ages 6–9 years.[10] At any given time, about 5–7% of children ages 5–8 have a 25-dB hearing loss, usually a self-limited complication of otitis media with effusion.[11] Only a small proportion of episodes of otitis media occurring in school-aged children result in serious long-term complications, usually due to chronic middle ear effusion or previously undetected sensorineural deficits.[11] The uncertainties of the population occurrence rates and causes of infant and childhood hearing loss have been emphasized.[81]

Hearing impairment creates further difficulties in adulthood. Adult hearing impairment has been correlated with social and emotional isolation, clinical depression, and limited activity.[2,12,13,16] Hearing loss acquired between adolescence and age 50 may be due to relatively uncommon causes such as Ménière's disease, trauma, otosclerosis, ototoxic drug exposure, and eighth cranial nerve tumors. Noise-induced hearing loss is a common cause of sensorineural hearing impairment in this age group. This is particularly true for the estimated 5 million Americans with occupational exposure to hazardous noise levels.[14] The prevalence of hearing impairment increases after age 50 years, with presbycusis being the most important contributor to this increase. Approximately 25% of patients between ages 51 and 65 years have hearing thresholds greater than 30 dB (normal range being 0–20 dB) in at least one ear.[15] An objective hearing loss can be identified in over 33% of persons aged 65 years and older and in up to half of patients ages 85 years and older.[16,17] Older persons with hearing impairment are particularly prone to suffering the associated social and emotional disabilities described earlier.[18,19]

Accuracy of Screening Tests

Multiple methods of audiologic testing are potentially suitable for evaluating possible hearing deficits. Test selection is usually dictated by patient age and occasionally by type of hearing loss in question (i.e., conductive vs. sensorineural). Cooperative children and adults are usually tested with pure-tone audiometry. With pure-tone thresholds in audiometric test booths used as a reference criterion, this technique has a reported sensitivity of 92% and a specificity of 94% in detecting sensorineural hearing impairment.[37] Comparable results have been obtained in recent studies using hand-held audiometers.[16,37] Audiometric results are, however, subject to error due to improper technique, background noise in the test area, and unintentional or intentional misreporting by the subject.[11,38] Efforts have been made to devise a sufficiently accurate test utilizing the pure-tone audiometer that is briefer and less costly than standard pure-tone audiometry, but clinical efficacy is not yet confirmed.[35]

Evaluation of neonates and infants below the age of 2–3 years with audiometry is more difficult or not feasible because it depends on developmental ability; it therefore usually requires some form of electrophysiologic and/or behavioral testing. Auditory brainstem response testing (ABR) is currently viewed as the standard for physiologic testing in infancy and the most accurate method available for determining hearing function.[1,2,5,20] Sensitivity rates have been reported to be 97–100% and specificity rates to be 86–96% in comparison with behavioral testing measures.[2,5,21]

In order to detect congenital or postnatally acquired hearing loss, some form of newborn screening performed prior to hospital discharge has been recommended as most efficacious for ensuring early identification and proper follow-up and treatment of hearing loss.[5,6,20,22] As a universal *screening* test, ABR (or modified ABR) is probably unsuitable because of the need for costly equipment and trained operators in all community hospitals and birthing centers. Another screening modality for neonates is the high-risk register (HRR), a specific list of clinical risk factors associated with higher rates of neonatal and infant hearing impairment.[23,24] Those who meet criteria then undergo more objective hearing evaluation, usually ABR. The HRR identifies 50% or more of unselected infants with hearing loss[24] and 75–80% of hearing-impaired neonates in the intensive care nursery.[5] Behavioral testing techniques have also been used for infant hearing screening, including the "crib-o-gram," auditory response cradle, and distraction testing.[29–32] The limited specificity and sensitivity of behavioral testing, as well as specialized equipment and training requirements, renders these methods less desirable than physiologic testing procedures.

Evoked otoacoustic emission (EOE) testing is a relatively new screening method suitable for neonatal and infant screening.[22,25–28] Otoacoustic emissions are sounds generated by normal cochlear hair cells and detectable with relatively simple instrumentation.[67] Data concerning normative standards and reproducibility are now becoming available.[68–73] Using a cutoff of 30 dB to designate hearing impairment, EOE testing has an overall agreement rate with ABR of 91%, with a sensitivity of 84% and specificity of 92%.[74,75] Statewide neonatal auditory screening programs have been devised using EOE, and the logistical issues of operating such a program have been described.[86] Studies of EOE testing suggest a high rate of false-positive screens relative to true-positive results, which would be expected when testing for a low-prevalence condition, and some failures of testability, necessitating retesting with EOE and ABR.[83] In one screening study, only 15% of positive EOE screening tests were confirmed on repeat EOE testing 4–6 weeks later; the proportion of infants with confirmed screening tests who actually had hearing loss is unknown, since the results of diagnostic follow-up tests were not available.[88] Based on the authors' estimates of true population prevalence, more than 90% of the positive neonatal EOE screening tests were false positives. Problems such as ambient noise in the newborn nursery and other factors that affect the technical conduct of EOE require solution before this technique can be applied widely.[83,84]

The majority of children with congenitally or neonatally acquired losses are identified by age 4–5 years.[1] Hearing loss in the preschool and school-aged group is largely related to acute or chronic otitis media with effusion (OME), of which the majority of cases resolve uneventfully.[11] Routine audiometry can often detect the mild conductive hearing loss associated with OME.[33] Accuracy for detecting hearing loss associated with OME by audiometry may be variable in this age group, however, because of the mild and changing nature of the conductive loss, varying patient cooperation, conditions that make testing difficult (e.g., mental retardation), and the fact that middle ear conduction deficits may be superimposed on previously undetected sensorineural hearing loss due to other conditions.

Routine screening of working-age adolescents and adults is usually limited to those in high-risk occupations involving exposure to excessive noise levels. Among older persons, however, in whom the rate of hearing impairment is high, recommended screening methods for detecting hearing loss have included written patient questionnaires, clinical history-taking and physical examination, audiometry with a hand-held device, and simple clinical techniques designed to assess for the presence of hearing impairment.[15,16,35,36] These screening tests have not been fully evaluated, however. For example, the whispered voice test is one simple clinical technique used to assess hearing. Reported sensitivities and specificities have been 70–100% using pure-tone audiometry as the reference standard, but there are inadequate data on interobserver variability.[16] The free-field voice, tuning fork, and finger rub tests have been criticized on similar grounds.[16] Self-assessment questionnaires to identify hearing impairment probably represent the most rapid and least expensive way to screen for hearing loss in the adult. Depending on audiometric criteria, these questionnaires are reported to be 70–80% accurate for identifying patients with hearing loss defined by pure-tone audiometry.[16,36,82]

Effectiveness of Early Detection

Assessing the effectiveness of screening for hearing impairment depends upon the evidence that (a) hearing loss leads to decreased function and affects the quality of life, (b) screening leads to earlier detection of hearing abnormalities than spontaneous clinical presentation or observation, (c) various forms of hearing loss can be treated effectively, and (d) effective treatment leads to improved function and well-being.

Theoretically, the greatest benefit from hearing screening comes from detection of moderate to severe hearing impairment between birth and age 3 years. Auditory stimuli during this period appear to be critical to development of speech and language skills,[2,46] although other factors undoubtedly also play an important role. If screening for hearing deficits is performed near the time of birth, followed by definitive diagnosis, the choice of treatment and treatment success will depend on the etiology of the hearing loss. For sensorineural impairment, depending on the degree of loss, treatment may range from amplification in the majority of cases to cochlear implantation in profoundly deaf children. In both cases, speech and hearing therapy has been promoted as a key component of treatment and the efficacy of such therapy has been claimed.[78,79] Cochlear implant technology continues to evolve for treatment of profound deafness in children. Several studies have demonstrated improved language development and communication skills in deaf infants following cochlear implantation.[47,48] Several nonrandomized, prospective studies have also demonstrated superior communication performance in prelingually deafened children who received implants as compared to similar children using more traditional tactile or acoustic hearing aids.[49,75,76]

Although the benefits of various treatments for hearing loss seem manifest, no controlled clinical trials have evaluated the effect of early screening on long-term functional and quality-of-life outcomes. Rather, studies of treatment efficacy are generally observational and retrospective, consisting of clinical series or case-control studies of highly selected patients, often with heterogeneous causes of hearing loss, and incompletely defined treatment regimens or protocols of uncertain compliance. Additionally, important confounders such as other patient characteristics (e.g., race or ethnic group, socioeconomic status, level and laterality of hearing loss, the presence of co-morbidity, disability, or developmental delay due to various causes), family characteristics, and the presence and nature of other therapeutic interventions are often not considered in the analysis. Thus, despite widespread professional opinion of general treatment efficacy, much more information is needed on the existence and level of treatment protocol efficacy. In many instances, however, it may understandably be deemed inappropriate to withhold any customary type of treatment in the research setting despite the limited evidence of treatment efficacy.[85]

Conductive hearing loss in the preschool-age group is most commonly due to self-limited cases of otitis media with effusion. Multiple studies have concluded that hearing impairment in infancy due to chronic or recurrent otitis media with effusion can impair language development.[39–41] Although these studies have come under methodologic criticism,[42,43] several authors believe that available evidence is adequate to substantiate this relationship.[8,44] Auditory thresholds in hearing-impaired children can be improved through amplification with hearing aids and frequency modulation radio devices. Auditory and language training can also improve communication skills.[12,75,76] While early detection and treatment of such hearing loss would therefore appear to be beneficial, there are no controlled studies comparing outcome of hearing-impaired persons identified through screening to those not screened. The fewer than 5% of infants with chronic otitis who do not respond spontaneously or with medical management are at further risk for more significant pathology including middle ear fibrosis or adhesions and cholesteatoma.[11] Myringotomy and pressure-equalizing tube placement can resolve the conductive loss and prevent reaccumulation of middle ear effusion.[50] No randomized or otherwise well-controlled study exists, however, demonstrating that infants or young children screened *with routine hearing tests* for chronic middle ear disease have a better outcome than those not screened in this manner. Nevertheless, if hearing loss is detected as part of the routine diagnosis or management of chronic OME, management of either sensorineural or conductive losses by standard regimens is indicated.

In older children, otitis media with effusion is responsible for the majority of hearing loss identified through screening.[3,11] As is the case in infants and toddlers, however, there is little evidence that asymptomatic children receiving hearing screening have better functional outcomes than those not screened. In fact, several studies of preschool and school-aged children who underwent audiometric screening demonstrated no significant difference in future audiometric performance between screened and unscreened children[51] nor any preventive benefit from screening.[4] Most hearing loss detected under these circumstances is self-limited and related to acute otitis media with effusion that resolves spontaneously within 6–8 weeks.[3,11] Since the critical period of language development has passed at this age, these individual episodes would appear to have little impact on educational performance. Studies have been unable to provide consistent evidence that clinical interventions for chronic OME (e.g., antibiotics, myringotomy, tympanostomy tubes) are able to achieve sufficient long-term improvement in hearing and language skills to justify the risk of complications.[41,43,51,53] A small portion of children routinely screened for hearing loss will demonstrate a protracted hearing impairment due to previously undetected, less severe, sensorineural losses as well as chronic and recurrent middle ear disease. These children may be at risk for educational and language problems,[1,52,53] although the evidence for this contention has been challenged.[42]

For adults between the ages of approximately 18 and 50 years, unrecognized hearing impairment is uncommon except for high-risk groups such as persons in occupations at risk for noise-induced hearing loss.[54,55] The incidence of hearing impairment, predominately due to presbycusis, rises quickly beyond age 50, however. No controlled study has proven the effectiveness of screening for hearing impairment in the adult population.[16] Two reviews cite numerous studies documenting the benefits of hearing amplification in these patients.[16,55] A 1990 randomized controlled trial demonstrated a measured improvement in social, cognitive, emotional, and communication function from hearing aid use in a group of elderly veterans with previously documented hearing loss.[56] The issue of patient compliance with recommendations to obtain hearing amplification has been raised as it relates to hearing screening,[15,55] but compliance rates of close to 40–60% can be achieved in some settings.[16] Patients receiving hearing aids have demonstrated improvement in communication and social function, as well as emotional status.[56]

Recommendations of Other Groups

The Joint Committee on Infant Hearing 1994 Position Statement, developed and approved by the American Speech-Language-Hearing Association (ASHA), American Academy of Otolaryngology-Head and Neck Surgery, American Academy of Audiology, American Academy of Pediatrics (AAP), and Directors of Speech and Hearing Programs in State health and welfare agencies, endorses the goal of universal detection of infants with hearing loss before 3 months of age.[59] When universal screening is not available, the committee recommends testing infants with indicators associated with sensorineural and/or conductive hearing loss, by 3 months of age. The high-risk indicators are similar to those described under *Clinical Intervention* (see below). The Bright Futures guidelines recommend hearing screening for all newborns prior to 3 months of age.[60] The National Institutes of Health recommends universal screening of all infants before age 3 months using evoked otoacoustic emission testing.[77] The Canadian Task Force on the Periodic Health Examination recommends regular assessment of hearing during well-baby visits during the first 2 years of life using parental questioning and the clap test.[80] The American Academy of Family Physicians (AAFP) recommends screening high-risk infants for hearing impairment; high-risk criteria are similar to those described under *Clinical Intervention* (see below).[65] The recommendations of the AAFP are currently under review.

The AAP recommends periodic historical inquiry regarding hearing throughout infancy and childhood and objective testing at ages 3, 4, 5, 10, 12, 15, and 18.[61] The Bright Futures guidelines recommend hearing screening at ages 3–6, 8, and 10, and yearly from ages 11–21 if the adolescent is exposed to loud noises, has recurring ear infections, or reports problems.[60] In 1990, ASHA reaffirmed its recommendation for annual audiometry for all children functioning at a developmental level of 3 years through grade 3 and for all children in high-risk groups.[62,63] ASHA also added tympanometry to their screening protocol for this age group as well as for any other patient undergoing screening audiometry up to age 40.

The Canadian Task Force on the Periodic Health Examination recommends against routine preschool screening for hearing problems.[80] The AAFP does not recommend routine hearing screening in children after age 3 years;[65] this recommendation is under review.

Recommendations for adults vary and also depend on age. Although ASHA proposes a screening protocol applicable to young adults, no guidelines are given regarding exactly who should be screened or what are optimal times for screening.[62] In the U.S., federal law mandates baseline and annual audiometry for workers of any age exposed to hazardous noise levels.[14] The Canadian Task Force recommends risk assessment for hearing loss by history and physical examination at age 16 and thereafter during clinical visits for any other reason.[64] The AAFP recommends screening for hearing impairment in adolescents and adults regularly exposed to excessive noise in recreational or other settings;[65] this recommendation is under review.

The Institute of Medicine recommended audiometric testing once each during ages 40–59, 60–74, and 75 and over.[66] The Canadian Task Force on the Periodic Health Examination recommends screening the elderly for hearing impairment, using a single question about hearing difficulty, whispered-voice out of the field of vision, or audioscope.[80] The AAFP recommends evaluation of hearing in persons aged 65 years and older, and hearing aids for patients found to have hearing deficits;[65] this recommendation is under review.

Discussion

While congenital hearing loss is a serious health problem associated with developmental delay in speech and language function, there is little evidence to support the use of routine, universal screening for all neonates. Although screening methods have reasonable sensitivity and specificity, a substantial number of infants will be misclassified because the prevalence of hearing impairment is low. Also, screening technology is evolving, and the costs and feasibility for universal application are not fully known. Most importantly, the evidence for efficacy of early intervention is incomplete. There have been no controlled clinical trials designed to test whether devices or complex protocols lead to superior speech and language outcomes in screened children. For older children, good quality evidence suggests little benefit from screening, while for adolescents and young and middle-aged adults there is limited evidence evaluating hearing impairment and treatment. Many older adults with clinical complaints of hearing loss or documented hearing deficits, however, benefit from hearing aids or other forms of amplification.

Treating deaf children with modalities such as cochlear implants has stimulated ethical concerns from some advocates for the deaf, a full discussion of which is beyond the scope of this chapter. Attitudes held by both physicians and by society toward deaf individuals have changed over time, and various associations now offer support for individuals affected by deafness, promote their full participation in society, and seek to preserve and expand deaf awareness, deaf culture, and deaf heritage efforts.[87]

CLINICAL INTERVENTION

Screening older adults for hearing impairment by periodically questioning them about their hearing, counseling them about the availability of hearing aid devices, and making referrals for abnormalities when appropriate, is recommended ("B" recommendation). The optimal frequency of such screening has not been determined and is left to clinical discretion. An otoscopic examination and audiometric testing should be performed on all persons with evidence of impaired hearing by patient inquiry. Although hand-held devices for audiometry testing (audioscopes) are also sensitive screening tools for hearing deficits, patient inquiry is likely to be a more rapid and less expensive way to screen for hearing loss in older adults. There is therefore insufficient evidence to recommend for or against routinely screening older adults for hearing deficits using audiometry testing ("C" recommendation).

There is insufficient evidence to recommend for or against routinely screening asymptomatic adolescents and working-age adults for hearing impairment ("C" recommendation). Recommendations against such screening, except for those exposed to excessive occupational noise levels, may be made on other grounds, including low prevalence, high cost, and the likelihood that hearing deficits in these individuals will present clinically. Screening of workers for noise-induced hearing loss should be performed in the context of existing worksite programs and occupational medicine guidelines.

Routine hearing screening of asymptomatic children beyond age 3 years is not recommended ("D" recommendation). It is recognized, however, that such testing often occurs outside the clinical setting. When this occurs, abnormal test results should be confirmed by repeat testing at appropriate intervals, and all confirmed cases identified through screening referred for ongoing audiologic assessment, selection of hearing aids, family counseling, psycho-educational management, and periodic medical evaluation.

There is insufficient evidence to recommend for or against routine screening of asymptomatic neonates for hearing impairment using evoked oto-acoustic emission (EOE) testing or auditory brainstem response (ABR) ("C" recommendation). Recommendations to screen high-risk infants may be made on other grounds, including the relatively high prevalence of hearing impairment, parental anxiety or concern, and the potentially beneficial effect on language development from early treatment of infants with moderate or severe hearing loss. For many high-risk conditions, hearing testing is commonly considered to be part of diagnostic evaluation and management. Risk factors for congenital or perinatally acquired hearing loss include family history of hereditary childhood sensorineural hearing loss; congenital perinatal infection with herpes, syphilis, rubella, cytomegalovirus, or toxoplasmosis; malformations involving the head or neck (e.g., dysmorphic and syndromal abnormalities, cleft palate, abnormal pinna); birth weight below 1,500 g; bacterial meningitis; hyperbilirubinemia requiring exchange transfusion; severe perinatal asphyxia (Apgar scores of 0–4 at 1 minute or 0–6 at 5 minutes, absence of spontaneous respirations for 10 minutes, or hypotonia at 2 hours of age); ototoxic medications; and findings associated with a syndrome known to include hearing loss. ABR testing may be useful for all infants who meet at least one of these high-risk criteria or for those who fail EOE testing. High-risk infants should ideally be screened prior to leaving the hospital after birth, but those not tested at birth should be screened before age 3 months with the goal being to initiate rehabilitation by age 6 months as clinically indicated. Clinicians examining any infant or young child should remain alert for symptoms or signs of hearing impairment, including parent/caregiver concern regarding hearing, speech, language, or developmental delay.

The draft update of this chapter was prepared for the U.S. Preventive Services Task Force by Robert Wallace, MD, MSc, and John Laurenzo, MD.

REFERENCES

1. Riko K, Hyde ML, Alberti PW. Hearing loss in early infancy: incidence, detection and assessment. Laryngoscope 1985;95:137–145.
2. Prager DA, Stone DA, Rose DN. Hearing loss screening in the neonatal intensive care unit: auditory brain stem response versus crib-o-gram; a cost-effectiveness analysis. Ear Hearing 1987;8:213–216.
3. Calogero B, Giannini P, Marciano E. Recent advances in hearing screening. Adv Otorhinolaryngol 1987;37:60–78.
4. Augustsson I, Nilson C, Ensgrand I. The preventive value of audiometric screening of preschool and young school-children. Int J Pediatr Otorhinolaryngol 1990;20:51–62.
5. Smith RJH, Zimmerman B, Connolly PK, et al. Screening audiometry using the high-risk register in a level III nursery. Arch Otolaryngol 1992;118:1306–1311.
6. Ruben RJ. Effectiveness and efficacy of early detection of hearing impairment in children. Acta Otolaryngol 1991; (Suppl 482):127–131.
7. Rach GH, Zielhuis GA, van den Broek P. The influence of chronic persistent otitis media with effusion on language development of 2- to 4-year olds. Int J Pediatr Otorhinolaryngol 1988;15:253–261.
8. Zinkus PW, Grottlieb MI. Patterns of perceptual and academic deficits related to early chronic otitis media. Pediatrics 1980;66:246–253.
9. Parving A. Hearing disorders in childhood: some procedures for detection, identification and diagnostic evaluation. Int J Pediatr Otorhinolaryngol 1985;9:31–57.
10. Daly KA. Epidemiology of otitis media. Otolaryngol Clin North Am 1991;24:775–786.
11. Cross AW. Health screening in schools. Part I. J Pediatr 1985;107:487–494.
12. Ruben RJ, Levine R, Fishman G, et al. Moderate to severe sensorineural hearing impaired child: analysis of etiology, intervention, and outcome. Laryngoscope 1982;92:38–46.

13. Stewart IF. After early identification—what follows? A study of some aspects of deaf education from an otolaryngological viewpoint. Laryngoscope 1984;94:784–799.
14. Department of Labor, Occupational Safety and Health Administration. Occupational noise exposure: hearing conservation amendment. Fed Reg 1981;46:4078–4180.
15. Davis A, Stephens D, Rayment A, et al. Hearing impairments in middle age: the acceptability, benefit and cost of detection (ABCD). Br J Audiol 1992;26:1–14.
16. Mulrow CD, Lichtenstein MJ. Screening for hearing impairment in the elderly: rationale and strategy. J Gen Intern Med 1991;6:249–258.
17. Havlik RJ. Aging in the eighties: impaired senses for sound and light in persons age 65 years and over. Preliminary data from the supplement on aging to the National Health Interview Survey: United States, January–June 1984. Advance data from vital and health statistics, no 125. Hyattsville, MD: National Center for Health Statistics, 1986. (Publication no. DHHS (PHS) 86-1250.)
18. Herbst KRG. Psychosocial consequences of disorders of hearing in the elderly. In: Hingchcliffe R, ed. Hearing and balance in the elderly. Edinburgh: Churchill-Livingstone, 1983.
19. Bess FH, Lichtenstein MJ, Logan SA, et al. Hearing impairment as a determinant of function in the elderly. J Am Geriatr Soc 1989;37:123–128.
20. Pettigrew AG, Edwards DA, Henderson-Smart DJ. Screening for auditory dysfunction in high risk neonates. Early Hum Dev 1986;14:109–120.
21. Hyde ML, Riko K, Malizia K. Audiometric accuracy of the click ABR in infants at risk for hearing loss. J Am Acad Audiol 1990;1:59–66.
22. Morgan DE, Canalis RF. Auditory screening of infants. Otolaryngol Clin North Am 1991;24:277–284.
23. Joint Committee Statement on Infant Hearing Screening. ASHA 1971;13:79.
24. Gerber SE. Review of a high risk register for congenital or early-onset deafness. Br J Audiol 1990;24:347–356.
25. Kennedy CR, Kimm L, Cafarelli Dees D, et al. Otoacoustic emissions and auditory brainstem responses in the newborn. Arch Dis Child 1991;66:1124–1129.
26. Kemp DT, Siobhan R. Otoacoustic emission tests in neonatal screening programmes. Acta Otolaryngol (Stockh) 1991;(Suppl 482):73–84.
27. Spektor Z, Leonard G, Kim DO, et al. Otoacoustic emissions in normal and hearing-impaired children and normal adults. Laryngoscope 1991;101:965–976.
28. Lonsbury-Martin BL, Whitehead ML, Martin GK. Clinical applications of otoacoustic emissions. J Speech Hearing Res 1991;34:964–981.
29. Webb KC, Krishnan V, Katzman G. Newborn hearing screening using the crib-o-gram. Arch Otolaryngol Head Neck Surg 1986;112:420–422.
30. Northern JL, Gerkin KP. New technology in infant hearing screening. Otolaryngol Clin North Am 1989;22:75–87.
31. Brown J, Watson E, Alberman E. Screening infants for hearing loss. Arch Dis Child 1989;64:1488–1495.
32. Hall DMB, Garner J. Feasibility of screening all neonates for hearing loss. Arch Dis Child 1988;63:652–653.
33. Margolis RH, Hunter LL. Audiologic evaluation of the otitis media patient. Otolaryngol Clin North Am 1991;24: 877–899.
34. *Deleted in proof.*
35. Schow RL. Considerations in selecting and validating an adult/elderly hearing screening protocol. Ear Hearing 1991; 12:337–348.
36. Sever JC, Harry DA, Rittenhouse TS. Using a self-assessment questionnaire to identify probable hearing loss among older adults. Percept Motor Skills 1989;69:511–514.
37. Frank T, Petersen DR. Accuracy of a 40 dB HL audioscope and audiometer screening for adults. Ear Hearing 1987;8:180–183.
38. Brooks DN. Audiology: state of the art. J Med Eng Tech 1986;10:167–179.
39. Teele DW, Klein JO, Rosner BA, Greater Boston Otitis Media Study Group. Otitis media with effusion during the first three years of life and development of speech and language. Pediatrics 1984;74: 282–287.
40. Sak RJ, Ruben RJ. Recurrent middle ear effusion in childhood: implications of temporary auditory deprivations for language and learning. Ann Otol Rhinol Laryngol 1981;90:546–551.
41. Rach GH, Zielhuis GA, Van Baarle PW, et al. The effect of treatment with ventilating tubes on language development in preschool children with otitis media with effusion. Clin Otolaryngol 1991;16:128–132.
42. Rapin I. Conductive hearing loss effects on children's language and scholastic skills: a review of the literature. Ann Otol Rhinol Laryngol 1979;88(Suppl 60)(5 pt 2):3–12.

43. Paradise JL. Otitis media during early life: how hazardous to development? A critical review of the evidence. Pediatrics 1981;68:869–873.
44. McDermott JC. Physical and behavioral aspects of middle ear disease in school children. J School Health 1983; 53:463–466.
45. *Deleted in proof.*
46. Bhattacharya J, Bennett MJ, Tucker SM. Long term follow up of newborns tested with the auditory response cradle. Arch Dis Child 1984;59:504–511.
47. Miyamoto RT, Osberger MJ, Robbins AM, et al. Longitudinal evaluation of communication skills of children with single- or multichannel cochlear implants. Am J Otol 1992;13:215–222.
48. Tobey EA, Angelette S, Murchison C, et al. Speech production performance in children with multichannel cochlear implants. Am J Otol 1991;12(suppl):165–173.
49. Geers A, Moog JS. Evaluating the benefits of cochlear implants in an education setting. Am J Otol 1991; 12(suppl):116–125.
50. Jung TTK, Ku Rhee C. Otolaryngologic approach to the diagnosis and management of otitis media. Otolaryngol Clin North Am 1991;24:931–945.
51. Feldman W, Milner R, Sackett B, et al. Effects of preschool screening for vision and hearing on prevalence of vision and hearing problems 6–12 months later. Lancet 1980;2:1014–1016.
52. National Center for Health Statistics. Prevalence of selected chronic conditions, United States, 1979–81. Vital and Health Statistics, series 10, no. 155. Washington, DC: Government Printing Office, 1986. (Publication no. DHHS(PHS) 86-1583.)
53. Callahan CW, Lazoritz S. Otitis media and language development. Am Fam Physician 1988;37:186–190.
54. Berwick DM. Screening in health fairs. JAMA 1985;254:1492–1498.
55. Bess FH, Lichtenstein MJ, Logan SA. Audiologic assessment of the elderly. In: Rintelmann WF, ed. Hearing assessment. Austin, TX: Pro-Ed, Inc., 1991:511–515.
56. Mulrow CD, Aguilar C, Endicott JE, et al. Quality of life changes and hearing impairment: results of a randomized trial. Ann Intern Med 1990;113:188–194.
57. *Deleted in proof.*
58. *Deleted in proof.*
59. Joint Committee on Infant Hearing. Joint Committee on Infant Hearing 1994 position statement. Pediatrics 1995;95: 152–156.
60. Green M, ed. Bright Futures: guidelines for health supervision of infants, children, and adolescents. Arlington, VA: National Center for Education in Maternal and Child Health, 1994.
61. American Academy of Pediatrics Committee on Practice and Ambulatory Medicine. Recommendations for preventive pediatric health care. Pediatrics 1995;96:373–374.
62. American Speech-Language-Hearing Association. Guidelines for screening for hearing impairments and middle ear disorders. ASHA 1990;32(Suppl 2):17–24.
63. American Speech-Language-Hearing Association. Guidelines for identification audiometry. ASHA 1985;27:49–52.
64. Canadian Task Force on the Periodic Health Examination. 1984 Update. Can Med Assoc J 1984;130: 1–16.
65. American Academy of Family Physicians. Age charts for periodic health examination. Kansas City, MO: American Academy of Family Physicians, 1994. (Reprint no. 510.)
66. National Academy of Sciences, Institute of Medicine, Ad Hoc Advisory Group on Preventive Services. Preventive services for the well population. Washington, DC: National Academy of Sciences, 1978.
67. Abdo MH, Feghali JG, Stapells DR. Transient evoked otoacoustic emissions: clinical applications and technical considerations. Int J Pediatr Otorhinolaryngol 1993;25:61–71.
68. Bonfils P, Dumont A, Marie P, et al. Evoked otoacoustic emissions in newborn hearing screening. Laryngoscope 1990;100:186–189.
69. Lafreniere D, Jung MD, Smurzynski J, et al. Distortion-product and click-evoked otoacoustic emissions in healthy newborns. Arch Otolaryngol 1991;117:1382–1389.
70. Chuang SW, Gerber SE, Thornton ARD. Evoked otoacoustic emissions in preterm infants. Int J Pediatr Otorhinolaryngol 1993;26:39–45.
71. Probst R, Harris FP. Transiently evoked and distortion-product otoacoustic emissions: comparison of results from normally hearing and hearing-impaired human ears. Arch Otolaryngol 1993;119:858–860.
72. Franklin DJ, McCoy MJ, Martin GK, et al. Test/retest reliability of distortion-product and transiently evoked otoacoustic emissions. Ear Hearing 1992;13:417–429.
73. Alpiner JG, McCarthy PA. Rehabilitative audiology: children. In: Rehabilitative audiology: children and adults. Baltimore: Williams & Wilkins, 1993:64–68.

74. Bonfils P, Uziel A, Pujol R. Screening for auditory dysfunction in infants by evoked otoacoustic emissions. Arch Otolaryngol 1988;114:887–890.
75. Osberger MJ, Robbins AM, Miyamoto RT, et al. Speech perception abilities of children with cochlear implants, tactile aids, or hearing aids. Am J Otol 1991;12(suppl):105–115.
76. Osberger MJ, Robbins AM, Berry SW, et al. Analysis of spontaneous speech samples of children with cochlear implants or tactile aids. Am J Otol 1991;12(suppl):151–164.
77. National Institutes of Health Consensus Statement. Early identification of hearing impairment in infants and young children. NIH Consensus Statement 1993;11:1–24.
78. Weiss KL, Goodwin MW, Moores DF. Characteristics of young deaf children and early intervention programs. Research Report 91. Department of HEW, Bureau of Education for the Handicapped, 1975.
79. Osberger MJ, Hesketh LJ. Speech and language disorders related to hearing impairment. In Lass NJ, et al, eds. Handbook of speech-language pathology and audiology. Toronto: BC Decker, 1988:858–885.
80. Canadian Task Force on the Periodic Health Examination. Canadian guide to clinical preventive health care. Ottawa: Canada Communication Group, 1994:258–266, 298–304, 954–963.
81. Todd NW. At-risk populations for hearing impairment in infants and children. Int J Pediatr Otorhinolaryngol 1994;29:11–21.
82. Koike KJ, Hurst MK, Wetmore SJ. Correlation between the American Academy of Otolaryngology-Head and Neck Surgery five-minute hearing test and standard audiologic data. Otolaryngol Head Neck Surg 1994;111:625–632.
83. Jacobson JT, Jacobson CA. The effects of noise on transient EOAE newborn nursery screening. Int J Pediatr Otorhinolaryngol 1994;29:235–248.
84. Vohr BR, White KR, Maxon AB, et al. Factors affecting the interpretation of transient evoked otoacoustic emission results in neonatal hearing screening. Semin Hearing 1993;14:57–72.
85. Laughton J. Models and current practices in early intervention with hearing-impaired infants. Semin Hearing 1994;15:148–159.
86. White KR, Vohr BR, Behrens TR. Universal newborn hearing screening using transient evoked otoacoustic emissions: results of the Rhode Island hearing assessment project. Semin Hearing 1993;14:18–29.
87. The National Association of the Deaf. Brochure. Silver Spring, MD: National Association of the Deaf, 1994.
88. Maxon AB, White KR, Behrens TR, et al. Referral rates and cost efficiency in a universal newborn hearing screening program using transient evoked otoacoustic emissions. J Am Acad Audiol 1995;6:271–277.

36. Screening Ultrasonography in Pregnancy

RECOMMENDATION

Routine third-trimester ultrasound examination of the fetus is not recommended. There is insufficient evidence to recommend for or against routine ultrasound examination in the second trimester in low-risk pregnant women (see *Clinical Intervention*).

Burden of Suffering

Ultrasonography is widely used in pregnancy in the U.S. According to 1992 U.S. natality data, 58% of mothers who had live births received ultrasonography in pregnancy, compared to 48% in 1989.[1] The highest rates occurred in white women and those ages 25–39 years. For asymptomatic low-risk women, a single scan in the second trimester may be used to estimate gestational age in women with unreliable dates of last menses and to detect multiple gestation and fetal malformations. A third-trimester scan may be used to screen for intrauterine growth retardation (IUGR) and fetal malpresentation as well as previously undetected multiple gestations and malformations.[2]

These conditions may be associated with increased maternal or perinatal morbidity and mortality. Inaccurate estimation of gestational age may lead to repeated testing of fetal well-being and induction of labor in pregnancies erroneously thought to be postterm.[3,4] About 25–45% of women are unable to provide an accurate menstrual history;[3,5,6] the estimated date of confinement derived from the last menstrual period differs by more than 2 weeks from the actual date of birth in nearly one quarter of pregnancies.[5] Multiple gestation is associated with increased perinatal mortality, preterm delivery, and other obstetric complications,[7] and it is more likely to result in cesarean delivery (56% compared to a baseline rate of 23%).[8] The ratio of multiple gestation births to all births (currently 24/1,000 live births) has risen steadily since 1972 and is the highest reported in the past 50 years.[1] Congenital anomalies are the leading cause of death before 1 year of age in the U.S., with a mortality rate of 1.7/1,000 live births, and are also important contributors to childhood morbidity and shortened life expectancy.[10,11] Fetal growth retardation has been associated with poor pregnancy outcomes, including fetal and neonatal death, reduced intelligence, seizures, and cerebral palsy, although most term growth-retarded infants develop normally.[12] Breech and other malpresentations may be associated with poor outcome and result in cesarean delivery in 84% of cases.[8] Malpresentation occurs in 38/1,000 live births, with the risk increasing with increasing age of the mother.[1]

Accuracy of the Screening Test

Real-time ultrasound consists of high-frequency sound waves that allow two-dimensional imaging of both structural and functional characteristics of the fetus, as well as the location and morphology of the placenta.[2] (This chapter will not address the topic of umbilical Doppler ultrasound[13]). Ultrasound is the recommended test for determination of gestational age in women with uncertain menstrual dates because measurement of the biparietal diameter, when performed early in the second trimester, has been shown to be accurate in determining gestational age.[5,6] Ninety percent of patients deliver within 2 weeks of the due date when gestational age is determined by early second-trimester ultrasound.[5]

Ultrasound can also detect multiple gestations, which are missed by clinical examination in nearly one third of cases.[14] One center that provided the only maternity services in its community reported that 98% of all twins were detected antenatally when routine ultrasound screening was performed.[4,6] The average gestational age at detection fell from 27 weeks to 20 weeks. Randomized controlled trials of routine ultrasound before 20 weeks found higher rates of early detection of multiple gestation with screening (83–100%) compared to unscreened controls (60–76%).[15–19] False-positive ultrasound diagnoses also occur, however, primarily in the first trimester; over 20% of multiple fetuses identified in the first trimester are either artifacts or die early in pregnancy.[20]

Many fetal structural malformations, including cardiac, gastrointestinal, renal, limb, and neural tube defects, can also be detected by current ultrasound techniques (for detailed discussion of ultrasound screening to detect chromosomal abnormalities and neural tube defects, see Chapters 41 and 42, respectively). Detection rates depend on the quality of the equipment and the expertise of the ultrasonographer. In a trial in low-risk pregnant women, routine serial ultrasonography at 15–22 and 31–35 weeks of gestation had a sensitivity of 35% for detecting fetuses with at least one major anomaly before delivery but only 17% for detection before the typical gestational-age limit for legal abortion (<24 weeks).[21] Only 4% of missed cases occurred in women who did not comply with scheduled screening ultrasounds. The sensitivity of selective ultrasound, performed only for obstetric or medical indications, was significantly lower than routine ultrasound: 11% before delivery and 5% before 24 weeks. In this study, the sensitivity of routine midtrimester ultrasound was significantly higher at tertiary compared to other scanning facilities (35% vs. 13%). False-positive diagnoses were reported for 7 cases, or 0.9/1,000 pregnant women scanned before 24 weeks, with most reported from other than tertiary facilities. In another trial, the rates of detection of major malformations by screening before 20 weeks (confirmed at abortion or delivery) were 36% and 77% at two hospitals.[19] Ten of the thirty cases with suspected major malformations were judged normal at follow-up ultrasound examinations at 20–36 weeks and an 11th was found to have only a minor anomaly at delivery; 2.7/1,000 pregnant women received a false diagnosis of a major fetal malformation. Large case series evaluating routine ultrasound in low-risk women have reported sensitivities ranging from 21% to 74% for detecting major fetal abnormalities prior to 22–24 weeks among women who were scanned in the second trimester.[22–24] False-positive rates of 0.2–1.0/1,000 women scanned were reported; in one study, 6 of 8 initially false-positive diagnoses were corrected on follow-up evaluation. Direct comparisons of the trials and series results are hampered by varying definitions of "fetal malformation."

The ultrasound examination is the most accurate means of detecting IUGR, although the lack of consensus on standards for the definition or diagnosis of IUGR[12] makes evaluating screening tests for this condition difficult. Measurements of the fetal abdomen and head, and indices that compare the relative sizes of these structures, are accurate in assessing fetal growth.[25–32] A small abdominal circumference, for example, the most commonly affected anatomic measurement,[3] has a sensitivity of 80–96% and a specificity of 80–90% in detecting growth-retarded fetuses in the third trimester.[3,26,33,34] The product of the crown-rump length and the trunk area has a sensitivity of 94% and a specificity of 90%.[35] Because of the relatively low risk of IUGR in the general population, however, the likelihood that an abnormal test indicates IUGR is relatively low. For example, an abnormal abdominal circumference at 34–36 weeks' gestation indicates IUGR in only 21–50% of cases.[26,33,36] The generalizability of these studies has also been questioned; many had small samples, used only expert ultrasonographers, and/or suffered from methodologic limitations.[26,37] In addition, the definitions commonly used in these studies may cause normal but constitutionally small fetuses to be labeled as IUGR.

Effectiveness of Early Detection

For routine ultrasonographic screening to be proven beneficial, evidence is needed that interventions in response to examination results lead to improved clinical outcome. Twelve randomized controlled trials have examined the effectiveness of routine ultrasound screening in improving maternal or neonatal outcomes. Four of these evaluated a single ultrasound before 20 weeks,[15–17,19] three trials assessed serial ultrasound at 18–20 weeks and 31–35 weeks,[18,21,38–40] three trials evaluated one or two ultrasounds between 32 and 37 weeks when all subjects received one ultrasound before 24 weeks,[35,41,42] and two tested multiple scans (plus Doppler flow studies in one trial) every 3–4 weeks beginning at 24–28 weeks, with all subjects receiving a single midtrimester scan.[43,44] In a 13th trial, all subjects received three ultrasounds, but the results of placental grading at 34–36 weeks were reported only for the experimental group.[45] In addition, four meta-analyses have been published, none of which included the U.S. RADIUS trial, the most recent and largest to date.[46–49] In most of the trials, large proportions of the controls also received ultrasound results, although not with the same timing or frequency as in the screened groups.

The most important potential benefit of ultrasound screening is reduced perinatal mortality. Among the seven trials that evaluated an ultrasound before 20 weeks (with or without additional late ultrasound), only the Helsinki trial[19] and a meta-analysis heavily influenced by that trial's results[47] were able to demonstrate a statistically significant benefit in lowering perinatal mortality. Two trials[17,40] showed nonsignificant reductions in mortality while the remaining four trials and another meta-analysis[48] showed no mortality benefit. In the Helsinki trial, the overall perinatal death rate was 4.6/1,000 deliveries (n = 18) in screened women versus 9.0/1,000 deliveries (n = 34) in unscreened women. In the experimental group, 11 induced abortions were performed because of ultrasound findings and two babies died with major anomalies, compared to no abortions and 10 deaths with anomalies in the control group. There was no difference in perinatal mortality when the induced abortions resulting from ultrasound detection of congenital anomalies were included as deaths in the analysis. The meta-analysis[47] that reported a significant mortality reduction included the four then-published trials[16–19] that compared routine to selective ultrasound scanning and that reported number of pregnancies, deliveries, and perinatal deaths. It also evaluated the live birth rate, which takes into account induced abortions for malformations, and found it to be identical in the screened and control groups. The largest trial to date, the RADIUS trial,[38] randomized 15,151 low-risk pregnant women to routine ultrasound scans at 15–22 and 31–35 weeks of gestation or to usual care, which included ultrasounds performed for indications that developed after randomization. The risk of fetal or neonatal death was the same in the screened (0.6%, n = 52) and control (0.5%, n = 41) groups. Including induced abortions for fetal anomalies (9 vs. 5 in the routinely and selectively screened groups, respectively) did not affect these estimates.

Effects on neonatal and maternal morbidity from a single second-trimester scan have also been evaluated. Most of the trials and meta-analyses showed no statistically significant benefit of prenatal ultrasound on neonatal morbidity (including low birth weight, admission to special care nursery, neonatal seizures, mechanical ventilation, and Apgar scores), or on maternal outcomes such as antenatal hospitalization.[15,17–19,46,47] In one randomized controlled trial of early second-trimester ultrasound,[16] babies born to screened women had a significantly greater mean birth weight (3,521 g vs. 3,479 g) than did those born to controls, with most of the benefit accruing to smokers. The Cochrane Database meta-analysis reported significantly fewer low birth weight singleton births and reduced risk of admission to special care nurseries with routine early ultrasound, but no effect on Apgar scores.[48] The RADIUS trial reported a slightly lower rate of tocolysis in screened women (3.4% vs. 4.2%), but no other differences in maternal outcomes (e.g., amniocentesis, external version, cesarean delivery, or days of hospitalization)[39] or in overall or individual indicators of perinatal morbidity.[38]

Accurate dates determined by second-trimester ultrasound might help prevent routine tests of fetal well-being and the induction of labor for fetuses thought to be postterm on the basis of erroneous dating.[3,4,26] Rates of induced labor for postterm pregnancy were significantly reduced in three trials[16,39,40] but were unaffected in two others;[17,18] meta-analysis demonstrated significantly decreased inductions for postterm pregnancy.[48] These trials may have underestimated such effects by including women with reliable dates, who are less likely to benefit from ultrasound dating. Trials and meta-analyses have not established whether overall rates of induced labor are reduced by a second-trimester ultrasound.[15–18,39,40,47,48] In the RADIUS trial, the significant decreases in induced labor for postterm pregnancy were completely offset by significant increases in inductions for IUGR.[39] Two meta-analyses[46,47] reported significant heterogeneity among the trials, suggesting that other factors, such as differences in obstetric management between countries or over time, may also influence this outcome. In one community, the incidence of postterm inductions fell from 8% to 2.6% after ultrasound screening was instituted,[4] but it was not proved that this trend was due specifically to improved accuracy of estimating gestational age. Two trials of second-trimester ultrasound reported other outcomes potentially related to inaccurate dates. The RADIUS trial found no significant effect of ultrasound screening on adverse perinatal outcomes among postdate pregnancies[38] or on the number of tests performed to assess fetal well-being.[39] Another trial reported significantly fewer days of inpatient neonatal care after treatment for "overdue pregnancy" among screened cases.[40]

Other potential benefits of prenatal ultrasound, including the early detection of multiple gestations and congenital anomalies, are often cited in support of screening. The early detection of multiple gestation, a risk factor for intrapartum and neonatal complications,[3] might allow improved antenatal surveillance and management, but direct evidence of clinical benefits from early detection, such as improved maternal or neonatal outcome, is lacking. No significant improvements in fetal, neonatal, or maternal outcomes in multiple gestations were reported in any of the screening trials, except for a small reduction in use of tocolytics in the RADIUS trial.[15–19,38,39] Numbers of multiple gestations were small in all trials, however, and power to detect improved outcomes from screening was generally inadequate. There is also no clear evidence that early intervention for identified multiple gestation, including routine hospital admission for bed rest, cervical cerclage, or prophylactic oral tocolysis, results in improved perinatal outcome.[50]

While ultrasound before 20 weeks allows earlier detection of fetal structural malformations, it is not clear that this results in improved outcome. In the Helsinki trial, early detection led to an increased rate of elective abortions (2.7/1,000 screened women vs. 0/1,000 control women) and therefore to reduced perinatal deaths (see above).[19] On the other hand, in the RADIUS trial,[38] screening had no statistically significant effect on the rate of induced abortion (n = 9 or 1.2/1,000 screened women compared to n = 4 or 0.5/1,000 controls). Although early detection might theoretically improve survival for infants with fetal anomalies if they could be delivered at tertiary care centers capable of immediate medical and surgical intervention, no significant effects of early detection on overall perinatal mortality, or on survival rates among infants born with acute life-threatening anomalies or with any major anomalies, were seen in the RADIUS trial.[21,38] Other trials of routine ultrasound before 20 weeks have detected too few (i.e., 0–2) malformations to allow meaningful comparisons of outcomes.[15–18,40] None of the trials has evaluated whether routine screening improves outcomes in newborns with nonlethal anomalies.

Eight randomized controlled trials and one meta-analysis have evaluated the effectiveness of routine third-trimester ultrasound focused on fetal anthropometry and morphology in improving outcomes.[18,35,38–44,49] Six trials involved low-risk patients or patients selected from the general population,[18,35,38–40,42,43] while two were restricted to women with suspected IUGR or at increased risk for IUGR or other complications (with results of the scan either released or withheld based on randomization).[41,44] Several of these trials had methodologic problems such as inadequate reporting of results,[40] use of hospital number for randomization,[35] and the revealing of test results for nearly one third of cases in the control group because of obstetrician requests.[41] These studies reported no significant reductions in low Apgar scores, admission to or length of stay in special care nursery, low birth weight or preterm delivery, perinatal morbidity, or perinatal mortality (excluding lethal malformations). There were also no consistent beneficial effects on antenatal hospitalization or induction of labor. The meta-analysis[49] reported that third-trimester ultrasound was associated with a significantly increased risk of antenatal hospital admission. One additional randomized controlled trial in unselected women, all of whom received ultrasounds at midtrimester and twice in the third trimester, evaluated whether reporting the result of placental grading by third-trimester ultrasound to the clinician responsible for care improved neonatal outcome.[45] Reporting the placental grading was associated with significant reductions in meconium staining in labor, low Apgar scores at 5 minutes, and perinatal mortality in normally formed babies. One previously cited trial[43] of serial third-trimester ultrasounds also assessed placental morphology and reported no beneficial effects of ultrasound on perinatal mortality or morbidity, but the method of assessing placental morphology was not described. Additional trials of third-trimester placental grading are needed to assess its effectiveness.

There is no clear evidence of important adverse effects related to screening ultrasonography reported from the published randomized controlled trials, although such effects might be difficult to detect given the small number of ultrasounds (usually one or two per patient) and the fact that the controls in many trials were also scanned, with results concealed. One randomized controlled trial compared routine multiple ultrasound scans plus Doppler flow studies to selective ultrasound for indications, with four or more scans being done in 91% of screened vs. 8% of control women.[43] The screened group had a significantly higher percentage of infants with birth weight below the 3rd and 10th percentiles. Although this was not a primary endpoint of the study, it suggests a possible adverse effect of frequent ultrasound examinations with Doppler studies on fetal growth, which is supported by several studies in mice and monkeys.[51–53] Long-term follow-up of singleton live births to age 8–9 years from the two Norwegian trials (in which only 19% of controls received ultrasound) was performed to evaluate possible adverse effects of ultrasound on neurologic development.[54,55] These two studies, with 83–89% response rates, found no differences between the two groups in school performance; deficits in attention, motor control, or perception (by parent questionnaire); development in infancy; or prevalence of dyslexia. Although false-positive diagnoses of major fetal malformations occurred in both the Helsinki trial (2.7/1,000 women in the screened group) and in the RADIUS trial (0.9/1,000), none of these pregnancies was electively aborted as a result.[19,21] Case reports have suggested adverse psychological effects of early and false-positive diagnoses of fetal abnormalities,[56–58] but no controlled studies that evaluated adverse effects of ultrasound diagnosis of fetal anomalies were found.

Recommendations of Other Groups

A National Institutes of Health consensus development conference recommended that ultrasound imaging during pregnancy be performed only for a specific medical indication and not for routine screening.[59] This is also the position of the American College of Obstetricians and Gynecologists.[2] The Canadian Task Force on the Periodic Health Examination found fair evidence to recommend a single second-trimester ultrasound examination in women with normal pregnancies, but concluded that there was insufficient evidence to recommend the inclusion or exclusion of routine serial ultrasound screening for IUGR in normal pregnancies.[60]

Discussion

Neither early, late, nor serial ultrasound in normal pregnancy has been proven to improve perinatal morbidity or mortality. Clinical trials show that a single midtrimester ultrasound examination detects multiple gestations and congenital malformations earlier in pregnancy, but there is currently insufficient evidence that early detection results in improved outcomes. In the U.S., it is not clear whether early detection of fetal anomalies by routine ultrasound leads to increased rates of induced abortion. In addition, many of the major fetal anomalies discoverable by routine ultrasound might be detected anyway during screening for Down syndrome (see Chapter 41) or neural tube defects (see Chapter 42). Routine second-trimester ultrasound can lower the rate of induction for presumed post-term pregnancy, a benefit likely to accrue primarily to women with unreliable dates, among whom ultrasound is more accurate than dates for predicting actual date of delivery. Early ultrasound has not been proven to reduce overall rates of induction, however, due to increases in inductions for other indications. It is also unclear whether the likeliest potential benefits of routine second-trimester ultrasound (reduced induction of labor for postterm pregnancy and increased induced abortions for fetal anomalies) would justify the significant economic implications of widespread testing. No benefits of routine ultrasound examination of the fetus in the third trimester have been demonstrated despite multiple randomized controlled trials. Additional trials of third-trimester placental grading are needed to adequately evaluate the potential benefits of screening for placental appearance. Further research to evaluate possible adverse effects of ultrasound and the cost-effectiveness of routine screening is also needed.

CLINICAL INTERVENTION

Routine ultrasound examination of the fetus in the third trimester is not recommended, based on multiple trials and meta-analyses showing no benefit for either the pregnant woman or her fetus ("D" recommendation). There is currently insufficient evidence to recommend for or against a single routine midtrimester ultrasound in low-risk pregnant women ("C" recommendation). These recommendations apply to routine screening

ultrasonography and not to diagnostic ultrasonography for specific clinical indications (e.g., follow-up evaluation of elevated maternal serum α-feto-protein). Recommendations regarding screening for Down syndrome appear in Chapter 41, and those for neural tube defects appear in Chapter 42.

The draft update of this chapter was prepared for the U.S. Preventive Services Task Force by Carolyn DiGuiseppi, MD, MPH, based in part on materials prepared for the Canadian Task Force on the Periodic Health Examination by Geoffrey Anderson, MD, PhD.

REFERENCES

1. Ventura SJ, Martin JA, Taffel SM, et al. Advance report of final natality statistics, 1992. Monthly vital statistics report; vol 43 no 5 (suppl). Hyattsville, MD: National Center for Health Statistics, 1994.
2. American College of Obstetricians and Gynecologists. Ultrasonography in pregnancy. Technical Bulletin no. 187. Washington, DC: American College of Obstetricians and Gynecologists, 1993.
3. Warsof SL, Pearce JM, Campbell S. The present place of routine ultrasound screening. Clin Obstet Gynecol 1983;10:445–457.
4. Persson PH, Kullander S. Long-term experience of general ultrasound screening in pregnancy. Am J Obstet Gynecol 1983;146:942–947.
5. Campbell S, Warsof SL, Little D, et al. Routine ultrasound screening for the prediction of gestational age. Obstet Gynecol 1985;65:613–620.
6. Grennert L, Persson PH, Gennser G. Benefits of ultrasonic screening of a pregnant population. Acta Obstet Gynecol 1978;78:5–14.
7. Klein L, Goldenberg RL. Prenatal care and its effect on preterm birth and low birth weight. In: Merkatz IR, Thompson JE, eds. New perspectives on prenatal care. New York: Elsevier, 1990:501–529.
8. Taffel SM. Cesarean delivery in the United States, 1990. National Center for Health Statistics. Vital Health Statistics, Series 21, no. 51. Washington, DC: Government Printing Office, 1994. (Publication no. DHHS (PHS) 94-1929.)
9. *Deleted in proof.*
10. National Center for Health Statistics. Annual summary of births, marriages, divorces, and deaths: United States, 1993. Monthly vital statistics report; vol 42 no 13. Hyattsville, MD: Public Health Service, 1994.
11. Powell-Griner E, Woolbright A. Trends in infant deaths from congenital anomalies: results from England and Wales, Scotland, Sweden and the United States. Int J Epidemiol 1990;19:391–398.
12. Goldenberg RL, Davis RO, Nelson KG. Intrauterine growth retardation. In: Merkatz IR, Thompson JE, eds. New perspectives on prenatal care. New York: Elsevier, 1990:461–478.
13. Giles W, Bisits A. Clinical use of Doppler ultrasound in pregnancy: information from six randomised trials. Fetal Diagn Ther 1993;8:247–255.
14. Farooqui MD, Grossman JH 3d, Shannon RA. A review of twin pregnancy and perinatal mortality. Obstet Gynecol Surv 1973;28(suppl):144–152.
15. Bennett MJ, Little G, Dewhurst J, et al. Predictive value of ultrasound measurement in early pregnancy: a randomized controlled trial. Br J Obstet Gynaecol 1982;89:338–341.
16. Waldenstrom U, Axelsson O, Nilsson S, et al. Effects of routine one-stage ultrasound screening in pregnancy: a randomised controlled trial. Lancet 1988;2:585–588.
17. Ewigman B, LeFevre M, Hesser J. A randomized trial of routine prenatal ultrasound. Obstet Gynecol 1990;76: 189–194.
18. Bakketeig LS, Eik-Nes SH, Jacobsen G, et al. Randomised controlled trial of ultrasonographic screening in pregnancy. Lancet 1984;2:207–211.
19. Saari-Kemppainen A, Karjalainen O, Ylostalo P, et al. Ultrasound screening and perinatal mortality: controlled trial of systematic one-stage screening in pregnancy. The Helsinki Ultrasound Trial. Lancet 1990;336:387–391.
20. Landy HJ, Weiner S, Corson SL, et al. The "vanishing twin": ultrasonographic assessment of fetal disappearance in the first trimester. Am J Obstet Gynecol 1986;155:14–19.
21. Crane JP, LeFevre ML, Winborn RC, et al. A randomized trial of prenatal ultrasonographic screening: impact on the detection, management and outcome of anomalous fetuses. The RADIUS Study Group. Am J Obstet Gynecol 1994;171:392–399.

22. Chitty LS, Hunt GH, Moore J, et al. Effectiveness of routine ultrasonography in detecting fetal structural abnormalities in a low-risk population. BMJ 1991;303:1165–1169.

23. Shirley IM, Bottomley F, Robinson VP. Routine radiographer screening for fetal abnormalities by ultrasound in an unselected low risk population. Br J Radiol 1992;65:564–569.

24. Levi S, Hyjazi Y, Schaaps J-P, et al. Sensitivity and specificity of routine antenatal screening for congenital anomalies by ultrasound: the Belgian Multicentric Study. Ultrasound Obstet Gynecol 1991;1:102–110.

25. Mintz MC, Landon MB. Sonographic diagnosis of fetal growth disorders. Clin Obstet Gynecol 1988; 31:44–52.

26. Geirsson RT, Persson PH. Diagnosis of intrauterine growth retardation using ultrasound. Clin Obstet Gynecol 1984; 11:457–479.

27. Pearce JM, Campbell S. A comparison of symphysis-fundal height and ultrasound as screening tests for light-for-gestational-age infants. Br J Obstet Gynaecol 1987;94:100–104.

28. Eik-Nes SH, Persson PH, Grottum P, et al. Prediction of fetal growth deviation by ultrasonic biometry. II. Clinical application. Acta Obstet Gynecol 1983;62:117–123.

29. Campbell S, Kurjak A. Comparison between urinary oestrogen assay and serial ultrasonic cephalometry in assessment of fetal growth retardation. BMJ 1972;2:336–340.

30. Campbell S, Dewhurst CJ. Diagnosis of the small-for-dates fetus by serial ultrasonic cephalometry. Lancet 1971; 2:1002–1006.

31. Persson PH, Grennert L, Gennser G. Diagnosis of intrauterine growth retardation by serial ultrasonic cephalometry. Acta Obstet Gynecol Scand [Suppl] 1978;78:40–48.

32. Secher NJ, Hansen PK, Lenstrup C, et al. On the evaluation of routine ultrasound screening in the third trimester for detection of light for gestation age (LGA) infants. Acta Obstet Gynecol Scand 1987; 66:463–471.

33. Brown HL, Miller JM, Gabert HA, et al. Ultrasonic recognition of the small-for-gestational-age fetus. Obstet Gynecol 1987;69:631–635.

34. Neilson JP, Whitfield CR, Aitchison TC. Screening for the small-for-dates fetus: a two-stage ultrasonic examination schedule. BMJ 1980;280:1203–1206.

35. Neilson JP, Munjanja SP, Whitfield CR. Screening for small-for-dates fetuses: a controlled trial. BMJ 1984;289: 1179–1182.

36. Warsof SL, Cooper DJ, Little D, et al. Routine ultrasound screening for antenatal detection of intrauterine growth retardation. Obstet Gynecol 1986;67:33–39.

37. Deter RL, Harrist RB, Hadlock FP, et al. The use of ultrasound in the detection of intrauterine growth retardation: a review. J Clin Ultrasound 1982;10:9–16.

38. Ewigman BG, Crane JP, Frigoletto FD, et al. Effect of prenatal ultrasound screening on perinatal outcome. The RADIUS Study Group. N Engl J Med 1993;329:821–827.

39. LeFevre ML, Bain RP, Ewigman BG, et al. A randomized trial of prenatal ultrasonographic screening: impact on maternal management and outcome. The RADIUS Study Group. Am J Obstet Gynecol 1993; 169:483–489.

40. Eik-Nes SH, Okland O, Aure JC, et al. Ultrasound screening in pregnancy: a randomised controlled trial. Lancet 1984;1:1347.

41. Secher NJ, Hansen PK, Lenstrup C, et al. A randomized study of fetal abdominal diameter and fetal weight estimation for detection of light-for-gestation infants in low-risk pregnancies. Br J Obstet Gynaecol 1987;94:105–109.

42. Duff GB. A randomized controlled trial in a hospital population of ultrasound measurement screening for the small-for-dates baby. Aust NZ J Obstet Gynaecol 1993;33:374–378.

43. Newnham JP, Evans SF, Michael CA, et al. Effects of frequent ultrasound during pregnancy: a randomised controlled trial. Lancet 1993;342:887–891.

44. Larsen T, Larsen JF, Petersen S, et al. Detection of small-for-gestational-age fetuses by ultrasound screening in a high-risk population: a randomized controlled study. Br J Obstet Gynaecol 1992;99:469–474.

45. Proud J, Grant AM. Third trimester placental grading by ultrasonography as a test of fetal wellbeing. BMJ 1987;294: 1641–1647.

46. Thacker SB. Quality of controlled clinical trials. The case of imaging ultrasound in obstetrics: a review. Br J Obstet Gynaecol 1985;92:437–444.

47. Bucher HC, Schmidt JG. Does routine ultrasound scanning improve outcome in pregnancy? Meta-analysis of various outcome measures. BMJ 1993;307:13–17.

48. Neilson JP. Routine ultrasound in early pregnancy. In: Enkin MW, Keirse MJNC, Renfrew MJ, Neilson JP, eds. Pregnancy and childbirth module, Cochrane database of systematic reviews, review no. 03872, June 1993. Oxford: Update Software, 1994, Disk Issue 1.

49. Neilson JP. Routine fetal anthropometry in late pregnancy. In: Enkin MW, Keirse MJNC, Renfrew MJ, Neilson JP, eds. Pregnancy and childbirth module, Cochrane database of systematic reviews, review no. 03873, March 1993. Oxford: Update Software, 1994, Disk Issue 1.

50. Klein L, Goldenberg RL. Prenatal care and its effect on preterm birth and low birth weight. In: Merkatz IR, Thompson JE, eds. New perspectives on prenatal care. New York: Elsevier, 1990;501–529.

51. O'Brien WD Jr. Dose dependent effect of ultrasound on fetal weight in mice. J Ultrasound Med 1983; 2:1–8.

52. Tarantal AF, Hendrickx AG. Evaluation of the bioeffects of prenatal ultrasound exposure in the Cynomolgus Macaque (Macaca fascicularis): I. Neonatal/infant observations. Teratology 1989;39: 137–147.

53. Tarantal AF, O'Brien WD, Hendrickx AG. Evaluation of the bioeffects of prenatal ultrasound exposure in the Cynomolgus Macaque (Macaca fascicularis): III. Developmental and hematologic studies. Teratology 1993;47: 159–170.

54. Salvesen KA, Bakketeig LS, Eik-Nes SH, et al. Routine ultrasonography in utero and school performance at age 8–9 years. Lancet 1992;339:85–89.

55. Salvesen KA, Vatten LJ, Eik-Nes SH, et al. Routine ultrasonography in utero and subsequent handedness and neurological development. BMJ 1993;307:159–164.

56. Griffiths DM, Gough MH. Dilemmas after ultrasonic diagnosis of fetal abnormality. Lancet 1985;i: 623–624.

57. Brereton RJ. Importance of surgical consultation after ultrasonic diagnosis. BMJ 1984;289:1618–1619.

58. Murphy S, Das P, Grant DN, et al. Importance of neurosurgical consultation after ultrasonic diagnosis of fetal hydrocephalus. BMJ 1984;289:1212–1213.

59. National Institutes of Health Consensus Development Conference. The use of diagnostic ultrasound imaging during pregnancy. JAMA 1984;252:669–672.

60. Canadian Task Force on the Periodic Health Examination. Canadian guide to clinical preventive health care. Ottawa: Canada Communication Group, 1994:4–14.

37. Screening for Preeclampsia

RECOMMENDATION

Screening for preeclampsia with blood pressure measurement is recommended for all pregnant women at the first prenatal visit and periodically throughout the remainder of pregnancy (see *Clinical Intervention*).

Burden of Suffering

Hypertension is a common medical complication of pregnancy, occurring in about 6–8% of all pregnancies.[1,2] It is seen in a group of disorders that include preeclampsia-eclampsia, latent or chronic essential hypertension, a variety of renal diseases, and transient (gestational) hypertension. The definitions used to distinguish these disorders are a matter of debate, leading to uncertainty about their exact prevalence, natural history, and response to treatment.[3,4] Based on 1992 birth certificate data, pregnancy-associated hypertension was noted in 3% of all pregnancies, and eclampsia in 0.4%.[4a]

Preeclampsia and eclampsia, once called toxemias of pregnancy, are the most dangerous of these disorders. Although definitions differ, many describe preeclampsia as acute hypertension (blood pressure greater than 140 mm Hg systolic or 90 mm Hg diastolic; or a rise of 30 mm Hg or 15 mm Hg above the usual systolic and diastolic pressures, respectively) presenting after the 20th week of gestation, accompanied by abnormal edema, proteinuria (more than 0.3 g/24 hours), or both.[4] Women with preeclampsia are at increased risk for such complications as abruptio placentae, acute renal failure, cerebral hemorrhage, disseminated intravascular coagulation, pulmonary edema, circulatory collapse, and eclampsia.[5] The fetus may become hypoxic, increasing its risk of low birth weight, premature delivery, or perinatal death.[6] Complications of pregnancy-induced hypertension, including eclampsia (the advanced stage of this disorder characterized by seizures), are major causes of maternal deaths in the U.S.[7] Women with preeclampsia are not at increased risk of developing chronic hypertension.[4] Individuals at increased risk of developing preeclampsia and eclampsia include primigravidas and women with multiple gestations, molar pregnancy or fetal hydrops, chronic hypertension or diabetes, or a personal or family history of eclampsia or preeclampsia.[8–10]

Other causes of hypertension during pregnancy include transient and chronic hypertension. Transient (gestational) hypertension is defined as the acute onset of hypertension in pregnancy or the early puerperium without proteinuria or abnormal edema and resolving within 10 days after delivery.[2] Chronic hypertension that had been latent prior to the pregnancy may also become evident during gestation. Pregnant women with latent chronic hypertension are also at increased risk for stillbirth, neonatal death, and other fetal complications, but the risk is much lower than that of women with preeclampsia or eclampsia. Women with transient or latent chronic hypertension are also more likely to develop chronic hypertension in later years.[3,4,8]

Accuracy of Screening Tests

Screening tests for preeclampsia are difficult to evaluate due to the absence of a "gold standard" to confirm the diagnosis. Glomerular endotheliosis, the renal lesion characteristic of preeclampsia, is present in only about half of patients who meet the clinical criteria for the disease;[11] diagnosis requires an invasive renal biopsy. In addition, the glomerular lesions of preeclampsia are not specific for preeclampsia, having been observed in association with other conditions, such as abruptio placentae and chronic renal disease.[11,12] For practical reasons, most studies of potential screening tests for preeclampsia have relied on clinical criteria to confirm the diagnosis.

Many proposed screening tests have been found unsuitable for early detection of preeclampsia. The appearance of edema and proteinuria alone is unreliable. Edema is common in normal pregnancies[13,14] and therefore lacks specificity. Measurable proteinuria usually occurs after hypertension is manifested and therefore is not useful for early detection.[2] In a prospective study of women between 24 and 34 weeks of gestation, a urine albumin concentration equal to or greater than 11 µg/mL had a sensitivity of 50% in predicting subsequent preeclampsia.[15] The conventional urine dipstick test is unreliable in detecting the moderate and highly variable elevations in albumin that occur early in the course of preeclampsia.[16,17] The definitive test for proteinuria, the 24-hour urine collection, is not practical for screening.[17] Because of these considerations, edema is no longer required to diagnose preeclampsia by some experts[5,9,14] and the inclusion of proteinuria is being reconsidered as well. Other tests that have been suggested include the angiotensin II infusion test and the supine pressor "rollover" examination, but these have also been found to be unsuitable, as the former is impractical and the latter lacks adequate sensitivity, specificity, and positive predictive value.[1,17]

The most promising screening test for preeclampsia is sphygmomanometry to detect elevated blood pressure, although there are several problems in relying on blood pressure readings as an accurate predictor. Common sources of measurement error associated with sphygmomanometry include instrument defects and examiner technique (see Chapter 3). In addition, maternal posture can significantly affect blood pressure in pregnant women;[17] the results can be erroneous, for example, if blood pressure is measured with the woman in the supine position. Measurements should be taken in the sitting position, after the patient's arm has rested at heart level for 5 minutes.[4] Most important, a single elevated blood pressure reading is neither diagnostic of nor a good predictor for preeclampsia.[1,18] Diagnosis utilizing only a change from baseline also has limited sensitivity (21–52% and 7–23% for the diastolic and systolic criteria, respectively) in predicting preeclampsia.[19] A combination of the blood pressure levels and the change from baseline may be more effective in identifying women at risk for preeclampsia,[20] and the trend in blood pressure over time is more important than a single isolated measurement.

In the middle trimester of pregnancy, the normal decline in blood pressure is often dampened or absent in women who subsequently develop preeclampsia.[6,21] Some experts therefore recommend using the middle trimester mean arterial pressure (MAP)—defined as (systolic pressure + [2 × diastolic pressure])/3)—as a screening test.[6] Studies indicate that a middle trimester MAP above 90 mm Hg has a sensitivity of 61–71% and a specificity of 62–74% in predicting preeclampsia,[6,22] and even higher sensitivity and specificity have been reported by some researchers.[23] Other studies report a much lower sensitivity of this test in detecting preeclampsia (22–35%) and suggest it is of little value in predicting eclampsia itself.[24] One review concluded that, due to inconsistencies in the definition of "preeclampsia" used in most of these studies (e.g., failure to require proteinuria for the diagnosis), elevations in second trimester blood pressure may be a better predictor of transient or chronic hypertension than of true preeclampsia.[25]

Effectiveness of Early Detection

The early detection of hypertension during pregnancy permits clinical monitoring and prompt therapeutic intervention for severe preeclampsia or eclampsia. The delivery of the fetus is considered to be the most definitive method to minimize preeclamptic complications, but other measures (e.g., bed rest and pharmacologic agents) have not been conclusively shown to improve outcome.[17,26] A randomized controlled trial found that antihypertensive therapy and hospitalization, when compared with hospitalization alone, did not improve maternal or fetal outcome.[27] There have been no clinical trials to determine whether hypertensive preeclamptic women treated early in pregnancy have a better prognosis than those who are not detected early.

Clinical experience, however, suggests that early detection and treatment of preeclampsia is beneficial to the patient and fetus.[1,5,9,14] This view is based in part on inferences drawn from the apparent effectiveness of regular prenatal care in reducing the complications of preeclampsia-eclampsia. Studies conducted as early as the 1940s suggested an inverse relationship between the extent of prenatal care and the incidence of eclampsia, perhaps reflecting benefits of early detection.[28] These findings do not provide direct evidence that better outcomes are due solely to blood pressure screening itself, rather than to other components of prenatal care or to the characteristics of women who receive regular prenatal care.

Recommendations of Other Groups

The American College of Obstetricians and Gynecologists recommends blood pressure measurements at the initial visit, every 4 weeks until 28 weeks' gestation, every 2–3 weeks until 36 weeks' gestation, and weekly thereafter.[29] The Canadian Task Force on the Periodic Health Examination recommends that systolic and diastolic blood pressures be measured on all obstetric patients at the first prenatal visit and periodically throughout the remainder of pregnancy.[30] A task force report to the U.S. Public Health Service recommended blood pressure measurements at a preconception visit, at the first prenatal visit (at 6–8 weeks' gestation, ideally) and at each prenatal visit after 24 weeks until delivery.[31]

Discussion

The most efficacious screening strategy for preeclampsia is the early detection of an abnormal blood pressure trend over time. Serial measurements during the second and third trimester increase the likelihood that a pathologic pattern or overt blood pressure elevation will be detected.[5,6,18,22,32] Although there is no direct proof that regular screening results in reduced maternal or perinatal morbidity and mortality, it is unlikely that a study will be conducted in which a control group does not receive blood pressure screening or treatment. Because the target condition is a common medical complication of pregnancy and the screening test is simple, inexpensive, and acceptable to patients, screening is indicated on an empirical basis.

Consistent attention should be given to using proper technique for measuring blood pressure.[4] Although the use of isolated specific blood pressure levels (e.g., above 140/90 mm Hg) has an important role in evaluating patients, more definitive data are needed to determine its positive predictive value in the diagnosis of preeclampsia.[20] Measurement of blood pressure and calculation of the MAP during the second trimester may also provide useful information prior to the development of preeclampsia-eclampsia, but more reliable data are needed to determine the positive predictive value of second trimester blood pressure and whether screening based on these criteria results in improved clinical outcome.

Several therapeutic agents are being investigated as preventive measures for preeclampsia. Aspirin prophylaxis for the prevention of preeclampsia and its complications is discussed elsewhere (see Chapter 70). Calcium supplementation is currently being evaluated.[4,5,14]

CLINICAL INTERVENTION

Screening for preeclampsia with blood pressure measurement is recommended for all pregnant women at the first prenatal visit and periodically throughout the remainder of pregnancy ("B" recommendation). The optimal frequency for measuring blood pressure in pregnant women has not been determined and is left to clinical discretion; it is most efficient to measure blood pressure on women who are being seen by their clinicians for other reasons. The collection of meaningful blood pressure data requires consistent use of correct technique and a cuff of appropriate size. In addition to the guidelines listed in Chapter 3, the patient should be in the sitting position and the blood pressure should be measured after the patient's arm has rested at heart level for 5 minutes.[4] Further diagnostic evaluation and clinical monitoring, including frequent blood pressure monitoring and urine testing for protein, are indicated if blood pressure does not decrease normally during the middle trimester, if the systolic pressure increases 30 mm Hg above baseline or the diastolic pressure increases 15 mm Hg above baseline, or if the blood pressure exceeds 140/90 mm Hg. Medical interventions should not be prescribed until the diagnosis of preeclampsia is confirmed. See Chapter 70 for recommendations on the use of aspirin prophylaxis in pregnancy.

The draft update of this chapter was prepared for the U.S. Preventive Services Task Force by Michelle Berlin, MD, MPH, and A. Eugene Washington, MD, MSc.

REFERENCES

1. DeVoe SF, O'Shaughnessy RW. Clinical manifestations and diagnosis of pregnancy-induced hypertension. Clin Obstet Gynecol 1984;27:836–853.
2. Chesley LC. History and epidemiology of preeclampsia-eclampsia. Clin Obstet Gynecol 1984;27:801–820.
3. World Health Organization. The hypertensive disorders of pregnancy: report of a WHO Study Group. Technical Report Series no. 758. Geneva: World Health Organization, 1987.
4. National High Blood Pressure Education Program Working Group. Report on high blood pressure in pregnancy. Am J Obstet Gynecol 1990;163:1691–1712.
4a. Ventura SJ, Martin JA, Taffel SM, et al. Advance report of final natality statistics, 1992. Monthly vital statistics report; vol 43 no 5 (suppl). Hyattsville, MD: National Center for Health Statistics, 1994.
5. Redman CWG, Roberts JM. Management of pre-eclampsia. Lancet 1993;341:1451–1454.
6. Page EW, Christianson R. The impact of mean arterial pressure in the middle trimester upon the outcome of pregnancy. Am J Obstet Gynecol 1976;125:740–746.

7. Atrash HK, Koonin LM, Lawson HW, et al. Maternal mortality in the United States, 1979–1986. Obstet Gynecol 1990;76:1055–1060.

8. Roberts JM, Redman CWG. Pre-eclampsia: more than pregnancy-induced hypertension. Lancet 1993;341: 1447–1451.

9. Cunningham FG, Lindheimer MD. Hypertension in pregnancy. N Engl J Med 1992;326:927–932.

10. Cunningham FG, MacDonald PC, Gant NF, et al. Hypertensive disorders of pregnancy. In: Williams obstetrics. 19th ed. Norwalk, CT: Appleton & Lange, 1993:763–817.

11. Fisher KA, Luger A, Spargo BH, et al. Hypertension in pregnancy: clinical-pathological correlations and remote prognosis. Medicine 1981;60:267–276.

12. Thomson D, Paterson WG, Smart GE, et al. The renal lesions of toxaemia and abruptio placentae studied by light and electron microscopy. J Obstet Gynaecol Br Commonw 1972;79:311–320.

13. Vollman RF. Study design, population and data characteristics. In: Friedman EA, ed. Blood pressure, edema and proteinuria in pregnancy. New York: Alan R. Liss, 1976:99.

14. Wallenburg HCS. Detecting hypertensive disorders of pregnancy. In: Chalmers I, Enkin M, Keirse MJNC, eds. Effective care in pregnancy and childbirth. Oxford: Oxford University Press, 1989:382–402.

15. Rodriguez MH, Masaki DI, Mestman J, et al. Calcium/creatinine ratio and microalbuminuria in the prediction of preeclampsia. Am J Obstet Gynecol 1988;159:1452–1455.

16. Irgens-Moller L, Hemmingsen L, Holm J. Diagnostic value of microalbuminuria in preeclampsia. Clin Chim Acta 1986;157:295–298.

17. Sibai BM. Pitfalls in diagnosis and management of preeclampsia. Am J Obstet Gynecol 1988;159:1–5.

18. Reiss RE, O'Shaughnessy RW, Quilligan TJ, et al. Retrospective comparison of blood pressure course during preeclamptic and matched control pregnancies. Am J Obstet Gynecol 1987;156:894–898.

19. Moutquin JM, Giroux L, Rainville C, et al. Does a threshold increase in blood pressure predict preeclampsia? Proceedings of 5th Congress International Society for the Study of Hypertension in Pregnancy. Nottingham, England, July 1986:108.

20. Redman CW, Jefferies M. Revised definition of pre-eclampsia. Lancet 1988;1:809–812.

21. Fallis NE, Langford HG. Relation of second trimester blood pressure to toxemia of pregnancy in the primigravid patient. Am J Obstet Gynecol 1963;87:123–125.

22. Moutquin JM, Rainville C, Giroux L, et al. A prospective study of blood pressure in pregnancy: prediction of preeclampsia. Am J Obstet Gynecol 1985;151:191–196.

23. Oney T, Kaulhausen H. The value of the mean arterial blood pressure in the second trimester (MAP-2 value) as a predictor of pregnancy-induced hypertension and preeclampsia. Clin Exp Hypertens 1983; 2:211–216.

24. Chesley LC, Sibai BM. Blood pressure in the midtrimester and future eclampsia. Am J Obstet Gynecol 1987;157:1258–1261.

25. Chesley LC, Sibai BM. Clinical significance of elevated mean arterial pressure in the second trimester. Am J Obstet Gynecol 1988;159:275–279.

26. Mathews DD, Shuttleworth TP, Hamilton EFB. Modern trends in management of non-albuminuric hypertension in late pregnancy. BMJ 1978;2:623–625.

27. Sibai BM, Gonzalez AR, Mabie WC, et al. A comparison of labetalol plus hospitalization versus hospitalization alone in the management of preeclampsia remote from term. Obstet Gynecol 1987;70:323–327.

28. Chesley LC. Eclampsia at the Margaret Hague Maternity Hospital. Bull Marg Hague Mat Hosp 1953;6: 2–11.

29. American Academy of Pediatrics and American College of Obstetricians and Gynecologists. Guidelines for perinatal care. 3rd ed. Washington, DC: American College of Obstetricians and Gynecologists, 1992.

30. Canadian Task Force on the Periodic Health Examination. Canadian guide to clinical preventive health care. Ottawa: Canada Communication Group, 1994:136–143.

31. National Institutes of Health. Caring for our future: the content of prenatal care. Washington, DC: Department of Health and Human Services, 1989. (Publication no. 90-3182.)

32. Page EW, Christianson R. Influence of blood pressure changes with and without proteinuria upon outcome of pregnancy. Am J Obstet Gynecol 1976;126:821–833.

38. Screening for D (Rh) Incompatibility

RECOMMENDATION

D (formerly Rh) blood typing and antibody screening is recommended for all pregnant women at their first prenatal visit. Repeat antibody screening at 24–28 weeks' gestation is recommended for unsensitized D-negative women (see *Clinical Intervention*).

Burden of Suffering

D incompatibility exists when a D-negative woman is pregnant with a D-positive fetus, which occurs in up to 9–10% of pregnancies, depending on race.[1,2] If no preventive measures are taken, 0.7–1.8% of these women will become isoimmunized antenatally, developing D antibody through exposure to fetal blood; 8–17% will become isoimmunized at delivery, 3–6% after spontaneous or elective abortion, and 2–5% after amniocentesis.[1–3] In subsequent D-positive pregnancies of isoimmunized women, maternal D antibody will cross the placenta into the fetal circulation and hemolyze red cells.[1] Without treatment, 25–30% of these offspring will have some degree of hemolytic anemia and hyperbilirubinemia, and another 20–25% will be hydropic and often will die either in utero or in the neonatal period.[4]

Since the introduction of routine postpartum prophylaxis in the 1960s, the crude incidence of D isoimmunization in the U.S. and Canada has fallen from 9.1–10.3 cases to 1.3 cases/1,000 total births.[5–9] Hemolytic disease of the fetus or newborn due to D isoimmunization (also called erythroblastosis fetalis) now accounts for only 4–5 deaths/100,000 total births,[6,10] although this may be an underestimate as early intrauterine deaths are not always reported.[10] Even before the introduction of prophylaxis, however, a decline in fetal and neonatal mortality from D hemolytic disease was occurring due to declines in both incidence and case fatality rates. It has been estimated that 30–40% of the recent decline in disease incidence is attributable to smaller family size, since the incidence of D hemolytic disease increases with increasing birth order.[11] Since the 1940s, the case fatality rate has fallen from about 50% to 2–6%.[8,9] This decline can be attributed in part to the trend toward smaller families, since the

425

first affected infant in a family generally has less severe disease.[1,5,9] The decline has also been associated with the introduction of interventions such as amniotic fluid spectrophotometry, exchange transfusion, amniocentesis, intrauterine fetal transfusion, and improved care of both the mother and the premature erythroblastotic infant.[1,9]

Accuracy of Screening Tests

Hemagglutination is the established reference standard for the determination of D blood type.[12] The indirect antiglobulin (Coombs) test (IAGT) is the reference standard for detecting anti-D antibody in women who are sensitized to D-positive blood.[12] The IAGT will also detect other maternal antibodies that may cause hemolytic disease.[13]

Effectiveness of Early Detection

The early detection of D-negative blood type in the pregnant woman is of substantial benefit if the patient is not yet isoimmunized and the father is not known to be D-negative. Administration of D immunoglobulin (or $Rh_o(D)$ immune globulin (human)) to an unsensitized D-negative woman after delivery of a D-positive fetus will prevent maternal isoimmunization and consequent hemolytic disease in subsequent D-positive offspring. The efficacy of D immunoglobulin prophylaxis was convincingly demonstrated in a series of controlled clinical trials in the early 1960s.[14-16] Despite a variety of minor flaws in study design, these trials showed that isoimmunization did not occur in any of the women who received a full dose of D immunoglobulin postpartum and who were unsensitized when it was administered. These findings led to the introduction of routine postpartum prophylaxis following licensure of D immunoglobulin in 1968. Time series studies have since shown a dramatic decline in the incidence of D isoimmunization, from 13–14% in the mid-1960s to 1–2% in the mid-1970s,[7,17] although as described above, at least some of this decline is probably attributable to smaller family size.

The most frequent cause of apparent failure of postpartum prophylaxis is antenatal isoimmunization, which happens in 0.7–1.8% of pregnant women at risk.[1,9,18] Although sample selection and other design features were not optimal, nonrandomized controlled trials have shown that the administration of D immunoglobulin at 28 weeks' gestation, when combined with postpartum administration, reduces the incidence of isoimmunization to 0.2% of women at risk.[19-21]

Since D isoimmunization during pregnancy is caused by transplacental hemorrhage, the risk of isoimmunization increases whenever such hemorrhage is likely to occur, including after abortion, amniocentesis, chorionic villus sampling (CVS), cordocentesis, ectopic pregnancy, fetal manipulation (e.g., external version procedures) or surgery, antepartum hemorrhage, antepartum fetal death, and stillbirth.[1,22–24] Studies documenting the effectiveness of D immunoglobulin prophylaxis are available for only a few of these indications, however. In a nonrandomized trial of D immunoglobulin after amniocentesis, control D-negative women delivering D-positive infants were more likely to become isoimmunized than were those receiving D immunoglobulin (5.2% vs. 0%), although because of small numbers this difference was not statistically significant.[25] Case series describing D immunoglobulin administration after amniocentesis have demonstrated isoimmunization rates as low as 0–0.5%.[26–28] In a case series of D immunoglobulin after induced abortion, isoimmunization occurred in 0.4%,[29] compared to 2.6% among a series of patients, described by the same authors, who did not receive D immunoglobulin.[30] The preliminary results from a randomized controlled trial of D immunoglobulin after CVS showed that among D-negative women delivering D-positive infants, similar rates of isoimmunization were seen in both intervention (2.3%) and control (1.1%) groups; insufficient details are provided to ensure baseline comparability between the two groups, however.[31] D-negative women who received D immunoglobulin experienced twice as many unintended fetal losses as did controls (6.9% vs. 3.8%), but this difference was not statistically significant. Results of the completed trial confirm the preliminary findings (S. Smidt-Jensen, Rigshospitalet, Copenhagen, Denmark; personal communication, January 1995), but have not yet been published. No studies evaluating the use of D immunoglobulin after other obstetric procedures or after obstetric complications were found.

The standard postpartum dose of D immunoglobulin (300 µg) contains sufficient D antibodies to prevent sensitization to at least 15 mL of D-positive fetal red blood cells (RBCs), or approximately 30 mL of fetal blood;[32] a "minidose" (50 µg) prevents sensitization to 2.5 mL of D-positive fetal RBCs. For women with transplacental hemorrhages >30 mL of fetal blood, the risk of D isoimmunization developing after the full postpartum D immunoglobulin dose is 30–35%.[3,33] The incidence of fetal-maternal hemorrhage >30 mL is 0.1–0.7% for all D-negative pregnancies,[1,33,34] but it is 1.7–2.5% after complicated vaginal and cesarean deliveries,[34,35] and 4.5% after stillbirth.[1] There are several available methods for detecting excess fetomaternal hemorrhage. Acid elution (Kleihauer-Betke) is both sensitive and specific when done correctly,[1,36] but it is subject to substantial laboratory and technologist error.[36] Flow cytometry is also highly sensitive and specific, but it is technically difficult to perform.[36] The erythrocyte rosette test is simple to perform and highly sensitive (99–100%) for the presence of ≥15 mL of D-positive fetal RBCs,[1,36] but its specificity is low[36,37] so positive results must be confirmed by more specific tests such as acid elution and flow cytometry.[1,36]

In clinical practice, combined antenatal and postnatal prophylaxis will prevent isoimmunization in 96% of women at risk.[21] The remaining cases are due to failure to give D immunoglobulin when indicated, isoimmunization that occurred before the widespread availability of D immunoglobulin, administration of an insufficient dose, or treatment failure (i.e., isoimmunization occurring before 28 weeks or transplacental hemorrhage too large or too late in pregnancy to be prevented by the standard antepartum dose).[3,38,39] Human error causes 22–50% of these cases.[6,21,39] While clinicians almost always administer D immunoglobulin postpartum or after induced abortion, administration rates have been documented to be lower for other obstetric procedures and complications: 81–88% after spontaneous abortion, 36–60% after ectopic pregnancy, 31% after antepartum hemorrhage, and 14% after amniocentesis.[2,40,41]

D immunoglobulin has few adverse effects.[1,42] Some fetuses will become weakly direct antiglobulin-positive following antenatal administration, but resulting anemia and hyperbilirubinemia in the newborn are very rare.[19] All plasma for D immunoglobulin production is screened for infectious diseases as required by the Food and Drug Administration; no cases of human immunodeficiency virus (HIV) infection from D immunoglobulin have been reported.[43] The evidence is therefore compelling that early detection and prophylaxis of the unsensitized D-negative woman is both safe and effective in preventing isoimmunization and thus in preventing D hemolytic disease.

Early detection is also beneficial for D-negative women who are already isoimmunized and are carrying D-positive offspring, because early intervention may improve clinical outcome. Decisions to intervene depend on the validity of screening tests in predicting the degree of fetal anemia. Obstetric history, maternal antibody titers, and ultrasound are currently used to determine the need for more invasive tests during isoimmunized pregnancies, but in the absence of hydrops none of these reliably distinguishes mild from severe hemolytic disease.[1,4,22,44] Immunologic tests on maternal serum show promise in predicting disease severity.[1,45,46] In the third trimester, serial amniotic fluid spectrophotometry has been found to correctly predict disease severity (i.e., cord hemoglobin and need for neonatal therapy) in 94–99% of cases.[47,48] In the second trimester, however, this test has insufficient sensitivity or specificity for predicting the need for intervention.[4,49,50] Determination of fetal hemoglobin and D blood type by ultrasound-guided cordocentesis, which can be performed in the second trimester, quantifies the degree of anemia, can be followed by transfusion if indicated, and allows referral of those with D-negative babies to routine care.[1,4] Case series, however, have demonstrated complication rates of 2–7% and procedure-related fetal mortality rates of 0.5–1%.[23,51,52] DNA amplification in amniotic cells and chorionic villus samples appears to be effective in determining fetal D blood type early in pregnancy, without the risk associated with invading the fetomaternal circulation.[53]

In the presence of severe fetal anemia, early intervention appears to offer substantial improvement in clinical outcome. Current perinatal survival after ultrasound-guided intravascular transfusion at experienced centers is 62–86% for hydropic fetuses and >90% for those without hydrops.[4,54,55] Once pulmonary maturity is established, the fetus can be delivered early and exchange transfusion performed with only 1% mortality risk.[56]

Recommendations of Other Groups

The American College of Obstetricians and Gynecologists (ACOG)[22] and the U.S. Public Health Service Expert Panel on the Content of Prenatal Care[57] recommend D blood typing and antibody screening at the first prenatal visit and repeat D antibody screening at 24–28 weeks of pregnancy for D-negative women. Both groups recommend offering D immunoglobulin to all unsensitized D-negative women at 28 weeks of gestation, and to those at increased risk of sensitization because of delivery of a D-positive infant, antepartum hemorrhage, spontaneous or induced abortion, amniocentesis, external version procedures, or ectopic pregnancy, within 72 hours of the event.[22,57] ACOG also recommends D immunoglobulin administration to unsensitized D-negative women who have CVS, cordocentesis, antepartum fetal death, fetal surgery, or transfusion of D-positive blood products.[22] ACOG recommends measuring fetal blood cell levels in the mother when antepartum placental hemorrhage occurs.[22] The Canadian Task Force on the Periodic Health Examination recommends D blood typing and antibody screening at the first prenatal visit, before elective procedures such as amniocentesis and therapeutic abortion in which there is the possibility of fetal bleed, between 24 and 28 weeks if the mother is D-negative, and within 72 hours of delivery. They recommend administration of D immunoglobulin to unsensitized women at 28 weeks and postpartum, and after amniocentesis or induced abortion.[58]

Discussion

Although the burden of suffering from this disease is now low, the incidence was at least 10/1,000 live births before the introduction of preventive measures in the 1960s.[9] There is excellent evidence for the efficacy and effectiveness of blood typing, anti-D antibody screening, and postpartum D immunoglobulin prophylaxis. Although antepartum prophylaxis offers some additional benefit, some critics argue that the total impact of antepartum prophylaxis on the incidence of D disease is relatively small, making it approximately 16 times less cost-effective than a program consisting only of postpartum treatment.[2,59,60] Other studies support the cost-effectiveness of antepartum prophylaxis.[21,61] The cost-effectiveness of D immunoglobulin after obstetric procedures and complications is unknown.

CLINICAL INTERVENTION

D blood typing and antibody testing is recommended for all pregnant women at their first prenatal visit, including visits for elective abortion ("A" recommendation). For purposes of blood typing and prophylaxis, D^u- and D-negative blood types should be considered equivalent.[22] Unless the father is known to be D-negative, a repeat D antibody test is recommended for all unsensitized D-negative women at 24–28 weeks' gestation, followed by the administration of a full (300 μg) dose of D immunoglobulin if they are antibody-negative ("B" recommendation). If a D- (or D^u-) positive infant is delivered, the dose should be repeated postpartum, preferably within 72 hours after delivery ("A" recommendation). Unless the father is known to be D-negative, a full dose of D immunoglobulin is recommended for all unsensitized D-negative women after elective abortion (50 μg before 13 weeks) and amniocentesis ("B" recommendation). There is currently insufficient evidence to recommend for or against the routine administration of D immunoglobulin after other obstetric procedures or complications such as chorionic villus sampling, ectopic pregnancy termination, cordocentesis, fetal surgery or manipulation (including external version), antepartum placental hemorrhage, antepartum fetal death, and stillbirth ("C" recommendation).

The draft update of this chapter was prepared for the U.S. Preventive Services Task Force by Carolyn DiGuiseppi, MD, MPH.

REFERENCES

1. Mollison PL, Engelfriet CP, Contreras M. Blood transfusion in clinical medicine. 8th ed. Oxford: Blackwell Scientific Publications, 1987.
2. Huchcroft S, Gunton P, Bowen T. Compliance with postpartum Rh isoimmunization prophylaxis in Alberta. Can Med Assoc J 1985;133:871–875.
3. Bowman JM. Controversies in Rh prophylaxis. Am J Obstet Gynecol 1985;151:289–294.
4. Tannirandorn Y, Rodeck CH. New approaches in the treatment of haemolytic disease of the fetus. Baillieres Clin Haematol 1990;3:289–320.
5. Centers for Disease Control. Rh hemolytic disease—Connecticut, United States, 1970–1979. MMWR 1981;30: 13–15.
6. Baskett TF, Parsons ML. Prevention of Rh(D) alloimmunization: a cost-benefit analysis. Can Med Assoc J 1990; 142:337–339.
7. Bowman JM, Pollock J. Rh immunization in Manitoba: progress in prevention and management. Can Med Assoc J 1983;129:343–345.
8. Wysowki DK, Flynt JW, Goldberg MF, et al. Rh hemolytic disease: epidemiologic surveillance in the United States, 1968 to 1975. JAMA 1979;242:1376–1379.
9. Bowman JM, Chown B, Lewis M. Rh isoimmunization, Manitoba, 1963–75. Can Med Assoc J 1977;116: 282–284.

10. Clarke CA. Preventing rhesus babies: the Liverpool research and follow up. Arch Dis Child 1989;64: 1734–1740.

11. Adams MM, Marks JS, Gustafson J, et al. Rh hemolytic disease of the newborn: using incidence observations to evaluate the use of Rh immune globulin. Am J Public Health 1981;71:1031–1035.

12. Walker RH, ed. Technical manual. 10th ed. Arlington, VA: American Association of Blood Banks, 1990.

13. American College of Obstetricians and Gynecologists. Management of isoimmunization in pregnancy. Technical Bulletin no. 148. Washington, DC: American College of Obstetricians and Gynecologists, 1990.

14. Chown B, Duff AM, James J, et al. Prevention of primary Rh immunization: first report of the Western Canadian Trial, 1966–1968. Can Med Assoc J 1969;100:1021–1024.

15. Pollack W, Gorman JG, Freda VJ, et al. Results of clinical trials of RhoGAM in women. Transfusion 1968;8:151–153.

16. Prevention of Rh-haemolytic disease: results of the clinical trial. A combined study from centres in England and Baltimore. BMJ 1966;2:907–914.

17. Freda VJ, Gorman JG, Pollack W. Prevention of Rh hemolytic disease: ten years' clinical experience with Rh immune globulin. N Engl J Med 1975;292:1014–1016.

18. Davey MG, Zipursky A. McMaster conference on prevention of Rh immunization. Vox Sang 1979;36: 50–64.

19. Bowman JM, Chown B, Lewis M. Rh isoimmunization during pregnancy: antenatal prophylaxis. Can Med Assoc J 1978;118:623–627.

20. Tovey LA, Stevenson BJ, Townley A. The Yorkshire antenatal anti-D immunoglobulin trial in primigravidae. Lancet 1983;2:244–246.

21. Trolle B. Prenatal Rh-immune prophylaxis with 300 µg immune globulin anti-D in the 28th week of pregnancy. Acta Obstet Gynecol Scand 1989;68:45–47.

22. American College of Obstetricians and Gynecologists. Prevention of D isoimmunization. Technical Bulletin no. 147. Washington, DC: American College of Obstetricians and Gynecologists, 1990.

23. Daffos F, Capella-Pavlovsky M, Forestier F. Fetal blood sampling during pregnancy with use of a needle guided by ultrasound: a study of 606 consecutive cases. Am J Obstet Gynecol 1985;153:655–660.

24. Blakemore KJ, Baumgarten A, Schoenfeld-Dimaio M, et al. Rise in maternal serum alpha-fetoprotein concentration after chorionic villus sampling and the possibility of isoimmunization. Am J Obstet Gynecol 1986;155:988–993.

25. Medical Research Council. An assessment of the hazards of amniocentesis. Br J Obstet Gynaecol 1978; 85(Suppl 2):1–42.

26. Crane JP, Rohland B, Larson D. Rh immune globulin after genetic amniocentesis: impact on pregnancy outcome. Am J Med Genet 1984;19:763–768.

27. Brandenburg H, Jahoda MGJ, Pijpers L, et al. Rhesus sensitization after midtrimester genetic amniocentesis. Am J Med Genet 1989;32:225–226.

28. Tabsh KMA, Lebherz TB, Crandall BF. Risks of prophylactic anti-D immunoglobulin after second-trimester amniocentesis. Am J Obstet Gynecol 1984;149:225–226.

29. Simonovits I. Efficiency of anti-D IgG prevention after induced abortion. Vox Sang 1974;26:361–367.

30. Simonovits I, Timar I, Bajtai G. Rate of Rh immunization after induced abortion. Vox Sang 1980;38: 161–164.

31. Smidt-Jensen S, Philip J. Comparison of transabdominal and transcervical CVS and amniocentesis: sampling success and risk. Prenat Diagn 1991;11:529–537.

32. Pollack W, Ascari WQ, Kochesky RJ, et al. Studies on Rh prophylaxis: 1. Relationship between doses of anti-Rh and size of antigenic stimulus. Transfusion 1971;11:333–339.

33. Bowman JM. Historical overview: hemolytic disease of the fetus and newborn. In: Kennedy MS, Wilson SM, Kelton JG, eds. Perinatal transfusion medicine. Arlington, VA: American Association of Blood Banks, 1990.

34. Ness PM, Baldwin ML, Niebyl JR. Clinical high-risk designation does not predict excess fetal-maternal hemorrhage. Am J Obstet Gynecol 1987;156:154–158.

35. Feldman N, Skoll A, Sibai B. The incidence of significant fetomaternal hemorrhage in patients undergoing cesarean section. Am J Obstet Gynecol 1990;163:855–858.

36. Bayliss KM, Keuck BD, Johnson ST, et al. Detecting fetomaternal hemorrhage: a comparison of five methods. Transfusion 1991;31:303–307.

37. Stedman CM, Baudin JC, White CA, et al. Use of the erythrocyte rosette test to screen for excessive fetomaternal hemorrhage in Rh-negative women. Am J Obstet Gynecol 1986;154:1363–1369.

38. Bowman JM, Pollock JM. Failures of intravenous Rh immune globulin prophylaxis: an analysis of the reasons for such failures. Transfus Med Rev 1987;1:101–112.

39. Tovey LAD. Haemolytic disease of the newborn—the changing scene. Br J Obstet Gynaecol 1986;93: 960–966.

40. Grimes DA, Ross WC, Hatcher RA. Rh immunoglobulin utilization after spontaneous and induced abortion. Obstet Gynecol 1977;50:261–263.

41. Grimes DA, Geary FH Jr, Hatcher RA. Rh immunoglobulin utilization after ectopic pregnancy. Am J Obstet Gynecol 1981;140:246–249.

42. Thornton JG, Page C, Foote G, et al. Efficacy and long term effects of antenatal prophylaxis with anti-D immunoglobulin. BMJ 1989;298:1671–1673.

43. Centers for Disease Control. Lack of transmission of human immunodeficiency virus through Rho(D) immune globulin (human). MMWR 1987;36:728–729.

44. Nicolaides KH, Fontanarosa M, Gabbe SG, et al. Failure of ultrasonographic parameters to predict the severity of fetal anemia in rhesus isoimmunization. Am J Obstet Gynecol 1988;158:920–926.

45. Nance SJ, Nelson JM, Horenstein J, et al. Monocyte monolayer assay: an efficient noninvasive technique for predicting the severity of hemolytic disease of the newborn. Am J Clin Pathol 1989;92:89–92.

46. Zupanska B, Brojer E, Richards Y, et al. Serological and immunological characteristics of maternal anti-Rh(D) antibodies in predicting the severity of haemolytic disease of the newborn. Vox Sang 1989;56: 247–253.

47. Bowman JM. Rh erythroblastosis fetalis 1975. Semin Hematol 1975;12:189–207.

48. Liley AW. Errors in the assessment of hemolytic disease from amniotic fluid. Am J Obstet Gynecol 1963;86:485–494.

49. Nicolaides KH, Rodeck CH, Mibashan RS, et al. Have Liley charts outlived their usefulness? Am J Obstet Gynecol 1986;155:90–94.

50. Ananth U, Queenan JT. Does midtrimester delta OD450 of amniotic fluid reflect severity of Rh disease? Am J Obstet Gynecol 1989;161:47–49.

51. Daffos F. Access to the other patient. Semin Perinatol 1989;13:252–259.

52. Pielet BW, Socol ML, MacGregor SN, et al. Cordocentesis: an appraisal of risks. Am J Obstet Gynecol 1988;159: 1497–1500.

53. Bennett PR, Le Van Kim C, Colin Y, et al. Prenatal determination of fetal RhD type by DNA amplification. N Engl J Med 1993;329:607–610.

54. Poissonnier MH, Brossard Y, Demedeiros N, et al. Two hundred intrauterine exchange transfusions in severe blood incompatibilities. Am J Obstet Gynecol 1989;161:709–713.

55. Harman CR, Bowman JM, Manning FA, et al. Intrauterine transfusion—intraperitoneal versus intravascular approach: a case-control comparison. Am J Obstet Gynecol 1990;162:1053–1059.

56. Watts DH, Luthy DA, Benedetti TJ, et al. Intraperitoneal fetal transfusion under direct ultrasound guidance. Obstet Gynecol 1988;71:84–88.

57. U.S. Public Health Service Expert Panel on the Content of Prenatal Care. Caring for our future: the content of prenatal care. Washington, DC: Public Health Service, Department of Health and Human Services, 1989. (NIH Publication No. 90–3182.)

58. Canadian Task Force on the Periodic Health Examination. Canadian guide to clinical preventive health care. Ottawa: Canada Communication Group, 1994:116–125.

59. Urbaniak SJ. Rh(D) haemolytic disease of the newborn: the changing scene. BMJ 1985;291:4–6.

60. Nusbacher J, Bove JR. Rh immunoprophylaxis: is antepartum therapy desirable? N Engl J Med 1980;303:935–937.

61. Torrance GW, Zipursky A. Cost-effectiveness of antepartum prevention of Rh immunization. Clin Perinatol 1984; 11:267–281.

39. Intrapartum Electronic Fetal Monitoring

RECOMMENDATION

Routine electronic fetal monitoring for low-risk women in labor is not recommended. There is insufficient evidence to recommend for or against intrapartum electronic fetal monitoring for high-risk pregnant women (see *Clinical Intervention*).

Burden of Suffering

Intrapartum fetal asphyxia is an important cause of stillbirth and neonatal death. In the U.S. in 1993, an estimated 700 infant deaths (17.3/100,000 live births) were attributed to intrauterine hypoxia and birth asphyxia.[1] Some neonates with intrauterine hypoxia require resuscitation and other aggressive medical interventions for such complications as acidosis and seizures. Asphyxia has also been implicated as a cause of cerebral palsy, although most cases of cerebral palsy occur in persons without evidence of birth asphyxia or other intrapartum events.[2–5] Most fetuses tolerate intrauterine hypoxia during labor and are delivered without complications, but assessments suggesting fetal distress are associated with an increased likelihood of cesarean delivery (63% compared to 23% for all births).[6] The exact incidence of fetal distress is uncertain; a rate of 42.9/1,000 live births was reported from 1991 U.S. birth certificate data, with the highest rates in infants born to mothers under age 20 or over age 40, and in blacks.[7]

Accuracy of the Screening Test

The principal screening technique for fetal distress and hypoxia during labor is the measurement of fetal heart rate. Abnormal decelerations in fetal heart rate and decreased beat-to-beat variability during uterine contractions are considered to be suggestive of fetal distress. The detection of these patterns during monitoring by auscultation or during electronic monitoring (cardiotocography) increases the likelihood that the fetus is in distress, but the patterns are not diagnostic. In addition, normal or equivocal heart rate patterns do not exclude the diagnosis of fetal distress.[5] Precise information on the frequency of false-negative and false-positive results is lacking, however, due in large part to the absence of an accepted definition of fetal distress.[8,9] For many years, acidosis and hypoxemia as determined by fetal scalp blood pH were used for this purpose in research and clinical practice, but it is now clear that neither finding is diagnostic of fetal distress.[5,10–12]

Electronic fetal heart rate monitoring can detect at least some cases of fetal distress, and it is often used for routine monitoring of women in labor. In 1991, the reported rate of electronic fetal monitoring in the U.S. was 755/1,000 live births.[7] The published performance characteristics of this technology, derived largely from research at major academic centers, may overestimate the accuracy that can be expected when this test is performed for routine screening in typical community settings. Two factors in particular that may limit the accuracy and reliability achievable in actual practice are the method used to measure fetal heart activity and the variability associated with cardiotocogram interpretations.

The measurement of fetal heart activity is performed most accurately by attaching an electrode directly to the fetal scalp, an invasive procedure requiring amniotomy and associated with occasional complications. This has been the technique used in most clinical trials of electronic fetal monitoring. Other noninvasive techniques of monitoring fetal heart rate, which include external Doppler ultrasound and periodic auscultation of heart sounds by clinicians, are more appropriate for widespread screening but provide less precise data than the direct electrocardiogram using a fetal scalp electrode. In studies comparing external ultrasound with the direct electrocardiogram, about 20–25% of tracings differed by at least 5 beats per minute.[13,14]

A second factor influencing the reliability of widespread fetal heart rate monitoring is inconsistency in interpreting results. Several studies have documented significant intra- and interobserver variation in assessing cardiotocograms even when tracings are read by experts in electronic fetal monitoring.[15–17] It would be expected that routine performance of electronic monitoring in the community setting with interpretations by less experienced clinicians would generate a higher proportion of inaccurate results and potentially unnecessary interventions than has been observed in the published work of major research centers.

Effectiveness of Early Detection

A potentially more important issue is whether electronic evidence of fetal distress during labor results in benefit to either the fetus or mother. Observational studies in the 1960s and 1970s suggested that electronic fetal monitoring during labor reduced the risk of intrapartum stillbirth, neonatal death, and developmental disability, but methodologic problems in these largely retrospective studies left the issue unsettled.[4,8] Ten randomized controlled trials and four meta-analyses of electronic fetal monitoring have since been published, all of which compared electronic monitoring, with or without fetal scalp blood sampling, to active clinical monitoring including intermittent auscultation by trained personnel. Three trials in low-risk women,[18-20] the largest of which involved nearly 13,000 patients,[18] compared continuous electronic monitoring to intermittent auscultation; where described, auscultation was performed at least every 15 minutes during the first stage of labor[18,20] and between each contraction during the second stage.[20] Two trials included scalp blood sampling.[19,20] These trials found no significant differences between the study groups in intrapartum or perinatal deaths, maternal or neonatal morbidity, Apgar scores, umbilical cord blood gases, the need for assisted ventilation, or admission to the special care nursery. The results of one of these trials[19] may have been biased by the method of randomization, however, which resulted in a large disparity in the distribution of primigravidae between the study groups. Similarly, no differences in clinical outcomes were reported in a subgroup analysis of low-risk women enrolled in a prospective study of nearly 35,000 pregnancies in which routine monitoring was compared with selective monitoring of high-risk pregnancies.[21,22] A controlled trial[23] that assigned intervention by week of admission also reported no effect of electronic fetal monitoring on low Apgar scores, admissions to special care nurseries, or neonatal infection. A trial from Greece carried out in predominantly low-risk pregnant women found no differences in most neonatal outcome measures, but reported a significant reduction in perinatal mortality rates (2.6 compared to 13/1,000 total births).[24] This study may not be generalizable to the U.S., however, given higher perinatal mortality and substantially lower cesarean delivery rates (<10%) than are typical in the U.S. In addition, the method of randomization and the large disparity in numbers between study and control group (746 vs. 682 women) raise the possibility of biased randomization.

The potential benefits of electronic fetal monitoring during labor have also been examined in high-risk pregnancies. Four clinical trials in developed countries found that electronic fetal heart rate monitoring in high-risk pregnancies, with or without scalp blood sampling, was of limited benefit when compared with intermittent auscultation during labor.[25-28] Neonatal death, Apgar scores, cord blood gases, and neonatal nursery morbidity were unchanged in three of the trials,[26-28] all of which performed intermittent auscultation systematically in control women: every 15 minutes in the first stage of labor and every 5 minutes in the second stage. The fourth trial found that continuous monitoring was associated with improved umbilical cord blood gases and neurologic symptoms and signs, and decreased need for intensive care.[25] This study has been criticized, however, because monitoring techniques in the control group were poorly described and one physician withdrew his patients from the control group after the trial began.[8,29] Results from a fifth trial in high-risk pregnant women in Zimbabwe are unlikely to be applicable to obstetric care in the U.S.[30]

Meta-analyses[31-33] that included all but the two most recently published randomized controlled trials[24,30] cited above reported no effect of electronic fetal monitoring on low Apgar scores, admissions to special care nurseries, or neonatal infection. With electronic fetal monitoring combined with scalp blood sampling, the relative risk of intrapartum death was 0.81 (95% confidence interval, 0.22 to 2.98) and of perinatal death was 0.98 (95% confidence interval, 0.58 to 1.64) when compared to intermittent auscultation. Relative risk of perinatal mortality when electronic fetal monitoring without blood sampling was used was 1.94 (95% confidence interval, 0.2 to 18.62). A meta-analysis of all trials from developed countries also reported no significant effect on overall perinatal mortality (typical odds ratio 0.87; 95% confidence interval, 0.57 to 1.33).[33a] The confidence intervals around these point estimates of the risk of perinatal death are wide, indicating that sample size is insufficient to exclude the possibility of clinically important increases or declines in mortality. One meta-analysis reported a significant reduction in perinatal mortality due to fetal hypoxia, but the method for attributing deaths to hypoxia was not standardized.[33a] The results appeared to be strongly influenced by the inclusion of one trial with questionable randomization methods and generalizability to the U.S. (see above);[24] a sensitivity analysis to examine the effect of excluding this trial from the meta-analysis was not reported.

Although most outcome measures in these studies were not influenced by electronic fetal monitoring, there is evidence that it reduces the incidence of neonatal seizures. This was suggested in early research[25,34] and confirmed in the Dublin trial of low-risk women.[20] This study reported a statistically significant reduction in the rate of neonatal seizures when continuous intrapartum fetal monitoring was compared with intermittent auscultation. Secondary analysis suggested that the reduced risk was limited to labors that were prolonged or induced or augmented with oxytocin. In a meta-analysis of the controlled trials that included scalp blood sampling as an adjunct, the odds of neonatal seizures were reduced by about one half with electronic monitoring.[31] A separate meta-analysis found no effect of electronic monitoring on neonatal seizures when no scalp blood sampling was performed,[32] raising the possibility that the benefit may have been due to the blood sampling rather than the electronic monitoring. What also remains unclear is the extent to which infants benefit from the prevention of neonatal seizures by monitoring. Seizures have been viewed by many as a poor prognostic indicator; in the Dublin trial, death occurred in 23% of the babies who experienced seizures, and autopsy confirmed that at least two thirds of these deaths were due to asphyxia during labor.[20] There are few prospective data on whether the prevention of neonatal seizures reduces the risk of neonatal death or long-term neurologic sequelae. The neonatal seizures prevented by electronic monitoring may not be those associated with long-term impairment.[20,31] At 4-year follow-up of survivors after seizures in the Dublin trial, the total number and rate with cerebral palsy (n = 3 and 0.5/1,000 enrolled subjects) were identical in the monitored and control groups.[35]

None of the three trials reporting longer term follow-up found that electronic fetal monitoring improved neurologic or developmental outcomes. A follow-up study of the growth and development at 9 months of age of infants involved in the second Denver trial[27] failed to show any long-term benefits of electronic fetal monitoring; the direction of the effect on mental and psychomotor development scores suggested increased risk in the monitored group.[36] In the Dublin trial,[20] the overall rates of cerebral palsy at 4-year follow-up were 1.8/1,000 in the electronically monitored group and 1.5/1,000 in the auscultation group.[35] Eighteen-month follow-up in a trial in high-risk women[28] revealed little difference in mean mental or psychomotor development scores on the Bayley Scales, but cerebral palsy and low mental development scores were both significantly more common in the electronically monitored group.[37] Cerebral palsy was associated with an increased duration of abnormal fetal heart rate patterns and time to delivery after diagnosis of such patterns in the electronically monitored group. Meta-analyses combining these three studies confirm little benefit from monitoring on adverse neurologic outcomes.[31,32]

Any potential benefit of intrapartum monitoring must be weighed against the potential risks associated both with diagnostic procedures and operative interventions for fetal distress. The insertion of fetal scalp electrodes, for example, is generally a safe procedure, but it may occasionally cause umbilical cord prolapse or infection due to early amniotomy; electrode or pressure catheter trauma to the eye, fetal vessels, umbilical cord, or placenta; and scalp infections with Herpes hominis type 2 or group B streptococcus.[10] Concerns have also been raised about the potential for enhancing transmission of human immunodeficiency virus (HIV) infection by the use of scalp electrodes.[38] Meta-analysis of randomized controlled trials indicates no increased risk of neonatal infection from electronic fetal monitoring compared to intermittent auscultation.[33] Perhaps the most important complication of intrapartum electronic fetal monitoring is the increased performance of cesarean delivery, an operation associated with maternal and neonatal morbidity and a small but measurable operative mortality.[39,40] Fetal distress is a common indication for cesarean delivery, and all trials showed a higher cesarean delivery rate in the electronically monitored group. The randomized controlled trials from the 1970s reported that cesarean delivery was performed significantly more frequently in association with electronic fetal monitoring.[18,19,25-27] In recent years, an effort has been made to lower the frequency of cesarean delivery, and four of five trials carried out in developed countries in the 1980s or 1990s reported no significant increase in the overall cesarean delivery rate with electronic fetal monitoring.[20,23,24,28] A fifth trial, comparing routine to selective electronic monitoring, reported a very small increase that was statistically but not clinically significant.[21] On the other hand, operative vaginal (e.g., forceps) deliveries were significantly increased in the newer trials,[20,23,24] suggesting an inverse relationship between cesarean and operative vaginal delivery. The meta-analyses[31,32,33a] previously cited reported a 1.3- to 2.7-fold increased likelihood of cesarean delivery and a 2.0- to 4.1-fold increased likelihood of cesarean delivery for fetal distress with continuous electronic fetal monitoring, with lower rates in the meta-analysis of studies that used scalp blood sampling. The likelihood of any operative delivery was increased by about 30% with electronic fetal monitoring. The meta-analyses also reported higher rates of both maternal infection and general anesthesia with electronic monitoring, presumably secondary to the higher rates of operative delivery.[31,32] Electronic monitoring may also have adverse psychological effects. In a comparison of subsamples from the randomized groups in one trial, women who had electronic fetal monitoring reported an increased likelihood of feeling "too restricted" during labor and were also more likely to report feeling left alone, although the latter difference was of only borderline significance.[41] On the other hand, in a subsample from a different trial, there were no differences between women in the two groups in their assessment of their monitoring experience, medical or nursing support, or the labor or delivery experience.[42]

Recommendations of Other Groups

The American College of Obstetricians and Gynecologists states that all patients in labor need some form of fetal monitoring, with more intensified monitoring indicated in high-risk pregnancies; the choice of technique (electronic fetal monitoring or intermittent auscultation) is based on various factors, including the resources available.[43] The Canadian Task Force on the Periodic Health Examination advises against routine electronic fetal monitoring in normal pregnancies but found poor evidence regarding the inclusion or exclusion of its routine use in high-risk pregnancies.[44]

Discussion

Electronic fetal monitoring has become an accepted standard of care in many settings in the U.S. for the management of labor.[4] Birth certificate data suggest that this technology was used in about three fourths of all live births in 1991;[7] in certain academic centers the rate may be as high as 86–100%.[4] As discussed above, there are important questions regarding the definition of fetal distress, as well as about the accuracy and reliability of electronic fetal monitoring in discriminating accurately between pregnancies with and without this disorder. It is also unclear whether the use of this technology results in significantly improved outcome for the baby when compared to active clinical monitoring. Adequately conducted trials generalizable to obstetric care in the U.S. have not reported a reduction in perinatal mortality, although sample sizes are not adequate to exclude a benefit. Evidence does support a reduced risk of neonatal seizures, but the benefit was mainly seen in women with complicated labors (i.e., induced, augmented with oxytocin, or prolonged), and it is not clear that there are long-term adverse effects associated with the types of seizures prevented. Follow-up of study subjects at 9 months to 4 years of age has not revealed any long-term neurologic benefits from electronic monitoring. If anything, effect estimates suggest an increased risk of cerebral palsy and low developmental scores in electronically monitored infants, possibly due to false reassurance and consequent delayed intervention.

In addition to the maternal risks associated with electronic fetal monitoring, including increased rates of cesarean or operative vaginal (e.g., forceps) delivery, general anesthesia and maternal infection, and the possible increased risk of adverse neonatal neurologic outcome, increased use of this technology is associated with increased costs of labor care. The widespread use of electronic fetal monitoring in low-risk pregnancies in the face of uncertain benefits, and certain maternal risks and costs, has been attributed to concerns about litigation.[8,45] It has been estimated that nearly 40% of all obstetric malpractice losses are due to fetal monitoring problems,[46] and this may be a major motivating factor behind the widespread use of electronic fetal monitoring during labor.

CLINICAL INTERVENTION

Routine electronic fetal monitoring is not recommended for low-risk women in labor when adequate clinical monitoring including intermittent auscultation by trained staff is available ("D" recommendation). There is insufficient evidence to recommend for or against electronic fetal monitoring over intermittent auscultation for high-risk pregnancies ("C" recommendation). For pregnant women with complicated labor (i.e., induced, prolonged, or oxytocin augmented), recommendations for electronic monitoring plus scalp blood sampling may be made on the basis of evidence for a reduced risk of neonatal seizures, although the long-term neurologic benefit to the neonate is unclear and must be weighed against the increased risk to the mother and neonate of operative delivery, general

anesthesia, and maternal infection, and a possible increased risk of adverse neurologic outcome in the infant. There is currently no evidence available to evaluate electronic fetal monitoring in comparison to no monitoring.

The draft update of this chapter was prepared for the U.S. Preventive Services Task Force by Carolyn DiGuiseppi, MD, MPH, based in part on materials prepared by Geoffrey Anderson, MD, PhD, for the Canadian Task Force on the Periodic Health Examination.

REFERENCES

1. National Center for Health Statistics. Annual summary of births, marriages, divorces, and deaths: United States, 1993. Monthly vital statistics report; vol 42, no 13. Hyattsville, MD: Public Health Service, 1994.
2. Freeman JM, Nelson KB. Intrapartum asphyxia and cerebral palsy. Pediatrics 1988;82:240–249.
3. Nelson KB, Ellenberg JH. Antecedents of cerebral palsy. Multivariate analysis of risk. N Engl J Med 1986;315:81–86.
4. Shy KK, Larson EB, Luthy DA. Evaluating a new technology: the effectiveness of electronic fetal heart rate monitoring. Ann Rev Public Health 1987;8:165–190.
5. Goodlin RC, Haesslein HC. When is it fetal distress? Am J Obstet Gynecol 1977;128:440–445.
6. Taffel SM. Cesarean delivery in the United States, 1990. National Center for Health Statistics. Vital Health Statistics, Series 21, no. 51. Washington, DC: Government Printing Office, 1994. (Publication no. DHHS (PHS) 94-1929.)
7. National Center for Health Statistics. Advance report of maternal and infant health data from the birth certificate, 1991. Monthly vital statistics report; vol 42, no 11. Hyattsville, MD: Public Health Service, 1994.
8. Prentice A, Lind T. Fetal heart rate monitoring during labour: too frequent intervention, too little benefit? Lancet 1987;2:1375–1377.
9. American College of Obstetricians and Gynecologists Committee on Obstetric Practice. Fetal distress and birth asphyxia. Committee Opinion no. 137. Washington, DC: American College of Obstetricians and Gynecologists, 1994.
10. Pritchard JA, MacDonald PC, Gant NF. Williams obstetrics, 17th ed. Norwalk, CT: Appleton-Century-Crofts, 1985: 281–293.
11. Perkins RP. Perinatal observations in a high-risk population managed without intrapartum fetal pH studies. Am J Obstet Gynecol 1984;149:327–334.
12. Clark SL, Paul RH. Intrapartum fetal surveillance: the role of fetal scalp blood sampling. Am J Obstet Gynecol 1985; 153:717–720.
13. Suidan JS, Young BK, Hochberg HM, et al. Observations on perinatal heart rate monitoring. II. Quantitative unreliability of Doppler fetal heart rate variability. J Reprod Med 1985;30:519–522.
14. Boehm FH, Fields LM, Hutchison JM, et al. The indirectly obtained fetal heart rate: comparison of first- and second-generation electronic fetal monitors. Am J Obstet Gynecol 1986;155:10–14.
15. Cohen AB, Klapholz H, Thompson MS. Electronic fetal monitoring and clinical practice: a survey of obstetric opinion. Med Decis Making 1982;2:79-95.
16. Beaulieu MD, Fabia J, Leduc B, et al. The reproducibility of intrapartum cardiotocogram assessments. Can Med Assoc J 1982;127:214–216.
17. Nielsen PV, Stigsby B, Nickelsen C, et al. Intra- and inter-observer variability in the assessment of intrapartum cardiotocograms. Acta Obstet Gynecol Scand 1987;66:421–424.
18. Kelso IM, Parsons RJ, Lawrence GF, et al. An assessment of continuous fetal heart rate monitoring in labor: a randomized trial. Am J Obstet Gynecol 1978;131:526–531.
19. Wood C, Renou P, Oats J, et al. A controlled trial of fetal heart rate monitoring in a low-risk obstetric population. Am J Obstet Gynecol 1981;141:527–534.
20. MacDonald D, Grant A, Sheridan-Pereira M, et al. The Dublin randomized controlled trial of intrapartum fetal heart rate monitoring. Am J Obstet Gynecol 1985;152:524–539.
21. Leveno KJ, Cunningham FG, Nelson S, et al. A prospective comparison of selective and universal electronic fetal monitoring in 34,995 pregnancies. N Engl J Med 1986;315:615–619.

22. Neilson JP. Liberal vs. restrictive use of EFM in labour (low-risk labours). In: Enkin MW, Keirse MJNC, Renfrew MJ, Neilson JP, eds. Pregnancy and childbirth module. Cochrane database of systematic reviews: review no. 03886, 12 May 1994, "Cochrane Updates on Disk." Oxford: Update Software, 1994, Disk Issue 1.
23. Neldam S, Osler M, Hansen PK, et al. Intrapartum fetal heart rate monitoring in a combined low- and high-risk population: a controlled clinical trial. Eur J Obstet Gynecol Reprod Biol 1986;23:1–11.
24. Vintzileos AM, Antsaklis A, Varvarigos I, et al. A randomized trial of intrapartum fetal heart rate monitoring versus intermittent auscultation. Obstet Gynecol 1993;81:899–907.
25. Renou P, Chang A, Anderson I, et al. Controlled trial of fetal intensive care. Am J Obstet Gynecol 1976;126:470–476.
26. Haverkamp AD, Thompson HE, McFee JG, et al. The evaluation of continuous fetal heart rate monitoring in high-risk pregnancy. Am J Obstet Gynecol 1976;125:310–317.
27. Haverkamp AD, Orleans M, Langendoerfer S, et al. A controlled trial of the differential effects of intrapartum fetal monitoring. Am J Obstet Gynecol 1979;134:399–409.
28. Luthy DA, Shy KK, van Belle G, et al. A randomized trial of electronic fetal monitoring in preterm labor. Obstet Gynecol 1987;69:687–695.
29. Thacker SB. The efficacy of intrapartum electronic fetal monitoring. Am J Obstet Gynecol 1987;156: 24–30.
30. Mahomed K, Nyoni R, Mulambo T, et al. Randomised controlled trial of intrapartum fetal heart rate monitoring. BMJ 1994;308:497–500.
31. Neilson JP. EFM + scalp sampling vs. intermittent auscultation in labour. In: Enkin MW, Keirse MJNC, Renfrew MJ, Neilson JP, eds. Pregnancy and childbirth module. Cochrane database of systematic reviews: review no. 03297, 4 May 1994, "Cochrane Updates on Disk." Oxford: Update Software, 1994, Disk Issue 1.
32. Neilson JP. EFM alone vs. intermittent auscultation in labour. In: Enkin MW, Keirse MJNC, Renfrew MJ, Neilson JP, eds. Pregnancy and childbirth module. Cochrane database of systematic reviews: review no. 03298, 4 May 1994, "Cochrane Updates on Disk." Oxford: Update Software, 1994, Disk Issue 1.
33. Neilson JP. EFM vs. intermittent auscultation in labour. In: Enkin MW, Keirse MJNC, Renfrew MJ, Neilson JP, eds. Pregnancy and childbirth module. Cochrane database of systematic reviews: review no. 03884, 4 May 1994, "Cochrane Updates on Disk." Oxford: Update Software, 1994, Disk Issue 1.
33a. Vintzileos AM, Nochimson DJ, Guzman ER, et al. Intrapartum electronic fetal heart rate monitoring versus intermittent auscultation: a meta-analysis. Obstet Gynecol 1995;85:149–155.
34. Chalmers I. Randomized controlled trials of intrapartum monitoring. In: Thalhammer O, Baumgarten KV, Pollak A, eds. Perinatal medicine. Stuttgart: Georg Thieme, 1979:260–265.
35. Grant A, O'Brien N, Joy M-T, et al. Cerebral palsy among children born during the Dublin randomised trial of intrapartum monitoring. Lancet 1989;ii:1233–1236.
36. Langendoerfer S, Haverkamp AD, Murphy J, et al. Pediatric follow-up of a randomized controlled trial of intrapartum fetal monitoring techniques. J Pediatr 1980;97:103–107.
37. Shy KK, Luthy DA, Bennett FC, et al. Effects of electronic fetal-heart-rate monitoring, as compared with periodic auscultation, on the neurologic development of premature infants. N Engl J Med 1990;322:588–593.
38. American College of Obstetricians and Gynecologists. Human immunodeficiency virus infections. Technical Bulletin no. 169. Washington, DC: American College of Obstetricians and Gynecologists, 1992.
39. American Academy of Pediatrics and American College of Obstetricians and Gynecologists. Guidelines for perinatal care. 3rd ed. Elk Grove Village, IL: American Academy of Pediatrics, 1992.
40. Pearson J, Rees G. Technique of caesarean section. In: Chalmers I, Enkin M, Keirse MJNC, eds. Effective care in pregnancy and childbirth, volume 2: childbirth. Oxford: Oxford University Press, 1989:1234–1269.
41. Garcia J, Corry M, MacDonald D, et al. Mothers' views of continuous electronic fetal heart monitoring and intermittent auscultation in a randomised controlled trial. Birth 1985;12:79–85.
42. Killien MG, Shy K. A randomized trial of electronic fetal monitoring in preterm labor: mothers' views. Birth 1989; 16:7–12.
43. American College of Obstetricians and Gynecologists. Intrapartum fetal heart rate monitoring. Technical Bulletin no. 132. Washington, DC: American College of Obstetricians and Gynecologists, 1989.
44. Canadian Task Force on the Periodic Health Examination. Canadian guide to clinical preventive health care. Ottawa: Canada Communication Group, 1994:158–165.
45. Cunningham AS. Electronic fetal monitoring in labour. J R Soc Med 1987;80:783.
46. Frigoletto FD Jr, Nadel AS. Electronic fetal heart rate monitoring: why the dilemma? Clin Obstet Gynecol 1988;31: 179–183.

40. Home Uterine Activity Monitoring

RECOMMENDATION

There is insufficient evidence to recommend for or against home uterine activity monitoring (HUAM) in high-risk pregnancies as a screening test for preterm labor, but recommendations against its use may be made on other grounds (see *Clinical Intervention*). HUAM is not recommended in normal-risk pregnancies.

Burden of Suffering

Preterm birth is a leading cause of perinatal morbidity and mortality in the U.S. Preterm neonates account for at least half of the mortality and morbidity among newborns without congenital anomalies.[1] These conditions represent a leading cause of years of potential life lost before age 65.[2] Preterm births generate large societal costs in providing neonatal intensive care and long-term treatment for complications.[3] Both primary and secondary preventive measures have been proposed for the prevention of prematurity. Primary prevention includes efforts to reduce risk factors for prematurity, such as cessation of tobacco, alcohol, and other drug use, and programs to improve nutrition, socioeconomic conditions, and prenatal care. Secondary prevention involves the early detection and treatment of preterm labor.

Accuracy of Screening Tests

The rationale behind screening for preterm labor is the assumption that the risk of preterm birth can be reduced significantly by the prompt initiation of treatment (e.g., rest, hydration, tocolytic therapy). These measures are of potential value in prolonging pregnancy only in those cases involving idiopathic preterm labor and not in medically indicated preterm births (e.g., preterm rupture of membranes, antepartum hemorrhage, fetal distress). Tocolytic medications are generally ineffective after substantial cervical dilation (>2–3 cm) and effacement have occurred. Because patients and physicians may have difficulty in recognizing the early signs of preterm labor, many patients arrive at the hospital with advanced cervical dilation and effacement and/or with ruptured membranes. Such delays in detection are thought to limit the effectiveness of tocolysis.

Screening for earlier detection of preterm labor has therefore been proposed. The principal screening tests are self-palpation and tocodynamometry. Programs to improve the early detection of preterm labor have centered on educating women about the symptoms of preterm labor and on teaching self-palpation to help them detect the increasing rate of uterine contractions which often precedes preterm labor.[4] Studies of these measures have produced mixed results. Some studies have shown that self-palpation has poor sensitivity in detecting preterm labor. One study reported that only 15% of contractions were detected by patients and that fewer than 11% of pregnant women were able to identify half of their recorded contractions.[5]

Although tocodynamometry is usually performed in the hospital, home uterine activity monitoring (HUAM) has been advocated as an ambulatory screening test for preterm labor in high-risk women. The home tocodynamometer consists of a pressure sensor that is held against the abdomen by a belt and a recording/storage device that is carried by a belt or hung from the shoulder. Uterine activity is typically recorded by the patient for 1 hour, twice daily, while performing routine activities. The stored data are transmitted via telephone to a practitioner, where a receiving device prints out the data. Patients are often contacted by, or have access to, personnel who can address monitoring problems.

The sensitivity and specificity of HUAM are uncertain, due to lack of data and the absence of a reference standard. External tocodynamometers, whether in the hospital or home, can produce inconsistent wave amplitudes when measuring uterine contractions, depending on the location of the instrument, the tension on the belt, thickness of adipose tissue, and other factors. Contractions of mild intensity can be confused with background noise. Studies suggest that HUAM performs similarly to monitoring devices used in the hospital, detecting 1.1–2.2 contractions for every contraction detected by conventional devices,[6,7] and there is good correlation between HUAM results and contractions detected by intrauterine pressure catheters.[8] There appears to be substantial variation among physicians in the interpretation of tocodynamometry tracings.[7,9]

Effectiveness of Early Detection

A nonrandomized observational study[10] and six randomized controlled trials[11–18] of women at risk for preterm labor have compared birth outcomes with and without the use of HUAM. Three trials[13,15,17] found no significant effect on the incidence of preterm birth or low birth weight, but sample size may have been inadequate to detect a difference. An observational study[10] and four other trials[14–16,18] reported a significant reduction in the incidence of preterm birth, neonatal morbidity and mortality, or low birth weight in pregnancies monitored by HUAM. In four of these studies,[10,14,16,18] HUAM-monitored women received more intensive nursing or telemetry personnel contact than did women in the control groups, making it unclear whether it was the device or the nursing contact that was responsible for the improved outcome. Overall, the studies showing benefit also lacked randomization, had high attrition and exclusion rates, or suffered from other design limitations.

Four studies[10,11,14,16] found that HUAM-monitored women were less likely to experience preterm cervical dilation, effacement, or ruptured membranes and were more likely to be eligible for long-term tocolysis. Reported reductions in these surrogate measures, however, are of uncertain value in inferring an effect on clinical outcomes. The overall evidence shows rather consistently that the combination of HUAM and frequent provider telephone contact produces better outcomes than standard care.

There are no known direct adverse effects from HUAM. The technology involves some inconvenience, and surveys suggest that some women reject the device because of its impact on their lifestyle.[19] There is little evidence of other adverse effects. Studies have shown that HUAM-monitored women attend no more than one extra physician visit per pregnancy than do unmonitored women.[10] Another theoretical adverse effect is unnecessary hospitalization or administration of tocolytic drugs to women who have abnormal home tocodynamometry data but are not in preterm labor. Objective evidence regarding the incidence of this problem is unavailable.

Recommendations of Other Groups

In 1989[20] and again in 1992,[21] the American College of Obstetricians and Gynecologists concluded that HUAM should remain investigational and should not be recommended for routine clinical use. That position was maintained in a recent technical bulletin.[21a] In 1989, the National Institute of Child Health and Human Development concluded that the existing evidence was not convincing that HUAM, independent of vigorous nursing support and other interventions, was effective in assessing the risk of preterm labor or in preventing preterm birth.[22] In a 1989 survey, 86% of the experts on an American Medical Association Diagnostic and Therapeutic Technology Assessment panel concluded that the effectiveness of HUAM was investigational, indeterminate, or unacceptable.[23] In 1991, the Food and Drug Administration licensed the marketing of a HUAM device for women who have had a previous preterm delivery.[24] A 1992 technology assessment by the Agency for Health Care Policy and Research concluded that current data did not support widespread use of HUAM or suggest its superiority over other methods for reducing the incidence of preterm births.[25]

Discussion

The cost implications of HUAM are potentially great but have been incompletely evaluated in published research. Some studies have reported that average charges for HUAM-monitored women are $5,000–$11,000 lower than those for unmonitored women, presumably because of savings achieved by reduced neonatal intensive care.[26–28] The cost-effectiveness of HUAM cannot fully be determined, however, until its clinical effectiveness has been demonstrated. Moreover, it remains unclear whether the money, personnel, and professional time required to provide this technology would divert resources from other potentially effective measures for the primary prevention of preterm births.

CLINICAL INTERVENTION

There is insufficient evidence to recommend for or against HUAM as a screening test for preterm labor in high-risk pregnancies (pregnancies with risk factors for preterm labor), but recommendations against its use may be made on other grounds, including its costs and inconvenience ("C" recommendation). HUAM is not recommended for normal-risk pregnancies (without risk factors for preterm labor) ("D" recommendation).

Note: See also the U.S. Preventive Services Task Force background paper on this topic: U.S. Preventive Services Task Force. Home uterine activity monitoring for preterm labor. JAMA 1993;270:369–376.

The draft of this chapter was prepared for the U.S. Preventive Services Task Force by Steven H. Woolf, MD, MPH, and Douglas B. Kamerow, MD, MPH.

REFERENCES
 1. Creasy RK. Preventing preterm birth. N Engl J Med 1992;325:727–729.
 2. Centers for Disease Control and Prevention. Years of potential life lost before age 65—United States, 1990 and 1991. MMWR 1993;42:251–253.
 3. Institute of Medicine. Preventing low birth weight. Washington, DC: National Academy Press, 1985.
 4. Katz M, Newman RB, Gill PJ. Assessment of uterine activity in ambulatory patients at high risk of preterm labor and delivery. Am J Obstet Gynecol 1986;154:44–47.
 5. Newman RB, Gill RJ, Wittreich P, Katz M. Maternal perception of prelabor uterine activity. Obstet Gynecol 1986;68:765–769.
 6. Katz M, Gill PJ. Initial evaluation of an ambulatory system for home monitoring and transmission of uterine activity data. Obstet Gynecol 1985;66:273–277.
 7. Hess LW, McCaul JF, Perry KG, et al. Correlation of uterine activity using the Term Guard monitor versus standard external tocodynamometry compared with the intrauterine pressure catheter. Obstet Gynecol 1990;76:52S–55S.
 8. Paul MJ, Smeltzer JS. Relationship of measured external tocodynamometry with measured internal uterine activity. Am J Perinatol 1991;8:417–420.
 9. Scheerer LJ, Campion S, Katz M. Ambulatory tocodynamometry data interpretation: evaluating variability and reliability. Obstet Gynecol 1990;76:67S–69S.
10. Katz M, Gill PJ, Newman RB. Detection of preterm labor by ambulatory monitoring of uterine activity: a preliminary report. Obstet Gynecol 1986;68:773–778.
11. Morrison JC, Martin JN, Martin RW, et al. Prevention of preterm birth by ambulatory assessment of uterine activity: a randomized study. Am J Obstet Gynecol 1987;156:536–543.

12. Iams JD, Johnson FF, O'Shaughnessy RW, et al. A prospective random trial of home uterine activity monitoring in pregnancies at increased risk of preterm labor. Part I. Am J Obstet Gynecol 1987;157: 638–643.

13. Iams JD, Johnson FF, O'Shaughnessy RW. A prospective random trial of home uterine activity monitoring in pregnancies at increased risk of preterm labor. Part II. Am J Obstet Gynecol 1988;159: 595–603.

14. Hill WC, Fleming AD, Martin RW, et al. Home uterine activity monitoring is associated with a reduction in preterm birth. Obstet Gynecol 1990;76:13S–18S.

15. Dyson DC, Crites YM, Ray DA, et al. Prevention of preterm birth in high-risk patients: the role of education and provider contact versus home uterine monitoring. Am J Obstet Gynecol 1991; 164:756–762.

16. Mou SM, Sunderji SG, Gall S, et al. Multicenter randomized clinical trial of home uterine activity monitoring for detection of preterm labor. Am J Obstet Gynecol 1991;165:858–866.

17. Blondel B, Breart G, Berthoux Y, et al. Home uterine activity monitoring in France: a randomized controlled trial. Am J Obstet Gynecol 1992;167:424–429.

18. Morrison JC, Martin JN Jr, Martin RW, et al. A program of uterine activity monitoring and its effect on neonatal morbidity. J Perinatol 1988;8:228–231.

19. Chibber G, Cohen AW, Lindenbaum CR, et al. Patient attitude toward home uterine activity monitoring. Obstet Gynecol 1990;76:90S–92S.

20. American College of Obstetricians and Gynecologists. Strategies to prevent prematurity: home uterine activity monitoring. Committee on Obstetrics: maternal and fetal medicine. Opinion no. 74. Washington, DC: American College of Obstetricians and Gynecologists, 1989.

21. American College of Obstetricians and Gynecologists. Home uterine activity monitoring. Committee Opinion no. 115. Washington, DC: American College of Obstetricians and Gynecologists, 1992.

21a. American College of Obstetricians and Gynecologists. Preterm labor. Technical Bulletin no. 206. Washington, DC: American College of Obstetricians and Gynecologists, 1995.

22. Rhoads GG, McNellis DC, Kessel SS. Home monitoring of uterine contractility: summary of a workshop sponsored by the National Institute of Child Health and Human Development and the Bureau of Maternal and Child Health and Resources Development, Bethesda, Maryland, March 29 and 30, 1989. Am J Obstet Gynecol 1991;165:2–6.

23. Diagnostic and Therapeutic Technology Assessment (DATTA). Home monitoring of uterine activity. JAMA 1989;261: 3027–3029.

24. Fed Reg 1990 Oct 23;55:427–479.

25. Holohan T, Green I. Health technology review of home uterine monitoring. Rockville, MD: Agency for Health Care Policy and Research, 1992. (AHCPR Publication no. 92-0064.)

26. Morrison JC, Martin JN Jr, Martin RW, et al. Cost effectiveness of ambulatory uterine activity monitoring. Int J Gynecol 1989;28:127–132.

27. Morrison JC, Pittman KP, Martin RW, et al. Cost/health effectiveness of home uterine activity monitoring in a Medicaid population. Obstet Gynecol 1990;76:76S–81S.

28. Kosasa TS, Abou-Sayf FK, Li-Ma G, et al. Evaluation of the cost-effectiveness of home monitoring of uterine contractions. Obstet Gynecol 1990;76:71S–75S.

41. Screening for Down Syndrome

RECOMMENDATION

The offering of amniocentesis or chorionic villus sampling (CVS) for chromosome studies is recommended for pregnant women at high risk for Down syndrome. The offering of screening for Down syndrome by serum multiple-marker testing is recommended for all low-risk pregnant women, and as an alternative to amniocentesis and CVS for high-risk women (see *Clinical Intervention*). This testing should be offered only to women who are seen for prenatal care in locations that have adequate counseling and follow-up services. There is currently insufficient evidence to recommend for or against screening for Down syndrome by individual serum marker testing or ultrasound examination, but recommendations against such screening may be made on other grounds (see *Clinical Intervention*).

Burden of Suffering

Down syndrome, a congenital syndrome caused by trisomy of all or part of chromosome 21, is the most common chromosome abnormality.[1] Population-based surveillance programs have reported a Down syndrome birth prevalence of 0.9/1,000 live births.[2] The incidence of Down syndrome is higher than the birth prevalence, however, since many fetuses are spontaneously aborted, some are recognized in utero and electively aborted, and some cases are not recognized at birth. Affected children are characterized by physical abnormalities that include congenital heart defects and other dysmorphisms, and varying degrees of mental and growth retardation. Although there are therapies for some of the specific malformations associated with Down syndrome, there are no proven therapies available for the cognitive deficits. Life expectancy for infants born with Down syndrome is substantially lower than that of the general population.[3] Based on 1988 cross-sectional data, the lifetime economic costs of Down syndrome have been estimated to be $410,000 per case.[4]

The risk for Down syndrome and certain other chromosome anomalies increases substantially with advancing maternal age.[1,5–10] Parents carrying chromosome-21 rearrangements are also at an increased risk of Down syndrome pregnancies,[11-13] with the risk being much higher if the mother carries the rearrangement than if the father does. Also at higher risk are those who have previously had an affected pregnancy, independent of advancing maternal age and chromosome rearrangements.[14,15]

Accuracy of Screening Tests

Down syndrome is diagnosed prenatally by determining karyotype in fetal cell samples obtained by amniocentesis or chorionic villus sampling (CVS). Because of their invasiveness, risks, and cost, these procedures are generally reserved for women identified as high-risk either by history (i.e., advanced maternal age, prior affected pregnancy, known chromosome rearrangement) or by screening maneuvers (e.g., serum markers, ultrasound). Chromosome analysis of fetal cells obtained by second-trimester amniocentesis has been demonstrated to be accurate and reliable for prenatal diagnosis of Down syndrome in a randomized controlled trial and several cohort studies.[16-19] CVS, a technique for obtaining trophoblastic tissue, is an alternative to amniocentesis for detecting chromosome anomalies. The advantages of this procedure include the ability to perform karyotyping as early as 10–12 weeks and more rapid cytogenetic analysis. Potential disadvantages of CVS include apparent discrepancies between the karyotype of villi and the fetus due to maternal cell contamination or placental mosaicism, and failure to obtain an adequate specimen, resulting in a repeat procedure (usually amniocentesis) in up to 5% of tested women.[20-22] In randomized controlled trials[20-22] and cohort studies[23-29] comparing CVS to amniocentesis, accurate prenatal diagnosis has been obtained in over 99% of high-risk women when CVS is accompanied by both direct and culture methods of cytogenetic examination and when amniocentesis is provided to clarify CVS diagnoses of mosaicism or unusual aneuploidy. Transabdominal CVS has been reported to have comparable accuracy to transcervical CVS in randomized controlled trials.[20,30,31] First-trimester amniocentesis (at 10–13 weeks) has been compared to CVS in one randomized controlled trial.[32] Success rates were the same for the two procedures (97.5%); early amniocentesis failures were primarily due to failed culture. First- and second-trimester amniocentesis have not been directly compared in controlled trials.

For low-risk women, the risks associated with prenatal diagnostic testing (see *Adverse Effects of Screening and Early Detection*, below) are generally considered to outweigh the potential benefits because of the low likelihood of diagnosing a Down syndrome gestation. If screening tests, such as measurement of maternal serum markers or ultrasound imaging, can identify women who are at high risk for carrying a Down syndrome fetus, the relative benefit of prenatal diagnostic testing increases, potentially justifying the more invasive diagnostic procedures. Reduced levels of maternal serum α-fetoprotein (MSAFP) and unconjugated estriol, and elevated levels of human chorionic gonadotropin (hCG), have each been associated with Down syndrome gestations. Intervention studies of screening have not been carried out with unconjugated estriol alone, while cohort intervention studies evaluating MSAFP and hCG have found them to have relatively poor discriminatory power as individual tests.[33–36] Multiple-marker screening uses results from two or three individual maternal serum marker tests, combined with maternal age, to calculate the risk of Down syndrome in the current gestation.[37,38] Amniocentesis and diagnostic chromosome studies are then offered to women whose screening test results suggest a high risk of Down syndrome, with high risk often defined as having the same or greater risk of an affected pregnancy that a 35-year-old woman has (i.e., 1 in 270).

Six interventional cohort studies that analyzed low-risk women younger than 35 years,[39–41] 36 years,[42] 37 years,[43] or 38 years,[44] and six that included women of any age desiring screening (90–95% ≤35 years),[45–50] have evaluated the proportion of Down syndrome pregnancies identified through double-marker (hCG and either MSAFP or estriol) or triple-marker screening in the midtrimester compared to the total number of such pregnancies identified. Interpretation of sensitivity is affected by incomplete ascertainment of karyotype and incomplete diagnosis at birth in these studies, although most had active surveillance systems for Down syndrome cases born to screened women. The reported sensitivity of multiple-marker screening for Down syndrome ranged from 48 to 91% (median 64.5%) and the false-positive rate (after revision of dates by ultrasound) ranged from 3% to 10%. The likelihood of Down syndrome given a positive screening test result was 1.2–3.8%, depending on the threshold for high risk used to define a positive test result. In these studies, the threshold chosen ranged from a 1 in 125 to a 1 in 380 chance of having an affected pregnancy given a positive test result. A young woman with a prescreen risk of about 1 in 1,000 who tested positive would have a postscreen risk similar to the risk in women of advanced age who are currently offered prenatal diagnosis.

Multiple-marker screening has also been evaluated in women 35 years of age or older, for whom prenatal diagnosis using amniocentesis or CVS is routinely recommended because of their increased risk of Down syndrome. Studies suggest that multiple-marker screening in these women might reduce the need for more invasive diagnostic tests. In a cohort study of 5,385 women ≥35 years of age with no other risk factors, all of whom were undergoing routine amniocentesis and chromosome studies (thus allowing complete ascertainment of chromosome abnormalities), estimates of the individual risk of Down syndrome were calculated based on maternal age in combination with the results of multiple-marker screening using

MSAFP, hCG, and unconjugated estriol.[51] If amniocentesis were performed only on older women with at least a 1 in 200 risk of carrying a fetus with Down syndrome based on triple-marker screening, 89% of affected fetuses would have been detected, 25% of women with unaffected fetuses would have been identified by screening as needing amniocentesis. A threshold of 1 in 300 (similar to risk based on age ≥35 years alone) did not add sensitivity but did increase the screen-positive rate to 34%. Thus, triple-marker screening could have avoided 75% of amniocenteses in older women, with their attendant risk of fetal loss, at a cost of missing 11% of cases of Down syndrome. In this study, performing amniocenteses only on women with postscreen risks of at least 1 in 200 for Down syndrome would also have detected 47% of fetuses with other autosomal trisomies, 44% of fetuses with sex aneuploidy, and 11% with miscellaneous chromosome abnormalities. In previously cited interventional cohort studies of double- or triple-marker screening that reported separate results for older women, the Down syndrome detection rate was reported as 80–100% for women ≥35 years[43,46,47,50] and 100% for women ≥36 years,[42,45] with false-positive screening results of 19–27%. Incomplete case ascertainment was possible, however, since screen-negative women rarely had diagnostic chromosome studies.

Although no controlled trials have directly compared double-marker to triple-marker screening, several cohort studies of triple-marker screening have reported the detection rates for double-marker screening with hCG and MSAFP only. Three markers appear to be somewhat more sensitive than two for detection of Down syndrome; the net difference in sensitivity ranged from –2 to +18% in these studies, depending on the false-positive rate and risk cut-off used.[43,48,50,51]

Ultrasonography is another potential screening test for Down syndrome. Abnormalities associated with Down syndrome (including intrauterine growth retardation, cardiac anomalies, hydrops, duodenal and esophageal atresia) and differences in long-bone length and nuchal fold thickness between Down syndrome and normal pregnancies observable on midtrimester ultrasound have been reviewed.[52] In prospective cohort studies of midtrimester ultrasound screening in high-risk women who were undergoing amniocenteses for chromosome studies, nuchal fold thickening identified 75% of Down syndrome fetuses; shortened humerus or femur length detected 31%; and an index based on thickened nuchal fold, major structural defect, and certain other abnormalities identified 69%.[53–55] The likelihood of Down syndrome given a positive result was 7–25% in these high-risk samples, but would be substantially lower in low-risk women. No published cohort studies have evaluated the accuracy of ultrasound screening for detection of chromosome abnormalities in low-risk women, nor have interventional cohort studies evaluated its efficacy as a screening tool in high-risk women. The use of ultrasound as a screening test for Down syndrome is limited by the technical difficulty of producing a reliable sonographic image of critical fetal structures.[56,57] Incorrect positioning of the transducer, for example, can produce artifactual images resembling a thickened nuchal skin fold in a normal fetus.[58] Sonographic indices are therefore subject to considerable variation. Imaging techniques require further standardization before routine screening by ultrasound for Down syndrome can be considered for the general population.[56,59,60] In addition, results obtained by well-trained and well-equipped operators in a research context may not generalize to widespread use. In a multicenter cohort study in high-risk women that involved a large number of ultrasonographers of varying ability, the sensitivity of nuchal fold thickening for Down syndrome was only 38%.[59] The false-positive rate in this study was 8.5%, many times higher than that reported in studies involving expert ultrasonographers.[55,61]

Effectiveness of Early Detection

The detection of Down syndrome and other chromosome anomalies in utero provides as its principal benefit the opportunity to inform prospective parents of the likelihood of giving birth to an affected child. Parents may be counseled about the consequences of the abnormality and can make more informed decisions about optimal care for their newborn or about elective abortion. No controlled trials have been performed to assess clinical outcomes for those using screening or prenatal diagnosis for Down syndrome compared to those who do not. Therefore, the usefulness of this information depends to a large extent on the personal preferences and abilities of the parents.[62] Whether or not parents choose to use prenatal screening or diagnosis is related both to their views on the acceptability of induced abortion and their perceived risk of the fetus being abnormal.[63] The perception of the harm or nature of the disability may play a greater role in the decision than the actual probability of its occurrence.[64–67]

Induced abortion is currently sought by the majority of women whose prenatal diagnostic studies (i.e., karyotyping) reveal fetuses with Down syndrome.[33–35,39,40,45,48,68] Estimates of the reduction in birth prevalence of Down syndrome associated with offering prenatal diagnosis to women 35 years and older range from 7.3% to 29% in the U.S. and other developed countries.[2,69–73] The effect of this approach on the total number of Down syndrome births is limited because older women have low birth rates and therefore account for a relatively small proportion of affected pregnancies despite their exponentially increased risk for having an affected pregnancy.[74] Limited data are available to estimate the impact of serum-marker screening in younger women on Down syndrome birth prevalence. In England and Wales, the proportion of all cytogenetically diagnosed Down syndrome cases detected prenatally (thus potentially preventable) increased from 31% to 46% after the introduction of screening by maternal serum analysis and ultrasound for low-risk women.[68] In cohort studies evaluating double- or triple-marker screening, when the proportions of screen-positive women who decided not to undergo amniocentesis or induced abortion were taken into account, the proportion of Down syndrome births to screened women that were actually prevented ranged from 36% to 62%.[39,40,45,48] Up to 25% of screen-positive women declined prenatal diagnosis by amniocentesis in these studies. The effectiveness of screening in preventing Down syndrome births may be further reduced by incomplete uptake of screening. In antenatal screening programs in which double- or triple-marker screening was offered to all women and amniocentesis or CVS was offered to women over 35 years of age, nearly 60% of all Down syndrome births were potentially preventable, the remainder either being missed by screening (14–23%) or occurring in women who were not screened (17–27%).[47,49] Neither study evaluated acceptance of induced abortion, however. In another population, offering double-marker screening to all women prevented 59% of all Down syndrome births.[45] This population had high rates of screening (89%), largely due to the fact that pregnant women had to specifically ask to be excluded. There was also high acceptance of amniocentesis in screen-positive women (89%), and of induced abortion of cytogenetically confirmed cases (91%). The birth prevalence of Down syndrome decreased from approximately 1.1/1,000 to 0.4/1,000 after initiation of prenatal screening in this population.

Other potential effects of prenatal detection of Down syndrome have not been adequately explored. In families at high risk of Down syndrome births, such as those with advanced maternal age, a previous affected pregnancy, or known carriage of translocations, the availability of prenatal diagnosis may reduce the induced abortion rate by identifying normal pregnancies that might otherwise be electively aborted. This benefit has been reported with screening for cystic fibrosis,[75] but it has not been evaluated for Down syndrome. The diagnosis of a chromosome abnormality may spare unsuspecting parents some of the trauma associated with delivering an abnormal infant, and may help parents to prepare emotionally. Studies evaluating these potential psychological benefits have not been reported, however. Prenatal diagnosis may also enable clinicians to better prepare for the delivery and care of the baby. Studies are lacking regarding the impact of these measures on neonatal morbidity and mortality.

An indirect benefit of testing to detect Down syndrome is the discovery during testing of abnormalities other than the target condition. Chromosome studies on specimens obtained by amniocentesis or CVS will detect other abnormalities besides Down syndrome. Autosomal trisomies other than Down syndrome are usually spontaneously aborted, so the principal benefit of screening may be avoidance of late fetal death.[76] The health consequences of sex aneuploidy are less significant than trisomies, but about half such pregnancies are nevertheless electively aborted when discovered prenatally.[77,78] Serum marker screening for Down syndrome will also identify some patients carrying fetuses with other chromosome abnormalities (e.g., Turner syndrome, trisomy-13 or -18); sensitivity is low,[51] however, because some of these abnormalities have different effects on serum markers than does Down syndrome, and require different risk thresholds.[50,79] Ultrasound screening for Down syndrome leads to a more accurate assessment of gestational age in women with uncertain dates, and some studies suggest that acting on this information may reduce the likelihood of induced labor for erroneously diagnosed postterm pregnancy (see Chapter 36). Multiple gestations and major congenital anomalies, such as diaphragmatic hernia, gastroschisis, nonimmune fetal hydrops, and obstructive uropathy, may also be detected by ultrasound. These discoveries permit antenatal treatment as well as delivery and neonatal care planning. Controlled trials proving that early detection by ultrasound of multiple gestations or congenital anomalies improves outcome have not been published, however (see Chapter 36).

Adverse Effects of Screening and Early Detection. The most important risks of early detection of Down syndrome include those to the fetus from amniocentesis and CVS performed as a primary or follow-up diagnostic test, the psychological effects of a positive test on the parents, and the complications resulting from induced abortion. The risks of amniocentesis include rare puncture of the fetus, bleeding, infection, and possibly isosensitization.[80,81] The procedure-related rate of fetal loss with current technique appears to be about 0.5–0.8%.[16,17,29] The best evidence on amniocentesis risks comes from a randomized controlled trial of screening,[16] which reported a procedure-related risk of fetal loss of 0.8% of pregnancies. This may nevertheless overestimate current rates of loss as techniques have improved. In a more recent series of patients undergoing amniocentesis as part of a clinical trial, the risk of fetal loss was 0.04%.[22] In a randomized controlled trial, neonatal respiratory distress syndrome and neonatal pneumonia were more frequent after amniocentesis, independent of birth weight and gestational age; the additional risk was about 1%.[16] A similar trend was seen in the Medical Research Council study,[18] but has not been confirmed in other studies. Infection has not been identified as a significant problem in any large studies. No clinically important effects on development, behavior, or physical status were identified in 4-year-old children whose mothers had undergone midtrimester amniocentesis.[83] Case series of women undergoing first-trimester amniocentesis suggest a procedure-related fetal loss rate of 3–7%.[84–87] In a randomized controlled trial, the total fetal loss rate with early amniocentesis was significantly higher than with CVS (5.9 vs. 1.2%).[32]

Several randomized controlled trials comparing amniocentesis and CVS have reported significantly higher fetal loss rates with CVS (1.0–1.5%) when compared with second-trimester amniocentesis.[20–22] Inexperience and the use of transcervical CVS appear related to a greater risk of fetal loss, although at least one trial found no significant difference in fetal loss rates between transcervical and transabdominal CVS (2.5% vs. 2.3%).[31] An increased risk of transverse limb reduction anomalies in infants born after CVS has been reported in case-control and case-series studies.[88–93b] Conflicting evidence from cohort studies may relate to varying methods of case ascertainment or classification.[94–99a] Decreasing risk and a trend from proximal to distal limb damage with increasing gestational age at CVS provide biologic plausibility for a true association with limb reduction defects.[93,99b] Current estimates for the overall risk of transverse limb deficiency from CVS range from 0.03% to 0.10% of procedures.[99a] Severe maternal complications from CVS are rarely reported, but the Canadian Collaborative Study suggested a higher risk of bleeding requiring intervention for women undergoing CVS compared to amniocentesis.[22] None of the CVS trials has reported increased risks of birth defects or major infant health problems, but sample size is inadequate in these trials to rule out rare adverse effects.

A positive screening test result can produce a harmful psychological effect on parents. This is especially important because the large majority of positive screening tests occur in normal pregnancies. Adverse psychological effects of screening tests include the fear of discovering an abnormal pregnancy as well as anxiety over possible complications from diagnostic and therapeutic procedures. Women who have been identified as being at high risk because of a positive serum-marker screening test may have greater distress than women who are identified as high risk because of advanced age.[100,101] Distress is reduced following a diagnostic procedure confirming a normal pregnancy, but some anxiety related to the false-positive screening test may persist.[102,103] Most women screened will have normal results, however, and this may have psychological benefits for the reassured parents.

The potential complications of induced abortion must also be considered, since this is the outcome of the majority of positive diagnostic test results. Morbidity from first-trimester induced abortion, including infection, hemorrhage, and injury, occurs in 2–3% of procedures, but serious complications are rare; in one series of 170,000 cases, 0.07% required hospitalization and none resulted in death.[104–107] Complication rates, including maternal case-fatality rates, are higher with second-trimester abortions, but remain uncommon.[108–110] The case-fatality rate from legally induced abortion, 0.4/100,000 procedures, is substantially lower than the risk of pregnancy-related death, which is 8–9/100,000 live births.[108,109,111,112] The most serious consequence of false-positive test results, the induced abortion of a normal pregnancy, was not reported in any of the trials, and appears to be rare with current techniques. The likelihood of diagnostic error is slightly higher with CVS than with amniocentesis, but the risk of induced abortion as a consequence has not been fully evaluated.

Recommendations of Other Groups

Most organizations recommend offering amniocentesis or CVS for prenatal diagnosis to all pregnant women who are aged 35 years and older or otherwise at high risk for chromosome abnormalities.[113–115] The Canadian Task Force on the Periodic Health Examination concluded that there is fair evidence to offer second-trimester triple-marker screening to all pregnant women less than 35 years of age, and as an alternative to prenatal diagnosis by karyotyping in women 35 years and older; such offering should be accompanied by education on its limited efficacy, as well as on the risks of second-trimester diagnosis and abortion, and on the psychological implications of screening and of a Down syndrome birth.[114] Offering multiple-marker screening between 15 and 18 weeks of gestation to low-risk women under 35 years of age to assess Down syndrome risk is also recommended by the American College of Obstetricians and Gynecologists (ACOG) and the American College of Medical Genetics (ACMG); neither group recommends a specific multiple-marker protocol.[115,116] Neither ACOG nor ACMG recommends prenatal cytogenic screening by multiple-marker testing in women 35 years and older; ACOG recommends that multiple-marker testing may be offered as an option for those women who do not accept the risk of amniocentesis or who wish to have this additional information prior to making a decision. No organizations currently recommend routine screening for Down syndrome by ultrasound. ACOG[117] and a National Institutes of Health consensus development conference[118] have recommended that ultrasound imaging be performed during pregnancy only in response to a specific medical indication.

Discussion

Prenatal diagnostic testing is accurate and reliable for detecting Down syndrome, but it is associated with a procedure-related fetal loss risk of about 0.5% for second-trimester amniocentesis and 1–1.5% for CVS, and a measurable risk of transverse fetal limb deficiency after CVS. The currently accepted medical practice of routinely offering amniocentesis or CVS for prenatal diagnosis to pregnant women aged 35 years and older or otherwise at high risk is based on the mother's increased risk of having a fetus with a chromosome abnormality balanced against the risk of fetal loss associated with these procedures, and therefore includes an element of judgment. It can be predicted from available data (odds of Down syndrome during the second trimester) that a program offering amniocentesis to all pregnant women at age 35 has the potential of exposing 200–300 normal fetuses to this procedure for every case detected.[10] With an estimated procedure-related fetal loss rate of 0.5%, one normal fetus would be lost by amniocentesis for every one to two chromosome anomalies detected in such women. For CVS, the number of normal fetuses lost per case detected would be higher, and for first-trimester amniocentesis, it may be higher still. The older the maternal age, the more favorable the ratio of affected fetuses to fetal loss. Most women who request such testing and receive a diagnosis of a Down syndrome pregnancy choose to abort the pregnancy, resulting in a measurable reduction in Down syndrome births. There is little good evidence of the effect on personal and family outcomes, however, or on the balance of risks and benefits for the group as a whole. Nevertheless, those women at high risk who desire prenatal diagnosis of Down syndrome may benefit substantially from it. Thus, there is fair evidence to support offering prenatal diagnosis to high-risk pregnant women who are identified by age, history, or screening tests when a comprehensive prenatal diagnosis program that includes education, interpretation, and follow-up is available.

In low-risk pregnant women, maternal serum multiple-marker screening in the second trimester can detect nearly two thirds of Down syndrome fetuses, but it will result in a large number of young women being offered amniocentesis who would not otherwise be subjected to its risks. The ratio of affected fetuses detected to procedure-related fetal loss in women with positive multiple-marker screening would be similar to or more favorable than that of women 35 years and older. The risk of fetal loss may be acceptable to parents with strong fears of having an affected child.[64,119–121] There is also evidence that multiple-marker screening in women 35 years and older can detect 80% or more of Down syndrome pregnancies while allowing the majority of such women to avoid the risks associated with invasive diagnostic testing. Multiple-marker screening is not supported by the same strength of evidence as is amniocentesis or CVS, however. Potential problems include the reduced sensitivity for Down syndrome and other chromosome abnormalities, the large proportion of false-positive tests, and the substantial number of women who refuse or do not receive follow-up amniocentesis and chromosome studies. This is of particular concern if such screening is offered to women 35 years and older who might otherwise receive amniocentesis or CVS. Nevertheless, in some older women, particularly those who may have had difficulty conceiving or carrying a pregnancy, the reduced likelihood of amniocentesis or CVS and consequent risk of fetal loss or injury may outweigh the reduced sensitivity of multiple-marker screening. There is therefore fair evidence to support offering multiple-marker screening to pregnant women of all ages when a comprehensive prenatal diagnosis program is available that includes education, interpretation, and follow-up.

There is a lack of sound evidence to support the use of individual maternal serum markers to screen for Down syndrome, and currently available evidence suggests that sensitivity is substantially lower than with multiple-marker screening. Similarly, ultrasonography has not been adequately evaluated as a routine screening test for Down syndrome, and there are important concerns about the measurement reliability and generalizability of this technology to widespread use. Since there is evidence supporting the effectiveness of other screening and diagnostic methods, neither individual serum markers nor ultrasonography can be recommended as screening tests for Down syndrome outside clinical trials.

Identification and selective abortion of Down syndrome pregnancies raises important ethical concerns, a full discussion of which is beyond the scope of this chapter. These concerns include the implicit message that Down syndrome is an undesirable state, the interpretation of induced abortion in eugenic terms by some persons, and societal and economic pressures that may stigmatize families with a Down syndrome member. Attitudes held by both physicians and by society toward individuals with Down syndrome have changed over time, and various Down syndrome associations now offer support for families and individuals with Down syndrome, promote their participation in society, and seek respect for them.[122,123] These issues highlight the importance of offering screening and prenatal diagnosis of Down syndrome in a value-sensitive fashion with emphasis on reliable information about Down syndrome itself as well as about the potential risks and benefits of screening procedures.

In these recommendations, primary consideration has been given to the prenatal detection of Down syndrome. Other chromosome anomalies (e.g., Turner syndrome, trisomy-18) are often detected during prenatal screening and diagnosis and many may consider their detection important. There are few studies directly addressing screening for these conditions, however, and screening protocols have not been sufficiently evaluated to warrant review at this point.

CLINICAL INTERVENTION

The offering of amniocentesis or CVS for chromosome studies to pregnant women aged 35 years and older and to those at high risk of Down syndrome for other reasons (e.g., previous affected pregnancy, known carriage of a chromosome rearrangement associated with Down syndrome) is recommended ("B" recommendation). In some circumstances,

depending on resources, preferences, and other factors, the selection of a different age threshold for offering prenatal diagnosis may be considered. Counseling before the procedure should include a comparison of the risks to the fetus from the procedure and the probability of a chromosome defect given the patient's age or other risk factors, as well as a full discussion of the potential outcomes associated with delivering a child with Down syndrome and of aborting a Down syndrome fetus.

The offering of screening for Down syndrome by maternal serum multiple-marker testing at 15–18 weeks of gestation is recommended for all pregnant women who have access to counseling and follow-up services, skilled high-resolution ultrasound and amniocentesis capabilities, and reliable, standardized laboratories ("B" recommendation). There is currently insufficient evidence to recommend a specific multiple-marker screening protocol. Counseling regarding screening should include information on the procedure itself, the likelihood of follow-up testing with amniocentesis and its associated risks, as well as a full discussion of the potential outcomes associated with delivering a child with Down syndrome and of aborting a Down syndrome fetus. Women with a positive screen should receive detailed information comparing the increased risk of trisomy and the risks of fetal loss from amniocentesis. For women aged 35 years and older, the choice of serum multiple-marker screening versus amniocentesis or CVS for chromosome studies depends on patient preferences and therefore requires a detailed discussion of the potential risks and benefits of each procedure. In particular, the patient should understand the reduced sensitivity of multiple-marker screening for Down syndrome and for other chromosome abnormalities compared to prenatal diagnosis by chromosome studies, and the increased risk of fetal loss or injury with amniocentesis and CVS.

There is currently insufficient evidence to recommend for or against routine ultrasound examination or the use of individual maternal serum markers in pregnant women as screening tests for Down syndrome ("C" recommendation). Recommendations against these tests may be made on other grounds, however, including the availability of other screening tests of proven effectiveness.

The draft update of this chapter was prepared for the U.S. Preventive Services Task Force by Carolyn DiGuiseppi, MD, MPH, based in part on material prepared for the Canadian Task Force on the Periodic Health Examination by Paul Dick, MDCM, FRCPC.

REFERENCES

1. National Center for Health Statistics Advance report of maternal and infant health data from the birth certificate, 1991. Monthly vital statistics report; vol 42, no 11 (suppl). Hyattsville, MD: Public Health Service, 1994.
2. Centers for Disease Control and Prevention. Down syndrome prevalence at birth—United States, 1983–1990. MMWR 1994;43:617–622.

3. Baird PA, Sadovnick AD. Life tables for Down syndrome. Hum Genet 1989;82:291–292.

4. Waitzman NJ, Romano PS, Scheffler RM. Estimates of the economic costs of birth defects. Inquiry 1994;31:188–205.

5. Hansen JP. Older maternal age and pregnancy outcome: a review of the literature. Obstet Gynecol 1986;41:726–742.

6. Ferguson-Smith M, Yates JRW. Maternal age specific rates for chromosome aberrations and factors influencing them: report of a collaborative European study on 52965 amniocenteses. Prenatal Diag 1984;4:5–44.

7. Hook EB. Rates of chromosome abnormalities at different maternal ages. Obstet Gynecol 1981;58:282–285.

8. Hook E, Topol BB, Cross PK. The natural history of cytogenetically abnormal fetuses detected at midtrimester amniocentesis: new data and estimates of the excess and relative risk of late fetal death associated with 47,+21 and some other abnormal karyotypes. Am J Hum Genetics 1989;45:855–861.

9. Cuckle HS, Wald NJ, Thompson SG. Estimating a woman's risk of having a pregnancy with Down's syndrome using her age and serum alpha-fetoprotein level. Br J Obstet Gynaecol 1987;94:387–402.

10. Palomaki GE, Haddow JE. Maternal serum alpha-fetoprotein, age, and Down syndrome risk. Am J Obstet Gynecol 1987;156:460–463.

11. Boue A, Gallano P. A collaborative study of the segregation of inherited chromosome structural rearrangements in 1356 prenatal diagnoses. Prenat Diagn 1984;4:45–67.

12. Stene J. Statistical inference on segregation ratios for D/G translocations, when the families are ascertained in different ways. Ann Hum Genet 1970;34:93–115.

13. Stene J. A statistical segregation analysis of (21q22q)- translocations. Hum Hered 1970;20:465–472.

14. Carter C, Evans KA. Risk of parents who have had one child with Down's syndrome (mongolism) having another child similarly affected. Lancet 1961;ii:785–788.

15. Stene J. Detection of higher recurrence risk for age dependent chromosome abnormalities with application to G1 (Down syndrome). Hum Hered 1970;20:112–122.

16. Tabor A, Madsen M, Obel EB, et al. Randomized controlled trial of genetic amniocentesis in 4606 low-risk women. Lancet 1986;i:1287–1292.

17. The NICHD National Registry for Amniocentesis Study Group. Midtrimester amniocentesis for prenatal diagnosis: safety and accuracy. JAMA 1976;236:1471–1476.

18. Medical Research Council Working Party on Amniocentesis. An assessment of the hazard of amniocentesis. Br J Obstet Gynaecol 1978;85(Suppl 2):1–41.

19. Simpson N, Dallaire L, Miller JR, et al. Prenatal diagnosis of genetic disease in Canada: report of a collaborative study. Can Med Assoc J 1976;115:739–748.

20. Smidt-Jensen S, Permin M, Philip J, et al. Randomized comparison of amniocentesis and transabdominal and trans-cervical chorionic villus sampling. Lancet 1992;340:1237–1244.

21. Medical Research Council Working Party on the Evaluation of Chorion Villus Sampling. Medical Research Council European trial of chorion villus sampling. Lancet 1991;337:1491–1499.

22. Lippman A, Tomkins DJ, Shime J, et al. Canadian multicentre randomized clinical trial of chorion villus sampling and amniocentesis. Final report. Prenat Diagn 1992;12:385–476.

23. Hogge WA, Schonberg SA, Golbus MS. Chorionic villus sampling: experience of the first 1000 cases. Am J Obstet Gynecol 1986;154:1249–1252.

24. Brambati B, Oldrini A, Ferrazzi E, et al. Chorionic villus sampling: an analysis of the obstetric experience of 1000 cases. Prenat Diag 1987;7:157–169.

25. Jahoda M, Piijpers L, Reuss A, et al. Evaluation of transcervical chorionic villus sampling with a completed follow-up of 1550 consecutive pregnancies. Prenat Diagn 1989;9:621–628.

26. Leschot N, Wolf H, Van Prooijen-Knegt AC, et al. Cytogenetic findings in 1250 chorionic villus samples obtained in the first trimester with clinical follow-up of the first 1000 pregnancies. Clin Genet 1989;96:663–670.

27. Simoni G, Gimelli G, Cuoco C, et al. First trimester fetal karyotyping: one thousand diagnoses. Hum Genet 1986;72:203–209.

28. Green J, Dorfmann A, Jones SL, et al. Chorionic villus sampling: experience with an initial 940 cases. Obstet Gynecol 1988;71:208–212.

29. Rhoads GG, Jackson LG, Schlesselman SE, et al. The safety and efficacy of chorionic villus sampling for early prenatal diagnosis of cytogenetic abnormalities. N Engl J Med 1989;320:609–617.

30. Brambati B, Terzian E, Tognoni G. Randomized clinical trial of transabdominal versus transcervical chorionic villus sampling methods. Prenat Diagn 1991;11:285–293.

31. Jackson L, Zachary JM. A randomized comparison of transcervical and transabdominal chorionic villus sampling. N Engl J Med 1992;327:594–598.

32. Nicolaides K, Brizot MD, Patel F, et al. Comparison of chorionic villus sampling and amniocentesis for fetal karyotyping at 10–13 weeks' gestation. Lancet 1994;344:435–439.

33. DiMaio MS, Baumgarten A, Greenstein RM, et al. Screening for fetal Down's syndrome in pregnancy by measuring maternal serum alpha-fetoprotein levels. N Engl J Med 1987;317:342–346.

34. New England Regional Genetics Group. Combining maternal serum alpha fetoprotein measurements and age to screen for Down syndrome in pregnant women under age 35. Am J Obstet Gynecol 1989; 160:575–581.

35. Lustig L, Clarke S, Cunningham G, et al. California's experience with low MS-AFP results. Am J Med Genet 1988;31:211–222.

36. Muller F, Boue A. A single chorionic gonadotropin assay for maternal serum screening for Down's syndrome. Prenat Diagn 1990;10:389–398.

37. Wald NJ, Cuckle HS, Densem JW, et al. Maternal serum screening for Down's syndrome in early pregnancy [published erratum appears in BMJ 1988;297:1029]. BMJ 1988;297:883–887.

38. Reynolds TM. Software for screening to assess risk of Down's syndrome [letter]. BMJ 1991;302:6782.

39. Wald NJ, Kennard A, Densem JW, et al. Antenatal maternal serum screening for Down's syndrome: results of a demonstration project. BMJ 1992;305:391–394.

40. Phillips OP, Elias S, Shulman LP, et al. Maternal serum screening for fetal Down syndrome in women less than 35 years of age using alpha-fetoprotein, hCG, and unconjugated estriol: a prospective 2-year study. Obstet Gynecol 1992;80:353–358.

41. Macri JN, Spencer K, Garver K, et al. Maternal serum free beta hCG screening: results of studies including 480 cases of Down syndrome. Prenat Diagn 1994;14:97–103.

42. Mancini G, Perona M, Dall'Amico D, et al. Maternal serum markers. Estimation of the risk of Down's syndrome: a prospective study. Int J Clin Lab Res 1994;24:49–53.

43. Cheng EY, Luthy DA, Zebelman AM, et al. A prospective evaluation of a second-trimester screening test for fetal Down syndrome using maternal serum alpha-fetoprotein, hCG, and unconjugated estriol. Obstet Gynecol 1993;81:72–77.

44. Herrou M, Leporrier N, Leymarie P. Screening for fetal Down syndrome with maternal serum hCG and oestriol: a prospective study. Prenat Diagn 1992;12:887–892.

45. Spencer K, Carpenter P. Prospective study of prenatal screening for Down's syndrome with free β human chorionic gonadotrophin. BMJ 1993;307:764–769.

46. Mooney RA, Peterson CJ, French CA, et al. Effectiveness of combining maternal serum alpha-fetoprotein and hCG in a second-trimester screening program for Down syndrome. Obstet Gynecol 1994;84: 298–303.

47. Crossley JA, Aitken DA, Berry E, et al. Impact of a regional screening programme using maternal serum α fetoprotein (AFP) and human chorionic gonadotrophin (hCG) on the birth incidence of Down's syndrome in the west of Scotland. J Med Screening 1994;1:180–183.

48. Haddow JE, Palomaki GE, Knight GJ, et al. Prenatal screening for Down's syndrome with use of maternal serum markers [see comments]. N Engl J Med 1992;327:588–593.

49. Piggott M, Wilkinson, J Bennett, et al. Implementation of an antenatal serum screening programme for Down's syndrome in two districts (Brighton and Eastbourne). J Med Screening 1994;1:45–49.

50. Burton BK, Prins GS, Verp MS. A prospective trial of prenatal screening for Down syndrome by means of maternal serum α-fetoprotein, human chorionic gonadotropin, and unconjugated estriol. Am J Obstet Gynecol 1993;169 :526–530.

51. Haddow JE, Palomaki GE, Knight GJ, et al. Reducing the need for amniocentesis in women 35 years of age or older with serum markers for screening. N Engl J Med 1994;330:1114–1118.

52. Lockwood JC, Lynch L, Berkowitz RL. Ultrasonographic screening for Down syndrome fetus. Am J Obstet Gynecol 1991;165:349–352.

53. Benacerraf BR, Nadel A, Bromley B. Identification of second-trimester fetuses with autosomal trisomy by use of a sonographic scoring index. Radiology 1994;193:135–140.

54. Nyberg DA, Resta RG, Luthy DA, et al. Humerus and femur length shortening in the detection of Down's syndrome. Am J Obstet Gynecol 1993;168:534-538.

55. Crane JP, Gray DL. Sonographically measured nuchal skinfold thickness as a screening tool for Down syndrome: results of a prospective clinical trial. Obstet Gynecol 1991;77:533–536.

56. Lockwood C, Benacerraf B, Krinsky A, et al. A sonographic screening method for Down syndrome. Am J Obstet Gynecol 1987;157:803–808.

57. Benacerraf BR, Gelman R, Frigoletto FD. Sonographic identification of second-trimester fetuses with Down's syndrome. N Engl J Med 1987;317:1371–1376.

58. Toi A, Simpson GF, Filly RA. Ultrasonically evident fetal nuchal skin thickening: is it specific for Down syndrome? Am J Obstet Gynecol 1987;156:150–153.

59. Grandjean H, Sarramon M-F, and the AFDPHE Study Group. Sonographic measurement of nuchal skin-fold thickness for detection of Down syndrome in the second-trimester fetus: a multicenter prospective study. Obstet Gynecol 1995;85:103–106.

60. Elias S, Annas GJ. Routine prenatal genetic screening. N Engl J Med 1987;317:1407–1409.

61. Benacerraf BR, Barss VA, Laboda LA. A sonographic sign for the detection in the second trimester of the fetus with Down syndrome. Am J Obstet Gynecol 1985;151:1078–1079.

62. Reed BD, Ratcliffe S, Sayres W. Maternal serum alpha-fetoprotein screening. J Fam Pract 1988;27:20–23.

63. Marteau T, Kidd J, Cook R, et al. Perceived risk not actual risk predicts uptake of amniocentesis. Br J Obstet Gynaecol 1991;98:282–286.

64. Thornton J, Lilford RJ, Howell D. Safety of amniocentesis [letter]. Lancet 1986;ii:225–226.

65. Evans M, Bottoms SF, Critchfield GC, et al. Parental perceptions of genetic risk: correlation with choice of prenatal diagnostic procedures. Int J Gynaecol Obstet 1990;31:25–28.

66. Ekwo E, Kim J, Gosselink CA. Parental perceptions of the burden of genetic disease. Am J Med Genet 1987;28: 955–963.

67. Drugan A, Greb A, Johnson P, et al. Determinants of parental decisions to abort for chromosomal abnormalities. Prenat Diagn 1990;10:483–490.

68. Morris JK, Mutton DE, Ide R, et al. Monitoring trends in prenatal diagnosis of Down's syndrome in England and Wales, 1989–92. J Med Screening 1994;1:233–237.

69. Bell J, Hilden J, Bowling F, et al. The impact of prenatal diagnosis on the occurrence of chromosome abnormalities. Prenat Diagn 1986;6:1–11.

70. Cuckle H, Nanchahal K, Wald N. Birth prevalence of Down's syndrome in England and Wales. Prenat Diagn 1991;11:29–34.

71. Walker S, Howard PJ. Cytogenetic prenatal diagnosis and its relative effectiveness in the Mersey Region and North Wales. Prenat Diagn 1986;6:13–23.

72. Wilson N, Bickley D, McDermott A. The prevention of Down's syndrome in the southwestern region of England 1975–1985. West Engl Med J 1990;105:15–17.

73. Youings S, Gregson N, Jacobs P. The efficacy of maternal age screening for Down's syndrome in Wessex. Prenat Diagn 1991;11:419–425.

74. Ventura SJ, Martin JA, Taffel SM, et al. Advance report of final natality statistics, 1992. Monthly vital statistics report; vol 43 no 5 (suppl). Hyattsville, MD: National Center for Health Statistics, 1994.

75. Borgo G, Fabiano T, Perobelli S, et al. Effect of introducing prenatal diagnosis on the reproductive behavior of families at risk for cystic fibrosis: a cohort study. Prenat Diagn 1992;12:820–830.

76. Hook EB, Cross PK, Schreinemachers DM. Chromosomal abnormality rates at amniocentesis and in live-born infants. JAMA 1983;249:2034–2038.

77. Robinson A, Bender BG, Linden MG. Decisions following the intrauterine diagnosis of sex chromosome aneuploidy. Am J Med Genet 1989;34:552–554.

78. Holmes-Siedle M, Ryynanen M, Lindenbaum RH. Parental decisions regarding termination of pregnancy following prenatal detection of sex chromosome abnormality. Prenat Diagn 1987;7:239–244.

79. Barkai G, Goldman B, Ries L, et al. Expanding multiple marker screening for Down's syndrome to include Edward's syndrome. Prenat Diagn 1993;13:843–850.

80. Campbell TL. Maternal serum alpha-fetoprotein screening: benefits, risks, and costs. J Fam Pract 1987;25:461–467.

81. Cuckle HS, Wald NJ, Lindenbaum RH. Maternal serum alpha-fetoprotein measurement: a screening test for Down syndrome. Lancet 1984;1:926–929.

82. *Deleted in proof.*

83. Finegan J, Quarrington BJ, Hughes HE, et al. Child outcome following mid-trimester amniocentesis: development, behavior, and physical status at age 4 years. Br J Obstet Gynaecol 1990;97:32–40.

84. Nevin J, Nevin NC, Dornan JC, et al. Early amniocentesis: experience of 222 consecutive patients, 1987–1988. Prenat Diagn 1990;10:79–83.

85. Stripparo L, Buscaglia M, Longatti L, et al. Genetic amniocentesis: 505 cases performed before the sixteenth week of gestation. Prenat Diagn 1990;10:359–364.

86. Penso CA, Sandstrom MM, Garber MF, et al. Early amniocentesis: report of 407 cases with neonatal follow-up. Obstet Gynecol 1990;76:1032–1036.

87. Hanson FW, Tennant F, Hune S, et al. Early amniocentesis: outcome, risks, and technical problems at 12.8 weeks. Am J Obstet Gynecol 1992;166:1707–1711.

88. Firth H, Boyd PA, Chamberlain P, et al. Severe limb abnormalities after chorion villus sampling at 56–66 days' gestation. Lancet 1991;337:762–763.

89. Mastroiacovo P, Botto LD, Cavalcanti DP, et al. Limb anomalies following chorionic villus sampling: a registry based case-control study. Am J Med Genet 1992;44:856–864.

90. Burton BK, Schulz CJ, Burd LI. Limb anomalies associated with chorionic villus sampling. Obstet Gynecol 1992;79: 726–730.

91. Brambati B, Simoni G, Travi M, et al. Genetic diagnosis by chorionic villus sampling before 8 gestational weeks: efficiency, reliability, and risks on 317 completed pregnancies. Prenat Diagn 1992;12: 789–799.

92. Hsieh FJ, Shyu MK, Sheu BC, et al. Limb defects after chorionic villus sampling. Obstet Gynecol 1995; 85:84–88.

93. Firth HV, Boyd PA, Chamberlain PF, et al. Analysis of limb reduction defects in babies exposed to chorionic villus sampling. Lancet 1994;343:1069–1071.

93a. Olney RS, Khoury MJ, Alo CJ, et al. Increased risk for transverse digital deficiency after chorionic villus sampling: results of the United States Multistate Case-Control Study, 1988–1992. Teratology 1995; 51:20–29.

93b. Dolk H, Bertrand F, Lechat MJ, for the EUROCAT Working Group. Chorionic villus sampling and limb abnormalities [letter]. Lancet 1992;339:876–877.

94. Mahoney JM. Limb abnormalities and chorionic villus sampling [letter]. Lancet 1991;337:1422–1423.

95. Jackson LG, Wapner RJ, Brambati B. Limb abnormalities and chorionic villus sampling [letter]. Lancet 1991; 337:1423.

96. Monni G, Ibba RM, Lai R, et al. Limb-reduction defects and chorion villus sampling [letter]. Lancet 1991; 337:1091.

97. Froster-Iskenius UG, Baird PA. Limb-reduction defects in over one million consecutive livebirths. Teratology 1989;39:127–135.

98. Froster UG, Baird PA. Limb-reduction defects and chorionic villus sampling [letter]. Lancet 1992;339:66.

99. Blakemore K, Filkins K, Luthy DA, et al. Cook obstetrics and gynecology catheter multicenter chorionic villus sampling trial: comparison of birth defects with expected rates. Am J Obstet Gynecol 1993; 169:1022–1026.

99a. Centers for Disease Control and Prevention. Chorionic villus sampling and amniocentesis: recommendations for prenatal counseling. MMWR 1995;44(RR-9):1–12.

99b. Olney RS, Khoury MJ, Botto LD, et al. Limb defects and gestational age at chorionic villus sampling [letter]. Lancet 1994;344:476.

100. Tunis S, Golbus MS, Copeland KL, et al. Patterns of mood states in pregnant women undergoing chorionic villus sampling or amniocentesis. Am J Med Genet 1990;37:191–199.

101. Abuelo D, Hopmann MR, Barsel-Bowers G, et al. Anxiety in women with low maternal serum alpha-fetoprotein screening results. Prenat Diagn 1991;11:381–385.

102. Burton B, Dillard RG, Clark EN. The psychological impact of false positive elevations of maternal serum alpha fetoprotein. Am J Obstet Gynecol 1985;151:77–82.

103. Robinson JO, Hibbard BM, Laurence KM. Anxiety during a crisis: emotional effects of screening for neural tube defects. J Psychosom Res 1984;28:163–169.

104. Hakim-Elahi E, Tovell HMM, Burnhill MS. Complications of first-trimester abortion: a report of 170,000 cases. Obstet Gynecol 1990;76:129–135.

105. Lawson H, Atrash HK, Franks AL. Fatal pulmonary embolism during legal induced abortion in the United States from 1972 to 1985. Am J Obstet Gynecol 1990;162:986–990.

106. Osborn JF, Arisi E, Spinelli A, et al. General anaesthesia, a risk factor for complication following induced abortion? Eur J Epidemiol 1990;6:416–422.

107. Stray-Pedersen B, Biornstad J, Dahl M, et al. Induced abortion: microbiological screening and medical complications. Infection 1991;19:305–308.

108. Lawson HW, Frye A, Atrash HK, et al. Abortion mortality, United States, 1972 through 1987. Am J Obstet Gynecol 1994;171:1365–1372.

109. Council on Scientific Affairs, American Medical Association. Induced termination of pregnancy before and after Roe v Wade. Trends in the mortality and morbidity of women. JAMA 1992;268: 3231–3239.

110. Mishell DR Jr. Contraception, sterilization, and pregnancy termination. In: Herbst AL, Mishell DR Jr, Stenchezer MA, Droegemueller W, eds. Comprehensive gynecology. 2nd ed. St. Louis, MO: Mosby-Year Book, 1992:295–361.

111. Kochanek KD, Hudson BL. Advance report of final mortality statistics, 1992. Monthly vital statistics report; vol 43, no 6 (suppl). Hyattsville, MD: National Center for Health Statistics, 1995.

112. Centers for Disease Control and Prevention. Differences in maternal mortality among black and white women—United States, 1990. MMWR 1995;44:6–7,13–14.

113. American Academy of Pediatrics and American College of Obstetricians and Gynecologists. Guidelines for perinatal care. 3rd ed. Elk Grove Village, IL: American Academy of Pediatrics, 1992.

114. Canadian Task Force on the Periodic Health Examination. Canadian guide to clinical preventive health care. Ottawa: Canada Communication Group, 1994:84–98.

115. American College of Medical Genetics Clinical Practice Committee. ACMG position statement on multiple marker screening in women 35 and older. American College of Medical Genetics Newsletter, Jan 1994, vol. 2.

116. American College of Obstetricians and Gynecologists. Down syndrome screening. Committee Opinion no. 141. Washington, DC: American College of Obstetricians and Gynecologists, 1994.

117. American College of Obstetricians and Gynecologists. Ultrasonography in pregnancy. Technical Bulletin no. 187. Washington, DC: American College of Obstetricians and Gynecologists, 1993.

118. National Institutes of Health Consensus Development Conference. The use of diagnostic ultrasound imaging during pregnancy. JAMA 1984;252:669–672.

119. Thornton JG, Lilford RJ. Prenatal diagnosis of Down's syndrome: a method for measuring the consistency of women's decisions. Med Decis Making 1990;10:288–293.

120. Brock DJH. Screening for Down syndrome [letter]. Lancet 1987;2:1083–1084.

121. Hershey DW. Screening for Down's syndrome. N Engl J Med 1988;318:927–928.

122. Haslam R, Milner R. The physician and Down syndrome: are attitudes changing? J Child Neurol 1992; 7:304–310.

123. Inglese C. Is the cultural approach towards Down's syndrome people changing? Am J Med Genet 1990;7:322–323.

42. Screening for Neural Tube Defects—*Including Folic Acid/Folate Prophylaxis*

RECOMMENDATION

The offering of screening for neural tube defects by maternal serum α-fetoprotein (MSAFP) measurement is recommended for all pregnant women who are seen for prenatal care in locations that have adequate counseling and follow-up services available (*see* Clinical Intervention). Screening with MSAFP may be offered as part of multiple-marker screening (see Chapter 41). There is insufficient evidence to recommend for or against the offering of screening for neural tube defects by midtrimester ultrasound examination to all pregnant women, but recommendations against such screening may be made on other grounds (also see Chapter 36). Daily multivitamins with folic acid to reduce the risk of neural tube defects are recommended for all women who are planning or capable of pregnancy (see *Clinical Intervention*).

Burden of Suffering

Neural tube defects, including anencephaly, encephalocele, and spina bifida, account for substantial morbidity and mortality. Anencephaly is almost always lethal, usually resulting either in stillbirth or death within hours or days of birth. Spina bifida can range from mild (spina bifida occulta) to severe (myelomeningocele). The manifestations of severe spina bifida may include infectious complications, paraplegia, bladder and bowel incontinence, Arnold-Chiari malformations, hydrocephalus, and, as a complication of hydrocephalus, diminished intelligence.[1] Aggressive surgical and medical care is often necessary for severely affected cases, along with special schooling and rehabilitative services for patients with permanent disabilities. Based on 1988 cross-sectional data, the estimated lifetime cost of spina bifida is $258,000 per case.[2]

The birth prevalence of neural tube defects has declined substantially over the past 60 years.[3,4] Neural tube defects are reported in 3.6–4.6/ 10,000 live births in the United States.[3,5] These rates underestimate true incidence, however, because affected pregnancies may be spontaneously or electively aborted and because not all cases are detected and reported at birth. Popu-

467

lation-based active surveillance programs that include prenatal diagnoses have reported neural tube defect rates of 7.2–15.6/10,000 live-born and still-born infants.[6] A personal or family history of a pregnancy affected by a neural tube defect is associated with an increased risk of having an affected pregnancy, as is maternal insulin-dependent diabetes, but about 90–95% of cases occur in the absence of any positive history.[7–9] The birth prevalence of neural tube defects in the U.S. is higher at younger maternal ages and is more than one third higher for whites than blacks.[5]

Accuracy of Screening Tests

Tests for neural tube defects include ultrasound examination and measurement of maternal serum α-fetoprotein (MSAFP), amniotic fluid α-fetoprotein (AFAFP), and amniotic fluid acetylcholinesterase (AFAChE). The latter two are used primarily as confirmatory tests and should not be regarded as part of routine screening of women at low risk for neural tube defects. Ultrasound examination is used both as a screening test and as a follow-up test after positive MSAFP screening.

An elevated MSAFP measured at 16–18 weeks' gestation is a good predictor of neural tube defects. Depending on the cutoff used to define an elevated level (usually 2–2.5 times the median value for gestational age, reported as multiples of the median or MoM), screening can detect between 56% and 91% of affected fetuses.[10–17] An elevated MSAFP occurs in about 1–5% of pregnant women,[9,14,15,17–20] but for a number of reasons, the likelihood of a neural tube defect given a positive screening test result is small. First, about one third of positive tests are not confirmed by a second MSAFP measurement.[9,19] Second, although the reported specificity of MSAFP when followed by appropriate diagnostic tests (i.e., high-resolution ultrasonography, AFAFP, AFAChE) approaches 100%,[12,18,21] MSAFP assays themselves are relatively nonspecific. About 90–95% of cases with confirmed elevated MSAFP are caused by conditions other than neural tube defects, such as an underestimated gestational age, other congenital anomalies, intrauterine growth retardation, multiple gestations, or fetal demise.[7,9,10,18,20,22] An ultrasound examination is necessary to rule out these explanations for an elevated MSAFP. If ultrasonography does not provide an explanation for the abnormal result (as occurs in about 50%),[10,14,15,17] an amniocentesis should be offered to measure AFAFP and/or AFAChE levels.[8] Less than 10% of these lead to the discovery of a neural tube or abdominal wall defect; the majority of the fetuses tested are normal.[9] In comparison with the number of women who must be tested, the actual number of neural tube defects detected through screening the general population is small (0.06–0.16% of pregnancies).[9,10,18,19]

Virtually all cases of anencephaly can be detected by ultrasound alone,[24] as can many closed neural tube defects that may escape detection by MSAFP measurement. Current ultrasound techniques are less sensitive, however, in detecting other neural tube defects such as small meningomyeloceles.[11] In addition, although the published sensitivities and specificities of sonographic detection of spina bifida are high (79–96% and 90–100%, respectively),[24–28] investigators have emphasized that these data were obtained from centers with special expertise.[24] They may overestimate the sensitivity that would be expected when prenatal ultrasound is conducted with older equipment or is performed by those with less complete training,[28] which has become increasingly common as more physicians perform their own ultrasound examinations.[29] In addition, many of the published studies were of high-risk women and may not be generalizable to screening in the low-risk population. Nevertheless, recent improvements in ultrasound diagnosis of neural tube defects, with sensitivity and specificity approaching 100% when performed by expert sonographers at major screening centers, has caused some experts to recommend the use of ultrasound instead of MSAFP in pregnancies at low risk for neural tube defects.[30,31] Ultrasound and MSAFP have not been directly compared as screening tests for neural tube defects.

Effectiveness of Early Detection

The detection of neural tube defects in utero provides as its principal benefit the opportunity to inform prospective parents of the likelihood of carrying an affected fetus. Parents may be counseled about the consequences of the malformation and can make more informed decisions about optimal care for their newborn or about elective abortion. The antenatal diagnosis of a severe and/or lethal malformation (e.g., anencephaly) may spare parents some of the trauma associated with delivering such an infant. No controlled trials have been performed to prove that those screened for neural tube defects have better outcomes compared to those not screened, however. Therefore, the usefulness of this information depends to a large extent on the personal preferences and abilities of the parents.[32] Whether or not parents choose to use prenatal screening is related both to their views on the acceptability of induced abortion and their perceived risk of the fetus being abnormal.[33]

Induced abortion is sought by the majority of women who choose to be screened and whose screening tests reveal neural tube defects, thus leading to a decreased birth prevalence of affected infants among screened women.[10,14,15,34–37] Time series from the United Kingdom, where screening by MSAFP and ultrasound is widespread, have reported a 49–50% decline in the birth prevalence of anencephaly and a 32–38% decline in the birth prevalence of spina bifida attributable to elective abortion for suspected central nervous system malformation.[38,39] The effectiveness of screening in reducing the number of infants born with neural tube defects is decreased by less than universal acceptance of screening, incomplete detection of affected fetuses, and varying decisions about elective abortion following early detection.[35]

Several interventional cohort studies have evaluated the effect of MSAFP programs on the birth incidence of neural tube defects. In one such study, MSAFP screening was offered to all pregnant women attending antenatal clinics during the study period (n = 15,687), of whom 70% were actually screened.[35] Of 66 total neural tube defects, 54 occurred in the screened group (4.9/1,000) and 12 occurred in the unscreened population (2.5/1,000). The higher incidence rate in the screened group suggests that women who elected screening may have been at higher risk. Offering screening resulted in the elective abortion of 56% (37/66) of all pregnancies with neural tube defects. In the screened group, 11 (20%) were not detected by screening. Six (11%) were detected but were not aborted because ultrasonography or tests on amniotic fluid mistakenly indicated an unaffected pregnancy. Screening resulted in fewer infants being born with neural tube defects (1.6/1,000 in screened women vs. 2.5/1,000 in unscreened women). In another cohort study of more than 18,000 women, MSAFP screening was accepted in approximately 85% of second-trimester pregnancies and detected 80% of open neural tube defects, all of which were electively aborted.[34] Screening in this population reduced the birth prevalence of anencephaly by 90% and of open spina bifida by 72%. In a third study, screening was performed in 72% of clinic patients and detected 59% of all affected pregnancies, 94% of which were aborted.[36] Offering screening therefore prevented the births of 55% of affected fetuses.

There is limited evidence evaluating ultrasound screening for neural tube defects. One randomized controlled trial of routine ultrasound examination in low-risk women reported increased prenatal detection of fetal malformations, but no differences in induced abortion rates, survival rates of anomalous fetuses, or other perinatal outcomes.[28,40] Neural tube defects were included among the anomalies detected, but the study was not designed to evaluate this outcome specifically and only 13 such defects occurred in the entire enrolled population. Of eight neural tube defects occurring in the screened group, seven were detected by screening and electively aborted, reducing the birth prevalence by 88%, to 0.13/1,000 screened women. In controls, three of five neural tube defects were detected prenatally, two of which were aborted, reducing the birth prevalence to 0.39/1,000. The numbers of fetuses affected by neural tube defects were too small for valid statistical comparison. Interventional cohort studies evaluating routine ultrasound examination as a screening test for detection of neural tube defects have not been published, so there is inadequate information available on the acceptability and impact of ultrasound screening, confirmatory tests, and induced abortion in the general population.

Early detection of neural tube defects may also help parents to prepare emotionally, although this potential benefit has not been evaluated. It may enable clinicians to provide more intensive obstetric care and to better prepare for the delivery and care of the baby. Studies are limited, however, regarding the impact of these measures on neonatal morbidity and mortality. In a series of 208 patients aged 2–18 years with meningomyeloceles, there were no statistically significant differences in motor or sensory level, or in ambulatory function, between those delivered vaginally compared to those who had cesarean delivery.[41] On the other hand, in a retrospective population-based study of 160 fetuses with uncomplicated meningomyelocele, cesarean delivery before the onset of labor resulted in better motor function at age 2 years than vaginal delivery or cesarean delivery after a period of labor.[42] Follow-up to 4 years of age was available for 85% of the original cohort.[43] The pre-labor cesarean group continued to have a significantly greater difference between the anatomic and motor spinal cord level compared to the vaginally delivered group. Motor function was not significantly better at 4 years, however. These types of studies have important design limitations. Controlled trials evaluating early cesarean delivery for neural tube defects have not yet been published.

Another potential benefit of MSAFP screening for neural tube defects is the discovery during testing of abnormalities other than the target condition. A raised level of MSAFP, even in the absence of a congenital defect, is a risk factor for low birth weight, preterm labor, preeclampsia, and abruptio placentae;[20,44,45] early obstetric intervention for these problems may be beneficial (see also Chapter 37). Reduced levels of MSAFP are associated with Down syndrome and certain other chromosomal anomalies; MSAFP is one component of multiple-marker screening, which is recommended for the early detection of Down syndrome (see Chapter 41). The ultrasound evaluation that follows the detection of raised MSAFP may lead to a diagnosis of twins or a more accurate assessment of gestational age, and some studies suggest that acting on this information may improve neonatal outcome (see Chapter 36). Other congenital anomalies, such as diaphragmatic hernia, gastroschisis, nonimmune fetal hydrops, and obstructive uropathy, may also be detected. Discovery of a fetus affected by one of these anomalies may be useful for parental decision making, allowing the options of elective abortion or of antenatal treatment if available, planning for delivery and appropriate neonatal care. Controlled trials have not proven that early detection of these anomalies improves outcome, however. Indeed, studies suggest that fetuses with diaphragmatic hernias detected in utero have poorer outcomes than those detected after birth,[46,47] perhaps in part because larger defects are more likely to be detected prenatally.

The potential benefits of early detection of neural tube defects must be weighed against the potential risks of screening. The most important risks include those to the fetus from amniocentesis, the psychological effects on the parents of a positive test, the complications resulting from induced abortion, and the risk of elective abortion of normal pregnancies due to false-positive test results. The risks of amniocentesis include miscarriage, puncture of the fetus, bleeding, infection, and possibly isosensitization.[9] The exact rate of fetal loss due to amniocentesis is uncertain, since women undergoing this procedure are already at increased risk of fetal loss. The procedure-related rate of fetal loss with current technique appears to be about 0.5–0.8%.[48–50] The best evidence on amniocentesis risks comes from a randomized controlled trial of screening,[48] which reported a procedure-related risk of fetal loss of 0.8% of pregnancies. This may nevertheless overestimate current rates of loss as techniques have improved. In a more recent series of patients undergoing amniocentesis as part of a clinical trial, the risk of fetal loss was 0.04%.[51] In a randomized controlled trial, neonatal respiratory distress syndrome and neonatal pneumonia were more frequent after amniocentesis, independent of birth weight and gestational age; the additional risk was about 1%.[48] A similar trend was seen in the Medical Research Council study,[52] but has not been confirmed in other studies. Infection has not been identified as a significant problem in any large studies. No clinically important effects on development, behavior, or physical status were identified in 4-year-old children whose mothers had undergone midtrimester amniocentesis.[53] Although MSAFP screening will increase the number of women undergoing amniocentesis, in cohort studies of screening programs fewer than 2% of MSAFP-screened women received amniocentesis.[10,14,15,17]

Another risk of screening is the harmful psychological effect on parents of a positive test result. This is especially important because the large majority of positive screening tests in low-risk pregnancies are false positives. There is evidence that expectant parents with normal fetuses who are informed of an abnormal MSAFP test suffer substantial anxiety during the weeks of diagnostic testing and waiting for definitive results.[54–57] The anxiety level of these women at delivery was the same as that of women who had normal screening test results, however. No published controlled trials have evaluated whether counseling and education prior to screening alleviates these psychological effects. Elective abortion of pregnancy because of a fetal anomaly may also have important psychological effects. In one small case-control study,[58] women who aborted fetuses with major malformations (including neural tube defects) experienced grief similar to those experiencing spontaneous perinatal loss, but no comparison was made to women delivering an infant with a severe anomaly, who may also grieve for the loss of a normal infant. Most women screened will have normal results, and this may have psychological benefits for the reassured parents.

The potential complications of induced abortion must also be considered, since this is the outcome of the majority of positive diagnostic test results. The maternal case-fatality rate from legal induced abortion is 0.4/100,000 procedures, which is substantially lower than the eight to nine maternal deaths per 100,000 live births due to pregnancy and childbirth.[59–62] Rates of other major maternal complications are also lower than in pregnancy and childbirth, occurring in an estimated 0.1% of legal abortions.[62] All maternal complication rates are higher with second-trimester than with first-trimester abortions.

The most serious consequence of false-positive results, the induced abortion of a normal pregnancy on the basis of erroneous diagnostic test results, appears to be very uncommon with current diagnostic techniques (i.e., high-resolution ultrasound, AFAFP, and AFAChE). Investigators have reported false-positive results leading to elective abortion of normal fetuses in 0.006–0.07% of women screened.[10,17,18,34,38,63,64]

Primary Prevention (Folic Acid/Folate Prophylaxis)

Randomized placebo-controlled trials[65,66] and nonrandomized controlled trials[67–69] in pregnant women with a prior pregnancy affected by a neural tube defect have demonstrated that folic acid supplements substantially reduce the risk of recurrent neural tube defects. In the international, multicenter British Medical Research Council (MRC) trial, involving nearly 1,200 high-risk women, 4 mg of folic acid daily at least 1 month before conception through the first trimester reduced the risk of recurrence of neural tube defects from 3.5% to 1.0%, for a relative risk of 0.28 (95% confidence interval, 0.12 to 0.71). The MRC and two other trials tested folic acid doses of 4–5 mg/day, but the 86% risk reduction seen in one nonrandomized trial[67] that used 0.36 mg of folic acid plus multivitamins daily suggests that lower doses may also be effective.

Several case-control studies have reported a reduced risk of neural tube defects in women without a prior affected pregnancy who took daily multivitamins during the periconceptional period (from 1–3 months before conception to 0.5–3 months after conception).[70–72] One of these analyzed the amount of folic acid the multivitamins contained, which was ≥0.4 mg for most women.[71] A similar study, on the other hand, reported no protective effect of either folic acid alone or multivitamins with folic acid.[73] Stronger evidence for a benefit of periconceptional multivitamins with folic acid in low-risk pregnant women comes from a cohort study of 22,715 women.[74] The risk of neural tube defects was significantly reduced, from

3.3/1,000 to 0.9/1,000 women, with daily intake of multivitamins containing 0.1–1.0 mg of folic acid during the first 6 weeks of pregnancy. In an unadjusted analysis, taking multivitamins with folic acid both in the 3 months before conception and in the first trimester was also protective against neural tube defects. In a random sample of the multivitamin users, about two thirds consumed multivitamins containing a daily dose of at least 0.4 mg of folic acid and 95% consumed at least 0.1 mg of folic acid daily. A randomized double-blind controlled trial of the efficacy of daily periconceptional multivitamin-multimineral supplements containing 0.8 mg of folic acid in preventing first occurrences of neural tube defects was conducted in Hungary, enrolling 4,753 women planning pregnancy.[75,76] Full supplementation was defined as taking them from 28 days before conception to at least the second missed menstrual period. The average daily consumption of dietary folate was 0.18 mg, which is similar to the estimated average intake of 0.2 mg/day by women aged 19 to 34 years in the United States.[77] The supplemented group experienced a significantly decreased prevalence of neural tube defects (0 of 2,104 vs. 6 of 2,052), congenital malformations as a whole (13.3 compared to 22.9/1,000), and major congenital abnormalities other than neural tube defects and genetic syndromes diagnosed by 8 months of age (14.7 vs. 28.3/1,000). Three observational studies provide limited evidence for the effectiveness of dietary folate at levels higher than 0.1–0.25 mg/day in preventing the occurrence of neural tube defects.[70,71,74] All three studies reported a protective effect of greater dietary folate intake, although not all results were statistically significant or adequately reported.

Research on adverse effects from folic acid supplementation is limited. Evidence that folic acid supplements in daily doses of 1–5 mg can mask the hematologic manifestations of vitamin B_{12} deficiency, possibly delaying its diagnosis and treatment thereby leading to permanent neurologic consequences, is limited to uncontrolled intervention studies[78–80] and case reports.[81–83] Hematologic improvement in pernicious anemia has also been reported in some patients taking folic acid doses <1 mg, but the response is not consistent, particularly at lower doses.[79,84–86] Nevertheless, this has been advanced as one reason to avoid universal supplementation or food fortification with folic acid. It has also been argued, however, that it is unreasonable to maintain anemia to make it easier to diagnose B_{12} deficiency while some neural tube defects occur that are potentially avoidable by supplementation.[87] Limited evidence supports independent associations of low-normal folate and B_{12} levels, and high homocysteine levels, with neural tube defects,[88,89] suggesting that a causal mechanism for these defects may be an abnormality in methionine synthase, a folate- and B_{12}-dependent enzyme. If these results are confirmed, supplementation with both folic acid and B_{12} may be appropriate to prevent neural tube defects. This could reduce the potential for adverse effects of folate supplementation in B_{12}-deficient patients.

Folic acid supplementation may also reduce intestinal absorption of zinc.[90] A randomized trial in which 50 women received either 10 mg folic acid or placebo daily showed no effect on plasma zinc concentrations after 2 and 4 months, however.[91] One cross-sectional study found a significant correlation between pregnancy complications and high folate and low zinc concentrations in the plasma of 450 pregnant women,[92] but confirmation is needed. Patients under therapy with medications that interfere with folic acid metabolism (e.g., treatments for cancer, asthma, arthritis, AIDS, and psoriasis) may be adversely affected by folic acid supplementation, but this risk has not been adequately assessed.[93] Folic acid supplementation might theoretically provoke convulsions in epileptic women by interfering with the activity of certain anticonvulsants; this potential risk has not been well studied.

None of the trials of healthy pregnant women reported serious adverse effects associated with folic acid supplementation. In the Hungarian trial,[94] infants born to women who received a multivitamin-multimineral supplement with folic acid did not differ from those born to women receiving only trace elements in mortality, somatic development, mental and behavioral development, or total serious or chronic disorders, at 8–21 months (mean 11 months) of age. The rate of atopic dermatitis, asthma, and wheezy bronchitis was significantly increased in the group whose mothers received multivitamins (16 vs. 5/1,000), but more affected infants in the supplemented group also had a positive family history for these disorders. This difference may also be a chance effect due to the large number of comparisons made. A series of 91 children born to women who had taken daily multivitamins containing 0.36 mg of folic acid to prevent neural tube defect recurrences revealed no adverse effects on health, auditory, visual, growth, or developmental status at age 7–10 years, compared with the general population.[95] The study found significant increases in neurotic traits, but whether this was attributable to folic acid or to other causes (e.g., increased parental anxiety related to having had a previously affected pregnancy) is unknown.

Recommendations of Other Groups

The American College of Obstetricians and Gynecologists (ACOG),[8] the American Society of Human Genetics,[96,97] the American Academy of Pediatrics (AAP),[98] the Canadian Task Force on the Periodic Health Examination,[99] and an international expert consensus conference[11] have recommended that MSAFP screening be offered to all pregnant women at

16–18 weeks' gestation, provided that it is accompanied by adequate counseling and follow-up and is performed in areas with qualified diagnostic centers (conventional and high-resolution ultrasound, amniocentesis) and high-quality standardized laboratories. The Canadian Task Force also recommends that high-resolution ultrasonography may be adequate for low-risk women.[99] The AAP and ACOG recommend that patients with a personal or family history of neural tube defects be offered amniocentesis at 15–16 weeks' gestation with AFAFP testing.[100] The recommendations of the American Academy of Family Physicians (AAFP) on screening for neural tube defects are currently under review.

The AAP,[101] Canadian Task Force,[99] and U.S. Public Health Service (USPHS)[102] recommend that all women of childbearing age who are capable of becoming pregnant take 0.4 mg of folic acid daily to reduce the risk of having a pregnancy affected with a neural tube defect. The AAP,[101] Canadian Task Force,[99] ACOG,[103] and the USPHS[104] recommend that patients who have had a previous pregnancy affected by a neural tube defect and who are planning to become pregnant should be offered treatment with 4 mg of folic acid daily starting 1–3 months prior to planned conception and continuing through the first 3 months of pregnancy. The recommendations of the AAFP on folate supplementation for the prevention of neural tube defects are currently under review.

Discussion

MSAFP is a sensitive screening test for neural tube defects. When positive results are followed by appropriate diagnostic tests, such as high-resolution ultrasound, AFAFP and AFAChE, MSAFP is highly specific as well. Early detection leads to a reduced birth prevalence of severely affected fetuses and may reduce complications due to labor and delivery in affected infants. It can also detect several other conditions, for some of which effective interventions exist. While MSAFP screening is a relatively safe procedure, neural tube defects are relatively uncommon, and in certain low-prevalence populations it is possible for the complication rate from screening and its follow-up diagnostic tests to equal or exceed the detection rate for the target condition. Some have expressed concern that the relatively small number of neural tube defects detected through screening may not justify the potential risks of amniocentesis and parental anxiety for the large majority of normal fetuses.[32] The increased risk may, nevertheless, be acceptable to parents with strong fears of having an abnormal child.[105] Whether or not to receive MSAFP screening therefore depends on the preferences of the individual patient, who must receive adequate counseling regarding potential risks and benefits of screening before being screened in order to make an informed decision. Ultrasonography performed by expert sonographers at major screening centers also appears to be a sensitive and specific screening tool, but these findings may not be generalizable to sonographers in other settings. Ultrasound has not yet been adequately evaluated as a routine screening test for neural tube defects.

Identification and abortion of pregnancies affected by neural tube defects raises important ethical concerns, a full discussion of which is beyond the scope of this chapter. These concerns include the implicit message that having a neural tube defect is an undesirable state, the interpretation of induced abortion in eugenic terms by some persons, and societal and economic pressures that may stigmatize families with a member who has a neural tube defect. These issues highlight the importance of offering screening and prenatal diagnosis of neural tube defects in a value-sensitive fashion with emphasis on reliable information about the defects themselves as well as about the potential risks and benefits of screening and diagnostic procedures.

For a woman who has had a previous pregnancy affected by a neural tube defect, there is good evidence that folic acid supplementation begun at least 1 month prior to conception and continued through the first trimester decreases the risk of recurrence. The only dosage adequately studied is a daily supplement of 4 mg, although some evidence suggests that lower dosages may be effective. For low-risk women who are planning pregnancy, a randomized controlled trial and several observational studies indicate that periconceptional intake of multivitamin-multimineral or multivitamin preparations containing 0.4–0.8 mg of folic acid can significantly reduce the risk of first occurrence of neural tube defects. All of these studies indicate the need to start supplementation at least 1 month before conception and to continue daily supplements through the first 2 to 3 months of pregnancy. There is limited evidence that dietary folate intake of greater than 0.1–0.3 mg/day reduces the risk of neural tube defects. No studies have directly compared the effectiveness of multivitamins with folic acid to increased dietary folate intake for the primary prevention of neural tube defects, but the evidence supporting use of multivitamins with folic acid is of higher quality. The current estimated average daily consumption of only 0.2 mg of dietary folate by American women aged 19–34 years[77] suggests that achieving adequate dietary intake may be more difficult for some women than taking supplements. It is unknown whether women who already have a diet that meets or exceeds 0.4 mg/day of folate would gain additional benefit from vitamin supplements. The effort required to assess dietary folate intake adequately may outweigh the costs and potential harms from routine supplementation.

Since half of pregnancies in the U.S. are unplanned,[106] all women capable of becoming pregnant would need to take multivitamins with folic acid (or increase their dietary folate intake) to maximize prevention of neural tube defects. It is likely that in the observational studies evaluating the association between multivitamins with folic acid and reduced risk of neural tube defects, many of the women evaluated had unplanned pregnancies, providing indirect evidence in support of this intervention. The ability of clinicians to convince women not contemplating pregnancy that they should take multivitamins with folic acid in order to prevent neural tube defects is unknown. Many women of childbearing age who are not planning pregnancy may not take supplements or pursue diets adequate in folate, particularly those who are poorer and less educated. Some authorities suggest that food fortification with folate has greater potential to reach the entire population at risk.[101-111]

The results of controlled trials indicate that folic acid supplementation will not prevent all neural tube defects. The Centers for Disease Control and Prevention estimates that low-dose folic acid supplementation of all women capable of pregnancy would reduce the incidence of neural tube defects in the U.S. by 50%.[102] Therefore, the use of periconceptional folic acid supplements does not preclude offering screening for neural tube defects, although the cost-effectiveness of such screening is likely to be reduced given a lower risk of occurrence.

CLINICAL INTERVENTION

The offering of screening for neural tube defects by maternal serum α-fetoprotein (MSAFP) measurement at 16–18 weeks' gestation is recommended for all pregnant women who are seen for prenatal care in locations that have adequate counseling and follow-up services, skilled high-resolution ultrasound and amniocentesis capabilities, and reliable, standardized laboratories ("B" recommendation). Women with elevated MSAFP levels should receive a second confirmatory test when time allows (i.e., before 18 weeks of gestation), and high-resolution ultrasound examination by an adequately trained and experienced examiner before amniocentesis is performed. Screening with MSAFP may be offered as part of multiple-marker screening (see Chapter 41). There is currently insufficient evidence to recommend for or against the offering of screening for neural tube defects by routine midtrimester ultrasound examination in pregnant women ("C" recommendation). Recommendations may be made against such screening, except when conducted by expert sonographers at major screening centers, based on its unproven accuracy in other settings, the availability and proven effectiveness of MSAFP screening, and cost. See Chapter 36 for additional recommendations regarding routine ultrasound examination in pregnancy. Pregnant women at high risk of neural tube defects (e.g., those with a previous affected pregnancy) should be referred to specialized centers for appropriate diagnostic evaluation, including high-resolution ultrasound and amniocentesis.

Folic acid supplementation at a dose of 4 mg/day beginning 1–3 months prior to conception and continuing through the first trimester is recommended for women planning pregnancy who have previously had a pregnancy affected by a neural tube defect, to reduce the risk of recurrence ("A" recommendation). It is also recommended that all women planning pregnancy take a daily multivitamin or multivitamin-multimineral supplement containing folic acid at a dose of 0.4–0.8 mg, beginning at least 1 month prior to conception and continuing through the first trimester, to reduce the risk of neural tube defects ("A" recommendation). Taking a daily multivitamin containing 0.4 mg of folic acid is also recommended for all women capable of becoming pregnant, to reduce the risk of neural tube defects in unplanned pregnancies ("B" recommendation). Women taking drugs that interfere with folate metabolism (e.g., methotrexate, pyrimethamine, trimethoprim, phenytoin), women at increased risk of vitamin B_{12} deficiency (e.g., vegans or persons with AIDS), and those with epilepsy whose seizures are controlled by anticonvulsant therapy, should consult with their clinician regarding potential risks and benefits prior to considering folic acid supplementation. There is currently insufficient evidence to recommend for or against counseling women planning or capable of pregnancy to increase their dietary folate consumption to 0.4 mg/day as an alternative to taking multivitamins with folic acid ("C" recommendation). Offering counseling to increase dietary folate intake to women who do not wish to take folic acid supplements may be recommended on other grounds, including low risk, low cost, and likely benefit.

The use of periconceptional multivitamins with folic acid does not necessarily obviate the need to offer screening for neural tube defects during pregnancy, since not all defects will be prevented by prophylaxis.

The draft update of this chapter was prepared for the U.S. Preventive Services Task Force by Carolyn DiGuiseppi, MD, MPH, based in part on background material prepared by Marie-Dominique Beaulieu, MD, MSc, and Brenda Beagan, MA, for the Canadian Task Force on the Periodic Health Examination.

REFERENCES

1. Hoffman HJ. Spinal dysraphism. Am Fam Physician 1987;36:129–136.
2. Waitzman NJ, Romano PS, Scheffler RM. Estimates of the economic costs of birth defects. Inquiry 1994; 31:188–205.
3. Flood T, Brewster M, Harris J, et al. Spina bifida incidence at birth—United States, 1983–1990. MMWR 1992;41: 497–500.
4. Windham GC, Edmonds LD. Current trends in the incidence of neural tube defects. Pediatrics 1982;70:333–337.
5. Ventura SJ, Martin JA, Taffel SM, et al. Advance report of final natality statistics, 1992. Monthly vital statistics report; vol 43, no 5 (suppl). Hyattsville, MD: National Center for Health Statistics, 1994.
6. Cragan JD, Roberts HE, Edmonds LD, et al. Surveillance for anencephaly and spina bifida and the impact of prenatal diagnosis—United States, 1985–1994. MMWR 1995;44(SS-4):1–13.
7. Macri JN. Critical issues in prenatal maternal serum alpha-fetoprotein screening for genetic anomalies. Am J Obstet Gynecol 1986;155:240–246.

8. American College of Obstetricians and Gynecologists. Alpha-fetoprotein. Technical Bulletin no. 154. Washington, DC: American College of Obstetricians and Gynecologists, 1991.

9. Campbell TL. Maternal serum alpha-fetoprotein screening: benefits, risks, and costs. J Fam Pract 1987;25:461–467.

10. Milunsky A, Alpert E. Results and benefits of a maternal serum alpha-fetoprotein screening program. JAMA 1984;252:1438–1442.

11. Maternal serum alpha-fetoprotein screening for neural tube defects: results of a consensus meeting. Prenat Diagn 1985;5:77–83.

12. Wald NJ, Cuckle H, Brock JH, et al. Maternal serum alpha-fetoprotein measurement in antenatal screening for anencephaly and spina bifida in early pregnancy. Report of U.K. collaborative study on alpha-fetoprotein in relation to neural tube defects. Lancet 1977;1:1323-1332.

13. Haddow JE, Kloza EM, Smith DE, et al. Data from an alpha-fetoprotein pilot screening program in Maine. Obstet Gynecol 1983;62:556–560.

14. Macri JN, Weiss RR. Prenatal serum alpha-fetoprotein screening for neural tube defects. Obstet Gynecol 1982;59: 633–639.

15. Burton BK, Sowers SG, Nelson LH. Maternal serum alpha-fetoprotein screening in North Carolina: experience with more than twelve thousand pregnancies. Am J Obstet Gynecol 1983;146:439–444.

16. Brock DJH, Barron L, Watt M, et al. Maternal plasma alpha-fetoprotein and low birthweight: a prospective study throughout pregnancy. Br J Obstet Gynaecol 1982;89:348–351.

17. Crandall BF, Robertson RD, Lebherz TB, et al. Maternal serum α-fetoprotein screening for the detection of neural tube defects. West J Med 1983;138:524–530.

18. Hooker JG, Lucas M, Richards BA, et al. Is maternal alpha-fetoprotein screening still of value in a low-risk area for neural tube defects? Prenat Diagn 1984;4:29–33.

19. Simpson JL, Baum LD, Marder R, et al. Maternal serum alpha-fetoprotein screening: low and high values for detection of genetic abnormalities. Am J Obstet Gynecol 1986;155:593–597.

20. Roop AP, Goughman JA, Blitzer MG. Study of the relationship between elevated maternal serum alpha-fetoprotein and adverse pregnancy outcome. Maryland Med J 1991;40:779–784.

21. Wald N, Cuckle H, Nanchahal K. Amniotic fluid acetylcholinesterase measurement in the prenatal diagnosis of neural tube defects. Second report of the Collaborative Acetylcholinesterase Study. Prenat Diagn 1989;9:813–829.

22. Daker M, Bobrow M. Screening for genetic disease and fetal anomaly during pregnancy. In: Chalmers I, Enkin M, Keirse MJNC, eds. Effective care in pregnancy and childbirth. Vol. 1: pregnancy. Oxford: Oxford University Press, 1989:366–381.

23. *Deleted in proof.*

24. Roberts CJ, Evans KT, Hibbard BM, et al. Diagnostic effectiveness of ultrasound in detection of neural tube defect: the South Wales experience of 2,509 scans (1977–1982) in high-risk mothers. Lancet 1983;2:1068–1069.

25. Tyrrell S, Howel D, Bark M, et al. Should maternal alpha-fetoprotein estimation be carried out in centers where ultrasound screening is routine? A sensitivity analysis approach. Am J Obstet Gynecol 1988;158:1092–1099.

26. Sabbagha RE, Sheikh Z, Tamura RK, et al. Predictive value, sensitivity, and specificity of ultrasonic targeted imaging for fetal anomalies in gravid women at high risk for birth defects. Am J Obstet Gynecol 1985;152:822–827.

27. Robinson HP, Hood VD, Adam AH, et al. Diagnostic ultrasound: early detection of fetal neural tube defects. Obstet Gynecol 1980;56:705–710.

28. Crane JP, LeFevre ML, Winborn RC, et al. A randomized trial of prenatal ultrasonographic screening: impact on the detection, management and outcome of anomalous fetuses. The RADIUS Study Group. Am J Obstet Gynecol 1994;171:392–399.

29. Sack RA, Maharry JM. Misdiagnoses in obstetric and gynecologic ultrasound examinations: causes and possible solutions. Am J Obstet Gynecol 1988;158:1260–1266.

30. Watson WJ, Chescheir NC, Katz VL, et al. The roles of ultrasound in evaluation of patients with elevated maternal serum alpha-fetoprotein: a review. Obstet Gynecol 1991;78:123–128.

31. Nadel AS, Green JK, Holmes LB, et al. Absence of need for amniocentesis in patients with elevated levels of maternal serum alpha-fetoprotein and normal ultrasonographic examinations. N Engl J Med 1990;323:557–561.

32. Reed BD, Ratcliffe S, Sayres W. Maternal serum alpha-fetoprotein screening. J Fam Pract 1988;27:20–23.

33. Marteau T, Kidd J, Cook R, et al. Perceived risk not actual risk predicts uptake of amniocentesis. Br J Obstet Gynaecol 1991;98:282–286.

34. Thom H, Campbell AGM, Farr V, et al. The impact of maternal serum alpha fetoprotein screening on open neural tube defect births in northeast Scotland. Prenat Diagn 1985;5:15–19.

35. Roberts CJ, Hibbard BM, Elder GH, et al. The efficacy of a serum screening service for neural-tube defects: the South Wales experience. Lancet 1983;1:1315–1318.

36. Wald NJ, Cuckle HS, Boreham J, et al. Antenatal screening in Oxford for fetal neural tube defects. Br J Obstet Gynaecol 1979;86:91–100.

37. EUROCAT Working Group. Prevalence of neural tube defects in 20 regions of Europe and the impact of prenatal diagnosis, 1980–1986. J Epidemiol Community Health 1991;45:52–58.

38. Cuckle HS, Wald NJ, Cuckle PM. Prenatal screening and diagnosis of neural tube defects in England and Wales in 1985. Prenat Diagn 1989;9:393–400.

39. Stone DH, Smalls MJ, Rosenberg K, et al. Screening for congenital neural tube defects in a high-risk area: an epidemiological perspective. J Epidemiol Community Health 1988;42:271–273.

40. Ewigman BG, Crane JP, Frigoletto FD, et al. Effect of prenatal ultrasound screening on perinatal outcome. N Engl J Med 1993;329:821–827.

41. Cochrane D, Aronyk K, Sawatzky B, et al. The effects of labor and delivery on spinal cord function and ambulation in patients with meningomyelocele. Child Nerv Syst 1991;7:312–315.

42. Luthy DA, Wardinsky T, Shurtleff DB, et al. Cesarean section before the onset of labor and subsequent motor function in infants with meningomyelocele diagnosed antenatally. N Engl J Med 1991;324: 662–666.

43. Shurtleff DB, Luthy DA, Nyberg DA, et al. Meningomyelocele: management in utero and postnatum. Ciba Found Symp 1994;181:270–280.

44. Robinson L, Grau P, Crandall BF. Pregnancy outcomes after increasing maternal serum alpha-fetoprotein levels. Obstet Gynecol 1989;74:17–20.

45. Williams MA, Hickok DE, Zingheim RW, et al. Elevated maternal serum alpha-fetoprotein levels and midtrimester placental abnormalities in relation to subsequent adverse pregnancy outcomes. Am J Obstet Gynecol 1992;167: 1032–1037.

46. Benacerraf BR, Adzick NS. Fetal diaphragmatic hernia: ultrasound diagnosis and clinical outcome in 19 cases. Am J Obstet Gynecol 1987;156:573–576.

47. Adzick NS, Harrison MR, Glick PL, et al. Diaphragmatic hernia in the fetus: prenatal diagnosis and outcome in 94 cases. J Pediatr Surg 1985;20:357–361.

48. Tabor A, Madsen M, Obel EB, et al. Randomized controlled trial of genetic amniocentesis in 6406 low-risk women. Lancet 1986;1:1287–1293.

49. The NICHD National Registry for Amniocentesis Study Group. Midtrimester amniocentesis for prenatal diagnosis: safety and accuracy. JAMA 1976;236:1471–1476.

50. Rhoads GG, Jackson LG, Schlesselman SE, et al. The safety and efficacy of chorionic villus sampling for early prenatal diagnosis of cytogenetic abnormalities. N Engl J Med 1989;320:609–617.

51. Lippman A, Tomkins DJ, Shime J, et al. Canadian multicentre randomized clinical trial of chorion villus sampling and amniocentesis. Final report. Prenat Diagn 1992;12:385–476.

52. Medical Research Council Working Party on Amniocentesis. An assessment of the hazard of amniocentesis. Br J Obstet Gynaecol 1978;85(Suppl 2):1–41.

53. Finegan J, Quarrington BJ, Hughes HE, et al. Child outcome following mid-trimester amniocentesis: development, behavior and physical status at age 4 years. Br J Obstet Gynaecol 1990;97:32–40.

54. Robinson JO, Hibbard BM, Laurence KM. Anxiety during a crisis: emotional effects of screening for neural tube defects. J Psychosom Res 1984;28:163–169.

55. Burton BK, Dillard RG, Clark EN. The psychological impact of false positive elevations of maternal serum alpha-fetoprotein. Am J Obstet Gynecol 1985;151:77–82.

56. Burton BK, Dillard RG, Clark EN. Maternal serum α-fetoprotein screening: the effect of participation on anxiety and attitude toward pregnancy in women with normal results. Am J Obstet Gynecol 1985; 152:540–543.

57. Frean J, Hibbard BM, Laurence KM, et al. Screening for neural tube defects and maternal anxiety. Br J Obstet Gynaecol 1982;89:218–222.

58. Zeanah CH, Dailey JV, Rosenblatt M-J, et al. Do women grieve after terminating pregnancies because of fetal anomalies? A controlled investigation. Obstet Gynecol 1993;82:270–275.

59. Lawson HW, Frye A, Atrash HK, et al. Abortion mortality, United States, 1972 through 1987. Am J Obstet Gynecol 1994;171:1365–1372.

60. Kochanek KD, Hudson BL. Advance report of final mortality statistics, 1992. Monthly vital statistics report; vol 43, no 6 (suppl). Hyattsville, MD: National Center for Health Statistics, 1995.

61. Centers for Disease Control and Prevention. Differences in maternal mortality among black and white women—United States, 1990. MMWR 1995;44:6–7, 13–14.

62. Council on Scientific Affairs, American Medical Association. Induced termination of pregnancy before and after Roe v Wade. Trends in the mortality and morbidity of women. JAMA 1992;268: 3231–3239.

63. Fuhrmann W, Weitzel HK. Maternal serum alpha-fetoprotein screening for neural tube defects. Hum Genet 1985;69:47–61.

64. Allen LC, Doran TA, Miskin M, et al. Ultrasound and amniotic fluid alpha-fetoprotein in the prenatal diagnosis of spina bifida. Obstet Gynecol 1982;60:169–173.

65. Laurence KM, James N, Miller M, et al. Double blind randomized controlled trial of folate treatment before conception to prevent recurrence of neural-tube defects. BMJ 1981;282:1509–1511.

66. MRC Vitamin Study Research Group. Prevention of neural tube defects: results of the Medical Research Council Vitamin Study. Lancet 1991;338:313–137.

67. Smithells RW, Seller MJ, Harris R, et al. Further experience of vitamin supplementation for prevention of neural tube defect recurrences. Lancet 1983;1:1027–1031.

68. Vergel RG, Sanchez LR, Heredero BL, et al. Primary prevention of neural tube defects with folic acid supplementation: Cuban experience. Prenat Diagn 1990;10:149–152.

69. Kirke PN, Daly LE, Elwood JH, et al. A randomised trial of low dose folic acid to prevent neural tube defects. Arch Dis Child 1992;67:1442–1446.

70. Bower C, Stanley FJ. Dietary folate as a risk factor for neural tube defects: evidence from a case-control study in Western Australia. Med J Aust 1989;150:613–619.

71. Werler MM, Shapiro S, Mitchel AA. Periconceptional folic acid exposure and risk of occurrence of neural tube defects. JAMA 1993;269:1257–1261.

72. Mulinare J, Cordero JF, Erickson JD, et al. Periconceptional use of multivitamins and the occurrence of neural tube defects. JAMA 1988;260:3141–3145.

73. Mills JL, Rhoads GG, Simpson JL, et al. The absence of a relation between the periconceptional use of vitamins and neural-tube defects. N Engl J Med 1989;321:430–435.

74. Milunsky A, Jick H, Jick SS, et al. Multivitamin/folic acid supplementation in early pregnancy reduces the prevalence of neural tube defects. JAMA 1989;262:2847–2852.

75. Czeizel AE, Dudas I. Prevention of the first occurrence of neural-tube defects by periconceptional vitamin supplementation. N Engl J Med 1992;327:1832–1835.

76. Czeizel AE. Prevention of congenital abnormalities by periconceptional multivitamin supplementation. BMJ 1993; 306:1645–1648.

77. Subar AF, Block G, James LD. Folate intake and food sources in the US population. Am J Clin Nutr 1989;50: 508–516.

78. Davidson LSP, Girdwood RH. Folic acid as therapeutic agent. BMJ 1947;1:587–591.

79. Hansen HA, Weinfeld A. Metabolic effects and diagnostic value of small dosages of folic acid and B_{12} in megaloblastic anemias. Acta Med Scand 1962;172:427–443.

80. Ross FJ, Belding H, Paegel BL. The development and progression of subacute combined degeneration of the spinal cord in patients with pernicious anaemia treated with synthetic pteroylglutamic (folic) acid. Blood 1948;3:68–90.

81. Allen RH, Stabler SP, Savage DG, et al. Diagnosis of cobalamin deficiency I: Usefulness of serum methylmalonic acid and total homocysteine concentrations. Am J Hematol 1990;34:90–98.

82. Cooper BA, Abe T. Variable response of bone marrow to feeding DL-5-formyltetrahydrofolate in pernicious anemia. Br J Haematol 1976;32:387–394.

83. Victor M, Lear AA. Subacute combined degeneration of the spinal cord. Am J Med 1956;20:896–911.

84. Baldwin JN, Dalessio DJ. Folic acid therapy and spinal-cord degeneration in pernicious anemia. N Engl J Med 1961;264:1339–1342.

85. Vilter RW, Will JJ, Wright T, et al. Interrelationships of vitamin B_{12}, folic acid, and ascorbic acid in the megaloblastic anemias. Am J Clin Nutr 1963;12:130–144.

86. Marshall RA, Jandl JH. Response to "physiologic" doses of folic acid in the megaloblastic anemias. Arch Intern Med 1960;105:352–360.

87. Wald NJ, Bower C. Folic acid, pernicious anaemia, and prevention of neural tube defects [commentary]. Lancet 1994;343:307.

88. Kirke PN, Molloy AM, Daly LE, et al. Maternal plasma folate and vitamin B_{12} are independent risk factors for neural tube defects. Q J Med 1993;86:703–708.

89. Mills JL, McPartlin JM, Kirke PN, et al. Homocysteine metabolism in pregnancies complicated by neural-tube defects. Lancet 1995;345:149–151.

90. Simmer K, Iles CA, James C, et al. Are iron-folate supplements harmful? Am J Clin Nutr 1987;45: 122–125.

91. Butterworth CE Jr, Hatch K, Cole P, et al. Zinc concentration in plasma and erythrocytes of subjects receiving folic acid supplementation. Am J Clin Nutr 1988;47:488–486.

92. Mukherjee MD, Sandstead HH, Ratnaparkhi MV, et al. Maternal zinc, iron, folic acid, and protein nutriture and outcome of pregnancy. Am J Clin Nutr 1984;40:496–507.

93. Butterworth CE Jr, Tamura T. Folic acid safety and toxicity: a brief review. Am J Clin Nutr 1989;50: 353–358.

94. Czeizel AE, Dobo M. Postnatal somatic and mental development after periconceptional multivitamin supplementation. Arch Dis Child 1994;70:229–233.

95. Holmes-Siedle M, Dennis J, Lindenbaum RH, et al. Long term effects of periconceptional multivitamin supplements for prevention of neural tube defects: a seven to 10 year follow up. Arch Dis Child 1992;67:1436–1441.

96. American Society of Human Genetics. Policy statement for maternal serum alpha-fetoprotein screening programs and quality control for laboratories performing maternal serum and amniotic fluid alpha-fetoprotein assays. Am J Hum Genet 1987;40:75–82.

97. Garver KL. Update on MSAFP policy statement from the American Society of Human Genetics. Am J Hum Genet 1989;45:332–334.

98. American Academy of Pediatrics, Committee on Genetics. Maternal serum α-fetoprotein screening. Pediatrics 1991;88:1282–1283.

99. Canadian Task Force on the Periodic Health Examination. Canadian guide to clinical preventive health care. Ottawa: Canada Communication Group, 1994:74–81.

100. American Academy of Pediatrics and American College of Obstetricians and Gynecologists. Antepartum and intrapartum care. In: Freeman RK, Poland RL. Guidelines for perinatal care. 3rd ed. Elk Grove Village, IL: American Academy of Pediatrics and Washington, DC: American College of Obstetricians and Gynecologists, 1992:49–90.

101. American Academy of Pediatrics. Folic acid for the prevention of neural tube defects. Pediatrics 1993;92:493–494.

102. Centers for Disease Control. Recommendations for the use of folic acid to reduce the number of cases of spina bifida and other neural tube defects. MMWR 1992;41(RR-14):1–7.

103. American College of Obstetricians and Gynecologists. Folic acid for the prevention of recurrent neural tube defects. Committee Opinion no. 120. Washington, DC: American College of Obstetricians and Gynecologists, 1993.

104. Centers for Disease Control. Use of folic acid for prevention of spina bifida and other neural tube defects—1983–1991. MMWR 1991;40:513–516.

105. Thornton JG, Lilford RJ, Howell D. Safety of amniocentesis. Lancet 1986;2:225–226.

106. National Center for Health Statistics. Healthy people 2000 review, 1992. Hyattsville, MD: Public Health Service, 1993:42.

107. Food and Drug Administration. Food standards: amendment to the standards of identity for enriched grain products to require addition of folic acid. Fed Reg 1993;58:53305–53312.

108. Food and Drug Administration. Food additives permitted for direct addition to food for human consumption: folic acid (folacin). Fed Reg 1993;58:53312–53317.

109. Food and Drug Administration. Food labeling: health claims and label statements; folate and neural tube defects. Fed Reg 1993;58:53254–53295.

110. Willett WC. Folic acid and neural tube defect: can't we come to closure? Am J Public Health 1992; 82:666–668.

111. Report from an Expert Advisory Group. Folic acid and the prevention of neural tube defects. London: Department of Health, 1992.

43. Screening for Hemoglobinopathies

RECOMMENDATION

Neonatal screening for sickle hemoglobinopathies is recommended to identify infants who may benefit from antibiotic prophylaxis to prevent sepsis. Whether screening should be universal or targeted to high-risk groups will depend on the proportion of high-risk individuals in the screening area, the accuracy and efficiency with which infants at risk can be identified, and other characteristics of the screening program. All screening efforts must be accompanied by comprehensive counseling and treatment services. Offering screening for hemoglobinopathies to pregnant women at the first prenatal visit is recommended, especially for those at high risk. There is insufficient evidence to recommend for or against routine screening for hemoglobinopathies in high-risk adolescents and young adults, but recommendations to offer such testing may be made on other grounds (see *Clinical Intervention*).

Burden of Suffering

Hemoglobin S is formed as the result of a single-gene defect causing substitution of valine for glutamic acid in position 6 of the β chain of adult hemoglobin. Persons homozygous for hemoglobin S (HbSS) have sickle cell anemia. Under conditions of low oxygen tension, hemoglobin S polymerizes, causing the red blood cells of persons with sickle cell anemia to assume a "sickled" shape. This deformity of red blood cells leads to the symptoms of sickle cell disease. Persons heterozygous for both hemoglobin S and hemoglobin C (HbSC) and persons heterozygous for both hemoglobin S and β-thalassemia (HbS/β-thal) also may experience sickle cell disease, although their symptoms tend to be less severe than those of persons homozygous for hemoglobin S.[1] Sickle cell disease affects an estimated 50,000 Americans[2-4] and affects persons of many racial and ethnic backgrounds. Among infants born in the U.S., sickle cell disease occurs in 1 in every 375 African Americans, 1 in 3,000 Native Americans, 1 in 20,000 Hispanics, and 1 in 60,000 whites.[4]

Compared to blacks in the general population, the average life expectancy of patients with sickle cell anemia is decreased by 25–30 years.[5] Symptom severity and life expectancy vary considerably, with some patients

485

surviving beyond middle age and others dying during infancy or child-hood. Mortality in children with sickle cell disease peaks between 1 and 3 years of age, and is chiefly due to sepsis caused by *Streptococcus pneumoniae.*[1] Pneumococcal septicemia occurs at a rate of approximately 8 episodes per 100 person-years of observation in children under the age of 3 years with sickle cell disease.[6,7] The case-fatality rate can be as high as 35%.[8] After infancy, patients with sickle cell disease are usually anemic and may experience painful crises and other complications, including acute chest syndrome, priapism, strokes, splenic and renal dysfunction, bone and joint disease, ischemic ulcers, cholecystitis, and hepatic dysfunction associated with cholelithiasis.[4,9] The causes of premature death in adults are varied, and include sudden death during acute pain episodes, stroke, infection, and chronic organ failure.[5] Treatment for sickle cell disease may be expensive. This chronic illness places a large economic and psychosocial burden on patients and their caretakers.[9]

About 2 million Americans are heterozygous for hemoglobin S and hemoglobin A (normal adult hemoglobin). This carrier state has been termed sickle cell trait and is present in 8% of the African American population.[3] Except for a slightly increased risk of exercise-related death under extreme conditions,[10] persons with sickle cell trait experience negligible morbidity.[11,12] Parents who are both carriers have a 25% probability with each pregnancy of having a child with sickle cell disease. One in every 150 African American couples in the U.S. is at risk of giving birth to a child with sickle cell disease (about 3,000 pregnancies per year).[13,14]

Certain thalassemias may also be detected by screening for hemoglobinopathies. Thalassemias result from genetic defects that cause reduced synthesis of the polypeptide globin chains that combine to form hemoglobin. The clinical severity of these syndromes is related to the degree of reduction of α- or β-globin synthesis.

The β-thalassemias occur primarily among individuals of Mediterranean, African, or Southeast Asian origin. β-Thalassemia minor occurs in persons heterozygous for a gene causing reduction in β-globin synthesis. Life expectancy is normal, and the clinical severity of this state is related to the specific defect and its effect on β-chain synthesis. β-Thalassemia major occurs in persons homozygous for genetic defects in β-globin synthesis. β-Globin synthesis in these individuals is markedly reduced or absent. They suffer from severe anemia and are transfusion dependent. Modern transfusion protocols and iron chelation therapy have greatly improved prognosis and some patients survive beyond the third decade of life.[15] β-Thalassemia major affects fewer than 1,000 Americans.[16]

α-Thalassemias are common in persons of Southeast Asian descent and also occur in persons of African and Mediterranean origin. α-Thalassemias result from deletions of one or more of the four genes responsible for α-globin synthesis. Patients with a four-gene deletion develop hydrops fetalis secondary to severe anemia and die before or shortly after birth. Mothers of these infants are at risk for toxemia during pregnancy, operative delivery, and postpartum hemorrhage.[17] The three-gene deletion is referred to as hemoglobin H disease and affects about 1% of Southeast Asians.[18] Three- and four-gene deletions are rare in African Americans. Persons with hemoglobin H disease experience chronic hemolytic anemia that is exacerbated by exposure to oxidants and may require transfusion. Persons with a two-gene deletion have microcytic red blood cells and occasionally mild anemia. The one-gene deletion is a "silent" carrier state. These latter two conditions are often called α-thalassemia trait. The exact prevalence of α-thalassemia trait is uncertain, but it is estimated to be 5–30% among African Americans and 15–30% among Southeast Asians.[18–20]

Hemoglobin E trait is the third most common hemoglobin disorder in the world and the most common in Southeast Asia, where its prevalence is estimated to be 30%.[18] Although hemoglobin E trait is associated with no morbidity, the offspring of individuals who carry this hemoglobin variant may exhibit thalassemia major (hemoglobin E/β-thalassemia) if the other parent has β-thalassemia trait and contributes that gene. This combination is the most common cause of transfusion-dependent thalassemia in areas of Southeast Asia.[18]

Accuracy of Screening Tests

Two-tier hemoglobin electrophoresis (cellulose acetate electrophoresis with confirmation by citrate agar electrophoresis) or thin-layer isoelectric focusing are widely used screening tests for hemoglobin disorders.[4,21] High-performance liquid chromatography (HPLC) is a newer technique that offers high resolution and is in use in at least one screening program.[22] Techniques employing monoclonal antibodies and recombinant DNA technology are not used widely.[23] Blood for screening is collected in heparinized tubes or, in the case of newborn screening, on filter paper (Guthrie paper blotter).[24]

Electrophoresis is highly specific in the detection of certain hemoglobin disorders, such as sickle cell disease. In one study, all 138 children with hemoglobin S identified by screening 3,976 African American newborns were found to have a sickling disorder when retested at age 3–5 years.[25] Another study of 131 infants detected by screening found only nine instances in which the sickling disorder required reclassification and no instance in which a child originally diagnosed as having sickle cell disease was found to have sickle cell trait.[26] Ten years' experience with universal screening of Colorado newborns (528,711 infants) using filter paper specimens and two-tier hemoglobin electrophoresis was reported in 1990.[27] Fifty infants with sickle cell diseases (HbSS, HbSC, HbS/β-thal) and 27 infants with other hemoglobin disorders were identified. Initial screening failed to identify four infants with sickle cell disease, but three of these were diagnosed on routine follow-up testing of infants suspected of having sickle cell trait. There were 32 false-positive results, 27 of which were confirmed to have a hemoglobinopathy trait on follow-up testing. The remaining five had normal hemoglobin. The test characteristics of HPLC may be superior to those of two-tier electrophoresis. Data are yet to be published.

The yield in screening pregnant women for hemoglobin disorders depends on the risk profile of the population being tested. In one study, electrophoresis in combination with a complete blood count was performed on 298 African American and Southeast Asian prenatal patients. Ninety-four women (31.5%) had a hemoglobin disorder (including sickle cell disease, sickle cell trait, hemoglobin E, α-thalassemia trait, β-thalassemia trait, hemoglobin H, and hemoglobin C).[19] In a larger study in a different community, similar tests were performed on 6,641 prenatal patients selected without regard to race or ethnic origin.[28] One hundred eighty-five women (3%) had sickle cell trait, 68 (1%) had hemoglobin C, 30 (0.5%) had β-thalassemia trait, and 17 (0.3%) had other disorders (hemoglobin E, α-thalassemia trait, hemoglobin H, hemoglobin E/β-thalassemia disease). These results were obtained by combining electrophoresis with red cell indices. When low mean corpuscular volume (MCV) was used as the only screening test to detect thalassemia, the yield was 0.3–0.5%.[29]

Prenatal diagnosis of sickle cell disease and other hemoglobinopathies in the fetus has been aided by advances in techniques of obtaining and analyzing specimens. Early tests involved the analysis of fetal blood obtained by fetoscopy or placental aspiration.[30] Genetic advances, however, have provided a safer[14] and more practical method in which amniocytes are obtained by amniocentesis and gene mutations are identified directly through recombinant DNA technology.[13] These techniques are highly accurate (error rate less than 1%) in detecting sickle cell disease and certain forms of thalassemia.[14,30–33] The principal disadvantage of using amniocentesis to obtain specimens is that it cannot be performed safely until about 16 weeks' gestation, thus delaying diagnosis and potential intervention until late in the second trimester. Chorionic villus sampling (CVS) is a means of obtaining tissue for DNA analysis as early as 10–12 weeks of gestation and is an established technique for prenatal diagnosis (see Chapter 41).[34,35]

Effectiveness of Early Detection

Screening for hemoglobin disorders is usually discussed with respect to two target populations: neonates and adults of reproductive age. Newborns

with sickle cell disease benefit from early detection through the early institution of prophylactic penicillin therapy to prevent pneumococcal sepsis. A
multicenter, randomized, double-blind, placebo-controlled trial demonstrated that the administration of prophylactic oral penicillin to infants and
young children with sickle cell disease reduced the incidence of pneumococcal septicemia by 84%.[36] Other benefits of identifying newborns with
sickle cell disease include prompt clinical intervention for infection or
splenic sequestration crises and education of caretakers about the signs
and symptoms of illness in these children. A 7-year longitudinal study reported lower mortality in children with sickle cell disease identified in the
newborn period than in children diagnosed after 3 months of age (2% vs.
8%), but the investigators did not account for confounding variables in the
control group.[37] A briefer longitudinal study (8–20 months) reported no
deaths in 131 newborns detected through screening.[26] In the Colorado experience described above, 47 of the 50 newborns with sickle cell disease
identified through screening remained in the state beyond 6 months of
age. None of the 47 died during the period of observation.[27]

Screening older children and adolescents is designed to detect carriers
with sickle cell trait, β-thalassemia trait, and other hemoglobin disorders
that have escaped detection during the first years of life. Identification of
carriers before childbearing allows them to make informed reproductive
choices by receiving genetic counseling about partner selection and the
availability of diagnostic tests in the event of pregnancy. There is some evidence that individuals who receive certain forms of counseling retain this information and may encourage other individuals, such as their partners, to
be tested.[28,38-40] A prospective study of 142 persons screened for β-thalassemia trait found that 62 (43%) encouraged other persons to be
screened.[38] Compared with controls, those who had received counseling
demonstrated significantly better understanding of thalassemia when tested
immediately after the session. There is no direct evidence, however, that individual genetic counseling by itself significantly alters reproductive behavior or the incidence of births of infants with hemoglobin disorders.[9,41]

Detection of carrier status during pregnancy provides prospective parents with the option of testing the fetus for a hemoglobinopathy. If the test
is positive, they have the time to discuss continuation of the pregnancy and
to plan optimal care for their newborn. Parents appear to act on this genetic information. About half of pregnant women with positive tests for
thalassemia refer their partners for testing and, if the father is positive,
about 60% consent to amniocentesis.[28] If sickle cell disease is diagnosed in
the fetus, about 50% of parents elect therapeutic abortion.[32,42] In a recent
study, 18,907 samples from pregnant women were screened for abnormal
hemoglobin including thalassemias and hemoglobin S. In 810 (4.3%), an
abnormal hemoglobin was identified; 66% occurred in mothers unaware

that they carried an abnormal hemoglobin, and 80% occurred in mothers unaware that they were at risk for giving birth to a child with a serious hematologic disorder. Eighty-six percent of mothers who received counseling said they wanted their partner tested and 55% of partners were tested. Seventy-seven pregnancies were identified as being at risk because the partner also was a carrier of an abnormal hemoglobin. Of these 77 pregnancies, the gestation was too advanced for prenatal diagnosis in 12 cases and the condition for which the pregnancy was at risk was too mild for this service to be offered in 12 others. Prenatal diagnosis was offered in the remaining 53 pregnancies and accepted by 25 couples (47%). Of 18 amniocenteses actually performed, 5 fetuses were found to have clinically significant hemoglobinopathies and one of these pregnancies was terminated.[43]

There is evidence from some European communities with a high prevalence of β-thalassemia that the birth rate of affected infants has declined significantly following the implementation of routine prenatal screening,[30] and there are data suggesting a similar trend in some North American communities that have introduced community education and testing for thalassemia.[16] Time series studies do not, however, prove that such trends are due specifically to the effects of prenatal screening.

Recommendations of Other Groups

Screening for sickle cell disease in all newborns, regardless of their race or ethnic origin, has been recommended by a National Institutes of Health consensus conference[8] and by a guideline panel convened by the Agency for Health Care Policy and Research.[4] Screening infants from high-risk groups (e.g., those of African, Caribbean, Latin American, Southeast Asian, Middle Eastern, or Mediterranean ethnicity) has been recommended by the World Health Organization,[44] the British Society for Haematology,[45] the American Academy of Family Physicians (AAFP),[46] and the Canadian Task Force on the Periodic Health Examination.[47] The recommendations of the AAFP are currently under review. The American Academy of Pediatrics[48] and Bright Futures[49] recommend routine screening for hemoglobinopathies as required by individual states. At present 29 states, Puerto Rico, and the District of Columbia mandate screening all newborns for hemoglobinopathies, and 12 states offer screening as an option.[50]

The American College of Obstetricians and Gynecologists,[51] the British Society for Haematology,[45] and the Canadian Task Force[47] recommend selective prenatal screening and counseling of pregnant women from high-risk ethnic groups. The Canadian Task Force[47] recommends that parents with established positive carrier status be offered prenatal DNA analysis of amniocentesis or CVS tissue sampling. No major organizations recommend routine screening of adolescents and young adults for carrier status.

Discussion

Hemoglobinopathies occur among all ethnic and racial groups. Efforts at targeting specific high-risk groups for newborn screening inevitably miss affected individuals due to difficulties in properly assigning race or ethnic origin in the newborn nursery. In one study of more than 500,000 newborns, parental race as requested on a screening form was found to be inaccurate or incomplete in 30% of cases.[27] Proponents of selective screening of high-risk populations emphasize that, especially in geographic areas with a small population at risk, cost-effectiveness is compromised and considerable expense incurred in screening large numbers of low-risk newborns to identify the rare individuals with sickle cell disease or other uncommon hemoglobin disorders.[52] Studies supporting this argument have compared universal screening to no screening, not targeted screening. Recent research that accounts for the additional procedural and administrative costs of targeted screening suggests that universal screening may be the more cost-effective alternative.[4] Whether to screen all infants (universal screening) or only those infants from ethnic groups known to be at relatively high risk of having sickle cell disease (targeted screening) is therefore a policy question to be addressed by individual screening programs, taking into consideration cost-effectiveness analyses, disease prevalence, and available resources.

There has been considerable debate over the value of screening for hemoglobinopathies in persons of reproductive age. Critics cite evidence that sickle cell screening programs in the past have failed to adequately educate patients and the public about the significant differences between sickle cell trait and sickle cell disease. This has resulted in unnecessary anxiety for carriers and inappropriate labeling by insurers and employers.[53] In addition, there is no evidence that counseling, however comprehensive, will be remembered throughout the individual's reproductive life, influence partner selection, alter use of prenatal testing, or ultimately reduce the rate of births of affected children.[9,29] Proponents argue that these outcomes should not be used as measures of effectiveness since the goal of genetic counseling is to facilitate informed decision making by prospective parents.[9,20,29] In this regard, clinicians are responsible for making the individual aware of the diagnosis, the risk to future offspring, and the recommended methods to reduce that risk, regardless of the strength of the evidence that such counseling reduces the number of affected offspring.

CLINICAL INTERVENTION

Screening newborn infants for hemoglobinopathies with hemoglobin electrophoresis or other tests of comparable accuracy on umbilical cord or heelstick blood specimens is recommended ("A" recommendation). In geographic areas with a very low incidence of hemoglobin disorders, selective screening of newborns may be more efficient than universal screening. Infants with sickle cell disease must receive prompt follow-up, including oral penicillin prophylaxis, diagnostic testing, immunizations, and regular evaluations of growth and nutritional status. Their families should receive genetic counseling regarding testing of family members and risks to future offspring, information about the disease, education about early warning signs of serious complications, and referrals for peer support groups and sources of medical and mental health services.

Offering screening for hemoglobinopathies with hemoglobin electrophoresis or other tests of comparable accuracy to pregnant women at the first prenatal visit is recommended ("B" recommendation), especially for those who are members of racial and ethnic groups with a high incidence of hemoglobinopathies (e.g., individuals of African, Caribbean, Latin American, Mediterranean, Middle Eastern, or Southeast Asian descent). Carriers identified through testing should be urged to have the father tested and should receive information on the availability of prenatal diagnosis if the father is positive and the fetus is at risk of having a clinically significant hemoglobinopathy.

There is insufficient evidence to recommend for or against screening for hemoglobinopathies in adolescents and young adults from ethnic and racial groups known to be at increased risk for sickle cell disease, thalassemias, and other hemoglobinopathies in order for them to be able to make informed reproductive choices ("C" recommendation). Recommendations to offer such testing may be made on other grounds, including burden of suffering and patient preference. If provided, testing should be accompanied by counseling, which should include a description of the significance of the disease, how it is inherited, the availability of a screening test, and the implications to individuals and their offspring of a positive result.

The draft update of this chapter was prepared for the U.S. Preventive Services Task Force by John Andrews, MD, MPH, and Modena Wilson, MD, MPH.

REFERENCES

1. Leikin SL, Gallagher D, Kinney TR, et al. Mortality in children and adolescents with sickle cell disease. Cooperative Study of Sickle Cell Disease. Pediatrics 1989;84:500–508.
2. Scott RB, Castro O. Screening for sickle cell hemoglobinopathies. JAMA 1979;241:1145–1147.
3. Motulsky AG. Frequency of sickling disorders in U.S. blacks. N Engl J Med 1973;288:31–33.
4. Agency for Health Care Policy and Research. Sickle cell disease: screening, diagnosis, management, and

counseling in newborns and infants. Clinical Practice Guideline no. 6. Rockville, MD: Agency for Health Care Policy and Research, 1993. (Publication no. 93-0562.)

5. Platt OS, Brambilla DJ, Rosse WF, et al. Mortality in sickle cell disease: life expectancy and risk factors for early death. N Engl J Med 1994;330:1639–1644.

6. Zarkowsky HS, Gallagher D, Gill F, et al. Bacteremia in sickle hemoglobinopathies. Cooperative Study of Sickle Cell Disease. J Pediatr 1986;109: 579–585.

7. Wong WY, Powars DR, Chan L, et al. Polysaccharide encapsulated bacterial infection in sickle cell anemia: a thirty-year epidemiologic experience. Am J Hematol 1992;39:176–182.

8. National Institutes of Health Consensus Development Conference Statement. Newborn screening for sickle cell disease and other hemoglobinopathies. JAMA 1987;258:1205–1209.

9. Bowman JE. Is a national program to prevent sickle cell disease possible? Am J Pediatr Hematol Oncol 1983; 5:367–372.

10. Kark JA, Posey DM, Schumacher HR, et al. Sickle-cell trait as a risk factor for sudden death in physical training. N Engl J Med 1987;317:781–787.

11. Sears DA. The morbidity of sickle cell trait: a review of the literature. Am J Med 1978;64:1021–1036.

12. Sullivan LW. The risks of sickle-cell trait: caution and common sense. N Engl J Med 1987;317:830–831.

13. Embury SH, Scharf SJ, Saiki RK, et al. Rapid prenatal diagnosis of sickle cell anemia by a new method of DNA analysis. N Engl J Med 1987;316:656–661.

14. Kazazian HH Jr, Boehm CD, Dowling CE. Prenatal diagnosis of hemoglobinopathies by DNA analysis. Ann NY Acad Sci 1985;445:337–348.

15. Ehlers KH, Giardina PJ, Lesser ML, et al. Prolonged survival in patients with beta thalassemia major treated with deferoxamine. J Pediatr 1991;118:540–545.

16. Pearson HA, Guiliotis DK, Rink L, et al. Patient age distribution in thalassemia major: changes from 1973 to 1985. Pediatrics 1987;80:53–57.

17. Wasi P. Hemoglobinopathies including thalassemia: Part 1. Tropical Asia. Clin Haematol 1981;10: 707–729.

18. Hurst D, Tittle B, Kleman KM, et al. Anemia and hemoglobinopathies in Southeast Asian refugee children. J Pediatr 1983;102:692–697.

19. Stein J, Berg C, Jones JA, et al. A screening protocol for a prenatal population at risk for inherited hemoglobin disorders: results of its application to a group of Southeast Asians and blacks. Am J Obstet Gynecol 1984;150:333–341.

20. Steinberg MH, Embury SH. Alpha-thalassemia in blacks: genetic and clinical aspects and interactions with the sickle hemoglobin gene. Blood 1986;68:985–990.

21. Kleman KM, Vichinsky E, Lubin BH. Experience with newborn screening using isoelectric focusing. Pediatrics 1989;83(5 pt 2):852–854.

22. Huisman THJ. Usefulness of cation exchange high performance liquid chromatography as a testing procedure. Pediatrics 1989;83(5 pt 2):849–851.

23. Garrick MD. Alternative methods for screening. Pediatrics 1989;83(5 pt 2):855–857.

24. Kinney TR, Sawtschenko M, Whorton M, et al. Techniques' comparison and report of the North Carolina experience. Pediatrics 1989;83(5 pt 2):843–848.

25. Kramer MS, Rooks Y, Johnston D, et al. Accuracy of cord blood screening for sickle hemoglobinopathies: three- to five-year follow-up. JAMA 1979;241:485–486.

26. Grover R, Shahidi S, Fisher B, et al. Current sickle cell screening program for newborns in New York City, 1979–1980. Am J Public Health 1983;73:249–251.

27. Githens JH, Lane PA, McCurdy RS, et al. Newborn screening in Colorado: the first ten years. Am J Dis Child 1990;144:466–470.

28. Rowley PT, Loader S, Walden ME. Toward providing parents the option of avoiding the birth of the first child with Cooley's anemia: response to hemoglobinopathy screening and counseling during pregnancy. Ann NY Acad Sci 1986;445:408–416.

29. Gehlbach DL, Morgenstern LL. Antenatal screening for thalassemia minor. Obstet Gynecol 1988;71: 801–803.

30. Alter BP. Advances in the prenatal diagnosis of hematologic diseases. Blood 1984;64:329–340.

31. Weatherall DJ, Mold J, Thein SL, et al. Prenatal diagnosis of the common haemoglobin disorders. J Med Genet 1985;22:422–430.

32. Boehm CD, Antonarakis SE, Phillips JA III, et al. Prenatal diagnosis using DNA polymorphisms: report on 95 pregnancies at risk for sickle-cell disease or beta-thalassemia. N Engl J Med 1983;308:1054–1058.

33. Orkin SH. Prenatal diagnosis of hemoglobin disorders by DNA analysis. Blood 1984;63:249–253.

34. Goosens M, Dumez Y, Kaplan L, et al. Prenatal diagnosis of sickle-cell anemia in the first trimester of pregnancy. N Engl J Med 1983;309:831–833.

35. Old JM, Fitches A, Heath C, et al. First-trimester fetal diagnosis for haemoglobinopathies: report on 200 cases. Lancet 1986;2:763–767.

36. Gaston MH, Verter JI, Woods G, et al. Prophylaxis with oral penicillin in children with sickle cell anemia: a randomized trial. N Engl J Med 1986;314:1593–1599.

37. Vichinsky E, Hurst D, Earles A, et al. Newborn screening for sickle cell disease: effect on mortality. Pediatrics 1988;81:749–755.

38. Lipkin M, Fisher L, Rowley PT, et al. Genetic counseling of asymptomatic carriers in a primary care setting: the effectiveness of screening and counseling for beta-thalassemia trait. Ann Intern Med 1986;105:115–123.

39. Whitten CF, Thomas JF, Nishiura EN. Sickle cell trait counseling: evaluation of counselors and counselees. Am J Hum Genet 1981;33:802–816.

40. Scriver CR, Bardanis M, Cartier L, et al. Beta-thalassemia disease prevention: genetic medicine applied. Am J Hum Genet 1984;36:1024–1038.

41. Rucknagel DL. A decade of screening in the hemoglobinopathies: is a national program to prevent sickle cell anemia possible? Am J Pediatr Hematol Oncol 1983;5:373–377.

42. Driscoll MC, Lerner N, Anyane-Yeboa K, et al. Prenatal diagnosis of sickle hemoglobinopathies: the experience of the Columbia University Comprehensive Center for Sickle Cell Disease. Am J Hum Genet 1987;40:548–558.

43. Rowley PT, Loader S, Sutera CJ, et al. Prenatal screening for hemoglobinopathies: I. A prospective regional trial. Am J Hum Genet 1991;48:439–446.

44. Treatment of haemoglobinopathies and allied disorders: report of a WHO scientific group. World Health Organization Technical Report Series no. 509. Geneva: World Health Organization 1972:33.

45. British Society for Haematology. Guidelines for haemoglobinopathy screening. Clin Lab Hematol 1988;10:87–94.

46. American Academy of Family Physicians. Age charts for the periodic health examination. Kansas City, MO: American Academy of Family Physicians, 1994. (Reprint no. 510.)

47. Canadian Task Force on the Periodic Health Examination. Canadian guide to clinical preventive health care. Ottawa: Canada Communication Group, 1994:206–218.

48. American Academy of Pediatrics Committee on Practice and Ambulatory Medicine. Recommendations for preventive pediatric health care. Pediatrics 1995;96:373–374.

49. Green M, ed. Bright Futures: guidelines for health supervision of infants, children and adolescents. Arlington, VA: National Center for Education in Maternal and Child Health, 1994.

50. Newborn Screening Committee, The Council of Regional Networks for Genetic Services (CORN). National newborn screening report—1991. New York: CORN, 1994.

51. American College of Obstetricians and Gynecologists. Hemoglobinopathies in pregnancy. Technical Bulletin no. 185. Washington, DC: American College of Obstetricians and Gynecologists, 1993.

52. Tsevat J, Wong JB, Pauker SG, Steinberg MH. Neonatal screening for sickle cell disease: a cost-effectiveness analysis. J Pediatr 1991;118:546–554.

53. Fost N. Ethical implications of screening asymptomatic individuals. FASEB J 1992;6:2813–2817.

44. Screening for Phenylketonuria

RECOMMENDATION

Screening for phenylketonuria (PKU) by measurement of phenylalanine level on a dried-blood spot specimen is recommended for all newborns prior to discharge from the nursery. Infants who are tested before 24 hours of age should receive a repeat screening test by 2 weeks of age. There is insufficient evidence to recommend for or against routine prenatal screening for maternal PKU, but recommendations against such screening may be made on other grounds.

Burden of Suffering

PKU is an inborn error of phenylalanine metabolism that occurs in 1 of every 12,000 births in North America.[1,2] In the absence of treatment during infancy, nearly all persons with this disorder develop severe, irreversible mental retardation. Many also experience neurobehavioral symptoms such as seizures, tremors, gait disorders, athetoid movements, and psychotic episodes with behaviors resembling autism.[3] These clinical manifestations of PKU have rarely developed in children born after the mid-1960s, when routine screening was legislated and early treatment for PKU became common. This has resulted in a cohort of healthy phenylketonuric women who have entered childbearing age. If dietary restriction of phenylalanine is not maintained during pregnancy, these women are at increased risk of giving birth to a child with mental retardation, microcephaly, congenital heart disease, and low birth weight.[4] The incidence of this maternal PKU syndrome is 1 of every 30,000–40,000 pregnancies.[5] In the absence of dietary control in women with PKU who become pregnant, it is estimated that exposure of the fetus to the teratogenic effects of maternal hyperphenylalaninemia could result in an increase in the incidence of PKU-related mental retardation to the level seen before PKU screening was established.[6]

Accuracy of Screening Tests

Blood phenylalanine determination by the Guthrie test has been the principal screening test for PKU for three decades.[7] Although well-designed evaluations of the sensitivity and specificity of the Guthrie test have never been performed,[8] sensitivity estimates[9,10] and international experience with its use in millions of newborns suggest that false-negative results are rare. Fluorometric assays, which can detect differences in blood phenylalanine levels as low as 0.1 mg/dL, are alternative forms of testing that also offer excellent sensitivity.[8] Most missed cases of PKU do not appear to be due to false-negative results of the screening tests, but to submission of an inadequate sample, clerical error involving the sample, or failure to follow up positive results.[9] Standards for adequate blood collection on filter paper for neonatal screening programs have been published.[10a]

False-positive as well as false-negative results can occur in PKU screening. In certain situations and population conditions, the ratio of false positives to true positives is as high as 32 to 1.[8] Although false positives have been viewed for many years as less important than false-negative results because they can be corrected easily by repeating the test, recalling patients for a second PKU test may generate considerable parental anxiety.[11,12]

The sensitivity of the Guthrie test is influenced by the age of the newborn when the sample is obtained. The current trend toward early discharge from the nursery (resulting in PKU screening being performed as early as 1 to 2 days of age) has raised concerns that test results obtained during this early period may have low sensitivity. This is because the blood level of phenylalanine is typically normal in affected neonates at birth and, with the initiation of protein feedings, increases progressively during the first days of life. Using the conventional cutoff of 4 mg/dL, diagnostic levels of phenylalanine may not be present in some phenylketonuric newborns tested in the first 24 hours of life. Prospective, longitudinal evaluations of serum phenylalanine levels in infants known to be at risk for PKU have demonstrated a variable rate of false-negative results when screening occurred within the first 24 hours of life.[13,14] The false-negative rates ranged from 2% to 31% for the first day of life, but decreased to 0.6% to 2% on the second day and to 0.3% by the third day.[8,13–16] Current rates may be lower due to the participation of many laboratories in a voluntary proficiency program run by the Centers for Disease Control and Prevention (CDC). The use of fluorometric assays, which offer more precise measurements of blood phenylalanine levels than the Guthrie test, result in lower false-negative rates as well.[8] Two additional solutions to improve sensitivity—repeat testing of all newborns after early discharge and lowering the cutoff value to reduce the false-negative rate—have encountered criticism for several reasons. Repeat testing would have low yield and reduced cost-effectiveness;[17,18] it has been estimated that detecting even one case of PKU in this manner would require performing an additional 600,000 to perhaps 6 million tests.[8,18] Lowering the cutoff value, on the other hand, improves sensitivity at the expense of specificity, thereby increasing the ratio of false positives to true positives.[8] As of 1991, nine of the 53 screening programs in the U.S. used a cutoff level of greater than 2 mg/dL to define abnormal.[19] The majority of labs continue to use a cutoff of 4 mg/dL or greater.

The development of a cloned phenylalanine hydroxylase gene probe has made possible the prenatal diagnosis of PKU in families with previously affected children by analyzing DNA isolated from cultured amniotic cells or samples of chorionic villi.[20–22] Through the use of polymerase chain reaction, 31 alleles of the phenylalanine hydroxylase gene have been identified.[1] This may eventually permit the screening of the general population for carriers of these alleles, thereby detecting at-risk families prior to the birth of an affected child.[21–23]

Routine screening of pregnant women for maternal PKU has been recommended as a means of preventing fetal complications.[2,5,24] This disorder is rare in the general population, however, and as a result of screening programs, many women with PKU are aware of their diagnosis. As the cohort of women born before implementation of routine newborn screening move out of their childbearing years, the yield from screening all pregnant women should be very low. In Massachusetts, routine screening of cord blood for 10 years detected only 22 mothers with previously undiagnosed hyperphenylalaninemia.[2,25]

Effectiveness of Early Detection

Before treatment with dietary phenylalanine restriction was recommended in the early 1960s, severe mental retardation was a common outcome in children with PKU. A review in 1953 reported that 85% of patients had an intelligence quotient (IQ) less than 40, and 37% had IQ scores below 10; less than 1% had scores above 70.[3] Since dietary phenylalanine restriction was introduced, however, over 95% of children with PKU have developed normal or near-normal intelligence.[26–29] A large longitudinal study reports a mean IQ of 100 in children who have been followed to 12 years of age,[30] and other reports show adolescent and young adult patients are functioning well in society.[31] Although the efficacy of dietary treatment has never been proven in a properly designed controlled trial, the contrast between children receiving dietary treatment and historical controls is compelling evidence of its effectiveness. Recognition of this prompted most Western governments to require routine neonatal screening as early as the late 1960s.

It is essential that phenylalanine restrictions be instituted shortly after birth to prevent the irreversible effects of PKU.[26,28,32,33] Traditionally, strict adherence to the diet was recommended for the first 4–8 years of life, after which liberalization of protein intake could occur without damage to the developed central nervous system.[26,28,32–34] Recent data, however, suggest that discontinuation of the diet may result in a deterioration of cognitive functioning, leading many to recommend continuation of the diet through adolescence and into adulthood.[35-37] Even if these precautions are taken, dietary treatment may not offer full protection from subtle effects of PKU. Intelligence scores in treated persons with PKU, although often in the normal range for the general population, are lower, on average, than those of siblings and parents,[26] and mild psychological deficits, such as perceptual motor dysfunction and attentional and academic difficulties, have been reported.[38-40]

Early detection of hyperphenylalaninemia in pregnant women may also be beneficial. The incidence of maternal PKU syndrome is increasing with the growing number of healthy phenylketonuric females now of childbearing age. Maternal hyperphenylalaninemia can produce teratogenic effects, even on normal fetuses who have not inherited PKU. If the mother with classic PKU does not follow a restricted phenylalanine diet during pregnancy, there is an overwhelming risk of birth of an abnormal child. This risk appears to increase as the average maternal levels of phenylalanine maintained during pregnancy increase.[41,42] Over 90% of these children will have mental retardation, 75% microcephaly, 40-50% intrauterine growth retardation, and 10-25% other birth defects.[4,5] Uncertainties exist, however, as to the extent these outcomes can be prevented by instituting treatment with dietary phenylalanine restriction during pregnancy.[4,43] Although some pregnant women under treatment have given birth to normal children, a number of investigators have found that dietary intervention during pregnancy fails to prevent fetal damage.[40,43-47] Preliminary evidence from the North American Collaborative Study of Maternal Phenylketonuria, on the other hand, suggests improved outcome if metabolic control is achieved by the 10th week of pregnancy.[48] Many believe dietary restrictions must be instituted prior to conception for them to be effective.[2,4,45,49] There are concerns, however, that the low-phenylalanine diet may produce deficiencies in calories, protein, and other nutrients that are needed for proper fetal growth.[5,43]

Recommendations of Other Groups

Every state has mandated that screening for PKU be provided to all newborns, but participation is not required by statute in Delaware, Maryland, North Carolina, or Vermont.[19] Testing for blood phenylalanine level after 24 hours of life and before 7 days is recommended by the American Academy of Pediatrics (AAP),[50] the American Academy of Family Physicians,[51] the American College of Obstetricians and Gynecologists (ACOG),[52] Bright Futures,[53] and the Canadian Task Force on the Periodic Health Examination.[54] All of these organizations recommend that infants who are not screened in the nursery should be screened by a physician by 3 weeks of age. As earlier hospital discharges (i.e., <24 hours) become the norm, eight states have mandated a second screening of all newborns between 1 and 6 weeks of age, and most other states recommend repeat specimens if first collected before 24–48 hours of age.[19] The AAP endorses a second test for those infants who were screened before 24 hours of age.[50]

No major organization recommends routine prenatal screening for maternal PKU. ACOG recommends taking a history for known inborn errors of metabolism at the initial evaluation of the pregnant woman.[55] The AAP recommends that female patients known to have hyperphenylalaninemia be referred to appropriate treatment centers prior to conceiving.[56]

Discussion

There is good evidence that early detection of PKU by neonatal screening substantially improves neurodevelopmental outcomes for affected persons. The evidence is less clear for a benefit from screening pregnant women for PKU. Available evidence has not proven that dietary restrictions during pregnancy occur early enough to prevent fetal damage, and such restrictions may have other adverse effects. In addition, the incidence of previously undiagnosed maternal hyperphenylalaninemia is low, since many women who are currently of childbearing age were born after the introduction of widespread PKU screening in the mid-1960s and are likely to have been detected as newborns. The cost-effectiveness of screening during pregnancy has not been established.

CLINICAL INTERVENTION

Screening for phenylketonuria by measurement of phenylalanine level on a dried-blood spot specimen, collected by heelstick and adsorbed onto filter paper,[10a] is recommended for all newborns before discharge from the nursery ("A" recommendation). Infants who are tested in the first 24 hours of age should receive a repeat screening test by 2 weeks of age. Premature infants and those with illnesses optimally should be tested at or near 7 days of age, but in all cases before newborn nursery discharge. All parents should be adequately informed regarding the indications for testing and the interpretation of PKU test results, including the probabilities of false-positive and false-negative findings.

There is insufficient evidence to recommend for or against routine prenatal screening for maternal PKU ("C" recommendation), but recommendations against such screening may be made on other grounds, including the rarity of previously undiagnosed maternal hyperphenylalaninemia, cost, and the potential adverse effects of dietary restriction.

The draft update of this chapter was prepared for the U.S. Preventive Services Task Force by Robert Baldwin, MD, and Modena Wilson, MD, MPH.

REFERENCES

1. O'Flynn ME. Newborn screening for phenylketonuria: thirty years of progress. Curr Probl Pediatr 1992;22:159–165.
2. Waisbren SE, Doherty LB, Bailey IV, et al. The New England Maternal PKU Project: identification of at-risk women. Am J Public Health 1988;78:789–792.
3. Jervis GA. Phenylpyruvic oligophrenia (phenylketonuria). Res Publ Assoc Res Nerv Ment Dis 1953;33: 259–282.
4. Lenke RR, Levy HL. Maternal phenylketonuria and hyperphenylalaninemia: an international survey of the outcome of untreated and treated pregnancies. N Engl J Med 1980;303:1202–1208.
5. Hanley WB, Clarke JTR, Schoonheyt W. Maternal phenylketonuria (PKU): a review. Clin Biochem 1987;20:149–156.
6. Kirkman HN. Projections of a rebound in frequency of mental retardation from phenylketonuria. Appl Res Ment Retard 1982;3:319–328.
7. Guthrie R, Susi A. A simple phenylalanine method for detecting phenylketonuria in large populations of newborn infants. Pediatrics 1963;32:338–343.
8. Kirkman HN, Carroll CL, Moore EG, et al. Fifteen-year experience with screening for phenylketonuria with an automated fluorometric method. Am J Hum Genet 1982;34:743–752.
9. Holtzman C, Slazyk WE, Cordero JF, et al. Descriptive epidemiology of missed cases of phenylketonuria and congenital hypothyroidism. Pediatrics 1986;78:553–558.
10. Holtzman NA, Meek AG, Mellits ED. Neonatal screening for phenylketonuria. JAMA 1974;229:667–670.
10a. National Committee for Clinical Laboratory Standards. Blood collection on filter paper for neonatal screening programs, 2nd ed; approved standard. Vol 12 no 13. Villanova, PA: NCCLS, 1992. (NCCLS document LA4-A2.)
11. Rothenberg MB, Sills EM. Iatrogenesis: the PKU anxiety syndrome. J Am Acad Child Psychiatry 1968;7:689–692.
12. Sorenson JR, Levy HL, Mangione TW, et al. Parental response to repeat testing of infants with false-positive results in a newborn screening program. Pediatrics 1984;73:183–187.
13. Meryash DL, Levy HL, Guthrie R, et al. Prospective study of early neonatal screening for phenylketonuria. N Engl J Med 1981;304:294–296.
14. Doherty LB, Rohr FJ, Levy HL. Detection of phenylketonuria in the very early newborn blood specimen. Pediatrics 1991;87:240–244.
15. Holtzman NA, McCabe ERB, Cunningham GC, et al. Screening for phenylketonuria [letter]. N Engl J Med 1981;304:1300–1301.
16. McCabe ERB, McCabe L, Mosher GA, et al. Newborn screening for phenylketonuria: predictive validity as a function of age. Pediatrics 1983;72:390–398.
17. Schneider AJ. Newborn phenylalanine/tyrosine metabolism: implications for screening for phenylketonuria. Am J Dis Child 1983;137:427–432.
18. Sepe SJ, Levy HL, Mount FW. An evaluation of routine follow-up blood screening of infants for phenylketonuria. N Engl J Med 1979;300:606–609.
19. Newborn Screening Committee, The Council of Regional Networks for Genetic Services (CORN). National Newborn Screening Report—1991. New York: CORN, July 1994.
20. Lidsky A, Guttler F, Woo S. Prenatal diagnosis of phenylketonuria by DNA analysis. Lancet 1985;1: 549–551.
21. Wulff K, Wehnert M, Schutz M, et al. Prenatal diagnosis of phenylketonuria by haplotype analysis. Prenat Diagn 1989;9:421–425.
22. Guttler F. Impact of medical genetics concerning phenylketonuria: accomplishments, status, and practical future possibilities. Clin Genet 1989;36:333–334.
23. Dockhorn-Dworniczak B, Dworniczak B, Brommelkamp L, et al. Non-isotopic detection of single strand conformation polymorphism (PCR-SSCP): a rapid and sensitive technique in the diagnosis of phenylketonuria. Nucleic Acids Res 1991;19:2500.
24. MacCready RA, Levy HL. The problem of maternal phenylketonuria. Am J Obstet Gynecol 1972;123:121–128.
25. Levy HL, Waisbren SE. Effects of untreated maternal phenylketonuria and hyperphenylalaninemia in the fetus. N Engl J Med 1983;309:1269–1274.

26. Berman PW, Waisman HA, Graham FK. Intelligence in treated phenylketonuric children: a developmental study. Child Dev 1966;37:731–747.
27. Hudson FP, Mordaunt VL, Leahy I. Evaluation of treatment begun in first three months of life in 184 cases of phenylketonuria. Arch Dis Child 1970;45:5–12.
28. Williamson ML, Koch R, Azen C, et al. Correlates of intelligence test results in treated phenylketonuric children. Pediatrics 1981;68:161–167.
29. Hsia DY. Phenylketonuria 1967. Dev Med Child Neurol 1967;9:531–540.
30. Azen CG, Koch R, Friedman EG, et al. Intellectual development in 12-year-old children treated for phenylketonuria. Am J Dis Child 1991;145:35–39.
31. Koch R, Yusin M, Fishler K. Successful adjustment to society by adults with phenylketonuria. J Inherit Metab Dis 1985;8:209–211.
32. Waisbren SE, Mahon BE, Schnell RR, et al. Predictors of intelligence quotient and intelligence quotient change in persons treated for phenylketonuria early in life. Pediatrics 1987;79:351–355.
33. Holtzman NA, Kronmal RA, van Doorninck W, et al. Effect of age at loss of dietary control on intellectual performance and behavior of children with phenylketonuria. N Engl J Med 1986;314:593–598.
34. Hackney IM, Hanley WB, Davidson W, et al. Phenylketonuria: mental development, behavior, and termination of low phenylalanine diet. J Pediatr 1968;72:646–655.
35. Seashore MR, Friedman E, Novelly R, et al. Loss of intellectual function in children with phenylketonuria after relaxation of dietary phenylalanine restriction. Pediatrics 1985;75:226–232.
36. Thompson AJ, Smith I, Brenton D, et al. Neurological deterioration in young adults with phenylketonuria. Lancet 1990;336:602–605.
37. Smith I, Beasley MG, Ades A. Effect on intelligence of relaxing the low phenylalanine diet in phenylketonuria. Arch Dis Child 1990;65:311–316.
38. Pennington BF, van Doorninck WJ, McCabe LL, et al. Neuropsychological deficits in early treated phenylketonuric children. Am J Ment Defic 1985;5:467–474.
39. Smith I, Beasley MG, Wolff OH, et al. Behavior disturbance in 8-year-old children with early treated phenylketonuria. Report from the MRC/DHHS Phenylketonuria Register. J Pediatr 1988;112: 403–408.
40. Faust D, Libon D, Pueschel S. Neuropsychological functioning in treated phenylketonuria. Int J Psych Med 1986–87;16:169–177.
41. Platt LD, Koch R, Azen C, et al. Maternal phenylketonuria collaborative study, obstetric aspects and outcome: the first six years. Am J Obstet Gynecol 1992;166:1150–1162.
42. Matalon R, Michals K, Azen C, et al. Maternal PKU collaborative study: the effect of nutrient intake on pregnancy outcome. J Inherit Metab Dis 1991;14:371–374.
43. Lenke RR, Levy HL. Maternal phenylketonuria: results of dietary therapy. Am J Obstet Gynecol 1982;142:548–553.
44. Murphy D, Saul I, Kirby M. Maternal PKU and phenylalanine-restricted diet: studies of seven pregnancies and of offspring produced. Ir J Med Sci 1985;154:66–70.
45. Scott TM, Fyfe WM, Hart DM. Maternal phenylketonuria: abnormal baby despite low phenylalanine diet during pregnancy. Arch Dis Child 1980;55:634–637.
46. Koch R, Hanley W, Levy H, et al. A preliminary report of the collaborative study of maternal phenylketonuria in the United States and Canada. J Inherit Metab Dis 1990;13:641–650.
47. Smith I, Glossop J, Beasley M. Fetal damage due to maternal phenylketonuria: effects of dietary treatment and maternal phenylalanine concentrations around the time of conception. J Inherit Metab Dis 1990;13:651–657.
48. Rohr FJ, Doherty LB, Waisbren SE, et al. The New England Maternal PKU Project: prospective study of untreated and treated pregnancies and their outcomes. J Pediatr 1987;110:391–398.
49. Koch R, Levy HL, Matalon R, et al. The North American Collaborative Study of Maternal Phenylketonuria. Status report 1993. Am J Dis Child 1993;147:1224–1230.
50. Committee on Genetics, American Academy of Pediatrics. Issues in newborn screening. Pediatrics 1992; 89:345–349.
51. American Academy of Family Physicians. Age charts for periodic health examination. Kansas City, MO: American Academy of Family Physicians, 1994. (Reprint no. 510.)
52. American Academy of Pediatrics and American College of Obstetricians and Gynecologists. Guidelines for perinatal care. 3rd ed. Washington, DC: American College of Obstetricians and Gynecologists, 1992.
53. Green M, ed. Bright Futures: guidelines for health supervision of infants, children, and adolescents. Arlington, VA: National Center for Education in Maternal and Child Health, 1994.

54. Canadian Task Force on the Periodic Health Examination. Canadian guide to clinical preventive health care. Ottawa: Canada Communication Group, 1994:180–188.

55. The American College of Obstetricians and Gynecologists. Standards for obstetric-gynecologic services. 7th ed. Washington, DC: The American College of Obstetricians and Gynecologists, 1989.

56. Committee on Genetics, American Academy of Pediatrics. Maternal phenylketonuria. Pediatrics 1991;88: 1284–1285.

45. Screening for Congenital Hypothyroidism

RECOMMENDATION

Screening for congenital hypothyroidism with thyroid function tests on dried-blood spot specimens is recommended for all newborns in the first week of life (see *Clinical Intervention*).

Burden of Suffering

In the U.S., congenital hypothyroidism occurs in 1 of 3,600–4,000 infants.[1,2] Clinical diagnosis occurs in <5% of newborns with hypothyroidism because symptoms and signs are often minimal.[1] Without prompt treatment, most affected children gradually develop growth failure, irreversible mental retardation, and a variety of neuropsychologic deficits, comprising the syndrome of cretinism.[1,2] These complications have become rare since the introduction in the 1970s of routine neonatal screening and early treatment of congenital hypothyroidism.

Accuracy of Screening Tests

In the U.S., screening for congenital hypothyroidism in neonates is almost always done by the radioimmunoassay of serum thyroxine (T_4) and thyroid-stimulating hormone (TSH) from dried-blood spot specimens collected by heelstick and adsorbed onto filter paper.[3,4] Laboratories in most of the U.S. measure T_4 on all specimens, and TSH only if the T_4 level is low; in several states, most of Europe, and elsewhere in the world, TSH is the initial screening test.[3,5] Simultaneous measurement of both T_4 and TSH has greater sensitivity for congenital hypothyroidism than either of the two sequential methods currently used,[6] but it is not considered cost-effective by most programs at this time.[5,7] The T_4 assay appears to have greater precision and reproducibility than the TSH assay, but false-negative rates are similar with the two methods.[6] Both types of screening may miss the 3–5% of cases of congenital hypothyroidism that are caused by pituitary dysfunction, as well as the 3–14% of cases in which patients present with hypothyroxinemia and delayed TSH elevation.[8–10] The primary T_4-supplemental TSH approach also misses some patients with residual thyroid tissue (i.e., ectopic gland) that results in initially normal T_4

with elevated TSH; sensitivity for these cases can be improved by repeat screening at 2–6 weeks.[11] Using a higher cutoff point to define abnormal T_4 results in fewer false negatives due to these biologic factors. In one population, using a cutoff of the lowest 5% of T_4 values to define "low" missed 3.5% of cases, whereas using the lowest 10% resulted in 1.5% being missed.[12] Only 0.2% of cases were missed using the lowest 20% as a cutoff, but at substantially increased cost in terms of repeat testing.

False negatives also occur due to screening errors. Such failures occur in specimen collection, laboratory procedures (e.g., failure to record an abnormal result), or follow-up.[13] Standards for adequate blood collection on filter paper for neonatal screening programs have been published.[13a] Infants at increased risk for false negatives from screening errors include those born at home, ill at birth, or transferred between hospitals early in life.[2] In North America, an estimated 6–12% of neonates with congenital hypothyroidism are not detected in screening programs as a result of biologic factors or screening errors.[8,13]

In established U.S. screening programs, there are 4–8 false positives for every proven case,[8] although follow-up testing readily corrects these. Screening with primary TSH instead of T_4-supplemental TSH may result in fewer false-positive tests.[8,14] False-positive results are more likely when screening is done in the first 24–48 hours of life, since normal TSH values in the first 2 days of life may exceed the standard cutoff used by most programs.[15] Evidence for long-term adverse psychologic effects from falsely positive screening test results is limited by methodologic flaws.[16–19]

Effectiveness of Early Detection

Most cases of congenital hypothyroidism present clinically during the first year of life.[20] Retrospective studies of patients with congenital hypothyroidism have reported that delay of diagnosis and treatment beyond the first 1–3 months of life is likely to result in irreversible neuropsychologic deficits.[21–25] More recent prospective studies show that screening neonates and treating affected infants within the first weeks of life results, on average, in normal or near-normal intellectual performance and growth at ages 5–12 years.[26–34] These children appear to have somewhat lower cognitive and motor development compared to sibling or classmate controls, however, and continue to manifest subtle deficits in language, perception, and motor skills.[27,28,31–35] Both age at onset of therapy and quality of therapeutic control achieved during the first year of life affect long-term intellectual outcome, supportive evidence for a benefit from earlier detection and treatment.[27,28,31–33,35] The reduced incidence of severe neuropsychologic effects observed with early, adequate treatment has prompted most Western governments to require routine screening for all neonates.

Screening at birth may, in fact, occur too late to prevent important neurodevelopmental deficits in some infants. Observational studies suggest that infants affected more severely in utero, as evidenced by greater delay in bone age at diagnosis, lower T_4 at screening, or a diagnosis of thyroid agenesis, have significantly poorer developmental outcomes compared to those with milder disease or to normal controls, even when detected and treated in the newborn period.[28,31-36]

Recommendations of Other Groups

Screening of newborns for hypothyroidism is offered in all states, but mandated in 46 states and the District of Columbia.[3] Five states and the District of Columbia require or strongly recommend a routine second screening test, from 1 to 4 weeks later.[3] Screening is recommended by the Canadian Task Force on the Periodic Health Examination,[37] the American Academy of Family Physicians,[38] Bright Futures,[39] and jointly by the American Academy of Pediatrics and the American Thyroid Association.[5]

Discussion

The natural history of congenital hypothyroidism has changed dramatically since newborn screening was instituted in this country.[2] Before screening was available, many children with this disorder were at least moderately, and sometimes profoundly, retarded, while recent prospective studies have demonstrated normal or near-normal intelligence in virtually all of those detected by screening and treated early in life. There is thus good evidence to support screening for congenital hypothyroidism in the newborn.

CLINICAL INTERVENTION

Screening for congenital hypothyroidism with thyroid function tests performed on dried-blood spot specimens is recommended for all newborns, optimally between days 2 and 6, but in all cases before newborn nursery discharge ("A" recommendation). Blood specimens should be collected by heelstick, adsorbed onto filter paper, and air dried using standard technique.[13a] The choice of which thyroid function test or tests to perform is generally determined by individual state requirements.[3] Testing procedures and follow-up treatment for abnormal results should follow current guidelines.[5] Care should be taken to ensure that those born at home, ill at birth, or transferred between hospitals in the first week of life are appropriately screened before 7 days of age. Normal newborn screening results should not preclude appropriate evaluation of infants presenting with clinical symptoms and signs suggestive of hypothyroidism.

The draft update of this chapter was prepared for the U.S. Preventive Services Task Force by Carolyn DiGuiseppi, MD, MPH.

REFERENCES

1. Committee on Genetics, American Academy of Pediatrics. Newborn screening fact sheets. Pediatrics 1989;83: 449–464.
2. Willi SM, Moshang T Jr. Diagnostic dilemmas: results of screening tests for congenital hypothyroidism. Pediatr Clin North Am 1991;38:555–566.
3. Newborn Screening Committee, The Council of Regional Networks for Genetic Services (CORN). National newborn screening report: 1991. New York: CORN, July 1994.
4. Therrell BL Jr, ed. Laboratory methods for neonatal screening. Washington, DC: American Public Health Association, 1993.
5. American Academy of Pediatrics and American Thyroid Association. Newborn screening for congenital hypothyroidism: recommended guidelines. Pediatrics 1993;91:1203–1209.
6. Dussault JH, Morissette J. Higher sensitivity of primary thyrotropin in screening for congenital hypothyroidism: a myth? J Clin Endocrinol Metab 1983;56:849–852.
7. Gruters A, Delange F, Giovanelli G, et al. Guidelines for neonatal screening programs for congenital hypothyroidism. European Society for Pediatric Endocrinology Working Group on Congenital Hypothyroidism. Horm Res 1994;41: 1–2.
8. Fisher DA. Effectiveness of newborn screening programs for congenital hypothyroidism: prevalence of missed cases. Pediatr Clin North Am 1987;34:881–890.
9. Hanna CE, Krainz PL, Skeels MR, et al. Detection of congenital hypopituitary hypothyroidism: ten-year experience in the Northwest Regional Screening Program. J Pediatr 1986;10:959–964.
10. de Zegher F, Vanderschueren-Lodeweyckx M, Heinrichs C, et al. Thyroid dyshormonogenesis: severe hypothyroidism after normal neonatal thyroid stimulating hormone screening. Acta Paediatr 1992;81:274–276.
11. LaFranchi SH, Hanna CE, Krainz PL, et al. Screening for congenital hypothyroidism with specimen collection at two time periods: results of the Northwest Regional Screening Program. Pediatrics 1985;76:734–740.
12. Verkerk PH, Buitendijk SE, Verloove-Vanhorick SP. Congenital hypothyroidism screening and the cutoff for thyrotropin measurement: recommendations from the Netherlands. Am J Public Health 1993;83:868–871.
13. Holtzman C, Slazyk WE, Cordero JF, et al. Descriptive epidemiology of missed cases of phenylketonuria and congenital hypothyroidism. Pediatrics 1986;78:553–558.
13a. National Committee for Clinical Laboratory Standards. Blood collection on filter paper for neonatal screening programs, 2nd ed; approved standard. Vol 12 no 13. Villanova, PA: NCCLS, 1992. (NCCLS document LA4-A2.)
14. Pharoah POD, Madden MP. Audit of screening for congenital hypothyroidism. Arch Dis Child 1992;67:1073–1076.
15. Allen DB, Sieger JE, Litsheim T, et al. Age-adjusted thyrotropin criteria for neonatal screening for hypothyroidism. J Pediatr 1990;117:309–312.
16. Fyro K, Bodegard G. Four-year follow-up of psychological reactions to false positive screening tests for congenital hypothyroidism. Acta Paediatr Scand 1987;76:107–114.
17. Fyro K, Bodegard G. Difficulties in psychological adjustment to a new neonatal screening programme. Acta Paediatr Scand 1988;77:226–231.
18. Bodegard G, Fyro K, Larsson A. Psychological reactions in 102 families with a newborn who has a falsely positive screening test for congenital hypothyroidism. Acta Paediatr Scand 1983;304 (suppl):1–21.
19. Fisher DA, Dussault JH, Foley TP, et al. Screening for congenital hypothyroidism: results of screening one million North American infants. J Pediatr 1979;94:700–705.
20. Alm J, Larsson A, Zetterstrom R. Congenital hypothyroidism in Sweden: incidence and age at diagnosis. Acta Paediatr Scand 1978;67:1–3.
21. Raiti S, Newns GH. Cretinism: early diagnosis and its relation to mental prognosis. Arch Dis Child 1971;46:692–694.
22. Alm J, Larsson A, Zetterstrom R. Congenital hypothyroidism in Sweden. Psychomotor development in patients detected by clinical signs and symptoms. Acta Paediatr Scand 1981;70:907–912.
23. Hulse JA. Outcome for congenital hypothyroidism. Arch Dis Child 1984;59:23–29.
24. Klein AH, Meltzer S, Kenny FM. Improved prognosis in congenital hypothyroidism treated before age three months. J Pediatr 1972;81:912–915.

25. Alm J, Hagenfeldt L, Larsson A, et al. Incidence of congenital hypothyroidism: retrospective study of neonatal laboratory screening versus clinical symptoms as indicators leading to diagnosis. BMJ 1984; 289:1171–1175.
26. New England Congenital Hypothyroidism Collaborative. Elementary school performance of children with congenital hypothyroidism. J Pediatr 1990;116:27–32.
27. Heyerdahl S, Kase BF, Lie SO. Intellectual development in children with congenital hypothyroidism in relation to recommended thyroxine treatment. J Pediatr 1991;118:850–857.
28. Toublanc JE, Rives S, Acosta A, et al. Le développement psychomoteur et intellectuel chez 52 enfants atteints d'hypothyroidie congénitale dépistée à la naissance: eléments susceptibles d'influer sur le pronostic. Arch Fr Pediatr 1990;47:191–195.
29. Ilicki A, Larsson A. Psychological development at 7 years of age in children with congenital hypothyroidism: timing and dosage of initial treatment. Acta Paediatr Scand 1991;80:199–200.
30. Aronson R, Ehrlich RM, Bailey JD, Rovet JF. Growth in children with congenital hypothyroidism detected by neonatal screening. J Pediatr 1990;116:33–37.
31. Glorieux J, Dussault J, Van Vliet G. Intellectual development at age 12 years of children with congenital hypothyroidism diagnosed by neonatal screening. J Pediatr 1992;121:581–584.
32. Rovet JF, Ehrlich RM, Sorbara DL. Neurodevelopment in infants and preschool children with congenital hypothyroidism: etiological and treatment factors affecting outcome. J Pediatr Psychol 1992; 17:187–213.
33. Kooistra L, Laane C, Vulsma T, et al. Motor and cognitive development in children with congenital hypothyroidism: a long-term evaluation of the effects of neonatal treatment. J Pediatr 1994;124: 903–909.
34. Fuggle PW, Grant DB, Smith I, et al. Intelligence, motor skills and behaviour at 5 years in early-treated congenital hypothyroidism. Eur J Pediatr 1991;150:570–574.
35. Virtanen M, Santavuori P, Hirvonen E, et al. Multivariate analysis of psychomotor development in congenital hypothyroidism. Acta Paediatr Scand 1989;78:405–411.
36. Chiovato L, Giusti L, Tonacchera M, et al. Evaluation of l-thyroxine replacement therapy in children with congenital hypothyroidism. J Endocrinol Invest 1991;14:957–964.
37. Canadian Task Force on the Periodic Health Examination. Canadian guide to clinical preventive health care. Ottawa: Canada Communication Group, 1994:190–194.
38. American Academy of Family Physicians. Age charts for periodic health examination. Kansas City, MO: American Academy of Family Physicians, 1994. (Reprint no. 510.)
39. Green M, ed. Bright Futures: guidelines for health supervision of infants, children and adolescents. Arlington VA: National Center for Education in Maternal and Child Health, 1994.

46. Screening for Postmenopausal Osteoporosis

RECOMMENDATION

There is insufficient evidence to recommend for or against routine screening for osteoporosis with bone densitometry in postmenopausal women. Recommendations against routine screening may be made on other grounds (see *Clinical Intervention*). All postmenopausal women should be counseled about hormone prophylaxis (see Chapter 68) and be advised of the importance of smoking cessation, regular exercise, and adequate calcium intake (see Chapters 54–56). For those high-risk women who would consider estrogen prophylaxis only to prevent osteoporosis, screening may be appropriate to assist treatment decisions (see *Clinical Intervention*).

Burden of Suffering

An estimated 1.3 million osteoporosis-related fractures occur each year in the U.S.[1] About 70% of fractures in persons aged 45 or older are types that are related to osteoporosis.[2] Most of these injuries occur in postmenopausal women. Over half of all postmenopausal women will develop a spontaneous fracture as a result of osteoporosis.[3] It has been estimated that about one quarter of all women over age 60 develop vertebral deformities and about 15% of women sustain hip fractures during their lifetime.[4,5] The annual cost of osteoporosis-related fractures in the U.S. has been estimated to be over $8 billion in direct and indirect costs.[6] Most fractures in elderly women are due in part to low bone mass; osteoporosis-related fractures commonly involve the proximal femur, vertebral body, and distal forearm.[7] Of these sites, the proximal femur (hip) has the greatest effect on morbidity and mortality; there is a 15–20% reduction in expected survival in the first year following a hip fracture.[8] Hip fractures are also associated with significant pain, disability, and decreased functional independence.[9] Among persons living at home at the time of a hip fracture, about half experience a deterioration in social function within 2.5 years.[10]

Low bone density is strongly associated with an increased risk of fracture.[11] By one estimate, a 50-year-old woman in the 10th percentile of bone density has a 25% lifetime risk of hip fracture (vs. 8% for those in the 90th percentile).[12] A World Health Organization study group has recommended that osteoporosis be defined as a bone density more than 2.5 standard deviations (SD) below the normal bone mass in young women, and that osteopenia (low bone mass) be defined as bone density 1–2.5 SD below the normal mean.[13] Risk of postmenopausal osteoporosis is a function of rate of bone loss as well as peak bone mass. The principal risk factors for osteoporosis are female sex, advanced age, Caucasian race, low body weight, and bilateral oophorectomy before menopause.[1,4] Other historical risk factors such as parity, lactation history, and caffeine intake have been shown to be poor predictors of bone mass.[14–16] Smoking is a probable risk factor for hip fracture, but it is a less reliable predictor of bone mass.[17] The lower weight and poorer health of smokers compared to nonsmokers may be responsible for the associations between smoking and bone mass and fracture risk.[18]

Accuracy of Screening Tests

A number of radiologic screening tests have been proposed for both clinical and research purposes to detect low bone mass in asymptomatic persons. These include conventional skeletal radiographs, quantitated computed tomography, single photon absorptiometry, dual photon absorptiometry, and dual energy x-ray absorptiometry. Although skeletal x-rays can detect focal bone disorders and fractures, they do not reliably detect bone loss of less than 20–30%, and they are of limited value in estimating bone mass.[19] The other techniques vary in their availability, cost, and convenience, and provide measures expressed as bone mineral content (BMC) in grams/cm, or as bone mineral density (BMD) in grams/cm^2.

Single photon absorptiometry (SPA), in which radioisotopes are the photon source, can measure BMC or BMD in cortical bone in the radius or calcaneus.[20] Dual photon absorptiometry (DPA), dual energy x-ray absorptiometry (DXA), and quantitative computed tomography (QCT) provide direct measures of BMD and are most useful in evaluating the trabecular bone density in locations beneath large amounts of soft tissue (e.g., lumbar vertebrae, proximal femur). DPA and DXA use radioisotopes (DPA) or x-rays (DXA) to emit photons at two different energy levels, thereby correcting for the effect produced by layers of soft tissues.[20–22] DXA is now widely used in the clinical setting, and provides more reproducible measures of bone density, with shorter examination times (5–10 vs. 20–40 minutes) than DPA.[20–22] The precision of DXA (variation in results on repeated measurement) is about 0.5–2%, compared to 1.5–4.0% for DPA.[23] Current data on the performance of these devices have been obtained primarily at specialized research centers, however. Most experts agree that DXA is a safe, accurate, and precise modality for measuring bone density that may be useful in the clinical setting.[24] Reproducibility of SPA is similar to DPA and DXA, but the cost per scan is significantly lower than DXA. Evidence suggests that SPA of the radius or calcaneus is also predictive for future risk of nonspine fracture.[25]

QCT is highly accurate in examining the anatomy and density of transverse sections and trabecular regions within the spine, but it is less practical as a routine screening test due to cost and higher radiation exposure. Ultrasound technology for assessing bone density and architecture is under development and may be of value in the future. Other screening tests under investigation include biochemical markers of bone turnover, which may be able to identify those women who will develop more significant bone loss.[26]

Effectiveness of Early Detection

There is little evidence from controlled trials that women who receive bone density screening have better outcomes (improved bone density or fewer fractures) than women who are not screened. The primary argument for screening is based on evidence that postmenopausal women with low bone density are at increased risk for subsequent fractures of the hip, vertebrae, and wrist,[27–35] and that interventions can slow the decline in bone density after menopause.

Prospective cohort studies have demonstrated the dose-response relationship between BMD and fracture risk.[11,36,37] In 2-year follow-up of 8,134 women over 65, annual risk of hip fracture for women in the lowest quartile of femoral neck BMD was approximately 1%, almost twice that of women in the second lowest quartile and more than 8 times that of women in the highest quartile.[11] Various studies have estimated that each standard deviation decrease in BMC or BMD is associated with a 1.5–2.8-fold increase in risk of fracture.[38] There are no studies, however, determining how well perimenopausal bone density predicts long-term risk of fracture. Because the rate of postmenopausal bone loss varies among women, bone mass at menopause correlates only moderately with bone mass 10–20 years later, when most fractures occur.[39]

Randomized trials have demonstrated that calcium supplementation and estrogen are effective in preserving bone density in postmenopausal women.[40–43] Due to the long delay between menopause and fracture, few prospective studies have been able to demonstrate directly that these interventions reduce fractures. Calcium plus vitamin D reduced hip fractures among very elderly women in France (mean age 84).[43] In a randomized trial in healthy postmenopausal women, calcium supplementation slowed bone loss and significantly reduced symptomatic fractures over 4 years.[43a] Numerous observational and nonrandomized experimental studies suggest that risk of fracture can be reduced 25–50% by estrogen replacement therapy (see Chapter 68). The benefits of hormone prophylaxis on bone mass and fracture risk appear greatest with treatment begun close to menopause (before the period of rapid bone loss), and continued for longer periods (>5 years). Benefits appear to wane after stopping estrogen.[44] As a result, preventing fractures in older postmenopausal women may require continuing hormone therapy indefinitely. Other agents that inhibit bone resorption (e.g., calcitonin, bisphosphonates) or stimulate bone formation (e.g., sodium fluoride) can preserve or increase bone mass, but their use in asymptomatic persons remains investigational.[40]

There is limited evidence that screening influences treatment decisions, and that women appreciate the more precise estimates of risk provided by BMD measurement. Women who had below average bone density were more likely to take calcium, vitamins, or estrogen than those with above average values (84% vs. 38%) in one study.[45] Compared to the low rates of compliance with hormone therapy in average women (see Chapter 68), 60% of women with low bone density detected by screening were still taking hormone therapy 8 months after screening.[46] The effect of BMD screening on long-term compliance is not known.

There are several important limitations to screening as a means of preventing fractures. In a single measure of bone density, there is a small risk of inaccurate values, and there is no value of BMD that discriminates well between patients who develop a fracture and those who do not.[44] Other risk factors that independently influence falls or bone strength may be more important than low BMD for identifying older women at high risk of fracture. In a prospective study of over 9,500 women over 65, the presence of multiple risk factors (e.g., age ≥80, fair/poor health, limited physical activity, poor vision, prior postmenopausal fracture, psychotropic drug use, among others) was a much stronger predictor of hip fracture than low bone density: incidence of first hip fracture in women with 5 or more risk factors was 19/1,000 woman-years versus 1.1/1,000 in women with two or fewer risk factors.[18] Screening perimenopausal women is less predictive of risk later in life, and even women with "normal" bone density are likely to benefit from measures to prevent postmenopausal bone loss. Equally important, there is no consensus on what interventions are indicated for any particular level of bone density. Hygienic measures such as adequate calcium and vitamin D intake, exercise, and smoking cessation can be recommended irrespective of bone density. The decision to begin estrogen, in contrast, often depends on factors other than risk of osteoporosis (see Chapter 68).

Screening could have adverse effects, if it leads to "labeling" in patients diagnosed with osteopenia or osteoporosis, or false reassurance in those with normal bone density. In one study of women referred for screening, women with low bone density were more likely to restrict their activities, and those with normal bone density were less likely to follow routine hygienic measures to prevent osteoporosis (e.g., calcium or vitamin D).[45] Interpreting and explaining the values obtained is complex and may require considerable time for patient counseling about the significance of an abnormal bone density. Although the absolute benefit of preserving bone mass may be greatest in women with low bone density, the overall balance of risks and benefits of hormone therapy in an individual patient is likely to depend on other factors.[39] If estrogen therapy is likely to be recommended on other grounds, the clinical usefulness of routine screening is limited.[47] If other more specific and expensive therapeutic modalities (e.g., bisphosphonates, calcitonin) are shown to be effective in reducing fractures in asymptomatic high-risk women, however, this may increase the role of screening to identify appropriate candidates for treatment.

Recommendations of Other Groups

Recommendations against routine radiologic screening for osteoporosis have been issued by the Canadian Task Force on the Periodic Health Examination[18] and the American College of Physicians (ACP)[48]; updated ACP guidelines are due out in 1996. Both of these organizations and a World Health Organization study group[49] concluded, however, that bone density measurements may be useful to guide treatment decisions in selected postmenopausal women considering hormone replacement therapy. The American Academy of Family Physicians recommends measuring BMC in women 40–64 years old with risk factors for osteoporosis (e.g., Caucasians, bilateral oophorectomy before menopause, slender build) and in women for whom estrogen replacement therapy would otherwise not be recommended; these recommendations are under review.[50] The American College of Obstetricians and Gynecologists does not recommend routine screening for osteoporosis.[51] The National Osteoporosis Foundation is in the process of revising its guidelines for screening for osteoporosis.[20]

Discussion

Routine bone densitometry of all postmenopausal women is likely to be time-consuming and very expensive. Screening times vary from 5–15 minutes for SPA and DXA to 20–45 minutes for QCT and DPA.[24] Average costs of screening have been estimated to be $75 with SPA, $75–100 with DXA, $100–150 with DPA, and $100–200 with QCT.[23,24] The costs and inconvenience of screening may be justified if screening reduces the burden of osteoporosis, but further research is necessary to demonstrate both the clinical effectiveness and cost-effectiveness of different screening and treatment strategies.[40,52]

Although routine screening may not be appropriate for asymptomatic women, measurement of bone density may be useful for identifying persons at high risk of fracture who might not otherwise consider effective treatments such as estrogen. Measures of bone density provide more reliable estimates of risk than clinical assessment, and they may help both the patient and the clinician make more informed decisions about the potential benefits and risks of therapies such as estrogen.[45] Women who have been identified as having low bone density may be more likely to take estrogen and comply with other preventive measures, but the effect of screening on long-term outcomes (compliance with therapy, bone density, or fracture) has not been adequately studied. The net benefit of screening may be small if high-risk women do not continue long-term therapy, or if screening causes those with normal BMD to forego preventive measures. There is little reason for screening if the information is not likely to influence decisions by the patient or provider. For most women, osteoporosis prevention is only one of many factors that go into the decision whether or not to take estrogen.

CLINICAL INTERVENTION

There is insufficient evidence to recommend for or against screening for osteoporosis or decreased bone density in asymptomatic, postmenopausal women ("C" recommendation). Recommendations against routine screening may be made on the grounds of the inconvenience and high cost of bone densitometry, and lack of universally accepted criteria for initiating treatment based on bone density measurements. All perimenopausal and postmenopausal women should be counseled about the potential benefits and risks of hormone prophylaxis (see Chapter 68). Although direct evidence of benefit is not available, selective screening may be appropriate for high-risk women who would consider hormone prophylaxis only if they knew they were at high risk for osteoporosis or fracture.

All women should also receive counseling regarding universal preventive measures related to fracture risk, such as dietary calcium and vitamin D intake (Chapter 56), weight-bearing exercise (Chapter 55), and smoking cessation (Chapter 54). Elderly persons should also receive counseling regarding preventive measures to reduce the risk of falls and the severity of fall-related injuries (Chapter 58).

The draft update of this chapter was prepared for the U.S. Preventive Services Task Force by Robert B. Wallace, MD, MPH, Denise Tonner, MD, and David Atkins, MD, MPH.

REFERENCES

 1. National Institutes of Health. Consensus conference: osteoporosis. JAMA 1984;252:799–802.
 2. Iskrant AP, Smith RW Jr. Osteoporosis in women 45 and over related to subsequent fractures. Public Health Rep 1969;84:33–38.
 3. Christiansen C, Riis BJ, Ridbro P. Prediction of rapid bone loss in postmenopausal women. Lancet 1987;1:1105–1108.
 4. Cummings SR, Kelsey JL, Nevitt C, et al. Epidemiology of osteoporosis and osteoporotic fractures. Epidemiol Rev 1985;7:178–208.
 5. Melton LJ III. Epidemiology of fractures. In: Riggs BL, Melton LJ III, eds. Osteoporosis: etiology, diagnosis, and management. New York: Raven Press, 1988.
 6. Peck WA, Riggs BL, Bell NH, Wallace RB, Johnston CC Jr, Gordon SL, Shulman LE. Research directions in osteoporosis. Am J Med 1991;84:275–282.
 7. Seeley DG, Browner WS, Nevitt MC, et al. Which fractures are associated with low appendicular bone mass in elderly women? Ann Intern Med 1991;115:837–842.
 8. Jensen GF, Christiansen C, Boesen J, et al. Epidemiology of postmenopausal spinal and long bone fractures: a unifying approach to postmenopausal osteoporosis. Clin Orthop 1982;166:75–81.
 9. Chrischilles EA, Butler CD, Davis CS, et al. A model of lifetime osteoporosis impact. Arch Intern Med 1991;151: 2026–2032.
10. Jensen JS, Baggar J. Long term social prognosis after hip fractures. Acta Orthop Scand 1982:53:97–101.
11. Cummings SR, Black DM, Nevitt MC, et al. Bone density at various sites for prediction of hip fractures. Lancet 1993; 341:72–75.
12. Black DM, Cummings SR, Melton LJ. Appendicular bone mineral and a woman's lifetime risk of hip fracture. J Bone Min Res 1992;7:639–646.
13. Kanis JA, Melton LJ, Christiansen C, et al. The diagnosis of osteoporosis. J Bone Min Res 1994;8:1137–1141.
14. Kelsey JL, Browner WE, Seeley DSG, et al. Risk factors for fractures of the distal forearm and proximal humerus. Am J Epidemiol 1992;135:477–489.
15. van Hemert AM, Vanderbroucke JP, Birkenhager JC, et al. Prediction of osteoporotic fractures in the general population by a fracture risk score. Am J Epidemiol 1990;132:123–135.
16. Cooper C, Shah S, Hand DJ (The Multicentre Vertebral Fracture Study Group). Screening for vertebral osteoporosis using individual risk factors. Osteoporosis Int 1991:2:48–53.
17. Slemenda CW, Hui SL, Longcope C, et al. Predictors of bone mass in perimenopausal women. Ann Intern Med 1990;112:96–101.
18. Cummings SR, Nevitt MC, Browner WS, et al. Risk factors for hip fracture in white women. N Engl J Med 1995;332: 767–773.
19. Canadian Task Force on the Periodic Health Examination. Canadian guide to clinical preventive health care. Ottawa: Canada Communication Group, 1994:620–631.
20. Johnston CC, Melton LJ, Lindsay R, et al. Clinical indications for bone mass measurement. A report from the Scientific Advisory Board of the National Osteoporosis Foundation. J Bone Min Res 1989; 4 (Suppl 2):1–28.
21. Johnston CC, Slemenda CW, Melton LJ. Clinical use of bone densitometry. N Engl J Med 1991;324:1105–1109.
22. Wahner HW, Dunn WL, Brown ML, et al. Comparison of dual energy absorptiometry and dual photon absorptiometry for bone mineral measurements of the lumbar spine. Mayo Clin Proc 1988;63:1075–1084.
23. Johnston CC, Slemenda CW. Measuring bone density and what it means. Endocrinologist 1991;1:83–87.
24. Kellie SE. Diagnostic and therapeutic technology assessment (DATTA). JAMA 1992;267:286–294.
25. Black DM, Cummings SR, Genant HK, et al. Axial and appendicular bone density predict fractures in older women. J Bone Min Res 1992;7:633–638.
26. Hansen MA, Kirsten O, Riis BJ, et al. Role of peak bone mass and bone loss in postmenopausal osteoporosis. BMJ 1991;303:961–964.
27. Krolner B, Nielsen SP. Bone mineral content of the lumbar spine in normal and osteoporotic women: cross-sectional and longitudinal studies. Clin Sci 1982;62:329–336.
28. Cann CE, Genant HK, Folb FO, et al. Quantitated computed tomography for prediction of vertebral fracture risk. Bone 1985;6:1–7.
29. Firooznia H, Golimbu C, Rafii M, et al. Quantitated computed tomography assessment of spinal trabecular bone. II. In osteoporotic women with and without vertebral fractures. J Comput Tomogr 1984;8:99–103.

30. Wasnich RD, Ross PD, Heilburn LK, et al. Prediction of postmenopausal fracture risk with use of bone mineral measurements. Am J Obstet Gynecol 1985;153:745–751.

31. Nillson BE, Westlin NE. The bone mineral content in the forearm of women with Colles' fracture. Acta Orthop Scand 1974;45:836–844.

32. Cummings S. Are patients with hip fractures more osteoporotic? Review of the evidence. Am J Med 1985;78:487–494.

33. Melton W, Wahner HW, Richelson LS, et al. Osteoporosis and the risk of hip fracture. Am J Epidemiol 1986;124:254–261.

34. Riggs BL, Wahner HW, Dunn WL, et al. Differential changes in bone mineral density of the appendicular and axial skeleton with aging. J Clin Invest 1981;67:328–335.

35. Ross PD, Davis JW, Epstein RS, et al. Pre-existing fractures and bone mass predict vertebral fracture incidence in women. Ann Intern Med 1991;114:919–923.

36. Hui SL, Slemenda CW, Johnston CC Jr. Age and bone mass as predictors of fracture in a prospective study. J Clin Invest 1988;81:1804–1809.

37. Gardsell P, Johnell O, Nilsson BE. The predictive value of bone loss for fragility fractures in women: a longitudinal study over 15 years. Calcif Tissue Int 1991;49:90–94.

38. Ross P, Davis J, Vagel J, et al. A critical review of bone mass and the risk of fractures in osteoporosis. Calcif Tissue Int 1990;46:149–161.

39. Cummings SR, Browner WS, Ettinger B. Should prescription of postmenopausal hormone therapy be based on the results of bone densitometry? Ann Intern Med 1990;113:565–567.

40. Riggs BL, Melton LJ. The prevention and treatment of osteoporosis. N Engl J Med 1992;327:620–627.

41. Cumming RG. Calcium intake and bone mass: a quantitative review of the evidence. Calcif Tissue Int 1990;47:194–201.

42. Aloia JH, Vaswani A, Yeh J, et al. Calcium supplementation with and without hormone replacement therapy to prevent postmenopausal bone loss. Ann Intern Med 1994;120:97–103.

43. Chapuy MC, Arlot ME, Delmas PD, et al. Effect of calcium and cholecalciferol treatment for three years on hip fractures in elderly women. BMJ 1994;308:1081–1082.

43a. Reid IR, Ames RW, Evans MC, et al. Long-term effects of calcium supplementation on bone loss and fractures in postmenopausal women: a randomized controlled trial. Am J Med 1995;98:331–335.

44. Law MR, Wald NJ, Meade TW. Strategies for prevention of osteoporosis and hip fracture. BMJ 1991;303:453–459.

45. Rubin SM, Cummings SR. Results of bone densitometry affect women's decisions about taking measures to prevent fractures. Ann Intern Med 1992;116:990–995.

46. Ryan PJ, Harrison R, Blake GM, et al. I. Compliance with hormone replacement therapy (HRT) after screening for postmenopausal osteoporosis. Br J Obstet Gynaecol 1992;99:325–328.

47. Hall FM, Davis MA, Baran DT. Bone mineral screening for osteoporosis. N Engl J Med 1987;316:212–214.

48. Melton LJ, Eddy DM, Johnston CC. Screening for osteoporosis. Ann Intern Med 1990;112:516–528.

49. Alexeera L, Burkhardt P, Christiansen C, et al. Assessment of fracture risk and application of screening for postmenopausal osteoporosis. World Health Organization Technical Report Series 843. Geneva: World Health Organization, 1994.

50. American Academy of Family Physicians. Age charts for periodic health examination. Kansas City, MO: American Academy of Family Physicians, 1994. (Reprint no. 510.).

51. American College of Obstetricians and Gynecologists. Guidelines for women's health care. Washington, DC: American College of Obstetricians and Gynecologists, 1996.

52. Tosteson AN, Rosenthal DI, Melton LJ, et al. Cost effectiveness of screening perimenopausal white women for osteoporosis: bone densitometry and hormone replacement therapy. Ann Intern Med 1990;113:594–603.

47. Screening for Adolescent Idiopathic Scoliosis

RECOMMENDATION

There is insufficient evidence to recommend for or against routine screening of asymptomatic adolescents for idiopathic scoliosis. Clinicians should remain alert for large spinal curvatures when examining adolescents.

Burden of Suffering

Scoliosis, a lateral spinal curve of 11° or greater, affects an estimated 500,000 adults in the United States.[1] Idiopathic scoliosis accounts for about 65% of cases of structural scoliosis,[2,3] and a large proportion of these cases develop during adolescence. A lateral spinal curve of 11° or greater is present in about 2–3% of adolescents at the end of their growth period. Curves greater than 20° occur in less than 0.5% of adolescents.[4] The potential adverse effects of scoliosis include the progressive development of unpleasant cosmetic deformities, back pain, social and psychological problems during both childhood (e.g., poor self-image, social isolation) and adulthood[5] (e.g., limited job opportunities, lower marriage rate), and the financial costs of treatment.

There is little firm evidence that persons with idiopathic scoliosis are at significantly greater risk of experiencing back complaints than is the general population; most existing epidemiologic studies have lost a large proportion of patients to follow-up and lack adequate statistical power to detect a difference.[6,7] Data on the psychosocial effects of scoliosis and poor cosmesis are also limited. Long-term studies suggest a poor correlation between the location or magnitude of curves and the extent of psychosocial complaints.[6] A number of surveys and uncontrolled long-term studies of scoliosis patients have reported low marriage rates in women and high rates of unemployment, disability, and poor self-esteem,[9–12] but these studies lacked internal control groups, and many patients in the cohorts had spinal conditions other than adolescent idiopathic scoliosis. Persons with severe curves are at increased risk of restrictive pulmonary disease and increased mortality, but such curves are usually early-onset and at least 100–120° in magnitude.[6,12–15] Severe curves of this magnitude have become uncommon in the United States and generally occur only as a consequence of severe, early-onset infantile or juvenile scoliosis.[17]

Only a subset of curves detected through screening are destined to progress to a point of potential clinical significance. The probability that curves will progress more than 5° can vary from 5% to 90%, depending on the patient's age, sex, and skeletal maturity, and the pattern and magnitude of the curve.[18–21] Progression is less likely in older children with greater skeletal maturity and with smaller curves. Depending on the patient population, between 25% and 75% of curves detected on screening may remain unchanged, and 3–12% of curves may improve.[21–24] The reported probability that curves less than 19° will progress is 10% in girls between age 13 and 15 and 4% in children over age 15.[18,19] In curves that progress, one study found that the probability was 34% that the curves would progress more than 10°, 18% that they would progress more than 20°, and 8% that they would progress more than 30°.[21] Another study of patients with untreated curves found that 25% ceased progression before reaching 25° and that 12% ceased progression before reaching 29°.[22]

Accuracy of Screening Tests

The principal screening test for scoliosis is the physical examination of the back, which includes upright visual inspection of the back and the Adams forward-bending test.[25] Patients with abnormal findings on initial physical examination are often then referred for a more thorough physical examination. Some physicians also obtain a standing roentgenogram to measure the degree of curvature (e.g., Cobb angle). Roentgenographic findings serve as the reference standard for estimating the sensitivity and specificity of screening tests. The reported 95% confidence interval for intraobserver and interobserver variability in measuring the Cobb angle on radiographs is 3–5° and 6–7°, respectively.[26,27]

A relatively large proportion of children screened in schools are found to be "positive" on initial examination, but only some of these cases are ultimately found to have scoliosis. In studies of school screening, 11–35% of screened children were classified as positive and were referred for further evaluation; in one study, 37% of those referred for orthopedic evaluation were found to have no abnormality.[24,28] The sensitivity and specificity of the physical examination depend on the skills of the examiner and the degree of spinal curve being sought. In one study, public health nurses with special training in school screening were able to detect all children (sensitivity of 100%) with a Cobb angle greater than 20°. The specificity of the examination was 91%. The sensitivity and specificity of the examination in detecting curves greater than 10° were 73.9% and 77.8%, respectively.[29]

The positive predictive value (PPV) of visual inspection and the forward-bending test varies with the degree of curvature by which a "true positive" is defined, the prevalence of scoliosis in the screened population, and the skills of the examiners. The magnitude of the PPV is inversely related to the degree of curvature used to define scoliosis, since the prevalence of small curves is greater than large curves. In an Australian study, the PPV was 78% for curves greater than 5° in a population with an estimated prevalence for this degree of curvature of 3%.[30] In another study, the PPV was 54% for curves greater than 10° (prevalence of 2%) and 24% for curves greater than 20° (prevalence of 1%). A Canadian study involving specially trained school nurses reported a PPV of 18% in detecting curves greater than 10° (prevalence of 1.7%) and a PPV of 4% in detecting curves greater than 20° (prevalence of 0.3%).[28]

Other scoliosis screening tests include the inclinometer[31,32] and Moire topography. The inclinometer has a reported sensitivity of 96–98%, specificity of 29–68%, and reliability coefficients of 0.86–0.97 in detecting a Cobb angle of 20° or more.[33] In some studies, Moire topography correlates poorly with the Cobb angle.[34] A study that combined Moire topography with the forward bending test found that Moire topography had a sensitivity of 95% and the forward bending test had a sensitivity of 46% in detecting curves of 10° or greater. The calculated PPV of the test was 29% (study prevalence of 4%).[35]

There is limited information about the value of repeated screening of children who have previously tested negative for scoliosis. Although the probability of false-positive results would be increased by such a practice, repeat screening could potentially detect cases in older adolescents that escaped detection in early puberty or that developed into significant curves after screening was performed. There are few data that confirm these benefits. In one study, 43% of the cases that were detected on screening during tenth grade had previously tested negative 2–3 years earlier.[30]

Effectiveness of Early Detection

Direct evidence of the effectiveness of scoliosis screening would require controlled prospective studies demonstrating that persons who receive screening experience better outcomes than those who are not screened. No such studies have ever been published, although there is some evidence that patients with advanced curves may be more likely to fail treatment (to progress further or undergo surgery) than patients with smaller curves.[36]

The effectiveness of screening has been inferred from temporal studies that compared outcomes in local communities before and after the institution of large screening programs. These studies reported an increase in the number of referrals to local scoliosis clinics, the proportion of curves detected by screening, and the use of braces; they also reported a decrease in the mean age of referred cases, mean curve size, number of curves progressing to 40°, proportion of cases requiring treatment, and the rate of spine fusions.[37–40] However, most of the studies provided limited information about the comparability of the "before" and "after" groups, making it difficult to determine whether the time trends were due to screening or to other temporal factors.

The rationale behind screening is the assumption that the early detection of curves permits prompt initiation of conservative therapeutic measures that may prevent progression of the curves and thereby avoid the complications of advanced scoliosis. The principal forms of conservative treatment for curves detected through screening include spinal orthoses (braces), electrical stimulation, and exercise therapy. Surgery may also be recommended for cases detected through screening, and it is argued that early surgery for large curves may produce better outcomes than surgery performed at later ages.

Braces are generally effective in providing immediate correction of curves; initial standing roentgenograms often demonstrate a 50–60% correction in the curve.[41] The effectiveness of braces in preventing progression is less certain. There have been no published controlled prospective studies establishing the effectiveness of brace treatment. A multicenter prospective controlled trial of brace therapy has recently been completed,[42] but the results were not published as of this writing. Most existing evidence regarding the effectiveness of brace therapy comes from uncontrolled case series reports. Early series with limited follow-up reported corrections in lateral curvature of as much as 50%. Although gradual loss of correction over the course of treatment was noted, follow-up 1–2 years after discontinuing brace treatment revealed significant improvement over pre-brace values in a large proportion of patients.[43] Mean rates of curve progression in braced patients were lower than rates expected from natural history data.[44] Long-term studies (more than 5 years of follow-up) have since demonstrated that the early post-treatment correction observed in these reports was often temporary. A gradual loss of correction was noted in the years following brace treatment, with mean overall improvement in such studies averaging 0–4° compared with pre-brace values.[45–47]

The absence of internal controls in most bracing studies limits inferences about the independent effects of braces on outcomes. Some investigators have relied on historical control groups to infer effectiveness. A recent review of over 1000 braced patients, for example, concluded that braces altered the natural history of the disease because treatment failures were significantly less common in this series than was observed in a 1984 study by the same authors.[48] A retrospective review that did include a control group of matched, untreated patients reported that braced patients had a lower rate of curve progression and a higher rate of curve regression than untreated patients.[49] The differences were not statistically significant, but the study may have lacked adequate sample size to detect a difference.

Another controlled study of similar design reported no statistically significant differences in any parameter of curve progression but also had a small sample size.[50]

Outcome measures in most bracing studies relate only to curve correction and provide little information on health outcomes (e.g., back pain, patient feelings about their appearance, psychosocial impact). Available evidence is limited to an uncontrolled study, which found that braced patients noted an improvement in back "surface shape," as determined by a computerized photogrammetric surface mapping procedure.[51] Compliance problems limit the effectiveness of brace treatment.[52] Braces are generally recommended to be worn for 23 hours/day, a program that is often difficult for adolescents to follow and that influences compliance.[53] One study reported that only 15% of patients were highly compliant and that patients wore their braces an average of 65% of the recommended time.[54] Another study reported that complaints were uncommon among adolescents who wore braces.[55]

Lateral electrical surface stimulation (LESS), in which surface electrodes are applied to the skin nightly for at least 8 hours until skeletal maturity is attained,[56] has only been evaluated in uncontrolled case series reports. Although early case series reports found low rates of progression (0–5%) in patients who received LESS,[57,58] subsequent studies found that 18–56% of patients progressed more than 10°.[59,60] A chart review of patients who had completed treatment with LESS and were fully compliant found that over two thirds of curves progressed at least 5°; 50% of the patients required fusion or ended treatment with a curve greater than 40°.[61]

Exercises have been advocated as prophylactic therapy to prevent the need for more extensive treatment (e.g., braces) and as adjunctive therapy to enhance the effectiveness of braces.[62] Scientific evidence to support either use of exercise therapy is limited. Exercise alone has historically demonstrated poor effectiveness in preventing curve progression,[62,63] although there have been few published studies in this area. A study of a school-based exercise program for adolescents with scoliosis found that curve progression after 1 year was not significantly different between the study group and a matched control group.[63] Supporting evidence includes a small randomized controlled trial (grade I evidence) of adolescents wearing a cast, which showed that exercise was more effective than traction in improving curves on lateral bending;[64] an uncontrolled cohort study that showed improved vital capacity in hospitalized scoliosis patients who received physiotherapy;[65] and an uncontrolled case series report, which found that some braced patients who performed a thoracic flexion exercise had reduced vertebral rotation and thoracic curves after exercise.[66] The study lacked controls, follow-up, and an assessment of clinical outcomes.

Surgery is generally not considered unless significant progression has occurred. Few clinical trials have compared surgery with no surgery to assess its efficacy; case series reports provide the largest body of evidence. In these studies, Harrington instrumentation and other surgical techniques appear to be effective in correcting scoliotic curves in the frontal plane— Cobb angles are corrected by 40–70%[67–71]—but thoracic hypokyphosis, deviations in axial rotation, and lordosis are often not corrected.[72] Reduced lumbar lordosis ("flat-back" deformity)[73] and "crankshaft" deformities (in skeletally immature patients with posterior arthrodeses)[74,75] can develop over time, although modifications in devices and techniques have reduced the risk of these complications. A small improvement in pulmonary function has also been reported.[76] Cotrel-Dubousset instrumentation appears to achieve correction in the frontal plane while maintaining normal sagittal contour, and some correction of axial rotation with improved cosmesis has also been reported.[77] Spinal decompensation due to torsional changes and spinal cord damage are potential complications of Cotrel-Dubousset instrumentation.[78,79] Another limitation to surgical techniques is loss of fixation, which can result in partial or total loss of correction. There is an estimated 10–25% loss of correction from Harrington instrumentation, but the risk may be lower in patients who are immobilized by a cast or brace.[80,81] Loss of correction appears to be uncommon with Cotrel-Dubousset instrumentation (loss of correction less than 2%), and the latter does not require immobilization.[82]

Few controlled studies have evaluated surgery in terms of clinical outcomes, such as back pain and functional status. Although spinal curves and axial rotations are influenced by surgery, they do not correlate well with the incidence of back pain or other symptoms.[83] Studies that have demonstrated effects on clinical outcomes have suffered from design limitations. An uncontrolled retrospective study of patients who underwent spinal fusion found that complaints of low back pain were lower than reported rates in the general population and in scoliotic patients who do not receive fusion.[84] This study did not include internal controls, and it was performed in the years before spinal instrumentation was introduced. Similarly, a review of 32 patients who underwent fusion reported that the preoperative prevalence of poor self-image (38%), uncomfortable sexual intercourse (35%), and frequent or constant back pain (53%) had decreased to zero when surveyed 24–50 months after surgery.[85] This study also lacked a control group. A retrospective cohort study found that surgically treated patients were less likely than nonsurgically treated patients to report pain and were more likely to be performing manual work.[86] The study and comparison groups were not selected randomly and there were important differences between groups in preoperative characteristics. A survey found that patients who had undergone Harrington instrumentation differed significantly from persons without scoliosis in terms of employment, activity levels, and complaints of back pain.[87] The control group did not consist of persons with scoliosis who did not receive surgery, and thus it is unclear whether observed differences were due to scoliosis or to the effects of surgery.

The adverse effects of screening itself are generally minor, but follow-up testing of abnormal findings may incur anxiety, inconvenience, work and school absenteeism for return visits, financial costs for visits and radiographic tests, and radiation exposure from follow-up roentgenograms (although roentgenograms are not routinely ordered on all follow-up evaluations and, when obtained, radiation exposure can be reduced by modern imaging and shielding techniques). Confirmed or suspected scoliosis may affect future health insurance and work eligibility. These postulated adverse effects have not been proven in controlled studies. Treatment may also incur adverse effects from follow-up visits (e.g., inconvenience, absenteeism, radiation exposure) and from treatment itself. Brace wear, for example, may produce skin irritation, disturbed sleep, restrictions on physical and recreational activities, and difficulty in finding clothes, but studies confirming these effects are lacking. Studies have shown an association between brace wear and adverse psychological effects, diminished self-esteem, and disturbed peer relationships.[88,89]

The potential adverse effects of surgery can include the general risks of surgery, such as anesthesia risks, pain, and postoperative complications (e.g., bleeding, infection, pulmonary embolism), although these have been reduced by modern surgical and anesthetic techniques.[90] The overall risk of spinal cord damage is about 1–3%,[71,91] but rates are thought to be lower in uncomplicated surgery or when somatosensory evoked potential spinal cord monitoring is performed.[92] Fusion at certain ages during adolescence may affect the longitudinal growth of the spine.[93] Hook dislodgement and laminar fracture are possible. Other adverse effects of surgery include financial costs, inconvenience and lost productivity associated with hospitalization and convalescence, and external immobilization with casts or braces, which may be required for a period of months after surgery. Potential long-term complications occur generally in adults and include the development of pain caudad to the level of fusion, bursitis, pseudo-arthrosis, kyphotic deformities, and loss of normal lumbar lordosis.[91,94] Often these complications require further surgery during adulthood.

Recommendations of Other Groups

The Scoliosis Research Society has recommended annual screening of all children aged 10–14 years.[95] The American Academy of Orthopedic Surgeons has recommended screening girls at ages 11 and 13 years and screening boys once at age 13 or 14 years.[96] The American Academy of Pediatrics has recommended scoliosis screening with the forward bending test at routine health supervision visits at ages 10, 12, 14, and 16 years; this recommendation is under review.[97] The Bright Futures guidelines recommend noting the presence of scoliosis during the physical examination of adolescents and children ≥8 years of age.[98] The Canadian Task Force on the Periodic Health Examination concluded that there was insufficient evidence to make a recommendation.[99] Scoliosis screening is required by law in some states.[100]

Discussion

The clinical logic behind screening for adolescent idiopathic scoliosis is based on a series of critical assumptions. The logic assumes that screening tests are accurate and reliable in detecting curves, that early detection of curves results in improved health outcomes, and that effective treatment modalities are available for cases detected through screening. Implicit in this causal pathway are the assumptions that small curves detected through screening are likely to progress to curves of potential clinical significance, that scoliosis causes important health problems, and that the benefits of early detection outweigh the potential adverse effects of screening and treatment. Scientific evidence to support these assumptions is limited.

The principal screening test for scoliosis, the physical examination of the back, has variable sensitivity and specificity, depending on the skills of the examiner and the size of the curve being sought. The positive predictive value in typical screening settings is low, due to the low prevalence of clinically significant curves. There is little evidence about the incremental value of repeat screening in children with previously normal results.

There have been no controlled studies to demonstrate whether adolescents who are screened routinely for idiopathic scoliosis have better outcomes than those who are not screened. Decreased curve size and surgery rates have been observed in communities that have adopted aggressive screening programs, but it is unclear whether the changes were due to screening or to other temporal factors. Beyond temporary correction of curves, there is inadequate evidence that braces limit the natural progression of the disease. The effectiveness of LESS and exercise has not been demonstrated convincingly in currently available research. Surgery is effective in reducing, but not eliminating, the lateral scoliotic curve. The scoliotic curves for which surgery is recommended (e.g., documented progression beyond 40–50°) are more likely to be detected without screening.

The natural history of idiopathic scoliosis is such that most cases detected at screening will not require treatment because they will not progress significantly. Indications for preventive treatment (e.g., braces) are therefore uncertain and can result in unnecessary treatment. Only a small proportion of adolescents with idiopathic scoliosis are currently considered candidates for treatment (e.g., those having progressive curves greater than 30°). Moreover, the burden of suffering associated with adolescent idiopathic scoliosis is uncertain. Cosmetic deformities and associated psychological and social effects have been difficult to evaluate in formal research. It is also unclear whether physical symptoms can be attributed to idiopathic scoliosis, except in severe cases. Finally, screening may result in mislabeling and the inconvenience, cost, and potential radiation exposure of follow-up evaluations. Both conservative treatment (e.g., braces) and surgery can be associated with medical, psychological, and social adverse effects.

In summary, there is insufficient evidence from clinical research that routine screening is effective in changing the outcome of adolescent idiopathic scoliosis. Limitations in the design of existing studies, however, also make it difficult to conclude that screening is ineffective or harmful. If screening for scoliosis is effective, discontinuation of school screening may have a disproportionate impact on disadvantaged adolescents. Adolescents who have access to primary care providers and to periodic health examinations have an opportunity outside the school setting to obtain back examinations. School screening may provide the only opportunity for back inspections of disadvantaged adolescents, including those from minority and low income families, who often lack access to such providers.

CLINICAL INTERVENTION

There is insufficient evidence to recommend for or against routine screening of asymptomatic adolescents for idiopathic scoliosis ("C" recommendation). The evidence does not support routine visits to clinicians for the specific purpose of scoliosis screening or for performing the examination at specific ages during adolescence. It is prudent for clinicians to include visual inspection of the back of adolescents when it is examined for other reasons. Additional specific inspection maneuvers to screen for scoliosis, such as the forward-bending test, are of unproven benefit.

Note: See the relevant background papers: U.S. Preventive Services Task Force. Screening for adolescent idiopathic scoliosis: policy statement. JAMA 1993;269:2664–2666; and U.S. Preventive Services Task Force. Screening for adolescent idiopathic scoliosis: review article. JAMA 1993;269:2667–2672.

The draft of this chapter was prepared for the U.S. Preventive Services Task Force by Steven H. Woolf, MD, MPH.

REFERENCES

1. AAOS Committee on Communications and Publications. A statement regarding school screening programs for the early detection of scoliosis. Park Ridge, IL: American Academy of Orthopedic Surgeons Bulletin 1984;32:27.
2. Berwick DM. Scoliosis screening. Pediatr Rev 1984;5:238–247.
3. Riseborough EJ, Herndon JH. Scoliosis and other deformities of the axial skeleton. Boston: Little, Brown, 1975:22.
4. Renshaw TS. Screening school children for scoliosis. Clin Orthop 1988;229:26–33.
5. Bengtsson G, Fallstrom K, Jansson B, Nachemson A. A psychological and psychiatric investigation of the adjustment of female scoliosis patients. Acta Psychiatr Scand 1974;50:50–59.
6. Weinstein SL. Adolescent idiopathic scoliosis: prevalence and natural history. Instr Course Lect 1989;38:115–128.
7. Weinstein SL, Zavala DC, Ponseti IV. Idiopathic scoliosis: long-term follow-up and prognosis in untreated patients. J Bone Joint Surg Am Vol 1981;63:702–712.
8. *Deleted in proof.*
9. Fowles JV, Drummond DS, L'Ecuyer S, Roy L, Kassab MT. Untreated scoliosis in the adult. Clin Orthop 1978;134:212–217.
10. Nilsonne U, Lundgren KD. Long-term prognosis in idiopathic scoliosis. Acta Orthop Scand 1968;39:456–465.
11. Nachemson A. A long-term follow-up study of non-treated scoliosis. Acta Orthop Scand 1968;39:466–476.
12. Kolind-Sorensen V. A follow-up study of patients with idiopathic scoliosis. Acta Orthop Scand 1973;44:98.
13. Smyth RJ, Chapman KR, Wright TA, Crawford JS, Rebuck AS. Ventilatory patterns during hypoxia, hypercapnia, and exercise in adolescents with mild scoliosis. Pediatrics 1986;77:692–697.
14. Davies G, Reid L. Effect of scoliosis on growth of alveoli and pulmonary arteries and on the right ventricle. Arch Dis Child 1971;46:623–632.
15. Branthwaite MA. Cardiorespiratory consequences of unfused idiopathic scoliosis. Br J Dis Chest 1986; 80:360–369.
16. Deleted in proof.
17. Dickson RA. Conservative treatment for idiopathic scoliosis. J Bone Joint Surg Br 1985;67:176–181.
18. Nachemson A, Lonstein JE, Weinstein SL. Report of the prevalence and natural history committee. Park Ridge, IL: Natural History Committee of Scoliosis Research Society, 1982.
19. Lonstein JE, Carlson MC. Prediction of curve progression in untreaed idiopathic scoliosis during growth. J Bone Joint Surg Am Vol 1984;66:1061–1071.
20. Bunnell WP. The natural history of idiopathic scoliosis before skeletal maturity. Spine 1986;11:773–776.
21. Lonstein JE. Natural history and school screening for scoliosis. Orthop Clin North Am 1988;19:227–237.
22. Willner S, Uden A. A prospective prevalence study of scoliosis in southern Sweden. Acta Orthop Scand 1982;53:233–237.
23. Rogala E, Drummond D, Gurr J. Scoliosis: incidence and natural history. J Bone Joint Surg Am 1978;60:173–176.
24. Gore DG, Passehl R, Sepic S, Dalton A. Scoliosis screening: results of a community project. Pediatrics 1981;67:196–200.
25. Renshaw TS. Screening school children for scoliosis. Clin Orthop 1988;229:26–33.
26. Morrissy RT, Goldsmith GS, Hall EC, Kehl D, Cowie GH. Measurement of the Cobb angle on radiographs of patients who have scoliosis. Evaluation of intrinsic error. J Bone Joint Surg Am 1990;72:320–327.
27. Pruijs JE, Hageman MA, Keesen W, van der Meer R, van Wieringen JC. Variation in Cobb angle measurements in scoliosis. Skel Radiol 1994;23:517–520.
28. Morais T, Bernier M, Turcotte F. Age- and sex-specific prevalence of scoliosis and the value of school screening programs. Am J Public Health 1985;75:1377–1380.
29. Viviani GR, Budgell L, Dok C, Tugwell P. Assessment of accuracy of the scoliosis school screening examination. Am J Public Health 1984;74:497–498.
30. Chan A, Moller J, Vimpani G, Paterson D, Southwood R, Sutherland A. The case for scoliosis screening in Australian adolescents. Med J Aust 1986;145:379–383.
31. Bunnell WP. An objective criterion for scoliosis screening. J Bone Joint Surg Am 1984;66:1381–1387.
32. Bunnell WP. Outcome of spinal screening. Spine 1993;18:1572–1580.

33. Amendt LE, Ause-Ellias KL, Eybers JL, Wadsworth CT, Nielsen DH, Weinstein SL. Validity and relability testing of the scoliometer. Phys Ther 1990;70:108–117.
34. Nissinen M, Heliovaara M, Ylikoski M, Poussa M. Trunk asymmetry and screening for scoliosis: a longitudinal cohort study of pubertal schoolchildren. Acta Paediatr 1993;82:77–82.
35. Laulund T, Sojbjerg, Horlyck E. Moire topography in school screening for structural scoliosis. Acta Orthop Scand 1982;53:765–768.
36. Focarile FA, Bonaldi A, Giarolo MA, Ferrari U, Zilioli E, Ottaviani C. Effectiveness of nonsurgical treatment for idiopathic scoliosis: overview of available evidence. Spine 1991;16:395–401.
37. Torell G, Nordwall A, Nachemson A. The changing pattern of scoliosis treatment due to effective screening. J Bone Joint Surg Am 1981;63:337–341.
38. Lonstein JE, Bjorklund S, Wanninger MH, Nelson RP. Voluntary school screening for scoliosis in Minnesota. J Bone Joint Surg Am 1982;64:481–488.
39. Ferris B, Edgar M, Leyshon A. Screening for scoliosis. Acta Orthop Scand 1988;59:417–418.
40. Montgomery F, Willner S. Screening for idiopathic scoliosis: comparison of 90 cases shows less surgery by early diagnosis. Acta Orthop Scand 1993;64:456–458.
41. Jonasson-Rajala E, Josefsson E, Lundberg B, Nilsson H. Boston thoracic brace in the treatment of idiopathic scoliosis: initial correction. Clin Orthop 1984;183:37–41.
42. Winter RB, Banta JV, Engler G. Screening for scoliosis [letter]. JAMA 1995;273:185–186.
43. Emans JB, Kaelin A, Bancel P, Hall JE, Miller ME. The Boston bracing system for idiopathic scoliosis: follow-up results in 295 patients. Spine 1986;11:792–801.
44. Bassett GS, Bunnell WP, MacEwen GD. Treatment of idiopathic scoliosis with the Wilmington brace. J Bone Joint Surg Am 1986;68:602–605.
45. Mellencamp DD, Blount WP, Anderson AJ. Milwaukee brace treatment of idiopathic scoliosis: late results. Clin Orthop 1977;126:47–57.
46. Carr W, Moe J, Winter R, Lonstein J. Treatment of idiopathic scoliosis in the Milwaukee brace. J Bone Joint Surg Am 1980;62:599–612.
47. Willers U, Normelli H, Aaro S, Svensson O, Hedlund R. Long-term results of Boston brace treatment on vertebral rotation in idiopathic scoliosis. Spine 1993;18:432–435.
48. Lonstein JE, Winter RB. The Milwaukee brace for the treatment of adolescent idiopathic scoliosis: a review of one thousand and twenty patients. J Bone Joint Surg Am 1994;76:1207–1221.
49. Miller JA, Nachemson AL, Schultz AB. Effectiveness of braces in mild idiopathic scoliosis. Spine 1984;9:632–635.
50. Goldberg CJ, Dowling FE, Hall JE, Emans JB. A statistical comparison between natural history of idiopathic scoliosis and brace treatment in skeletally immature adolescent girls. Spine 1993;18:902–908.
51. Weisz I, Jefferson RJ, Carr AJ, et al. Back shape in brace treatment of idiopathic scoliosis. Clin Orthop 1989;240:157–162.
52. Wynne EJ. Scoliosis: to screen or not to screen. Can J Public Health 1984;75:277–280.
53. Kehl DK, Morrissy RT. Brace treatment in adolescent idiopathic scoliosis: an update on concepts and technique. Clin Orthop 1988;229:34–43.
54. DiRaimondo CV, Green NE. Brace-wear compliance in patients with adolescent idiopathic scoliosis. J Pediatr Orthop 1988;8:143–146.
55. Gratz RR, Papalia-Finlay D. Psychosocial adaptation to wearing the Milwaukee brace for scoliosis. J Adolesc Health Care 1984;5:237–242.
56. Francis EE. Lateral electrical surface stimulation treatment for scoliosis. Ped Nurs 1987;13:157–160.
57. Axelgaard J, Brown JC. Lateral electrical surface stimulation for the treatment of progressive idiopathic scoliosis. Spine 1983;8:242–260.
58. McCollough NC. Nonoperative treatment of idiopathic scoliosis using surface electrical stimulation. Spine 1986;11: 802–804.
59. Bradford DS, Tanguy A, Vanselow J. Surface electrical stimulation in the treatment of idiopathic scoliosis: preliminary results in 30 patients. Spine 1983;8:757–764.
60. Sullivan JA, Davidson R, Renshaw TS, Emans JB, Johnston C, Sussman M. Further evaluation of the Scolitron treatment of idiopathic adolescent scoliosis. Spine 1986;11:903–906.
61. O'Donnell CS, Bunnell WP, Betz RR, Bowen JR, Tipping CR. Electrical stimulation in the treatment of idiopathic scoliosis. Clin Orthop 1988;229:107–113.
62. Farady JA. Current principles in the nonoperative management of structural adolescent idiopathic scoliosis. Phys Ther 1983;63:512–523.

63. Stone B, Beekman C, Hall V, Guess V, Brooks HL. The effect of an exercise program on change in curve in adolescents with minimal idiopathic scoliosis. Phys Ther 1979;59:759–763.

64. Dickson RA, Leatherman KD. Cotrel traction, exercises, casting in the treatment of idiopathic scoliosis: a pilot study and prospective randomized controlled clinical trial. Acta Orthop Scand 1978;49:46–48.

65. Weiss HR. The effect of an exercise program on vital capacity and rib mobility in patients with idiopathic scoliosis. Spine 1991;16:88–93.

66. Miyasaki RA. Immediate influence of the thoracic flexion exercise on vertebral position in Milwaukee brace wearers. Phys Ther 1980;60:1005–1009.

67. Akbarnia BA. Selection of methodology in surgical treatment of adolescent idiopathic scoliosis. Orthop Clin North Am 1988;19:319–329.

68. Willers U, Hedlund R, Aaro S, Normelli H, Westman L. Long-term results of Harrington instrumentation in idiopathic scoliosis. Spine 1993;18:713–717.

69. Jeng CL, Sponseller PD, Tolo VT. Outcome of Wisconsin instrumentation in idiopathic scoliosis: minimum 5-year follow-up. Spine 1993;18:1584–1590.

70. Schlenzka D, Poussa M, Muschik M. Operative treatment of adolescent idiopathic scoliosis: Harrington-DTT versus Cotrel-Dubousset instrumentation. Clin Orthop Relat Res 1993;297:155–160.

71. Richards BS, Herring JA, Johnston CE, Birch JG, Roach JW. Treatment of adolescent idiopathic scoliosis using Texas Scottish Rite Hospital instrumentation. Spine 1994;19:1598–1605.

72. Stokes IA, Ronchetti PJ, Aronsson DD. Changes in shape of the adolescent idiopathic scoliosis curve after surgical correction. Spine 1994;19:1032–1037.

73. La Grone MO. Loss of lumbar lordosis: a complication of spinal fusion for scoliosis. Orthop Clin North Am 1988;19:383–393.

74. Mullaji AB, Upadhyay SS, Luk KD, Leong JC. Vertebral growth after posterior spinal fusion for idiopathic scoliosis in skeletally immature adolescents: the effect of growth on spinal deformity. J Bone Joint Surg Br 1994;76:870–876.

75. Sanders JO, Herring JA, Browne RH. Posterior arthrodesis and instrumentation in the immature (Risser-grade-0) spine in idiopathic scoliosis. J Bone Joint Surg Am 1995;77:39–45.

76. Kinner WJ, Johnston ID. Does Harrington instrumentation improve pulmonary function in adolescents with idiopathic scoliosis? A meta-analysis. Spine 1993;18:1556–1559.

77. Suk SI, Lee CK, Chung SS. Comparison of Zielke ventral derotation system and Cotrel-Dubousset instrumentation in the treatment of idiopathic lumbar and thoracolumbar scoliosis. Spine 1994;19:419–429.

78. Thompson JP, Transfeldt EE, Bradford DS, Ogilvie JW, Boachie-Adjei O. Decompensation after Cotrel-Dubousset instrumentation of idiopathic scoliosis. Spine 1990;15:927–931.

79. Been HD, Kalkman CJ, Traast HS, Ongerboer de Visser BW. Neurologic injury after insertion of laminar hooks during Cotrel-Dubousset instrumentation. Spine 1994;19:1402–1405.

80. Mielke CH, Lonstein JE, Denis F, Vandenbrink K, Winter RB. Surgical treatment of adolescent idiopathic scoliosis: a comparative analysis. J Bone Joint Surg Am 1989;71:1170–1177.

81. Christodoulou AG, Prince HG, Webb JK, et al. Adolescent idiopathic scoliosis. J Bone Joint Surg Br 1987;69:13–16.

82. Shufflebarger HL, Crawford AH. Is Cotrel-Dubousset instrumentation the treatment of choice for idiopathic scoliosis in the adolescent who has an operative thoracic curve? Orthopedics 1988;11:1579–1588.

83. Poitras B, Mayo NE, Goldberg MS, Scott S, Hanley J. The Ste-Justine Adolescent Idiopathic Scoliosis Cohort Study. Part IV: Surgical correction and back pain. Spine 1994;19:1582–1588.

84. Moskowitz A, Moe JH, Winter RB, Binner H. Long-term follow-up of scoliosis fusion. J Bone Joint Surg Am 1980;62:364–376.

85. Moskowitz A, Trommanhauser S. Surgical and clinical results of scoliosis surgery using Zielke instrumentation. Spine 1993;18:2444–2451.

86. Edgar MA, Mehta MH. Long-term follow-up of fused and unfused idiopathic scoliosis. J Bone Joint Surg Br 1988;70:712–716.

87. Dickson JH, Erwin WD, Rossi D. Harrington instrumentation and arthrodesis for idiopathic scoliosis: a twenty-one year follow-up. J Bone Joint Surg Am 1990;72:678–683.

88. Kahanovitz N, Snow B, Pinter I. The comparative results of psychologic testing in scoliosis patients treated with electrical stimulation or bracing. Spine 1984;9:442–444.

89. Fallstrom K, Cochran T, Nachemson A. Long-term effects on personality development in patients with adolescent idiopathic scoliosis: influence of type of treatment. Spine 1986;11:756–758.
90. Guay J, Haig M, Lortie L, Guertin MC, Poitras B. Predicting blood loss in surgery for idiopathic scoliosis. Can J Anaesth 1994;41:775–781.
91. Kostuik JP. Operative treatment of idiopathic scoliosis. J Bone Joint Surg Am1990;72:1108–1113.
92. Nuwer MR, Dawson EG, Carlson LG, Kanim LE, Sherman JE. Somatosensory evoked potential spinal cord monitoring reduces neurologic deficits after scoliosis surgery: results of a large multicenter survey. Electroencephal Clin Neurophysiol 1995;96:6–11.
93. Hsu LC, Upadhyay SS. Effect of spinal fusion on growth of the spine and lower limbs in girls with adolescent idiopathic scoliosis: a longitudinal study. J Pediatr Orthop 1994;14:564–568.
94. Renshaw TS. The role of Harrington instrumentation and posterior spine fusion in the management of adolescent idiopathic scoliosis. Orthop Clin North Am 1988;19:257–267.
95. Scoliosis Research Society. Scoliosis: a handbook for patients. Park Ridge, IL: Scoliosis Research Society, 1986.
96. American Academy of Orthopedic Surgeons. Position statement: school screening programs for the early detection of scoliosis. Park Ridge, IL: American Academy of Orthopedic Surgeons, Bulletin, January 1993:6.
97. American Academy of Pediatrics. Guidelines for health supervision II. Elk Grove Village, IL: American Academy of Pediatrics, 1988.
98. Green M, ed. Bright Futures: guidelines for health supervision of infants, children, and adolescents. Arlington, VA: National Center for Education in Maternal and Child Health, 1994.
99. Canadian Task Force on the Periodic Health Examination. Canadian guide to clinical preventive care. Ottawa: Canada Communication Group, 1994:346–354.
100. Asher M, Beringer GB, Orrick J, Halverhout N. The current status of scoliosis screening in North America, 1986: results of a survey by mailed questionnaire. Spine 1989;14:652–662.

48. Screening for Dementia

RECOMMENDATION

There is insufficient evidence to recommend for or against routine screening for dementia with standardized instruments in asymptomatic persons. Clinicians should remain alert for possible signs of declining cognitive function in older patients and evaluate mental status in patients who have problems performing daily activities (see *Clinical Intervention*).

Burden of Suffering

Dementia is usually defined as global impairment of cognitive function that interferes with normal activities.[1,2] Although impaired short- and long-term memory are typical of dementia, deficits in other cognitive functions in addition to memory (e.g., abstract thinking, judgment, speech, coordination, planning or organization) are required for the diagnosis of dementia.[2,3] Alzheimer's disease accounts for most cases of dementia in North America (50–85%),[4,5] with an additional 10–20% attributed to vascular ("multi-infarct") dementia. The relative importance of vascular dementias is higher in populations where hypertension and stroke are more common (Asians, African Americans, persons over 85).[6–8] Other important causes of dementia include alcoholism, Parkinson's disease, metabolic disorders (vitamin B_{12} deficiency, hypothyroidism), central nervous system infections (e.g., HIV, neurosyphilis), intracranial lesions, and other illnesses.[4,9]

The prevalence of dementia increases steadily with age, roughly doubling every 5 years.[10] Studies of community-dwelling elderly in North America have reported dementia in 0.8–1.6% of persons 65–74 years old, 7–8% of persons 75–84 years old, and 18–32% of persons over 85.[5,8,11,12] The substantially higher prevalence reported from a community survey in East Boston[13]—19% for ages 75–84, 47% in those over 85—may reflect the inclusion of cases with milder impairment.[4] Estimates of the annual incidence of dementia in community-based studies are 0.6–1% for ages 65–74, 2–3% for ages 75–84, and 4–8% for ages 85 or older;[14,14a] many incident cases have only mild cognitive impairment, however. Dementia is common among institutionalized elderly[11] and is present in one half to two thirds of the 1.3 million American nursing home residents.[13] Estimates of the number of Americans over 65 currently affected by Alzheimer's disease range from 1.4–4 million.[15,16] This number is projected to increase dramatically as the population of older (over 65) and very old (over 85) men and women increases in the U.S.[15]

Family history is consistently associated with an increased risk of Alzheimer's disease, with an estimated 3-fold higher risk among first-degree relatives.[17] Genetic risk factors for Alzheimer's disease have been identified[18,19] but are of uncertain value in clinical practice. A variety of other possible risk factors (e.g., lower educational level,[20] prior head trauma, family history of Down syndrome) and protective factors (e.g., smoking, estrogen replacement) for Alzheimer's disease have been reported, but the nature of each these associations remains uncertain.[4,5]

Alzheimer's disease progresses over a period of 2–20 years, causing increasing functional impairment and disability due to acute medical illnesses, depression, wandering, incontinence, adverse drug reactions, poor personal hygiene, and unintentional injuries (falls, burns, etc.).[21,22] Survival is reduced in patients with Alzheimer's disease[23] and in patients with any cognitive impairment;[24] mortality is strongly associated with severity of dementia. Dementia is estimated to account for about 120,000 deaths annually.[25] Care of the demented patient imposes an enormous psychosocial and economic burden on family and other caretakers. The annual costs of treating Alzheimer's disease alone, including medical and nursing costs and lost productivity, have been estimated to be $67 billion.[15]

Accuracy of Screening Tests

Dementia is easily recognized in its advanced stages, but numerous studies indicate that clinicians often overlook the early signs of dementia.[26–29a] The significance of early symptoms, whose onset is insidious, may be underestimated; patients and clinicians alike may mistakenly attribute changes to "normal aging."[29] Other patients, fearing a label of Alzheimer's disease, deliberately minimize their symptoms, and patients with more advanced dementia may not be aware of their deficits. Clinicians fail to detect an estimated 21% to 72% of patients with dementia, especially when the disease is early in its course.[26–29a] Conversely, clinicians may mistakenly attribute the symptoms of depression or drug toxicity in older subjects to irreversible dementia.

The routine physical examination and patient history is not sensitive for dementia, especially if family members are not present to corroborate patient self-report. Many clinicians include only a cursory examination of mental status as part of the routine history and physical. The inability to recall the correct date or place is reasonably specific (92–100%), but highly insensitive (15–53%) for dementia.[30,31] Neurologic findings, such as re-

lease signs, gait disorders, and impaired stereognosis, are usually late findings and are not sufficiently sensitive or specific to screen for dementia.[32]

The usual diagnostic standard for dementia consists of detailed assessment of mental status and careful investigation to rule out other causes of
cognitive impairment. A variety of abbreviated instruments have been examined for their ability to screen for dementia in the outpatient setting.[33]
The most widely studied of these instruments is the Mini-Mental State Examination (MMSE), a short, structured examination that takes 5–10 minutes to administer.[34] The MMSE contains 30 items and is reproducible
using a standardized version.[35] Various studies suggest that an MMSE score
of less than 24 of 30 has a reasonable sensitivity (80–90%) and specificity
(80%) for discriminating between dementia cases and normal controls.[36]
There are only limited data, however, on its performance as a screening
test for early dementia among a representative population of outpatients.
The positive predictive value (PPV) of MMSE for dementia depends on
the definition of an abnormal score and the prevalence of dementia.
Based on its performance in one community study,[37] a MMSE score of 20
or less has a PPV of only 48% when the prevalence of dementia is 10%
(e.g., a population of 75–84-year-olds), but a much higher PPV (73%)
when prevalence of dementia is 25% (e.g., age over 85).[31] The predictive
value of intermediate MMSE scores (21–25) appears to be low (21–44%)
for dementia in most populations.[31]

Recent data suggest that level of education and cultural differences
have important effects on the range of MMSE scores in a given population.
Among individuals with only 5–8 years of education versus those with college education, the cutpoints that identified the lowest 25% on MMSE were
23 and 29, respectively.[38] Spanish-speaking persons scored significantly
lower than did English speakers on several MMSE items in one community-
based study.[39] These data suggest that applying a uniform MMSE cutoff
may miss significant changes among well-educated patients (false-negative
result) and generate more frequent false-positive results among persons
who are less educated or from different cultures.[40] Shorter screening instruments such as the Short Portable Mental Status Questionnaire[41] and
the Clock Drawing Test[42] seem to be reasonably sensitive and specific for
moderate to severe dementia, but they have not been adequately studied as
screening tests in asymptomatic outpatients. Because they each examine a
lesser range of cognitive function, they are not likely to be as sensitive as the
MMSE or more comprehensive tests for detecting early dementia.

An alternative to screening for cognitive problems is to screen for functional impairment, which is a diagnostic criterion for dementia.[2] The Instrumental Activities of Daily Living (IADL) assesses level of function in
eight common tasks.[43] When IADL was administered to a random sample
of community-living persons over 65 (prevalence of dementia 2%), sub-

jects who reported difficulty using the telephone, using public transportation, taking medications, or handling finances were 12 times more likely to be diagnosed with dementia.[44] The Functional Activities Questionnaire, which scores function in 10 activities, also seems to be useful in measuring impairment and diagnosing dementia.[45,46] While these instruments generally rely on other informants (spouse, etc.), one recent study suggests that patients with mild dementia can reliably describe their functional status.[47] Because nondementing illnesses also interfere with daily activities, neither screen is specific for dementia.

The low predictive value of most screening tests for dementia raises the possibility that unselective screening may have adverse effects. Many asymptomatic patients with abnormal results on MMSE or other screening tests will not have dementia; these patients may be subjected to further tests (e.g., neuropsychological testing, blood tests, lumbar puncture, computed tomography [CT]) to confirm the diagnosis, rule out other reasons for altered mental status, and assign a cause of dementia. Comprehensive follow-up, although posing little risk to patients, will be time-consuming and expensive. If clinicians make a diagnosis based on screening alone, patients may be incorrectly diagnosed as having a progressive, incurable illness. Nonetheless, in the absence of screening, misdiagnosis of dementia is common in outpatient practice.[26] In one study in which general practice doctors administered a brief (10–15 minutes) standardized assessment to all patients over age 80, they revised their initial impression of cognitive function for 32 of 174 (18%) patients.[48] Interestingly, 16 patients initially diagnosed as "possibly demented" were reclassified as "not demented" after screening.

Effectiveness of Early Detection

There are several potential benefits of detecting dementia before patients are severely impaired: reversible causes of dementia may be identified and treated, treatments to slow the progression of disease can be instituted, measures can be taken to reduce the morbidity associated with dementia, and patients and their family members can anticipate and prepare for problems that will arise as dementia progresses.

Although early reports suggested that a substantial proportion of dementia was potentially reversible,[49] the number of patients who experience long-term improvements is relatively small. An overview of earlier studies concluded that only 11% of dementing illnesses improved in older patients, and only 3% resolved completely.[50] The most common correctable causes were drug intoxication, depression, and metabolic abnormalities. Among 36 cases of dementia evaluated in one community-based screening study, no cases of reversible dementia were found.[51] Among 85-year-old residents of Gothenburg, Sweden, only 3 of 147 cases of dementia were potentially reversible.[7]

Various treatments to improve cognitive function in Alzheimer patients have been examined in randomized clinical trials. Drugs that increase central levels of acetylcholine, such as tetrahydroaminoacridine (tacrine), have shown the most promise. Although several studies reported no benefit,[52,53] the three largest trials suggested a significant but modest benefit of tacrine in patients with mild to moderate dementia (average MMSE scores 16–19) over 6–30 weeks.[54–56] In one trial, the benefit of tacrine on cognitive test results was comparable to delaying disease progression by 5 months.[54] Improvements in overall clinical function have been small and inconsistent[54] but increase at higher doses.[55] The usefulness of tacrine is limited by high cost (over $100 per month) and frequent gastrointestinal side effects: up to 25% of patients taking lower doses, and two thirds of those on high doses, stopped therapy due to nausea, vomiting, or elevated liver enzymes.[53–56] Dihydroergotoxine (hydergine) improved some measures of cognitive function in previous trials, but does not produce important clinical benefits.[53,57] Other therapies under investigation include chelation therapy,[58] neuroprotective agents, and growth factors, but consistent evidence of clinical benefits is lacking.[5,53]

Early detection of vascular dementia may prompt better control of risk factors for cerebrovascular disease (treatment of hypertension, smoking cessation, aspirin therapy).[59] The effect of these measures on progression of vascular dementia, however, is not known. In a 2-year follow-up of 52 patients with multi-infarct dementia, smoking cessation was associated with improving cognitive function, but low blood pressure was associated with worsening function.[60] About one half of elderly demented patients manifest at least one coexisting illness, and treatment of associated disorders may improve function in patients with dementia.[61,62]

Identifying patients with early cognitive problems allows patients and their families to take measures to reduce the medical morbidity caused by progressive dementia. Patients are at increased risk of falls and automobile accidents as dementia progresses.[63] Effective interventions to prevent falls or accidents in patients with dementia have not been determined, however (see also Chapters 57 and 58). Comprehensive geriatric assessment has been shown to increase the number of older patients able to live independently at home,[64] but it is not possible to separate the benefits of cognitive assessment from other components (e.g., medical evaluation, social evaluation, drug management, follow-up).

An early diagnosis also permits care providers, especially family and friends of the patient, to benefit from support and self-help strategies in order to minimize the financial, emotional, and medicolegal pressures that will occur throughout the patient's illness. The psychiatric symptoms (depression, delirium or disruptive behavior) accompanying dementia can be anticipated and treated with psychotropic drugs and/or counseling.[65]

Decisions about durable power of attorney and advance directives can be made while the patient is still competent to participate. These benefits of early detection are based on clinical experience, but there are no data to prove that routine screening improves these outcomes.

An early diagnosis of dementia may also have adverse consequences: patients may have difficulty obtaining health or life insurance and may be excluded from retirement communities or long-term care facilities. Negative attitudes toward patients with dementia have been documented among professionals and lay people.[66]

Recommendations of Other Groups

There are no formal recommendations for routine screening for cognitive impairment or dementia. The Canadian Task Force on the Periodic Health Examination concluded that there was insufficient evidence to recommend for or against screening for asymptomatic cognitive impairment, but they advised that clinicians should remain alert for clues suggesting deteriorating cognitive function.[67] The American Academy of Family Physicians recommends that physicians include questions about functional status in the patient history of patients over 65, and remain alert for evidence of changes in cognitive function.[68] A National Institutes of Health consensus development conference concluded that no single test can diagnose dementia and urged clinicians to take the time necessary to conduct a thorough clinical evaluation.[1] Guidelines on the recognition and early assessment of dementia prepared by an expert panel convened by the Agency for Health Care Policy and Research (AHCPR), U.S. Public Health Service, are due to be released in 1996.

Discussion

Dementia is responsible for an enormous and growing burden on affected patients, their family members, and the clinicians who care for them. Early signs of dementia are often overlooked in routine encounters, and a variety of brief tests of mental status are available to help clinicians assess cognitive function more accurately in their patients. In the absence of more effective treatments to improve prognosis in patients with dementia, however, it is uncertain whether routine use of these instruments in all older patients will be of sufficient benefit to justify the inconvenience, costs, and possible harms of unselective screening. The predictive value of available screening tests is relatively low in the general population of asymptomatic older adults. Administering tests such as the MMSE to all older patients, and further evaluating those with positive results, will be time-consuming and expensive. Some patients may be incorrectly diagnosed with dementia on the basis of screening tests alone. Although there are many plausible benefits of early detection, there are few studies demonstrating that routine screening actually reduces the medical, psychological, and social consequences of dementia. Other appropriate interventions (treating hypertension, correcting underlying illnesses, and taking precautions to prevent accidents) can be recommended for older patients with or without dementia.

Despite the limitations of unselective screening, clinicians can improve the timely diagnosis of dementia by being alert to suggestive signs and symptoms in their older patients (trouble with daily activities, concerns voiced by family members), and by using standardized instruments to evaluate cognitive function in those suspected of having dementia. A positive screening test is more meaningful in patients when there is prior reason to suspect dementia (due to the higher prevalence of disease), and normal mental status test results may provide reassurance. Screening tests, however, should not be used in isolation to diagnose dementia.

CLINICAL INTERVENTION

There is insufficient evidence to recommend for or against routine screening for dementia in asymptomatic elderly persons ("C" recommendation). Clinicians should periodically ask patients about their functional status at home and at work, and they should remain alert to changes in performance with age. When possible, information about daily activities should be solicited from family members or other persons. Brief tests such as the MMSE should be used to assess cognitive function in patients in whom the suspicion of dementia is raised by restrictions in daily activities, concerns of family members, or other evidence of worsening function (e.g., trouble with finances, medications, transportation). Possible effects of education and cultural differences should be considered when interpreting results of cognitive tests. The diagnosis of dementia should not be based on results of screening tests alone. Patients suspected of having dementia should be examined for other causes of changing mental status, including depression, delirium, medication effects, and coexisting medical illnesses.

The draft update of this chapter was prepared for the U.S. Preventive Services Task Force by David Atkins MD, MPH, with contributions from materials prepared for the Canadian Task Force on the Periodic Health Examination by Christopher Patterson MD, FRCP and materials prepared for the AHCPR Panel on Recognition and Initial Assessment of Alzheimer's and Related Dementia.

REFERENCES

1. National Institutes of Health Consensus Development Conference. Differential dignosis of dementing diseases. JAMA 1987;258:3411–3416.
2. American Psychiatric Association. Diagnostic and statistical manual of mental disorders. 4th ed. Washington, DC: American Psychiatric Association, 1994.

3. McKhann G, Drachman D, Folstein M, et al. Clinical diagnosis of Alzheimer's disease: a report of the NINCDS-ADRDA Work Group under the auspices of the Department of Health and Human Services Task Force on Alzheimer's Disease. Neurology 1984;34:939–944.

4. Larson EB, Kukull WA, Katzman RL. Cognitive impairment: dementia and Alzheimer's disease. Annu Rev Public Health 1992;13:431–449.

5. Breteler MMB, Claus JJ, van Duijn CM, et al. Epidemiology of Alzheimer's disease. Epidemiol Rev 1992;14:59–82.

6. Heyman A, Fillenbaum G, et al. Estimated prevalence of dementia among elderly black and white community residents. Arch Neurol 1991;48:594–598.

7. Skoog I, Nillson L, Palmertz B, et al. A population-based study of dementia in 85-year-olds. N Engl J Med 1993;328:153–158.

8. Aronson MK, Ooi WL, Geva DL, et al. Dementia. Age-dependent incidence, prevalence, and mortality in the old old. Arch Intern Med 1991;151:989–992.

9. Beck JC, Benson DF, Scheibel AB, et al. Dementia in the elderly: the silent epidemic. Ann Intern Med 1982;97: 231–241.

10. Jorm AF, Korten AE, Henderson AS. The prevalence of dementia: a quantitative integration of the literature. Acta Psychiatr Scand 1987;76:456–479.

11. Canadian Study of Health and Aging Working Group. Canadian Study of Health and Aging: study methods and prevalence of dementia. Can Med Assoc J 1994;150:899–913.

12. Bachman DL, Wolf PA, Linn R, et al. Prevalence of dementia and probable senile dementia of the Alzheimer type in the Framingham Study. Neurology 1992;42:115–119.

13. Evans DA, Funkenstein HH, Albert MS, et al. Prevalence of Alzheimer's disease in a community population of older persons. JAMA 1989;262:2551–2556.

14. Bickel H, Cooper B. Incidence and relative risk of dementia in an urban elderly population: findings of a prospective field study. Psychol Med 1994;24:179–192.

14a. Hebert LE, Scherr PA, Beckett LA, et al. Age-specific incidence of Alzheimer's disease in a community population. JAMA 1995;273:1354–1359.

15. Ernst RL, Hay JW. The US economic and social costs of Alzheimer's disease revisited. Am J Public Health 1994;84:1261–1264.

16. Evans DA. Estimated prevalence of Alzheimer's disease in the United States. Milbank Q 1990;68: 267–289.

17. van Duijn CM, Clayton D, Chandra V, et al. Familial aggregation of Alzheimer's disease and related disorders: a collaborative re-analysis of case-control studies. Int J Epidemiol 1991;20(Suppl 2): S13–S20.

18. Alzheimer's Disease Collaborative Group. Apolipoprotein E genotype and Alzheimer's disease. Lancet 1993;342: 737–738.

19. Small GW, Mazziotta JC, Collins MT, et al. Apolipoprotein E type 4 allele and cerebral glucose metabolism in relatives at risk for familial Alzheimer disease. JAMA 1995;273:942–947.

20. Mortimer JA, Graves AB. Education and other socioeconomic determinants of dementia and Alzheimer's disease. Neurology 1993;43(Suppl 4):S39–S44.

21. Larson EB, Buchner DM, Uhlmann RF, et al. Caring for elderly patients with dementia. Arch Intern Med 1986;146:1909–1910.

22. Teri L, Larson EB, Reifler BV. Behavioral disturbance in dementia of the Alzheimer's type. J Am Geriatr Soc 1988;36:1–6.

23. Walsh JS, Welch HG, Larson EB. Survival of outpatients with Alzheimer-type dementia. Ann Intern Med 1990;113:429–434.

24. Kelman HR, Thomas C, Kennedy GJ, et al. Cognitive impairment and mortality in older community residents. Am J Public Health 1994;84:1255–1260.

25. Jordan BD, Schoenberg BS. Mortality from presenile and senile dementia in the United States. South Med J 1986;79:529–531.

26. Pinholt EM, Kroenke K, Hanley JF, et al. Functional assessment of the elderly: a comparison of standard instruments with clinical judgement. Arch Intern Med 1987;147:484–488.

27. Roca RP, Klein LE, Kirby SM, et al. Recognition of dementia among medical patients. Arch Intern Med 1984;144:73–75.

28. World Health Organization. Dementia in later life: research and action: report of a WHO scientific group on senile dementia. Technical Report Series 730. Geneva: World Health Organization, 1986:40–47.

29. German PS, Shapiro S, Skinner EA, et al. Detection and management of mental health problems of older patients by primary care providers. JAMA 1987;257:489–493.

29a. Callahan CM, Hendrie HC, Tierney WM. Documentation and evaluation of cognitive impairment in elderly primary care patients. Ann Intern Med 1995;122:422–429.

30. Klein LE, Roca RP, McArthur J, et al. Diagnosing dementia: univariate and multivariate analyses of the mental status examination. J Am Geriatr Soc 1985;33:483–488.

31. Siu AL. Screening for dementia and investigating its causes. Ann Intern Med 1991;115:122–132.

32. Huff FJ, Boller F, Lucchelli F, et al. The neurologic examination in patients with probable Alzheimer's disease. Arch Neurol 1987;44:929–932.

33. Ritchie K. The screening of cognitive impairment in the elderly: a critical review of current methods. J Clin Epidemiol 1988;41:635–643.

34. Folstein MF, Folstein SE, McHugh PR. Mini-mental state: a practical method for grading the cognitive state of patients for the clinician. J Psychiatr Res 1975;12:189–198.

35. Molloy DW, Alemayehu E, Roberts R. Reliability of a standardized Mini-Mental State Examination compared with the traditional Mini-Mental State Examination. Am J Psychiatry 1991;148:102–105.

36. Tombaugh TN, McIntyre NJ. The Mini-Mental State Examination: a comprehensive review. J Am Geriatr Soc 1992;40:922–935.

37. Kay DW, Henderson AS, Scott R, et al. Dementia and depression among the elderly living in the Hobart community: the effect of diagnostic criteria on prevalence rates. Psychol Med 1985;15:771–788.

38. Crum RM, Anthony JC, Bassett SS, Folstein MF. Population-based norms for the Mini-Mental State Examination by age and education level. JAMA 1993;269:2386–2391.

39. Escobar J, Buirman A, Karns M, et al. Use of the Mini-Mental State Examination (MMSE) in a community population of mixed ethnicity: cultural and linguistic artifacts. J Nerv Ment Dis 1986;174:607–614.

40. Cummings JL. Mini-Mental State Examination. Norms, normals, and numbers. JAMA 1993;269:2420–2421.

41. Pfeiffer E. A short portable mental status questionnaire for the assessment of organic brain deficit in elderly patients. J Am Geriatr Soc 1975;23:433–441.

42. Tuokko H, Hadjistravropoulos T, Miller JA, et al. The Clock test: a sensitive measure to differentiate normal elderly from those with Alzheimer's disease. J Am Geriatr Soc 1992;40:579–584.

43. Applegate WB, Blass JP, Williams TF. Instruments for the functional assessment of older patients. N Engl J Med 1990;322:1207–1214.

44. Barberger-Gateau P, Commenges D, Gagnon M, et al. Instrumental activities of daily living as a screening tool for cognitive impairment and dementia in elderly community dwellers. J Am Geriatr Soc 1992;40:1129–1134.

45. Pfeffer RI, Kurosaki TT, Harrah CH, et al. Measurement of functional activities in older adults in the community. J Gerontol 1982;37:323–329.

46. Hershey LA, Jaffe DF, Greenough PG, et al. Validation of cognitive and functional assessment instruments in vascular dementia. Int J Psychiatry Med 1987;17:183–192.

47. Weinberger M, Samsa GP, Schmader K, et al. Comparing proxy and patients' reports of functional status: results from an outpatient geriatric clinic. J Am Geriatr Soc 1992;40:585–588.

48. O'Connor DW, Fertig A, Grande MJ, et al. Dementia in general practice: the practical consequences of a more positive approach to diagnosis. Br J Gen Pract 1993;43:185–188.

49. Larson EB, Reifler BV, Featherstone HJ, et al. Dementia in elderly outpatients: a prospective study. Ann Intern Med 1984;100:417–423.

50. Clarfield AM. The reversible dementias: do they reverse? Ann Intern Med 1988;109:476–486.

51. Folstein MF, Anthony JC, Parhad I, et al. The meaning of cognitive impairment in the elderly. J Am Geriatr Soc 1985;33:228–235.

52. Gauthier S, Bouchard R, Lamontagne A, et al. Tetrahydroaminoacridine-lecithin combination treatment in patients with intermediate-stage Alzheimer's disease. N Engl J Med 1990;322:1272–1276.

53. Schneider LS, Tariot PN. Emerging drugs for Alzheimer's disease. Med Clin North Am 1994;78:911–934.

54. Farlow M, Gracon SI, Hershey LA, et al. A controlled trial of tacrine in Alzheimer's disease. JAMA 1992;268:2523–2529.

55. Davis KL, Thal LJ, Gamzu ER, et al. A double-blind, placebo-controlled multicenter study of tacrine for Alzheimer's disease. N Engl J Med 1992;327:1253–1259.

56. Knapp MJ, Knopman DS, Solomon PR, et al. A 30-week randomized controlled trial of high-dose tacrine in patients with Alzheimer's disease. JAMA 1994;271:985–991.

57. Thompson TL, Filley CM, Mitchell WD, et al. Lack of efficacy of hydergine in patients with Alzheimer's disease. N Engl J Med 1990;323:445–448.

58. Crapper McLachlan DR, Dalton AJ, Kruck TP, et al. Intramuscular desferrioxamine in patients with Alzheimer's disease [Published erratum in Lancet 1991;337:1618]. Lancet 1991;337:1304–1308.

59. Hachinski V. Preventable senility: a call for action against the vascular dementias. Lancet 1992;340:645–648.

60. Meyer JS, Judd BW, Tawaklna T, et al. Improved cognition after control of risk factors for multi-infarct dementia. JAMA 1986;256:2203–2209.

61. Larson EB, Reifler BV, Sumi SM, et al. Diagnostic evaluation of 200 elderly outpatients with suspected dementia. J Gerontol 1985;40:536–543.

62. Reifler BV, Larson E. Excess disability in demented elderly outpatients: the rule of halves. J Am Geriatr Soc 1988;36:82–83.

63. Drachman DA, Swearer JM. Driving and Alzheimer's disease: the risk of crashes. Neurology 1993;43:2448–2456.

64. Stuck AE, Siu AL, Wieland GD, et al. Comprehensive geriatric assessment: a meta-analysis of controlled trials. Lancet 1993;342:1032–1036.

65. Small GW. Psychopharmacological treatment of elderly demented patients. J Clin Psychiatry 1988; 49 (suppl):8–13.

66. Cyrus-Lutz C, Gaitz CM. Psychiatrists' attitudes toward the aged and aging. Gerontologist 1972;12:163–167.

67. Canadian Task Force on the Periodic Health Examination. Canadian guide to clinical preventive health care. Ottawa: Canada Communication Group, 1994:902–909.

68. American Academy of Family Physicians. Age charts for periodic health examination. Kansas City, MO: American Academy of Family Physicians, 1994. (Reprint no. 510.)

49. Screening for Depression

RECOMMENDATION

There is insufficient evidence to recommend for or against the routine use of standardized questionnaires to screen for depression in asymptomatic primary care patients. Clinicians should maintain an especially high index of suspicion for depressive symptoms in those persons at increased risk for depression (see *Clinical Intervention*). Physician education in recognizing and treating affective disorders is recommended (see Chapter 50).

Burden of Suffering

Depression is a common and costly mental health problem, seen frequently in general medical settings.[1] Major depressive disorder, diagnosed by structured psychiatric interviews and specific diagnostic criteria, is present in 5–13% of patients seen by primary care physicians.[2–7] The prevalence of this disease in the general population is about 3–5%.[8] The annual economic burden of depression in the U.S. (including direct care costs, mortality costs, and morbidity costs) has been estimated to total almost $44 billion.[9] Depression is more common in persons who are young, female, single, divorced, separated, seriously ill, or who have a prior history or family history of depression.[10]

Major depressive disorder can result in serious sequelae. The suicide rate in depressed persons is at least 8 times higher than that of the general population.[11] In 1993, 31,230 suicide deaths were reported, although the actual number is probably much higher.[12] Most persons who commit suicide have a mental disorder, with depression associated with about half of suicides.[9,11] The incidence of documented suicides by adolescents and young adults has tripled in the last 25 years, with 5,000 youths committing suicide each year and perhaps as many as 500,000–1,000,000 making an attempt[13] (see Chapter 50).

On a population basis, the most important effect of major depression may be on quality of life and productivity rather than suicide. This effect is widespread and has been shown to be comparable to that associated with major chronic medical conditions such as diabetes, hypertension, or coronary heart disease.[14,15] Also, depressed persons frequently present with a variety of physical symptoms—three times the number of somatic symptoms of controls in one study.[16] If their depression is not recognized, these patients may be subjected to the risks and costs of unnecessary diagnostic testing and treatment.[17,18]

Accuracy of Screening Tests

The prevailing standard for the diagnosis of depression is the opinion of an examining psychiatrist that a patient's symptoms meet the criteria described in the fourth edition of the Diagnostic and Statistical Manual of Mental Disorders (DSM-IV).[19] For research purposes, psychiatric diagnoses have been operationalized through the development of structured diagnostic interview instruments such as the Diagnostic Interview Schedule (DIS).[20]

To aid in the detection of this important disorder, screening questionnaires have been proposed to predict a patient's risk of depression. Several brief (2–5 minutes) questionnaires have been tested for routine use by primary care providers. These include the Beck Depression Inventory (BDI),[21] the Center for Epidemiologic Studies Depression scale (CES-D),[22] and the Zung Self-Rating Depression Scale (SDS).[23] These three instruments have been shown to detect adult patients with depressive symptoms fairly accurately in primary care settings, with sensitivities and specificities that vary depending on the cutoff score selected. For example, when compared to the diagnosis of major depression in primary care patients using a standardized psychiatric instrument such as the DIS, the BDI had a sensitivity of 100% and a specificity of 89% at a cutoff score of 16;[6] the CES-D had a sensitivity of 89% and a specificity of 70% at a cutoff score of 27;[2] and the SDS had a sensitivity of 97% and a specificity of 63% at a cutoff score of 50.[24] A recent meta-analysis of 18 studies that compared various depression screening instruments to accepted diagnostic criteria in primary care patients estimated an overall sensitivity of 84% and specificity of 72% for these tests.[27a] The authors calculated that screening 100 primary care patients (prevalence of major depression 5%) would identify 31 patients with a positive screen, 4 of whom actually have major depression.

Depression screening questionnaires developed specifically for children and adolescents include the Center for Epidemiologic Studies Depression Scale for Children (CES-DC)[25] and the Children's Depression Inventory (CDI).[26] They have been validated against structured diagnostic interview instruments developed for children and adolescents. At a cutoff of 15, the CES-DC had a sensitivity of 71% and a specificity of 57% for major depressive disorder.[25] In addition, the adult CES-D and BDI have been tested on adolescents, with a sensitivity of 84% and a specificity of 75% for the CES-D at a cutoff of 24 and a sensitivity of 84% and a specificity of 81% for the BDI at a cutoff of 11.[27]

It should be noted that the usual nomenclature used in the assessment of screening tests for asymptomatic persons is not strictly applicable to depression screening, because the diagnosis of depression is itself based on symptoms. A patient cannot truly be asymptomatic and have major depressive disorder. Thus, these screening questionnaires are actually being evaluated for their ability to detect unrecognized, rather than strictly asymptomatic, depressive symptoms (sleeplessness, loss of appetite, etc.) and disease.

Effectiveness of Early Detection

It has been repeatedly documented that primary care providers do not recognize major depression in approximately half of their adult patients with this disorder.[2,28–31] Because the majority of persons with depression are seen by nonpsychiatrist physicians,[32] and because effective treatments—drugs, psychotherapy, or a combination of the two—are available for the treatment of depression,[33] it has been proposed that routine depression screening could result in improved recognition and earlier treatment of depression with improved patient outcome.

Clinical trials have shown that the use of depression screening tests in primary care settings can increase clinician detection of depression.[31,34–36] A randomized controlled trial of screening with SDS found increased recognition and increased treatment of depression in the patients detected by screening.[37] A prospective controlled study found that providing SDS scores to the physician and prescribing a 4-week course of antidepressants to those with elevated scores resulted in lower patient SDS scores than in controls in whom SDS results were withheld and who received unspecified care.[38] This study had several design limitations, however, including confounding variables, different data collection techniques for controls, short follow-up, and the use of questionnaire scores as outcome measures.

These and other studies have established that depression screening can lead to increased recognition and, in some studies, treatment of depression in primary care patients. Separate research has found that the treatment of depressed patients leads to improved outcome.[33] Taken together, however, these studies still constitute insufficient evidence to conclude that routine depression screening is indicated in unselected patients, because it has not been shown that the early detection and treatment of depression in primary care leads to improved outcome when compared to routine diagnosis and treatment of this disorder when symptoms appear and are detected. While there is evidence that the initiation of treatment in the early stages of a recurrent episode of depression in psychiatric settings results in a better outcome than intervention when the traditional symptoms of depression become conspicuous,[39] data are not available demonstrating a similar advantage of early detection and treatment for the initial onset of depression or for the typically less severe depression seen in primary care. No published studies have shown improvement in rigorously assessed psychiatric outcome in primary care patients screened, treated, and compared to controls, although a study of this type is currently under way with an adult population.[40]

No studies to date have demonstrated that screening asymptomatic children or adolescents for depression leads to improved outcomes.

Recommendations of Other Groups

The Canadian Task Force on the Periodic Health Examination found fair evidence to exclude the use of depression detection tests from the periodic health examination of asymptomatic people.[41] The Depression Guideline Panel sponsored by the Agency for Health Care Policy and Research recommended that providers maintain a high index of suspicion for depression and evaluate risk factors, detecting depressive symptoms with a clinical interview.[42] The American Academy of Family Physicians advises physicians to remain alert for depressive symptoms in adolescents and adults;[43] this policy is under review. The American Medical Association recommends that all adolescents be asked annually about behaviors or emotions that indicate recurrent or severe depression.[44] Bright Futures recommends annual screening of adolescents for behaviors or emotions that may indicate recurrent or severe depression or risk of suicide.[45]

Discussion

At present, available depression questionnaires lack the evidence necessary to support their routine use as screening tools in the periodic health examination for primary care patients.[27a] Emerging research, both on current screening questionnaires[40] and on new primary care mental disorder diagnostic tools,[46] may change this situation. The enormous burden of suffering from this disease, its high prevalence in primary care settings, and its frequent presentation with somatic symptoms that lead to extensive medical testing and interventions all argue for better awareness of depressive symptoms by primary care physicians so that fewer cases of depression will escape detection. It is also important that depressed persons who are identified receive adequate follow-up care.

CLINICAL INTERVENTION

There is insufficient evidence to recommend for or against the routine use of standardized questionnaires to screen for depression in asymptomatic primary care patients ("C" recommendation). Clinicians should, however, maintain an especially high index of suspicion for depressive symptoms in adolescents and young adults, persons with a family or personal history of

depression, those with chronic illnesses, those who perceive or have experienced a recent loss, and those with sleep disorders, chronic pain, or multiple unexplained somatic complaints. Physician education in recognizing and treating affective disorders is recommended (see Chapter 50). Persons with depressive symptoms should be evaluated further and, if diagnosed with major depressive disorder, either treated or referred for treatment.

The draft update of this chapter was prepared for the U.S. Preventive Services Task Force by Douglas B. Kamerow, MD, MPH.

REFERENCES

1. Katon W, Schulberg H. Epidemiology of depression in primary care. Gen Hosp Psychiatry 1992;14:237–247.
2. Schulberg HC, Saul M, McClelland M, Ganguli M, Christy W, Frank R. Assessing depression in primary medical and psychiatric practices. Arch Gen Psychiatry 1985;42:1164–1170.
3. Von Korff M, Shapiro S, Burke JD. Anxiety and depression in a primary care clinic. Arch Gen Psychiatry 1987;44:152–156.
4. Barrett JE, Barrett JA, Oxman TE, Gerber PD. The prevalence of psychiatric disorders in a primary care practice. Arch Gen Psychiatry 1988;45:1100–1106.
5. Coulehan JL, Schulberg HC, Block MR, Janosky JE, Arena VC. Medical comorbidity of major depressive disorder in a primary medical practice. Arch Intern Med 1990;150:2363–2367.
6. Zich JM, Attkisson CC, Greenfield TK. Screening for depression in primary care clinics: the CES-D and the BDI. Int J Psychiatry Med 1990;20:259–277.
7. Coyne JC, Fechner-Bates S, Schwenk TL. Prevalence, nature, and comorbidity of depressive disorders in primary care. Gen Hosp Psychiatry 1994;16:267–276.
8. Myers JK, Weissman MM, Tischler GE, et al. Six-month prevalence of psychiatric disorders in three communities. Arch Gen Psychiatry 1984;41:959–970.
9. Greenberg PE, Stiglin LE, Finkelstein SN, Berndt ER. The economic burden of depression in 1990. J Clin Psychiatry 1993;54:405–418.
10. Weissman MM. Advances in psychiatric epidemiology: rates and risks for depression. Am J Public Health 1987;77: 445–451.
11. Monk M. Epidemiology of suicide. Epidemiol Rev 1987;9:51–68.
12. National Center for Health Statistics. Advance report of final mortality statistics, 1993. Monthly vital statistics report; vol 42 no 13 (suppl). Hyattsville, MD: Public Health Service, 1994.
13. Greydanus DE. Depression in adolescence: a perspective. J Adolesc Health Care 1986;7:109S–120S.
14. Wells KB, Stewart A, Hays RD, et al. The functioning and well-being of depressed patients: results from the Medical Outcomes Study. JAMA 1989;262:914–919.
15. Broadhead WE, Blazer DG, George LK, Tse CK. Depression, disability days, and days lost from work in a prospective epidemiologic survey. JAMA 1990;264:2524–2528.
16. Waxman HM, McCreary G, Weinrit RM, Carner EA. A comparison of somatic complaints among depressed and nondepressed older persons. Gerontologist 1985;25:501–507.
17. Katon W, Russo J. Somatic symptoms and depression. J Fam Pract 1989;29:65–69.
18. Katon W, Berg AO, Robins AJ, Risse S. Depression: medical utilization and somatization. West J Med 1986;144:564–568.
19. American Psychiatric Association. Diagnostic and statistical manual of mental disorders. 4th ed. Washington, DC: American Psychiatric Association, 1994:339–345.
20. Robins LN, Helzer JE, Croughan J, Ratcliff KS. National Institute of Mental Health Diagnostic Interview Schedule: its history, characteristics, and validity. Arch Gen Psychiatry 1981;38:381–389.
21. Beck AT, Rial WY, Rickels K. Short form of depression inventory: cross validation. Psychol Rep 1974;34:1184–1186.
22. Radloff LS. The CES-D Scale: a self-report depression scale for research in the general population. Appl Psychol Meas 1977;1:385–401.

23. Zung WWK. A self-rating depression scale. Arch Gen Psychiatry 1965;12:63–70.
24. Zung WWK, Magruder-Habib K, Velez R, Alling W. The comorbidity of anxiety and depression in general medical patients: a longitudinal study. J Clin Psychiatry 1990;51(6 Suppl):77–80.
25. Fendrich M, Weissman MM, Warner V. Screening for depressive disorder in children and adolescents: validating the Center for Epidemiologic Studies Depression Scale for Children. Am J Epidemiol 1990;131:538–551.
26. Saylor CF, Finch AJ, Spirito A. The Children's Depression Inventory: a systematic evaluation of psychometric properties. J Consult Clin Psychol 1984;52:955–967.
27. Roberts RE, Lewinsohn PM, Seeley JR. Screening for adolescent depression: a comparison of depression scales. J Am Acad Child Adolesc Psychiatry 1991;30:58–66.
27a. Mulrow CD, Williams JW, Gerety MB, et al. Case-finding instruments for depression in primary care settings. Ann Intern Med 1995;122:913–921.
28. Borus JF, Howes MJ, Devins NP, Rosenberg R, Livingston WW. Primary health care providers' recognition and diagnosis of mental disorders in their patients. Gen Hosp Psychiatry 1988;10:317–321.
29. Wells KB, Hays RD, Burnam MA, Rogers W, Greenfield S, Ware JE. Detection of depressive disorder for patients receiving prepaid or fee-for-service care: results from the Medical Outcomes Study. JAMA 1989;262:3298–3302.
30. Coyne JC, Schwenk TL, Smolinski M. Recognizing depression: a comparison of family physicians ratings, self-report, and interview measures. J Am Board Fam Pract 1991;4:207–215.
31. Attkisson CC, Zich JM, eds. Depression in primary care: screening and detection. New York: Routledge, 1990.
32. Regier DA, Narrow WE, Rae DS, et al. The de facto US mental and addictive disorders service system: Epidemiologic Catchment Area prospective 1-year prevalence rates of disorders and services. Arch Gen Psychiatry 1993;50:85–94.
33. Elkin I, Shea T, Watkins JT, et al. National Institute of Mental Health treatment of depression collaborative research program: general effectiveness of treatments. Arch Gen Psychiatry 1989;46:971–982.
34. Moore JT, Lilimperi DR, Bobula JA. Recognition of depression by family medicine residents: the impact of screening. J Fam Pract 1978;7:509–513.
35. Linn LS, Yager J. The effect of screening, sensitization, and feedback on notation of depression. J Med Educ 1980;55:942–949.
36. Zung WWK, Magill M, Moore JT, George DT. Recognition and treatment of depression in a family medicine practice. J Clin Psychiatry 1983;44:3–6.
37. Magruder-Habib K, Zung WWK, Feussner JR. Improving physicians' recognition and treatment of depression in general medical care: results from a randomized clinical trial. Med Care 1990;28:239–250.
38. Zung WWK, King RE. Identification and treatment of masked depression in a general medical practice. J Clin Psychiatry 1983;44:365–368.
39. Kupfer DJ, Frank E, Perel JM. The advantage of early treatment intervention in recurrent depression. Arch Gen Psychiatry 1989;46:771–775.
40. Schulberg HC, Coulehan J, Block M, et al. Clinical trials of primary care treatments for major depression: issues in design, recruitment, and treatment. Int J Psychiatry Med 1993;23:29–42.
41. Canadian Task Force on the Periodic Health Examination. Canadian guide to clinical preventive health care. Ottawa: Canada Communication Group, 1994:450–455.
42. Depression Guideline Panel. Depression in primary care: vol 1. Detection and diagnosis. Clinical practice guideline no. 5. Rockville, MD: Department of Health and Human Services, Public Health Service, Agency for Health Care Policy and Research. (Publication no. 93-0550.)
43. American Academy of Family Physicians. Age charts for periodic health examination. Kansas City, MO: American Academy of Family Physicians, 1994. (Reprint no. 510.)
44. American Medical Association. Guidelines for adolescent preventive services (GAPS): recommendations and rationale. Chicago: American Medical Association, 1994:131–139.
45. Green M, ed. Bright Futures: guidelines for health supervision of infants, children, and adolescents. Arlington, VA: National Center for Education in Maternal and Child Health, 1994.
46. Spitzer RL, Williams JBW, Kroenke K, et al. Utility of a new procedure for diagnosing mental disorders in primary care: the PRIME-MD 1000 Study. JAMA 1994;272:1749–1756.

50. Screening for Suicide Risk

RECOMMENDATION

There is insufficient evidence to recommend for or against routine screening by primary care clinicians to detect suicide risk in asymptomatic persons (see *Clinical Intervention*). Clinicians should be alert to signs of suicidal ideation in persons with established risk factors. The training of primary care clinicians in recognizing and treating affective disorders is recommended. Clinicians should be alert to signs and symptoms of depression (see Chapter 49) and should routinely ask patients about their use of alcohol and other drugs (Chapters 52 and 53).

Burden of Suffering

In 1993, the age-adjusted rate of suicide in the U.S. was approximately 11.2/100,000 persons; 31,230 suicide deaths were reported.[1] The actual incidence is uncertain because suicidal intent is often difficult to prove after the fact; uniform criteria for declaring a death due to suicide have only recently been developed.[2] An estimated 210,000 persons attempt suicide each year, resulting in over 10,000 permanent disabilities, 155,500 physician visits, 259,200 hospital days, over 630,000 lost work days, and over $115 million in direct medical expenses.[3] The highest rate of completed suicide is among men aged 65 years and older, but suicide attempts are more commonly reported among women and among men and women aged 20–24 years.[4] The suicide rate in American teenagers has increased substantially in recent years.[5] Suicide is the third leading cause of death in persons 15–24 years old[1] as well as a leading cause of years of potential life lost.[6] Suicides among young persons may also lead to suicide clusters, in which a number of other adolescents in the same community commit suicide.[7]

The most important risk factor for suicide is psychiatric illness. The majority of suicide victims have affective, substance abuse, personality or other mental disorders.[8–9a] Persons with a history of one or more psychiatric hospital admissions carry a particularly high risk of suicide.[10] Other risk factors for suicide and attempted suicide, particularly in persons with underlying mental or substance abuse disorders, include social adjustment problems, serious medical illness, living alone, recent bereavement, personal or family history of suicide attempt, family history of completed suicide, divorce, separation, and unemployment.[4,8,11,12]

Firearms are used in about 60% of all suicides.[1,4,8,9,13] Firearm-related deaths accounted for nearly all the increase in suicide rates during the 1980s.[14] Case-control studies have demonstrated that the risk of suicide is almost five times higher for persons who live in a household where at least one firearm is kept, when compared with persons who live in a household free of guns.[14a–16] The second most common means of suicide among males is hanging, whereas among females it is poisoning (drug overdose).[4] Alcohol intoxication is associated with at least 25–50% of all suicides[9] and is especially common in suicides involving firearms.[4]

Accuracy of Screening Tests

About one half to two thirds of persons who commit suicide visit physicians less than 1 month before the incident, and 10–40% visit in the preceding week.[9,17] It is often difficult, however, for physicians to identify suicidal patients accurately. Direct questions about suicidal intent may have low yield; only 3–5% of persons threatening suicide express unequivocal certainty that they want to die.[18] Nearly 30% of American high school students report having seriously thought about committing suicide,[19,20] making it unlikely that suicidal thoughts alone would be a useful index of suspicion in this population. Although the clinician can identify established risk factors in the medical history (e.g., psychiatric illness, prior suicide attempt, access to firearms, substance abuse, recent life event such as death or divorce), the majority of patients with these characteristics do not intend to kill themselves.[21,22] Asking general medical patients about sleep disturbance, depressed mood, guilt, and hopelessness correctly identified 84% of those who had experienced suicidal thoughts within the previous year.[22a] The study was not designed to assess actual suicide risk, however, and has not been replicated in the clinical setting. If validated, these questions may identify patients who may benefit from in-depth evaluation for suicide risk.

Researchers have attempted to identify specific risk factors that are the strongest predictors of suicidal behavior. Many studies have shown, however, that structured instruments to assess these risk factors misclassified many persons as high risk who did not subsequently attempt suicide and (with some instruments) identified many as low risk who did commit suicide.[23–28] For example, one scoring system,[25] based on 4–6 years of longitudinal data from 4,800 psychiatric patients, was able to identify correctly 35 of 63 (56%) subsequent suicides, but it generated 1,206 false positives (positive predictive value less than 3%).

Also, physicians may not effectively assess risk factors for suicide, such as previous suicide attempts or psychiatric illness. In one study of completed suicides,[29] over two thirds of victims had made previous attempts or threats, but only 39% of their physicians were aware of this history. Although psychological autopsy studies (retrospective psychiatric evaluation based on interviews with survivors) reveal that nearly all victims have evidence of previous psychiatric diagnoses (e.g., depression, bipolar disorder, alcohol and other drug abuse, schizophrenia) and previous psychiatric treatment,[17,21,30] many primary care clinicians fail to recognize the presence of mental illness. Several studies have shown that depression is frequently overlooked (see Chapter 49), as is substance abuse (see Chapters 52 and 53). Improved early detection of these conditions might help persons at risk for suicide, but further research is needed to evaluate its effectiveness in reducing suicide rates.

Recent studies have identified evidence of altered serotonin activity in patients who complete suicide, particularly those with depression and schizophrenia.[31–33] No studies have evaluated these biochemical markers as screening tools in the general population.

Effectiveness of Early Detection

Suicide is a relatively rare event, and large samples and lengthy follow-up would be needed for studies to demonstrate significant reduction in suicide rates as a result of a specific intervention such as mental health counseling and hospitalization, limitation of access to potential instruments of suicide, and treatment of underlying conditions.[18] Although these measures seem to be clinically prudent, no direct evidence that they reduce suicide rates was found. Effects on less specific outcome measures, such as feelings of hopelessness,[34] have been reported. Even in the setting of attempted suicide, there is limited and conflicting evidence that intervention is beneficial; but there is also no conclusive evidence that it is not. Surveys indicate that patients receiving psychiatric consultation for attempted suicide find the therapy to be of limited benefit,[35] and 35–40% choose not to remain in treatment.[36,37] One study of hospitalized patients admitted for poisoning or self-inflicted injury reported fewer subsequent suicide attempts in persons who received psychiatric counseling than in controls who were discharged prematurely before seeing a psychiatrist.[38] Another cohort study of patients hospitalized for self-poisoning found no difference in subsequent suicide attempts among patients who attended psychiatric outpatient follow-up and those who did not.[39] Among suicide attempters without immediate psychiatric or medical needs randomized to receive hospital admission or discharge home, there were no differences in psychological testing or further suicide attempts between the two groups at 1 week; long-term follow-up was not evaluated, however.[40] Some selection biases were apparent in all of these studies, thereby limiting the generalizability of their results to all suicide attempters. Findings from these studies may not be applicable to successful suicide because people who attempt and those who complete suicide may differ. Involuntary hospitalization can be of immediate benefit to persons planning suicide and is often required for medicolegal reasons in persons with suspected suicidal ideation,[41,42] but no reliable data on the long-term effectiveness of this measure were found.

Another potential intervention is limiting access to the most common instruments of suicide, such as firearms and drugs. Although there is no direct evidence that removal of firearms can prevent suicide, studies have shown that geographic locations with reduced availability of these weapons have lower suicide rates among adolescents and young adults.[8,43] Studies of deaths by drug overdose have found that, in over half of cases, the ingested drugs were either prescribed by a physician within the preceding week or were provided in a refillable prescription.[44] There is little information, however, on how the physician can best identify persons who require nonlethal quantities of prescription drugs, or whether these measures will prevent subsequent suicide. Legislation in one country restricting the prescription of sedatives may have been associated with a reduced rate of suicide, but the evidence was not conclusive.[45]

Since it has been estimated that as many as 90% of persons who commit suicide suffer from psychiatric disorders, it is possible that treatment of these underlying illnesses may prevent suicide.[34] Indirect evidence suggests that patients with affective disorders who receive comprehensive psychiatric care have lower suicide rates than most persons with psychiatric illnesses,[46,47] but studies with control groups are needed to exclude the possibility of selection bias in these results. A Swedish population-based time series study evaluated suicide rates before and 1 year after all postgraduate physicians in a community were trained to recognize and manage affective disorders appropriately.[48] The suicide rate in the community decreased 50% in the year following the program, which was significant compared to previous trends in that community and to national rates in Sweden. Repetition of these results in a controlled trial with longer follow-up is needed. As many as 50% of persons who kill themselves are intoxicated with alcohol or other drugs,[9] and a significant proportion also suffer from a substance abuse disorder.[8] Early detection and treatment of alcohol and other drug abuse has the potential to prevent suicide, but firm evidence of this effect is lacking.

Recommendations of Other Groups

The American Academy of Pediatrics recommends asking all adolescents about suicidal thoughts during the routine medical history.[49] The American Medical Association[50] and Bright Futures[51] recommend that providers screen adolescents annually to identify those at risk for suicide.

The Canadian Task Force on the Periodic Health Examination found insufficient evidence to recommend for or against the inclusion of suicide risk evaluation in the periodic health examination. Based on the high burden of suffering, however, they recommend that clinicians routinely evaluate the risk of suicide among persons in high-risk groups, particularly if there is evidence of psychiatric disorder (especially psychosis), depression, or substance abuse, or if the patient has recently attempted suicide or has a family member who committed suicide.[52] The recommendations of the American Academy of Family Physicians are currently under review.

Discussion

Suicide is a leading cause of death in the U.S., but there is no evidence that screening the general population for suicide risk is effective in reducing suicide rates. Routine medical history is often not sufficient to recognize suicide risk or suicidal intent. Several screening instruments have been developed to identify risk factors, but these do not accurately predict the likelihood of suicide. Even when a risk factor or suicidal intent is detected, there is weak evidence that interventions effectively reduce suicide rates. Several studies have evaluated treatment of those who attempt suicide, but results were conflicting, and these studies may not be generalizable to the population of those who complete suicide. Training primary care clinicians to recognize and treat appropriately underlying mental health problems such as depression and substance abuse may be effective, but long-term controlled studies have yet to be performed.

CLINICAL INTERVENTION

There is insufficient evidence to recommend for or against routine screening by primary care clinicians to detect suicide risk in asymptomatic persons ("C" recommendation). Clinicians should be alert to evidence of suicidal ideation when the history reveals risk factors for suicide, such as depression, alcohol or other drug abuse, other psychiatric disorder, prior attempted suicide, recent divorce, separation, unemployment, and recent bereavement. Patients with evidence of suicidal ideation should be questioned regarding the extent of preparatory actions (e.g., obtaining a weapon, making a plan, putting affairs in order, giving away prized possessions, preparing a suicide note). It may also be prudent to question the person's family members regarding such actions. Persons with evidence of suicidal intent should be offered mental health counseling and possibly hospitalization.

The training of primary care clinicians in recognizing and treating affective disorders in order to prevent suicide is recommended ("B" recommendation). Clinicians should be alert to signs of depression (see Chapter 49) and other psychiatric illnesses, and they should routinely ask patients about their use of alcohol and other drugs (see Chapters 52 and

53). Patients who are judged to be at risk should receive evaluation for possible psychiatric illness, including substance abuse, and counseling and referral as needed.

Patients who are recognized as having suicidal ideation, or patients who suspect suicidal thoughts in their relatives or friends, should be made aware of available community resources such as local mental health agencies and crisis intervention centers. Parents and homeowners should also be counseled to restrict unauthorized access to potentially lethal prescription drugs and to firearms within the home (also see Chapters 58 and 59).

The draft update of this chapter was prepared for the U.S. Preventive Services Task Force by S. Patrick Kachur, MD, MPH, and Carolyn DiGuiseppi, MD, MPH.

REFERENCES

1. National Center for Health Statistics. Annual summary of births, marriages, divorces, and deaths: United States, 1993. Monthly vital statistics report; vol 42 no 13. Hyattsville, MD: Public Health Service, 1994.
2. Centers for Disease Control. Operational criteria for determining suicide. MMWR 1988;37:773–774, 779–780.
3. Rosenberg ML, Gelles RJ, Holinger PC, et al. Violence: homicide, assault, and suicide. In: Amler RW, Dull BH, eds. Closing the gap: the burden of unnecessary illness. New York: Oxford University Press, 1987:164–178.
4. Baker SP, O'Neill B, Ginsburg MG, et al. The injury fact book. New York: Oxford University Press, 1992:65–77.
5. Centers for Disease Control and Prevention. Suicide among children, adolescents, and young adults— United States, 1980–1991. MMWR 1995;44:289–291.
6. Centers for Disease Control and Prevention. Years of potential life lost before age 65—United States, 1990 and 1991. MMWR 1993;42:251–253.
7. Gould MS, Wallenstein S, Kleinman MH. Time-space clustering of teenage suicide. Am J Epidemiol 1990;131: 71–78.
8. Monk M. Epidemiology of suicide. Epidemiol Rev 1987;9:51–69.
9. Blumenthal SJ. Suicide: a guide to risk factors, assessment, and treatment of suicidal patients. Med Clin North Am 1988;72:937–971.
9a. Brent DA, Perper JA, Moritz G, et al. Psychiatric risk factors for adolescent suicide: a case-control study. J Am Acad Child Adolesc Psychiatry 1993;32:521–529.
10. Allebeck P, Allgulander C. Psychiatric diagnoses as predictors of suicide; a comparison of diagnoses at conscription and in psychiatric care in a cohort of 50,465 young men. Br J Psychiatry 1990;157:339–344.
11. Lewinsohn PM, Rohde P, Seeley JR. Psychosocial characteristics of adolescents with a history of suicide attempt. J Am Acad Child Adolesc Psychiatry 1993;32:60–68.
12. Pfeffer CR, Klerman GL, Hurt SW, et al. Suicidal children grow up: rates and psychosocial risk factors for suicide attempts during follow-up. J Am Acad Child Adolesc Psychiatry 1993;32:106–113.
13. Moscicki EK, Boyd JH. Epidemiological trends in firearm suicides among adolescents. Pediatrician 1983–85;12: 52–62.
14. Centers for Disease Control and Prevention. Surveillance summary report: suicide in the United States, 1980–1990. Atlanta, GA: Centers for Disease Control and Prevention, 1994.
14a. Brent DA, Perper JA, Moritz G, et al. Firearms and adolescent suicide: a community case-control study. Am J Dis Child 1993;147:1066–1071.
15. Brent DA, Perper JA, Allman CJ, et al. The presence and accessibility of firearms in the homes of adolescent suicides, a case-control study. JAMA 1991;266:2989–2995.
16. Kellerman AL, Rivara FP, Somes G, et al. Suicide in the home in relation to gun ownership. N Engl J Med 1992;327: 467–472.
17. Robins E, Murphy GE, Wilkinson RH Jr, et al. Some clinical considerations in the prevention of suicide based on a study of 134 successful suicides. Am J Public Health 1959;49:888–899.

18. Pfeffer CR. Suicide prevention: current efficacy and future promise. Ann NY Acad Sci 1986;487:341–350.
19. Centers for Disease Control. Attempted suicide among high school students—United States, 1990. MMWR 1991; 40:1–3.
20. Shaffer D, Garland A, Gould M, et al. Preventing teenage suicide: a critical review. J Am Acad Child Adolesc Psychiatry 1988;27:675–687.
21. Mann JJ. Psychobiologic predictors of suicide. J Clin Psychiatry 1987;48(Suppl 12):39–43.
22. Murphy GE. On suicide prediction and prevention. Arch Gen Psychiatry 1983;40:343–344.
22a. Cooper-Patrick L, Crum RM, Ford DE. Identifying suicidal ideation in general medical patients. JAMA 1994;272: 1757–1762.
23. Motto JA, Heilbron DC, Juster RP. Development of a clinical instrument to estimate suicide risk. Am J Psychiatry 1985;142:680–686.
24. Erdman HP, Greist JH, Gustafson DH, et al. Suicide risk prediction by computer interview: a prospective study. J Clin Psychiatry 1987;48:464–467.
25. Pokorny AD. Prediction of suicide in psychiatric patients: report of a prospective study. Arch Gen Psychiatry 1983;40:249–257.
26. Beck AT, Brown G, Berchick RJ, et al. Relationship between hopelessness and ultimate suicide: a replication with psychiatric outpatients. Am J Psychiatry 1990;147:190–195.
27. Rydin E, Asberg M, Edman G, et al. Violent and nonviolent suicide attempts—a controlled Rorschach study. Acta Psychiatr Scand 1990;82:30–39.
28. Goldstein RB, Black DW, Nasrallah A, et al. The prediction of suicide: sensitivity, specificity, and predictive value of a multivariate model applied to suicide among 1906 patients with affective disorders. Arch Gen Psychiatry 1991;48: 418–422.
29. Murphy GE. The physician's responsibility for suicide. II. Errors of omission. Ann Intern Med 1975; 82:305–309.
30. Rich CL, Young D, Fowler RC. San Diego suicide study. I. Young vs. old subjects. Arch Gen Psychiatry 1986;43: 577–582.
31. Pandey GN, Pandey SC, Janicak PG, et al. Platelet serotonin-2 receptor binding sites in depression and suicide. Biol Psychiatry 1990;28:215–222.
32. Wetzler S, Kahn RS, Asnis GM, et al. Serotonin receptor sensitivity and aggression. Psychiatry Res 1991;37: 271–279.
33. Cooper SJ, Kelley CB, King DJ. 5-Hydroindoleacetic acid in cerebrospinal fluid and prediction of suicidal behavior in schizophrenia. Lancet 1992;340:940–941.
34. Blumenthal SJ, Kupfer DJ. Generalizable treatment strategies for suicidal behavior. Ann NY Acad Sci 1986;487: 327–339.
35. Hengleveld MW, Kerkof AJFM, van der Wal J. Evaluation of psychiatric consultations with suicide attempters. Acta Psychiatr Scand 1988;77:283–289.
36. Morgan HG, Barton J, Pottle S, et al. Deliberate self-harm: a follow-up study of 279 patients. Br J Psychiatry 1976;128:361–368.
37. van Aalst JA, Shotts SD, Vitsky JL, et al. Long-term follow-up of unsuccessful violent suicide attempts: risk factors for subsequent attempts. J Trauma 1992;33:457–464.
38. Greer S, Bagley C. Effect of psychiatric intervention in attempted suicide: a controlled study. BMJ 1971;1:310–312.
39. Ojehagen A, Danielsson M, Traskman-Bendz L. Deliberate self-poisoning: a treatment follow-up of repeaters and nonrepeaters. Acta Psychiatr Scand 1992;85:370–375.
40. Waterhouse J, Platt S. General hospital admission in the management of parasuicide; a randomized controlled trial. Br J Psychiatry 1990;156:236–242.
41. Waltzer H. Malpractice liability in a patient's suicide. Am J Psychother 1980;34:89–98.
42. Wise TN, Berlin R. Involuntary hospitalization: an issue for the consultation-liaison psychiatrist. Gen Hosp Psychiatry 1987;9:40–44.
43. Sloan JH, Rivara FP, Reay DT, et al. Firearm regulations and rates of suicide: a comparison of two metropolitan areas. N Engl J Med 1990;322:369–373.
44. Murphy GE. The physician's responsibility for suicide. I. An error of commission. Ann Intern Med 1975;82:301–304.
45. Goldney RD, Katsikitas M. Cohort analysis of suicide rates in Australia. Arch Gen Psychiatry 1983;40:71–74.
46. Martin RL, Cloninger R, Guxe SB, et al. Mortality in a follow-up of 500 psychiatric outpatients. Arch Gen Psychiatry 1985;42:58–66.

47. Jamison KR. Suicide and bipolar disorders. Ann NY Acad Sci 1986;487:301–315.
48. Rutz W, von Knorring L, Walinder J. Frequency of suicide on Gotland after systematic postgraduate education of general practitioners. Acta Psychiatr Scand 1989;80:151–154.
49. American Academy of Pediatrics, Committee on Adolescence. Suicide and suicide attempts in adolescents and young adults. Pediatrics 1988;81:322–324.
50. American Medical Association. Guidelines for adolescent preventive services (GAPS): recommendations and rationale. Chicago: American Medical Association, 1994:131–143.
51. Green M, ed. Bright Futures: guidelines for health supervision of infants, children, and adolescents. Arlington, VA: National Center for Education in Maternal and Child Health, 1994.
52. Canadian Task Force on the Periodic Health Examination. Canadian guide to clinical preventive health care. Ottawa: Canada Communication Group, 1994:456–470.

51. Screening for Family Violence

RECOMMENDATION

There is insufficient evidence to recommend for or against the use of specific screening instruments to detect family violence, but recommendations to include questions about physical abuse when taking a history from adult patients may be made on other grounds (see *Clinical Intervention*). Clinicians should be alert to the various presentations of child abuse, spouse and partner abuse, and elder abuse.

Burden of Suffering

Family violence is a serious public health problem for many Americans. Family violence includes **child abuse** (physical and sexual abuse), **domestic violence** (physical or sexual abuse of spouse or intimate partner), and **elder abuse** (abuse or neglect of older persons).[1] Because many cases of family violence go unreported, the true magnitude of the problem can only be estimated.[2]

Child Abuse. In 1993, child protective service agencies substantiated maltreatment of over 1 million children in the U.S. (a rate of 14/1,000 children); over 1,028 deaths due to child maltreatment were reported in 1993.[3] Intentional injury is the leading cause of injury-related death in children under 1 year of age.[4] Parents or other relatives are responsible for over 90% of reported cases of child maltreatment.[3] In addition to physical injuries, children who have been victims of or witnesses to violence often experience abnormal physical, social, and emotional development; adolescents and adults who were abused as children are more likely to abuse tobacco and alcohol, attempt suicide, and exhibit violent or criminal behavior.[2,5–7]

Approximately 140,000 cases of child sexual abuse were reported in 1993,[3] but the true incidence has been estimated to be as high as 450,000 cases per year.[8] In sexual abuse cases where the abuser was known to the child, over two thirds involved abuse by family members.[9] Girls are victims of sexual abuse two and a half times more frequently than boys.[10] Child sexual abuse often results in severe psychological trauma,[11] has been associated with a variety of psychological problems persisting into adulthood, and can cause medical complications such as sexually transmitted diseases. Teens who had been sexually abused were significantly more likely than nonabused controls to be sexually active, to abuse alcohol or drugs, and to have attempted suicide.[7,12]

A number of parental and family characteristics have been identified as risk factors or risk markers for child physical abuse—poor social support, low socioeconomic status, single parent family, and unplanned or unwanted pregnancy[13]—but abuse is usually the result of multiple interacting factors.[14] Abuse of drugs or alcohol, although not clearly an independent risk factor, often coexists with conditions (poverty, social isolation, etc.) that increase the risk of abuse.[15] Abusive mothers are often themselves victims of physical violence by their spouse or partner,[16] and abusive parents often experienced abuse as children. A poor understanding of normal child development, poor anger control, and use of physical punishment as a discipline technique are more common among abusive parents.[13] In contrast, demographic or family characteristics are of little value in predicting risk of child sexual abuse.[17]

Domestic Violence. Estimates of the prevalence of domestic violence among couples vary depending on the source of data and definition of violence.[18] A national survey of 50,000 households conducted in 1992 and 1993 estimated that over 1 million women (9.3/1,000) and nearly 150,000 men (1.4/1,000) are victims each year of assault, robbery, or rape committed by their spouse, ex-spouse, or intimate partner;[19] over half of these incidents result in minor injury, and 3% in serious injury (broken bones, loss of consciousness, hospitalization, etc.).[20] This estimate may be conservative due to underreporting. In a comprehensive survey of family violence, involving detailed interviews of a total of 8,145 families in 1975 and 1985, 16% of couples reported instances of violence in the previous year (including shoving, slapping, or grabbing); 40% of these episodes involved more serious actions such as kicking, punching, or use of a weapon.[21,22] In recent surveys, 2–3% of women reported being kicked, bitten, or hit with fist or some other object by their partner in the preceding year.[22,23] Family studies indicate that both men and women engage in violence against partners, but women are the primary victims of chronic battering and episodes leading to injury.[24] In 95% of episodes of domestic violence leading to criminal investigation,[20] and 59% of spouse murders,[25] women were the victims. The prevalence of domestic violence is also high among female patients in clinical settings: 15% of women visiting an emergency department[26] and 12–23% of women in family practice settings[27,28] reported having been physically abused or threatened by their partner within the last year. Domestic violence tends to be repetitive—female victims reported an average of six violent incidents per year.[22] The psychological consequences of abuse can be as important as physical injuries: abused women may suffer from posttraumatic stress disorder, and they are more likely than nonabused women to be depressed, attempt suicide, abuse alcohol or drugs, and transfer their aggression to their children.[29,30]

Violence between spouses or partners can occur in families from all demographic and economic strata of society,[22] but risk of physical assault appears higher for some groups of women. Women who are under age 35, have not attended college, are of lower socioeconomic status, or are unmarried are more likely to report being victims of domestic violence.[20] A review of 52 studies found that only one risk marker—witnessing parental violence as a child or adolescent—was consistently associated with being a battered spouse.[31] Childhood family violence and alcohol problems are more common among abusive partners.[22] In general, however, the primary care physician is not able to predict reliably which patients are likely to be affected by domestic partner violence.[32]

Pregnant women are also at risk from domestic violence.[33,34] In surveys of pregnant women (primarily from urban, public clinics), 7–18% of women reported physical abuse (including forced sexual activity) during the current pregnancy.[35-38] Many studies have reported an association between violence and worse outcomes in pregnancy. Battered women are more likely to register late for care, suffer preterm labor or miscarriage, or have low birth weight infants than nonabused controls.[35-39]

Elder Abuse. Elderly persons are also vulnerable to physical or psychological abuse or neglect by family members or other caregivers.[40,41] Community surveys in Boston and Canada estimated that 3–4% of persons over age 65 are victims of physical abuse, neglect, or regular verbal abuse.[42,43] Factors that appear to increase vulnerability to abuse among older persons include poor or failing health, cognitive impairment, and lack of family, financial, or community support.[41] The abuser is usually a relative, most often the spouse.[44] Family members who have a history of substance abuse, mental illness, or violence, or who are financially dependent on the elder person, are more likely to be abusive.[41] Accurate estimates of the medical consequences of elderly abuse (patient visits, hospitalizations, or costs of care) are not available.[42] It is estimated that less than 1 in 5 cases of elder abuse is reported, due to denial or minimization of the problem by the victim, abuser, or health professionals.[45] In one report, up to 60% of elder abuse victims admitted for acute medical care remained permanently institutionalized.[46] The incidence of mistreatment of elders in institutions is not known. A survey of nursing home staff revealed that 36% of the staff had witnessed physical abuse, and 81% had witnessed psychological abuse of patients.[47]

Accuracy of Screening Tests

Family violence may come to attention when it results in severe injuries, but ongoing abuse often goes unrecognized in the clinical setting. The clinician can identify victims of domestic violence through the patient interview, use of a standardized questionnaire, or the physical examination.

There are few reliable techniques for screening for child abuse. Questionnaires can identify risk factors for child abuse and neglect, but the potential to falsely label families as "potential abusers" is a limitation to their use in clinical practice.[48] Eliciting evidence of child physical or sexual abuse through patient interview is difficult. Young children may not be able to answer reliably, both child and parent may be ashamed or fearful of admitting to abuse, and some abusive parents may not regard their use of physical punishment as abuse. Most authorities recommend exploring for potential problems with open-ended, nonjudgmental questions about parenting and discipline (e.g., "What do you do when he misbehaves? Have you ever been worried that someone was going to hurt your child?").[14,49] The value of standardized questions or screening instruments to improve the detection of child abuse is not known. Physical findings suggestive of abuse noted during routine or symptomatic examinations have been described.[50] Burns, bruises, and other lesions can be suggestive due to their appearance (e.g., patterns resembling hands, belts, cords, and other weapons) or location (buttocks, lower back, upper thighs, and face). Multiple traumatic injuries without a plausible explanation are also suspicious. At the same time, accidental injuries may produce similar findings in children, and many abused children (especially victims of sexual abuse) have no obvious physical findings. In a survey of studies of sexually abused children, normal examinations were reported in up to 73% of girls and 82% of boys.[51] Neither the sensitivity nor specificity of screening for abuse with physical examination is known.

Some studies report that less than 10% of battered women are accurately diagnosed by physicians, even in hospitals with an established protocol for this problem.[30,33] The routine patient interview often fails to detect abuse in adult patients, in large part because physicians do not routinely ask about domestic violence. Only a third of physicians in one survey felt that routine questions on abuse should be part of the annual examination.[52] Many physicians are reluctant to ask about abuse, out of fear of offending their patients, inability to "fix" abusive relationships, frustration in dealing with resistant patient behavior, and lack of time to deal with the problem.[53] Both victim and abuser may deny abuse for a variety of reasons—embarrassment, psychologic repression, or fear of reprisal, abandonment, or legal consequences.

Consistent use of screening protocols significantly improves the detection of abuse as a cause of trauma,[54] and similar measures have been shown to increase the detection of domestic violence affecting pregnant and nonpregnant outpatients. The large majority of abuse victims favored routine questions about abuse, and half indicated that they would volunteer information about domestic violence only if specifically asked.[52] Directly asking individuals about the occurrence of abuse has been shown to elicit more positive reports (29% vs. 7%) than the use of a written self-report.[55] The Abuse Assessment Screen, containing five questions on the frequency and severity of past and current physical abuse and forced sexual activity, has been validated against more comprehensive instruments in pregnant women.[56] Incorporation of this instrument into the standard social service interview of pregnant patients significantly increased the detection of recent abuse compared to historical controls (15% vs. 3%).[35]

There are fewer studies on screening for elder abuse. The value of the patient interview may be limited if the abuser is present. A 15-item instrument for detecting elder abuse had a sensitivity of 64% and specificity of 91% in a pilot study, but has not been validated for screening in routine practice.[57]

Effectiveness of Early Detection

The repetitive nature of family violence suggests that early detection may be important in preventing future problems from abuse. Specifically, patients can be counseled about the nature and course of family violence, given information about available resources (community counseling and support groups, shelters, protective service agencies, etc.), and counseled about means to prevent further abuse. Psychological counseling, by either the primary care clinician or a mental health professional, may help the patient terminate personal relationships with violent individuals. The clinician may also identify individuals who are at increased risk of committing abuse in the future. Such persons may be referred for psychiatric counseling or family therapy to learn stress management and nonviolent alternatives for conflict resolution. Finally, the clinician is able (in many instances, required) to report suspected cases of abuse and neglect to appropriate protective service agencies for further evaluation and intervention.

Intervention studies in child abuse have concentrated on primary prevention.[48] Two randomized clinical trials have shown that home visits to high-risk families decrease the rate of child abuse and the need for medical visits early in life.[58,59] Interventions may need to be ongoing to retain effectiveness: extended follow-up of one of these trials found no effect of intervention on the rate of abuse and neglect later in life (ages 25–50 months).[60] Unfortunately, most clinicians do not have the option of providing this level of intervention. Studies evaluating the effectiveness of treatments for abused children are limited, and their results have been mixed.[61] Recurrent abuse despite interventions may occur in up to 60% of cases.[62] The effectiveness of treating sexual abusers of children remains controversial; one outpatient program reduced recidivism by half.[63]

The effectiveness of early intervention for domestic violence is also difficult to determine. Most interventions for spouse abuse (e.g., shelters, legal action) are crisis oriented and have been directed at women who have already been injured by domestic violence. The options available to women are often limited by associated factors common in abusive relationships: financial dependence on an abusive partner, fear of retribution, alcohol or drug problems, or psychological vulnerability.[22,64] As a result, many abused women decline offers of help.[65] For women who do attempt to terminate an abusive relationship, the available resources to assist them are often limited and temporary. In a controlled study of battered women leaving a shelter, women who received services of an advocate for 4–6 hours per week reported better overall quality of life, but no significant difference in levels of physical abuse, compared to controls.[66] Whether treatment of abusive men is effective in reducing domestic violence remains controversial. A randomized trial of group therapy (vs. standard care) for convicted wife-abusers showed that repeat abuse was significantly lower for the treatment group.[67] Effective approaches to couples who engage in mutual, less severe violence (pushing, shoving, etc.) have not been developed. A large controlled study is under way to examine whether an integrated program to improve detection and management of domestic violence in the primary care setting leads to better clinical outcomes.[68]

Effective interventions for elder abuse may also be limited, in large part because the abuser is often the primary caregiver to the victim.[41] If the only alternative is nursing home placement, victims may be reluctant to give up their independence in order to escape abuse. A review of elder physical abuse victims in Illinois reported that most victims received few tangible services from social service agencies other than case management (primarily monitoring).[69] Among abused elders, an advocate program decreased social isolation and improved services, but a reduction in subsequent abuse was not demonstrated.[70]

Recommendations of Other Groups

The American Academy of Pediatrics,[71] American Medical Association,[72,73] American Academy of Family Physicians (AAFP),[74] and the Bright Futures guidelines[49] all recommend that physicians remain alert for the signs and symptoms of child physical abuse and child sexual abuse in the routine examination. Bright Futures suggests including questions about child discipline, and abuse of the child or parents, at the discretion of the clinician. The AMA's Guidelines for Adolescent Preventive Services (GAPS) recommend that teens should be asked annually about a history of emotional, physical, and sexual abuse.[75] The use of screening devices to identify families at risk for child maltreatment is not recommended by the Canadian Task Force on the Periodic Health Examination (CTF).[48] Legislation in all states requires health care professionals to report suspected cases of child abuse.[73]

The American College of Obstetricians and Gynecologists (ACOG),[76] the U.S. Surgeon General,[77] the American College of Physicians,[78] and the AAFP[74] all recommend that clinicians be alert to the possibility of domestic violence as a causal factor in illness and injury. ACOG and AMA guidelines on domestic violence recommend that physicians routinely ask women direct, specific questions about abuse.[79,80] ACP and AAFP guidelines are currently under review. An expert panel convened by the National Research Council and the Institute of Medicine (Washington, DC) to evaluate the effectiveness of family violence interventions is scheduled to publish its findings in 1996. Healthy People 2000, a report of national health objectives,[81] and the Joint Commission on Accreditation of Healthcare Organizations[82] recommend that all emergency departments use protocols to improve the detection and treatment of victims of domestic violence.

The CTF determined that there was insufficient evidence to include or exclude case-finding for elder abuse as part of the periodic health examination, but recommended that physicians be alert for indicators of abuse and institute measures to prevent further abuse.[44] The AMA recommends that physicians routinely ask elderly patients direct, specific questions about abuse.[83] Many states require reporting of domestic violence[84] and elder abuse.[41]

Discussion

Family violence is an important cause of physical and psychological harm in children and adults, yet it often goes undetected by clinicians. Identifying victims of domestic violence provides important information to clinicians and may allow early intervention to reduce the risk from future abuse. Although the benefit of routine screening has not been directly assessed, several factors support greater efforts by clinicians to detect domestic violence between spouses or sexual partners: the substantial prevalence of violent behavior among couples, the repetitive nature of domestic violence, and its high medical and societal costs.[1] Contrary to common perceptions, most patients appreciate being asked about possible abuse, and direct questioning may substantially increase reporting of episodes of domestic violence.

At the same time, clinicians face important obstacles in preventing violence or sexual abuse within the family. The etiology of domestic violence is multifactorial and is a function of social conditions, family conflict, cultural attitudes, and biologic factors. Interventions for physical or sexual abuse, mostly outside of the medical domain, vary greatly in effectiveness.

Although crisis interventions (arrests, referral to shelters) are appropriate to protect victims in specific cases, there are few adequately controlled studies to determine the effect of counseling or referral on the long-term outcome of family violence. Appropriate screening methods for child abuse and elder abuse are also uncertain. Screening for abuse through the patient history is problematic with young children, may be unreliable if the abuser is also present, and can be complicated by denial in all age groups. Errors in diagnosing abuse are of great concern because of the serious emotional, legal, and societal implications of either failing to take action in cases of abuse or of incorrectly accusing innocent persons.

Despite the limited and imperfect options for detecting and intervening in domestic violence, the benefits are substantial for those families where the cycle of abuse can be interrupted. It is also important for clinicians to maintain a high index of suspicion when examining other persons at risk of physical or sexual abuse (e.g., children and the elderly), to assess potential risk factors for domestic violence, and to refer abuse victims and perpetrators to other professionals and community services to help prevent future incidents.

CLINICAL INTERVENTION

There is insufficient evidence to recommend for or against the use of specific screening instruments for family violence, but including a few direct questions about abuse (physical violence or forced sexual activity) as part of the routine history in adult patients may be recommended on other grounds ("C" recommendation). These other grounds include the substantial prevalence of undetected abuse among adult female patients, the potential value of this information in the care of the patient, and the low cost and low risk of harm from such screening. All clinicians examining children and adults should be alert to physical and behavioral signs and symptoms associated with abuse and neglect. Various guidelines are available to help clinicians in recognizing abuse and neglect in children,[71-73] spouses/partners,[80] and elders.[81] In all states, suspected cases of child abuse or neglect must be reported to local child protective services agencies. In most states, suspected elder abuse must also be reported.[41] All individuals who present with multiple injuries and an implausible explanation should be evaluated with attention to possible abuse or neglect. Injured pregnant women and elderly patients should receive special consideration for this problem. Suspected cases of abuse should receive proper documentation of the incident and physical findings (e.g., photographs, body maps); treatment of physical injuries; arrangements for counseling by a skilled mental health professional; and the telephone numbers of local crisis centers, shelters, and protective service agencies. The safety of children of victims of abuse should also be ensured.

The draft update of this chapter was prepared for the U.S. Preventive Services Task Force by Craig F. Thompson, MD, MPH, and David Atkins, MD, MPH, with contributions from materials prepared by Christopher Patterson, MD, FRCPC, Harriet L. MacMillan, MD, FRCPC, James H. MacMillan, MSc, and David R. Offord, MD, FRCPC, for the Canadian Task Force on the Periodic Health Examination.

REFERENCES

1. McAfee RE. Physicians and domestic violence: can we make a difference? JAMA 1995;273:1790–1791.
2. Van Hasselt VB, Morrison RL, Bellack AS, et al., eds. Handbook of family violence. New York: Plenum Press, 1988.
3. U.S. Department of Health and Human Services, National Center on Child Abuse and Neglect. Child maltreatment 1993: reports from the states to the National Center on Child Abuse and Neglect. Washington, DC: Government Printing Office, 1995.
4. Waller AE, Baker SP, Szocka A. Childhood injury deaths: national analysis and geographic variations. Am J Public Health 1989;79:310–315.
5. Reece RM, ed. Child abuse: medical diagnosis and management. Philadelphia: Lea & Febiger, 1994.
6. Wissow LS. Child abuse and neglect. N Engl J Med 1995;332:1425–1431.
7. Riggs S, Alario AJ, McHorney. Health risk behaviors and attempted suicide in adolescents who report prior maltreatment. J Pediatr 1990;116:815–821.
8. National Committee for Prevention of Child Abuse. National incidence and prevalence of child abuse and neglect. Washington, DC: American Humane Association, 1987.
9. Berkowitz CD. Sexual abuse of children and adolescents. Adv Pediatr 1987;34:275–312.
10. Finkelhor D, Baron L. High-risk children. In: Finkelhor D, ed. Sourcebook on child sexual abuse. Beverly Hills, CA: Sage, 1986:60–88.
11. Kendall-Tackett KA, Williams LM, Finkelhor D. Impact of sexual abuse on children: a review and synthesis of recent empirical studies. Psychol Bull 1993;113:164–180.
12. Nagy S, Adcock AG, Nagy MC. A comparison of risky health behaviors of sexually active, sexually abused, and abstaining adolescents. Pediatrics 1994;93:570–575.
13. Biller HB, Solomon RS. Child maltreatment and parental deprivation: a manifesto for research, prevention and treatment. Lexington, MA: Lexington Books, 1986.
14. Dubowitz H. Pediatrician's role in preventing child maltreatment. Pediatr Clin North Am 1990;37:989–1001.
15. Bays J. Substance abuse and child abuse. Pediatr Clin North Am 1990;37:881–904.
16. McKibben L, De Vos E, Newberger EH. Victimization of mothers of abused children. Pediatrics 1989;84:531–535.
17. Finkelhor D. Epidemiological factors in the clinical identification of child sexual abuse. Child Abuse Neglect 1993;17:67–70.
18. Brott AA. Battered-truth syndrome. Washington Post, July 31,1994:C1–C2.
19. Bachman R, Saltzman LE. Violence against women: estimates from the redesigned survey. Bureau of Justice Statistics special report. Washington, DC: U.S. Department of Justice, 1995. (Publication no. NCJ-154348.)
20. Bachman R. Violence against women: a National Crime Victimization Survey report. Bureau of Justice Statistics report. Washington, DC: U.S. Department of Justice, 1994. (Publication no. NCJ-145325.)
21. Straus MA, Gelles RJ, Steinmetz SK. Behind closed doors: a survey of family violence in America. New York: Doubleday, 1980.
22. Straus MA, Gelles RJ. Physical violence in American families. New Brunswick, NJ: Transaction Publishers, 1990.
23. The Commonwealth Fund Survey of Women's Health. New York: Commonwealth Fund, 1993.
24. Cascardi M, Langhinrichsen J, Vivian D. Marital aggression. Impact, injury, and health correlates for husbands and wives. Arch Intern Med 1992;152:1178–1184.
25. Dawson JM, Langan PA. Murder in families. Bureau of Justice Statistics special report. Washington, DC: U.S. Department of Justice, 1994. (Publication no. NCJ-143498.)
26. Abbott J, Johnson R, Koziol-McLain J, et al. Domestic violence against women: incidence and prevalence in an emergency department population. JAMA 1995;273:1763–1767.

27. Hamberger LK, Saunders DG, Hovey M. Prevalence of domestic violence in community practice and rate of physician inquiry. Fam Med 1992;24:382–387.

28. Elliott BA, Johnson MM. Domestic violence in a primary care setting. Arch Fam Med 1995;4:113–119.

29. Plichta S. The effects of woman abuse on health care utilization and health status: a literature review. Women's Health Issues 1992;2:1154–1173.

30. Stark E, Flitcraft A, Zuckerman D, et al. Wife abuse in the medical setting: an introduction for health personnel. Monograph no. 7, Washington, DC: Office of Domestic Violence, 1981.

31. Hotaling GT, Sugarman DB. An analysis of risk markers in husband to wife violence: the current state of knowledge. Violence Vict 1986;1:101–124.

32. Sassetti MR. Domestic violence. Primary Care 1993;20:289–305.

33. Mehta P, Dandrea LA. The battered woman. Am Fam Phys 1988;37:193–199.

34. Campbell JC, Poland ML, Waller JB, Ager J. Correlates of battering during pregnancy. Res Nurs Health 1992;15: 219–226.

35. Norton LB, Peipert JF, Zieler S, et al. Battering in pregnancy: an assessment of two screening methods. Obstet Gynecol 1995;85:321–325.

36. Amaro H, Fried LE, Cabral H, et al. Violence during pregnancy and substance use. Am J Public Health 1990;80: 575–579.

37. Berenson AB, Wiemann CM, Wilkinson GS, et al. Perinatal morbidity associated with violence experienced by pregnant women. Am J Obstet Gynecol 1994;170:1760–1769.

38. Parker B, McFarlane J, Soeken K. Abuse during pregnancy: effects on maternal complications and birth weight in adults and teenage women. Obstet Gynecol 1994;84:323–328.

39. Schei B, Samuelsen SO, Bakketeig LS. Does spousal physical abuse affect the outcome of pregnancy? Scand J Soc Med 1991;19:26–31.

40. Council on Scientific Affairs. Elder abuse and neglect. JAMA 1987;257:966–971.

41. Lachs MS, Pillemer K. Abuse and neglect of elderly persons. N Engl J Med 1995;332:437–443.

42. Pillemer K, Finkelhor D. The prevalence of elder abuse: a random sample survey. Gerontologist 1988;28:51–57.

43. Podnieks E. National survey on abuse of the elderly in Canada. J Elder Abuse Neglect 1992;4:5–58.

44. Canadian Task Force on the Periodic Health Examination. Canadian guide to clinical preventive health care. Ottawa: Canada Communication Group, 1994:922–929.

45. Wolf RS, Pillemer K. Helping elderly victims: the reality of elder abuse. New York: Columbia University Press, 1989.

46. Faulkner LR. Mandating the reporting of suspected cases of elder abuse: an inappropriate, ineffective and ageist response to the abuse of older adults. Fam Law Q 1982;16:69–91.

47. Pillemer K, Moore DW. Abuse of patients in nursing homes: findings from a survey of staff. Gerontologist 1989;29: 314–320.

48. Canadian Task Force on the Periodic Health Examination. Canadian guide to clinical preventive health care. Ottawa: Canada Communication Group, 1994:320–332.

49. Green M, ed. Bright Futures: guidelines for health supervision of infants, children and adolescents. Arlington VA: National Center for Education in Maternal and Child Health, 1994.

50. Johnson CF. Inflicted injury versus accidental injury. Pediatr Clin North Am 1990;37:791–814.

51. Bays J, Chadwick D. Medical diagnosis of the sexually abused child. Child Abuse Neglect 1993;17:91–110.

52. Friedman LS, Samet JH, Roberts MS, et al. Inquiry about victimization experiences: a survey of patient preferences and physician practices. Arch Intern Med 1992;152:1186–1190.

53. Sugg NK, Inui T. Primary care physicians' response to domestic violence: opening Pandora's box. JAMA 1992;267: 3157–3160.

54. McLeer SV, Anwar RAH. The role of the emergency physician in the prevention of domestic violence. Ann Emerg Med 1987;16:1155–1161.

55. McFarlane J, Christoffel K, Bateman L, et al. Assessing for abuse: self-report versus nurse interview. Public Health Nurs 1991;8:245–250.

56. McFarlane J, Parker B, Soeken K, et. al. Assessing for abuse during pregnancy: severity and frequency of injuries and associated entry into prenatal care. JAMA 1992;267:3176–3178.

57. Neale AV, Hwalek MA, Scott RO, et al. Validation of the Hwalek-Sengstock elder abuse screening test. J Applied Gerontol 1991;10:406–418.

58. Olds DL, Henderson CR, Chamberlin R, et. al. Preventing child abuse and neglect: a randomized trial of nurse home visitation. Pediatrics 1986;78:65–78.

59. Hardy JB, Streett R. Family support and parenting education in the home: an effective extension of clinic-based preventive health care services for poor children. J Pediatr 1989;115:927–931.

60. Olds DL, Henderson CR, Kitzman H. Does prenatal and infancy nurse home visitation have enduring effects on qualities of parental caregiving and child health at 25 to 50 months of life? Pediatrics 1994;93:89–98.
61. Dubowitz H. Costs and effectiveness of interventions in child maltreatment. Child Abuse Neglect 1990;14:177–186.
62. Jones DPH. The untreatable family. Child Abuse Neglect 1987;11:409–420.
63. Marshall WL, Barbaree HE. An outpatient treatment program for child molesters. Ann NY Acad Sci 1988;528:205–214.
64. Campbell J, Fishwick N. Abuse of female partners. In: Campbell J, Humphreys J, eds. Nursing care of victims of family violence. St. Louis: CV Mosby, 1993.
65. Bergman BK, Larsson GE, Brismar BG, et. al. Battered women—their susceptibility to treatment. Scand J Soc Med 1988;16:155–160.
66. Sullivan CM, Campbell R, Angelique H, et al. An advocacy intervention program for women with abusive partners: six-month follow-up. Am J Community Psychol 1994;22:101–122.
67. Palmer SE, Brown RA, Barrera ME. Group treatment program for abusive husbands: long-term evaluation. Am J Orthopsychiatry 1992;62:276–283.
68. Agency for Health Care Policy and Research. AHCPR funds study to identify and treat victims of domestic violence. Research Activities no. 184. Rockville, MD: Agency for Health Care Policy and Research, May 1995. (Publication no. 95-0063.)
69. Sengstock MC, Hwalek M, Petrone S. Services for aged abuse victims: service types and related factors. J Elder Abuse Neglect 1989;1:37–56.
70. Filinson R. An evaluation of a program of volunteer advocates for elder abuse victims. J Elder Abuse Neglect 1993;5:77–93.
71. American Academy of Pediatrics, Committee on Child Abuse and Neglect. Guidelines for the evaluation of sexual abuse of children. Pediatrics 1991;87:254–260.
72. American Medical Association. Diagnostic and treatment guidelines on child sexual abuse. Chicago: American Medical Association, 1992.
73. American Medical Association. Diagnostic and treatment guidelines on child physical abuse and neglect. Chicago: American Medical Association, 1992.
74. American Academy of Family Physicians. Age charts for periodic health examination. Kansas City, MO: American Academy of Family Physicians, 1994. (Reprint no. 510.)
75. American Medical Association. Guidelines for adolescent preventive services (GAPS): recommendations and rationale. Chicago: American Medical Association, 1994.
76. American College of Obstetricians and Gynecologists. The battered woman. Technical Bulletin no. 124. Washington, DC: American College of Obstetricians and Gynecologists, 1989.
77. Raymond C. Campaign alerts physicians to identify, assist victims of domestic violence. JAMA 1989;261:963–964.
78. American College of Physicians. Domestic violence: position paper of the American College of Physicians. Philadelphia: American College of Physicians, 1986.
79. American Medical Association. Diagnostic and treatment guidelines on domestic violence. Chicago: American Medical Association, 1992.
80. American College of Obstetricians and Gynecologists. The obstetrician gynecologist and primary preventive health care. Washington, DC: ACOG, 1993.
81. U.S. Department of Health and Human Services. Healthy People 2000: national health promotion and disease prevention objectives. Washington, DC: Public Health Service, 1991:237–238. (Publication no. PHS 91-50212.)
82. Joint Commission on Accreditation of Healthcare Organizations. Accreditation manual for hospitals. Vol 1, standards. Oakbrook Terrace, IL: Joint Commission of Accreditation of Healthcare Organizations, 1992:21–22.
83. American Medical Association. Diagnostic and treatment guidelines on elder abuse and neglect. Chicago: American Medical Association, 1992.
84. Hyman A, Schillinger D, Lo B. Laws mandating reporting of domestic violence: do they promote patient well-being? JAMA 1995;273:1781–1787.

52. Screening for Problem Drinking

RECOMMENDATION

Screening to detect problem drinking is recommended for all adult and adolescent patients. Screening should involve a careful history of alcohol use and/or the use of standardized screening questionnaires (see *Clinical Intervention*). Routine measurement of biochemical markers is not recommended in asymptomatic persons. Pregnant women should be advised to limit or cease drinking during pregnancy. Although there is insufficient evidence to prove or disprove harms from light drinking in pregnancy, recommendations that women abstain from alcohol during pregnancy may be made on other grounds (see *Clinical Intervention*). All persons who use alcohol should be counseled about the dangers of operating a motor vehicle or performing other potentially dangerous activities after drinking alcohol.

Burden of Suffering

Over half a million Americans are under treatment for alcoholism, but there is growing recognition that alcoholism (i.e., alcohol dependence) represents only one end of the spectrum of "problem drinking."[1] Many problem drinkers have medical or social problems attributable to alcohol (i.e., alcohol abuse or "harmful drinking") without typical signs of dependence,[2,3] and other asymptomatic drinkers are at risk for future problems due to chronic heavy alcohol consumption or frequent binges (i.e., "hazardous drinking"). Heavy drinking (more than 5 drinks per day, 5 times per week) is reported by 10% of adult men and 2% of women.[4] In large community surveys using detailed interviews,[5–8] the prevalence of alcohol abuse and dependence in the previous year among men was 17–24% among 18–29-year-olds, 11–14% among 30–44-year-olds, 6–8% among 45–64-year-olds, and 1–3% for men over 65; among women in the corresponding age groups, prevalence of abuse or dependence was 4–10%, 2–4%, 1–2%, and less than 1%, respectively. Problem drinking is even more common among patients seen in the primary care setting (8–20%).[9]

Medical problems due to alcohol dependence include alcohol withdrawal syndrome, psychosis, hepatitis, cirrhosis, pancreatitis, thiamine deficiency, neuropathy, dementia, and cardiomyopathy.[10] Nondependent heavy drinkers, however, account for the majority of alcohol-related morbidity and mortality in the general population.[1] There is a dose-response relationship between daily alcohol consumption and elevations in blood pressure and risk of cirrhosis, hemorrhagic stroke, and cancers of the oropharynx, larynx, esophagus, and liver.[11-13] A number of studies have reported a modest increase in breast cancer among women drinking 2 drinks per day or more, but a causal connection has not yet been proven.[14] Three large cohort studies, involving over 500,000 men and women, observed increasing all-cause mortality beginning at 4 drinks per day in men[11,12] and above 2 drinks per day in women.[15] Women achieve higher blood alcohol levels than do men, due to smaller size and slower metabolism.[11,15] Compared to nondrinkers and light drinkers, overall mortality was 30–38% higher among men, and more than doubled among women, who drank 6 or more drinks per day.[11,12] Of the more than 100,000 deaths attributed to alcohol annually, nearly half are due to unintentional and intentional injuries,[16] including 44% of all traffic fatalities in 1993[17] and a substantial proportion of deaths from fires, drownings, homicides, and suicides (see Chapters 50, 51, 57, 58, and 59).

The social consequences of problem drinking are often as damaging as the direct medical consequences. Nearly 20% of drinkers report problems with friends, family, work, or police due to drinking.[10] Persons who abuse alcohol have a higher risk of divorce, depression, suicide, domestic violence, unemployment, and poverty (see Chapters 49–51).[10] Intoxication may lead to unsafe sexual behavior that increases the risk of sexually transmitted diseases, including human immunodeficiency virus (HIV). Finally, an estimated 27 million American children are at risk for abnormal psychosocial development due to the abuse of alcohol by their parents.[25]

Moderate alcohol consumption has favorable effects on the risk of coronary heart disease (CHD).[18-23] CHD incidence and mortality rates are 20–40% lower in men and women who drink 1–2 drinks/day than in nondrinkers.[15,21,22] A meta-analysis of epidemiologic studies suggests little additional benefit of drinking more than 0.5 drinks per day.[20] The exact mechanism for the protective effect of alcohol is not known but may involve increases in high-density lipoprotein[23] and/or fibrinolytic mediators.[24]

Alcohol Use during Pregnancy. The proportion of pregnant women who report drinking has declined steadily in the U.S.[26] Recent surveys indicate 12–14% of pregnant women continue to consume some alcohol,[27,28] with most reporting only occasional, light drinking (median: 4 drinks per month).[26] Binge drinking or daily risk drinking (usually defined as 2 drinks per day or greater) is reported by 1–2% of pregnant women,[27-29] but higher rates (4–6%) have been reported in some screening studies.[30,31] Excessive use of alcohol during pregnancy can produce the fetal alcohol syndrome (FAS), a constellation of growth retardation, facial deformities, and central nervous system dysfunction (microcephaly, mental retardation, or behavioral abnormalities).[32] Other infants display growth retardation or neurologic involvement in the absence of full FAS (i.e., fetal alcohol effects [FAE]).[10] FAS has been estimated to affect approximately 1 in 3,000 births in the U.S. (1,200 children annually), making it a leading treatable cause of birth defects and mental retardation.[33,34]

The level of alcohol consumption that poses a risk during pregnancy remains controversial.[10,35] FAS has only been described in infants born to alcoholic mothers, but the variable incidence of FAS among alcoholic women (from 3–40%)[33] suggests that other factors (e.g., genetic, nutritional, metabolic, or temporal) may influence the expression of FAS.[10] The reported incidence of FAS is higher in Native Americans and blacks than in whites.[33,36] Most studies report an increased risk of FAE among mothers who consume 14 drinks per week or more,[35,37–39] but the effects of lower levels of drinking have been inconsistent.[35,40,41] Modest developmental effects have been attributed to light drinking (7 drinks per week) in some studies, but underreporting by heavy drinkers and confounding effects of other important factors (nutrition, environment, etc.) make it difficult to prove or disprove a direct effect of light drinking.[10,35,42] Timing of exposure and pattern of drinking may be important, with greater effects proposed for exposure early in pregnancy and for frequent binge drinking.[10]

Alcohol Use by Adolescents and Young Adults. Use of alcohol by adolescents and young adults has declined over the past decade, but remains a serious problem.[43] Among 12–17-year-olds surveyed in 1993, 18% had used alcohol in the last month, and 35% in the last year.[4] In a separate 1993 survey, 45% and 33%, respectively, of male and female 12th graders reported "binge" drinking (5 or more drinks on one occasion) within the previous month.[44] The leading causes of death in adolescents and young adults—motor vehicle and other unintentional injuries, homicides, and suicides—are each associated with alcohol or other drug intoxication in about half of the cases. Driving under the influence of alcohol is more than twice as common in adolescents than in adults.[45] Binge drinking is especially prevalent among college students: half of all men and roughly one third of all women report heavy drinking within the previous 2 weeks.[43,46] Most frequent binge drinkers report numerous alcohol-related problems, including problems with school work, unplanned or unsafe sex, and trouble with police.[46]

Accuracy of Screening Tests

Accurately assessing patients for drinking problems during the routine clinical encounter is difficult. The diagnostic standard for alcohol dependence or abuse (Diagnostic and Statistical Manual of Mental Disorders [DSM] IV)[2] requires a detailed interview and is not feasible for routine screening. Physical findings (hepatomegaly, skin changes, etc.) are only late manifestations of prolonged, heavy alcohol abuse.[47] Asking the patient about the quantity and frequency of alcohol use is an essential component of assessing drinking problems, but it is not sufficiently sensitive or specific by itself for screening. In one study, drinking 12 or more drinks a week was specific (92%) but insensitive (50%) for patients meeting DSM criteria for an active drinking disorder.[48] The reliability of patient report is highly variable and dependent on the patient, the clinician, and individual circumstances. Heavy drinkers may underestimate the amount they drink because of denial, forgetfulness, or fear of the consequences of being diagnosed with a drinking problem.

A variety of screening questionnaires have been developed which focus on consequences of drinking and perceptions of drinking behavior. The 25-question Michigan Alcoholism Screening Test (MAST)[49] is relatively sensitive and specific for DSM-diagnosed alcohol abuse or dependence (84–100% and 87–95%, respectively)[49,50] but it is too lengthy for routine screening. Abbreviated 10- and 13-item versions are easier to use but are less sensitive and specific in primary care populations (66–78% and 80%, respectively).[51,52] The four-question CAGE instrument[a] is the most popular screening test for use in primary care[53] and has good sensitivity and specificity for alcohol abuse or dependence (74–89% and 79–95%, respectively) in both inpatients[54,55] and outpatients.[56–58] The CAGE is less sensitive for early problem drinking or heavy drinking, however (49–73%).[58,59] Both the CAGE and MAST questionnaires share important limitations as screening instruments in the primary care setting: an emphasis on symptoms of dependence rather than early drinking problems, lack of information on level and pattern of alcohol use, and failure to distinguish current from lifetime problems.[52]

Some of these weaknesses are addressed by the Alcohol Use Disorders Identification Test (AUDIT), a 10-item screening instrument developed by the World Health Organization (WHO) in conjunction with an international intervention trial. The AUDIT incorporates questions about drinking quantity, frequency, and binge behavior along with questions about consequences of drinking.[60] For the study population in which it was derived, a score of 8 of 40 on the AUDIT had high sensitivity and specificity for "harmful and hazardous drinking" (92% and 94%, respectively) as as-

---

[a]C: "Have you ever felt you ought to Cut down on drinking?"

A: "Have people Annoyed you by criticizing your drinking?"

G: "Have you ever felt bad or Guilty about your drinking?"

E: "Have you ever had a drink first thing in the morning to steady your nerves or get rid of a hangover (Eye opener)?

sessed by more extensive interview.[60] Validation studies have reported more variable performance of the AUDIT. Sensitivity and specificity for current abuse/dependence were high (96% and 96%, respectively) in an inner-city clinic;[61] among rural outpatients, AUDIT was less sensitive and specific (61% and 90%) for current drinking problems but superior to the Short MAST-13.[51] Because it focuses on drinking in the previous year, however, AUDIT is less sensitive for past drinking problems.[62] Further validation studies in other populations are under way.

Brief screening tests may be less sensitive or less specific in young persons: sensitivity of the CAGE for problems due to alcohol among college freshmen was 42% in men and 25% in women.[63] Only 38% of college students with an AUDIT score of 8 or greater met DSM criteria for abuse or dependence;[64] many of these "false-positive" results were due to drinking patterns (frequent binge drinking) that would be considered hazardous. Alternative screens have been developed for adolescents, such as the Perceived-Benefit-of-Drinking scale[65] and the Problem Oriented Screening Instrument for Teenagers (POSIT),[66] but they have not yet been adequately validated in the primary care setting.

Instruments that focus on alcohol dependency (e.g., CAGE or MAST) are not sensitive for levels of drinking considered dangerous in pregnancy.[67] Women may underreport alcohol consumption while pregnant,[68] and direct questions about drinking may provoke denial.[69] Brief instruments that incorporate questions about tolerance to alcohol ("How many drinks does it take to make you feel high?" or "How many drinks can you hold?") were more sensitive than the CAGE (69–79% vs. 49%) for risk-drinking in pregnancy (2 drinks per day or greater).[30,70] Women who require 3 or more drinks to feel high, or who can drink more than 5 drinks at a time, are likely to be at risk.[71]

Laboratory tests are generally insensitive and nonspecific for problem drinking. Elevations in hepatocellular enzymes, such as aspartate aminotransferase (AST), or the erythrocyte mean corpuscular volume (MCV) are found in less than 10% and 30% of problem drinkers, respectively.[72] Serum γ-glutamyl transferase (GGT) is more sensitive (33–60%) in various studies,[54,55,72] but elevations in GGT may be due to other causes (medications, trauma, diabetes, and heart, kidney, or biliary tract disease). Even when the prevalence of problem drinking is high (30%), the predictive value of an elevated GGT has been estimated at only 56%.[72]

Effectiveness of Early Detection

Numerous studies demonstrate that clinicians are frequently unaware of problem drinking by their patients.[10] Early detection and intervention may alleviate ongoing medical and social problems due to drinking and reduce the future risks from excessive alcohol use.

Nondependent Drinkers. A number of randomized trials have now demonstrated the efficacy of brief outpatient counseling (5–15 minutes) for nondependent problem drinkers. In four Scandinavian studies, which enrolled patients with elevated GGT and heavy alcohol consumption, brief counseling to reduce drinking and regular follow-up produced significant improvements (decreased GGT and/or decreased alcohol consumption) in treated versus control subjects;[73–76] counseling reduced reported sick days in one study.[74] In the longest of these studies, patients receiving counseling had fewer hospitalizations and 50% lower mortality after 5 years.[73] Some of this benefit, however, may have been due to the close medical follow-up (every 1–3 months) in the intervention group rather than the initial counseling.

Additional trials have demonstrated that brief interventions can reduce alcohol consumption in problem drinkers identified by screening questionnaires or self-reported heavy drinking.[77–79] Most recently, an international WHO study examined the effects of 5 or 20 minutes of counseling about drinking in 1,500 "at-risk" male and female drinkers: >35 drinks per week for men; >21 drinks per week for women; or intoxicated twice per month; or self-perceived drinking problem.[80] After 9 months, self-reported alcohol consumption among men was reduced 32–38% in the intervention groups and 10% in controls. Among women, alcohol consumption declined significantly (>30%) among both treated and control groups. A meta-analysis of six brief-intervention trials estimated that interventions reduced average alcohol consumption by 24%.[81] Although self-reported consumption may be subject to bias, reported changes in drinking correlated with objective measures (GGT, blood pressure) in most studies. Two additional studies demonstrated significant reductions in blood pressure as a result of advice to stop drinking or substitution of nonalcoholic beer.[82,83]

Pregnancy. There are no definitive controlled trials of treatments for excessive drinking in pregnancy.[84] In several uncontrolled studies, a majority of heavy-drinking pregnant women who received counseling reduced alcohol consumption,[32,85,86] and reductions in drinking were associated with lower rates of FAS.[32,86] Many women spontaneously reduce their drinking while pregnant, however, and women who continue to drink differ in many respects from women who cut down (e.g., heavier drinking, poorer prenatal care and nutrition). As a result, it is difficult to determine precisely the benefit of screening and counseling during pregnancy. In two trials that employed a control group, the proportions of women abstaining or reducing consumption were similar in intervention and control groups.[87,88]

Adolescents. A 1990 Institute of Medicine (IOM) report concluded that specific recommendations for the treatment of alcohol problems in young persons were impossible, due to disagreement over what constitutes a drinking problem in adolescents, the wide variety of interventions employed, and the absence of any rigorous evaluation of different treatments.[1] Alcohol interventions in adolescents have focused on primary prevention of alcohol use.[10] Recent reviews of school-based programs found that most effects were inconsistent, small, and short-lived; programs that sought to develop social skills to resist drug use seem to be more effective than programs that emphasize factual knowledge.[89,90]

Alcohol-Dependent Patients. Patients with alcohol dependence usually receive more intensive treatment. A 1989 report of the IOM[91] reviewed a variety of alcohol treatment modalities and concluded that various treatments were effective, but there was no single superior treatment for all patients, and few treatments were effective for the majority of patients. They found no evidence that residential versus nonresidential programs, or long- versus short-duration programs, were more effective for the average patient, and no studies existed that adequately evaluated the independent effect of Alcoholics Anonymous (AA). In a subsequent trial among employees referred for alcohol problems, patients who received inpatient treatment and mandatory AA follow-up were more likely to be abstinent at 2-year follow-up (37% vs. 16%) than patients assigned to mandatory AA only.[92]

Two short-term (12 weeks) randomized trials demonstrated a significant benefit of naltrexone, an opioid antagonist, as an adjunct to treatment of alcohol dependence. In one study, patients receiving naltrexone and supportive psychotherapy had significantly higher abstinence rates than did subjects receiving placebo (61% vs. 19%).[93] In the second, men receiving naltrexone reported less alcohol craving and fewer drinking days than placebo-treated men.[94] In both trials, naltrexone significantly reduced the likelihood of relapse (heavy drinking or steady drinking) among subjects who did not achieve complete abstinence. The benefits of alcohol-sensitizing agents, however, remain uncertain.[10] Disulfiram (i.e., Antabuse) did not improve long-term abstinence rates in a controlled trial, but it did reduce drinking days among patients receiving the highest dose.[95]

In a 10-year follow-up of 158 patients completing inpatient treatment, 61% reported complete or stable remission of alcoholism.[96] Completing an extended inpatient program was associated with significantly lower mortality among alcoholic patients in a second study.[97] Many such studies of alcohol treatment, however, suffer from important methodologic limitations: inadequate control groups, insufficient or selective follow-up, and selection bias due to the characteristics of patients who successfully complete voluntary treatment programs.[91,98,99] Since spontaneous remission occurs in as many as 30% of alcoholics,[100,101] reduced consumption may be inappropriately attributed to treatment. Successful treatment is likely to represent a complex interaction of patient motivation, treatment characteristics, and the posttreatment environment (family support, stress, etc.).[1,10] The IOM review concluded that treatment of other life problems (e.g., with antidepressant medication, family or marital therapy, or stress management) and empathetic therapists were likely to improve treatment outcomes.[91]

Recommendations of Other Groups

There is a consensus among professional groups such as the American Medical Association (AMA)[102] and the American Academy of Family Physicians (AAFP)[103] that clinicians should be alert to the signs and symptoms of alcohol abuse and should routinely discuss patterns of alcohol use with all patients. AAFP recommendations are under review. The Canadian Task Force on the Periodic Health Examination (CTF)[104] and a 1990 IOM panel[1] recommended screening adults for problem drinking, using patient inquiry or standardized instruments, and offering brief counseling to nondependent problem drinkers.

The American Academy of Pediatrics (AAP),[105] AMA Guidelines for Adolescent Preventive Services (GAPS),[106] the Bright Futures guidelines,[107] and the AAFP[103] all recommend careful discussion with all adolescents regarding alcohol use and regular advice to abstain from alcohol. The AAP also advises physicians to counsel parents regarding their own use of alcohol in the home. Recommendations of the U.S. Surgeon General,[108] the American College of Obstetricians and Gynecologists,[109] and the AAP[109,110] advise counseling all women who are pregnant or planning pregnancy that drinking can be harmful to the fetus and that abstinence is the safest policy. The CTF recommends that all women be screened for problem drinking and advised to reduce alcohol use during pregnancy.[104]

Several organizations have made recommendations about "safe" levels of alcohol consumption for nonpregnant adults. The National Institute on Alcohol Abuse and Alcoholism,[111] the U.S. Surgeon General,[112] and dietary guidelines produced jointly by the U.S. Departments of Health and Human Services and Agriculture[113,114] recommend no more than 2 drinks per day for men and 1 drink per day for nonpregnant women. Slightly higher limits were proposed by national health authorities in the U.K.[115]

Discussion

Alcohol problems are common in the primary care setting, but they often go undetected by clinicians. Although imperfect, asking patients direct questions about the quantity, frequency, and pattern of their drinking is an important way to identify those who are most likely to experience problems due to alcohol. Questions about tolerance to the effects of alcohol may circumvent denial among pregnant women and heavy drinkers. The CAGE and other brief screening instruments are useful supplements to the standard patient history, but they may be less sensitive for early problems and hazardous drinking. The AUDIT may detect a broader range of current drinking problems, but its performance in the primary care setting needs further evaluation. Although laboratory tests such as GGT are not sufficiently sensitive or specific for routine screening, they may be useful in selected high-risk patients to confirm clinical suspicion or to motivate changes in drinking. Neither questionnaires nor laboratory tests should be considered diagnostic of problem drinking without more detailed evaluation (see *Clinical Intervention*).

Detecting early problem drinkers is important, because they account for a large proportion of all alcohol problems and they are more likely to respond to simple interventions than patients with alcohol dependency. There is now good evidence that brief counseling can reduce alcohol consumption in problem drinkers, and several trials have also reported improved clinical outcomes. Since the risks from alcohol rise steadily at higher levels of consumption, reducing drinking should also benefit heavy drinkers (i.e., hazardous drinkers) who do not yet manifest problems due to drinking. Early attention to problem drinking is especially important in young adults: hazardous drinking is common, adverse effects of alcohol increase with duration of use, and few persons initiate drinking after age 30.[116] Early detection is also important for alcohol-dependent patients, but effective treatment requires more intensive and sustained efforts to promote abstinence.

Uncertainties remain about optimal screening methods and interventions during pregnancy, but screening is justified by the strong evidence of the adverse effects of alcohol on the fetus. Although the risks of occasional, light drinking during pregnancy have not been established, abstinence can be recommended as a prudent approach for pregnant women. At the same time, women concerned about the effects of previous moderate drinking early in pregnancy can be reassured that important harms have not been demonstrated from such limited exposures. Because exposure early in pregnancy may be most important, screening and advice should be directed toward women contemplating pregnancy and those at risk for unintended pregnancy, not just women who are already pregnant.

There is insufficient evidence to make precise recommendations about desirable levels of drinking, but the strong association between heavy alcohol use and risk of future complications justifies advising all drinkers to drink moderately and avoid frequent intoxication, even in the absence of current problems (see below).

CLINICAL INTERVENTION

Screening to detect problem drinking and hazardous drinking is recommended for all adult and adolescent patients ("B" recommendation). Screening should involve a careful history of alcohol use and/or the use of

standardized screening questionnaires. Patients should be asked to describe the quantity, frequency, and other characteristics of their use of wine, beer, and liquor, including frequency of intoxication and tolerance to the effects of alcohol. One drink is defined as 12 ounces of beer, a 5-ounce glass of wine, or 1.5 fluid ounces (one jigger) of distilled spirits. Brief questionnaires such as the CAGE or AUDIT may help clinicians assess the likelihood of problem drinking or hazardous drinking (see Table 52.1). Responses suggestive of problem drinking should be confirmed with more extensive discussions with the patient (and family members where indicated) about patterns of use, problems related to drinking, and symptoms of alcohol dependence.[2] Routine measurement of biochemical markers, such as serum GGT, is not recommended for screening purposes. Discussions with adolescents should be approached with discretion to establish a trusting relationship and to respect the patient's concerns about the confidentiality of disclosed information.

All pregnant women should be screened for evidence of problem drinking or risk drinking (2 drinks per day or binge drinking) ("B" recommendation). Including questions about tolerance to alcohol may improve detection of at-risk women. All pregnant women and women contemplating pregnancy should be informed of the harmful effects of alcohol on the fetus and advised to limit or cease drinking. Although there is insufficient evidence to prove or disprove harms from occasional, light drinking during pregnancy, abstinence from alcohol can be recommended on other grounds: possible risk from even low-level exposure to alcohol, lack of harm from abstaining, and prevailing expert opinion ("C" recommendation). Women who smoke should be advised that the risk of low birth weight is greatest for mothers who both smoke and drink.

Patients with evidence of alcohol dependence should be referred, where possible, to appropriate clinical specialists or community programs specializing in the treatment of alcohol dependence. Patients with evidence of alcohol abuse or hazardous drinking should be offered brief advice and counseling. Counseling should involve feedback of the evidence of a drinking problem, discussion of the role of alcohol in current medical or psychosocial problems, direct advice to reduce consumption, and plans for regular follow-up. Problems related to alcohol (e.g., physical symptoms, behavioral or mood problems, or difficulties at work and home) should be monitored to determine whether further interventions are needed. There is no single definition of "hazardous" drinking in asymptomatic persons, but successful intervention trials have generally defined 5 drinks per day in men, 3 drinks per day in women, or frequent intoxication to identify persons at risk. Several U.S. organizations have suggested lower limits for "safe" drinking: 2 drinks per day in men and 1 drink per day in women.[18] All persons who drink should be informed of the dangers of dri-

Table 52.1
AUDIT Structured Interview[a]

Question	Score				
	0	1	2	3	4
How often do you have a drink containing alcohol?	Never	Monthly or less	2–4 times/mo	2–3 times/wk	4 or more times/wk
How many drinks do you have on a typical day when you are drinking?	None	1 or 2	3 or 4	5 or 6	7–9*
How often do you have 6 or more drinks on one occasion?	Never	Less than monthly	Monthly	Weekly	Daily or almost daily
How often during the last year have you found that you were unable to stop drinking once you had started?	Never	Less than monthly	Monthly	Weekly	Daily or almost daily
How often during the last year have you failed to do what was normally expected from you because of drinking?	Never	Less than monthly	Monthly	Weekly	Daily or almost daily
How often during the last year have you needed a first drink in the morning to get yourself going after a heavy drinking session?	Never	Less than monthly	Monthly	Weekly	Daily or almost daily
How often during the last year have you had a feeling of guilt or remorse after drinking?	Never	Less than monthly	Monthly	Weekly	Daily or almost daily
How often during the last year have you been unable to remember what happened the night before because you had been drinking?	Never	Less than monthly	Monthly	Weekly	Daily or almost daily
Have you or someone else been injured as a result of your drinking?	Never	Yes, but not in last year (2 points)		Yes, during the last year (4 points)	
Has a relative, doctor, or other health worker been concerned about your drinking or suggested you cut down?	Never	Yes, but not in last year (2 points)		Yes, during the last year (4 points)	

[a]Score of greater than 8 (out of 41) suggests problem drinking and indicates need for more in-depth assessment. Cut-off of 10 points recommended by some to provide greater specificity.

*5 points if response is 10 or more drinks on a typical day.

ving or other potentially dangerous activities after drinking (see Chapter 57). The use of alcohol should be discouraged in persons younger than the legal age for drinking ("B" recommendation), although the effectiveness of alcohol abstinence messages in the primary care setting is uncertain.

The draft update of this chapter was prepared for the U.S. Preventive Services Task Force by David Atkins, MD, MPH, with contributions from materials prepared for the Canadian Task Force on the Periodic Health Examination by Deborah L. Craig, MPH, and Jean L. Haggerty, MSc.

REFERENCES

1. Institute of Medicine. Broadening the base of treatment for alcohol problems: report of a study by a committee of the Institute of Medicine, Division of Mental Health and Behavioral Medicine. Washington, DC: National Academy Press, 1990.
2. American Psychiatric Association. Diagnostic and statistical manual of mental disorders. 4th ed. Washington, DC: American Psychiatric Association, 1994.
3. World Health Organization. International classification of diseases, 10th revision. Geneva: World Health Organization, 1992.
4. Substance Abuse and Mental Health Administration. National Household Survey on Drug Abuse: population estimates 1993. Rockville, MD: U.S. Department of Health and Human Services, Substance Abuse and Mental Health Administration, 1994. (Publication no. (SMA) 94-3017.)
5. Grant BF, Harford TC, Chou P, et al. Epidemiologic Bulletin no. 27: Prevalence of DSM-III-R alcohol abuse and dependence: United States, 1988. Alcohol Health Res World 1991;15:91–96.
6. Helzer JE, Burnam A, McEvoy LT. Alcohol abuse and dependence. In: Robins LN, Regier DA, eds. Psychiatric disorders in America: the Epidemiologic Catchment Area Study. New York: Free Press, 1991:81–115.
7. Grant BF, Harford TC, Dawson D, et al. Prevalence of DSM-IV alcohol abuse and dependence: United States, 1992. Alcohol Health Res World 1994;18:243–248.
8. Kessler RC, McGonagle KA, Zhao S, et al. Lifetime and 12-month prevalence of DSM-III-R psychiatric disorders in the United States: results from the National Comorbidity Survey. Arch Gen Psychiatry 1994;51:8–19.
9. Bradley KA. The primary care provider's role in the prevention and management of alcohol problems. Alcohol Health Res World 1994;18:97–104.
10. National Institute on Alcohol Abuse and Alcoholism. Alcohol and health: eighth special report to the U.S. Congress from the Secretary of Health and Human Services. Rockville, MD: U.S. Department of Health and Human Services, National Institutes of Health, 1993. (NIH Publication no. 94-3699.)
11. Klatsky AL, Armstrong AA, Friedman GD. Alcohol and mortality. Ann Intern Med 1992;117:646–654.
12. Boffetta P, Garfinkel L. Alcohol drinking and mortality among men enrolled in an American Cancer Society prospective study. Epidemiology 1990;1:342–348.
13. Anderson P, Cremona A, Paton A, et al. The risk of alcohol. Addiction 1993;88:1493–1508.
14. Rosenberg L, Metzger LS, Palmer JR. Alcohol consumption and risk of breast cancer: a review of the epidemiologic evidence. Epidemiol Rev 1993;15:133–168.
15. Fuchs CS, Stampfer MJ, Colditz GA, et al. Alcohol consumption and mortality among women. N Engl J Med 1995;332:1245–1250.
16. Centers for Disease Control. Alcohol-related mortality and years of potential life lost—United States, 1987. MMWR 1990;39:173–178.
17. National Highway Traffic Safety Administration. Traffic safety facts 1993: alcohol. Washington, DC: U.S. Department of Transportation, National Highway Traffic Safety Administration, National Center for Statistics and Analysis, 1994.
18. Bradley KA, Donovan DM, Larson EB. How much is too much? Advising patients about safe levels of alcohol consumption. Arch Intern Med 1993;153:2734–2740.

19. Stampfer MJ, Rimm EB, Walsh DC. Commentary: alcohol, the heart, and public policy. Am J Public Health 1993;83:801–804.
20. Maclure M. Demonstration of deductive meta-analysis: ethanol intake and risk of myocardial infarction. Epidemiol Rev 1993;15:328–351.
21. Klatsky AL, Armstrong AA, Friedman GD. Risk of cardiovascular mortality in alcohol drinkers, ex-drinkers and non-drinkers. Am J Cardiol 1990;66:1237–1242.
22. Stampfer MJ, Colditz GA, Willett WC, et al. A prospective study of moderate alcohol consumption and the risk of coronary disease and stroke in women. N Engl J Med 1988;319:267–273.
23. Gaziano JM, Buring JE, Breslow JL, et al. Moderate alcohol intake, increased levels of high-density lipoprotein and its subfractions, and decreased risk of myocardial infarction. N Engl J Med 1993;329:1829–1835.
24. Ridker PM, Vaughan DE, Stampfer MJ, et al. Association of moderate alcohol consumption and plasma concentration of endogenous tissue-type plasminogen activator. JAMA 1994;272:929–933.
25. Sher KJ, ed. Children of alcoholics: a critical appraisal of theory and research. Chicago: University of Chicago Press, 1991.
26. Serdula M, Williamson DF, Kendrick J, et al. Trends in alcohol consumption by pregnant women: 1985 through 1988. JAMA 1991;265:876–879.
27. Goodwin MM, Bruce C, Zahniser SC, et al. Behavioral risk factors before and during pregnancy. In: Wilcox LS, Marks JS, eds. From data to action: CDC's public health surveillance for women, infants, and children. Washington, DC: Department of Health and Human Services, 1994:93–104.
28. Centers for Disease Control and Prevention. Frequent alcohol consumption among women of child-bearing age—Behavioral Risk Factor Surveillance System, 1991. MMWR 1994;43:328–329, 335.
29. Centers for Disease Control and Prevention. Sociodemographic and behavioral characteristics associated with alcohol consumption during pregnancy—United States, 1988. MMWR 1995;44:261–264.
30. Sokol RJ, Martier SS, Ager JW. The T-ACE questions: practical prenatal detection of risk-drinking. Am J Obstet Gynecol 1989;160:863–870.
31. Russell M, Martier SS, Sokol RJ, et al. Screening for pregnancy risk-drinking. Alcohol Clin Exp Res 1994;18: 1156–1161.
32. Rosett HL, Weiner L, Edelin KC. Treatment experience with pregnant problem drinkers. JAMA 1983;249:2029–2033.
33. Abel EA, Sokol RJ. A revised conservative estimate of the incidence of FAS and its economic impact. Alcohol Clin Exp Res 1991;15:514–524.
34. Centers for Disease Control and Prevention. Fetal alcohol syndrome—United States, 1979–1992. MMWR 1993;42:339–341.
35. Russell M. Clinical implications of recent research on the fetal alcohol syndrome. Bull NY Acad Sci 1991;67: 207–222.
36. Burd L, Moffatt ME. Epidemiology of fetal alcohol syndrome in American Indians, Alaskan Natives, and Canadian Aboriginal peoples: a review of the literature. Public Health Rep 1994;109:688–693.
37. Virji SK. The relationship between alcohol consumption during pregnancy and infant birthweight: an epidemiologic study. Acta Obstet Gynecol Scand 1991;303–308.
38. Forrest F, Florey CDV, Taylor D, et al. Reported social alcohol consumption during pregnancy and infants' development at 18 months. BMJ 1991;303:22–26.
39. Verkerk PH, Noord-Zaadstra BMV, Florey CDV, et al. The effect of moderate maternal alcohol consumption on birth weight and gestational age in a low risk population. Early Hum Dev 1993;32:121–129.
40. Jacobson JL, Jacobson SW, Sokol RJ, et al. Teratogenic effects of alcohol on infant development. Alcohol Clin Exp Res 1993;17:174–183.
41. Streissguth AP, Barr HM, Sampson PD. Moderate prenatal alcohol exposure: effects on child IQ and learning problems at age 7.5 years. Alcohol Clin Exp Res 1990;14:662–669.
42. Knupfer G. Abstaining for fetal health: the fiction that even light drinking is dangerous. Br J Addict 1991;86: 1063–1073.
43. National Institute on Drug Abuse. National survey results on drug use from the Monitoring the Future Study, 1975–1992. Vols 1 and 2. Rockville, MD: Department of Health and Human Services, National Institute on Drug Abuse, 1993. (NIH Publications nos. 93-3596 and 3597.)
44. Centers for Disease Control and Prevention. Youth Risk Behavior Surveillance—United States, 1993. MMWR 1995;44(SS-1):1–56.
45. Centers for Disease Control. Drinking and driving and binge drinking in selected states, 1982 and 1985: the Behavioral Risk Factor Surveys. MMWR 1987;35:788–791.

46. Wechsler H, Davenport A, Dowdall G, et al. Health and behavioral consequences of binge drinking in college: a national survey of students at 140 campuses. JAMA 1994;272:1672–1677.

47. Glaze LW, Coggan PG. Efficacy of an alcoholism self-report questionnaire in a residency clinic. J Fam Pract 1987; 25:60–64.

48. Buchsbaum DG, Welsh J, Buchanan RG, et al. Screening for drinking problems by patient self-report: even "safe" levels may indicate a problem. Arch Intern Med 1995;155:104–108.

49. Selzer ML. The Michigan Alcoholism Screening Test: the quest for a new diagnostic instrument. Am J Psychiatry 1971;127:1653–1658.

50. Pokorny AD, Miller BA, Kaplan HB. The Brief MAST: a shortened version of the Michigan Alcoholism Screening Test. Am J Psychiatry 1972;129:342–345.

51. Barry K, Fleming M. The Alcohol Use Disorders Identification Test (AUDIT) and the SMAST-13: predictive validity in a rural primary care sample. Alcohol Alcohol 1993;28:33–42.

52. Chan AWK, Pristach EA, Welte JW, et al. Use of the TWEAK test in screening for alcoholism/heavy drinking in three populations. Alcohol Clin Exp Res 1993;17:1188–1192.

53. Ewing JA. Detecting alcoholism: the CAGE questionnaire. JAMA 1984;252:1905–1907.

54. Bernadt MW, Mumford J, Taylor C, et al. Comparison of questionnaire and laboratory tests in the detection of excessive drinking and alcoholism. Lancet 1982;1:325–328.

55. Bush B, Shaw S, Cleary P, et al. Screening for alcohol abuse using the CAGE questionnaire. Am J Med 1987;82:231–235.

56. King M. At risk drinking among general practice attenders: validation of the CAGE questionnaire. Psychol Med 1986;16:213–217.

57. Buchsbaum DG, Buchanan RG, Centor RM, et al. Screening for alcohol abuse using CAGE scores and likelihood ratios. Ann Intern Med 1991;115:774–777.

58. Chan AWK, Pristach EA, Welte JW. Detection by the CAGE of alcoholism or heavy drinking in primary care outpatients and the general population. J Subst Abuse 1994;6:123–135.

59. Hays JT, Spickard WA. Alcoholism: early diagnosis and intervention. J Gen Intern Med 1987;2:420–427.

60. Saunders JB, Aasland OG, Babor TF, et al. Development of the Alcohol Use Disorders Identification Test (AUDIT): WHO collaborative project on early detection of persons with harmful alcohol consumption—II. Addiction 1993;88:791–804.

61. Isaacson JH, Butler R, Zacharek M, et al. Screening with the Alcohol Use Disorders Identification Test (AUDIT) in an inner-city population. J Gen Intern Med 1994;9:550–553.

62. Schmidt A, Barry K, Fleming MF. Detection of problem drinkers: the Alcohol Use Disorders Identification Test (AUDIT). Southern Med J 1995;88:52–59.

63. Werner MJ, Walker LS, Greene JW. Screening for problem drinking among college freshmen. J Adolesc Health 1994;15:303–310.

64. Fleming MF, Barry KL, MacDonald R. The Alcohol Use Disorders Identification Test (AUDIT) in a college sample. Int J Addict 1991;26:1173–1185.

65. Petchers MK, Singer MI. Perceived-benefit-of-drinking Scale: approach to screening for adolescent alcohol abuse. J Pediatr 1987;110:979–981.

66. National Institute on Drug Abuse. Problem oriented screening instrument for teenagers. In: Rahdert E, ed. The adolescent assessment/referral system manual. Rockville, MD: National Institute on Drug Abuse, 1990:5–9.

67. Waterson EJ, Murray-Lyon IM. Screening for alcohol-related problems in the antenatal clinic. Alcohol Alcohol 1989;24:21–30.

68. Jacobson SW, Jacobson JL, Sokol RJ, et al. Maternal recall of alcohol, cocaine, and marijuana use during pregnancy. Neurotoxicol Teratol 1991;13:535–540.

69. Ernhart CB, Morrow-Tlucak M, Sokol RJ, et al. Underreporting of alcohol use in pregnancy. Alcohol Clin Exp Res 1988;12:506–511.

70. Russell M, Martier SS, Sokol RJ, et al. Screening for pregnancy risk-drinking. Alcohol Exp Clin Res 1994;18: 1156–1161.

71. Russell M. New assessment tools for risk drinking during pregnancy: T-ACE, TWEAK, and others. Alcohol Health Res World 1994;18:55–61.

72. Hoeksema HL, de Bock GH. The value of laboratory tests for the screening and recognition of alcohol abuse in primary care patients. J Fam Pract 1993;37:268–276.

73. Kristenson H, Trell E, Hood B. Serum glutamyl-transferase in screening and continuous control of heavy drinking in middle-aged men. Am J Epidemiol 1981;114:862–872.

74. Persson J, Magnusson PH. Early intervention in patients with excessive consumption of alcohol: a controlled study. Alcohol 1989;6:403–408.

75. Romelsjo A, Andersson L, Barrner H, et al. A randomized study of secondary prevention of early stage problem drinkers in primary health care. Br J Addict 1989;84:1319–1327.

76. Nilssen O. The Tromso Study: identification of and a controlled intervention on a population of early-stage risk drinkers. Prev Med 1991;20:518–528.

77. Chick J, Lloyd G, Crombie E. Counselling problem drinkers in medical wards: a controlled study. BMJ 1985;290:965–967.

78. Wallace P, Cutler S, Haines A. Randomized controlled trial of general practitioner intervention in patients with excessive alcohol consumption. BMJ 1988;297:663–668.

79. Heather N, Kissoon-Singh J, Fenton GW. Assisted natural recovery from alcohol problems: effects of a self-help manual with and without supplementary telephone contact. Br J Addict 1990;85:1177–1185.

80. Babor TF, Grant M, eds. Project on identification and management of alcohol-related problems. Report on Phase II: a randomized clinical trial of brief interventions in primary health care. Geneva: World Health Organization, 1992.

81. Brief interventions and alcohol use. Effective Health Care, bulletin no. 7. Leeds, UK: Nuffield Institute for Health Care, University of Leeds, 1993.

82. Maheswaran R, Beevers M, Beevers DG. Effectiveness of advice to reduce alcohol consumption in hypertensive patients. Hypertension 1992:19:79–84.

83. Cox KL, Puddey IB, Morton AR, et al. The combined effects of aerobic exercise and alcohol restriction on blood pressure and serum lipids: a two-way factorial study in sedentary men. J Hypertens 1993;11:191–201.

84. Schorling JB. The prevention of prenatal alcohol use: a critical analysis of intervention studies. J Stud Alcohol 1993;54:261–267.

85. Larson G. Prevention of fetal alcohol effects. Acta Obstet Gynecol Scand 1983;62:171–178.

86. Halmesmaki E. Alcohol counselling of 85 pregnant problem drinkers: effect on drinking and fetal outcome. Br J Obstet Gynaecol 1988;95:243–247.

87. Waterson EJ, Murray-Lyon IM. Preventing fetal alcohol effects: a trial of three methods of giving information in the antenatal clinic. Health Educ Res 1990;5:53–61.

88. Meberg A, Halvorsen B, Holter B, et al. Moderate alcohol consumption—need for intervention programs in pregnancy? Acta Obstet Gynecol Scand 1986;65:861–864.

89. Ennett ST, Tobler NS, Ringwalt CL, et al. How effective is drug abuse resistance education? A meta-analysis of project DARE outcome evaluations. Am J Public Health 1994;84:1394–1401.

90. Hansen WB. School-based substance abuse prevention: a review of the state of the art in curriculum, 1980–1990. Health Educ Res 1992;7:403–430.

91. Institute of Medicine. Prevention and treatment of alcohol problems: research opportunities. Washington, DC: National Academy Press, 1989.

92. Walsh DC, Hingson RW, Merrigan DM, et al. A randomized trial of treatment options for alcohol-abusing workers. N Engl J Med 1991;325:775–782.

93. O'Malley SS, Jaffe AJ, Chang G, et al. Naltrexone and coping skills therapy for alcohol dependence: a controlled study. Arch Gen Psychiatry 1992;49:881–887.

94. Volpicelli JR, Alterman AI, Hayashida M, et al. Naltrexone in the treatment of alcohol dependence. Arch Gen Psychiatry 1992;49:876–880.

95. Fuller RK, Branchey L, Brightwell DR, et al. Disulfiram treatment of alcoholism: A Veterans Administration study. JAMA 1986;256:1449–1455.

96. Cross GM, Morgan CW, Mooney AJ, et al. Alcoholism treatment: a ten-year follow-up study. Alcohol Clin Exp Res 1990;14:169–173.

97. Bunn JY, Booth BM, Loveland Cook CA, et al. The relationship between mortality and intensity of inpatient alcoholism treatment. Am J Public Health 1994;84:211–214.

98. Thurstin AH, Alfano AM, Sherer M. Pretreatment MMPI profiles of A.A. members and nonmembers. J Stud Alcohol 1986;47:468–471.

99. Emrick CD. Alcoholics Anonymous: affiliation processes and effectiveness as treatment. Alcohol Clin Exp Res 1987;11:416–423.

100. Smart R. Spontaneous recovery in alcoholics: a review and analysis of the available research. Drug Alcohol Depend 1975/76;1:277.

101. Saunders WM, Kershaw PW. Spontaneous remission from alcoholism: a community study. Br J Addict 1979;74: 251–265.

102. American Medical Association, Council on Scientific Affairs. Guidelines for alcoholism diagnosis, treatment and referral. Chicago: American Medical Association, 1979.
103. American Academy of Family Physicians. Age charts for periodic health examination. Kansas City, MO: American Academy of Family Physicians, 1994. (Reprint no. 510.)
104. Canadian Task Force on the Periodic Health Examination. Canadian guide to clinical preventive health care. Ottawa: Canada Communication Group, 1994:52–61, 826–836.
105. American Academy of Pediatrics, Committee on Adolescence. Alcohol use and abuse: a pediatric concern. Pediatrics 1995;95:439–442.
106. American Medical Association. Guidelines for adolescent preventive services (GAPS): recommendations and rationale. Chicago: American Medical Association, 1994.
107. Green M, ed. Bright Futures: guidelines for health supervision of infants, children and adolescents. Arlington VA: National Center for Education in Maternal and Child Health, 1994.
108. Surgeon General's Advisory on alcohol and pregnancy. FDA Drug Bull 1981;11:9–10.
109. American Academy of Pediatrics and American College of Obstetricians and Gynecologists. Guidelines for perinatal care. 3rd ed. Washington, DC: American Academy of Pediatrics and American College of Obstetricians and Gynecologists, 1992.
110. American Academy of Pediatrics, Committee on Substance Abuse and Committee on Children with Disabilities. Fetal alcohol syndrome and fetal alcohol effects. Pediatrics 1993;91:1004–1006.
111. National Institute on Alcohol Abuse and Alcoholism. Moderate drinking. Alcohol Alert no. 16. Bethesda: U.S. Department of Health and Human Services, 1992.
112. U.S. Department of Health and Human Services. The Surgeon General's report on nutrition and health. Washington, DC: Government Printing Office, 1988. (Publication no. PHS-88-50210.)
113. U.S. Department of Agriculture and U.S. Department of Health and Human Services. Dietary guidelines for Americans. Washington, DC: Department of Agriculture, 1990.
114. Dietary Guidelines Advisory Committee. Report of the Dietary Guidelines Advisory Committee on the dietary guidelines for Americans, 1995, to the Secretary of Health and Human Services and the Secretary of Agriculture. Washington, DC: U.S. Department of Agriculture, 1995.
115. Secretary of State for Health. The Health of the Nation: a strategy for health in England. London: Her Majesty's Stationery Office, 1992.
116. Chen K, Kandel D. The natural history of drug use from adolescence to mid-thirties in a general population sample. Am J Public Health 1995;85:41–47.

53. Screening for Drug Abuse

RECOMMENDATION

There is insufficient evidence to recommend for or against routine screening for drug abuse with standardized questionnaires or biologic assays. Including questions about drug use and drug-related problems when taking a history from all adolescent and adult patients may be recommended on other grounds (see *Clinical Intervention*). All pregnant women should be advised of the potential adverse effects of drug use on the development of the fetus. Clinicians should be alert to signs and symptoms of drug abuse in patients and refer drug abusing patients to specialized treatment facilities where available.

Burden of Suffering

The abuse of both illicit and legal drugs remains an important medical problem in the U.S. Although casual (i.e., occasional) use of illicit drugs declined steadily in the general population from 1979 to 1992, drug use appears to be increasing since then, especially among teenagers and young adults.[1,2] Moreover, there has been little improvement in the numbers of persons using drugs on a regular basis.[3,4] In a 1991 survey of over 8,000 persons aged 15–54 years, 3.6% met diagnostic criteria for drug dependence or drug abuse in the past year,[5] and drug-related emergency visits in the U.S. reached all-time highs in 1993.[6] An estimated 5.5 million Americans, half of whom are in the criminal justice system, are affected by drug abuse or dependence.[7]

In a national household survey in 1993, 14% of adults ages 18–25 and 3% of those over 35 reported using illicit drugs within the last month.[2] Occasional use of marijuana accounts for a large proportion of reported drug use, but many drug users used other illicit drugs (cocaine, heroin, phencyclidine, methaqualone, hallucinogens, etc.), legal drugs not prescribed by a physician (e.g., amphetamines, benzodiazepines, barbiturates, and anabolic steroids), or inhalants (amyl and butyl nitrite, gasoline, nitrous oxide, glue, and other solvents). An estimated 5 million Americans smoke marijuana regularly (at least once a week), almost 500,000 use cocaine weekly, and over 500,000 used heroin or other injectable drug in the past year.[2] Others have estimated that up to 500,000 Americans are addicted to heroin and 1–1.6 million currently use injection drugs.[8] Drug use is more common among men, the unemployed, adults who have not completed high school, and urban residents. The overall prevalence of drug use does not differ greatly among white, African American, and Hispanic populations, but patterns of drug use may differ.[4]

Adverse effects of drug use are greatest in heavy users and those dependent on drugs, but some can occur from even occasional drug use. Cocaine can produce acute cardiovascular complications (e.g., arrhythmias, myocardial infarction, cerebral hemorrhage, and seizures), nasal and sinus disease, and respiratory problems (when smoked).[9,10] Dependence on cocaine produces diminished motivation, psychomotor retardation, irregular sleep patterns, and other symptoms of depression.[11] "Crack," a popular and cheaper smokeable form of cocaine, is also highly addictive. Mortality among injection drug users (IDUs) is high from overdose, suicide, violence, and medical complications from injecting contaminated materials (e.g., human immunodeficiency virus [HIV] infection, hepatitis, bacterial endocarditis, chronic glomerulonephritis, and pulmonary emboli); in some cities, up to 40% of IDUs are infected with HIV.[12] Although the extent of adverse effects of marijuana use is controversial, chronic use may be associated with respiratory complications or amotivational syndrome.[13,14] In a 1991 survey, 8% of cocaine users and 21% of marijuana users reported daily use for 2 weeks or more.[15]

The indirect medical and social consequences of drug use are equally important: criminal activities related to illegal drugs take a tremendous toll in many communities, use of injection drugs and crack are major factors in the spread of HIV infection[16,17] (see Chapter 28), and drugs play a role in many homicides, suicides, and motor vehicle injuries (see Chapters 50, 57, and 59). Nearly half of all users of cocaine or marijuana reported having driven a car shortly after using drugs.[13,15]

Drug Use During Pregnancy. A national probability sample of 2,613 women giving birth in 1992–1993 estimated that 5.5% used some illicit drug during pregnancy: the most frequently used drugs were marijuana (2.9%) and cocaine (1.1%).[18] Anonymous urine testing of nearly 30,000 women giving birth in California in 1992 detected illicit drugs in 5.2%: marijuana (1.9%), opiates (1.5%), and cocaine (1.1%) were the most frequently detected substances.[19] Prevalence of drug use is generally higher among mothers who smoke or drink, are unmarried, are not working, have public or no insurance, live in urban areas, or receive late or no prenatal care.[18–20] Anonymous urine testing detected cocaine use in 7–15% of pregnant women from high-risk, urban communities[21,22] and in 0.2–1.5% of mothers in private clinics and rural areas.[23,24] The most important forms of substance abuse during pregnancy are the use of alcohol and tobacco, however (see Chapters 52 and 54).[25]

Drug use during pregnancy has been associated with a variety of adverse outcomes, but problems associated with drug use (e.g., use of alcohol or cigarettes, poverty, poor nutrition, and inadequate prenatal care) may be more important than the direct effects of drugs.[26,27] Regular use of cocaine and opiates is associated with poor weight gain among pregnant women, impaired fetal growth, and increased risk of premature birth; cocaine appears to increase the risk of abruptio placentae.[28] The effects of social use of cocaine in the first trimester are uncertain.[29,30] Cocaine has been blamed for some congenital defects,[27] but the teratogenic potential of cocaine has not been definitively established. Infants exposed to drugs in utero may exhibit withdrawal symptoms due to opiates, or increased tremors, hyperexcitability, and hypertonicity due to cocaine.[27,31] Possible long-term neurologic effects of drug exposure are difficult to separate from the effects of other factors that influence development among disadvantaged children.[27,32,33] The effects of marijuana on the fetus remain controversial.[34-36]

Drug Use in Children and Adolescents. Drug use and abuse remain important problems among adolescents.[37] After more than 10 years of decreasing trends, drug use among high school students increased in 1993 and 1994.[1,38] Use of illicit drugs may interfere with school, increase the risk of injuries, contribute to unsafe sex, and progress to more harmful drug use. Among high school seniors in 1994, 22% reported using an illicit drug in the past month: marijuana (19%), stimulants (4%), inhalants (3%), and hallucinogens (3%) were more common than cocaine (1.5%) or heroin (0.3%).[1] Abuse of inhalants is a leading drug problem in younger adolescents[1] and can cause asphyxiation or neurologic damage with chronic abuse.[39] Abuse of anabolic steroids in adolescent boys and young men can cause psychiatric symptoms and has been associated with hepatic, endocrine, and cardiovascular problems.

Accuracy of Screening Tests

The diagnostic standard for drug abuse and dependence is the careful diagnostic interview.[40] Important information from the patient history includes the quantity, frequency, and pattern of drug use; adverse effects of drugs on work, health, and social relationships; and any symptoms of dependence.[41] Clinicians often have trouble accurately identifying drug use and drug abuse among their patients in routine clinical encounters, however. Time may be too limited to take a careful history, some patients may not acknowledge drug problems due to denial, and many others are reluctant to admit to using drugs, for fear of discrimination by health care providers or concerns about confidentiality. It is common for adolescents to distrust authority figures such as clinicians, and young persons may be especially concerned about their drug use becoming known to family members, school officials, or the police.[42]

There are few data to determine whether or not the use of standardized screening questionnaires can increase the detection of potential drug problems among patients. Brief alcohol screening instruments such as the CAGE or MAST (see Chapter 52) can be modified to assess the consequences of drug use in a standardized manner,[41,43] but these instruments have not been compared to routine history or clinician assessment. Questionnaires which include items about personal problems, outlook, and high-risk behaviors can identify adolescents at increased risk for drug use, but they have not been validated in prospective studies.[44] Other instruments such as the Addiction Severity Index[45] are useful for evaluating treatment needs but are too long for screening.

Toxicologic tests can provide objective evidence of drug use. The most common tests employ radioimmunoassays (RIA), enzymatic immunoassay (EIA), fluorescence polarization immunoassay (FPI), or thin-layer chromatography (TLC) to measure concentrations of specific drugs and their metabolites in urine specimens.[46] Sensitivity of these tests is generally above 99% compared with reference standards;[47] sensitivity for detecting drug use in individuals, however, depends directly on timing of drug use and the urinary excretion of drug metabolites. Marijuana may be detected for up to 14 days after repeated use, but evidence of cocaine, opiates, amphetamines, and barbiturates is present for only 2–4 days after use. Various techniques may be employed by drug users who wish to avoid detection that further reduce the sensitivity of urine testing: water loading, diuretic use, ingestion of interfering substances, or adulterating urine samples. Most importantly, toxicologic tests do not distinguish between occasional users and individuals who are dependent on or otherwise impaired by drug use.

False-positive results from urine drug screening are possible due to cross-reaction with other medications or naturally occurring compounds in foods.[48] To prevent falsely implicating persons as users of illegal drugs, screen-positive samples are usually confirmed with more specific (and expensive) techniques such as gas chromatography-mass spectroscopy (GC-MS). These procedures reduce, but do not eliminate, the possibility of false-positive results due to cross-reactions, contamination, or mislabeled specimens. Proficiency testing of nearly 1,500 urine specimens sent to 31 U.S. laboratories produced no false-positive results and 3% false-negative results.[49] A similar study of 120 clinical laboratories in the U.K. demonstrated higher error rates (4% false-positive, 8% false-negative), largely due to laboratories that did not use confirmatory tests.[50]

Screening Pregnant Women and Newborn Infants. A careful history taken by trusted clinicians remains the most sensitive means of detecting drug use and abuse,[51,52] but many pregnant women conceal use of illicit drugs, since it may provide grounds for action by child welfare agencies. Clinicians often selectively screen for drug use, based on preconceptions of the typical drug-using mother. Studies using sensitive toxicologic tests suggest that only one in four pregnant women who have used opiates, cocaine, or marijuana are identified as drug users in the medical record.[51] Patient history identified only 40–60% of pregnant women with urine tests positive for illicit drugs.[21,53] Detection of drug use is increased by use of a standard protocol for assessing drug use in patients, rather than screening based on the discretion of the clinician.[54,55]

Testing of newborn specimens can identify infants exposed to drugs in utero. Assays of infant urine are most common but are not sensitive for drug use early in pregnancy. Among mothers admitting drug use during pregnancy, RIA of infant urine had a sensitivity of 52%, versus 88% for RIA of meconium.[51] Among 39 women who used cocaine, RIA of infant hair was more sensitive (78%) than RIA of infant urine (38%) or meconium (52%).[52] These more sensitive tests are not widely available, however, and have not yet been sufficiently validated for screening purposes.[56] Moreover, clinical history may be more useful than toxicologic testing for identifying newborns at risk: among drug-exposed infants identified by meconium testing, adverse outcomes were limited to infants born to mothers who admitted to drug use.[51]

Adverse Effects of Screening. Drug testing is frequently performed without informed consent in the clinical setting on the grounds that it is a diagnostic test intended to improve the care of the patient. Because of the significance of a positive drug screen for the patient, however, the rights of patients to autonomy and privacy have important implications for screening of asymptomatic persons.[57] If confidentiality is not ensured, test results may affect a patient's employment, insurance coverage, or personal relationships.[58] Testing during pregnancy is especially problematic, because clinicians may be required by state laws to report evidence of potentially harmful drug or alcohol use in pregnant patients.

Effectiveness of Early Detection

Early intervention has the potential to avert some of the serious consequences of drug abuse, including injuries, legal problems, and medical complications. Although various treatments have been proven effective in drug-dependent patients (see below), they have largely been studied in patients who have already developed medical, social, or legal problems due to their drug use. There is much less evidence that systematic screening and earlier intervention is effective in improving clinical outcomes among asymptomatic persons, who may be less motivated to undergo treatment than more severely impaired drug users.

The evidence supporting the effectiveness of treatment for drug abuse and dependence was reviewed in 1990 by the Institute of Medicine.[7] The most consistent evidence supports the clinical benefits of methadone maintenance in persons addicted to heroin. Several studies, including two randomized controlled trials, have shown that heroin addicts who remain in methadone maintenance programs have reduced heroin consumption, lower rates of HIV infection, decreased criminality and unemployment, and lower mortality than subjects who are not treated or treated for only short periods.[7,59] Over the short term, methadone treatment is associated with a 95% reduction in self-reported heroin use and a 57–68% reduction in self-reported cocaine use,[60] but some persons switch from heroin to other drugs while on treatment.[61] Moreover, results may be biased due to reliance on patient self-report and loss to follow-up of patients who drop out of treatment.[62]

Drug abusers are frequently enrolled in residential treatment programs, often as part of a court order related to drug offenses. Patients entering such programs experience lower rates of drug use, imprisonment, and unemployment than drug users who do not enroll.[7] Longer programs seem to be more effective than short (<3 months) programs.[63] However, attrition rates from residential programs can reach 75%,[64] and selection bias may contribute to the improved outcomes in subjects who complete programs.[65] Less intensive outpatient programs also seem to be effective for drug users, but the wide variation in interventions used limits the conclusions that can be drawn. Attrition is highest in outpatient, nonresidential programs.[7] There are fewer data on long-term (>1 year) outcomes of drug treatment; recidivism is high and many patients suffer from other problems (psychiatric disorders, unemployment, homelessness) which reinforce drug use and are often not addressed by drug treatment.[7]

Treatment of adolescent substance abusers has been recently reviewed for nearly 1,500 primarily middle-class adolescents aged 12–19 years who entered inpatient or residential treatment programs.[66] Compared to use before treatment, there was a significant reduction in regular drug use (weekly or more) 1 year after treatment (85% vs. 29%), and 50% of teens had been abstinent for 6 months. Increasing parental participation in treatment was associated with greater levels of abstinence. High school primary prevention programs which emphasize "life skills" have reduced tobacco or alcohol use over the short term (1 year),[67] but long-term effects on illicit drug use have not been well studied. In a 6-year randomized trial among 3,597 high school students, a prevention curriculum delivered in grades 7–9 significantly reduced smoking and alcohol use, but not marijuana use, in high school seniors; a subgroup of students who received a more complete intervention were less likely to use marijuana regularly (5% vs. 9%).[68]

Treatment of Pregnant Drug Abusers. There are few controlled trials of interventions for pregnant women who use illicit drugs. Women who use crack and other forms of cocaine account for the largest group of pregnancies at risk from illicit drugs, but optimal treatment for cocaine users is uncertain. In two observational studies, risk of low birth weight decreased substantially with increasing number of prenatal visits.[69,70] Women who reduced use of cocaine during pregnancy, or used cocaine infrequently, had outcomes similar to nonusers in several studies.[30,34] Methadone maintenance is the usual treatment for pregnant women addicted to opiates: withdrawal during pregnancy is dangerous, and the regular contact required for methadone treatment may encourage women to receive regular prenatal care.[27] Methadone can be safely withdrawn after delivery but it prolongs withdrawal in the infant. Because the most seriously impaired drug users often present late for care, if at all, options for improving the course of drug-exposed pregnancies are often limited.

Recommendations of Other Groups

The American Medical Association (AMA)[71] and the American Academy of Family Physicians (AAFP)[72] advise physicians to include an in-depth history of substance abuse as part of a complete health examination for all patients. The AAFP,[72] AMA Guidelines for Adolescent Preventive Services (GAPS),[73] Bright Futures recommendations,[74] and American Academy of Pediatrics[75,76] suggest that clinicians discuss the dangers of drug use with all children and adolescents and include questions about substance abuse as a part of routine adolescent visits. The American College of Obstetricians and Gynecologists recommends that clinicians take a thorough history of substance use and abuse in all obstetric patients, and remain alert to signs of substance abuse in all women.[77,78]

The AMA supports drug testing (in conjunction with rehabilitation and treatment) as part of preemployment examinations for jobs affecting the health and safety of others.[71] The AMA and most other medical organizations endorse urine testing when there is reasonable suspicion of substance abuse, but none of these groups recommends routine drug screening in the absence of clinical indications.

Discussion

Many Americans face substantial health risks from illicit drugs and the nonmedical use of other drugs, but questions remain about appropriate methods for screening for drug abuse among asymptomatic patients. The routine use of screening instruments or laboratory tests has not yet been proven effective in reducing harmful drug use. Nonetheless, information about drug use is an important component of the medical interview, especially for adolescents and young adults, and a careful history remains the best way to identify those who need treatment. Despite frequent treatment failures, the medical and social benefits of treating drug abuse are substantial for patients who achieve long-term abstinence. Reducing drug use is also likely to have important benefits to society in reducing criminal activity and the spread of HIV.[7]

Urine testing is sensitive and specific for recent drug use but has many limitations as a routine screening test: it does not distinguish occasional use from drug abuse or dependence; sensitivity and specificity vary with timing of drug use; and the effectiveness of early intervention has not been examined in asymptomatic drug users detected by toxicologic screening.[79] Routine screening in asymptomatic individuals also poses important risks: testing without informed consent may violate patient autonomy; the predictive value of positive test results may be low in populations with a low prevalence of drug use; and patients may be discriminated against if confidentiality of results is not ensured.

Efforts to screen for drug use in pregnancy have been prompted by concern about the adverse effects on the developing fetus, the impact of parental drug use on child safety and welfare, and the realization that many drug-using mothers go undetected by routine patient history. Use of standardized clinical assessment in all pregnant women can increase the identification of drug use, but there is little evidence that routine urine screening in asymptomatic women reduces drug use during pregnancy or results in better perinatal outcomes. Treatment services for pregnant, drug-abusing women are often scarce, testing may not identify those pregnancies at highest risk, and positive tests have direct legal and social consequences for the mother and child.[80] Where clinicians must report drug use in pregnancy, routine testing may lead some women to avoid needed prenatal care.

CLINICAL INTERVENTION

There is insufficient evidence to recommend for or against routine screening for drug abuse with standardized questionnaires or biologic assays ("C" recommendation). Including questions about drug use when taking a history from adolescent and adult patients may be recommended on other grounds, including the prevalence of drug use and the serious consequences of drug abuse and dependence. Clinicians should be alert to signs and symptoms of drug abuse and ask about the use of illicit drugs and legal drugs of abuse (e.g., sedatives, stimulants); use of inhalants should be considered in older children, adolescents, and young adults. The quantity, frequency, patterns of consumption, and adverse consequences of drug use (e.g., interference with school or work, evidence of dependence) should be assessed for all patients who report drug use. Clinicians should establish a trusting relationship with patients, approach discussion of drug use in a nonjudgmental manner, and respect the patient's concerns about the confidentiality of disclosed information.

All pregnant women should be advised about the potential risks to the fetus of drug use during pregnancy and the potential to transmit drugs to infants through breastfeeding. Routine drug testing of urine or other body fluids is not recommended as the primary method of detecting drug use in pregnant women or other asymptomatic adults. Selective use of urine testing during pregnancy may be appropriate when the possibility of drug use is suggested by clinical signs and symptoms (e.g., growth retardation, inadequate weight gain, inadequate prenatal care); periodic testing can also help monitor and encourage abstinence in women who have used drugs. Pregnant women who abuse drugs should be advised of the importance of regular prenatal care and be referred for treatment, where available.

Patients should give consent prior to drug testing and be informed of any legal obligations on the part of the clinician to report drug use to child protective agencies or other authorities. Both positive and negative results should be interpreted with understanding of the kinetics of drug metabolism and the limitations of testing methods, and positive screening tests should be confirmed by more reliable methods.

All patients who report potentially harmful use of drugs should be informed of the risks associated with their drug use and advised to cut down or stop. Decisions about treatment should be based on evidence of drug abuse or drug dependence obtained through careful patient interview, including discussion with friends or family members where appropriate. A treatment plan should be developed for the patient and family that is tailored to the drug of abuse and the needs of the patient. Patients with evidence of drug dependence should be referred to appropriate drug-treatment providers and community programs specializing in the treatment of drug dependencies. Persons who continue to inject drugs should be screened periodically for HIV infection and advised of measures that may reduce the risk of infections due to drug use: use a new sterile syringe with each use, never share or re-use injection equipment, use clean (sterile, if possible) water to prepare drugs, clean the injection site with alcohol prior to injection, and safely dispose of syringes after use (see Chapters 28 and 62). Drug-using patients should be informed of available resources for sterile injection equipment.

The draft update of this chapter was prepared for the U.S. Preventive Services Task Force by David Atkins, MD, MPH.

REFERENCES

1. National Institute on Drug Abuse. Monitoring the Future Study, 1975–1994: national high school senior drug abuse survey. NIDA Capsules, November 1994. Rockville, MD: National Institute on Drug Abuse, 1994.
2. Substance Abuse and Mental Health Services Administration. National Household Survey on Drug Abuse: population estimates, 1993. Rockville, MD: Department of Health and Human Services, Substance Abuse and Mental Health Services Administration, 1994. (DHHS Publication no. (SMA) 94-3017.)

3. Substance Abuse and Mental Health Services Administration. Preliminary estimates from the 1992 National Household Survey on Drug Abuse. Advance Report no. 3. Rockville, MD: U.S. Department of Health and Human Services, Substance Abuse and Mental Health Services Administration, 1993.

4. National Institute on Drug Abuse. Epidemiologic trends in drug abuse. Vol. I–II. Rockville, MD: National Institute on Drug Abuse, National Institutes of Health, 1994. (NIH Publication nos. 94-3745, 3746.)

5. Kessler RC, McGonagle KA, Zhao S, et al. Lifetime and 12-month prevalence of DSM-III-R psychiatric disorders in the United States: results from the National Comorbidity Survey. Arch Gen Psychiatry 1994;51:8–19.

6. Substance Abuse and Mental Health Services Administration. Preliminary estimates from the Drug Abuse Warning Network: 1993 preliminary estimates of drug-related emergency department episodes. Advance Report no. 8. Rockville, MD: U.S. Department of Health and Human Services, Substance Abuse and Mental Health Services Administration, 1994.

7. Gerstein DR, Harwood HJ, eds. Treating drug problems. Committee for the Substance Abuse Coverage Study, Institute of Medicine. Washington, DC: National Academy Press, 1990.

8. Centers for Disease Control and Prevention, Division of STD/HIV Prevention. 1993 annual report. Atlanta: Centers for Disease Control and Prevention, 1994.

9. Perper JA, Van Thiel DH. Cardiovascular complications of cocaine abuse. Recent Dev Alcohol 1992;10:343–361.

10. Warner EA. Cocaine abuse. Ann Intern Med 1993;119:226–235.

11. Gold MS, Washton AM, Dackis CA. Cocaine abuse: neurochemistry, phenomenology, and treatment. Natl Inst Drug Abuse Res Monogr Ser 1985;61:130–150.

12. National Center for Infectious Diseases, Division of HIV/AIDS. National HIV Serosurveillance summary—results through 1992. Vol 3. Atlanta: Centers for Disease Control and Prevention, 1993. (Publication no. HIV/NCID/11-93/036.)

13. Schwartz RH. Marijuana: an overview. Pediatr Clin North Am 1987;34:305–317.

14. Jones RT. Marijuana: health and treatment issues. Psychiatr Clin North Am 1984;7:703–712.

15. Keer DW, Colliver JD, Kopstein AN, et al. Restricted activity days and other problems associated with use of marijuana or cocaine among persons 18–44 years of age: United States, 1991. Advance data from vital and health statistics; no 246. Hyattsville, MD: National Center for Health Statistics, 1994.

16. Centers for Disease Control and Prevention. Update: acquired immunodeficiency syndrome—United States, 1994. MMWR 1995;44:64–67.

17. Edlin BR, Irwin KL, Faruque S, et al. Intersecting epidemics—crack cocaine use and HIV infection among inner-city young adults: Multicenter Crack Cocaine and HIV Infection Team. N Engl J Med 1994;331:1422–1427.

18. National Institute on Drug Abuse. NIDA press briefing, September 12, 1994. Rockville, MD: National Institute on Drug Abuse, 1994.

19. Vega WA, Kolodny B, Hwang J, Noble A. Prevalence and magnitude of perinatal substance exposures in California. N Engl J Med 1993;329:850–854.

20. Moser JM, Jones VH, Kuthy ML. Use of cocaine during immediate prepartum period by childbearing women in Ohio. Am J Prev Med 1993;9:85–91.

21. Colmorgen GHC, Johnson C, Zazzarino MA, et al.Routine urine drug screening at the first prenatal visit. Am J Obstet Gynecol 1992;166:588–590.

22. Schulman M, Morel M, Karmen A, et al. Perinatal screening for drugs of abuse: reassessment of current practice in a high-risk area. Am J Perinatol 1993;10:374–377.

23. Sloan LB, Gay JW, Snyder S, et al. Substance abuse during pregnancy in a rural population. Obstet Gynecol 1992;79:245–248.

24. Burke MS, Roth D. Anonymous cocaine screening in a private obstetric population. Obstet Gynecol 1993;81: 354–356.

25. Chasnoff IJ, Landress HJ, Barrett ME. The prevalence of illicit-drug or alcohol use during pregnancy and discrepancies in mandatory reporting in Pinellas County, Florida. N Engl J Med 1990;322:1202–1206.

26. Mayes LC, Granger RH, Bornstein MH, et al. The problem of prenatal cocaine exposure. A rush to judgment. JAMA 1992;267:406–408.

27. Robins LN, Mills JL, eds. Effects of in utero exposure to street drugs. Am J Public Health 1993;83 (suppl):1–32.

28. Volpe JJ. Effect of cocaine use on the fetus. N Engl J Med 1992;327:399–407.

29. Graham K, Dimitrakoudis D, Pellegrini E, et al. Pregnancy outcomes following first trimester exposure to cocaine in social users in Toronto, Canada. Vet Hum Toxicol 1989;31:143–148.

30. Chasnoff IJ, Griffith DR, MacGregor S, et al. Temporal patterns of cocaine use in pregnancy. JAMA 1989;261: 1741–1744.

31. Hutchings DE. Methadone and heroin during pregnancy: a review of behavioral effects in human and animal offspring. Neurobehav Toxicol Teratol 1982;4:429–434.

32. Frank DA, Bresnahan K, Zuckerman BS. Maternal cocaine use: impact on child health and development. Adv Pediatr 1993;40:65–99.

33. Chasnoff IJ, Griffith DR, Freier C, Murray J. Cocaine/polydrug use in pregnancy: two year follow-up. Pediatrics 1992;89:284–289.

34. Zuckerman B, Frank DA, Hingson R, et al. Effects of maternal marijuana and cocaine use on fetal growth. N Engl J Med 1989;320:762–768.

35. Day NL, Richardson GA. Prenatal marijuana use: epidemiology, methodologic issues, and infant outcomes. Clin Perinatol 1991;18:77–91.

36. Bell GL, Lau K. Perinatal and neonatal issues in substance abuse. Pediatr Clin North Am 1995;42:261–281.

37. O'Malley PM, Johnston LD, Bachman JG. Adolescent substance abuse: epidemiology and implications for public policy. Pediatr Clin North Am 1995;42:241–260.

38. National Institute of Drug Abuse. National survey results on drug use from Monitoring the Future Study, 1975–1992. Vol 1. Secondary school students. Washington, DC: Government Printing Office, 1993. (Publication no. NIH 93-3597.)

39. Sharp CW. Introduction to inhalant abuse. Inhalant abuse: a volatile research agenda. Natl Inst Drug Abuse Res Monogr 1992;129:1–10.

40. American Psychiatric Association. Diagnostic and statistical manual of mental disorders. 4th ed. Washington, DC: American Psychiatric Association, 1994.

41. Trachtenberg AI, Fleming MF. Diagnosis and treatment of drug abuse in family practice. American Family Physician monograph, Summer 1994. Kansas City, MO: American Academy of Family Physicians, 1994.

42. Cogswell BE. Cultivating the trust of adolescent patients. Fam Med 1985;17:254–258.

43. Skinner HA. The drug abuse screening test. Addict Behav 1982;7:363–371.

44. Schwartz RH, Wirtz PW. Potential substance abuse. Detection among adolescent patients. Clin Pediatr 1990;29: 38–43.

45. McLellan AT, Luborsky L, Woody GE, et al. An improved diagnostic evaluation instrument for substance abuse patients. The Addiction Severity Index. J Nerv Ment Dis 1980;168:26–33.

46. Catlin D, Cowan D, Donike M, et al. Testing urine for drugs. Clin Chim Acta 1992;207:S13–S26.

47. Armbruster DA, Schwarzoff RH, Hubster EC, et al. Enzyme immunoassay, kinetic microparticle immunoassay, radioimmunoassay, and fluorescence polarization immunoassay compared for drugs-of-abuse screening. Clin Chem 1993;39:2137–2142.

48. ElSohly HN, ElSohly MA. Poppy seed ingestion and opiates urinalysis: a closer look. J Anal Toxicol 1990;14:308–310.

49. Frings CS, Bataglia DJ, White RM. Status of drugs-of-abuse testing in urine under blind conditions: an AACC study. Clin Chem 1989;35:891–894.

50. Burnett D, Lader S, Richens A, et al. A survey of drugs of abuse testing by clinical laboratories in the United Kingdom. Ann Clin Biochem 1990;27:213–222.

51. Ostrea EM, Brady M, Gause S, et al. Drug screening of newborns by meconium analysis: a large-scale, prospective epidemiologic study. Pediatrics 1992;89:107–113.

52. Callahan CM, Grant TM, Phipps P, et al. Measurement of gestational cocaine exposure: sensitivity of infants' hair, meconium, and urine. J Pediatr 1992;120:763–768.

53. McCalla S, Minkoff HL, Feldman J, et al. Predictors of cocaine use in pregnancy. Obstet Gynecol 1992;79:641–644.

54. Chasnoff IJ. Drug use and women: establishing a standard of care. Ann NY Acad Sci 1989;562:208–210.

55. Slutsker L, Smith R, Higginson G, et al. Recognizing illicit drug use by pregnant women: reports from Oregon birth attendants. Am J Public Health 1993;83:61–64.

56. Ostrea EM, Welch RA. Detection of prenatal drug exposure in the pregnant woman and her newborn infant. Clin Perinatol 1991;18:629–645.

57. Merrick JC. Maternal substance abuse during pregnancy. Policy implications in the United States. J Legal Med 1993;14:57–71.

58. Rosenstock L. Routine urine testing for evidence of drug abuse in workers: the scientific, ethical, and legal reasons not to do it. J Gen Intern Med 1987;2:135–137.

59. Gunne LM, Gronbladh L. The Swedish methadone maintenance program: a controlled study. Drug Alcohol Depend 1981;7:249–256.

60. Chaisson RE, Bacchetti P, Osmond D, et al. Cocaine use and HIV infection in intravenous drug users in San Francisco. JAMA 1989;261:561–565.

61. Condelli WS, Fairbank JA, Dennis ML, et al. Cocaine use by clients of methadone programs: significance, scope, and behavioral interventions. J Subst Abuse Treat 1991;8:203–212.

62. Greenstein RA, Resnick RB, Resnick E. Methadone and naltrexone in the treatment of heroin dependence. Psychiatr Clin North Am 1984;7:671–679.

63. Charuvastra VC, Dalali ID, Cassuci M, et al. Outcome study: comparison of short-term vs. long-term treatment in a residential community. Int J Addict 1992;27:15–23.

64. Wickizer T, Maynard C, Atherly A, et al. Completion rates of clients discharged from drug and alcohol treatment programs in Washington state. Am J Public Health 1994;84:215–221.

65. Power R, Hartnoll R, Chalmers C. Help-seeking among illicit drug users: some differences between a treatment and non-treatment sample. Int J Addict 1992;27:887–904.

66. Bergmann PE, Smith MB, Hoffman NG. Adolescent treatment. Implications for assessment, practice guidelines, and outcome management. Pediatr Clin North Am 1995;42:453–472.

67. Botvin GJ, Botvin EM. School-based and community based prevention approaches. In: Lowinson JH, Ruiz P, Millman RB, eds. Substance abuse: a comprehensive textbook. Baltimore: Williams & Wilkins, 1992:910–927.

68. Botvin GJ, Baker E, Dusenbury L, et al. Long-term follow-up results of a randomized drug abuse prevention trial in a white, middle-class population. JAMA 1995;273:1106–1112.

69. Racine A, Joyce T, Anderson R. The association between prenatal care and birth weight among women exposed to cocaine in New York City. JAMA 1993;270:1581–1586.

70. Feldman J, Minkoff HL, McCalla S, et al. A cohort study of the impact of perinatal drug use on prematurity in an inner-city population. Am J Public Health 1992;82:726–728.

71. American Medical Association. Drug abuse in the United States: a policy report. Report of the Board of Trustees. Chicago: American Medical Association, 1988.

72. American Academy of Family Physicians. Age charts for periodic health examination. Kansas City, MO: American Academy of Family Physicians, 1994. (Reprint no. 510.)

73. American Medical Association. Guidelines for adolescent preventive services (GAPS): recommendations and rationale. Chicago: American Medical Association, 1994.

74. Green M, ed. Bright Futures: national guidelines for health supervision of infants, children, and adolescents. Arlington, VA: National Center for Education in Maternal and Child Health, 1994.

75. American Academy of Pediatrics. Screening for drugs of abuse in children and adolescents. Pediatrics 1989;84:396–398.

76. American Academy of Pediatrics, Committee on Substance Abuse. Role of the pediatrician in prevention and management of substance abuse. Pediatrics 1993;91:1010–1013.

77. American College of Obstetricians and Gynecologists. Substance abuse. Technical Bulletin no. 194. Washington, DC: American College of Obstetricians and Gynecologists, July 1994.

78. American College of Obstetricians and Gynecologists. Substance abuse in pregnancy. Technical Bulletin no. 195. Washington, DC: American College of Obstetricians and Gynecologists, July 1994.

79. Greenblatt DJ, Shader RI. Say "no" to drug testing. J Clin Psychopharmacol 1990;10:157–159.

80. Chavkin W. Mandatory treatment for drug use during pregnancy. JAMA 1991;266:1556–1561.

section two

COUNSELING

54. Counseling to Prevent Tobacco Use

RECOMMENDATION

Tobacco cessation counseling on a regular basis is recommended for all persons who use tobacco products. Pregnant women and parents with children living at home also should be counseled on the potentially harmful effects of smoking on fetal and child health. The prescription of nicotine patches or gum is recommended as an adjunct for selected patients. Antitobacco messages are recommended for inclusion in health promotion counseling of children, adolescents, and young adults (see _Clinical Intervention_).

Burden of Suffering

Smoking accounts for one out of every five deaths in the U.S.[1] It is the most important modifiable cause of premature death, responsible annually for an estimated 5 million years of potential life lost.[1,2] About 420,000 Americans die each year as a result of smoking.[1] Since early studies in the 1950s and 1960s, a large body of epidemiologic evidence has accumulated regarding the health effects of smoking. Major cohort studies, many case-control studies, and other data sources provide consistent, convincing evidence linking the use of tobacco with a variety of serious pulmonary, cardiovascular, and neoplastic diseases. The scope of this report does not permit an examination of each study of the health effects of smoking or the nature of the risk relationship (e.g., relative risk, dose-response relationship) between smoking and each disease. Detailed reviews of this extensive literature have been published elsewhere.[1-6] A number of consistent findings from this body of evidence are well established. First, tobacco is one of the most potent of human carcinogens, causing an estimated 148,000 deaths among smokers annually due to smoking-related cancers.[1] The majority of all cancers of the lung, trachea, bronchus, larynx, pharynx, oral cavity, and esophagus are attributable to the use of smoked or smokeless tobacco.[2,6] Smoking also accounts for a significant but smaller proportion of cancers of the pancreas,[3,7-9] kidney,[2] bladder,[3,10] and cervix.[3,11-13] Second, smoking promotes atherosclerosis and is a leading risk factor for myocardial infarction and coronary artery, cerebrovascular, and peripheral vascular disease.[2,3] It is responsible for about 100,000 deaths from coronary heart disease and 23,000 deaths due to cerebrovascular disease each year.[1] Third, smoking is an important risk factor for respiratory illnesses, causing 85,000 deaths per year from pulmonary diseases such as chronic obstructive pulmonary disease (COPD) and pneumonia.[1,3] Children and adolescents who are active smokers have an increased prevalence and severity of respiratory symptoms and illnesses, decreased physical fitness, and potential retardation of lung growth.[14] Fourth, the nicotine in tobacco is an addictive drug, and the pharmacologic and behavioral processes that determine nicotine addiction are similar to those that determine addiction to drugs such as heroin and cocaine.[15,16] The initiation of tobacco use at an early age is associated with more severe addiction as an adult. Fifth, tobacco use may be associated with an increased risk of osteoporosis.[17,18] Sixth, smoking affects the health of nonsmokers. Smoking during pregnancy causes about 5–6% of perinatal deaths, 17–26% of low-birth-weight births, and 7–10% of preterm deliveries,[2,3] and it increases the risk of miscarriage and fetal growth retardation.[3] It may also increase the risk for sudden infant death syndrome (SIDS).[19,20] Passive smoking (or environmental tobacco smoke) increases the risk of lung cancer in nonsmokers,[4,21] causing approximately 3,000 lung cancer deaths each year.[4] It may also increase the risk of coronary heart disease in otherwise healthy nonsmokers.[22–25] Environmental tobacco smoke exposure increases the frequency of middle ear effusions and lower respiratory infections in children, causing an estimated 150,000–300,000 cases of lower respiratory tract infections leading to 7,500–15,000 hospitalizations.[4] In children, passive smoking is also associated with a small but measurable reduction in lung function[4] and exacerbates asthma,[4,26,27] causing symptoms in 200,000 to 1,000,000 asthmatics in addition to as many as 8,000–26,000 new cases of asthma a year.[4] Passive smoking has also been associated with an increased risk of SIDS.[19,20,27a] Finally, cigarettes are responsible for about 25% of deaths from residential fires, causing some 1,000 fire-related deaths and 3,300 injuries each year.[28] Estimated smoking-attributable costs for medical care in 1993 were $50 billion,[29] and excess lifetime medical expenditures for the current cohort of smokers may be as high as $500 billion.[30]

Although smoking has declined in the past three decades, 25% of adults in the U.S. continue to smoke.[31] Among adults, cigarette smoking is more common among men, Native Americans and Alaska Natives, and persons of low socioeconomic status or with 9–11 years of education.[31] Due to an increase in smoking by women during the period between 1940 and the early 1960s, lung cancer mortality in females has risen steadily since the mid-1960s; lung cancer is now the leading cause of cancer death in women.[32] Two thirds of female smokers continue to smoke during pregnancy.[33] Most smokers begin tobacco use as teenagers.[14] Currently, 19% of all high school seniors smoke on a regular basis; among black high school seniors, however, only 4% smoke regularly.[33a] Of persons aged 18–24, 26% are current smokers.[31] Smokeless tobacco is regularly used by 3% of adults (5.3 million persons)[34] and by about 20% of male high school seniors.[14]

Efficacy of Risk Reduction

There is a large body of evidence from prospective cohort and case-control studies showing that many of these health risks can be reduced by smoking cessation. Smokers who quit smoking before the age of 50 have up to half the risk of dying in the next 15 years that continuing smokers have; evidence suggests that the risk of dying is reduced substantially even among persons who stop smoking after age 70.[3] After 10 years of abstinence, the risk of lung cancer is 30–50% lower than that of continuing smokers; the risk of oral and esophageal cancer is halved as soon as 5 years after cessation.[3,7–9,35] Compared to current smokers, former smokers also have a lower risk of cervical and bladder cancer.[3,13] One year after quitting, the risk of myocardial infarction and death from coronary heart disease is reduced by one half, and after 15 years it approaches that of nonsmokers.[3,35a] The risk and complications of peripheral artery disease decrease after smoking cessation.[3] As early as 2 years after quitting, the risk of stroke starts to decrease, and within 5–15 years it returns to (or near to) that of persons who have never smoked.[3,36,36a] Relative to continuing smokers, smokers who quit have decreased COPD mortality rates; respiratory symptoms such as cough, sputum production, and wheezing; and infections such as bronchitis and pneumonia.[3] Pregnant women who stop smoking by the 30th week of gestation have infants with higher birth weights than infants born to women who smoke throughout pregnancy.[3]

Effectiveness of Counseling

Clinicians have both the opportunity and the means to modify smoking behavior and address nicotine dependency in their patients. It has been estimated that about 70% of the 46 million adult smokers in the U.S. could be counseled by clinicians during the course of ongoing medical care.[31,37] The effectiveness of tobacco cessation counseling in improving clinical outcomes has been demonstrated in several studies in pregnant women. In two randomized controlled trials, smoking cessation counseling with self-help materials significantly increased mean birth weight and decreased the incidence of intrauterine growth retardation.[38,39] For nonpregnant individuals, evidence of improved clinical outcomes is more limited. Among otherwise healthy middle-aged smokers with spirometric evidence of early COPD, an intensive smoking cessation program combining behavior modification and nicotine gum significantly reduced the age-related decline in forced expiratory volume in 1 second (FEV1).[39a] In middle-aged men, smoking cessation counseling alone[40] or in combination with dietary advice and/or hypertension management[41,42] decreased coronary heart disease morbidity and mortality, although results were statistically significant in only one trial.[41]

A number of clinical trials have demonstrated the effectiveness of certain forms of clinician[43-48] and group[47,49,50] counseling in changing the smoking behavior of patients. In pregnant women, randomized controlled trials have reported improvements in abstinence rates of 5–23% between intervention and control groups.[38,39,51-53] The intervention groups received individual counseling sessions at the time of the first prenatal visit, self-help manuals that targeted pregnant women, and mail or phone follow-up, while control groups received advice alone. A meta-analysis of 39 clinical trials in nonpregnant adults examined different types of clinical smoking cessation techniques involving various combinations of counseling, distribution of literature, and nicotine replacement therapy. It found higher cessation rates in the intervention compared to the control groups, with the differences in cessation rates averaging 6% after 1 year.[47] Subsequent published trials have demonstrated increases in abstinence rates of 3–7% in patients receiving clinician counseling[43-46,48] and of 8–25% with group counseling, compared to controls.[49,50] The key elements of effective counseling seem to be providing reinforcement through consistent and repeated advice from a team of providers to stop smoking, setting a specific "quit date," and scheduling follow-up contacts or visits. Using additional modalities, such as self-help materials, referral to group counseling, advice from more than one clinician, or chart reminders identifying patients who smoke, seems to further enhance effectiveness.[47,48,54-56]

One controlled trial that evaluated the effectiveness of counseling in changing smokeless tobacco use found significantly higher abstinence rates at 12-month follow-up in patients receiving personalized advice and explanation of oral lesions by dental hygienists, self-help materials, and encouragement to set a quit date, compared to those receiving usual care.[57,57a] Another controlled trial in professional baseball team players found that compared to those receiving usual care, patients who received counseling (similar to that in the trial cited above) plus nicotine gum, and who were shown photographs of oral cancer-associated facial disfigurement had significantly higher smokeless tobacco cessation rates.[58]

As adjuncts to counseling, the prescription of nicotine products can facilitate smoking cessation.[59-71a] Randomized controlled trials have found that 12-month cessation rates after brief clinician counseling and multiple follow-up visits double from 4–9% with placebo to 9–25% with the nicotine patch.[64,65,69,71] When used correctly and in combination with clinician advice to stop smoking, nicotine gum increases long-term smoking cessation rates by about one third.[72,73] The higher dose nicotine gum (4 mg) has proven to be more effective than the 2 mg dose in highly nicotine-dependent subjects.[73] (Nicotine dependence is commonly measured by the number of cigarettes smoked daily or by the Fagerström Test for Nicotine Dependence.[74]) Nicotine inhalers and nasal sprays are new modalities that have been found to be effective in clinical trials, but studies in primary care settings are needed before widespread use can be recommended.[75–76a] No trials have directly compared the effectiveness of the various adjuncts. Two meta-analyses of controlled trials of nicotine replacement therapies found a significant benefit for all modalities with no modality being significantly better than another.[73,77] Nicotine gum, however, was found to be effective in patients with high but not low nicotine dependence, while there was no difference in the efficacy of the nicotine patch by severity of nicotine dependence.[73] The evidence suggests that nicotine products are most effective as adjuncts to ongoing smoking cessation counseling.[77,78] Furthermore, patients need proper instruction on how to use the nicotine replacement therapies. Patients have been reported to use nicotine patches and gum without discontinuing smoking, thus increasing the risk of nicotine toxicity.[79,80] The most common adverse effects of nicotine gum include hiccups, flatulence, nausea, and indigestion, while the nicotine patch commonly causes local skin reactions and insomnia.[73,78] The nicotine inhaler and nasal spray are associated with irritation of the throat and coughing, and with nasal soreness, respectively.[75,76]

Clonidine has also been investigated as an adjunct to smoking cessation counseling. Four of five randomized trials with follow-ups of 3–12 months have reported improved abstinence rates of 8–21%.[81–85] Only one result was statistically significant,[83] but sample sizes may have been inadequate in the other three trials that showed nonsignificant benefits.[82,84,85] Side effects, including drowsiness and dry mouth, occurred in 5–25% of those receiving clonidine, resulting in significantly higher rates of discontinuation of clonidine compared to placebo.[81,83,84]

The prevention of initiation of tobacco use by children and adolescents is an important role for the clinician. Nearly all current initiation of tobacco use occurs before high school graduation.[14] Approximately 25% of 12–13-year-old children report having experimented with cigarettes, and 4% are regular smokers.[86] There have been no published trials that have adequately evaluated interventions by clinicians in preventing tobacco use initiation. Since the mid-1970s, however, over 90 controlled trials of school-based tobacco use prevention interventions have been published.[14] School-based programs reduce the incidence[87,88] and prevalence[89–91] of tobacco use in adolescents at 2–4-year follow-up. Longer follow-up has shown little long-term benefit, however, suggesting that program effects need to be reinforced.[92,93] The most successful of these programs involve teaching the skills to resist social pressures to use tobacco, along with the short- and long-term consequences of using tobacco (see *Clinical Interven-tion*).[94]

Recommendations of Other Groups

All major health care organizations and authorities recommend routine clinician counseling of adults, pregnant women, parents, and adolescents to avoid or discontinue smoking and use of smokeless tobacco.[95–108]

Discussion

Although the significant health hazards of tobacco use and the benefits of cessation are well established, studies suggest that many clinicians fail to counsel patients (or their parents) who smoke to stop tobacco use.[37,109,110] This reluctance to intervene may be the result of a number of variables, in-cluding lack of confidence in the ability to provide adequate counseling, lack of patient interest, lack of financial reimbursement or personal re-ward, insufficient time, and inadequate staff support.[111] As described above, however, a number of studies have shown that clinician counseling can change behavior, even when the intervention is relatively brief. Nearly 50% of all living individuals who have ever smoked have stopped,[31] and 30% of quitters report being urged to quit by a physician.[113] Approxi-mately 90% of successful quitters have quit without intensive counseling but by stopping abruptly or with the help of quitting manuals.[113] More-over, even a modest decrease in smoking rates can have significant public health implications when multiplied by the more than 30 million smokers seen annually by U.S. clinicians.[37] A cost-effectiveness study supports the clinical value of offering smoking cessation counseling during the routine office visit of patients who smoke.[114]

Although there are no data on the effectiveness of clinician counseling in preventing the initiation of tobacco use by children, school-based pro-grams are effective in reducing the prevalence of smoking among children for up to 4 years. Clinicians can provide leadership and support that may enhance both school-based programs and community-based efforts such as restrictions on tobacco advertising, enforcement of laws that prevent mi-nors' access to tobacco, and tax increases on tobacco products to decrease the demand among children.[14]

CLINICAL INTERVENTION

A complete history of tobacco use, and an assessment of nicotine depen-dence among tobacco users, should be obtained from all adolescent and adult patients. Tobacco cessation counseling is recommended on a regular basis for all patients who use tobacco products ("A" recommendation). Pregnant women and parents with children living at home also should be

counseled on the potentially harmful effects of smoking on fetal and child health ("A" recommendation). The optimal frequency for performing counseling to prevent tobacco use has not been determined with certainty, but repeated messages over long periods of time are associated with the greatest success in helping patients achieve abstinence.[47] The prescription of nicotine patches or gum is recommended as an adjunct for selected patients ("A" recommendation). There is insufficient evidence to recommend for or against clonidine as an effective adjunct to tobacco cessation counseling ("C" recommendation).

Certain strategies can increase the effectiveness of counseling against tobacco use (also see published guidelines[104,105,107,115–118]):

- **Direct, face-to-face advice and suggestions.** The most effective clinician message is a brief, unambiguous, and informative statement on the need to stop using tobacco. If possible, the clinician should also review the short- and long-term health, social, and economic benefits of quitting and foster the tobacco user's belief in his or her ability to stop. The message should address the patient's concerns and any barriers presented by age, social environment, nicotine dependence, and general health. If the patient is not contemplating cessation, then the clinician should try to motivate the patient again at the next visit. If the patient is contemplating stopping, then the clinician should try to get agreement on a specific "quit date" and should prepare the patient for withdrawal symptoms. Patients who have experienced a relapse after previous quit attempts should be reassured that most smokers achieve long-term cessation only after several unsuccessful attempts.
- **Reinforcement.** Schedule "support visits" or follow-up telephone calls, especially during the first 2 weeks when relapse is common.[119]
- **Office reminders.** Use a register system or chart stickers for tobacco users to increase the probability that an anti-tobacco message is delivered at each visit.
- **Self-help materials.** Dispense a variety of effective self-help packages to motivate and aid the majority of tobacco users who quit on their own. These materials are listed in reference works[120] and are available from voluntary organizations in most communities.
- **Community programs for additional help in quitting.** Local hospitals, health departments, community health centers, work sites, commercial services, and voluntary organizations frequently offer smoking cessation programs to which patients can be referred. Clinicians should not, however, refer patients to programs providing treatment of unproven efficacy (e.g., electric shock therapy).[121]
- **Drug therapy.** The prescription of nicotine products as adjuncts to counseling may facilitate cessation by relieving withdrawal symptoms. Persons using the nicotine patch or gum should be advised to stop all tobacco use completely before starting the medication and to carefully store and dispose of products to prevent accidental ingestion by children or pets. The patch should be used on clean, dry, non-hairy skin sites that are alternated daily. A skin site should not be used more frequently than once a week.[122] The patch

is generally prescribed for 6–8 weeks over which time the dosage of nicotine is weaned.[78] Those using nicotine gum should be instructed to chew the gum slowly and intermittently to allow proper absorption by the buccal mucosa. While using nicotine gum, patients should not drink or eat acidic substances such as coffee, colas, or citrus juices, which impair nicotine absorption.[123] Nicotine gum is used as needed for up to 3 months, when the risk of relapse is greatest, and then tapered over the next 3 months.[122] In pregnant or nursing patients or patients with a recent myocardial infarction, severe or worsening angina, serious arrhythmias, or vasospastic or endocrine disorders, the potential risks of nicotine adjuncts must be weighed carefully against the known adverse effects of tobacco. Nicotine adjuncts should also be used with caution in persons with peptic ulcer disease, claudication, renal or hepatic insufficiency, or accelerated hypertension. Nicotine gum is contraindicated in patients with active temporomandibular joint disease.[122]

Anti-tobacco messages should be included in health promotion counseling of children, adolescents, and young adults based on the proven efficacy of risk reduction from avoiding tobacco use ("A" recommendation), although the evidence for the effectiveness of clinical counseling to prevent the initiation of tobacco use is less clear ("C" recommendation).

Because school-based programs have been shown to delay initiation of tobacco use, clinicians should support such programs in their communities. Effective school-based programs teach children skills to recognize and resist social pressure to smoke, dip, or chew tobacco as well as to understand the short-term (e.g., bad breath, cost, decreased athletic ability, cough, phlegm production, and shortness of breath) and long-term adverse consequences of tobacco use. Examples of support that clinicians can provide include: becoming aware of programs already in place in local schools and reinforcing their messages with patients and their parents, alerting parents to the existence of such programs, and encouraging parental participation and involvement; serving as a consultant to local schools that implement such programs; developing a list of referrals for tobacco cessation programs for youths; and serving as a community advocate to keep effective programs in place (L.A. Maiman and D. Haynie, National Institutes of Health, personal communication, March 1994).

The draft update of this chapter was prepared for the U.S. Preventive Services Task Force by Mary Jo Trepka, MD, MPH, and Carolyn DiGuiseppi, MD, MPH, based in part on a background paper on smoking and pregnancy prepared for the Canadian Task Force on the Periodic Health Examination by Susan E. Moner, MD.

REFERENCES

1. Centers for Disease Control and Prevention. Cigarette smoking—attributable mortality and years of potential life lost—United States, 1990. MMWR 1993;42:645–649.
2. Department of Health and Human Services. Reducing the health consequences of smoking: 25 years of progress. A report of the Surgeon General. Rockville, MD: Department of Health and Human Services, 1989. (Publication no. DHHS (CDC) 89-8411.)

3. Department of Health and Human Services. The health benefits of smoking cessation: a report of the Surgeon General. Rockville, MD: Department of Health and Human Services, 1990. (Publication no. DHHS (CDC) 90-8416.)

4. U.S. Environmental Protection Agency. Respiratory health effects of passive smoking: lung cancer and other disorders. Washington, DC: Environmental Protection Agency, Office of Health and Environmental Assessment, Office of Research and Development, 1992. (Publication no. EPA/600/6-90/ 006F.)

5. National Cancer Institute. Smokeless tobacco or health: an international perspective. Bethesda: National Institutes of Health, 1993. (Publication no. DHHS (NIH) 93-3461.)

6. Department of Health and Human Services. The health consequences of smokeless tobacco: a report of the advisory committee to the Surgeon General. Washington, DC: Government Printing Office, 1986. (Publication no. DHHS (PHS) 86-2874.)

7. Ghadirian P, Simard A, Baillargeon J. Tobacco, alcohol and coffee and cancer of the pancreas: a population-based, case-control study in Quebec, Canada. Cancer 1991;67:2664–2670.

8. Howe GR, Jain M, Burch JD, et al. Cigarette smoking and cancer of the pancreas: evidence from a population-based case-control study in Toronto, Canada. Int J Cancer 1991;47:323–328.

9. Bueno de Mesquita HB, Maisonneuve P, Moerman CJ, et al. Life-time history of smoking and exocrine carcinoma of the pancreas: a population-based case-control study in the Netherlands. Int J Cancer 1991;49:816–822.

10. Hartge P, Silverman DT, Schairer C, et al. Smoking and bladder cancer risk in blacks and whites in the United States. Cancer Causes Control 1993;4:391–394.

11. Coker AL, Rosenberg AJ, McCann MF, et al. Active and passive cigarette smoke exposure and cervical intraepithelial neoplasia. Cancer Epidemiol Biomarkers Prev 1992;1:349–356.

12. Sood AK. Cigarette smoking and cervical cancer: meta-analysis and critical review of recent studies. Am J Prev Med 1991;7:208–213.

13. Gram IT, Austin H, Stalsberg H. Cigarette smoking and the incidence of cervical intraepithelial neoplasia, grade III, and cancer of the cervix uteri. Am J Epidemiol 1992;135:341–346.

14. Department of Health and Human Services. Preventing tobacco use among young people: a report of the Surgeon General. Washington, DC: Government Printing Office, 1994. (Publication no. S/N 017-001-00491-0.)

15. Department of Health and Human Services. The health consequences of smoking: nicotine addiction. A report of the Surgeon General, 1988. Rockville, MD: Department of Health and Human Services, 1988. (Publication no. DHHS (CDC) 88-8406.)

16. Henningfield JE, Cohen C, Pickworth WB. Psychopharmacology of nicotine. In: Orleans CT, Slade J, eds. Nicotine addiction. New York: Oxford University Press, 1994:24–45.

17. Hopper JL, Seeman E. The bone density of female twins discordant for tobacco use. N Engl J Med 1994;330: 387–392.

18. Seeman E, Melton LJ, O'Fallon WM, et al. Risk factors for spinal osteoporosis in men. Am J Med 1983;75: 977–983.

19. Mitchell EA, Ford RPK, Steward AW, et al. Smoking and the sudden infant death syndrome. Pediatrics 1993;91: 893–896.

20. Schoendorf KC, Kiely JL. Relationship of sudden infant death syndrome to maternal smoking during and after pregnancy. Pediatrics 1992;90:905–908.

21. Stockwell HG, Goldman AL, Lyman GH, et al. Environmental tobacco smoke and lung cancer risk in nonsmoking women. J Natl Cancer Inst 1992;84:1417–1422.

22. Hole DJ, Gillis CR, Chopra C, et al. Passive smoking and cardiorespiratory health in a general population in the west of Scotland. BMJ 1989;299:423–427.

23. Helsing KJ, Sandler DP, Comstock GW, et al. Heart disease mortality in nonsmokers living with smokers. Am J Epidemiol 1988;127:915–922.

24. Humble C, Croft J, Gerber A, et al. Passive smoking and 20-year cardiovascular disease mortality among nonsmoking wives, Evans County, Georgia. Am J Public Health 1990;80:599–601.

25. Svendson KH, Kuller LH, Martin MJ, et al. Effects of passive smoking in the Multiple Risk Factor Intervention Trial. Am J Epidemiol 1987;126:783–795.

26. Chilmonczyk BA, Salmun LM, Megathlin KN, et al. Association between exposure to environmental tobacco smoke and exacerbations of asthma in children. N Engl J Med 1993;328:1665–1669.

27. Sherrill DL, Martinez FD, Lebowitz MD, et al. Longitudinal effects of passive smoking on pulmonary function in New Zealand children. Am Rev Respir Dis 1992;145:1136–1141.

27a. Klonoff-Cohen HS, Edelstein SL, Lefkowitz ES, et al. The effect of passive smoking and tobacco exposure through breast milk on sudden infant death syndrome. JAMA 1995;273:795–798.

28. Miller AL. The U.S. smoking-material fire problem through 1991: the role of lighted tobacco products in fire. Quincy, MA: National Fire Protection Association, 1993.

29. Centers for Disease Control and Prevention. Medical-care expenditures attributable to cigarette smoking—United States, 1993. MMWR 1994;43:469–472.

30. Hodgson TA. Cigarette smoking and lifetime medical expenditures. Milbank Q 1992;70:81–125.

31. Centers for Disease Control and Prevention. Cigarette smoking among adults—United States, 1993. MMWR 1994;43:925–930.

32. Centers for Disease Control and Prevention. Mortality trends for selected smoking-related cancers and breast cancer—United States, 1950–90. MMWR 1993;42:857–866.

33. National Center for Health Statistics. Health United States 1992 and Healthy People 2000 Review. Hyattsville, MD: Department of Health and Human Services, 1993. (Publication no. DHHS (PHS) 93-1232.)

33a. Giovino GA, Schooley MW, Zhu B-P, et al. Surveillance for selected tobacco-use behaviors, United States, 1900–1994. In: CDC surveillance summaries, November 18, 1994. MMWR 1994;43(SS-3):1–43.

34. Centers for Disease Control and Prevention. Use of smokeless tobacco among adults—United States, 1991. MMWR 1993;42;263–266.

35. Yu MC, Garabrant DH, Peters JM, et al. Tobacco, alcohol, diet, occupation, and carcinoma of the esophagus. Cancer Res 1988;48:3843–3848.

35a. Negri E, La Vecchia C, D'Avanzo B, et al. Acute myocardial infarction: association with time since stopping smoking in Italy. GISSI-EFRIM Investigators. J Epidemiol Community Health 1994;48:129–133.

36. Kawachi I, Colditz GA, Stampfer MJ, et al. Smoking cessation and decreased risk of stroke in women. JAMA 1993;269:232–236.

36a. Wannamethee SG, Shaper AG, Whincup PH, et al. Smoking cessation and the risk of stroke in middle-aged men. JAMA 1995;274:155–160.

37. Centers for Disease Control and Prevention. Physician and other health-care professional counseling of smokers to quit—United States, 1991. MMWR 1993;42:854–857.

38. Ershoff DH, Quinn VP, Mullen PD, et al. Pregnancy and medical cost outcomes of a self-help prenatal smoking cessation program in an HMO. Public Health Rep 1990;105:340–347.

39. Sexto M, Hebel JR. A clinical trial of change in maternal smoking and its effect on birth weight. JAMA 1984;251:911–915.

39a. Anthonisen NR, Connett JE, Kiley JP, et al. Effects of smoking intervention and the use of an inhaled anticholinergic bronchodilator on the rate of decline of FEV1. The Lung Health Study. JAMA 1994; 272:1497–1505.

40. Rose G, Hamilton PJS, Colwell L, et al. A randomised controlled trial of anti-smoking advice: 10-year results. J Epidemiol Community Health 1982;36:102–108.

41. Hjermann I, Velve Byre K, Holme I, et al. Effect of diet and smoking intervention on the incidence of coronary heart disease. Report from the Oslo Study Group of a randomised trial in healthy men. Lancet 1981;2:1303–1310.

42. Multiple Risk Factor Intervention Trial Research Group. Mortality rates after 10.5 years for participants in the Multiple Risk Factor Intervention Trial: findings related to a priori hypotheses of the trial [published erratum in JAMA 1990;263:3151]. JAMA 1990;263:1795–1801.

43. Wilson DM, Taylor DW, Gilbert JR, et al. A randomized trial of a family physician intervention for smoking cessation. JAMA 1988;260:1570–1574.

44. Okene JK, Kristeller J, Goldberg R, et al. Increasing the efficacy of physician-delivered smoking interventions: a randomized clinical trial. J Gen Intern Med 1991;6:1–8.

45. Bronson DL, Flynn BS, Solomon LJ, et al. Smoking cessation counseling during periodic health examinations. Arch Intern Med 1989;149:1653–1656.

46. Hollis JF, Lichtenstein E, Vogt TM, et al. Nurse-assisted counseling for smokers in primary care. Ann Intern Med 1993;118:521–525.

47. Kottke TE, Battista RN, DeFriese GH, et al. Attributes of successful smoking cessation interventions in medical practice: a meta-analysis of 39 controlled trials. JAMA 1988;259:2882–2889.

48. Cohen SJ, Stookey GK, Katz BP, et al. Encouraging primary care physicians to help smokers quit: a randomized, controlled trial. Ann Intern Med 1989;110:648–652.

49. Curry SJ, Marlatt GA, Gordon J, et al. A comparison of alternative theoretical approaches to smoking cessation and relapse. Health Psychol 1988;7:545–556.

50. Stevens VJ, Hollis JF. Preventing smoking relapse, using an individually tailored skills-training technique. J Consult Clin Psychol 1989;57:420–424.
51. Hjalmarson AIM, Hahn L, Svanberg B. Stopping smoking in pregnancy: effect of a self-help manual in controlled trial. Br J Obstet Gynaecol 1991;98:260–264.
52. Windsor RA, Lowe JB, Perkins LL, et al. Health education for pregnant smokers: its behavioral impact and cost benefit. Am J Public Health 1993;83:201–206.
53. Mayer JKP, Hawkins B, Todd R. A randomized evaluation of smoking cessation interventions for pregnant women at a WIC clinic. Am J Public Health 1990;80:76–78.
54. Russell MAH, Wilson C, Taylor C, et al. Effect of general practitioners' advice against smoking. BMJ 1979;2: 231–235.
55. Janz NK, Becker MH, Kirscht MK, et al. Evaluation of a minimal contact smoking cessation intervention in an outpatient setting. Am J Public Health 1987;77:805–808.
56. Sanders D, Fowler G, Mant D, et al. Randomized controlled trial of anti-smoking advice by nurses in general practice. J R Coll Gen Pract 1989;39:273–276.
57. Little SJ, Stevens VJ, Severson HH, et al. An effective smokeless tobacco intervention for dental hygiene patients. J Dent Hyg 1992;66:185–190.
57a. Stevens VJ, Severson H, Lichtenstein E, et al. Making the most of a teachable moment: a smokeless-to-bacco cessation intervention in the dental office. Am J Public Health 1995;85:231–235.
58. Greene JC, Walsh MM, Masouredis C. A program to help major league baseball players quit using spit tobacco: report of a pilot study. J Am Dent Assoc 1994;124:559–568.
59. Lam W, Sze PC, Sacks HS, et al. Meta-analysis of randomised controlled trials of nicotine chewing-gum. Lancet 1987;2:27–30.
60. Jarvis MJ, Raw M, Russell MAH, et al. Randomised controlled trial of nicotine chewing gum. BMJ 1982;285:537–540.
61. Jackson PH, Stapleton JA, Russell MAH, et al. Predictors of outcome in a general practitioner intervention against smoking. Prev Med 1986;15:244–253.
62. Tonnesen P, Fryd V, Hansen M, et al. Effect of nicotine chewing gum in combination with group counseling on the cessation of smoking. N Engl J Med 1988;318:15–18.
63. Hughes JR, Gust SW, Kennan RM, et al. Nicotine vs placebo gum in general medical practice. JAMA 1989;261:1300–1305.
64. Tonnesen P, Norregaard J, Simonsen K, et al. A double-blind trial of a 16-hour transdermal nicotine patch in smoking cessation. N Engl J Med 1991;325:311–315.
65. Stapleton JA, Russell MA, Feyerabend C, et al. Dose effects and predictors of outcome in a randomized trial of transdermal nicotine patches in general practice. Addiction 1995;90:31–42.
66. Transdermal Nicotine Study Group. Transdermal nicotine for smoking cessation: six-month results from two multicenter controlled clinical trials. JAMA 1991;266:3133–3138.
67. Daughton DM, Heatley SA, Prendergast JJ, et al. Effect of transdermal nicotine delivery as an adjunct to low-intervention smoking cessation therapy: a randomized, placebo-controlled, double-blind study. Arch Intern Med 1991; 151:749–752.
68. Muller P, Abelin T, Ehrsam R, et al. The use of transdermal nicotine in smoking cessation. Lung 1990; 168(suppl):445–453.
69. Sachs DPL, Sawe U, Leischow SJ. Effectiveness of a 16-hour transdermal nicotine patch in a medical practice setting, without intensive group counseling. Arch Intern Med 1993;153:1881–1890.
70. Fiore MC, Kenford SL, Jorenby DE, et al. Two studies of the clinical effectiveness of the nicotine patch with different counseling treatments. Chest 1994;105:524–533.
71. Hurt RD, Dale LC, Fredrickson PA, et al. Nicotine patch therapy for smoking cessation combined with physician advice and nurse follow-up: one-year outcome and percentage of nicotine replacement. JAMA 1994;271:595–600.
71a. Fiore MC, Smith SS, Jorenby DE, et al. The effectiveness of the nicotine patch for smoking cessation. A meta-analysis. JAMA 1994;271:1940–1947.
72. Oster G, Huse DM, Delea TE, et al. Cost-effectiveness of nicotine gum as an adjunct to physician's advice against cigarette smoking. JAMA 1986;256:1315–1318.
73. Tang JL, Law M, Wald N. How effective is nicotine replacement therapy in helping people to stop smoking? BMJ 1994;308:21–26.
74. Fagerström KO, Heatherton TF, Kozlowski LT. Nicotine addiction and its assessment. Ear Nose Throat J 1992;69: 763–767.

75. Tonnesen P, Norregaard J, Mikkelsen K, et al. A double-blind trial of a nicotine inhaler for smoking cessation. JAMA 1993;269:1268–1271.

76. Sutherland G, Stapleton JA, Russell MA, et al. Randomised controlled trial of nasal nicotine spray in smoking cessation. Lancet 1992;340:324–329.

76a. Hjalmarson A, Franzon M, Westin A, et al. Effect of nicotine nasal spray on smoking cessation. A randomized, placebo-controlled, double-blind study. Arch Intern Med 1994;154:2567–2572.

77. Silagy C, Mant D, Fowler G, et al. Meta-analysis on efficacy of nicotine replacement therapies in smoking cessation. Lancet 1994;343:139–142.

78. Fiore MC, Jorenby DE, Baker TB, et al. Tobacco dependence and the nicotine patch: clinical guidelines for effective use. JAMA 1992;268:2687–2694.

79. Johnson RE, Steven VJ, Hollis JF, et al. Nicotine chewing gum use in the outpatient care setting. J Fam Pract 1992;34:61–65.

80. Orleans CT, Resch N, Noll E, et al. Use of transdermal nicotine in a state-level prescription plan for the elderly: a first look at "real-world" patch users. JAMA 1994;271:601–607.

81. Prochazka AV, Petty TL, Nett L, et al. Transdermal clonidine reduced some withdrawal symptoms but did not increase smoking cessation. Arch Intern Med 1992;152:2065–2069.

82. Wei H, Young D. Effect of clonidine on cigarette cessation and in the alleviation of withdrawal symptoms. Br J Addict 1988;83:1221–1226.

83. Glassman AH, Stetner F, Walsh T, et al. Heavy smokers, smoking cessation, and clonidine: results of a double-blind, randomized trial. JAMA 1988;259:2863–2866.

84. Davison R, Kaplan K, Fintel D, et al. The effect of clonidine on the cessation of cigarette smoking. Clin Pharmacol Ther 1988;44:265–267.

85. Hilleman DE, Mohiuddin SM, Delcore MG, et al. Randomized, controlled trial of transdermal clonidine for smoking cessation. Ann Pharmacother 1993;27:1025–1028.

86. Moss AJ, Allen KF, Giovino GA, et al. Recent trends in adolescent smoking, smoking-update correlates, and expectations about the future. Advance data from vital and health statistics, no. 221. Hyattsville, MD: National Center for Health Statistics, 1992.

87. Hansen WB, Johnson CA, Flay BR, et al. Affective and social influences approaches to the prevention of multiple substance abuse among seventh-grade students: results from Project SMART. Prev Med 1988;17:135–154.

88. Abernathy TJ, Bertrand LD. Preventing cigarette smoking among children: results of a four-year evaluation of the PAL program. Can J Public Health 1992;83:226–229.

89. Elder JP, Wildey M, de Moor C, et al. The long-term prevention of tobacco use among junior high school students: classroom and telephone interventions. Am J Public Health 1993;83:1239–1244.

90. Schinke SP, Gilchrist LD, Snow WH. Skills intervention to prevent cigarette smoking among adolescents. Am J Public Health 1985;75:665–667.

91. Botvin GJ, Dusenbury L, Tortu S, et al. Preventing adolescent drug abuse through a multimodal cognitive-behavioral approach: results of a three-year study. J Consult Clin Psychol 1990;58:437–446.

92. Flay BR, Koepke D, Thomson SJ, et al. Six-year follow-up of the first Waterloo School Smoking Prevention Trial. Am J Public Health 1989;79:1371–1376.

93. Murray DM, Pirie P, Luepker RV, et al. Five- and six-year follow-up results from four seventh-grade smoking prevention strategies. J Behav Med 1989;12:207–218.

94. Bruvold WH. A meta-analysis of adolescent smoking prevention programs. Am J Public Health 1993;83:872–880.

95. American College of Physicians, Health and Public Policy Committee. Methods for stopping cigarette smoking. Ann Intern Med 1986;105:281–295.

96. American Academy of Family Physicians. Age charts for periodic health examination. Kansas City, MO: American Academy of Family Physicians, 1994. (Reprint no. 510.)

97. American Academy of Pediatrics. Tobacco-free environment: an imperative for the health of children and adolescents. Pediatrics 1994;93:866–868.

98. American Academy of Pediatrics. Guidelines for health supervision II. Elk Grove Village, IL: American Academy of Pediatrics, 1988.

99. American College of Obstetricians and Gynecologists. Smoking and reproductive health. Technical Bulletin no. 180. Washington, DC: American College of Obstetricians and Gynecologists, 1993:1–6.

100. Manley M, Epps RP, Husten C, et al. Clinical interventions in tobacco control: a National Cancer Institute training program for physicians. JAMA 1991;266:3172–3173.

101. American Medical Association. Policy compendium. Chicago: American Medical Association, 1993: 432–435.

102. American Dental Association. Transaction 1992:26.

103. Canadian Task Force on the Periodic Health Examination. Canadian guide to clinical preventive health care. Ottawa: Canada Communication Group, 1994:26–36, 500–513.

104. National Institutes of Health. Clinical interventions to prevent tobacco use by children and adolescents: a supplement to: How to help your patients stop smoking: a National Cancer Institute manual for physicians. Bethesda: National Institutes of Health, 1989. (Publication no. DHHS (NIH) 89-3064.)

105. American Medical Association. Guidelines for adolescent preventive services (GAPS): recommendations and rationale. Chicago: American Medical Association, 1994:107–116.

106. American Academy of Otolaryngology–Head and Neck Surgery. Smokeless tobacco. Washington, DC: American Academy of Otolaryngology–Head and Neck Surgery, 1992.

107. National Institutes of Health. Tobacco and the clinician: interventions for medical and dental practice. Bethesda: National Institutes of Health, 1994. (Publication no. DHHS (NIH) 94-3693.)

108. Green M, ed. Bright Futures: guidelines for health supervision of infants, children, and adolescents. Arlington, VA: National Center for Education in Maternal and Child Health, 1994.

109. Anda RF, Remington PL, Sienko DG, et al. Are physicians advising smokers to quit? The patient's perspective. JAMA 1987;257:1916–1919.

110. Frankowski BL, Secker-Walker RH. Advising parents to stop smoking: opportunities and barriers in pediatric practice. Am J Dis Child 1989;143:1091–1094.

111. Kottke TE, Willms DG, Solberg LI, et al. Physician-delivered smoking cessation advice: issues identified during ethnographic interviews. Tobacco Control 1994;3:46–49.

112. *Deleted in proof.*

113. Fiore MC, Novotny TE, Pierce JP, et al. Methods used to quit smoking in the United States. Do cessation programs help? [published erratum appears in JAMA 1991;265:358]. JAMA 1990;263:2760–2765.

114. Cummings SR, Rubin SM, Oster G. The cost-effectiveness of counseling smokers to quit. JAMA 1989; 261:75–79.

115. National Institutes of Health. Clinical opportunities for smoking intervention: a guide for the busy physician. Bethesda: National Institutes of Health, 1986. (Publication no. DHHS (NIH) 86-2178.)

116. National Institutes of Health. How to help your patients stop smoking: a National Cancer Institute manual for physicians. Bethesda: National Institutes of Health, 1989. (Publication no. DHHS (NIH) 89-3064.)

117. American Academy of Family Physicians. AAFP stop smoking program. Kansas City, MO: American Academy of Family Physicians, 1987.

118. American Medical Association. How to help patients stop smoking: guidelines for diagnosis and treatment of nicotine dependence. Chicago: American Medical Association, 1994.

119. Kenford SL, Fiore MC, Jorenby DE. Predicting smoking cessation: who will quit with and without the nicotine patch. JAMA 1994;271:589–594.

120. U.S. Public Health Service. Clinician's handbook of preventive services. Washington, DC: Public Health Service, 1994:117, 333–336.

121. Orleans CT. Understanding and promoting smoking cessation: overview and guidelines for physician intervention. Annu Rev Med 1985;36:51–61.

122. Physicians' desk reference. 47th ed. Montvale, NJ: Medical Economics Data, 1993:1264–1267, 1380–1387, 6765–6769.

123. Henningfield JE, Radzius A, Cooper TM, et al. Drinking coffee and carbonated beverages blocks absorption of nicotine from nicotine polacrilex gum. JAMA 1990;264:1560–1564.

55. Counseling to Promote Physical Activity

RECOMMENDATION

Counseling patients to incorporate regular physical activity into their daily routines is recommended to prevent coronary heart disease, hypertension, obesity, and diabetes. This recommendation is based on the proven benefits of regular physical activity; the effectiveness of clinician counseling to promote physical activity is not established (see *Clinical Intervention*).

Burden of Suffering

In 1985, national survey data revealed that 56% of men and 61% of women in the U.S. either never engaged in physical activity or did so on an irregular basis.[1] Surveillance data from 1991 suggests the prevalence of sedentary lifestyle (58% overall) has not changed.[2] Coronary heart disease (CHD), the predominant risk associated with a sedentary lifestyle, is the leading cause of mortality in the U.S.[3] In the sedentary, an estimated 35% of the excess CHD could be eliminated by becoming more physically active.[4] The excess CHD risk attributable to sedentary lifestyle, and the societal costs of this excess risk, are higher than those attributed individually to obesity, hypertension, and smoking.[4,5] The total burden of suffering attributable to sedentary lifestyle in the U.S. is unknown but is probably large.

Efficacy of Risk Reduction

Evidence exists that physical activity and fitness reduce morbidity and mortality for at least six chronic conditions: coronary heart disease, hypertension, obesity, diabetes, osteoporosis, and mental health disorders. Evidence linking sedentary lifestyle with other conditions exists but is not reviewed here.[6–9] Moderate physical activity comprises activities that can be comfortably sustained for at least 60 minutes (e.g., walking, slow biking, raking leaves, cleaning windows, light restaurant work). Vigorous activity describes those of an intensity sufficient to result in fatigue within 20 minutes (e.g., shoveling snow).[10]

Coronary Heart Disease. There are no prospective intervention trials of physical activity for the primary prevention of CHD. Evidence from cohort studies, however, has shown a consistent association between physical activity and reduced incidence of CHD.[9,11–15] A relative risk of death from CHD of 1.9 (95% confidence interval, 1.6 to 2.2) for sedentary persons compared with the physically active was calculated in a meta-analysis of studies on primary prevention of CHD.[11] A relative risk of 1.9 was also reported in an earlier comprehensive review.[12] In a cohort of men, beginning moderately vigorous sports activity was associated with a 41% lower risk of death from CHD, which was comparable to the risk reduction associated with smoking cessation (44%).[15] In another cohort study, initially unfit men who subsequently became fit had a 52% reduction in cardiovascular disease mortality compared with those who remained unfit.[16] The absolute reduction in the age-adjusted death rate from cardiovascular disease was 34/10,000 man-years. Similar benefits from exercise have been reported in older men.[14,17] Physiologically, the response to physical activity in women appears similar to that in men.[18] Epidemiologic data sufficient to confirm a primary preventive role of physical activity for CHD in women are not yet available, however.[9,19]

One reason that those who are physically active may be at decreased risk for CHD is self-selection—persons who choose to exercise may be healthier and have fewer overall risk factors for CHD. Studies controlling for such confounding variables, however, have found that the effects of exercise are independent of other CHD risk factors, and that the cardiovascular benefits may even be augmented in the presence of other risk factors for CHD.[9,15,20] Moreover, the type of individual who adopts athletic behavior is not protected from CHD if regular exercise is discontinued (e.g., college athletes who are sedentary later in adult life).[21]

Although observational data cannot prove causal associations, the strength, consistency, and coherence of the evidence and presence of a biologic gradient, clearly suggest that both physical activity and fitness influence risk for CHD. Inference of a causal relationship between increased physical activity and decreased CHD is supported by demonstrated physiologic effects which suggest plausible biologic mechanisms (e.g., enhanced fibrinolysis, decreased platelet adhesiveness, improved lipoprotein profile, and lessened adrenergic response to stress).[8,22]

Hypertension. Cohort studies suggest that physically inactive persons have a 35–52% greater risk of developing hypertension than those who exercise, independent of other risk factors for hypertension.[23,24] A graded inverse relationship between increasing fitness quartile and blood pressure was noted in a large cohort.[25] Randomized controlled trials of primary prevention of hypertension to date, however, have been either nonspecific (i.e., exercise grouped together with diet and weight loss)[26,27] or limited in sample size. Inconsistencies in results between studies of secondary prevention[28,29] suggest that certain subsets of individuals (e.g., women and individuals with diastolic elevations) may be more responsive to the blood pressure-lowering effects of physical activity than others.[31,32] A meta-analysis of controlled longitudinal studies found a weighted net drop in systolic over diastolic blood pressure with endurance training of 3/3, 6/7, and 10/8 mm Hg in normotensive, borderline, and hypertensive subjects, respectively.[32] A similar effect on blood pressure appears across ages 15–80 years,[33,34] in different social groups, and in both men and women.[30] Low- to moderate-intensity endurance training or circuit weight training may be at least as effective in lowering blood pressure as are high-intensity endurance training and resistance training primarily for muscle strength.[22,32,35,36] A sigmoidal relationship between physical activity and blood pressure benefit may exist, and the threshold of activity necessary for significant effect may be lower than that necessary for cardiovascular fitness or improvement in lipid profile.[31] A possible mechanism is the attenuation of elevated sympathetic nervous system activity from hyperinsulinemia via the effects of exercise.[32,37]

Obesity. Data from prospective population studies suggest an increased risk for the development of significant weight gain for persons in lower leisure-time physical activity categories compared to those in higher physical activity categories.[38–40] Experimental data on secondary prevention of obesity confirm such a relationship.[40,41] Physical activity can influence the development of obesity (e.g., assist in long-term maintenance of isocaloric or balanced energy state) and increase the chances of success in initial and long-term weight loss.[40] This influence stems from increased total energy output, preservation of lean body mass, changes in substrate utilization and fat distribution, and possible reversal of diet-induced suppression of basal metabolic rate, as well as psychologic reinforcement.[9,42–44] An association between low levels of leisure time physical activity and insulin resistance with resultant hyperinsulinemia may link obesity (especially abdominal) with hypertension, hyperlipidemia, and CHD in some individuals.[37,45] Morbidity and mortality in prospective cohort data have been lower in overweight individuals who are physically active even if they remain overweight.[9,22,40,46,47] Normalization of the metabolic profile (e.g., glucose tolerance, insulin, lipids) is a plausible mechanism for such a decrease in morbidity and mortality.[48]

Non-Insulin-Dependent Diabetes Mellitus. Prospective cohort data reveal an inverse relationship between the level of physical activity and the risk of developing non-insulin-dependent diabetes mellitus (NIDDM).[49–51] This effect is pronounced among overweight men,[49] but it is also seen in women.[50] The age-adjusted risk of NIDDM is reduced by 6% for each 500-

kcal increment in energy expenditure per week.[51] The protective effect of physical activity is especially pronounced in persons at highest risk for NIDDM (i.e., those with positive family history, obesity, or hypertension).[51] In one cohort study, cardiopulmonary fitness appeared to attenuate mortality at each level of glycemic control.[52] Possible mechanisms for these primary and secondary preventive effects are reviewed elsewhere,[22,53] but decreased insulin resistance seems to play an important role. Both the onset of positive effects of physical activity on glycemic control and the loss of these effects upon its discontinuation are rapid.[53–55]

Osteoporosis. Nonrandomized controlled interventional data,[56–58] confirmed by limited randomized controlled trial data,[59] support earlier studies suggesting that postmenopausal women can retard bone loss through physical activity.[60] Cross-sectional studies examining exercise history[61] and fitness level[62] reveal higher bone mass in the more active and fit, respectively. Some prospective data,[63,64] along with cross-sectional data comparing the bone density of athletic women with that of nonathletic premenopausal women,[60,61] suggest that physical activity can also reduce the rate of bone loss in premenopausal women with a normal hormonal milieu.

Direct evidence that physical activity reduces the incidence of hip fractures includes a recent large case-control study.[65] This study found a reduction in the risk of hip fracture in women who were active in the past, as well as in those with recent moderate activity.[65] Prior studies focused on recent activity[66] or were cross-sectional in study design.[67] A plausible biologic mechanism is suggested by a large cohort study that substantiated an inverse relationship between bone mineral density and hip fractures.[68,69] Some studies have suggested that skeletal loads generating muscle pull or resistance rather than gravity or weight bearing alone may provide greater benefit to bone mineral density.[63,70] Inconsistencies in the literature exist, however.[71] Important questions remain unanswered, such as the role and relative impact of physical activity with respect to estrogen replacement. Furthermore, the percentage of variance in bone mineral density attributable to differences in activity is thought to be modest (20%) compared with the genetic contribution.[70]

Mental Health Disorders. Some consistent findings have emerged from controlled trials assessing problems with affect, such as depression and anxiety, before and after various forms of physical activity. First, improvements are greatest in those who are more depressed and more anxious at the onset of the study.[72,73] Second, improved cardiovascular fitness is not necessary for mood enhancement.[74] Third, several recent studies have shown diminished gain at high intensity compared to moderate intensity physical activity.[75–77] Prospective cohort data suggest physical activity also has a preventive effect.[78] Study methodologies to date may lack the sensitivity to detect decreased prevalence in those without preexisting affect disorders, however.[77,79-81] Healthy individuals may derive a preventive effect from physical activity, while those with mild to moderate affect disorders derive a therapeutic benefit.[73,82]

General well-being can apparently be enhanced with physical activity.[73,80] Research on self-esteem and physical activity has been criticized as being overly simplistic.[83] A more complex model was postulated, giving rise to several new terms that may be considered dimensions of self-esteem, e.g., self-efficacy (capacity to produce a desired effect), self-acceptance, self-concept, physical competence.[82,83] Exercise-induced increases in self-efficacy may have an important role in successful maintenance of physical activity habits.[84] Study results are mixed as to whether aerobic or anaerobic exercise imparts a greater increase in these components of self-esteem.[85-87] Furthermore, the relative importance of perceived improvements in areas of life not quantified by standard psychometric batteries (e.g., sleep patterns, sex life) remains to be determined.[88] Cognition does not appear to be improved significantly with physical activity.[82,89] Mechanisms for psychologic benefit remain undefined,[90,91] and the role of β-endorphins requires further study.[92,93]

Quantity and Intensity of Physical Activities. To improve cardiovascular fitness, exercise cannot be performed occasionally or seasonally,[94] nor can one expect protection from CHD simply by having exercised regularly in the past.[21] Beginning moderately vigorous physical activity during adulthood, however, may reduce the risk of CHD to the level of those who have been active for many years.[15] Among previously unfit men, achieving fitness, which requires regular physical activity, substantially reduces the risk of both all-cause and cardiovascular disease mortality.[16] In a recent cohort study, participating in increasing levels of vigorous activity was associated with decreasing total mortality in a graded relationship.[95] Clearly, regular vigorous physical activity sufficient to achieve physical fitness is associated with important health benefits.

While regular vigorous physical activity is likely to be most beneficial, prior recommendations for developing and maintaining cardiorespiratory fitness[96] may inadequately address the potential benefits of low to moderate levels of physical activity and subsequent risk factor modification, particularly for unfit and sedentary individuals. Moderate physical activities have higher compliance rates than vigorous exercise activities, mesh better with daily lifestyle, and are well maintained over time.[9,97,98] Studies with at least three levels of physical activity exposure uniformly reveal a reduction in CHD risk from the lowest to the next-to-lowest activity level.[12] It is not that more modest amounts of physical activity will provide the maximum reduction in CHD risk, but rather that those at greatest risk (i.e., the sedentary and least fit) may derive substantial benefits from initiating even some activity.[8,99] No clear minimal intensity of physical activity required for benefit has been defined. Intensity can convey an absolute or relative amount (e.g., what might be low intensity to one might be high intensity to another).[99] A linear dose-response relationship (except for the most vigorous levels or more than 3,000 kcal/week) seems to exist between physical activity and health (both lower incidence of disease and improved functional capability).[8] Modifications in the physical activity message may be required to accommodate those with differing interests, limitations, or cultural milieu as well as those with disability[100] (especially when mobility is reduced).

A trial of middle-aged men compared the training effect of 30 minutes of moderate physical activity with three 10-minute bouts per day of equivalent activity separated by at least 4 hours. Over an 8-week study period, both groups achieved similar results.[101] Also, cohort studies of physical activity exposure have assessed the amounts of activity performed per day and time devoted per week, not duration of specific workouts, and achieved significant results.[15,47] Thus, attention to total energy expenditure per day and per week is warranted.[8] How the expenditure is accumulated is secondary and dependent more on personal preference, musculoskeletal tolerance, and available facilities.

Potential Adverse Effects of Physical Activity. The benefits of physical activity must be weighed against its potential adverse effects, which include injury, osteoarthritis, myocardial infarction, and, rarely, sudden death. Data remain scarce on the incidence of injury during most noncompetitive physical activity.[102] One exception is running, with an annual risk of injury of 35–65%; risk is positively related to the level of exposure to the activity and to prior injury.[102] Aerobic dance participation also carries a relatively high risk, which increases with the frequency of classes.[102] One trial randomly assigned 70–79-year-old men and women to strength training, walk/jog, or control groups. Injury rates were 8.7% for the strength training group during the full 26 weeks, 4.8% for the walk group during weeks 1–13, and 57% for those who jogged during weeks 14–26 and had walked during the first 14 weeks.[103] In cohort data, physical activity in men and women was also associated with an increased risk of orthopedic problems.[104] Most exercise-induced injuries are preventable. They often occur as a result of excessive levels of physical activity, sudden dramatic increases in activity level (especially in persons with poor baseline fitness), and improper exercise techniques or equipment. Intense exercise training can also result in the interruption of menstrual function, bone loss (partly reversible), and an increased fracture risk.[70,71]

Long-term physical activity probably does not accelerate the development of osteoarthritis (OA) in major weight-bearing joints (e.g., hips, knees). Case-control data revealed no significant difference in knee OA among groups with varying leisure-time physical activity; OA patients were significantly more likely to have been obese at 20 years of age or had prior knee injury.[105] In a 5-year longitudinal cohort with a mean age of 63, runners were matched with controls and followed radiographically and clinically; acceleration of OA in runners was not found.[106] Graduated activity that allows cartilage adaptation is less likely to induce OA than painful or mechanically improper motion that places infrequent but excessive stress on joints.[107] Available data suggest that moderate physical activity performed within the limits of comfort while putting joints through normal motions will not, in the absence of joint abnormality, inevitably lead to joint injury.[108]

Adverse cardiovascular events are perhaps the greatest concern about vigorous exercise. Two recent large studies provide estimates of the relative risk of triggering myocardial infarctions within 1 hour of heavy physical activity compared with less strenuous or no exertion. These relative risks are 2.1 (95% confidence interval, 1.6 to 3.1)[109] and 5.9 (4.6–7.7),[110] respectively. A protective effect was seen with regular physical activity in both studies, however. As the frequency of exercise per week increased, the relative risk of infarction during vigorous activity dropped.[109,110] The risk of sudden death is known to be increased during vigorous physical activity.[111] This risk appears greater in sedentary persons who engage in vigorous activity as compared to those who are habitually active.[112] In those over 35 years of age, more than 80% of sudden deaths during or shortly after exercise are from CHD.[113] Exercise as a cause of sudden cardiac death was reviewed recently.[114] The overall risk of sudden death is lower, however, for those who are habitually active, despite the transient increase in risk during the actual physical activity, when compared with sedentary counterparts.[112,113]

Effectiveness of Counseling

The rationale and evidence for effectiveness of physical activity counseling have been reviewed.[60] Prior studies that have demonstrated benefits from counseling provide little information about long-term compliance and are of limited generalizability, because the form of counseling, delivery (e.g., inclusion of community health promotion[115]), type of patients, or clinical setting have not been representative of typical primary care clinician counseling of healthy patients. A recent randomized controlled trial contained similar limitations; the frequency of physical activity was not significantly increased and follow-up was limited to 1 month.[116] A nonrandomized controlled trial of brief physician counseling plus one brief follow-up phone call demonstrated significant increases in both self-reported and objectively measured (using an electronic monitor) physical activity; there were important study limitations, however, including self-selection to the intervention group, use of patient volunteers, and follow-up of only 4–6 weeks.[117] A multicenter cohort study using pre- and postintervention surveys to assess changes in several behaviors over 1 year did find an increase in beginning regular physical activity.[118] Thus, sufficient published evidence concerning the efficacy of physical activity counseling is lacking.

Recommendations of Other Groups

The American College of Sports Medicine and the Centers for Disease Control and Prevention recommend that every adult accumulate 30 minutes or more of moderate-intensity physical activity on most, preferably all, days of the week.[119] The American Heart Association[120] and the American Academy of Family Physicians (AAFP)[121] recommend that physicians counsel patients in selecting an exercise program and promote regular exercise. The policy of the AAFP is currently under review. The American College of Obstetricians and Gynecologists has issued guidelines on counseling women about regular exercise.[122] The Canadian Task Force on the Periodic Health Examination (CTF) recommends that moderate-level physical activity be performed consistently to accumulate 30 minutes or more most days of the week.[123] The CTF found insufficient evidence to recommend for or against including physical activity counseling in the periodic health examination.

The American Academy of Pediatrics recommends teaching the importance of regular, moderate to vigorous physical activity as a way to prevent illness in adult life, and encouraging parents to serve as role models by participating in regular physical activity.[124] The Bright Futures guidelines recommend that children and adolescents participate in regular physical activity, and that parents encourage such activity.[125] The American Medical Association recommends that all adolescents receive annual guidance about the benefits of exercise and encouragement to engage in safe exercise on a regular basis.[126]

Discussion

Direct evidence is limited that clinician counseling can increase the physical activity of asymptomatic patients, but other considerations warrant devoting time to this intervention. First, given the sizable independent relative risk for impaired health in sedentary individuals together with the large population at risk,[8] even modest increases in physical activity levels could have great public health impact.[127] Second, consideration of the total societal cost[4] associated with the sedentary lifestyle and its disproportionate burden[128] is also relevant. Third, the success of counseling in other settings and for other behavioral risk factors deserves consideration.[60]

Clinician counseling may reinforce several other important interventions (e.g., school-based emphasis on lifelong activity patterns, reduction of barriers to physical activity at work and in the community) that can change sedentary behavior.

CLINICAL INTERVENTION

Counseling to promote regular physical activity is recommended for all children and adults. This recommendation is based on the proven efficacy of regular physical activity in reducing the risk for coronary heart disease, hypertension, obesity, and diabetes ("A" recommendation), although there is currently insufficient evidence that counseling asymptomatic primary care patients to incorporate physical activity into their daily routines will have a positive effect on their behavior ("C" recommendation). Clinicians should determine each patient's activity level, ascertain barriers specific to that individual, and provide information on the role of physical activity in disease prevention. The clinician may then assist the patient in selecting appropriate types of physical activity. Factors that should be considered include medical limitations and activity characteristics that both improve health (e.g., increased caloric expenditure, enhanced cardiovascular fitness, low potential adverse effects) and enhance compliance (e.g., low perceived exertion, minimal cost, and convenience).

An emphasis on regular, moderate-intensity physical activity rather than on vigorous exercise is reasonable in sedentary persons. This emphasis encourages a variety of self-directed, moderate-level physical activities (e.g., walking or cycling to work, taking the stairs, raking leaves, mowing the lawn with a power mower, cycling for pleasure, swimming, racket sports)[119] that can be more easily incorporated into an individual's daily routine. An appropriate short-term goal is activity that is a small increase over current levels. Over a period of several months, progression to a level of activity that achieves cardiovascular fitness (e.g., 30 minutes of brisk walking most days of the week) would be ideal. Development and maintenance of muscular strength and joint flexibility is also desirable. Sporadic exercise, especially if extremely vigorous in an otherwise sedentary individual, should be discouraged in favor of moderate-level activities performed consistently.

The draft update of this chapter was prepared for the U.S. Preventive Services Task Force by John Burress, MD, MPH, David Christiani, MD, MPH, and Donald M. Berwick, MD, MPP.

REFERENCES

1. Caspersen CJ, Christenson GM, Pollard RA. Status of 1990 physical fitness and exercise objectives—evidence from NHIS 1985. Public Health Rep 1986;101:587–592.

2. Centers for Disease Control and Prevention. Prevalence of sedentary lifestyle—behavioral risk factor surveillance system, United States, 1991. MMWR 1993;42:576–579.

3. Kochanek KD, Hudson BL. Advance report of final mortality statistics, 1992. Monthly vital statistics report; vol 43 no 6 (suppl). Hyattsville, MD: National Center for Health Statistics, 1994.

4. Centers for Disease Control and Prevention. Public health focus: physical activity and the prevention of coronary heart disease. MMWR 1993;42:669–672.

5. Hahn RA, Teutsch SM, et al. Excess deaths from nine chronic diseases in the U.S., 1986. JAMA 1990;264: 2654–2659.

6. Bouchard C, Shepard RJ, Stephens T, eds. Physical activity, fitness, and health. Champaign, IL: Human Kinetics, 1994.

7. Lee IM. Physical activity, fitness, and cancer. In: Bouchard C, Shepard RJ, Stephens T, eds. Physical activity, fitness, and health. Champaign, IL: Human Kinetics, 1994.

8. Blair SN, Kohl HW, Gordon NF. How much physical activity is good for health? Annu Rev Public Health 1992;13:99–126.

9. Blair SN, Kohl HW, Paffenbarger RS Jr, et al. Physical fitness and all-cause mortality: a prospective study of healthy men and women. JAMA 1989;262:2395–2401.

10. American College of Sports Medicine. Guidelines for exercise testing and prescription. Philadelphia: Lea & Febiger, 1991.

11. Berlin JA, Colditz GA. A meta-analysis of physical activity in the prevention of coronary heart disease. Am J Epidemiol 1990;132:612–628.

12. Powell KE, Thompson PD, Caspersen CJ, et al. Physical activity and the incidence of coronary heart disease. Annu Rev Public Health 1987;8:253–287.

13. Leon AS, Connett J. Physical activity and 10.5 year mortality in the Multiple Risk Factor Intervention Trial (MRFIT). Int J Epidemiol 1991;20:690–695.

14. Donahue RP, Abbott RD, Reed DM, et al. Physical activity and coronary heart disease in middle-aged and elderly men: the Honolulu Heart Program. Am J Public Health 1988;78:683–685.

15. Paffenbarger RS Jr, Hyde RT, Wing AL, et al. The association of changes in physical-activity level and other lifestyle characteristics with mortality among men. N Engl J Med 1993;328:538–545.

16. Blair SN, Kohl HW III, Barlow CE, et al. Changes in physical fitness and all-cause mortality: a prospective study of healthy and unhealthy men. JAMA 1995;273:1093–1098.

17. Morris JN, Pollard R, Everitt MG, et al. Vigorous exercise in leisure-time: protection against coronary events. Lancet 1980;2;1207–1210.

18. Mitchell JH, Tate C, Raven P, et al. Acute response and chronic adaptation to exercise in women. Med Sci Sports Exerc 1992;24:S258–S265.

19. Douglas PS, Clarkson TB, et al. Exercise and atherosclerotic heart disease in women. Med Sci Sports Exerc 1992;24:S266–S275.

20. Siscovick DS, Weiss NS, Fletcher RH, et al. Habitual exercise and primary cardiac arrest: effect of other risk factors on the relationship. J Chronic Dis 1984;37:625–631.

21. Paffenbarger RS Jr, Hyde RT, Wing AL. A natural history of athleticism and cardiovascular health. JAMA 1984;252: 491–495.

22. Haskell WL, Leon AS, Caspersen CJ, et al. Cardiovascular benefits and assessment of physical activity and physical fitness in adults. Med Sci Sports Exerc 1992;24:S201–S220.

23. Paffenbarger RS Jr, Thorne MC, et al. Physical activity and incidence of hypertension in college alumni. Am J Epidemiol 1983;117:245–257.

24. Blair SN, Goodyear NN, et al. Physical fitness and incidence of hypertension in healthy normotensive men and women. JAMA 1984;252:487–490.

25. Ekelund LG, Haskell WA, et al. Physical fitness as a predictor of cardiovascular mortality in asymptomatic North American men. The Lipid Research Clinics mortality follow-up study. N Engl J Med 1988; 319:1379–1384.

26. Hypertension Prevention Collaborative Research Group. The effects of nonpharmacologic interventions on blood pressure of persons with high normal levels. JAMA 1992;267:1213–1220.

27. Stamler R, Stamler J, Gosch CF, et al. Primary prevention of hypertension by nutritional-hygienic means: final report of a randomized clinical trial. JAMA 1989;262:1801–1807.

28. Gordon NF, Scott CB, et al. Exercise and mild essential hypertension: recommendations for adults. Sports Med 1990;10:390–404.

29. Blumenthal JA, Siegel WC, Appelbaum M. Failure of exercise to reduce blood pressure in patients with mild hypertension: results of a randomized controlled trial. JAMA 1991;266:2098–2104.

30. *Deleted in proof.*

31. Jennings GL, Deakin G, et al. What is the dose-response relationship between exercise training and blood pressure? Ann Med 1991;23:313–318.

32. Fagard RH, Tipton CM. Physical activity, fitness, and hypertension. In: Bouchard C, Shepard RJ, Stephens T, eds. Physical activity, fitness, and health. Champaign, IL: Human Kinetics, 1994.

33. Cononie CC, Graves JE, Pollock ML, et al. Effect of exercise training on blood pressure in 70- to 79-yr-old men and women. Med Sci Sports Exerc 1991;23:505–511.

34. Hagberg JM, Montain SJ, Martin WH, et al. Effect of exercise training on 60–69 year-old persons with essential hypertension. Am J Cardiol 1989;64:348–353.

35. American College of Sports Medicine. Position stand: physical activity, physical fitness, and hypertension. Med Sci Sports Exerc 1993;25:i–x.

36. National High Blood Pressure Education Program Working Group. Report on primary prevention of hypertension. Arch Intern Med 1993;153:186–208.

37. Johnson D, Prud'homme D, et al. Relation of abdominal obesity to hyperinsulinemia and high blood pressure in men. Int J Obesity 1992;16:881–890.

38. Rissanen AM, Heliovaara M, et al. Determinants of weight gain and overweight in adult Finns. Eur J Clin Nutr 1991;45:419–430.

39. Williamson DF, Madans J, et al. Recreational physical activity and ten-year weight change in a U.S. national cohort. Int J Obesity 1993;17:279–286.

40. Blair SN. Evidence for success of exercise in weight loss and control. Ann Intern Med 1993;119: 702–706.

41. Bouchard C, Tremblay A, Nadeau A, et al. Long-term exercise training with constant energy intake. 1. Effect on body composition and selected metabolic variables. Int J Obesity 1990;14:57–73.

42. Stefanick ML. Exercise and weight control. In: Holloszy JO, ed. Exercise and sports medicine reviews. Baltimore: Williams & Wilkins, 1993;21:363–396.

43. Despres JP, Pouliot MC, et al. Loss of abdominal fat and metabolic response to exercise training obese women. Am J Physiol 1991;261:E159–E167.

44. King AC, Frey-Hewitt, Dreon DM, et al. Diet vs. exercise in weight maintenance: the effects of minimal intervention strategies on long-term outcomes in men. Arch Intern Med 1989;149:2741–2746.

45. Defronzo RA, Ferrannini E. Insulin resistance. A multifaceted syndrome responsible for NIDDM, obesity, hypertension, dyslipidemia, and atherosclerotic cardiovascular disease. Diabetes Care 1991;14:173–191.

46. Morris JN, Clayton DG, et al. Exercise in leisure time: coronary attack and death rate. Br Heart J 1990;63:325–334.

47. Paffenbarger RS Jr, Hyde RT, et al. Physical activity, all-cause mortality, and longevity of college alumni. N Engl J Med 1986;314:605–613.

48. Tremblay A, Despres JP, et al. Normalization of the metabolic profile in obese women by exercise and a low fat diet. Med Sci Sports Exerc 1991;23:1326–1331.

49. Manson JE, Nathan DM, et al. A prospective study of exercise and incidence of diabetes among US male physicians. JAMA 1992;268:63–67.

50. Manson JE, Rimm EB, et al. Physical activity and incidence of non-insulin dependent diabetes mellitus in women. Lancet 1991;338:774–778.

51. Helmrich SP, Ragland DR, Leung RW, et al. Physical activity and reduced occurrence of non-insulin dependent diabetes mellitus. N Engl J Med 1991;325:147–152.

52. Kohl HW, Gordon NF, et al. Cardiorespiratory fitness, glycemic status, and mortality risk in men. Diabetes Care 1992;15:184–192.

53. Wallberg-Henriksson H. Exercise and diabetes mellitus. In: Holloszy JO, ed. Exercise and sport sciences review. 1992;20:339–368.

54. Rogers MA, Yamamoto C, et al. Improvement in glucose tolerance after 1 week of exercise in patients with mild NIDDM. Diabetes Care 1988;11:613–618.

55. King DS, Dalsky GP, et al. Effects of lack of exercise on insulin secretion and action in trained subjects. Am J Physiol 1988;254:E537–E542.

56. Smith EL, Gilligan C, et al. Deterring bone loss by exercise intervention in premenopausal and postmenopausal women. Calcif Tissue Int 1989;44:312–321.

57. Dalsky GP, Stocke KS, et al. Weight-bearing exercise training and lumbar bone mineral content in postmenopausal women. Ann Intern Med 1988;108:824–828.

58. Bloomfield SA, Williams NI, et al. Non-weightbearing exercise may increase lumbar spine bone mineral density in healthy postmenopausal women. Am J Phys Med Rehab 1993;72:204–209.

59. Chow R, Harrison JE, Notarius C. Effect of two randomized exercise programs on bone mass of healthy postmenopausal women. BMJ 1987;295:1441–1444.
60. Harris SS, Caspersen CJ, et al. Physical activity counseling for healthy adults as a primary preventive intervention in the clinical setting. JAMA 1989;261:3590–3598.
61. Jacobson PC, Beaver W, Grubb SA. Bone density in women: college athletes and older athletic women. J Orthop Res 1984;2:8–32.
62. Chow RK, Harrison JE, et al. Physical fitness effect on bone mass in postmenopausal women. Arch Phys Med Rehab 1986;67:231–234.
63. Marcus R, Drinkwater B, et al. Osteoporosis and exercise in women. Med Sci Sports Exerc 1992;24:S301–S307.
64. Snow-Harter C, Bouxsein ML, Lewis BT, et al. Effects of resistance and endurance exercise on bone mineral status of young women: a randomized exercise intervention trial. J Bone Min Res 1992;7:761–769.
65. Jaglal SB, Kreiger N, Darlington G. Past and recent physical activity and the risk of hip fracture. Am J Epidemiol 1993;138:107–118.
66. Paganini-Hill A, Ross RK, Henderson BE, et al. Menopausal estrogen therapy and hip fractures. Ann Intern Med 1981:95:28–31.
67. Chalmers J, Ho KC. Geographic variations in senile osteoporosis: the association of physical activity. J Bone Joint Surg 1970;52:371–378.
68. Cummings SR, Black DM, et al. Appendicular bone density and age predict hip fracture in women. The Study of Osteoporotic Fractures Research Group. JAMA 1990;263:665–668.
69. Seeley DG, Browner WS, et al. Which fractures are associated with low appendicular bone mass in elderly women? The Study of Osteoporotic Fractures Research Group. Ann Intern Med 1991;115: 837–842.
70. Snow-Harter C, Marcus R. Exercise, bone mineral density, and osteoporosis. Exerc Sport Sci Rev 1991; 19:351–388.
71. Drinkwater B. Physical activity, fitness and osteoporosis. In: Bouchard C, Shepard RJ, Stephens T, eds. Physical activity, fitness, and health. Champaign, IL: Human Kinetics, 1994.
72. Landers DM, Petruzzello SJ. Physical activity, fitness, and anxiety. In: Bouchard C, Shepard RJ, Stephens T, eds. Physical activity, fitness, and health. Champaign, IL: Human Kinetics, 1994.
73. Morgan WP. Physical activity, fitness, and depression. In: Bouchard C, Shepard RJ, Stephens T, eds. Physical activity, fitness, and health. Champaign, IL: Human Kinetics, 1994.
74. LaFontaine TP, DiLorenzo TM, et al. Aerobic exercise and mood: a brief review, 1985–1990. Sports Med 1992;13:160–170.
75. Thirlaway K, Benton D. Participation in physical activity and cardiovascular fitness have different effects on mental health and mood. J Psychosom Res 1992;36:657–666.
76. Moses J, Steptoe A, et al. The effects of exercise training on mental well-being in the normal population: a controlled trail. J Psychosom Res 1989;33:47–61.
77. Steptoe A, Edwards S, et al. The effects of exercise training on the mood and perceived coping ability in anxious adults from the general population. J Psychosom Res 1989;33:537–547.
78. Farmer ME, Locke BZ, et al. Physical activity and depressive symptomatology: the NHANES I epidemiologic follow-up study. Am J Epidemiol 1988;128:1340–1351.
79. King AC, Taylor CB, et al. Influence of regular aerobic exercise on psychological health: a randomized, controlled trial of healthy middle-aged adults. Health Psychol 1989;8:305–324.
80. Cramer SR, Nieman DC, Lee JW. The effects of moderate exercise training on psychological well-being and mood state in women. J Psychosom Res 1991;35:437–449.
81. Blumenthal JA, Emery CF, et al. Long-term effects of exercise on psychological functioning in older men and women. J Gerontol 1991;46:352–361.
82. Raglin JS. Exercise and mental health: beneficial and detrimental effects. Sports Med 1990;9:323–329.
83. Sonstroem RJ, Morgan WP. Exercise and self-esteem: rationale and model. Med Sci Sports Exerc 1989;21: 329–337.
84. McAuley E. Self-efficacy and the maintenance of exercise participation in older adults. J Behav Med 1993;16: 103–113.
85. Caruso CM, Gill DL. Strengthening physical self-perceptions through exercise. J Sports Med Phys Fitness 1992;32: 416–427.
86. Stein PN, Motta RW. Effects of aerobic and nonaerobic exercise on depression and self-concept. Percept Mot Skills 1992;74:79–89.

87. Ossip-Klein DJ, Doyne EJ, et al. Effects of running or weight training on self-concept in clinically depressed women. J Consult Clin Psychol 1989;57:158–161.

88. Emery CF, Blumenthal JA. Perceived change among participants in an exercise program for older adults. Gerontologist 1990;30:516–521.

89. Hill RD, Storandt M, Malley M. The impact of long-term exercise training on psychological function in older adults. J Gerontol 1993;48:P12–P17.

90. Dunn AL, Dishman RK. Exercise and the neurobiology of depression. Exerc Sport Sci Rev 1991;19: 41–98.

91. Berger BG, Owen DR. Mood alteration with yoga and swimming: aerobic exercise may not be necessary. Percept Mot Skills 1992;75:1331–1343.

92. Schwarz L, Kindermann W. Changes in β-endorphin levels in response to aerobic and anaerobic exercise. Sports Med 1992;13:25–36.

93. Daniel M, Martin AD, Carter J. Opiate receptor blockade by naltrexone and mood state after acute physical activity. Br J Sports Med 1992;26:111–115.

94. Magnus K, Matroos A, Strackee J. Walking, cycling, gardening with or without seasonal interruption in relation to acute coronary events. Am J Epidemiol 1979;110:724–733.

95. Lee I-M, Hsieh C-C, Paffenbarger RS Jr. Exercise intensity and longevity in men: the Harvard Alumni Health Study. JAMA 1995;273:1179–1184.

96. American College of Sports Medicine. The recommended quantity and quality of exercise for developing and maintaining cardiorespiratory and muscular fitness in healthy adults. Med Sci Sports Exerc 1990;22:256–274.

97. King AC, Haskell WL, Taylor CB, et al. Group- vs home-based exercise training in healthy older men and women: a community-based clinical trial. JAMA 1991;266:1535–1542.

98. Duncan JJ, Gordon NF, Scott CB. Women walking for health and fitness: how much is enough? JAMA 1991;266: 3295–3299.

99. Blair SN, Powell KE, Bazzarre TL, et al. Physical inactivity: workshop V. Circulation 1993;88: 1402–1405.

100. Fletcher BJ, Dunbar SB, Felner JM, et al. Exercise testing and training in physically disabled men with clinical evidence of coronary artery disease. Am J Cardiol 1994;73:170–174.

101. Debusk RF, Stenestrand U, Sheehan M, et al. Training effects of long versus short bouts of exercise in healthy subjects. Am J Cardiol 1990;65:1010–1013.

102. Pate RR, Macera CA. Risks of exercising: musculoskeletal injuries. In: Bouchard C, Shepard RJ, Stephens T, eds. Physical activity, fitness, and health. Champaign, IL: Human Kinetics, 1994.

103. Pollock ML, Carroll JF, et al. Injuries and adherence to walk/jog and resistance training programs in the elderly. Med Sci Sports Exerc 1991;23:1194–1200.

104. Macera CA, Jackson KL, Hagenmaier GW, et al. Age, physical activity, physical fitness, body composition, and incidence of orthopedic problems. Res Q Exerc Sport 1989;60:225–233.

105. Kohatsu ND, Schurman DJ. Risk factors for the development of osteoarthrosis of the knee. Clin Orthop 1990;246: 242–246.

106. Lane NE, Michel B, Bjorkengren A, et al. The risk of osteoarthritis with running and aging: a 5-year longitudinal study. J Rheumatol 1993;20:461–468.

107. Swann AC, Seedhom BB. The stiffness of normal articular cartilage and the predominant acting stress levels: implications for the aetiology of osteoarthrosis. Br J Rheumatol 1993;32:16–25.

108. Panush RS. Physical activity, fitness, and osteoarthritis. In: Bouchard C, Shepard RJ, Stephens T, eds. Physical activity, fitness, and health. Champaign, IL: Human Kinetics, 1994.

109. Willich SN, Lewis M, et al. Physical exertion as a trigger of acute myocardial infarction. N Engl J Med 1993;329:1684–1690.

110. Mittleman MA, Maclure M, et al. Triggering of acute myocardial infarction by heavy physical exertion-protection against triggering by regular exertion. N Engl J Med 1993;329:1677–1683.

111. Thompson PD, Fink EJ, et al. Incidence of death through jogging in Rhode Island from 1975–1980. JAMA 1982;247: 2535–2538.

112. Siscovick DS, Weiss NS, et al. The incidence of primary cardiac arrest during vigorous exercise. N Engl J Med 1984;311:874–877.

113. Kohl HW, Powell KE, et al. Physical activity, physical fitness, and sudden cardiac death. Epidemiol Rev 1992;14: 37–58.

114. Thompson PD, Fahrenbach MC. Risks of exercising: cardiovascular, including sudden cardiac death. In: Bouchard C, Shepard RJ, Stephens T, eds. Physical activity, fitness, and health. Champaign, IL: Human Kinetics, 1994.

115. Campbell MJ, Browne D, Waters WE. Can general practitioners influence exercise habits? Controlled trial. BMJ 1985;290:1044–1046.
116. Lewis B, Lynch W. The effect of physician advice on exercise behavior. Prev Med 1993;22:110–121.
117. Calfas KJ, Long BJ, Sallis JF, et al. A controlled trial of physician counseling to promote the adoption of physical activity. Prev Med 1996 (in press).
118. Logsdon DN, Lazaro CM, Meier RV. The feasibility of behavioral risk reduction in primary medical care. Am J Prev Med 1989;5:249–256.
119. Pate RR, Pratt M, Blair SN, et al. Physical activity and health: a recommendation from the Centers for Disease Control and Prevention and the American College of Sports Medicine. JAMA 1995;273:402–407.
120. American Heart Association. Statement on exercise: benefits and recommendations for physical activity programs for all Americans. Circulation 1992;86:340–343.
121. American Academy of Family Physicians. Age charts for periodic health examination. Kansas City, MO: American Academy of Family Physicians, 1994. (Reprint no. 510.)
122. American College of Obstetricians and Gynecologists. Women and exercise. Technical Bulletin no. 173. Washington, DC: American College of Obstetricians and Gynecologists, 1992.
123. Canadian Task Force on the Periodic Health Examination. Canadian guide to clinical preventive care. Ottawa: Canada Communication Group, 1994:560–569.
124. American Academy of Pediatrics. Assessing physical activity and fitness in the office setting. Pediatrics 1994:93: 686–689.
125. Green M, ed. Bright Futures: guidelines for health supervision of infants, children, and adolescents. Arlington, VA: National Center for Education in Maternal and Child Health, 1994.
126. American Medical Association. Guidelines for adolescent preventive services (GAPS): recommendations and rationale. Chicago: American Medical Association, 1994.
127. Centers for Disease Control and Prevention. Surveillance for diabetes mellitus—United States, 1980–89. MMWR 1993;42(SS-2):1–20.
128. Dishman RK, Sallis JF. Determinants and interventions for physical activity and exercise. In: Bouchard C, Shepard RJ, Stephens T, eds. Physical activity, fitness, and health. Champaign, IL: Human Kinetics, 1994.

56. Counseling to Promote a Healthy Diet

RECOMMENDATION

Counseling adults and children over age 2 to limit dietary intake of fat (especially saturated fat) and cholesterol, maintain caloric balance in their diet, and emphasize foods containing fiber (i.e., fruits, vegetables, grain products) is recommended. There is insufficient evidence to recommend for or against counseling the general population to reduce dietary sodium intake or increase dietary intake of iron, beta-carotene, or other antioxidants to improve health outcomes, but recommendations to reduce sodium intake may be made on other grounds. Women should be encouraged to consume recommended quantities of calcium (see *Clinical Intervention*). Parents should be encouraged to breastfeed their infants. Providing pregnant women with specific nutritional guidelines to enhance fetal and maternal health is recommended. Although there is insufficient evidence to recommend for or against special assessment of the dietary needs and habits of older adults, recommendations to do so can be made on other grounds. There is insufficient evidence that nutritional counseling by physicians has an advantage over counseling by dietitians or community interventions in changing the dietary habits of patients. See Chapter 22 regarding the role of iron during pregnancy and in the diets of newborns and young children, and Chapter 42 regarding the use of folic acid by women of childbearing age. See Chapter 61 regarding intake of refined sugars and adherent carbohydrates that may affect dental health. Counseling regarding alcohol consumption is discussed in Chapter 52.

Burden of Suffering

Diseases associated with dietary excess and imbalance rank among the leading causes of illness and death in the U.S. Major diseases in which diet plays a role include coronary heart disease, some types of cancer, stroke, hypertension, obesity, and non-insulin-dependent diabetes mellitus.[1] Heart disease is the leading cause of death in the U.S.,[2] with coronary heart disease accounting for up to 1.5 million myocardial infarctions and nearly 500,000 deaths each year.[2,3] Cancer of the colon, breast, and prostate, the three forms of cancer most closely associated epidemiologically with nutritional risk factors, together, cause over 140,000 deaths annually.[4] Cerebrovascular disease, the third leading cause of death, accounted for about 150,000 deaths in 1993.[2] Hypertension, another disease with nutritional risk factors, occurs in about 43 million Americans.[5] Caloric intake, when it exceeds energy expenditure, can also lead to overweight and obesity, which affects about 58 million American adults aged 20 and older.[6] Obesity is a risk factor for a number of serious disorders (see Chapter 21), including both hypertension and adult-onset diabetes mellitus. An estimated 14 million persons in the U.S. have diabetes mellitus, which accounts for over 55,000 deaths each year and is a leading cause of neuropathy, peripheral vascular disease, renal failure, and blindness.[2,7]

Nutritional factors have also been linked to osteoporosis, constipation, diverticular disease, iron deficiency anemia (see Chapter 22), oral disease, and malnutrition. An estimated 40% of women in the U.S. will suffer from osteoporosis-related fractures by the time they reach age 70.[8] Hip fractures in particular are associated with significant pain and disability, decreased functional independence, and high mortality; there is a 15–20% reduction in expected survival in the first year following a hip fracture.[9] Constipation is a complaint of over 4.5 million Americans,[10] and intestinal diverticular disease is reported by nearly 1.5 million persons.[11] The average schoolchild has at least one cavity in permanent teeth by age 9, three cavities by age 12, and eight by age 17.[12] The average adult in the U.S. has 10–17 decayed, missing, or filled permanent teeth and one untreated decayed permanent tooth.[13] Disorders of both overeating and undereating are common among older adults, up to 40% of whom have inadequate dietary intake of three or more nutrients.[14] Many older adults suffer from protein-calorie malnutrition—up to 50% of nursing home residents in the U.S. may be malnourished,[15] and an additional number suffer from marginal malnutrition that is less clinically evident.

Efficacy of Risk Reduction

Eating habits over a lifetime can have a significant impact on the incidence and severity of many health disorders. The complete body of literature regarding the health effects of foods is beyond the scope of this report and has been the subject of extensive reviews.[1,16] In summary, it is clear that a direct relationship exists between nutritional risk factors and certain key diseases. It is well established, for example, that caloric imbalance (intake exceeding expenditure) can lead to overweight and obesity. Persons who are overweight are at increased risk of glucose intolerance, hypertension, high blood cholesterol, and other disorders (see Chapter 21); reduction of body weight has been shown to reduce these risks.[17–20] The average person is likely to benefit from dietary practices and physical activity (see Chapter 55) that keep caloric intake commensurate with daily energy expenditures.

In addition to the overall objective of caloric balance, modified intake of specific dietary factors may also help prevent certain diseases.

Reduced intake of **dietary fat**, especially saturated fats (and, possibly, partially hydrogenated vegetable fats), appears to reduce the risk of developing coronary heart disease. A large body of epidemiologic evidence links serum cholesterol levels to the development of coronary atherosclerosis.[21–23] Serum cholesterol levels can in turn be modified by dietary measures. Clinical trials incorporating reduced total or saturated fat intake, either as a sole intervention or as part of a multifactorial intervention, have reported mixed results in reducing serum cholesterol levels and in decreasing the incidence of cardiac events, such as myocardial infarction and sudden death.[24–32] Intake of saturated fat correlates more closely with serum cholesterol levels than does total fat intake. Clinical trials have also found that serum cholesterol-lowering drugs can reduce the incidence of coronary heart disease in asymptomatic middle-aged men with hyperlipidemia.[33–38] These studies found that the incidence of cardiac events in such men is decreased by an average of 2% for every 1% reduction in serum cholesterol (see Chapter 2). (Evidence regarding benefits in persons with preexisting coronary heart disease is reviewed in Chapter 2.)

Modeling studies based on these data suggest that coronary heart disease mortality rates in the U.S. could be lowered by 5–20% if all Americans restricted their fat intake to less than 30% of total calories but that increases in life expectancy among low-risk persons might be modest.[39–41] Two randomized controlled trials reported that a low-fat diet does not increase high-density lipoprotein (HDL) cholesterol levels unless coupled with physical activity,[42,43] and one meta-analysis of 27 trials suggested that substantial reductions in dietary fat intake might lower HDL cholesterol levels.[44] Some observational studies also suggest a possible association between intake of *trans*-isomers of fatty acids (formed in the partial hydrogenation of vegetable oils) and unfavorable changes in low-density lipoprotein (LDL) and HDL cholesterol[45,46] and in the risk of coronary heart disease;[47–49] others suggest an association between fatty acids found primarily in fish oils and reduced risk of cardiovascular disease.[50–52] Dietary cholesterol intake may also influence serum cholesterol levels, especially LDL cholesterol levels, but the association appears to be weaker and more variable than that of dietary saturated fat intake.[1] Finally, prospective cohort data suggest that a diet with increased intake of fruits and vegetables is associated with decreased risk of stroke, but further study is needed.[53]

The association between foods high in dietary fat and certain forms of cancer is currently under investigation. An effect of dietary fat on carcinogenesis has been demonstrated in animal research. Furthermore, international comparisons of cancer incidence and most case-control studies have revealed an epidemiologic correlation between dietary fat consumption and the incidence of cancer of the breast, colon, prostate, and lung.[54–63] Within more homogenous populations, however, cohort studies to date have been unable to provide consistent evidence of a causal relationship between increased dietary fat consumption and the incidence of breast, prostate, colon, or other cancers.[64–74] Similarly, inconsistent results have been reported in epidemiologic studies of the link between low blood cholesterol and cancer.[75,76] Clinical trials are now in progress to examine further the relationship between dietary fat and cancer.[77] These and other studies may help elucidate whether low-fat diets reduce cancer risk because of decreased fat intake or because of increased intake of fruits, vegetables, or fiber (see below).

A diet emphasizing the consumption of foods high in **complex carbohydrates** and fiber (e.g., whole grain foods and cereal products, vegetables [including dried beans and peas], and fruits) is an important means of lowering dietary fat consumption by replacing caloric intake from fat. Foods high in complex carbohydrates and fiber and low in fat content also have lower average caloric density, and they are therefore preferred for maintaining caloric balance and healthful body weight.[1,78,79] There are other health benefits associated with the replacement of foods high in simple carbohydrates (e.g., table sugar, honey, corn sweeteners) with those containing starch and fiber. In addition to improving caloric balance, reduced intake and less frequent consumption of refined sugars may lower the risk of developing dental caries (see also Chapter 61),[80–85] and the avoidance of highly refined grain products reduces the contribution of "empty calories" to the diet.[86]

Increased intake of **dietary fiber** improves gastrointestinal function.[87] Certain types of dietary fiber may also be helpful in the treatment of glucose intolerance, weight reduction, and the control of lipid disorders.[87,88] The consumption of foods containing large amounts of soluble fiber (e.g., dried beans, oat products) appears to lower levels of LDL cholesterol (independent of their replacement of foods high in saturated fat and cholesterol).[89,90] An insoluble high-fiber diet (most plant foods) may be effective in reducing intracolonic pressure and preventing diverticular disease.[91] The risk of developing colorectal cancer may also be influenced by dietary fiber intake. At least 15 cross-cultural studies have shown an inverse relationship between dietary fiber consumption and the incidence of colon cancer.[92,93] Such studies do not, however, provide direct evidence that high dietary fiber intake, rather than other population dietary characteristics (e.g., low fat intake), is directly responsible for the lower cancer incidence rate. Case-control studies have produced inconsistent results regarding the association between dietary fiber and colon cancer.[94–97] Meta-analyses of these studies, however, suggest an overall benefit from dietary fiber.[98,99] Observational studies also suggest an association between intake of vegetables and fruits and lower risk of cancer.[86] Cohort studies to date that have examined the relationship between dietary fiber and cancer have produced inconsistent results and suffer from methodologic limitations, including the difficulty of determining whether observed benefits were due to fiber itself or to its substitution of foods high in saturated fats.[73,100–103]

Reduced intake of **dietary sodium** may be of clinical benefit to persons who either have sodium-dependent hypertension or are likely to develop it in the future.[104] A number of clinical trials and recent meta-analyses have demonstrated the ability of dietary sodium restriction to lower blood pressure by at least several millimeters of mercury in some hypertensive and normotensive individuals.[105–118] In addition, cross-cultural studies have shown a correlation between the sodium intake of different populations and the incidence of hypertension.[119–121] A multinational study involving 52 sites also demonstrated an association between sodium excretion and the rate of change of blood pressure with age.[122] However, controlled prospective studies will ultimately be necessary to provide definitive evidence that normotensive persons who practice dietary sodium restriction are at lower risk of developing hypertension over time than are those with more typical sodium consumption.

Many American women and adolescent girls consume less **dietary calcium** than is recommended by major groups (men: 1,000 mg/day; adolescents and young adults, 1,200–1,500 mg/day; women 25–50 years of age, 1,000 mg/day; postmenopausal women, 1,000–1,500 mg/day; pregnant and nursing women, 1,200–1,500 mg/day).[123] Population and cross-sectional studies suggest that reduced calcium intake among women, especially young women, may be an important risk factor for bone mineral loss and postmenopausal osteoporosis,[124,125] and studies suggest that calcium supplementation in adolescence and early adulthood may increase bone mineral density.[126,127] Prospective studies of asymptomatic postmenopausal women have produced inconsistent results about the efficacy of increasing dietary calcium intake as a means of slowing bone loss. Although some studies have reported that a daily intake of 750–1,700 mg/day can reduce significantly the rate of bone loss in asymptomatic postmenopausal women,[128–130] other controlled studies have shown either no effect or an effect only on compact bone with doses as high as 1,800–2,000 mg/day.[131–134] A meta-analysis of intervention and observational studies concluded that 1,000 mg of calcium daily would prevent about 1% of bone loss per year.[135] Clinical trials suggest that calcium supplementation may reduce the risk of fractures in postmenopausal women.[135a,135b] In such women, however, estrogen replacement therapy may be a more effective form of chemoprophylaxis than calcium supplementation (see Chapter 68). (See also the discussion of the relationship between exercise and bone density in Chapter 55.) There appears to be little significant risk for women who moderately increase their consumption of dietary calcium. Gross and prolonged use of calcium supplements may, under unusual circumstances, result in milk alkali syndrome or an increased occurrence of kidney stones, although direct evidence of the latter is lacking.[136]

Adequate **dietary iron** intake may be important for menstruating women and for young children to maintain iron stores and prevent iron deficiency anemia. This topic is discussed in detail in Chapter 22. Although infants and young children may benefit from iron supplementation (see below), there is little evidence from prospective studies of older children and menstruating women that mild anemia in the absence of symptoms is a direct cause of increased morbidity or mortality. It may be clinically prudent, however, to recommend diets including iron-rich foods (e.g., lean meats, certain beans, iron-enriched and whole grain products) for persons at increased risk of iron deficiency.

Current research is exploring the potential health benefits of other minerals and vitamins. For example, evidence suggests that women of childbearing age who take folic acid supplements may be less likely to give birth to children with neural tube defects (see Chapter 42).[137] The role of beta-carotene, vitamins (e.g., vitamin A, vitamin C, vitamin E), and other antioxidants in reducing the risk of cancer, atherosclerosis, and other chronic diseases is currently being studied.[138-143]

Special Populations

Infants and Children. Infants require breast milk or appropriate alternatives (e.g., infant formulas) to provide adequate nutrition. Nutritional status remains important throughout childhood to facilitate normal growth and development.[144] Epidemiologic evidence and randomized prospective studies suggest that infant consumption of breast milk for at least 6 months may reduce the risk of otitis media, lower respiratory tract illness, meningitis, allergic illness, diarrhea, hospital admissions, and abnormal cognitive development in the child.[145-147] Breast-fed infants often have higher blood cholesterol levels than formula-fed infants, but current evidence, with the exception of one cohort study,[148] suggests that these elevations resolve with weaning[149] and are not linked to adult blood cholesterol levels or increased risk of heart disease. Iron deficiency anemia during infancy may also be associated with impaired infant neurologic and cognitive development,[150] and infants may therefore benefit from iron-fortified formula and foods to replace depleted iron stores.

The benefits of reduced dietary fat intake during childhood are uncertain. There is some epidemiologic evidence of tracking (persistence of childhood elevations of blood cholesterol into adulthood) and autopsy evidence of atherosclerotic disease among children and young adults with elevated cholesterol levels,[151,152] but evidence of improved health outcomes from lowering blood cholesterol during childhood is lacking. Observational studies provide evidence that children can achieve statistically significant reductions in total and LDL cholesterol levels through dietary fat reduction.[153,154] A potential risk of such interventions is that excessive low-fat diets may not provide children with sufficient nutrients for healthy growth and development,[155] but direct evidence of this adverse effect is limited to extreme cases of dietary restriction. A cross-sectional study found that 10-year-old children with low fat intake had no significant differences in anthropometric measurements, but they were more likely to be deficient in the Recommended Dietary Allowances for calcium, phosphorus, magnesium, iron, and certain vitamins.[156] A recent randomized controlled trial involving children aged 8–10 reported that a diet providing 28% of energy from total fat achieved statistically significant reductions in LDL cholesterol levels with no significant effects on height, ferritin levels, or selected psychometric indices.[157]

Pregnant Women. Nutritional status is especially important during pregnancy. Studies have shown that low birth weight and neonatal mortality are more common in pregnant women with very poor nutritional status[158,159] and in those who fail to gain adequate weight during pregnancy,[160–163] although factors other than nutrient intake may account for these outcomes. Prenatal programs providing nutritional support for pregnant women have been associated with improved perinatal outcomes.[164] Pregnancy brings increased requirements for energy and specific nutrients, such as protein, calcium, folic acid, and iron.[162,165,166] Oral iron supplements may be beneficial in preventing iron deficiency anemia in pregnancy, and they are often prescribed routinely as part of prenatal health care. Although an association between moderate to severe iron deficiency anemia and adverse obstetric outcomes has been demonstrated in some observational studies, there is little direct evidence that routine iron supplementation during pregnancy (in the absence of documented anemia or iron deficiency) results in improved clinical outcome for the mother or fetus.[167]

Older Adults. The elderly can also have special nutritional requirements. Depending on the patient's nutritional status, underlying medical disorders, functional status, dentition, and therapeutic drug regimens, it can be important to modify recommended daily intake levels of calories, sodium, calcium, water, dietary fat, fiber, protein, and other nutrients to reduce the risk of complications.[168] Observational data suggest that older adults benefit to some extent by reducing elevated blood cholesterol levels.[169] It is unclear from current evidence whether women who have already developed clinical evidence of postmenopausal osteoporosis benefit from calcium supplementation.[170–173] Clinical recognition of protein-calorie malnutrition, especially when manifested by clinically subtle findings, is often delayed among older adults. This has prompted the introduction of nutritional screening initiatives in this population,[174] but direct evidence of clinical benefit from screening is currently lacking.

Effectiveness of Counseling

The effectiveness of nutritional counseling in changing the dietary habits of patients has been demonstrated in a number of clinical trials.[175] For example, randomized controlled trials have shown that dietary counseling of patients with high blood cholesterol can lower serum lipids in both patients and their families[176] and that regular reinforcement can enhance compliance with dietary recommendations.[177] Tailored printed materials distributed in primary care settings have also been effective in lowering dietary fat consumption.[178] Other measures that may enhance compliance with low-fat diets include setting strict limits on fat intake, frequent (e.g., monthly) monitoring, involvement of family in nutritional counseling sessions, and group sessions.[179] Studies have confirmed the effectiveness of nutritional counseling among pregnant women[180] and the important role of parental guidance in modifying the diets of children.[181]

In most studies of nutritional counseling, however, the counselor was not a physician, but rather a nurse, nutritionist, registered dietitian, health educator, or psychologist. Many of the interventions tested in these studies were part of highly specialized or community-wide programs. Such interventions are not easily reproduced in the typical physician-patient clinical encounter. Although physicians can often provide general guidelines on proper nutrition, many lack the time and skills to obtain a thorough dietary history, to address potential barriers to changes in eating habits, and to offer specific guidance on food selection.[182] Patients may also have difficulty with long-term compliance,[183] especially if food selection and preparation for recommended diets are perceived as unappealing or inconvenient. Fat-containing foods, in particular, are a popular component of the American diet.[184] It is possible, however, that physicians can overcome many of these limitations by expanding the content of the nutritional information they provide to patients, by emphasizing to the patient the health benefits of good nutrition, and by referring those requiring help with dietary changes to qualified registered dietitians, nutritionists, health educators, nurses, or other providers with greater nutrition expertise.

Recommendations of Other Groups

Dietary guidelines for the general population have been issued by the Department of Agriculture and the Department of Health and Human Services[185] and reaffirmed by the Surgeon General,[1] in the Year 2000 Objectives for the Nation,[186] and in the "Food Guide Pyramid" released in 1992 by the Department of Agriculture.[187] The Food and Nutrition Board of the National Research Council has published Recommended Dietary Allowances (RDAs) for specific nutrients,[165] and it has released an extensive report on diet and chronic disease risk.[16] Recommendations for nutritional counseling of patients have been issued by the American Medical Association,[188] the American College of Physicians,[189] the Canadian Task Force,[203] and the American Heart Association.[144,190] Guidelines for dietary practices to reduce the risk of cancer have been issued by the National Research Council,[191] the American Cancer Society,[192] and the National Cancer Institute.[193] Recommendations on nutritional counseling to reduce cardiac risk factors have been issued by panels convened by the National Heart, Lung, and Blood Institute[194] and by the National High Blood Pressure Education Program[195] and National Cholesterol Education Program,[196,197] which are endorsed by over 40 organizations and government agencies. Dietary recommendations for children have been issued by the American Academy of Pediatrics[198,199] and National Cholesterol Education Program.[200] Dietary guidelines for pregnant women have been issued by the American College of Obstetricians and Gynecologists[201] and the Institute of Medicine.[162] Recommendations on the use of folic acid supplementation by women have been issued by the U.S. Public Health Service.[202] Dietary guidelines for Americans were updated in 1995.[204]

CLINICAL INTERVENTION

Adults and children over age 2 should limit dietary intake of fat (especially saturated fat) ("A" recommendation) and cholesterol ("B" recommendation), maintain caloric balance in their diet ("B" recommendation), and emphasize fruits, vegetables, and grain products containing fiber ("B" recommendation). Both diet and exercise should be designed to achieve and maintain a desirable weight by keeping caloric intake balanced with energy expenditures. Adolescents and adults, in particular, should reduce total fat intake to less than 30% of total calories and dietary cholesterol to less than 300 mg/day. Saturated fat consumption should be reduced to less than 10% of total calories. To achieve these goals, patients should emphasize consumption of fish, poultry prepared without skin, lean meats, and low-fat dairy products. They should be encouraged to eat a variety of foods, with emphasis on the consumption of whole grain products and cereals, legumes, vegetables, and fruits. Current recommendations from the U.S. Department of Health and Human Services are for at least five servings of fruits and vegetables and at least six servings of breads, cereals, or legumes each day. Detailed food selection guidelines for healthy eating are published elsewhere.[185]

There is insufficient evidence that, for the general population, reducing dietary sodium intake or increasing dietary intake of iron, beta-carotene, or other antioxidants results in improved health outcomes ("C" recommendation); recommendations to reduce sodium intake may be made on other grounds, including the potential beneficial effects on blood pressure in salt-sensitive persons. See Chapter 61 for information regarding intake of refined sugars and dental health. Women should be encouraged to consume recommended quantities of calcium (adolescents and young adults, 1,200–1,500 mg/day; adults aged 25–50, 1,000 mg/day; postmenopausal women, 1,000–1,500 mg/day; pregnant and nursing women, 1,200–1,500 mg/day[123]) ("B" recommendation). Parents should be encouraged to offer breastfeeding to their infants ("A" recommendation). Pregnant women should receive specific nutritional guidelines to enhance fetal and maternal health. See Chapter 22 regarding the role of iron during pregnancy and in the diets of newborns and young children, and see Chapter 42 regarding the use of folic acid by women of childbearing age. There is insufficient evidence to recommend for or against the special assessment of dietary needs and habits of older adults ("C" recommendation), but recommendations to do so can be made on other grounds, such as the increased prevalence of nutrition-related disorders in this age group. Counseling regarding alcohol consumption is discussed in Chapter 52.

There is insufficient evidence that nutritional counseling by physicians, as opposed to counseling by dietitians or community interventions, is effective in changing the dietary habits of patients ("C" recommendation). Clinicians who lack the time or skills to perform a complete dietary history, to address potential barriers to changes in eating habits, and to offer specific guidance on meal planning and food selection and preparation, should either have patients seen by other trained providers in the office or clinic or should refer patients to a registered dietitian or qualified nutritionist for further counseling.

The draft update of this chapter was prepared for the U.S. Preventive Services Task Force by Steven H. Woolf, MD, MPH.

REFERENCES

1. Department of Health and Human Services. The Surgeon General's report on nutrition and health. Washington, DC: Government Printing Office, 1988. (Publication no. DHHS (PHS) 88-50210.)
2. National Center for Health Statistics. Annual summary of births, marriages, divorces, and deaths: United States, 1993. Monthly vital statistics report; vol 42, no 13. Hyattsville, MD: Public Health Service, 1994.
3. American Heart Association. Heart and stroke facts: 1995 statistical supplement. Dallas, TX: American Heart Association, 1995.
4. Wingo PA, Tong T, Bolden S. Cancer statistics, 1995. CA Cancer J Clin 1995;45:8–30.
5. Burt VL, Whelton P, Roccella EJ, et al. Prevalence of hypertension in the US adult population: results from the Third National Health and Nutrition Examination Survey, 1988–1991. Hypertension 1995;25:305–313.

6. Kuczmarski RJ, Flegal KM, Campbell SM, et al. Increasing prevalence of overweight among US adults. JAMA 1994;272:205–211.

7. Geiss LS, Herman WH, Goldschmid MG, et al. Surveillance for diabetes mellitus: United States, 1980–1989. MMWR CDC Surv Summ 1993;42:1–20.

8. Audran MJ. Epidemiology, etiology, and diagnosis of osteoporosis. Curr Opin Rheum 1992;4: 394–401.

9. Jensen GF, Christiansen C, Boesen J, et al. Epidemiology of postmenopausal spinal and long bone fractures: a unifying approach to postmenopausal osteoporosis. Clin Orthop 1982;166:75–81.

10. Johanson JF, Sonnenberg A, Koch TR. Clinical epidemiology of chronic constipation. J Clin Gastroenterol 1989;11: 525–536.

11. National Center for Health Statistics. Prevalence of selected chronic conditions, United States, 1979–81. Vital and health statistics; series 10, no 155. Washington, DC: Government Printing Office, 1986. (Publication no. DHHS (PHS) 86-1583.)

12. Public Health Service. Oral health of United States children: the national survey of dental caries in U.S. school children: 1986–1987. National and regional findings. Bethesda: National Institutes of Health, 1989. (NIH Publication no. 89-2247.)

13. National Institute of Dental Research. Oral health of United States adults, the national survey of oral health in U.S. employed adults and seniors: 1985–86. Bethesda: National Institute of Dental Research, 1987. (Publication no. DHHS (NIH) 87-2868.)

14. Posner BM, Jette AM, Smith KW, et al. Nutrition and health risks in the elderly: the Nutrition Screening Initiative. Am J Public Health 1993;83:972–978.

15. Goodwin JS. Social, psychological, and physical factors affecting the nutritional status of elderly subjects: separating cause and effect. Am J Clin Nutr 1989;50:1201–1209.

16. Food and Nutrition Board, National Research Council. Diet and health; implications for reducing chronic disease. Washington, DC: National Academy Press, 1989.

17. Henry RR, Schaeffer L, Olefsky, JM. Glycemic effects of intensive caloric restriction and isocaloric refeeding in noninsulin-dependent diabetes mellitus. J Clin Endocrinol Metab 1985;61:917–925.

18. Henry RR, Wiest-Kent TA, Schaeffer L, et al. Metabolic consequences of very-low-calorie diet therapy in obese noninsulin-dependent diabetic and nondiabetic subjects. Diabetes 1986;35:155–164.

19. MacMahon S, Cutler J, Brittain E, et al. Obesity and hypertension: epidemiological and clinical issues. Eur Heart J [Suppl B] 1987;8:57–70.

20. Rifkind BM, Goor R, Schucker B. Compliance and cholesterol-lowering in clinical trials: efficacy of diet. In: Schettler FG, Gotto AM, Middelhoff G, et al, eds. Atherosclerosis VI. Proceedings of the Sixth International Symposium. New York: Springer-Verlag, 1983:306–310.

21. Grundy SM. Cholesterol and coronary heart disease: a new era. JAMA 1986;256:2849–2858.

22. Posner BM, Cobb JL, Belanger AJ, et al. Dietary lipid predictors of coronary heart disease in men: the Framingham Study. Arch Intern Med 1991;151:1181–1187.

23. Menotti A, Keys A, Kromhout D, et al. Twenty-five-year mortality from coronary heart disease and its prediction in five cohorts of middle-aged men in Finland, the Netherlands, and Italy. Prev Med 1990;19:270–278.

24. Dayton S, Pearce ML, Hashimoto S, et al. A controlled clinical trial of a diet high in unsaturated fat in preventing complications of atherosclerosis. Circulation 1969;40(Suppl 2):1–63.

25. Hjermann I, Holme I, Velve Byre K, et al. Effect of diet and smoking intervention on the incidence of coronary heart disease. Report from the Oslo Study Group of a randomized trial in healthy men. Lancet 1981;2:1303–1310.

26. Multiple Risk Factor Intervention Trial Research Group. Multiple Risk Factor Intervention Trial: risk factor changes and mortality results. JAMA 1982;248:1465–1477.

27. World Health Organization European Collaborative Group. European collaborative trial of multifactorial prevention of coronary heart disease: final report on the 6-year results. Lancet 1986;1: 869–872.

28. Rinzler S. Primary prevention of coronary heart disease by diet. Bull NY Acad Med 1968;44:936–949.

29. Turpeinen O, Karvonen MJ, Pekkarinen M, et al. Dietary prevention of coronary heart disease: the Finnish Mental Hospital Study. Int J Epidemiol 1979;8:99–118.

30. Miettinen M, Turpeinen O, Karvonen MJ, et al. Effect of cholesterol-lowering diet on mortality from coronary heart disease and other causes: a twelve-year clinical trial in men and women. Lancet 1972;2:835–838.

31. Stamler J. Acute myocardial infarction, progress in primary prevention. Br Heart J 1971;33:145–164.

32. Frantz ID Jr, Dawson EA, Ashman PL, et al. Test of effect of lipid lowering by diet on cardiovascular risk: the Minnesota Coronary Survey. Arteriosclerosis 1989;9:129–135.

33. Report from the Committee of Principal Investigators. A cooperative trial in the primary prevention of ischaemic heart disease using clofibrate. Br Heart J 1978;40:1069–1118.

34. Report of the Committee of Principal Investigators. W.H.O. cooperative trial on primary prevention of ischaemic heart disease using clofibrate to lower serum cholesterol: mortality follow-up. Lancet 1980;2:379–385.

35. Report of the Committee of Principal Investigators. W.H.O. cooperative trial on primary prevention of ischaemic heart disease with clofibrate to lower serum cholesterol: final mortality follow-up. Lancet 1984;2:600–604.

36. The Lipid Research Clinics Coronary Primary Prevention Trial Results. I. Reduction in incidence of coronary heart disease. JAMA 1984;251:351–364.

37. The Lipid Research Clinics Coronary Primary Prevention Trial Results. II. The relationship of reduction in incidence of coronary heart disease to cholesterol lowering. JAMA 1984;251:365–374.

38. Frick MH, Elo O, Haapa K, et al. Helsinki Heart Study: primary prevention trial with gemfibrozil in middle-aged men with dyslipidemia. Safety of treatment, changes in risk factors, and incidence of coronary heart disease. N Engl J Med 1987;317:1237–1245.

39. Browner WS, Westenhouse J, Tice JA. What if Americans ate less fat? A quantitative estimate of the effect on mortality. JAMA 1991;265:3285–3291.

40. Taylor W, Pass T, Shepard D, et al. Cholesterol reduction and life expectancy: a model incorporating multiple risk factors. Ann Intern Med 1987;106:605–614.

41. Grover SA, Abrahamowicz M, Joseph L, et al. The benefits of treating hyperlipidemia to prevent coronary heart disease: estimating changes in life expectancy and morbidity. JAMA 1992;267:816–822.

42. Wood PD, Stefanick ML, Williams PT, et al. The effects on plasma lipoproteins of a prudent weight-reducing diet, with or without exercise, in overweight men and women. N Engl J Med 1991;325:461–466.

43. Singh RB, Sircar AR, Singh RG, et al. Dietary modulators of lipid metabolism in the Indian Diet-Heart Study. Int J Vitam Nutr Res 1992;62:73–82.

44. Mensink RP, Katan MB. Effect of dietary fatty acids on serum lipids and lipoproteins: a meta-analysis of 27 trials. Arterioscler Thromb 1992;12:911–919.

45. Mensink RP, Katan MB. Effect of dietary trans fatty acids on high-density and low-density lipoprotein cholesterol levels in healthy subjects. N Engl J Med 1990;323:439–445.

46. Judd JT, Clevidence BA, Muesing RA, et al. Dietary trans fatty acids: effects on plasma lipids and lipoproteins of healthy men and women. Am J Clin Nutr 1994;59:861–868.

47. Siguel EN, Lerman RH. Trans-fatty acid patterns in patients with angiographically documented coronary artery disease. Am J Cardiol 1993;71:916–920.

48. Willett WC, Stampfer MJ, Manson JE, et al. Intake of trans fatty acids and risk of coronary heart disease among women. Lancet 1993;341:581–585.

49. Ascherio A, Hennekens CH, Buring JE, et al. Trans-fatty acids intake and risk of myocardial infarction. Circulation 1994;89:94–101.

50. Dolecek TA. Epidemiological evidence of relationships between dietary polyunsaturated fatty acids and mortality in the Multiple Risk Factor Intervention Trial. Proc Soc Exp Biol Med 1992;200:177–182.

51. Kromhout D, Bosschieter EB, deLezenne-Coulander C. The inverse relation between fish consumption and 20-year mortality from coronary heart disease. N Engl J Med 1985;312:1205–1209.

52. Shekelle RB, Paul O, Shryock AM, et al. Fish consumption and mortality from coronary heart disease. N Engl J Med 1985;313:820.

53. Gillman MW, Cupples LA, Gagnon D, et al. Protective effect of fruits and vegetables on development of stroke in men. JAMA 1995;273:1113–1117.

54. Rose DP, Boyar AP, Wynder EL. International comparisons of mortality rates for cancer of the breast, ovary, prostate, and colon, and per capita food consumption. Cancer 1986;58:2363–2371.

55. Kakar F, Henderson M. Diet and breast cancer. Clin Nutr 1985;4:119–130.

56. Kolonel LN, Hankin JH, Nomura AM. Multiethnic studies of diet, nutrition, and cancer in Hawaii. In: Hayashi Y, ed. Diet, nutrition, and cancer. Tokyo: Japan Science Society Press, 1986:29–40.

57. Toniolo P, Riboli E, Protta F, et al. Calorie-providing nutrients and risk of breast cancer. J Natl Cancer Inst 1989;81:278–286.

58. Kesteloot H, Lesaffre E, Joossens JV. Dairy fat, saturated animal fat, and cancer risk. Prev Med 1991; 20:226–236.

59. Mettlin CJ, Schoenfeld ER, Natarajan N. Patterns of milk consumption and risk of cancer. Nutr Cancer 1990;13: 89–99.

60. West DW, Slattery MLI, Robison LM, et al. Adult dietary intake and prostate cancer risk in Utah: a case-control study with special emphasis on aggressive tumors. Cancer Causes Control 1991;2:85–94.

61. Hursting SD, Thornquist M, Henderson MM. Types of dietary fat and the incidence of cancer at five sites. Prev Med 1990;19:242–253.

62. Whittemore AS, Wu-Williams AH, Lee M, et al. Diet, physical activity, and colorectal cancer among Chinese in North America and China. J Natl Cancer Inst 1990;82:915–926.

63. Howe GR, Hirohata T, Hislop TG, et al. Dietary factors and risk of breast cancer: combined analysis of 12 case-control studies. J Natl Cancer Inst 1990;82:561–569.

64. Hirayama T. Epidemiology of breast cancer with special reference to the role of diet. Prev Med 1978;7:173–195.

65. Snowden DA, Phillips RL, Choi W. Diet, obesity, and risk of fatal prostate cancer. Am J Epidemiol 1984;120: 244–250.

66. Willett WC, Stampfer MJ, Colditz GA, et al. Dietary fat and the risk of breast cancer. N Engl J Med 1987;316:22–28.

67. Jones DY, Schatzkin A, Green SB, et al. Dietary fat and breast cancer in the National Health and Nutrition Examination Survey. I. Epidemiological follow-up study. J Natl Cancer Inst 1987;79:465–471.

68. Giovannucci E, Rimm EB, Colditz GA, et al. A prospective study of dietary fat and risk of prostate cancer. J Natl Cancer Inst 1993;85:1571–1579.

69. Hsing AW, McLaughlin JK, Schuman LM, et al. Diet, tobacco use, and fatal prostate cancer: results from the Lutheran Brotherhood Cohort Study. Cancer Res 1990;50:6836–6840.

70. Severson RK, Nomura AMY, Grove JS, et al. A prospective study of demographics, diet, and prostate cancer among men of Japanese ancestry in Hawaii. Cancer Res 1989;49:1857–1860.

71. Mills PK, Beeson WL, Phillips RL, Cohort study of diet, lifestyle, and prostate cancer in Adventist men. Cancer 1989;64:598–604.

72. Hunter DJ, Willett WC. Diet, body size, and breast cancer. Epidemiol Rev 1993;15:110–132.

73. Willett WC, Hunter DJ, Stampfer MJ, et al. Dietary fat and fiber in relation to risk of breast cancer: an 8-year follow-up. JAMA 1992;268:2037–2044.

74. Willett WC, Stampfer MJ, Colditz GA, et al. Relation of meat, fat, and fiber intake to the risk of colon cancer in a prospective study among women. N Engl J Med 1990;323:1664–1672.

75. Kritchevsky SB. Dietary lipids and the low blood cholesterol-cancer association. Am J Epidemiol 1992;135: 509–520.

76. Jacobs D, Blackburn H, Higgins M, et al. Report of the conference on low blood cholesterol: mortality associations. Circulation 1992;86:1046–1060.

77. Chlebowski RT, Grosvenor M. The scope of nutrition intervention trials with cancer-related endpoints. Cancer 1994;74(9 Suppl):2734–2738.

78. Miller WC, Lindeman AK, Wallace J, et al. Diet composition, energy intake, and exercise in relation to body fat in men and women. Am J Clin Nutr 1990;52:426–430.

79. Alford BB, Blankenship AC, Hagen RD. The effects of variations in carbohydrate, protein, and fat content of the diet upon weight loss, blood values, and nutrient intake of adult obese women. J Am Diet Assoc 1990;90:534–540.

80. Gustafsson BE, Quensel CE, Lanke LS, et al. The Vipeholm dental caries study: the effect of different levels of carbohydrate intake on caries activity in 436 individuals observed for 5 years. Acta Odontol Scand 1954;11:232–364.

81. Harris R. Biology of the children of Hopewood House, Bowral, Australia. IV. Observations of dental caries experience extending over five years (1957–1961). J Dent Res 1963;42:1387–1398.

82. Sundin B. Caries and consumption of sweets in 15- and 18-year-olds interviewed with visualization. Scand J Dent Res 1990;98:96–101.

83. Akpata ES, Al-Shammery AR, Saeed HI. Dental caries, sugar consumption and restorative dental care in 12–13-year-old children in Riyadh, Saudi Arabia. Community Dent Oral Epidemiol 1992;20:343–346.

84. Frostell G, Birkhed D, Edwardsson S, et al. Effect of partial substitution of invert sugar for sucrose in combination with Duraphat treatment on caries development in preschool children: the Malmo study. Caries Res 1991;25: 304–310.

85. Holt RD. Foods and drinks at four daily time intervals in a group of young children. Br Dent J 1991;170:137–143.

86. Willett WC. Diet and health: what should we eat? Science 1994;264:532–537.
87. Federation of American Societies for Experimental Biology. Physiological effects and health consequences of dietary fiber. Report to the Food and Drug Administration. Bethesda: Federation of American Societies for Experimental Biology, 1987.
88. Bolton-Smith C, Woodward M, Smith WCS, et al. Dietary and non-dietary predictors of serum total and HDL-cholesterol in men and women: results from the Scottish Heart Health Study. Int J Epidemiol 1991;20:95–104.
89. Glore SR, Van Treeck D, Knehans AW, et al. Soluble fiber and serum lipids: a literature review. J Am Diet Assoc 1994;94:425–436.
90. Jenkins DJA, Wolever TMS, Rao AV, et al. Effect on blood lipids of very high intakes of fiber in diets low in saturated fat and cholesterol. N Engl J Med 1993;329:21–26.
91. Painter N. Diverticular disease of the colon. In: Trowell H, Burkitt D, Heaton K, eds. Dietary fibre, fibre-depleted foods and disease. New York: Academic Press, 1985:145–160.
92. Irving D, Drasar BS. Fibre and cancer of the colon. Br J Cancer 1973;28:462–463.
93. McKeown-Eyssen GE, Bright-See E. Dietary factors in colon cancer: international relationships. Nutr Cancer 1984;6:160–170.
94. Modan B, Barrell V, Lubin F, et al. Low-fiber intake as an etiologic factor in cancer of the colon. J Natl Cancer Inst 1975;55:15–18.
95. Jain M, Cook GM, Davis FG, et al. A case-control study of diet and colorectal cancer. Int J Cancer 1980;26: 757–768.
96. Potter JD, McMichael AJ. Diet and cancer of the colon and rectum: a case-control study. J Natl Cancer Inst 1986; 76:557–569.
97. Sandler RS, Lyles CM, Peipins LA, et al. Diet and risk of colorectal adenomas: macronutrients, cholesterol, and fiber. J Natl Cancer Inst 1993;85:884–891.
98. Trock B, Lanza E, Greenwald P. Dietary fiber, vegetables, and colon cancer: critical review and meta-analyses of the epidemiologic evidence. J Natl Cancer Inst 1990;82:650–661.
99. Howe GR, Benito E, Castelleto R, et al. Dietary intake of fiber and decreased risk of cancers of the colon and rectum: evidence from the combined analysis of 13 case-control studies. J Natl Cancer Inst 1992;84:1887–1896.
100. Hirayama T. A large-scale cohort study on the relationship between diet and selected cancers of the digestive organs. In: Bruce WR, Correa P, Lipkin M, et al, eds. Banbury Report 7. Gastrointestinal cancer: endogenous factors. Cold Spring Harbor, NY: Cold Spring Harbor Laboratory, 1981:409–429.
101. Kromhout D, Bosschieter EB, de Lezenne Coulander C. Dietary fibre and 10-year mortality from coronary heart disease, cancer, and all causes: the Zutphen Study. Lancet 1982;2:518–522.
102. Phillips RL, Snowden DA. Dietary relationships with fatal colorectal cancer among Seventh-Day Adventists. J Natl Cancer Inst 1985;74:307–317.
103. Graham S, Zielezny M, Marshall J, et al. Diet in the epidemiology of postmenopausal breast cancer in the New York State Cohort. Am J Epidemiol 1992;136:1327–1337.
104. Stamler J. Dietary salt and blood pressure. Ann NY Acad Sci 1993;676:122–156.
105. Grobbee DE, Hofman A. Does sodium restriction lower blood pressure? BMJ 1986;293:27–29.
106. Parijs J, Joosens JV, Van der Linden L, et al. Moderate sodium restriction and diuretics in the treatment of hypertension. Am Heart J 1973;85:22–34.
107. MacGregor GA, Markandu N, Best F, et al. Double-blind, randomized, crossover trial of moderate sodium restriction in essential hypertension. Lancet 1982;1:351–355.
108. Langford HG, Blaufox MD, Oberman A, et al. Dietary therapy slows the return of hypertension after stopping prolonged medication. JAMA 1985;253:657–664.
109. Morgan T, Adams W, Gillies A, et al. Hypertension treated by salt restriction. Lancet 1978;1:227–230.
110. Beard TC, Cooke HM, Gray WR, et al. Randomized, controlled trial of a no-added-sodium diet for mild hypertension. Lancet 1982;2:455–458.
111. Weinberger MH, Cohen SJ, Miller JZ, et al. Dietary sodium restriction as adjunctive treatment of hypertension. JAMA 1988;259:2561–2565.
112. Miller JZ, Daugherty SA, Weinberger MH, et al. Blood pressure response to dietary sodium restriction in normotensive adults. Hypertension 1983;5:790–795.
113. Forte JG, Miguel JM, Miguel MJ, et al. Salt and blood pressure: a community trial. J Hum Hypertens 1989;3: 179–184.
114. Elliott P. Sodium and blood pressure: a review of the evidence from controlled trials of sodium reduction and epidemiological studies. Klin Wochenschr 1991;69:3–10.

115. Cutler J, Follman D, Elliott P, et al. An overview of randomised trials of sodium reduction and blood pressure. Hypertension 1991;17(Suppl I):I27–I33.

116. Law MR, Frost CD, Wald NJ. By how much does salt restriction lower blood pressure? I. Analysis of observational data among populations. II. Analysis of data from trials of salt reduction. BMJ 1991;302:811–824.

117. The Trials of Hypertension Prevention Collaborative Research Group. The effects of nonpharmacologic interventions on blood pressure of persons with high normal levels: results of the Trials of Hypertension, Phase I. JAMA 1992;267:1213–1220.

118. Mascioli S, Grimm R Jr, Launer C, et al. Sodium chloride raises blood pressure in normotensive subjects: the study of sodium and blood pressure. Hypertension 1991;17(Suppl I):I21–I26.

119. Page LB, Damon A, Moellering RC Jr. Antecedents of cardiovascular disease in six Solomon Island societies. Circulation 1974;49:1132–1146.

120. Kaminer B, Lutz WPW. Blood pressure in bushmen of the Kalahari Desert. Circulation 1960;22:289–295.

121. Saunders GM, Bancroft H. Blood pressure studies on negro and white men and women living in the Virgin Islands of the United States. Am Heart J 1942;23:410–423.

122. Intersalt Cooperative Research Group. Intersalt: an international study of electrolyte excretion and blood pressure. Results for 24 hour urinary sodium and potassium excretion. BMJ 1988;297:319–328.

123. National Institutes of Health Consensus Development Panel on Optimal Calcium Intake. Optimal calcium intake. JAMA 1994;272:1942–1948.

124. Turner JG, Gilchrist NL, Ayling EM, et al. Factors affecting bone mineral density in high school girls. NZ Med J 1992;105:95–96.

125. Murphy S, Khaw KT, May H, et al. Milk consumption and bone mineral density in middle-aged and elderly women. BMJ 1994;308:939–941.

126. Johnston CC Jr, Miller JZ, Slemenda CW, et al. Calcium supplementation and increases in bone mineral density in children. N Engl J Med 1992;327:82–87.

127. Lloyd T, Andon MB, Rollings N, et al. Calcium supplementation and bone mineral density in adolescent girls. JAMA 1992;270:841–844.

128. Horsman A, Gallagher JC, Simpson M, et al. Prospective trial of oestrogen and calcium in postmenopausal women. BMJ 1977;2:789–792.

129. Recker RR, Saville PD, Heaney RP. Effect of estrogens and calcium carbonate on bone loss in postmenopausal women. Ann Intern Med 1977;87:649–655.

130. Aloia JF, Vaswani A, Yeh JK, et al. Calcium supplementation with and without hormone replacement therapy to prevent postmenopausal bone loss. Ann Intern Med 1994;120:97–103.

131. Ettinger B, Genant HK, Cann CE. Postmenopausal bone loss is prevented by treatment with low-dosage estrogen with calcium. Ann Intern Med 1987;106:40–45.

132. Riis B, Thomsen K, Christiansen C. Does calcium supplementation prevent postmenopausal bone loss? A double-blind, controlled clinical study. N Engl J Med 1987;316:173–177.

133. Nilas L, Christiansen C, Rodbro P. Calcium supplementation and postmenopausal bone loss. BMJ 1984;289: 1103–1106.

134. Stevenson JC, Whitehead MI, Padwick M, et al. Dietary intake of calcium and postmenopausal bone loss. BMJ 1988;297:15–17.

135. Cumming RG. Calcium intake and bone mass: a quantitative review of the evidence. Calcif Tissue Int 1990;47: 194–201.

135a. Chapuy MC, Arlot ME, Delmas PD, et al. Effect of calcium and cholecalciferol treatment for three years on hip fractures in elderly women. BMJ 1994;308:1081–1082.

135b. Reid IR, Ames RW, Evans MC, et al. Long-term effects of calcium supplementation on bone loss and fractures in postmenopausal women: a randomized controlled trial. Am J Med 1995;98:331–335.

136. Curhan GC, Willett WC, Rimm EB, et al. A prospective study of dietary calcium and other nutrients and the risk of symptomatic kidney stones. N Engl J Med 1993;328:833–838.

137. Czeizel AE, Dudas I. Prevention of the first occurrence of neural-tube defects by periconceptional vitamin supplementation. N Engl J Med 1992;327:1832–1835.

138. Comstock GW, Bush TL, Helzlsouer K. Serum retinol, beta-carotene, vitamin E, and selenium as related to subsequent cancer of specific sites. Am J Epidemiol 1992;135:115–121.

139. Manson JE, Buring JE, Satterfield S, et al. Baseline characteristics of participants in the Physicians' Health Study: a randomized trial of aspirin and beta-carotene in U.S. physicians. Am J Prev Med 1991;7:150–154.

140. Stahelin HB, Gey KF, Eichholzer M, et al. Plasma antioxidant vitamins and subsequent cancer mortality in the 12-year follow-up of the prospective Basel study. Am J Epidemiol 1991;133:766–775.

141. Ziegler RG, Subar AF, Craft NE, et al. Does beta-carotene explain why reduced cancer risk is associated with vegetable and fruit intake? Cancer Res 1992;52(7 Suppl):2060S–2066S.

142. Stampfer MJ, Hennekens CH, Manson JE, et al. Vitamin E consumption and the risk of coronary disease in women. N Engl J Med 1993;328:1444–1449.

143. Hodis HN, Mack WJ, LaBree L, et al. Serial coronary angiographic evidence that antioxidant vitamin intake reduces progression of coronary artery atherosclerosis. JAMA 1995;273:1849–1854.

144. American Heart Association. Diet in the healthy child: Task Force Committee of the Nutrition Committee and the Cardiovascular Disease in the Young Council. Circulation 1983;67:1411A–1414A.

145. Cunningham AS, Jelliffe DB, Jelliffe EFP. Breastfeeding and health in the 1980s: a global epidemiologic review. J Pediatr 1991;118:659–665.

146. Lucas A, Brooke OG, Morley R, et al. Early diet of preterm infants and development of allergic or atopic disease: randomized prospective study. BMJ 1990;300:837–840.

147. Lucas A, Morley R, Cole TJ, et al. Breast milk and subsequent intelligence quotient in children born pre-term. Lancet 1992;339:199–248.

148. Fall CHD, Barker DJP, Osmond C, et al. Relation of infant feeding to adult serum cholesterol concentration and death from ischaemic heart disease. BMJ 1992;304:801–805.

149. Jooste PL, Rossouw LJ, Steenkamp HJ, et al. Effect of breast feeding on the plasma cholesterol and growth of infants. J Pediatr Gastroenterol Nutr 1991;13:139–142.

150. Lozoff B, Jimenez E, Wolf AW. Long-term developmental outcome of infants with iron deficiency. N Engl J Med 1991;325:687–694.

151. Webber LS, Srinivasan SR, Wattigney WA, et al. Tracking of serum lipids and lipoproteins from childhood to adulthood: the Bogalusa heart study. Am J Epidemiol 1991;133:884–899.

152. Berenson GS, Wattigney WA, Tracy RE, et al. Atherosclerosis of the aorta and coronary arteries and cardiovascular risk factors in persons aged 6 to 30 years and studied at necropsy (the Bogalusa heart study). Am J Cardiol 1992;70:851–858.

153. Quivers ES, Driscoll DJ, Garvey CD, et al. Variability in response to a low-fat, low-cholesterol diet in children with elevated low-density lipoprotein cholesterol levels. Pediatrics 1992;89:925–929.

154. Viikari J, Akerblom HK, Rasanen L, et al. Cardiovascular risk in young Finns. Acta Paediatr Scand Suppl 1990;365:13–19.

155. Hardy SC, Kleinman RE. Fat and cholesterol in the diet of infants and young children: implications for growth, development, and long-term health. J Pediatr 1994;125:S69–S77.

156. Nicklas TA, Webber LS, Koschak ML, et al. Nutrient adequacy of low fat intakes for children: the Bogalusa heart study. Pediatrics 1992;89:221–228.

157. The Writing Group for the DISC Collaborative Research Group. Efficacy and safety of lowering dietary intake of fat and cholesterol in children with elevated low-density lipoprotein cholesterol: the Dietary Intervention Study in Children (DISC). JAMA 1995;273:1429–1435.

158. Antonov AN. Children born during the siege of Leningrad in 1942. J Pediatr 1947;30:250–295.

159. Stein A, Susser M, Saenger G, et al. Famine and human development: the Dutch hunger winter of 1944/45. New York: Oxford University Press, 1974.

160. Singer JE, Westphal M, Niswander K. Relationship of weight gain during pregnancy to birthweight and infant growth and development in the first year of life: a report from the collaborative study of cerebral palsy. Obstet Gynecol 1968;31:417.

161. Abrams BF, Laros RD. Prepregnancy weight, weight gain, and birthweight. Am J Obstet Gynecol 1986;154:503.

162. Institute of Medicine, Subcommittee on Nutritional Status and Weight Gain During Pregnancy. Nutrition during pregnancy. Washington, DC: National Academy Press, 1990.

163. Worthington-Roberts BS. Nutrition, fertility, and family planning. In: Worthington-Roberts BS, Williams SR, eds. Nutrition in pregnancy and lactation. 5th ed. St. Louis: CV Mosby, 1993:34–63.

164. Rush D, Leighton J, Sloan NL, et al. The National WIC evaluation: evaluation of the Special Supplemental Food Program for Women, Infants, and Children. II. Review of past studies of WIC. Am J Clin Nutr 1988;48:394–411.

165. National Research Council, Food and Nutrition Board. Recommended dietary allowances. 10th ed. Committee on Dietary Allowances. Washington, DC: National Academy Press, 1989.

166. Institute of Medicine. Preventing low birthweight. Washington, DC: National Academy Press, 1985.

167. U.S. Preventive Services Task Force. Routine iron supplementation during pregnancy: review article. JAMA 1993; 270:2848–2854.

168. Ahmed FE. Effect of nutrition on the health of the elderly. J Am Diet Assoc 1992;92:1102–1108.

169. Kronmal RA, Cain KC, Ye Z, et al. Total serum cholesterol levels and mortality risk as a function of age: a report based on the Framingham data. Arch Intern Med 1993;153:1065–1073.

170. Nordin BEC, Horsman A, Crilly RG, et al. Treatment of spinal osteoporosis in postmenopausal women. BMJ 1980; 280:451–454.

171. Riggs BL, Seeman E, Hodgson SF, et al. Effect of the fluoride/calcium regimen on vertebral fracture occurrence in postmenopausal women: comparison with conventional therapy. N Engl J Med 1982;306:446–450.

172. Resnick NM, Greenspan SL. Senile osteoporosis reconsidered. JAMA 1989;261:1025–1029.

173. Fujita T, Fukase M, Miyamoto H, et al. Increase of bone mineral density by calcium supplement with oyster shell electrolysate. Bone Mineral 1990;11:85–91.

174. Dwyer JT. Screening older Americans' nutritional health: current practices and future possibilities. Washington, DC: Nutrition Screening Initiative, 1991.

175. Glanz K. Nutrition education for risk factor reduction and patient education: a review. Prev Med 1985;14:721–752.

176. Knutsen SF, Knutsen R. The Tromso Survey: The Family Intervention Study—the effect of intervention on some coronary risk factors and dietary habits, a 6-year follow-up. Prev Med 1991;20:197–212.

177. Milkereit J, Graves JS. Follow-up dietary counseling benefits attainment of intake goals for total fat, saturated fat, and fiber. J Am Diet Assoc 1992;92:603–605.

178. Campbell MK, DeVellis BM, Strecher VJ, et al. Improving dietary behavior: the effectiveness of tailored messages in primary care settings. Am J Public Health 1994;84:783–787.

179. Barnard ND, Akhtar A, Nicholson A. Factors that facilitate compliance to lower fat intake. Arch Fam Med 1995;4: 153–158.

180. Kafatos AG, Vlachonikolis IG, Codrington CA. Nutrition during pregnancy: the effects of an educational intervention program in Greece. Am J Clin Nutr 1989;50:970–979.

181. Klesges RC, Stein RJ, Eck LH, et al. Parental influence on food selection in young children and its relationships to childhood obesity. Am J Clin Nutr 1991;53:859–864.

182. Wechsler H, Levine S, Idelson RK, et al. The physician's role in health promotion: a survey of primary-care practitioners. N Engl J Med 1983;308:97–100.

183. Randall DE, Marshall JR, Brasure J, et al. Patterns in food use and compliance with NCI dietary guidelines. Nutr Cancer 1991;15:141–158.

184. Drewnowski A. Dietary fats: perceptions and preferences. J Am Coll Nutr 1990;9:431–435.

185. Department of Agriculture, Department of Health and Human Services. Dietary guidelines for Americans. 3rd ed. Bulletin no. 232. Washington, DC: Department of Agriculture, 1990.

186. Department of Health and Human Services. Healthy People 2000: national health promotion and disease prevention objectives. Washington, DC: Department of Health and Human Services. (DHHS Publication no. 91-50212.)

187. Food Guide Pyramid: A Guide to Daily Food Choices. Home and Garden Bulletin no. 232. Washington, DC: Department of Agriculture, 1992.

188. Council on Scientific Affairs. Medical evaluation of healthy persons. Chicago: American Medical Association, 1983.

189. American College of Physicians. Nutrition: position paper. Washington, DC: American College of Physicians, 1985.

190. American Heart Association. Dietary guidelines for healthy American adults: a statement for physicians and health professionals by the Nutrition Committee, American Heart Association. Circulation 1988;77:721A–724A.

191. National Research Council, Committee on Diet, Nutrition, and Cancer. Diet, nutrition, and cancer. Washington, DC: National Academy Press, 1982.

192. Nixon DW. Nutrition and cancer: American Cancer Society guidelines, programs, and initiatives. CA Cancer J Clin 1990;40:71–75.

193. National Cancer Institute. Diet, nutrition, and cancer prevention: the good news. Washington, DC: Government Printing Office, 1986. (Publication no. DHHS (NIH) 87-2878.)

194. National Heart, Lung, and Blood Institute. Heart to heart: a manual on nutritional counseling for the reduction of cardiovascular disease risk factors. Bethesda: National Heart, Lung, and Blood Institute, 1983. (Publication no. DHHS (NIH) 85-1528.)

195. National High Blood Pressure Education Program. Working Group Report on primary prevention of hypertension. Bethesda: National Institutes of Health, 1993 (Publication no. 93-2669.)

196. National Cholesterol Education Program. Report of the Expert Panel on Population Strategies for Blood Cholesterol Reduction: executive summary. Arch Intern Med 1991;151:1071–1084.

197. Summary of the Second Report of the National Cholesterol Education Program (NCEP) Expert Panel on Detection, Evaluation, and Treatment of High Blood Cholesterol in Adults (Adult Treatment Panel II). JAMA 1993; 269:3015–3023.

198. American Academy of Pediatrics Committee on Nutrition. Statement on cholesterol. Pediatrics 1992; 90:469–473.

199. American Academy of Pediatrics. Pediatric nutrition handbook. 3rd ed. Elk Grove Village, IL: American Academy of Pediatrics, 1993.

200. National Cholesterol Education Program. Report of the Expert Panel on Blood Cholesterol Levels in Children and Adolescents. Bethesda: National Institutes of Health, 1991. (Publication no. 91-2732.)

201. American College of Obstetricians and Gynecologists. Nutrition in pregnancy. Technical Bulletin no. 179. Washington, DC: American College of Obstetricians and Gynecologists, 1993.

202. Centers for Disease Control and Prevention. Recommendations for the use of folic acid to reduce the number of cases of spina bifida and other neural tube defects. MMWR 1992;41:RR-14.

203. Canadian Task Force on the Periodic Health Examination. Canadian guide to clinical preventive health care. Ottawa: Canada Communication Group, 1994:586–599.

204. U.S. Department of Health and Human Services and U.S. Department of Agriculture. Nutrition and your health: dietary guidelines for Americans. 4th ed. Washington, DC: Government Printing Office, 1995.

57. Counseling to Prevent Motor Vehicle Injuries

RECOMMENDATION

Counseling all patients, and the parents of young patients, to use occupant restraints (lap/shoulder safety belts and child safety seats), to wear helmets when riding motorcycles, and to refrain from driving while under the influence of alcohol or other drugs is recommended (see *Clinical Intervention*). There is currently insufficient evidence to recommend for or against counseling patients to prevent pedestrian injuries. See Chapter 58 for recommendations on the prevention of bicycling injuries.

Burden of Suffering

In 1993, motor vehicle crash-related injuries were the eighth leading cause of death in the U.S.[1] Motor vehicle injuries are a leading cause of death in children and young adults,[2] and the leading cause of years of potential life lost before age 65.[3] A total of 40,115 Americans died in motor vehicle crashes in 1993 (15.6/100,000 population), and more than 3 million suffered nonfatal injuries (1,212/100,000).[4] Over 3,200 of those killed were children under age 16 years.[4] In the same year, 2,444 motorcycle occupants were killed.[4] The motorcycle occupant fatality rate is nearly 20 times higher than for passenger car occupants (25.1 vs. 1.3/100 million vehicle miles traveled).[4] More than 5,600 pedestrians were also killed in 1993 (2.2/100,000).[4] The annual number of motor vehicle fatalities has decreased since the late 1960s, despite an increase in annual number of vehicle miles traveled.[5] Motor vehicle crashes during 1990 resulted in an estimated total lifetime economic cost of $137.5 billion.[6] They account for about one-third of the total lifetime cost of injury in the U.S.[7]

Motor vehicle fatality rates are highest for young and elderly adults, while injury rates peak in young adulthood.[1,4] In 1992, motor vehicle crashes accounted for 30% of all deaths in persons aged 15–24.[1] The high mortality rate in older adults reflects a high case-fatality rate, probably due to increased likelihood of developing serious complications after motor vehicle injuries, as drivers 65 years of age and older have the lowest rate of crashes per 100,000 licensed drivers.[4,8,9] Motor vehicle fatality rates for males are more than twice that for females.[1,4] Although alcohol-related traffic fatality rates have declined by more than one third since 1979,[10] alcohol use remains an important risk factor for motor vehicle injuries. An estimated 17,461 persons were killed in alcohol-related motor vehicle crashes in 1993, accounting for 44% of total traffic fatalities for the year.[4] About one third of drivers killed in crashes in 1993 were intoxicated by alcohol (typically defined in U.S. law as blood alcohol concentration [BAC] ≥ 0.10 g/dL).[4] The proportion of fatally injured drivers having BAC above 0.10 g/dL is highest for those aged 21–44.[4] In 1992, 1.6 million persons were arrested for driving under the influence of alcohol or drugs.[11] Alcohol-involved crashes have been estimated to account for 40% of comprehensive motor vehicle crash costs in the U.S.[12]

Efficacy of Risk Reduction

Driving while impaired by alcohol or drugs and failing to use occupant protection (e.g., safety belts, child safety seats, motorcycle helmets) are two of the most important risk factors for motor vehicle injury. (Screening for potential impairment due to medical conditions such as diabetes or epilepsy will not be addressed in this chapter.[13,14]) Case series have reported that up to half of fatally injured drivers have BAC of 0.10 g/dL or higher (although the proportion has declined in recent decades).[4,9,15] Controlled studies have shown that drivers involved or injured in crashes are more likely to have a BAC of at least 0.10 g/dL than are other drivers.[16–18] BAC at or below 0.05 g/dL are also associated with impaired driving skills performance and an increased risk of motor vehicle crash involvement and fatality, particularly for younger drivers.[19–22] In addition to its role as a risk factor for causing motor vehicle crashes, alcohol use may increase the risk of death or serious injury during a crash;[23,24] this association may be partially confounded by other high-risk behaviors associated with alcohol use, such as failing to use safety belts and motorcycle helmets.[25–27] Alcohol can also limit the ability of the victim to escape from the vehicle.[15,23] Alcohol-intoxicated survivors with severe brain injuries appear to have longer hospitalizations and more persistent neurologic impairment than those who were not intoxicated.[28] Evidence that reducing drinking and driving decreases the risk of motor vehicle injury comes from multiple time series studies demonstrating that raising the legal drinking age or lowering legal blood alcohol limits can significantly reduce alcohol-related fatal crashes.[29–33]

Many alcohol-related motor vehicle crashes may be attributable to problem drinkers. Persons dying in alcohol-related traffic crashes are significantly more likely to have alcohol-related arrest histories or autopsy findings suggestive of alcoholism.[4,34–36] In a cohort of Swedish men followed for 20 years, the relative risk of dying in a traffic crash among heavy drinkers was 2.3 times higher than for moderate drinkers and 8 times higher than for nondrinkers.[37] One study has also suggested that alcoholic drivers, when compared to the general driving population, have more motor vehicle crashes per capita and per vehicle mile driven and more frequent convictions for impaired driving.[38] Screening for problem drinking followed by a brief counseling intervention has been proven to reduce alcohol consumption (see Chapter 52). Therefore, such screening is likely to be efficacious in reducing motor vehicle injuries and fatalities.

It has been estimated that drugs (such as marijuana, cocaine, and tranquilizers) may be present in 10–32% of drivers injured in traffic crashes,[39–43] although not all studies have been able to separate the effects of these drugs from those of alcohol and the presence of such drugs does not necessarily indicate impairment. In case series that tested drivers injured in traffic crashes for both substances, almost half who tested positive for illicit drugs had negative BAC.[41–43] One study evaluated 175 consecutive subjects stopped by police for reckless driving who were not felt to be alcohol-impaired based on a negative breath analysis, lack of odor of alcohol, or both.[44] Urine testing was performed on 150 (86%), of whom 88 (59%) tested positive for marijuana, cocaine, or both, while 5% tested positive for alcohol. Whether the illicit drugs caused reckless driving, or were simply associated with it in persons disposed to multiple high-risk behaviors, is not established. Simulated driving tests suggest impairment of certain abilities by marijuana and other drugs, similar to that produced by alcohol.[45–47] Thus, evidence indicates that impairment with drugs other than alcohol may also play an important role in traffic injuries and deaths, although the relationship is not as well defined as for alcohol.

Use of occupant restraints has been shown to reduce the risk of motor vehicle injury and death. The efficacy of safety belts has been demonstrated in a variety of study designs that include laboratory experiments (using human volunteers, cadavers, and anthropomorphic crash dummies), postcrash comparisons of injuries sustained by restrained and unrestrained occupants, and postcrash judgments by crash analysts regarding the probable effects of restraints had they been used.[48–53] It has been estimated on the basis of such evidence that the proper use of lap and shoulder belts can decrease the risk of moderate to serious injury to front seat occupants by up to 55%[49,53,54] and can reduce crash mortality by 40–50%.[53,54] When brought to the hospital, crash victims who were wearing safety belts at the time of the crash have less severe injuries, are less likely to require admission, and have lower hospital charges.[50,52] Multiple time series studies evaluating mandatory seat belt laws have reported significant reductions in motor vehicle-related injuries, hospital admissions, and fatalities after implementation of such laws.[55–59]

Child safety seats are also effective. It has been reported that unrestrained children are over 10 times as likely to die in a motor vehicle crash as are restrained children,[60,61] although these data come from studies with important design limitations. More recent studies suggest that child safety seats can reduce serious injury by up to 67% and mortality by as much as 71%.[62–64] A 20–25% decline in head and extremity injuries for children under age 4 has been reported in States after enactment of mandatory child restraint legislation.[65] Child restraints may also reduce noncrash injuries (e.g., those due to sudden stops) to child passengers by preventing both falls within the vehicle and ejections.[66] The efficacy of child safety seats may be reduced by improper use; such misuse has been reported in up to two thirds of children.[67] The safety of child safety seats used in combination with air bags is unknown. Laboratory crash test data indicate a potential for injury to an infant placed in a rear-facing car seat in the front seat of a vehicle equipped with a passenger-side air bag.[68]

Beginning with the model year 1998, all new passenger cars in the U.S. will be required to have driver- and passenger-side air bags.[69] A review by the National Highway Traffic Safety Administration estimated that air bags increase the effectiveness of lap/shoulder belts by about 5–10%.[70] Recent modeling[71] and observational[72] studies estimate that air bags prevent 18–19% of all automobile driver fatalities and 13% of right front passenger fatalities, over and above the fatality reduction due to seat belt use. The estimated reduction in driver fatalities was about 21% for unbelted drivers and 9% for belted drivers.[72] Air bags are designed to be a supplemental restraint system, and they do not deploy in low-speed, rear, side, or rollover crashes. Most reported adverse effects of air bag deployment are minor (e.g., erythema, abrasions, and contusions), although more serious injuries such as facial fractures have also been reported.[73,74]

By wearing safety helmets, persons who operate or ride on motorcycles can reduce their risk of injury or death from head trauma in the event of a crash. Head injury rates are reduced by about 40–75% among motorcyclists who wear safety helmets.[75–77] Multiple time series studies have reported that rates of fatal and nonfatal injuries have declined significantly in states that have passed mandatory helmet laws.[9,78–81] In one large study, a motorcycle helmet use law was associated with a 37.5% reduction in fatalities (from 523 in 1991 to 327 in 1992), a 26.5% reduction in motorcycle fatality rates (from 70.1 to 51.5/100,000 per year), and similar reductions in admitted and emergency department-treated riders with motorcycle crash injuries.[82] Observed helmet use during the first year of the law was over 99%, compared to 46% helmet usage before the law.[83] States that have repealed mandatory motorcycle helmet laws have experienced significant increases in motorcycle fatalities.[75,84]

The epidemiology of pedestrian injury varies by age group. Child pedestrian injuries most often occur close to home and the majority of events involve children darting out into traffic at mid-block.[85,86] Risk factors for child pedestrian injury are being male and age 5–9 years,[4] presumably due to both increased exposure and developmentally related limitations in pedestrian skills.[85,87] In a population-based New Zealand study, child pedestrian injury hospitalization rates were 1.7/1 million road crossings and 72/100,000 population at age 5 years, declining to about 0.6 and 40, respectively, by age 9 years with little change thereafter.[88] One of the most important risk factors for adult pedestrian injury is alcohol intoxication. In 1993, 36% of fatally injured pedestrians over 14 years of age had BAC of at least 0.10 g/dL.[88a] Elderly persons have the highest pedestrian death rate, despite studies showing that they may exhibit the most cautious street-crossing behavior.[89,90] Reduced mobility[91] and sensory deficits associated with aging may contribute to their increased risk. As with motor vehicle crash injuries, however, the high death rate in elderly persons to a large extent reflects a high case-fatality rate.

There is no evidence to date that changes in any of the risk factors for the different age groups reduces pedestrian injury. Studies have shown that parents of young children may overestimate the pedestrian skills of their children, implying that teaching parents about developmental limitations on pedestrian skills might decrease injuries.[92,93] Observational studies suggest that pedestrian visibility affects the risk of motor vehicle-pedestrian crashes.[94,95] Several small experiments have reported that wearing reflective or brightly colored clothing increases pedestrian visibility and motorists' yielding to pedestrians,[96–98] but these studies have important design limitations. Whether wearing such clothing would reduce the risk of pedestrian injury has not been studied.

Effectiveness of Counseling

Although the rate of alcohol-related driver fatalities has decreased in recent years, as many as 1.6 million persons continue to be arrested annually for driving under the influence of alcohol or other drugs;[11] this substantially underestimates the total number of persons who drive while impaired, since only a small proportion are arrested.[98a] Similarly, while the use of occupant protection systems and motorcycle helmets has increased substantially in recent years,[69,99–101] at least half of all Americans, and presumably many patients seen by clinicians, either do not use occupant restraints or do not use them correctly when driving or riding in a motor vehicle. Thus, it is likely that many patients could potentially benefit from clinician counseling to modify their behaviors as drivers and passengers in motor vehicles. Since motor vehicle crashes represent a leading cause of death and nonfatal injury in the U.S., even modest successes through clinical interventions could have major public health value.

In actual practice, however, little is known about how effectively clinicians can alter any of these behaviors. Although there is some evidence that persons involved in motor vehicle crashes while intoxicated demonstrate lower recidivism with alcohol treatment interventions[102] and that community-based educational interventions to reduce alcohol-impaired driving may be effective,[103] there is generally little information from clinical studies on the ability of clinicians to influence patients to refrain from driving while impaired by alcohol or other drugs. There is good evidence, however, that brief clinician counseling can reduce alcohol consumption in problem drinkers (see Chapter 52), which may, in turn, result in reduced drinking and driving.

There have been few studies examining the effectiveness of clinician counseling to increase safety belt use. Most of the available studies have evaluated counseling parents to increase seat belt use by their children.[104] One controlled trial found increased self-reported safety belt use with pediatrician counseling compared to mailed information; the interval to outcome assessment was not specified.[105] A second trial found that pediatrician counseling resulted in an immediate increase in observed safety belt use, but there was no difference in self-reported usage rates between the study group and controls at 1-year follow-up.[106] In the same study, however, observed seat belt use was highly correlated with the physician's own estimate of the proportion of visits during which he counseled parents about seat belts.[106] A nonrandomized controlled trial involving adult patients evaluated the effect of improved physician delivery of clinical preventive services after an intervention that included physician training, physician use of prevention protocols, and reimbursement for counseling.[107] The proportion of patients reporting that they "began always using seat belts" was significantly higher in the intervention group at 1-year follow-up. In a questionnaire survey, patients claimed to have increased their use of safety belts as a result of a brief statement by their physician during a routine office visit,[108] but the study lacked controls and may have been biased by the patients selected. Other measures that have been proven successful in motivating persons to use safety belts, such as community educational programs and intensive psychological strategies,[109] may not be generalizable to the clinical practice setting.

Stronger evidence that clinician counseling can be effective comes from randomized and other controlled trials in which parents of newborns and infants were encouraged to use infant safety seats before this practice became widely mandated by law. These trials often used other types of interventions in addition to clinician counseling, including written materials, videos, or free or loaner car seats. Results from such trials indicate that significant immediate or short-term (up to 3 months) improvements in car seat use are possible.[110–118] One randomized controlled trial involving parents of children ages 1–17 years found no effect of clinician counseling and additional interventions on the use of occupant protection,[119] but most of the children were already using restraints prior to the intervention.

The long-term efficacy of clinician counseling is less clear. One randomized controlled trial in a military population showed increased reported car seat use at 9–12 months and increased car seat sales for 10 months after the intervention,[112] but in several other trials that included clinician counseling, significant immediate or short-term increases in car seat use were not maintained at longer follow-up.[113,116–118] A time series study in which nurses conducted educational sessions in the prenatal period, postpartum period, and at 2-month intervals after discharge found that proper use of child safety seats had improved compared with rates in the previous year, suggesting that periodic reinforcement is necessary to maintain high use rates.[120]

Direct evidence that physician counseling combined with community education programs can reduce motor vehicle-related injuries to young children comes from a nonrandomized controlled trial.[121] This trial reported a 54% decrease in motor vehicle-related injuries among children aged 0–5 living in the intervention communities compared to children in the control communities, despite no difference in self-reported overall restraint use. In a separate analysis in which persons in both communities were combined, reported car seat use was 12% higher in households exposed to "participatory" prevention programs (i.e., received specific counseling, materials, or other interventions), compared to those not exposed. Persons in the intervention communities were significantly more likely to have such "participatory" exposure than were those in control communities (55% vs. 34%). The authors were unable to distinguish between the effects of the various interventions; a similar proportion of subjects reported exposure to pediatrician counseling (21%) and to community education programs (17%).

Studies of the effectiveness of school-based programs to teach pedestrian skills to children have shown some improvement in their attitudes and skills,[122–124] and one researcher has reported reductions in child pedestrian crash involvement through safety education films and other materials.[125,126] There is no evidence to indicate whether or not such interventions are generalizable to the clinical setting.

Recommendations of Other Groups

Mandatory safety belt laws were in effect in 43 states, the District of Columbia, and Puerto Rico in 1993.[4] Child safety seat use is required by law in all 50 states, the District of Columbia, and Puerto Rico.[4] Recommendations specifically urging clinicians to counsel patients to use occupant restraints (child safety seats or fitted lap/shoulder belts, as appropriate for age) have been issued by a number of groups. These include the American Medical Association,[127,128] the American College of Physicians,[129,130] the American Academy of Family Physicians (AAFP),[131] the American Academy of Pediatrics (AAP),[132] the Bright Futures project,[133] the American College of Obstetricians and Gynecologists,[134] the Canadian Task Force on the Periodic Health Examination,[135] the Public Health Service,[135a] and the National Highway Traffic Safety Administration.[136] The AAP has instituted special parent-oriented educational programs ("Every Ride, Safe Ride") in which pediatricians encourage the use of child occupant protection beginning with the ride home from the hospital and continuing throughout childhood.[137] The AAP, Centers for Disease Control and Prevention, and the Society of Automotive Engineers recommend against the use of rear-facing child restraints in the front seat of cars with passenger-side air bags.[68]

In 1993, twenty-five states, the District of Columbia, and Puerto Rico had universal motorcycle helmet laws; an additional 22 states required only that persons under a specified age (usually 18) wear a helmet.[138] The AAFP,[131] the AMA,[128,139] and Bright Futures[133] recommend that physicians counsel their patients who are motorcyclists to use approved helmets. The Canadian Task Force found insufficient evidence to recommend for or against counseling patients to wear motorcycle helmets.[135]

In 36 states and the District of Columbia, driving a motor vehicle with a BAC of 0.10 g/dL is a criminal offense; in 10 states, the limit is 0.08 g/dL.[4] In addition, all states prohibit the purchase of alcohol by persons under the age of 21.[140] The AAP,[141] the AAFP,[131] the AMA,[128] Bright Futures,[133] and the Centers for Disease Control and Prevention[142] recommend counseling patients to abstain from intoxicants when driving. The AAP also advises parents and children to discuss the use of alcohol at teen parties, and suggest alternatives to driving while intoxicated or riding in a vehicle operated by an intoxicated driver.[141] The Canadian Task Force found insufficient evidence to recommend for or against counseling patients to avoid drinking and driving.[135]

Bright Futures and the AAP recommend teaching pedestrian safety to children.[132,133]

Discussion

There is good evidence that persons who use occupant protection devices or avoid driving while alcohol or drug impaired are at significantly decreased risk of injury or death from motor vehicle crashes. The evidence is less extensive that counseling by clinicians to adopt these practices is effective in changing the behavior of motorists or passengers. Since motor vehicle injury represents one of the leading causes of death in the U.S. and years of potential life lost, however, interventions of even modest effectiveness are likely to have enormous public health benefit. Most of the available evidence supports a relatively short-term effect of clinician counseling on the use of occupant restraints, indicating the need for periodic reinforcement of this message.

There is little published evidence evaluating whether changing pedestrian behavior leads to reductions in motor vehicle-related injuries or whether clinician counseling can influence pedestrian behavior. Further study is also needed on environmental controls (e.g., barriers that prevent pedestrians from crossing in the middle of dangerous roadways) that have the potential to reduce pedestrian injuries.

CLINICAL INTERVENTION

Clinicians should regularly urge their patients to use lap/shoulder belts for themselves and their passengers, and for their children who have outgrown safety seats, whenever driving or riding in an automobile, including automobiles equipped with air bags ("A" recommendation for wearing seat belts; "B" recommendation for counseling). Operators of vehicles carrying infants and toddlers should be urged to install and regularly use federally approved child safety seats in accordance with the manufacturer's instructions and the child's size ("A" recommendation for child safety seat use; "B" recommendation for counseling parents). Passengers should not ride in the cargo beds of pickup trucks. Passengers also should not ride in the cargo areas of station wagons or vans except when those areas are fitted with passenger seats and passengers are properly restrained in them with seat belts or child safety seats as appropriate for age. Clinicians may wish to inform their patients of the effectiveness of air bags as a supplement to lap/shoulder belt use in reducing motor vehicle crash-related morbidity and mortality. Rear-facing infant seats should not be placed in the front seat of a car equipped with a passenger-side air bag. Although forward-facing infant seats can be used in this situation, clinicians may wish to inform parents that the safest seating position in the car is the middle of the rear seat. Those who operate or ride on motorcycles should be counseled to wear approved safety helmets; this recommendation is based on the proven efficacy of risk reduction from wearing helmets ("A" recommendation), although the effectiveness of clinician counseling to increase helmet use has not yet been evaluated ("C" recommendation). Recommendations for bicyclists appear in Chapter 58.

All patients should be counseled regarding the dangers of operating a motor vehicle while under the influence of alcohol or other drugs, as well as the risks of riding in a vehicle operated by someone who is under the influence of these substances. This recommendation is based on the proven efficacy of risk reduction ("A" recommendation) and the effectiveness of counseling problem drinkers to reduce alcohol consumption ("B" recommendation) (see Chapter 52); the effectiveness of counseling patients to avoid drinking and driving has not been evaluated ("C" recommendation). Adolescents and young adults in particular should be encouraged to avoid using alcohol or other drugs when driving is anticipated and to discuss with their families transportation alternatives for social activities where alcohol and other drugs are used (also see Chapters 52 and 53). The optimal frequency for counseling patients about motor vehicle injury has not been determined and is left to clinical discretion. Counseling is most important for those at increased risk of motor vehicle injury, such as adolescents and young adults, persons who use alcohol or other drugs, and patients with medical conditions that may impair motor vehicle safety.

There is currently insufficient evidence to recommend for or against counseling patients or their parents in order to reduce pedestrian injuries ("C" recommendation). Recommendations for such counseling for elderly patients and for the parents of school-age and younger children may be made on other grounds, including high burden of suffering, low cost, and lack of adverse effects. One measure that may reduce pedestrian injury risk is wearing brightly colored or reflective clothing to increase visibility to motorists. Educating parents to recognize the developmental limitations on the pedestrian skills of young children and provide appropriate supervision in situations that place children at risk for pedestrian injuries may also be effective in reducing pedestrian injury risk. Although there is insufficient evidence to recommend for or against counseling regarding problem drinking and alcohol use specifically to prevent pedestrian injury ("C" recommendation), such counseling can be recommended on other grounds (see Chapter 52).

The draft update of this chapter was prepared for the U.S. Preventive Services Task Force by Natalie Smith, MD, MPH, and Carolyn DiGuiseppi, MD, MPH.

REFERENCES

1. National Center for Health Statistics. Annual summary of births, marriages, divorces, and deaths: United States, 1993. Monthly vital statistics report; vol 42, no 13 (suppl). Hyattsville, MD: Public Health Service, 1994.
2. National Highway Traffic Safety Administration. Traffic safety facts 1993. Washington, DC: Department of Transportation, 1994. (Publication DOT HS 808 169.)
3. Desenclos JA, Hahn RA. Years of potential life lost before age 65, by race, Hispanic origin, and sex—United States, 1986–1988. MMWR 1992;41(SS-6):13–23.
4. National Highway Traffic Safety Administration. Traffic safety facts 1992: a compilation of motor vehicle crash data from the Fatal Accident Reporting System and the General Estimates System. Washington, DC: Department of Transportation, 1994. (Publication DOT HS 808 022.)
5. Centers for Disease Control and Prevention. Deaths resulting from firearm- and motor-vehicle-related injuries—United States, 1968–1991. MMWR 1994;43:37–42.
6. Centers for Disease Control and Prevention. Economic impact of motor-vehicle crashes—United States, 1990. MMWR 1993;42:443–448.

7. Max W, Rice DP, MacKenzie EJ. The lifetime cost of injury. Inquiry 1990;27:332–343.
8. Barr RA. Recent changes in driving among older adults. Hum Factors 1991;33:597–600.
9. Baker SP, O'Neill B, Ginsburg MJ, et al. The injury fact book. New York: Oxford University Press, 1992.
10. Zobeck TS, Grant BF, Stinson FS, et al. Alcohol involvement in fatal traffic crashes in the United States: 1979–90. Addiction 1994;89:227–231.
11. Federal Bureau of Investigation. Uniform crime reports for the United States, 1992. Washington, DC: Government Printing Office, 1993:216–217. (Publication no. 342-498/94321.)
12. Miller TR, Blincoe JL. Incidence and cost of alcohol-involved crashes in the United States. Accid Anal Prev 1994;26:583–591.
13. Doege TC, Engelberg AL, eds. Medical conditions affecting drivers. Chicago: American Medical Association, 1986.
14. Fisher RS, Parsonage M, Beaussart M, et al. Epilepsy and driving: an international perspective. Epilepsia 1994;35: 675–684.
15. Waller JA. Injury control: a guide to causes and prevention of trauma. Lexington, MA: DC Heath, 1985.
16. McCarroll JR, Haddon W Jr. A controlled study of fatal automobile accidents in New York City. J Chronic Dis 1962;15:811–826.
17. Hurst PM. Epidemiological aspects of alcohol in driver crashes and citations. J Safety Res 1973;5:130–148.
18. National Highway Traffic Safety Administration. Alcohol and traffic safety: a review of the state of knowledge, 1978. Washington, DC: Department of Transportation, 1979. (Publication DOT HS 805 172.)
19. Howat P, Sleet D, Smith I. Alcohol and driving: is the 0.05% blood alcohol concentration limit justified? Drug Alcohol Rev 1991;10:151–166.
20. National Highway Traffic Safety Administration. Consensus report on impaired driving. Washington, DC: U.S. Department of Transportation, 1989. (Publication DOT HS-807-390.)
21. Zador PL. Alcohol-related relative risk of fatal driver injuries in relation to driver age and sex. J Stud Alcohol 1991;52:302–310.
22. Mayhew DR, Donelson AC, Beirness DJ, et al. Youth, alcohol and relative risk of crash involvement. Accid Anal Prev 1986;18:273–287.
23. AMA Council on Scientific Affairs. Alcohol and the driver. JAMA 1986;255:522–527.
24. Waller PF, Stewart JR, Hansen AR, et al. The potentiating effects of alcohol on driver injury. JAMA 1986;256: 1461–1466.
25. Andersen JA, McLellan BA, Pagliarello G, et al. The relative influence of alcohol and seatbelt usage on severity of injury from motor vehicle crashes. J Trauma 1990;30:415–417.
26. Nelson D, Sklar D, Skipper B, et al. Motorcycle fatalities in New Mexico: the association of helmet nonuse with alcohol intoxication. Ann Emerg Med 1992;21:279–283.
27. Foss RD, Beirness DJ, Sprattler K. Seat belt use among drinking drivers in Minnesota. Am J Public Health 1994;84:1732–1737.
28. Kraus JF, Morgenstern H, Fife D, et al. Blood alcohol tests, prevalence of involvement, and outcomes following brain injury. Am J Public Health 1989;79:294–299.
29. Hingson R, Heeren T, Winter M. Lower legal blood alcohol limits for young drivers. Public Health Rep 1994;109: 738–744.
30. O'Malley P, Wagenaar A. Effects of minimum drinking age laws on alcohol use, related behaviors and traffic crash involvement among American youth, 1976–1987. J Stud Alcohol 1991;52:478–491.
31. Jones NE, Pieper CF, Robertson LS. The effect of legal drinking age on fatal injuries of adolescents and young adults. Am J Public Health 1992;82:112–115.
32. Williams A, Zador P, Harris S, et al. The effect of raising the legal minimum drinking age on involvement in fatal crashes. J Leg Stud 1983;XII:169–179.
33. Smith DI. Effect on traffic safety of introducing a 0.05% blood alcohol level in Queensland, Australia. Med Sci Law 1988;28:165–170.
34. Waller JA, Turkel HW. Alcoholism and traffic deaths. N Engl J Med 1966;275:532–536.
35. Fine EW, Scoles P. Secondary prevention of alcoholism using a population of offenders arrested for driving while intoxicated. Ann NY Acad Sci 1976;273:637–645.
36. Brewer RD, Morris PD, Cole TB, et al. The risk of dying in alcohol-related automobile crashes among habitual drunk drivers. N Engl J Med 1994;331:513–517.
37. Andreasson S, Romelsjo A, Allebeck P. Alcohol, social factors and mortality among young men. Br J Addict 1991; 86:877–887.

38. Schmidt W, Smart RG, Popham RE. The role of alcoholism in motor vehicle accidents. Traffic Safety Res 1962;6: 21–27.

39. Williams AF, Peat MA, Crouch DJ, et al. Drugs in fatally injured young male drivers. Public Health Rep 1985;100: 19–25.

40. National Highway Traffic Safety Administration. Use of controlled substances and highway safety: a report to Congress. Washington, DC: Department of Transportation, 1988. (Publication DOT HS 807 261.)

41. Marzuk PM, Tardiff K, Leon AC. Prevalence of recent cocaine use among motor vehicle fatalities in New York City. JAMA 1990;263:250–256.

42. Kirby JM, Maull KI, Fain W. Comparability of alcohol and drug use in injured drivers. South Med J 1992;85: 800–802.

43. Soderstrom CA, Trifillis AL, Shankar BS, et al. Marijuana and alcohol use among 1023 trauma patients: a prospective study. Arch Surg 1988;123:733–737.

44. Brookoff D, Cook CS, Williams C, et al. Testing reckless drivers for cocaine and marijuana. N Engl J Med 1994;331: 518–522.

45. Rafaelson OJ, Bech P, Christiansen J, et al. Cannabis and alcohol: effects on simulated car driving. Science 1973;179:920–923.

46. Moskowitz H, Hulbert S, McGlothin WH. Marijuana: effects on simulated driving performance. Accid Anal Prev 1976;8:45–50.

47. Smily A, Moskowitz HM, Ziedman K, et al. Effects of drugs on driving: driving simulator tests of secobarbital, diazepam, marijuana, and alcohol. Washington, DC: Department of Health and Human Services, 1985. (Publication no. (ADM) 85-1386.)

48. Newman RJ. A prospective evaluation of the protective effect of car seatbelts. J Trauma 1986;26: 561–564.

49. Campbell BJ. Safety belt injury reduction related to crash severity and front seated position. J Trauma 1987;27: 733–739.

50. Orsay EM, Turnbull TL, Dunne M, et al. Prospective study of the effect of safety belts on morbidity and health care costs in motor-vehicle accidents. JAMA 1988;260:3598–3603.

51. McGee DL, Rhodes P. Estimating trends in the effectiveness of seat belts in saving lives, 1975–1985. Stat Med 1989;8:379–385.

52. Marine WM, Kerwin EM, Moore EE, et al. Mandatory seatbelts: epidemiologic, financial, and medical rationale from the Colorado matched pairs study. J Trauma 1994;36:96–100.

53. Cooper PJ. Estimating overinvolvement of seat belt nonwearers in crashes and the effect of lap/shoulder restraint use on different crash severity consequences. Accid Anal Prev 1994;26:263–275.

54. Department of Transportation. Final regulatory impact assessment on amendments to Federal Motor Vehicle Safety Standard 208, Front Seat Occupant Protection. Washington, DC: Department of Transportation, 1984. (Publication DOT HS 806 572.)

55. Reinfurt DW, Campbell BJ, Stewart JR, et al. Evaluating the North Carolina safety belt wearing law. Accid Anal Prev 1990;22:197–210.

56. States JD, Annechiarico RP, Good RG, et al. A time comparison study of the New York State safety belt use law utilizing hospital admission and police accident report information. Accid Anal Prev 1990;22:509–521.

57. Wagenaar AC, Margolis LH. Effects of a mandatory safety belt law on hospital admissions. Accid Anal Prev 1990; 22:235–261.

58. Campbell BJ, Stewart JR, Reinfurt DW. Change in injuries associated with safety belt laws. Accid Anal Prev 1991; 23:87–93.

59. Lestina DC, Williams AF, Lund AK, et al. Motor vehicle crash injury patterns and the Virginia seat belt law. JAMA 1991;265:1409–1413.

60. Decker MD, Dewey MJ, Hutcheson RH, et al. The use and efficacy of child restraint devices: the Tennessee experience, 1982 and 1983. JAMA 1984;252:2571–2575.

61. Scherz R. Fatal motor vehicle accidents of child passengers from birth through 4 years of age in Washington State. Pediatrics 1981;68:572–575.

62. Kahane C. An evaluation of child passenger safety: the effectiveness and benefits of safety seats. Washington, DC: Department of Transportation, 1986. (Publication DOT HS 806 890.)

63. Centers for Disease Control. Child passenger restraint use and motor-vehicle-related fatalities among children—United States, 1982–1990. MMWR 1991;40:600–602.

64. Johnston C, Rivara FP, Soderberg R. Children in car crashes: analysis of data for injury and use of restraints. Pediatrics 1994;93:960–965.
65. Margolis LH, Wagenaar AC, Liu W, et al. The effects of mandatory child restraint law on injuries requiring hospitalization. Am J Dis Child 1988;142:1099–1103.
66. Agran PF, Dunkle DE, Winn DG. Motor vehicle childhood injuries caused by noncrash falls or ejections. JAMA 1985;253:2530–2533.
67. Margolis LH, Wagenaar AC, Molnar LJ. Use and misuse of automobile child restraint devices. Am J Dis Child 1992;146:361–366.
68. American Academy of Pediatrics, Society of Automotive Engineers and Centers for Disease Control and Prevention. Warning on interaction between air bags and rear-facing child restraints. MMWR 1993;42:280–282.
69. National Highway Traffic Safety Administration. Traffic safety facts 1993: occupant protection. Washington, DC: U.S. Department of Transportation, 1994.
70. Federal motor vehicle safety standard occupant crash protection: final rule. Fed Reg 1984;49:28962–29010.
71. Evans L. Restraint effectiveness, occupant ejection from cars, and fatality reductions. Accid Anal Prev 1990;22:167–175.
72. Zador PL, Ciccone MA. Automobile driver fatalities in frontal impacts: air bags compared to manual belts. Am J Public Health 1993;83:661–666.
73. Smith GR, Gulash EC, Baker RG. Human volunteer and anthropomorphic dummy tests of driver air cushion system. Clin Plast Surg 1975;2:35–45.
74. Huelke DF, Moore JL. Field investigations of the performance of air bag deployments in frontal collisions. Accid Anal Prev 1993;25:717–730.
75. National Highway Traffic Safety Administration. A report to the Congress on the effect of motorcycle helmet use repeal—a case report for helmet use. Washington, DC: Department of Transportation, 1980.
76. Offner PJ, Rivara FP, Maier RV. The impact of motorcycle helmet use. J Trauma 1992;32:636–641.
77. Rutledge R, Stutts J. The association of helmet use with the outcome of motorcycle crash injury when controlling for crash/injury severity. Accid Anal Prev 1993;25:347–353.
78. McSwain NE, Belles A. Motorcycle helmets—medical costs and the law. J Trauma 1990;30:1189–1197.
79. Sosin DM, Sacks JJ, Holmgreen P. Head injury-associated deaths from motorcycle crashes. JAMA 1990;264: 2395–2399.
80. Sosin DM, Sacks JJ. Motorcycle helmet-use laws and head injury prevention. JAMA 1992;267:1649–1651.
81. Fleming NS, Becker ER. The impact of the Texas 1989 motorcycle helmet law on total and head-related fatalities, severe injuries, and overall injuries. Med Care 1992;30:832–845.
82. Kraus JF, Peek C, McArthur DL, et al. The effect of the 1992 California motorcycle helmet use law on motorcycle crash fatalities and injuries. JAMA 1994;272:1506–1511.
83. Kraus JF, Peek C, Williams A. Compliance with the 1992 California motorcycle helmet use law. Am J Public Health 1995;85:96–99.
84. Chenier TC, Evans L. Motorcyclist fatalities and the repeal of mandatory helmet wearing laws. Accid Anal Prev 1987;19:133–139.
85. Malek M, Guyer B, Lescohier I. The epidemiology and prevention of child pedestrian injury. Accid Anal Prev 1990;22:301–313.
86. Pitt R, Guyer B, Hsieh C, et al. The severity of pedestrian injuries in children: an analysis of the pedestrian injury causation study. Accid Anal Prev 1990;22:549–559.
87. Rivara FP. Child pedestrian injuries in the United States. Am J Dis Child 1990;144:692–696.
88. Roberts IG, Keall MD, Frith WJ. Pedestrian exposure and the risk of child pedestrian injury. J Paediatr Child Health 1994;30:220–223.
88a. National Highway Traffic Safety Administration and Centers for Disease Control and Prevention. Motor vehicle-related deaths involving intoxicated pedestrians—United States, 1982–1992. MMWR 1994;43:249–253.
89. Harrell WA. Perception of risk and curb standing at street corners by older pedestrians. Percept Motor Skill 1990;70:1363–1366.
90. Harrell WA. Precautionary street crossing by elderly pedestrians. Int J Aging Hum Dev 1991;32: 65–80.
91. Hoxie RE, Rubenstein LZ. Are older pedestrians allowed enough time to cross intersections safely? J Am Geriatr Soc 1994;42:241–244.

92. Rivara FP, Bergman AB, Drake C. Parental attitudes and practices toward children as pedestrians. Pediatrics 1989;84:1017–1021.

93. Dunne RG, Asher KN, Rivara FP. Behavior and parental expectations of child pedestrians. Pediatrics 1992;89:486–490.

94. Hazlett RD, Allen MJ. The ability to see a pedestrian at night: the effects of clothing, retroreflectorization and driver intoxication. Am J Optom Arch Am Acad Optom 1968;45:246–257.

95. Ferguson SA, Preusser DF, Lund AK, et al. Daylight saving time and motor vehicle crashes: the reduction in pedestrian and vehicle occupant fatalities. Am J Public Health 1995;85:92–96.

96. Shinar D. Actual versus estimated nighttime pedestrian visibility. Ergonomics 1984;27:863–871.

97. Shinar D. The effects of expectancy, clothing reflection and detection criterion on nighttime pedestrian visibility. Hum Factors 1985;27:327–333.

98. Harrell WA. Effects of pedestrians' visibility and signs on motorists' yielding. Percept Motor Skills 1994;78:355–362.

98a. Smith PF, Remington PL. The epidemiology of drinking and driving: results from the behavioral risk factor surveillance system, 1986. Health Educ Q 1989;16:345–358.

99. National Highway Traffic Safety Administration. Nineteen-city safety belt and child safety seat use observational survey. Washington, DC: Department of Transportation, February 1989.

100. Centers for Disease Control. Child passenger restraint use and motor-vehicle-related fatalities among children—United States, 1982–1990. MMWR 1991;40:600–602.

101. National Highway Traffic Safety Administration. Traffic safety facts 1992—motorcycles. Washington, DC: Department of Transportation, 1993.

102. Colquitt M, Fielding LP, Cronan JF. Drunk drivers and medical and social injury. N Engl J Med 1987;317: 1262–1266.

103. Worden JK, Flynn BS, Merrill DG, et al. Preventing alcohol-impaired driving through community self-regulation training. Am J Public Health 1989;79:287–290.

104. Bass JL, Christoffel KK, Widome M, et al. Childhood injury prevention counseling in primary care settings: a critical review of the literature. Pediatrics 1993;92:544–550.

105. Bass JL, Wilson TR. The pediatrician's influence in private practice measured by a controlled seat belt study. Pediatrics 1964;33:700–704.

106. Macknin ML, Gustafson C, Gassman J, et al. Office education by pediatricians to increase seat belt use. Am J Dis Child 1987;141:1305–1307.

107. Logsdon DN, Lazaro CM, Meier RV. The feasibility of behavioral risk reduction in primary medical care. Am J Prev Med 1989;5:249–256.

108. Kelly RB. Effect of a brief physician intervention on seat belt use. J Fam Pract 1987;24:630–632.

109. Weinstein ND, Grubb PD, Vautier JS. Increasing automobile seat belt use: an intervention emphasizing risk susceptibility. J Appl Psychol 1986;71:285–290.

110. Allen DB, Bergman AB. Social learning approaches to health education: utilization of infant auto restraint devices. Pediatrics 1976;58:323–328.

111. Kanthor HA. Car safety for infants: effectiveness of prenatal counseling. Pediatrics 1976;58:320–322.

112. Scherz RG. Restraint systems for the prevention of injury to children in automobile accidents. Am J Public Health 1976;66:451–455.

113. Reisinger KS, Williams AF, Wells JK, et al. Effect of pediatricians' counseling on infant restraint use. Pediatrics 1981;67:201–206.

114. Kelly B, Sein C, McCarthy PL. Safety education in a pediatric primary care setting. Pediatrics 1987; 79:818–824.

115. Greenberg LW, Coleman AB. A prenatal and postpartum safety education program: influence on parental use of infant car restraints. J Dev Behav Pediatr 1982;3:32–34.

116. Christophersen ER, Sullivan MA. Increasing the protection of newborn infants in cars. Pediatrics 1982;70:21–25.

117. Robitaille Y, Legault J, Abbey H, et al. Evaluation of an infant car seat program in a low-income community. Am J Dis Child 1990;144:74–78.

118. Reisinger KS, Williams AF. Evaluation of programs to increase the protection of infants in cars. Pediatrics 1978;62:280–287.

119. Miller JR, Pless IB. Child automobile restraints: evaluation of health education. Pediatrics 1977;59:907–911.

120. Berger LR, Saunders S, Armitage K, et al. Promoting the use of car safety devices for infants: an intensive health education approach. Pediatrics 1984;74:16–19.
121. Guyer B, Gallagher SS, Chang BH, et al. Prevention of childhood injuries: evaluation of the Statewide Childhood Injury Prevention Program (SCIPP). Am J Public Health 1989;79:1521–1527.
122. Rivara FP, Booth CL, Bergman AB, et al. Prevention of pedestrian injuries to children: effectiveness of a school training program. Pediatrics 1991;88:770–775.
123. Renaus L, Suissa S. Evaluation of the efficacy of simulation games in traffic safety education of kindergarten children. Am J Public Health 1989;79:307–309.
124. Yeaton WH, Bailey JS. Teaching pedestrian safety skills to young children: an analysis and one-year followup. J Appl Behav Anal 1978;11:315–329.
125. Preusser DF, Blomberg RD. Reducing child pedestrian accidents through public education. J Safety Res 1984;15: 47–56.
126. Preusser DF, Lund AK. And Keep on Looking: a film to reduce pedestrian crashes among 9 to 12 year olds. J Safety Res 1988;19:177–185.
127. American Medical Association. Resolution no. 62 (A-84): seat belts and survival in auto accidents. Chicago: American Medical Association, 1984.
128. American Medical Association. Guidelines for adolescent preventive services (GAPS). Chicago: American Medical Association, 1994.
129. American College of Physicians. Health promotion/disease prevention: seat belt use. Philadelphia: American College of Physicians, 1984.
130. Hayward RS, Steinberg EP, Ford DE, et al. Prevention care guidelines: 1991. Ann Intern Med 1991;114:758–783.
131. American Academy of Family Physicians. Age charts for periodic health examination. Kansas City, MO: American Academy of Family Physicians, 1994. (Reprint no. 510.)
132. Committee on Injury and Poison Prevention, American Academy of Pediatrics. Office-based counseling on injury prevention. Pediatrics 1994;94:566–567.
133. Green M, ed. Bright Futures: national guidelines for health supervision of infants, children, and adolescents. Arlington, VA: National Center for Education in Maternal and Child Health, 1994.
134. American College of Obstetricians and Gynecologists. Automobile passenger restraints for children and pregnant women. Technical Bulletin no. 151. Washington, DC: American College of Obstetricians and Gynecologists, 1991.
135. Canadian Task Force on the Periodic Health Examination. Canadian guide to clinical preventive health care. Ottawa: Canada Communication Group, 1994:514–524.
135a. U.S. Department of Health and Human Services. Healthy People 2000: national health promotion and disease prevention objectives. Washington, DC: Public Health Service, 1991. (DHHS Publication no. (PHS) 91-50212.)
136. Steed D. The case for safety belt use. JAMA 1988;260:3651.
137. Committee on Accident and Poison Prevention, American Academy of Pediatrics. Safe transportation of newborns discharged from the hospital. Pediatrics 1990;86:486–487.
138. National Highway Traffic Safety Administration. Facts about motorcycle crashes and safety helmet use. Washington, DC: Department of Transportation, 1994. (Publication no. NTS-23.)
139. Council on Scientific Affairs, American Medical Association. Helmets and preventing motorcycle- and bicycle-related injuries. JAMA 1994;272:1535–1538.
140. National Highway Traffic Safety Administration. Alcohol involvement in fatal traffic crashes—1992. Washington, DC: Department of Transportation, 1994. (Publication DOT HS 808 094.)
141. Committee on Adolescence. Alcohol use and abuse: a pediatric concern. Pediatrics 1987;79:450–453.
142. Brewer RD, Sleet DA. Alcohol and injuries: time for action. Arch Fam Med 1995;4:499–500.

58. Counseling to Prevent Household and Recreational Injuries

RECOMMENDATION

Periodic counseling of the parents of children on measures to reduce the risk of unintentional household and recreational injuries is recommended. Counseling to prevent household and recreational injuries is also recommended for adolescents and adults based on the proven efficacy of risk reduction, although the effectiveness of counseling these patients to prevent injuries has not been adequately evaluated. Persons with alcohol or drug problems should be identified, counseled, and monitored (see Chapters 52 and 53). Those who use alcohol or illicit drugs should be warned against engaging in potentially dangerous activities while intoxicated. Counseling elderly patients on specific measures to prevent falls is recommended based on fair evidence that these measures reduce the risk of falls, although the effectiveness of counseling elders to prevent falls has not been adequately evaluated. More intensive individualized multifactorial intervention is recommended for high-risk elderly patients in settings where adequate resources to deliver such services are available. There is insufficient evidence to recommend for or against the use of external hip protectors to prevent fall injuries. Counseling to prevent motor vehicle and pedestrian injuries is discussed in Chapter 57.

Burden of Suffering

Unintentional injuries accounted for nearly 89,000 deaths (34.4/100,000 population) in the U.S. in 1993, making them the fifth leading cause of death.[1] Although the age-adjusted unintentional injury death rate has declined by 28% since 1979,[2] such injuries remain the leading cause of death in all age groups from 1 to 34 years[1] and the leading cause of years of potential life lost before age 65.[3] In the U.S. in 1992, injuries accounted for 2.7 million hospitalizations (10.7/1,000 population),[4] 34 million emergency department visits,[5] and 62 million visits to office-based physicians and hospital outpatient departments (nearly 10% of all such visits).[6,7] The lifetime economic cost for injuries that occurred in the U.S. in 1985, updated to 1988, has been estimated at $182 billion.[8] Almost half of all unintentional injury-related deaths occur in motor vehicle crashes (see Chapter 57).[1] The remainder, about 48,000 each year,[1] are household, recreational, and other unintentional injuries. Falls, poisoning, fires and burns, drowning, suffocation and aspiration, firearms, and bicycling cause nearly two thirds of these deaths.[9] Almost 90% of deaths relating to sports and recreation occur during swimming, boating, bicycling, riding off-road vehicles such as all-terrain vehicles (ATVs), or using firearms.[9]

Each year about 12,000 Americans, primarily older persons, die as a result of **falls**.[9] Falls are the second leading cause of unintentional injury death in the U.S. (after motor vehicle injuries) and the leading cause of nonfatal injuries.[5,9,10] The death rate due to falls in the general population is 5.1/100,000 persons, increasing to 10.2/100,000 for those aged 65–74 and to 147.0/100,000 for persons aged 85 and over.[10] Population-based studies of community-dwelling elderly persons have estimated an annual total injurious fall rate of 229/1,000 persons,[11] serious fall injury rate of 84–96/1,000,[12] and fall injury hospitalization rate of 13.5/1,000.[13] Half of serious fall injury events in elderly persons result in discharge to a nursing home.[12] Hip fractures are an especially grave complication of falls in older adults, resulting in more hospital admissions than any other injury, and accounting for 254,000 hospital admissions in 1988.[9] There is a 10–20% reduction in expected survival in the first year following a hip fracture,[14–17] and roughly half of survivors never recover normal function.[15]

Unintentional **poisonings**, the third leading cause of unintentional injury deaths, account for 5,300 deaths each year, the vast majority of these among adults.[9] The mortality rate for poisonings among children 0–4 years of age was 0.2/100,000 in 1988, a >90% decline from 1960.[9] **Fires and burns** are the fourth leading cause of unintentional injury death in the U.S. Each year, fires and burns are responsible for at least 5,000 deaths and 1.4 million injuries.[9] Residential fires account for 73% of these deaths. The lifetime cost of fire and burn injuries occurring in 1985 was estimated to be $3.8 billion.[8] Nearly 5,000 Americans die each year by **drowning**, including 1,000 boating-related drownings.[9] Death rates from drowning are highest in children <5 years old and in young men aged 15–24 years.[10,18,19] It has been estimated that for each childhood drowning fatality, about 4 children are hospitalized and 14 are seen in the emergency department and released.[19] From 1971 to 1988, drowning rates declined substantially among older children and adolescents, but declined only slightly in toddlers and actually increased in infants.[18] Some 4,700 deaths attributable to **mechanical suffocation** (e.g., strangulation on clothing) and **aspiration** of food and other foreign materials occur annually, most of these in infants and in elderly persons.[9] **Firearm injuries** resulted in 1,740 unintentional deaths (5% of all firearm fatalities) in 1993,[1] and cause 12,000 to 30,000 nonfatal injuries each year.[9,20,21] BB guns and other air-powered firearms are estimated to injure an additional 19,500–34,500 people each year.[21] **Bicycling injuries** accounted for about 550,000 emergency room visits and 1,000 deaths annually between 1984 and 1988, mostly in children and adolescents.[22] The injury rate has been estimated at 187/100,000 and the head injury rate at 51–75/100,000, with peak rates occurring among children aged 5–14 years.[22,23] Data regarding bicyclists involved in traffic crashes suggest declines in both injuries and fatalities in the last 5 years.[24] Between 1982 and 1988 more than 1,100 fatalities and 400,000 emergency room-treated injuries related to ATVs were reported to the Consumer Product Safety Commission.[25]

Efficacy of Risk Reduction

Certain injury-specific risk factors have been identified for household and recreational injuries. These are discussed below. In general, injury control strategies based on these risk factors are derived from evidence of association observed in retrospective studies rather than from prospective trials demonstrating efficacy. There have been only a few cohort studies or clinical trials measuring the impact on injury rates of eliminating risk factors for household and recreational injuries.

Children. **Fires and burns** were the second leading cause of unintentional injury-related death among children aged 0–9 years in 1991.[26] Most injuries and 75–90% of deaths from fires occur in residential fires.[27,28] The risk of fatality in the event of a house fire is significantly increased when children <5 years old are present in the household.[29] Smoke detectors are effective in preventing deaths in residential fires. Death in a residential fire is 2–3 times more likely in homes without smoke detectors than in those with such devices.[29–31] Smoke detectors often fail to operate, however, due to incorrect installation or inadequate testing.[28,32] Correct installation and periodic testing are necessary to ensure proper operation.

Measures to prevent residential fires from occurring are also important for reducing fire and burn injuries. Residential fires occur more frequently in the winter, associated with the use of portable heaters, fireplaces, and Christmas trees.[26,29] Some attention has been given to the hazards of certain stoves and heaters,[33] but the effectiveness of clinical intervention to reduce these hazards has not been evaluated. Cigarette smoking by household members is a leading cause of residential fires, many of which may be preventable (see *Adolescents and Adults,* below). A large proportion of residential fire deaths in children <5 years of age is caused by children playing with matches and lighters.[26] The development of child-resistant cigarette lighters has been proposed as a preventive measure.[34] For children, wearing flame-retardant clothing is effective in reducing injury from clothing ignition due to, for example, residential fires, cigarettes, matches, or lighters.[10,35,36]

Hot tap water burns, which account for 2,600 hospitalizations each year and 24% of all scald burn hospitalizations in children, are preventable by setting household water heaters at or below 120–130°F.[10,37–39] Anti-scald devices can be installed to cut off water flow when the water temperature exceeds 120°F, although their efficacy in reducing burn rates has not been evaluated adequately. In one pilot study, 85% of such devices had been removed within 9 months of installation because of sediment build-up, and there were too few outcomes to assess any impact on scald burn rates.[40]

The causes of **drowning**, and thus preventive strategies, depend on the age of the patient. In small children, 40–90% of drownings (depending on locale) occur in swimming pools, usually located in the victim's backyard.[41–47] In about two thirds of these cases, the children are supervised by one or both parents at the time of drowning and the adult caretakers are unaware that the toddler has wandered near the pool or entered the water.[42,46,48] Observational studies suggest that 50–80% of such drownings can be prevented by enclosing swimming pools with 4-foot, four-sided fences with self-latching, self-closing gates that isolate the pool from the house and yard ("isolation fences") to protect children from wandering into the pool area.[42,48–52a] Some have recommended infant and toddler swimming lessons as a means of improving survival after submersion. The effectiveness of lessons at this age has never been proved convincingly, however;[53] their safety has been questioned on the basis of case reports of water intoxication and hyponatremia.[54] Bathtub-related drowning is an important problem in children <5 years old.[55] The majority of infant drownings occur in bathtubs.[46,47] These drownings are often associated with a history of inadequate supervision.[46,47,55] Interventions to improve bathing supervision have not been evaluated, however. Immediate initiation of cardiopulmonary resuscitation (CPR) in children with submersion injury has been associated with improved outcome,[44,48,56,57] suggesting that CPR training for pool owners, parents, and children's caretakers may reduce the likelihood of drowning or neurologic injury after submersion.

Among children under 15 years, 35–40% of **firearm** deaths are unintentional.[21] Over 90% of firearm incidents involving children occur at home; a study in children aged 0–14 years found that 40% involved a firearm stored in the room where the shooting occurred.[58] Persons who keep guns for the purpose of protection are more likely to keep their guns loaded,[59] but for each case of a firearm being successfully used for self-protection (i.e., shooting an intruder), firearms in the home are estimated to be 1.3–6 times more likely to cause an unintentional fatality and 10 times more likely to cause an unintentional injury, many of these in children.[21,60] The U.S. General Accounting Office estimated that nearly one third of unintentional firearm deaths might be prevented by the use of trigger locks and loading indicators.[61] These and other potential clinical preventive strategies to prevent firearm injuries (e.g., removing guns from the home, storing weapons unloaded and in a locked compartment) would appear to be effective but have not been studied adequately. Receipt of firearm training (usually covering firearm storage) has been associated with an increased likelihood of storing guns loaded and unlocked.[59] It is unknown whether this increase was because the training was ineffective, did not teach appropriate storage, or was received by persons who were inherently less likely to store firearms safely than were those who did not receive training. The association between firearm availability and violent injury is discussed in Chapters 50 and 59.

A substantial proportion of childhood **poisonings** can be prevented by keeping medications in child-resistant containers. Federal legislation requiring such containers for aspirin, acetaminophen, prescription drugs, and household chemicals has been associated with a subsequent decrease in childhood poisoning from these substances.[62–64] Poisoning with children's aspirin has also been reduced by limiting the number of tablets packaged in each bottle.[62,65] In contrast, poison-warning labels designed for children do not appear to be efficacious. Controlled trials have demonstrated that poison warning stickers (such as the "Mr. Yuk" series) do not deter children from playing with medication containers[66] or reduce the rate of childhood poisoning.[67] The use of aversive bittering agents may reduce ingestion of the substance to which the agent was added,[68,69] but the ability of these agents to reduce the incidence or severity of childhood poisoning is unproven.[70]

Bicycling injuries are important causes of morbidity and mortality, particularly among school-age children.[22] Nearly half of all Americans and 80–90% of U.S. children ride bicycles.[71,71a] Potential interventions include wearing safety helmets, having bicycle safety training, and avoiding riding near motor vehicle traffic. Between 50% and 85% of bicycle fatalities and hospitalizations are the result of head trauma.[22,72,73] Cross-sectional studies of persons involved in bicycling crashes suggest that bicycle helmets reduce head injuries by at least 40%.[74–77] Case-control studies estimate that the risk of head injury among bicyclists is reduced by 63–85% by the use of bicycle helmets.[78,79] Control for factors such as estimated crash severity, motor vehicle involvement, non-head injury severity, rider experience or age, or other sociodemographic characteristics, did not eliminate the protective effect of bicycle helmets found in these studies.[78,79] In multiple time-series studies, mandatory bicycle helmet use laws and community-based education programs have been associated with substantial increases in helmet use and with reductions in bicycle-related fatalities, head-injuries, and hospitalizations.[80–84] These studies provide strong support for the routine use of helmets while bicycling.

An additional potential intervention to prevent bicycling injuries, bicycle safety training, is suggested by surveys showing that many bicycle crashes among children result from cyclist error.[79,85–87] One small controlled trial in children aged 8–9 years reported a positive short-term effect of training on bicycling behavior,[88] but no controlled studies have evaluated the effectiveness of formal training in preventing crashes or injury. A recommendation for counseling bicyclists to avoid riding near motor vehicle traffic is based on evidence that some 95% of bicycle fatalities occur as a result of a collision with a motor vehicle.[72,73] Efforts to separate bicyclists from motor vehicle traffic, such as designated bicycle lanes and paths, have met with some success in reducing bicycle crashes,[89] although a meta-analysis based on cross-sectional and before-after studies suggested that bicycle paths may increase the risk to bicyclists at certain intersections.[90]

In children under age 5, **falls** are a common cause of injury, although few of these injuries lead to death or permanent sequelae.[9,91] These injuries often involve falls from stairs or furniture.[92] Baby walkers are an important cause of injuries in young children, many of which result from falls down stairs.[93–95] Collapsible gates have been advocated as a means of protecting children from stairways,[92] although the efficacy of stairway gates has not been studied. Children can fall from windows even when there are screens in place. There is evidence that window guards can reduce child falls from apartment windows.[96]

Adolescents and Adults. Intoxication with **alcohol or other drugs** and problem drinking are important risk factors for injuries and injury deaths.[9,29,97–104] In addition to its role in motor vehicle crashes, which has been most thoroughly studied (see Chapter 57), alcohol intoxication is involved in 40% of all fatal fires and burns and an estimated 25–50% of adolescent and adult deaths from drowning, boating mishaps, and shootings, and is also associated with asphyxiation by choking.[9,10,47,105–108] Problem drinking by mothers has been associated with increased risk of serious injury in their children.[108a] Chronic alcohol abuse is a risk factor for poorer health outcome when trauma does occur.[109] In national surveys, 30% of all high-school students had had five or more drinks on at least one occasion (i.e., episodic heavy drinking) during the preceding 30 days,[110] and 5% of adults reported regular heavy drinking (more than five drinks per day more than five times per week).[111] The large body of evidence linking alcohol intoxication to injuries, and the high prevalence of heavy drinking, argues strongly for screening for problem drinking (see Chapter 52) and for counseling on the safe use of alcohol as important measures to prevent injuries.

The highest unintentional **poisoning** mortality rate occurs in young adult men (20–39 years of age), who account for 40% of unintentional poisoning deaths.[112] A large proportion of these deaths are attributable to overdoses of alcohol, heroin, and cocaine,[9,112] at least some of which may be preventable by identification and treatment of problem drinking and illicit drug abuse (see Chapters 52 and 53). Intentional self-poisoning is discussed in Chapter 50.

Drownings of adolescents and adults are most common among young males, and occur under different circumstances from those of toddlers.[18,19,47,113] Most such drowning occurs in lakes, rivers, and ponds in association with water activities, including swimming, diving, boating, and fishing.[47,113,114] The highest rate of fatal recreational boating incidents occurs in adolescents (8.1/million operator-hours compared to 1.0/million for all ages).[115] Intoxication by alcohol or other drugs is common in both drowning and boating mishaps; about 25–50% of all victims have a significant blood alcohol level, and as many as 10% have evidence of other drugs with central nervous system effects.[47,113,116,117] In a national survey of adolescents and adults who participated in aquatic activities, 42% had used alcohol during such activities, with males aged 16–20 reporting the highest level of alcohol consumption.[118] Discouraging swimming or boating while intoxicated would therefore appear to be appropriate, but there has been little research on the impact of such a clinical intervention. More than three fourths of boating-related drownings are associated with nonuse of personal flotation devices,[119] but there are few data on the impact of promoting the use of these devices. Higher rates of fatal recreational boating incidents have been associated with fewer hours of operator experience, suggesting that supervised experience and training programs might be beneficial in preventing drowning, but these have not been evaluated.[115] Swimming lessons may also offer some protection against drowning, but this has never been proved convincingly.

Most unintentional injuries from **firearms** involve adolescent and young adult males, with the highest rate of unintentional firearm deaths (3.4/100,000) occurring in males aged 15–24.[1,21] Unintentional firearm death rates are 4 times higher in rural compared with suburban and urban settings,[9] which probably reflects increased gun ownership for hunting and recreation.[120] After the home, where at least 65% of unintentional firearm injuries occur (see *Children*, above), the most common location for unintentional firearm injuries is the hunting site.[10] In 1987, 9.2 firearm injuries were reported per 100,000 hunting licenses sold.[121] These incidents often involve members of the same hunting party and result from accidental discharge or unsafe handling of the firearm, and from the victim being out of sight or mistaken for game.[53,123] In a small sample of unintentional self-inflicted hunting fatalities, one third of victims had positive blood alcohol concentrations.[123] National data suggest that one-fourth of injured hunters are <21 years of age.[121] One population-based study found that 40% of shooters in hunting accidents were less than 20 years of age and fewer than half were supervised by adults; unsafe hunting practices such as carrying the firearm incorrectly were significantly more common in shooters who were 8–19 years of age.[123] Hunting firearm injuries might be reduced by adult supervision of child and adolescent hunters and by wearing fluorescent orange clothing while hunting to increase visibility, but the effectiveness of these measures has not been studied adequately. Education programs for hunters on the safe use of firearms have had mixed effects on fatality rates.[53]

Cigarette smoking is a leading cause of **fire and burn** injuries and fatalities.[29,124,124a] Cigarette smoking causes about 25% of residential fires, usually through unintentional ignition of bedding or upholstery. Smoke detectors are effective interventions for preventing fire and burn injuries and deaths in adults as well as children (see *Children*, above). Many advocate counseling regarding careless smoking practices and the promotion of self-extinguishing cigarettes, neither of which has been adequately evaluated.

Bicycle deaths and head injuries remain an important problem in older adolescents and young adults, with nearly 400 deaths and more than 150,000 injuries occurring each year among persons aged 15–39.[22] Use of bicycle helmets is an effective preventive intervention (see *Children*, above), yet only 7% of older adolescents and 18% of all bicyclists wear bicycle helmets sometimes or always.[110,124b] ATV injuries primarily occur in adolescence and young adulthood. A multivariate analysis based on nationally reported data on ATV injuries suggested that given a crash resulting in injury, helmet use reduces the risk of death by about 42%.[125] Similar analyses have reported reduced risks from ATVs with smaller engines and four rather than three wheels.[125,126] In 1987, the marketing and sale of three-wheeled ATVs was banned (although those already in use were not recalled), changes were made in marketing to reduce sales of larger-engined machines to children and adolescents, and educational features such as safety warnings and rebates for safety education were introduced.[127] These interventions have been associated with a decline in injury rates (but not fatalities).[127]

Elderly Adults. **Falls** are the leading cause of nonfatal injuries and unintentional injury deaths in older persons in the U.S.[9,10] Physiological changes with age and environmental agents are the principal risk factors for falls in older persons. Among the physiological factors that have been associated with falls are postural instability, gait disturbances, diminished muscle strength and proprioception, poor vision, cognitive impairment, number of medications, and the use of psychoactive and antihypertensive drugs.[11,128–136] Frail elderly persons, who have multiple physiologic deficiencies, are at significantly increased risk for falls compared with vigorous older persons.[137] Environmental risk factors identified retrospectively by fallers as contributory include stairs, pavement irregularities, slippery surfaces (including loose rugs), inadequate lighting, unexpected objects, low chairs, and incorrect footwear.[128,129,138-140] Controlled studies have not consistently reported significant associations between falls and environmental hazards when adjustments are made for other risk factors;[128-130,137] several studies suggest that risk from home hazards may vary with underlying functional status.[137,141] Among the risk factors associated with injury after a fall are osteoporosis (see Chapter 46), syncope, impaired cognitive function, use of diuretics or vasodilators, and falling on hard surfaces such as concrete.[129,134,142] These physiological and environmental risk factors for falls and fall injuries serve as the basis for potential preventive interventions: exercise programs to enhance strength, balance and mobility; external protection against falls on hard surfaces; monitoring and adjustment of medications; correction of environmental hazards; and measures to increase bone density (see Chapters 46 and 68). Several trials have evaluated the ability of various measures to reduce falls or risk factors for falls. The efficacy of these measures in preventing fall injuries and consequent deterioration in ambulatory function has not been fully evaluated.

Randomized controlled trials of exercise programs for elderly persons have generally shown improved strength and mobility; effects on balance have been less consistent.[143-148] Two controlled trials of exercise programs for elderly ambulatory or institutionalized persons found no reduction in falls (although this was not a primary outcome in the latter study).[143,144] These exercise programs may have been inadequate, however, since neither study reported significantly improved strength or balance as a result of the intervention. A preplanned meta-analysis of individual data from seven randomized controlled trials concluded that interventions that included an exercise component reduced the adjusted risk of falling by 10% in elderly subjects.[149] Of the exercise components studied (resistance, balance, endurance, flexibility), only balance training had a significant individual effect on risk of falls. The types and modes of exercise were not standardized across trials, however. Since fall assessment was based on self-report and patients were not blinded to the intervention, the possibility of biased results exists. The meta-analysis suggested a slight nonsignificant increase in the risk of injurious falls with exercise; neither the individual trials nor the meta-analysis had sufficient sample size to assess adequately the effect of exercise on injurious falls.

Only one study has evaluated external protection against falls on hard surfaces. In a trial evaluating external hip protectors fixed in special undergarments, the risk of hip fracture was reduced by 56% among elderly men and women who were resident on nursing home wards that were randomly assigned to receive the protectors.[150] None of the eight intervention subjects who had a hip fracture wore the protectors at the time of the fracture; compliance with regular wearing was only 24%. Ward assignment of new arrivals could have been influenced by knowledge of the ward intervention status, potentially invalidating the randomization. There were no differences in non-hip fracture rates in the two groups, however, or in the rates of falls or falls on hips in a subset of intervention and control wards that used a prospective falls register, supporting the validity of the results.

Several trials have evaluated multifactorial interventions to reduce falls and fall injury rates in elderly adults, targeted to a variety of physiologic and environmental risk factors. In a randomized controlled trial in community-dwelling persons aged 70 or older, the intervention group received medication review and adjustment, behavioral instruction and training, environmental alterations (e.g., installation of grab bars), and exercise to improve gait, balance, and strength; the interventions were delivered during multiple home visits by a nurse practitioner and a physical therapist over a 3-month period.[151] Controls received a similar number of structured home visits from social-work students. At 1-year follow-up, the intervention group had a significantly longer time to first fall, smaller proportion of subjects who fell (35% vs. 47%), and lower incidence of falls (0.012 vs. 0.018 falls/person-week), with favorable trends for falls requiring medical care and falls resulting in serious injury. In multivariate analysis, the risk of falling declined by 11% for each 1.0 decrease in the number of fall-related risk factors. No adverse effects from the intervention were reported except self-limited musculoskeletal symptoms in 7% of subjects. In the institutional setting, multidisciplinary postfall assessment designed to address a variety of risk factors for falls substantially reduced subsequent falls in a small uncontrolled experiment.[152] A randomized controlled trial of postfall assessment in a nursing home, however, found little effect on falls.[153] The assessment did significantly reduce hospitalizations and hospital days, suggesting that falls served mainly as a marker for treatable underlying disorders. Additional trials related to preventing falls and fall injuries in elderly persons are currently under way.[154]

Another leading cause of unintentional injury death in persons over 65 years of age is **asphyxiation** by choking from foreign materials in the respiratory tract, with 2,500 deaths annually, including 270 in institutions.[9] Poor dentition, use of sedative drugs, dementia, and reduced motor coordination may contribute to this high rate.[9] Interventions such as correcting denture fit, adjusting medications, dietary changes related to food size and consistency, and training those who care for elderly persons in use of the Heimlich maneuver and cardiopulmonary resuscitation may be effective interventions, but data evaluating these or other interventions to prevent aspiration and asphyxiation are lacking.

Fires and burns are also leading causes of death in older adults.[9,155] Compared with younger hospitalized burn victims, the mortality rate is higher for elderly hospitalized burn patients (0.4 vs. 2.6 deaths/100,000 person-years).[156] The risk of fatality in the event of a house fire is significantly increased when persons over 65 years old are present in the household.[29] Older persons may be at increased risk of dying in residential fires because of impaired vision, hearing, mobility, or mental status, which can lead to greater difficulty in avoiding burns.[29] More than three fourths of deaths from clothing ignition occur among persons aged 65 and older, which may be due in part to decreased coordination in handling cigarettes, lighters, etc.[9,155] Smoking materials have been implicated in 10% of severe burn injuries and 33% of residential-fire deaths among elderly persons.[26,156] Scald burns account for 42% of hospitalizations for burn injuries in persons aged 65 years and older and primarily involve hot tap water, food, and drinks.[156] Interventions similar to those discussed for children and younger adults are likely to be effective in preventing fire and burn injuries in elderly adults (see above). Efforts to improve mobility, coordination, and sensory function may also be effective in reducing burn injuries, although these have not been evaluated.

Effectiveness of Counseling

The most effective measures to control injuries are passive interventions, those that do not rely on the potential victim to adopt new behaviors voluntarily. Examples of effective passive interventions include window guards in high-rise apartments, nonflammable sleepwear, automatic sprinkler systems, and child-resistant packaging to prevent poisoning.[157] Since injury prevention advice from clinicians usually requires active cooperation from patients (e.g., changing smoking practices in bed, installing and testing smoke detectors), counseling faces inherent limitations. It is therefore not surprising that counseling is most effective in combination with other measures that promote compliance, such as safety regulations.[96,158]

Children. Clinical counseling by itself appears to be of some benefit when offered to parents of young children.[159] Only a few studies have evaluated the effects of counseling on injury rates as well as on knowledge and behavior. A small randomized controlled trial found that parents who received an individualized course on child safety during well-baby visits demonstrated greater knowledge about home hazards and had fewer hazards in the home when tested 1 month after the last visit; there was no difference in the rate of injuries reported by the parents or recorded in hospital records.[160] A nonrandomized controlled trial found that infants of mothers who received counseling on fall prevention had fewer falls over the course of a year than did those whose mothers were not counseled.[161] In a controlled demonstration project, clinical counseling resulted in significantly improved knowledge and behavior related to poisoning prevention, but had no effect on poisoning rates.[162] In a well-designed prospective cohort study, the children of urban, adolescent mothers who reported having received home safety information at 3 months postpartum were half as likely to have been injured at follow-up about 1 year later.[163] There was a dose-response relationship between the number of home safety information sources and reduced injury risk; 71% reported receiving their information from health professionals. Several ecologic studies that included both primary care and community interventions have reported improvements in safety knowledge and behavior compared to control communities; significant improvements or favorable trends in injury rates were also reported in the intervention communities.[164–166]

A number of other trials have assessed behavioral outcomes related to injury prevention. A randomized controlled trial found that couples who received information on burn prevention during well-child care classes were more likely to have their hot water heaters set at 130°F or lower when checked by investigators during a home visit.[167] In a nonrandomized trial, parents who received counseling along with the opportunity to purchase a smoke detector at cost were more likely to have an operational smoke detector 4–6 weeks later, compared with controls.[168] In another small nonrandomized trial of low-income parents, those who received detailed safety advice during a home visit by a health worker were found to have corrected significantly more home hazards compared to controls.[169] Education has also been shown to motivate parents to obtain syrup of ipecac, to display poison control center telephone numbers, and to learn more about the proper use of ipecac.[170–172] Thus, the evidence supports a beneficial effect of clinician counseling on safety-related knowledge and behavior. It is less clear from direct evidence whether counseling results in lower injury rates.

Not all studies have found counseling parents to be effective in promoting safety. One randomized controlled trial found that a program providing mothers with counseling on household hazards, a safety booklet, and free safety devices was unsuccessful in changing either the knowledge of the subjects or the number of home hazards detected in an unannounced home visit, although in this study the counseling was administered by a research assistant rather than a clinician.[173] To be effective, safety counseling may have to be provided by the patient's own clinician, as suggested by one descriptive study.[174] A population-based nonrandomized controlled trial found little effect on preventive behaviors of a brief nurse counseling intervention, but contamination of the comparison group may have occurred because the same nurses saw study and control groups in alternating weeks.[175] The limited benefit from parent counseling reported in these studies may therefore have been due to their methodologic limitations.

Some researchers have attempted to prevent childhood injuries through free distribution of injury control devices during the clinic visit. When free smoke detectors were made available in one program, 92% of the recipients installed the devices and 88% of these were found to be operational 4–9 months later.[176] Distributing a liquid-crystal thermometer along with office counseling increased the likelihood of testing tap water temperature compared to counseling alone, but both groups were equally likely to report lowering the thermostat.[177] In another study, free distribution of cabinet locks and electrical outlet covers resulted in increased use of outlet covers, which are easy to apply, but no increase in the installation of cabinet locks, a more inconvenient task requiring minimal carpentry skills.[178] Similarly, providing a free slide-style cabinet lock and telephone stickers significantly increased their use, while a discount coupon for syrup of ipecac (which required a visit to a pharmacy to purchase) did not increase the likelihood of having ipecac on hand.[179]

Adolescents and Adults. Evidence on counseling to prevent household and recreational injuries to adolescents and young or middle-aged adults is quite limited. Two randomized controlled trials directed to young adolescents and their parents evaluated brief physician counseling addressing awareness of bicycling injury risk and helmet efficacy and found only a slight, nonsignificant increase in bicycle helmet purchases.[180,181] The counseling intervention was designed primarily to increase awareness and was probably inadequate to induce behavioral change (see Chapter iv). A comprehensive review revealed no other studies specifically evaluating household or recreational injury prevention counseling of adolescents or younger adults in the primary care setting. Counseling middle-aged men who were heavy drinkers to reduce alcohol consumption substantially reduced hospital days for accidents and injuries at 2–5-year follow-up of a randomized controlled trial,[182] although it is not clear whether this was due to a reduction in injury events or in complications once an injury occurred. The effectiveness of identifying and counseling persons with problem drinking is described in detail in Chapter 52.

Elderly Adults. A number of trials have evaluated counseling elders to reduce the risk of household and other unintentional injuries, although none involved counseling within the context of the routine office visit. A randomized controlled trial enrolling public health clients ≥65 years compared the effects of safety education (including falls prevention and fire safety) delivered during a public health nurse home visit to control (influenza) education delivered in the same manner.[183] At 2–3-month follow-up, there were no differences between the two groups in the proportion of subjects reporting they had made safety changes in the home (22% vs. 18%) or in the mean number of safety changes made (0.35 vs. 0.26). Effects on injuries were not assessed. Three randomized controlled trials have evaluated the effects of counseling interventions on falls and fall injuries, one involving home visits and two conducted among elderly volunteers belonging to health maintenance organizations (HMOs). A large trial conducted within a general practice randomly assigned all households with patients aged 70 years and older to usual care or to receive a home health visit at least once a year that included risk assessment for falls; counseling on diet, medications, syncope, and environmental hazards; referrals as needed; and weekly fitness classes.[184] At 4-year follow-up, there were no differences between intervention and control groups in the proportions who reported falls (28% vs. 20%) or fractures due to falls (5% vs. 4%) during the study period. One HMO trial evaluated the effects of four weekly, 90-minute group counseling sessions led by a health behaviorist and a physical therapist and focused on exercise and measures to reduce environmental hazards and behavioral risks, followed by quarterly maintenance sessions; financial and technical assistance to make safety repairs was also offered.[185] The intervention reduced the odds of falling by 15%, but had little effect on the probability or number of injury falls or of falls requiring medical treatment. Neither the odds of falling nor number of falls was significantly related to the number of sessions attended by intervention subjects, but analysis suggested that those with a higher underlying fall risk were more likely to attend. The other HMO trial randomly assigned 1559 elderly volunteers to one of three groups: usual care, a 60–90-minute visit with a nurse to discuss chronic disease prevention, or a 60–90-minute visit with a nurse/educator who performed fall-related risk assessment and screening, developed tailored recommendations for preventing falls (e.g., medication review, exercise, alcoholism treatment, home safety inspection), and made 1–2 follow-up calls.[186] Compared to usual care, the intervention significantly reduced the percentage of subjects reporting falls and injurious falls, with favorable trends for medically attended and hospitalized falls, at 1-year follow-up, but differences disappeared by the end of 2 years. It is unclear how much of the reduction in falls at 1-year follow-up can be attributed to the intervention: similar reductions were seen in the control nurse visit group, and the intervention had no effect on the prevalence of any fall-related behaviors except the receipt of a home safety inspection. Whether the effects of home visits or of fairly intensive interventions in volunteers who belong to HMOs can be extrapolated to routine clinician counseling in the office setting is unclear. In all three of the trials assessing fall outcomes, falls were self-reported, possibly leading to biased reporting of falls due to knowledge of intervention assignment.

Adverse Effects of Injury Prevention Counseling. Injury prevention counseling has not been associated with adverse effects in any trials. Concern has been raised that injury control counseling may be harmful in some patients, such as adolescents.[53] Several investigators have hypothesized that adolescents who favor risk-taking behavior may respond to certain health information (i.e., drug and sex education) by performing activities that increase risk,[187–189] but no direct evidence to support this hypothesis, either for injury or other conditions, was found.

Recommendations of Other Groups

Specific recommendations for office-based counseling on household and recreational injury prevention have been issued by the American Academy of Pediatrics,[190] the American Academy of Family Physicians,[191] the Bright Futures project,[192] the American Medical Association Guidelines for Adolescent Preventive Services (GAPS),[193] and the Public Health Service.[193a] Clinicians are advised by these groups to provide age-specific injury prevention counseling, which may include the following: install and maintain smoke detectors in the home, safely store matches and lighters and avoid smoking near bedding or upholstery; set hot water temperatures to 120–130°F; install window and stairway guards/gates and discourage use of infant walkers; supervise young children in the bathtub and all children when swimming, install isolation fences around swimming pools, learn CPR, learn how to swim, and avoid alcohol use during water-related activities; avoid keeping guns or keep guns unloaded and stored in locked cabinets separate from ammunition; purchase and use bicycle helmets; safely store medicines and household products and acquire syrup of ipecac; correct home hazards related to falls; and follow other recommendations on injury prevention. The American College of Obstetricians and Gynecologists recommends injury prevention counseling on safety helmets, recreational hazards, and firearms for all women.[193b] The Centers for Disease Control and Prevention recommends that all persons wear bicycle helmets whenever and wherever they ride a bicycle.[194] The Canadian Task Force on the Periodic Health Examination recommends counseling parents to recognize home hazards, use smoke detectors and nonflammable sleepwear, reduce hot water thermostat settings, keep ipecac on hand, and know the poison control center telephone number, but it found insufficient evidence to recommend parent counseling to prevent drowning or bicycling injuries.[195] The Canadian Task Force found insufficient evidence to recommend for or against counseling adults (other than parents) to prevent household and recreational injuries.

Discussion

There is good evidence from controlled trials that counseling the parents of young children can increase safety-related behaviors (e.g., lowering hot water temperatures, reducing home hazards, installing smoke detectors), and fair evidence from multiple observational studies that certain safety behaviors are associated with reduced childhood injuries. A chain of evidence can thus be constructed to support a recommendation that parents of children be counseled to prevent household and recreational injuries, even though the evidence is less strong for a direct effect of clinician safety counseling on injury rates. There is clearly room for substantial improvement in the implementation of childhood injury prevention measures: in a national survey of households with children, only 67% had functional smoke detectors, 50% knew the Poison Control Center number, 26% had ipecac on hand, and 9% had hot water temperature known to be below 125°F.[196] The prevalence of all these measures decreased with decreasing level of education and income. High cost and limited access to recommended protective devices,[197] the need for technical skills to install certain devices, and living in rental units should be recognized as important barriers to implementing childhood injury prevention advice that particularly affect low-income households.

No trials of counseling or other interventions in elderly adults have demonstrated significant reductions in serious fall injuries, but there is strong observational evidence of the association between falls and mortality and serious morbidity in the elderly, indicating that interventions that reduce falls are likely to improve clinical outcomes. A meta-analysis of randomized controlled trials indicates that exercise (especially balance training) can reduce the risk of falls in elderly persons by about 10%. An intensive multifactorial intervention that directly addressed physiologic and environmental risk factors during regular home visits also reduced the likelihood of falling in high-risk community-dwelling elders, although substantial resources were required that may not be available in all settings. Whether clinician advice to exercise or to address fall risk factors will reduce falls or fall injuries is less clear. Weekly group counseling sessions or detailed individualized counseling by health workers trained to address physiological, behavioral, and environmental risk factors leads to modest short-term reductions in fall risk. These interventions may not be generalizable to brief advice delivered in the office setting, however, and direct evidence of a reduction in fall injuries with counseling is lacking. Periodic counseling of elderly persons to exercise and to address environmental and behavioral risk factors for falls is thus supported by fair evidence that these measures will reduce falls and thereby reduce fall-related injuries, although the effectiveness of counseling patients to exercise and to address these risk factors has not been established. There is fair evidence to recommend an intensive multifactorial fall prevention intervention for community-dwelling elders at high risk for falls, in settings where adequate resources to deliver this intervention are available.

In institutionalized elderly persons, there is evidence from one trial that the use of external hip protectors reduces hip fracture rates. Confirmation of these results is needed, but the large potential benefit and lack of adverse effects support their use. At present, such protectors are not widely available nor have these devices been approved by the Food and Drug Administration. Compliance with wearing the protectors was poor in institutionalized elderly. Whether community-dwelling elders would comply with wearing similar protectors is questionable; further research to address compliance is therefore necessary. Postfall assessment and multifactorial intervention for institutionalized elderly does not appear to reduce falls, but can be recommended on the basis of other significant health benefits unrelated to injuries.

Although there are few injury control measures for adolescents and younger adults for which there is conclusive evidence of efficacy, and the effectiveness of injury control counseling of adults is largely unstudied, counseling by physicians on these matters may be justified because of the enormous burden of suffering associated with injuries. Thus, even minor reductions in their incidence can have large public health benefits. The cost of physician time to deliver injury prevention counseling may be kept to a minimum by conducting counseling during clinical encounters and focusing attention on specific injuries for which the patient is at greatest risk and on preventive strategies for which the strongest evidence of efficacy is available. For adolescents and adults, intoxication by alcohol and other drugs appears to be most strongly associated with the risk of unintentional injury or death, and there is fair evidence that counseling for problem drinking is effective (see Chapter 52). Additional measures likely to prevent household and recreational injuries to adolescents and adults include smoking cessation (see Chapter 54), proper installation and testing of smoke detectors, and wearing bicycle and ATV safety helmets.

The solutions to many injury problems may require intervention both at the individual level (i.e., in the clinical setting) and at the community, state or national level. There are numerous examples of public health education programs and legislation that have proved effective in promoting safe behavior and preventing injuries.[36,39,64,80,81,84,96,198,199] Measures likely to be even more effective in preventing injuries involve re-engineering the household environment or products (e.g., residential sprinkler systems, hot water heaters preset to 125° at the factory[32,34]), because these measures do not depend on voluntary behavior changes. Such re-engineering can also be achieved through legislation. In many communities, physicians and other health professionals have provided leadership for effective community programs and legislation to reduce injury morbidity and mortality.[39,64,200,201] Clinicians may wish to consider playing an advocacy role as a means of preventing household and recreational injuries, while continuing to support behavior change with clinical interventions.

CLINICAL INTERVENTION

Counseling the parents of children on measures to reduce the risk of unintentional injuries from residential fires and hot tap water, drowning, poisoning, bicycling, firearms, and falls is recommended ("B" recommendation). Persons with alcohol or drug problems should be identified, counseled, and monitored, and referred for treatment as appropriate (see Chapters 52 and 53); all adolescents and adults who use alcohol or other drugs should be advised to avoid engaging in potentially dangerous activities (e.g., swimming, boating, handling of firearms, smoking in bed, hunting, bicycling) while intoxicated ("B" recommendation). Counseling regarding other measures to prevent household and recreational injuries is recommended for adolescent and adult (including elderly) patients based on fair evidence for the efficacy of risk reduction ("B" recommendation), although the effectiveness of such counseling has not been adequately evaluated ("C" recommendation). The need to prevent household or recreational injuries should be discussed regularly with patients, although the optimal frequency for such counseling has not been determined and is left to clinical discretion. Clinicians should remain alert to the possibility of abuse or neglect as the etiology of certain household and recreational injuries (see Chapter 51). Illicit drug use, an important risk factor for adolescent and adult poisonings, is discussed in Chapter 53. See also Chapter 50 (suicide), Chapter 57 (motor vehicle and pedestrian injuries), and Chapter 59 (violent injuries).

Specific recommendations to prevent injuries to children include the following measures, many of which are also likely to be effective in preventing injuries to adolescents and adults (including elderly persons). Homeowners should be advised to install smoke detectors in appropriate locations and to test the devices periodically to ensure proper operation. Infants and children should wear flame-resistant nightwear during sleep. Smokers should be advised to cease or reduce smoking (see Chapter 54). Hot water heaters should be set at 120–130°F. Parents, grandparents, or other patients with children in the home should be advised to keep a 1-ounce bottle of syrup of ipecac, to display the telephone number of the local poison control center, and to place all medications, toxic substances, and matches in child-resistant containers. Bicyclists and parents of children who ride bicycles should be counseled about the importance of wearing approved safety helmets[194] and avoiding riding in motor vehicle traffic. Children and adolescents who ride all-terrain vehicles, and their parents, should be advised to use approved safety helmets and four-wheeled (rather than three-wheeled) machines with smaller engines. Families should be encouraged to install 4-foot four-sided isolation fences with self-latching, self-closing gates around swimming pools, and window guards on windows in buildings that pose high risk for falls. Swimming pool owners and individuals living with or caring for young children or elderly persons should be encouraged to learn cardiopulmonary resuscitation and maneuvers to manage choking incidents. Although there is at present only limited evidence to support removing firearms from the home or keeping them unloaded in a locked compartment for the prevention of unintentional injuries, this intervention can be recommended based on its efficacy for the prevention of violent injuries (see Chapters 50 and 59). Additional interventions likely to be effective but for which there is currently limited evidence of benefit include: avoiding smoking near bedding or upholstery and unsafe handling of smoking materials, installing collapsible gates or other barriers to stairway entrances, observing safe boating practices and wearing personal flotation devices while boating, and wearing orange fluorescent clothing while hunting. Poison-warning stickers intended to deter children from playing with containers of medicine or other poisons (e.g., "Mr. Yuk" stickers) have been found to be ineffective and are not recommended ("D" recommendation).

Counseling elderly patients on measures to reduce the risk of falling, including exercise (particularly training to improve balance), safety-related skills and behaviors, and environmental hazard reduction, along with monitoring and adjusting medications, is recommended based on fair evidence that these measures reduce the likelihood of falling ("B" recommendation), although the effectiveness of routinely counseling elders to prevent falls has not been adequately evaluated ("C" recommendation). Recommendations for regular physical activity in elderly patients without contraindications can also be made based on other proven benefits (see Chapter 55). Intensive individualized home-based multifactorial intervention to reduce the risk of falls is recommended for high-risk elderly patients in settings where adequate resources are available to deliver such services ("B" recommendation). Elderly persons at high risk for falls include those aged 75 years and older; or aged 70–74 with one or more additional risk factors including: use of certain psychoactive and cardiac medications (e.g., benzodiazepines, antihypertensives); use of ≥4 prescription medications; impaired cognition, strength, balance, or gait. There is insufficient evidence to recommend for or against the routine use of external hip protectors to prevent fall injuries ("C" recommendation). Once these devices become generally available, recommendations for their use in institutionalized elderly may be made on other grounds, including the large potential benefit and limited adverse effects. There is insufficient evidence to recommend for or against postfall assessment and intervention in institutionalized elderly persons in order to prevent falls ("C" recommendation), but recommendations for such interventions may be made on the basis of other benefits, including reduced hospitalizations and hospital days unrelated to falls. For other recommendations relevant to fall injuries in the elderly, see Chapter 33 (screening for visual impairment), Chapter 46 (screening for postmenopausal osteoporosis), Chapter 48 (screening for dementia), Chapter 55 (counseling to promote physical activity), and Chapter 68 (hormone replacement therapy).

The draft update of this chapter was prepared for the U.S. Preventive Services Task Force by Carolyn DiGuiseppi, MD, MPH.

REFERENCES

1. National Center for Health Statistics. Annual summary of births, marriages, divorces, and deaths: United States, 1993. Monthly vital statistics report; vol 42, no 13. Hyattsville, MD: National Center for Health Statistics, 1994.
2. Centers for Disease Control and Prevention. Mortality patterns—United States, 1991. MMWR 1993;42:891, 897–900.
3. Centers for Disease Control and Prevention. Years of potential life lost before age 65—United States, 1990 and 1991. MMWR 1993;42:251–253.
4. Graves EJ. 1992 summary: National hospital discharge survey. Advance data from vital and health statistics; no 249. Hyattsville, MD: National Center for Health Statistics, 1994.
5. Burt CW. Injury-related visits to hospital emergency departments: United States, 1992. Advance data from vital and health statistics; no 261. Hyattsville, MD: National Center for Health Statistics, 1995.
6. Schappert SM. National ambulatory medical care survey: 1992 summary. Advance data from vital and health statistics; no 253. Hyattsville, MD: National Center for Health Statistics, 1994.
7. McCaig LF. Outpatient department summary: national hospital ambulatory medical care survey, 1992. Advance data from vital and health statistics; no 248. Hyattsville, MD: National Center for Health Statistics, 1994.
8. Max W, Rice DP, MacKenzie EJ. The lifetime cost of injury. Inquiry 1990;27:332–343.
9. Baker SP, O'Neill B, Ginsburg MJ, et al, eds. The injury fact book. 2nd ed. New York: Oxford University Press, 1992.
10. Centers for Disease Control. Public health surveillance of 1990 injury control objectives for the nation. CDC surveillance summary. MMWR 1988;37(SS-1):1-68.
11. O'Loughlin JL, Robitaille Y, Boivin J-F, et al. Incidence of and risk factors for falls and injurious falls among the community-dwelling elderly. Am J Epidemiol 1993;137:342–354.
12. Sattin RW, Lambert Huber DA, DeVito CA, et al. The incidence of fall injury events among the elderly in a defined population. Am J Epidemiol 1990;131:1028–1037.
13. Alexander BH, Rivara FP, Wolf ME. The cost and frequency of hospitalization for fall-related injuries in older adults. Am J Public Health 1992;82:1020–1023.
14. Jensen GF, Christiansen C, Boesen J, et al. Epidemiology of postmenopausal spinal and long bone fractures: a unifying approach to postmenopausal osteoporosis. Clin Orthop 1982;166:75–81.
15. Cummings SR, Kelsey J, Nevitt M, et al. Epidemiology of osteoporosis and osteoporotic fractures. Epidemiol Rev 1985;7:178–208.
16. Magaziner J, Simonsick EM, Kashner TM, et al. Survival experience of aged hip fracture patients. Am J Public Health 1989;79:274–278.
17. Lu-Yao GL, Baron JA, Barrett JA, et al. Treatment and survival among elderly Americans with hip fractures: a population-based study. Am J Public Health 1994;84:1287–1291.

18. Brenner RA, Smith GS, Overpeck MD. Divergent trends in childhood drowning rates, 1971 through 1988. JAMA 1994;271:1606–1608.
19. Wintemute GJ. Childhood drowning and near-drowning in the United States. Am J Dis Child 1990;144:663–669.
20. Mercy JA. The public health impact of firearm injuries. Am J Prev Med 1993;9(Suppl 1):8–11.
21. Lee RK, Harris MJ. Unintentional firearm injuries: the price of protection. Am J Prev Med 1993; 9(Suppl 1):16–20.
22. Sacks JJ, Holmgreen P, Smith SM, et al. Bicycle-associated head injuries and deaths in the United States from 1984 through 1988. How many are preventable? JAMA 1991;266:3016–3018.
23. Thompson DC, Thompson RS, Rivara FP. Incidence of bicycle-related injuries in a defined population. Am J Public Health 1990;80:1388–1389.
24. National Highway Traffic Safety Administration. Traffic safety facts 1992. Washington, DC: Department of Transportation, 1994. (Publication no. DOT HS 808 022.)
25. Newman R. Update of all-terrain vehicle deaths and injuries. Washington, DC: U.S. Consumer Product Safety Commission, 1988.
26. Centers for Disease Control and Prevention. Deaths resulting from residential fires—United States, 1991. MMWR 1994;43:901–904.
27. Federal Emergency Management Agency. Fire in the United States: 1983–1990. Emmitsburg, MD: U.S. Fire Administration, 1993. (Publication no. USFA/FA-140.)
28. Centers for Disease Control. Regional distribution of deaths from residential fires—United States, 1978–1984. JAMA 1987;258:2355–2356.
29. Runyan CW, Bangdiwala SI, Linzer MA, et al. Risk factors for fatal residential fires. N Engl J Med 1992;327: 859–863.
30. Budnick EK. Estimating effectiveness of state-of-the-art detectors and automatic sprinklers on life safety in residential occupancies. Washington, DC: Department of Commerce, National Bureau of Standards, National Engineering Laboratory, Center for Fire Research, 1984. (Publication no. NBSIR 84-2819.)
31. Hall JR Jr. A decade of detectors: measuring the effect. Fire 1985;79:37–43.
32. Council on Scientific Affairs, American Medical Association. Preventing death and injury from fires with automatic sprinklers and smoke detectors. JAMA 1987;257:1618–1620.
33. Harwood B, Kluge P. Hazards associated with the use of wood- or coal-burning stoves or free-standing fireplaces. Washington, DC: U.S. Consumer Product Safety Commission, 1985.
34. McLoughlin E, McGuire A. The causes, cost, and prevention of childhood burn injuries. Am J Dis Child 1990;144: 677–683.
35. Anonymous. Accident prevention in childhood. Lancet 1979;2:564–565.
36. McLoughlin E, Clarke N, Stahl K, et al. One pediatric burn unit's experiences with sleepwear-related injuries. Pediatrics 1977;60:405–409.
37. Katcher ML. Prevention of tap water scald burns: evaluation of a multi-media injury control program. Am J Public Health 1987;77:1195–1197.
38. Feldman KW, Schaller RT, Feldman JA, et al. Tap water scald burns in children. Pediatrics 1978;62:1–7.
39. Erdmann TC, Feldman KW, Rivara FP, et al. Tap water burn prevention: the effect of legislation. Pediatrics 1991;88: 572–577.
40. Fallat ME, Rengers SJ. The effect of education and safety devices on scald burn prevention. J Trauma 1993;34: 560–564.
41. Centers for Disease Control. Aquatic deaths and injuries—United States. MMWR 1982;31:417–419.
42. Pitt WR. Increasing incidence of childhood immersion injury in Brisbane. Med J Aust 1986;144:683–685.
43. Pearn J, Nixon J, Wilkey I. Freshwater drowning and near-drowning accidents involving children. Med J Aust 1976;2:942–946.
44. Wintemute GJ, Kraus JF, Teret SP, et al. Drowning in childhood and adolescence: a population-based study. Am J Public Health 1987;77:830–832.
45. O'Carroll PW, Alkin E, Weiss B. Drowning mortality in Los Angeles County, 1976 to 1984. JAMA 1988;260: 380–383.
46. Jensen LR, Williams SD, Thurman DJ, et al. Submersion injuries in children younger than 5 years in urban Utah. West J Med 1992;157:641–644.
47. Quan L, Gore EJ, Wentz K, et al. Ten-year study of pediatric drowning and near-drowning in King County, Washington: lessons in injury prevention. Pediatrics 1989;83:1035–1040.
48. Present P. Child drowning study: a report on the epidemiology of drowning in residential pools to children under age five. Washington, DC: Directorate for Epidemiology, US Consumer Product Safety Commission, 1987.

49. Pearn JH, Wong RYK, Brown J III, et al. Drowning and near-drowning involving children: a five-year population study from the city and county of Honolulu. Am J Public Health 1979;69:450–454.

50. Pearn J, Brown J III, Hsia EY. Swimming pool drowning and near-drowning involving children: a total population study from Hawaii. Mil Med 1980;145:15–18.

51. Milner N, Pearn J, Guard R. Will fenced pools save lives? A 10-year study from Mulgrave Shire, Queensland. Med J Aust 1980;2:510–511.

52. Rodgers GB. Factors contributing to child drowning and near-drowning in residential swimming pools. Hum Factors 1989;31:123–132.

52a. Centers for Disease Control. Child drownings and near drownings associated with swimming pools— Maricopa, Arizona, 1988 and 1989. MMWR 1990;39:441–442.

53. Halperin SF, Bass JL, Mehta KA, et al. Unintentional injuries among adolescents and young adults: a review and analysis. J Adolesc Health Care 1983;4:275–281.

54. Spyker DA. Submersion injury: epidemiology, prevention, and management. Pediatr Clin North Am 1985;32: 113–123.

55. Budnick LD, Ross DA. Bathtub-related drowning in the United States, 1979–81. Am J Public Health 1985;75: 630–633.

56. Kyriacou DN, Arcinue EL, Peek C, et al. Effect of immediate resuscitation on children with submersion injury. Pediatrics 1994;94:137–142.

57. Orlowski JP. Prognostic factors in pediatric cases of drowning and near-drowning. JACEP 1979;8:176–179.

58. Wintemute GJ, Teret SP, Kraus JF, et al. When children shoot children: 88 unintended deaths. JAMA 1987;257: 3107–3109.

59. Hemenway D, Solnick SJ, Azrael DR. Firearm training and storage. JAMA 1995;273:46–50.

60. Kellermann AL, Reay DT. Protection or peril? An analysis of firearm-related deaths in the home. N Engl J Med 1986;314:1557–1560.

61. U.S. General Accounting Office. Accidental deaths: many deaths and injuries caused by firearms could be prevented. Washington, DC: U.S. General Accounting Office, 1991. (Publication no. GAO/PEMD-91-9.)

62. Centers for Disease Control. Unintentional poisoning among young children—United States. MMWR 1983;32: 117–118.

63. Palmisano P. Targeted intervention in the control of accidental overdoses in children. Public Health Rep 1981;96: 150–156.

64. Walton WW. An evaluation of the Poison Prevention Packaging Act. Pediatrics 1982;69:363–370.

65. Clarke A, Walton WW. Effect of safety packaging on aspirin ingestion by children. Pediatrics 1979;63: 687–693.

66. Vernberg K, Culver-Dickinson P, Spyker DA. The deterrent effect of poison-warning stickers. Am J Dis Child 1984; 138:1018–1020.

67. Fergusson DM, Horwood LJ, Beautrais AL, et al. A controlled field trial of a poisoning prevention method. Pediatrics 1982;69:515–520.

68. Sibert JR, Frude N. Bittering agents in the prevention of accidental poisoning: children's reactions to denatonium benzoate (Bitrex). Arch Emerg Med 1991;8:1–7.

69. Berning CK, Griffith JF, Wild JE. Research on the effectiveness of denatonium benzoate as a deterrent to liquid detergent ingestion by children. Fundam Appl Toxicol 1982;2:44–48.

70. Rodgers GC. The role of aversive bittering agents in the prevention of pediatric poisonings. Pediatrics 1994;93: 68–69.

71. Rivara FP. Traumatic deaths of children in the United States: currently available prevention strategies. Pediatrics 1985;75:456–462.

71a. Waller JA. Bicycle ownership, use, and injury patterns among elementary school children. Pediatrics 1971;47: 1042–1050.

72. Friede AM, Azzara CV, Gallagher SS, et al. The epidemiology of injuries to bicycle riders. Pediatr Clin North Am 1985;32:141–151.

73. Spence LJ, Dykes EH, Bohn DJ, et al. Fatal bicycle accidents in children: a plea for prevention. J Pediatr Surg 1993;28:214–216.

74. McDermott FT, Lane JC, Brazenor GA, et al. The effectiveness of bicyclist helmets: a study of 1710 casualties. J Trauma 1993;34:834–845.

75. Spaite DW, Murphy M, Criss EA, et al. A prospective analysis of injury severity among helmeted and nonhelmeted bicyclists involved in collisions with motor vehicles. J Trauma 1991;31:1510–1516.

76. Wasserman RC, Buccini RV. Helmet protection from head injuries among recreational bicyclists. Am J Sports Med 1990;18:96–97.
77. Maimaris C, Summers CL, Browning C, et al. Injury patterns in cyclists attending an accident and emergency department: a comparison of helmet wearers and non-wearers. BMJ 1994;308:1537–1540.
78. Thompson RS, Rivara FP, Thompson DC. A case-control study of the effectiveness of bicycle safety helmets. N Engl J Med 1989;320:1361–1367.
79. Thomas S, Acton C, Nixon J, et al. Effectiveness of bicycle helmets in preventing head injury in children: case-control study. BMJ 1994;308:173–176.
80. Centers for Disease Control and Prevention. Mandatory bicycle helmet use—Victoria, Australia. MMWR 1993;42: 359–363.
81. Cooke CT, Margolius KA, Cadden GA. Cycling fatalities in Western Australia. Med J Aust 1993;159:783–785.
82. DiGuiseppi CG, Rivara FP, Koepsell TD, et al. Bicycle helmet use by children: evaluation of a community-wide helmet campaign. JAMA 1989;262:2256–2261.
83. Centers for Disease Control and Prevention. Bicycle helmet promotion programs—Canada, Australia, and United States. MMWR 1993;42:203, 209–210.
84. Rivara FP, Thompson DC, Thompson RS, et al. The Seattle children's bicycle helmet campaign: changes in helmet use and head injury admissions. Pediatrics 1994;93:567–569.
85. Begg DJ, Langley JD, Chalmers DJ, et al. Bicycle road crashes during the fourteenth and fifteenth years of life. NZ Med J 1991;104:60–61.
86. Cushman R, Down J, MacMillan N, et al. Bicycle-related injuries: a survey in a pediatric emergency department. Can Med Assoc J 1990;143:108–112.
87. Simpson AHRW, Mineiro J. Prevention of bicycle accidents. Injury 1992;23:171–173.
88. Van Schagen INLG, Brookhuis KA. Training young cyclists to cope with dynamic traffic situations. Accid Anal Prev 1994;26:223–230.
89. Organization for Economic Cooperation and Development. Traffic safety of children. Report of OECD Scientific Expert Group. Paris: Organization for Economic Cooperation and Development, 1983.
90. Garder P, Leden L, Thedeen T. Safety implications of bicycle paths at signalized intersections. Accid Anal Prev 1994;26:429–439.
91. Kraus JF, Rock A, Hemyari P. Brain injuries among infants, children, adolescents, and young adults. Am J Dis Child 1990;144:684–691.
92. Garrettson LK, Gallagher SS. Falls in children and youth. Pediatr Clin North Am 1985;32:153–162.
93. Coats TJ, Allen M. Baby walker related injuries—a continuing problem. Arch Emerg Med 1991;8:52–55.
94. Kavanagh CA, Banco L. The infant walker—a previously unrecognized hazard. Am J Dis Child 1982;136:205–206.
95. Fazen LE, Felizberto PI. Baby walker injuries. Pediatrics 1982;70:106–109.
96. Spiegel CN, Lindaman FC. Children can't fly: a program to prevent childhood morbidity and mortality from window falls. Am J Public Health 1977;67:1143–1147.
97. Kozararevic DJ, Vojvodic N, Gordon T, et al. Drinking habits and death: the Yugoslavia Cardiovascular Disease Study. Int J Epidemiol 1983;12:145–150.
98. Boffetta P, Garfinkel L. Alcohol drinking and mortality among men enrolled in an American Cancer Society prospective study. Epidemiology 1990;1:342–348.
99. Anda RF, Williamson DF, Remington PL. Alcohol and fatal injuries among U.S. adults: findings from the NHANES I epidemiologic follow-up study. JAMA 1988;260:2529–2542.
100. Klatsky AL, Armstrong MA, Friedman GD. Alcohol and mortality. Ann Intern Med 1992;117:646–654.
101. Blose JO, Holder HD. Injury-related medical care utilization in a problem drinking population. Am J Public Health 1991;81:1571–1575.
102. Cherpitel CJ. Alcohol consumption among emergency room patients: comparison of county/community hospitals and an HMO. J Stud Alcohol 1993;54:432–440.
103. Cherpitel CJ. Alcohol, injury, and risk-taking behavior: data from a national sample. Alcohol Clin Exp Res 1993;17: 762–766.
104. Rivara FP, Koepsell TD, Jurkovich GJ, et al. The effects of alcohol abuse on readmission for trauma. JAMA 1993;270:1962–1964.
105. Brodzka W, Thornhill HL, Howard S. Burns: causes and risk factors. Arch Phys Med Rehabil 1985;66:746–752.
106. Centers for Disease Control. Fatal injuries to children—United States, 1986. MMWR 1990;39: 442–445, 451.

107. Li G, Baker SP. Alcohol in fatally injured bicyclists. Accid Anal Prev 1994;26:543–548.

108. Plueckhahn VD. Alcohol consumption and death by drowning in adults: a 24-year epidemiological analysis. J Stud Alcohol 1982;43:445–452.

108a. Bijur PE, Kurzon M, Overpeck MD, et al. Parental alcohol use, problem drinking, and children's injuries. JAMA 1992;267:3166–3171.

109. Jurkovich GJ, Rivara FP, Gurney JG, et al. The effect of acute alcohol intoxication and chronic alcohol abuse on outcome from trauma. JAMA 1993;270:51–56.

110. Kann L, Warren CW, Harris WA, et al. Youth risk behavior surveillance—United States, 1993. CDC surveillance summaries, March 24, 1995. MMWR 1995;44(SS-1):1–56.

111. Substance Abuse and Mental Health Services Administration. Preliminary estimates from the National Household Survey on Drug Abuse. Advance report no. 3. Washington, DC: Department of Health and Human Services, 1993.

112. Centers for Disease Control. Unintentional poisoning mortality—United States, 1980–1986. MMWR 1989;38: 153–157.

113. Wintemute GJ, Kraus JF, Teret SP, et al. The epidemiology of drowning in adulthood: implications for prevention. Am J Prev Med 1988;4:343–348.

114. Press E, Walker J, Crawford I. An interstate drowning study. Am J Public Health 1968;12:2275–2289.

115. Molberg PJ, Hopkins RS, Paulson J, et al. Fatal incident risk factors in recreational boating in Ohio. Pub Health Rep 1993;108:340–346.

116. Howland J, Hingson R. Alcohol as a risk factor for drowning: a review of the literature (1950–1985). Accid Anal Prev 1988;20:19–25.

117. Dietz PE, Baker SP. Drowning: epidemiology and prevention. Am J Public Health 1974;64:303–312.

118. Centers for Disease Control. Alcohol use and aquatic activities—United States, 1991. MMWR 1993;42:675, 681–683.

119. U.S. Coast Guard. Boating statistics, 1993. Washington, DC: U.S. Coast Guard, 1994. (Commandant publication 16754.7.)

120. Senturia YD, Christoffel KK, Donovan M. Children's household exposure to guns: a pediatric practice-based survey. Pediatrics 1994;93:469–475.

121. North American Association of Hunter Safety Coordinators. Hunting accident report, with graphics of 1983–1987 data. Seattle: Outdoor Empire Publishing, 1987.

122. *Deleted in proof.*

123. Cole TB, Patetta MJ. Hunting firearm injuries, North Carolina. Am J Public Health 1988;78:1585–1586.

124. Ballard JE, Koepsell TD, Rivara F. Association of smoking and alcohol drinking with residential fire injuries. Am J Epidemiol 1992;135:26–34.

124a. Miller AL. The U.S. smoking-material fire problem through 1990: the role of lighted tobacco products in fire. Quincy, MA: National Fire Protection Association, 1993.

124b. Rodgers GB. Bicycle and bicycle helmet use patterns in the United States: a description and analysis of national survey data. Washington, DC: U.S. Consumer Product Safety Commission, 1993.

125. Rodgers GB. The effectiveness of helmets in reducing all-terrain vehicle injuries and deaths. Accid Anal Prev 1990;22:47–58.

126. Rodgers GB, Rubin, PH. Cost-benefit analysis of all-terrain vehicles at the CPSC. Risk Anal 1989;9:63–69.

127. Widome MD. Pediatric injury prevention for the practitioner. Curr Prob Pediatr 1991;21:428–468.

128. Tinetti ME, Speechley M, Ginter SF. Risk factors for falls among elderly persons living in the community. N Engl J Med 1988;319:1701–1707.

129. Nevitt MC, Cummings SR, Hudes ES. Risk factors for injurious falls: a prospective study. J Gerontol 1991;46: M164–M170.

130. Teno J, Kiel DP, Mor V. Multiple stumbles: a risk factor for falls in community-dwelling elderly. A prospective study. J Am Geriatr Soc 1990;38:1321–1325.

131. Campbell AJ, Borrie MJ, Spears GF. Risk factors for falls in a community-based prospective study of people 70 years and older. J Gerontol 1989;44:M112–M117.

132. Robbins AS, Rubenstein LZ, Josephson KR, et al. Predictors of falls among elderly people. Results of two population-based studies. Arch Intern Med 1989;149:1628–1633.

133. Jantti PO, Pyykko VI, Hervonen ALJ. Falls among elderly nursing home residents. Public Health 1993;107:89–96.

134. Myers AH, Baker SP, Van Natta ML, et al. Risk factors associated with falls and injuries among elderly institutionalized persons. Am J Epidemiol 1991;133:1179–1190.

135. Lord SR, Clark RD, Webster IW. Physiological factors associated with falls in an elderly population. J Am Geriatr Soc 1991;39:1194–1200.
136. Lord SR, Sambrook PN, Gilbert C, et al. Postural stability, falls and fractures in the elderly: results from the Dubbo Osteoporosis Epidemiology Study. Med J Aust 1994;160:684–691.
137. Northridge ME, Nevitt MC, Kelsey JL, et al. Home hazards and falls in the elderly: the role of health and functional status. Am J Public Health 1995;85:509–515.
138. Archea J. Falls in the elderly: environmental risk factors associated with stair accidents by the elderly. Clin Geriatr Med 1985;1:555–569.
139. Campbell AJ, Borrie MJ, Spears GF, et al. Circumstances and consequences of falls experienced by a community population 70 years and over during a prospective study. Age Ageing 1990;19:136–141.
140. Hornbrook MC, Wingfield DJ, Stevens VJ, et al. Falls among older persons: antecedents and consequences. In: Weindruch R, Hadley E, Ory M, eds. Reducing frailty and falls in older persons. Springfield, IL: Charles C Thomas, 1991:106–125.
141. Speechley M, Tinetti ME. Falls and injuries in frail and vigorous community elderly persons. J Am Geriatr Soc 1991; 39:46–52.
142. Nevitt MC, Cummings SR, and the Study of Osteoporotic Fractures Research Group. Type of fall and risk of hip and wrist fractures: the Study of Osteoporotic Fractures. J Am Geriatr Soc 1993;41:1226–1234.
143. Reinsch S, MacRae P, Lachenbruch PA, et al. Attempts to prevent falls and injury: a prospective community study. Gerontologist 1992;32:450–456.
144. Mulrow CD, Gerety MB, Kanten D, et al. A randomized trial of physical rehabilitation for very frail nursing home residents. JAMA 1994;271:519–524.
145. Johansson G, Jarnlo G-B. Balance training in 70-year-old women. Physiother Theory Pract 1991;7:121–125.
146. Crilly RG, Willems DA, Trenholm KJ, et al. Effect of exercise on postural sway in the elderly. Gerontologist 1989;35:137–143.
147. Nelson ME, Fiatarone MA, Morganti CM, et al. Effects of high-intensity strength training on multiple risk factors for osteoporotic fractures: a randomized controlled trial. JAMA 1994;272:1909–1914.
148. Fiatarone MA, O'Neill EF, Ryan ND, et al. Exercise training and nutritional supplementation for physical frailty in very elderly people. N Engl J Med 1994;330:1769–1775.
149. Province MA, Hadley EC, Hornbrook MC, et al. The effects of exercise on falls in elderly patients: a pre-planned meta-analysis of the FICSIT trials. JAMA 1995;273:1341–1347.
150. Lauritzen JB, Petersen MM, Lund B. Effect of external hip protectors on hip fractures. Lancet 1993;341:11–13.
151. Tinetti ME, Baker DI, McAvay G, et al. A multifactorial intervention to reduce the risk of falling among elderly people living in the community. N Engl J Med 1994;331:821–827.
152. Wolf-Klein GP, Silverstone FA, Basavaraju N, et al. Prevention of falls in the elderly population. Arch Phys Med Rehabil 1988;69:689–691.
153. Rubenstein LZ, Robbins AS, Josephson KR, et al. The value of assessing falls in an elderly population: a randomized clinical trial. Ann Intern Med 1990;113:308–316.
154. Ory MG, Schechtman KB, Miller JP, et al. Frailty and injuries in later life: the FICSIT trials. J Am Geriatr Soc 1993;41:283–296.
155. Gulaid JA, Sacks JJ, Sattin RW. Deaths from residential fires among older people, United States, 1984. J Am Geriatr Soc 1989;37:331–334.
156. Rossignol AM, Locke JA, Boyle CM, et al. Consumer products and hospitalized burn injuries among elderly Massachusetts residents. J Am Geriatr Soc 1985;33:768–772.
157. Centers for Disease Control. Childhood injuries in the United States. Am J Dis Child 1990;144:627–646.
158. Gallagher SS, Hunter P, Guyer B. A home injury prevention program for children. Pediatr Clin North Am 1985;32: 95–112.
159. Bass JL, Christoffel KK, Widome M, et al. Childhood injury prevention counseling in primary care settings: a critical review of the literature. Pediatrics 1993;92:544–550.
160. Kelly B, Sein C, McCarthy PL. Safety education in a pediatric primary care setting. Pediatrics 1987;79:818–824.
161. Kravitz H, Grove M. Prevention of accidental falls in infancy by counseling mothers. Ill Med J 1973;144:570–573.
162. Steele P, Spyker DA. Poisonings. Pediatr Clin North Am 1985;32:77–86.
163. Jordan EA, Duggan AK, Hardy JB. Injuries in children of adolescent mothers: home safety education associated with decreased injury risk. Pediatrics 1993;91:481–487.

164. Guyer B, Gallagher SS, Chang B-H, et al. Prevention of childhood injuries: evaluation of the statewide childhood injury prevention program (SCIPP). Am J Public Health 1989;79:1521–1527.

165. Bass JL, Mehta KA, Ostrovsky M. Childhood injury prevention in a suburban Massachusetts population. Public Health Rep 1991;106:437–442.

166. Tellnes G. An evaluation of an injury prevention campaign in general practice in Norway. Fam Pract 1985;825–827.

167. Thomas KA, Hassanein RS, Christophersen ER. Evaluation of group well-child care for improving burn prevention practices in the home. Pediatrics 1984;74:879–882.

168. Miller RE, Reisinger KS, Blatter MM, et al. Pediatric counseling and subsequent use of smoke detectors. Am J Public Health 1982;72:392–393.

169. Colver AF, Hutchinson PJ, Judson EC. Promoting children's home safety. BMJ 1982;285:1177–1180.

170. Dershewitz RA, Posner M, Paichel W. The effectiveness of health education on home use of ipecac. Clin Pediatr 1983;22:268–270.

171. Woolf A, Lewander W, Fillipone G, et al. Prevention of childhood poisoning: efficacy of an educational program carried out in an emergency clinic. Pediatrics 1987;80:359–363.

172. Alpert JJ, Levine MD, Kosa J. Public knowledge of ipecac syrup in the management of accidental poisonings. J Pediatr 1967;71:890–894.

173. Dershewitz RA, Williamson JW. Prevention of childhood household injuries: a controlled clinical trial. Am J Public Health 1977;67:1148–1153.

174. Phillips WR, Little TL. Continuity of care and poisoning prevention education. Patient Counsel Health Educ 1980; 4:170–173.

175. Vineis P, Ronco G, Ciccone G, et al. Home injuries in children: a population-based intervention trial. Epidemiology 1994;5:349–351.

176. Gorman RL, Charney E, Holtzman NA, et al. A successful city-wide smoke detector giveaway program. Pediatrics 1985;75:14–18.

177. Katcher ML, Landry GL, Shapiro MM. Liquid-crystal thermometer use in pediatric office counseling about tap water burn prevention. Pediatrics 1989;83:766–771.

178. Dershewitz RA. Will mothers use free household safety devices? Am J Dis Child 1979;133:61–64.

179. Woolf AD, Saperstein A, Forjuoh S. Poisoning prevention knowledge and practices of parents after a childhood poisoning incident. Pediatrics 1992;90:867–870.

180. Cushman R, James W, Waclawik H. Physicians promoting bicycle helmets for children: a randomized trial. Am J Public Health 1991;81:1044–1046.

181. Cushman R, Down J, MacMillan N, et al. Helmet promotion in the emergency room following a bicycle injury: a randomized trial. Pediatrics 1991;88:43–47.

182. Kristenson H, Ohlin H, Hulten-Nosslin M-B, et al. Identification and intervention of heavy drinking in middle-aged men: results and follow-up of 24–60 months of long-term study with randomized controls. Alcohol Clin Exp Res 1983;7:203–209.

183. Ploeg J, Black ME, Hutchison BG, et al. Personal, home and community safety promotion with community-dwelling elderly persons: response to a public health nurse intervention. Can J Public Health 1994;85:188–191.

184. Vetter NJ, Lewis PA, Ford D. Can health visitors prevent fractures in elderly people? BMJ 1992;304:888–890.

185. Hornbrook MC, Stevens VJ, Wingfield DJ, et al. Preventing falls among community-dwelling older persons: results from a randomized trial. Gerontologist 1994;34:16–23.

186. Wagner EH, LaCroix AZ, Grothaus L, et al. Preventing disability and falls in older adults: a population-based randomized trial. Am J Public Health 1994;84:1800–1806.

187. Stuart RB. Teaching facts about drugs: pushing or preventing? J Educ Psych 1974;66:189–201.

188. Tennant FS, Weaver SC, Lewis CE. Outcomes of drug education: four case studies. Pediatrics 1973;52:246–251.

189. Chilton LA. Potential benefit vs. risks of current attempts in health education among adolescents. J Pediatr 1977; 90:163–164.

190. Committee on Injury and Poison Prevention, American Academy of Pediatrics. Office-based counseling for injury prevention. Pediatrics 1994;94:566–567.

191. American Academy of Family Physicians. Age charts for periodic health examination. Kansas City, MO: American Academy of Family Physicians, 1994. (Reprint no. 510.)

192. Green M, ed. Bright Futures: guidelines for health supervision of infants, children, and adolescents. Arlington, VA: National Center for Education in Maternal and Child Health, 1994.

193. American Medical Association. Guidelines for adolescent preventive services (GAPS): recommendations and rationale. Chicago: American Medical Association, 1994.

193a. U.S. Department of Health and Human Services. Healthy People 2000: national health promotion and disease prevention objectives. Washington, DC: Public Health Service, 1991:286–287. (DHHS Publication no. (PHS) 91 50212.)

193b. American College of Obstetricians and Gynecologists. The obstetrician-gynecologist and primary preventive care. Washington, DC: American College of Obstetricians and Gynecologists, 1993.

194. Centers for Disease Control and Prevention. Injury-control recommendations: bicycle helmets. MMWR 1995; 44(RR-1):1–16.

195. Canadian Task Force on the Periodic Health Examination. Canadian guide to clinical preventive health care. Ottawa: Canada Communication Group, 1994:306–317, 526–537, 912–920.

196. Mayer M, LeClere FB. Injury prevention measures in households with children in the United States, 1990. Advance data from vital and health statistics; no 250. Hyattsville, MD: National Center for Health Statistics, 1994.

197. Paul CL, Redman S, Evans D. The cost and availability of devices for preventing childhood injuries. J Paediatr Child Health 1992;28:22–26.

198. Schwarz DF, Grisso JA, Miles C, et al. An injury prevention program in an urban African-American community. Am J Public Health 1993;83:675–680.

199. Cote TR, Sacks JJ, Lambert-Huber DA, et al. Bicycle helmet use among Maryland children: effect of legislation and education. Pediatrics 1992;89:1216–1220.

200. Scheidt PC, Wilson MH, Stern MS. Bicycle helmet law for children: a case study of activism in injury control. Pediatrics 1992;89:1248–1250.

201. Sanders RS. How Tennessee pediatricians led the fight for child restraint legislation. Traffic Safety 1977;77:8–9, 34–35.

59. Counseling to Prevent Youth Violence

RECOMMENDATION

There is insufficient evidence to recommend for or against clinician counseling of asymptomatic adolescents and adults to prevent morbidity and mortality from youth violence. Adolescent and adult patients should be screened for problem drinking (see Chapter 52). Clinicians should also be alert for symptoms and signs of drug abuse and dependence (see Chapter 53), the various presentations of family violence (see Chapter 51), and suicidal ideation in persons with established risk factors (see Chapter 50).

Burden of Suffering

Violence has enormous individual and public health consequences. Victims of violence suffer psychological trauma, physical injuries, disability, and death. The most serious manifestations of violent behavior are homicide and suicide (the latter is discussed in Chapter 50).[a] Homicide is the 10th leading cause of death in the U.S.,[1] and because of the young age of its victims is a leading cause of years of potential life lost.[2,3] More than 25,000 Americans (10.0/100,000 population) were murdered in 1992.[1] The age-adjusted homicide rate increased 25% between 1985 and 1991;[4] a decrease of 3.7% occurred between 1991 and 1992.[1] In the 1991 National Crime Victimization Survey, the rate of aggravated (i.e., involving a weapon) assault was 780/100,000 persons over 12 years of age, while the rate for all nonfatal crimes of violence (including attempted and completed rape, robbery, and assault) was 3,130/100,000.[5] In 1 year, aggravated assaults alone accounted for 355,000 hospitalizations, 4 million lost workdays, and $638 million in medical costs.[6]

Persons at greatest risk of violence victimization include young males, minorities (including non-Hispanic black, Hispanic, and Native Amer-

---

[a]Domestic violence, including spouse, child, and elder abuse, is an important cause of violent injury that is discussed in detail in Chapter 51 and will not be addressed directly in this chapter. It is recognized that interventions targeted toward reducing injuries from youth violence (e.g., reduced gun ownership, training in conflict resolution) also have the potential to reduce injuries due to domestic violence.

ican), persons with a history of delinquent or criminal behavior or of violence victimization, and persons living in poor urban communities.[1,6-15] Nearly half of all homicide victims in 1991 were males aged 15–34 years; most of the increase in homicide rates between 1985 and 1991 was attributable to increased rates in this age group.[4] Young African Americans are at especially high risk for violent injury. Homicide is the leading cause of death in black men and women aged 15–24.[1] In an urban African-American population, the average annual rate of interpersonal violence-related injuries resulting in emergency room visits or death was 3,930/100,000; this rate increased 42% between 1987 and 1990.[16] Interpersonal violence-related injury rates were highest for persons aged 10–39 years, with annual rates ranging from 4,780 to 9,290/100,000. In this study, 41% of 20–29-year-olds had at least one interpersonal intentional injury in the 4-year study period.

Risk factors for violence perpetration are similar to those for victimization, including young age, male sex, minority race, poverty and urbanization, and prior exposure to and victimization by violence.[7,17] These risk factors are highly correlated; for example, minority race is most likely a marker for other factors, such as low socioeconomic status and urban residence, that strongly influence violent behavior. Assailants risk injury to themselves, disrupted personal lives, damaging criminal records, extended imprisonment, and, in some cases, capital punishment. In 1992, 55% of those arrested for murder were under 25 years of age and 15% were under 18.[7] Between 1983 and 1992, the number of juveniles (less than 18 years of age) arrested for murder increased 128% compared to a 7% increase for adults, and the number arrested for aggravated assault (58,000) doubled, compared to a 69% increase in adults.[7]

Firearms, most often handguns, were used in 7 of every 10 murders committed in the U.S. in 1992, and in 25% of aggravated assaults.[7] Because firearm-related homicide rates have increased markedly among teenaged and young adult populations, years of potential life lost attributable to firearm-related homicide has increased by 16% since 1980.[18] Firearm-related assaults account for an estimated 22.4 nonfatal injuries requiring emergency department treatment per 100,000 population per year.[19] In a nationwide survey of high school students, 22% reported that they had carried a weapon and 8% reported carrying a gun during the 30 days preceding the survey.[20]

Efficacy of Risk Reduction

The etiology of youth violence is multifactorial, with complex interactions among personal, family, community, and societal problems.[21-23] While multifaceted community programs to address risk factors such as poverty, unemployment, and poor schools are likely to be most effective in combating youth violence (see *Discussion*), several risk factors may be amenable to interventions by the individual clinician acting in the office setting. These risk factors include the ready availability of weapons, particularly handguns, that increase the lethality of violent behavior, and inadequate social problem-solving skills and abuse of alcohol and illicit drugs, which may increase the incidence of violent behavior.

Firearm-related violence typically results in more severe injury than violence involving other weapons or no weapons. Evidence that reducing gun availability might reduce the risk of violent injury and death comes primarily from ecologic and observational studies. In national and international comparisons, an increased concentration of firearms (as measured by gun permits issued, gun prevalence indices, new firearms for sale, or surveys of gun ownership) is associated with increased rates of firearm robbery, assault, and homicide, and increased overall rates of homicide and robbery-related homicide.[24–28] Several of these studies suggest a dose-response relationship between gun density and violent outcomes. It is difficult to determine from these types of comparisons what, if any, portion of the association is accounted for by social, cultural, and economic differences among populations. The results of several ecologic studies suggest that race and urbanization may modify the association between gun ownership and homicide.[24,29] This modification might be attributable to factors such as poverty, drugs, and other problems characteristic of urban environments, since in a population-based case-control study of homicides in the home, there were no racial differences in the association between homicide and gun ownership after control for other covariates.[30]

These findings in ecologic studies may have several explanations. People may own or carry guns due to an increased risk of violence victimization; if this were the case, gun ownership or carrying would necessarily be associated with higher rates of violent injury. Many persons give self-defense as one of the most important reasons for owning or carrying a gun, particularly a handgun.[31–34] There are no controlled studies evaluating the effect of youths' carrying guns outside the home on their risk of violence victimization, but several studies have evaluated the risks related to guns in the home. In a prospective case series of home invasion crimes, three victims (1.5%) employed a firearm in self-protection, while in one case (0.5%) the homeowner's gun was used against her; the total proportion of victims who kept guns in the home was not recorded, however.[35] In a case series of gunshot deaths (excluding suicides), guns kept in the home were 18 times more likely to be involved in the death of a household member than in the death of an intruder.[36] Stronger evidence for an adverse effect of gun ownership comes from a population-based case-control study, which demonstrated that keeping a gun in the home significantly increased the risk for homicide after adjustment for other covariates.[30] Nearly 90% of the guns used in these homicides were handguns. No published studies have evaluated whether there is a reduced risk of assault or homicide when people voluntarily relinquish the firearms they own or carry.

While guns may predispose to violence, it also may be that those predisposed to violence are more likely to obtain a gun. In cross-sectional surveys and case-control studies among adolescents, gun possession has been associated with more violent attitudes, increased likelihood of being involved in and starting fights, and prior delinquent or illegal behavior.[37–41] A study of inner-city junior high school students reported significant associations between gun carrying and having been arrested, knowing more victims of violence, starting fights, and being willing to justify shooting someone, suggesting that gun-carrying may be a component of aggressive delinquency, rather than purely defensive behavior.[38] Among suburban youths, gun carrying was associated with having been threatened with a gun, but also with drug and violent criminal activities;[41] involvement in such activities is likely to increase the risk of receiving such threats. Reducing gun accessibility is unlikely to reduce the risk of violence among youth predisposed to violent behavior, but it has the potential to reduce the lethality of this behavior when it occurs.

Legislative approaches to reducing gun availability and use have yielded mixed effects on violent injury. A 1978 Government report on various handgun control laws found no evidence of decreased levels of violence because of gun control measures.[42] In one study, a law banning handguns in an urban area was associated with significantly decreased gun-related homicides and annual firearm homicide mortality rates compared to non-firearm-related cases, and to rates in surrounding suburbs without such a law.[43] This study did not assess other trends and differences between populations that might have contributed to the reported effect, however, nor were long-term effects evaluated. Additional studies are needed to replicate these results and determine their generalizability to other populations.

Increasing the punishment for crimes committed with firearms is another legislative prevention strategy. Multiple time series studies of mandatory sentencing for illegally carrying, concealing, or using a firearm have reported small decreases in firearm violence, generally without compensatory increases in non-firearm violence, although not all such series showed statistically significant effects.[44–46] This type of legislation is unlikely to have a large impact on mortality, however, because most homicides are not committed during the course of other criminal activities.

In 1992, almost half of murder victims were related to or acquainted with their assailants, and arguments, brawls, or other interpersonal conflict caused at least one third of all murders.[7] Case-control, cross-sectional, and case series studies of homicide and assault victims suggest that interpersonal conflict with family and acquaintances increases the risk of violent injury.[30,47–49] In large cross-sectional surveys of middle and high school students, violent or aggressive attitudes and behaviors have been associated with an increased risk of being involved in physical fights.[37,50] For example, students previously involved in a physical fight were less likely to believe that apologizing or walking away was an effective way to avoid fights. Violent juvenile offenders have been reported to be more inclined to hold beliefs supporting aggression and to have less extensive skills in social problem-solving compared to control adolescents.[51] These data have led some experts to suggest that changing violent or aggressive attitudes and improving conflict resolution skills might reduce the risk of violent injuries.[52–54] Because attitudes toward violence, social behaviors, and interpersonal problem-solving strategies begin to develop in early childhood,[54] however, it is unclear whether skills training directed to adolescents or young adults will have important effects on their behavior. There have been no evaluations of conflict resolution skills training in the clinical setting, so the effectiveness of such interventions for reducing violent injuries remains unproven.

Case series in the U.S. and in other nations show that about half (range 22–60%) of homicide victims have positive blood alcohol levels at the time of death, and that there is also substantial alcohol involvement among perpetrators.[55–66] Most case-control and cross-sectional studies report that individuals who consume alcohol or who are problem drinkers are at greater risk of violence perpetration and victimization,[58,61,62,67–73] although many of these studies did not evaluate other variables that might confound this association. The strongest evidence in support of an association between alcohol and violence in adults comes from a large population-based prospective cohort study using multivariate analysis, in which heavy drinkers (≥6 drinks per day) were 7 times more likely to be homicide victims than were lifelong abstainers.[74] There was also a 4-fold greater risk in those consuming 3–5 drinks per day and a 2-fold greater risk in light drinkers, but these were not statistically significantly different from abstainers. There were insufficient numbers to assess the risk of homicide in ex-drinkers, although the risk for any unnatural death in ex-drinkers was similar to that of light drinkers and abstainers. Similar to gun owners versus non-owners, alcohol drinkers are likely to differ from nondrinkers in other ways, and a causal relationship between alcohol and violence is not established. Nevertheless, these data suggest that there may be a benefit of reducing alcohol intake in preventing violent injury.

Legislative interventions aimed at reducing alcohol intake in young persons by raising the legal drinking age have not reduced homicide rates,[75,76] but appear to have had little effect on alcohol consumption in the targeted population.[75] In one evaluation of legal drinking age laws, homicide rates increased more than expected in the year drinking became legal, and increased (rather than decreased) as drinking experience increased.[76] Thus, a higher legal drinking age might delay the onset of heavy drinking and associated homicides, but reductions of earlier years may be more than offset by increased homicide rates once access to alcohol becomes legal.

Many victims of violence have evidence of other drugs besides alcohol on toxicologic testing, including cocaine (13–33%), barbiturates (8%), and heroin (3–5%).[15,57,77–79] Adolescent, young adult, and minority homicide victims are more likely to have positive drug screens at autopsy.[15,60,77,78] Evidence for a causal relationship with violence is more limited for illicit drugs than for alcohol. One case-control study found that homicide victims killed in their own home were more likely to have a history of individual or household use of illicit drugs compared with neighborhood matched controls.[30] Several large surveys of high school students have reported associations between illicit drug use and involvement (as victims or perpetrators) in violence.[11,47] In an epidemiologic analysis of homicides in Baltimore, drugs or drug trafficking was involved in 42% of homicides.[80] While it is reasonable to conclude that treatment and referral for substance abuse might contribute to reduced violence, this has not been studied.

Effectiveness of Counseling

Potential victims or perpetrators of violence can be counseled by the clinician in an attempt to prevent future injuries or killings. Specifically, patients can be advised about risk factors, such as possession of firearms and alcohol and substance abuse, that may increase the likelihood of intentional injuries. Persons identified as at increased risk of committing intentional injuries in the future might also be counseled (or referred for counseling) to learn nonviolent approaches to conflict resolution. The efficacy of these measures is largely unstudied, however, and the available evidence is inadequate to determine whether any one of these strategies is successful in preventing subsequent violent injury. An ongoing trial evaluating clinician counseling combined with referral to community resources for adolescent victims of violence (personal communication, D. Stone, June 1994) may provide useful information on the efficacy of clinical counseling to prevent violence.

There is limited evidence regarding the effectiveness of community- and school-based interventions for preventing violence.[81] A number of schools have begun conflict resolution skills curricula, but additional evaluation is needed to determine their effectiveness.[82] In one school-based program in inner-city schools, the program produced improvements in knowledge and some attitudes related to aggressive behavior; injury outcomes were not evaluated.[83] A 3-year community and school-based intervention in Central Harlem that targeted both intentional and unintentional injuries was associated with a significant decline in assault injuries in the targeted community, without a corresponding decrease in the control community.[84] There was little apparent effect of the intervention on overall injury rates because of declines in unintentional injuries in the control community.

Recommendations of Other Groups

The American Academy of Pediatrics (AAP) recommends that all clinicians promote the responsibility of the family to create a gun-safe home environment, including counseling patients, parents, and relatives on the dangers of having a gun in the home, and advising removal or secured storage of guns in the household[85] ". . . emphasis should be placed on high-risk homes—those with alcohol or drug-prone or drug-addicted individuals—and those with adolescent boys."[86] The AAP also supports attempts to identify adolescents at highest risk, including those with a history of violence victimization or family or peer violence, substance abuse, depression, or carrying of weapons.[85] The American Academy of Family Physicians (AAFP) recommends counseling adolescents about alcohol and other drug abuse, and counseling adolescents and young adults, especially males, on violent behavior and firearms.[87] The AAFP policy is under review. The American College of Physicians urges physicians to inform patients about the dangers of keeping firearms, particularly handguns, in the home and to advise them on ways to reduce the risk for injury.[88] The College further supports counseling patients to keep guns away from children and recommending the voluntary removal of the gun from the home. The 1985 Surgeon General's Workshop on Violence and Public Health Report recommended education on the association of alcohol with violence, and education of health professionals in identification, treatment, and/or referral of victims, perpetrators, and persons at high risk for interpersonal violence.[89] In 1992, the Assistant Secretary for Health, U.S. Public Health Service, recommended that clinicians offer counsel on the risks of firearms and on conflict resolution skills.[90]

Discussion

Violent injuries and death exact a terrible toll on adolescents and young adults in this country, yet there is surprisingly little evidence on effective interventions. Although youth violence has been associated with alcohol and substance abuse, availability and ownership of guns, and interpersonal conflict, it is not clear whether these factors predispose to violence, or whether those already predisposed to violence are more likely to obtain a gun, use alcohol and illicit drugs, and become involved in conflict. Most evidence suggests a complex, multifactorial relationship among violent attitudes and behaviors, guns, substance abuse, and violent injury. The ability of clinician counseling to change these behaviors is largely unstudied, however.

There is fair evidence that keeping a gun in the home substantially increases the risk of homicide among those living in or visiting the home. Given that guns in the home are also associated with increased risks of suicide (see Chapter 50) and of unintentional injury deaths (see Chapter 58), removal or secured storage of guns in the home is likely to be an effective intervention for reducing injury-related mortality. Current evidence is insufficient to determine whether clinician advice will influence patients to remove or safely store guns, however.

Although the effectiveness of screening followed by brief counseling to reduce problem drinking has not been evaluated in adolescents and young adults, such screening can be recommended based on its proven efficacy in middle-aged adults (see Chapter 52), the limited adverse effects from such screening, and the large potential impact on both intentional and unintentional injuries, including youth violence, suicide (see Chapter 50), motor vehicle injuries (Chapter 57), and household and recreational injuries (Chapter 58).

As with domestic violence (see Chapter 51), the etiology of youth violence is multifactorial, related to social conditions, cultural attitudes, and personal and family characteristics that begin their influence early in childhood.[21-23] Therefore, the clinician acting alone in the medical setting will have difficulty in preventing violent injuries among adolescents and young adults. Comprehensive prevention programs that address multiple contributors to violence are more likely to be effective in combating morbidity and mortality from youth violence but are beyond the scope of this report. Evaluations of a number of multifaceted violence prevention interventions and programs, including several sponsored by the National Center for Injury Prevention and Control, Centers for Disease Control and Prevention, are ongoing. These projects involve such diverse elements as adult mentoring, job training and placement, peer mediation training among "natural leaders" in schools, social skills training, parenting skills training for the parents of at-risk youths, training of neighborhood violence prevention advocates, school-based conflict resolution programs, counseling and education for violence victims, and schoolwide antiviolence campaigns (T. Thornton, personal communication, 1994).[52,81,84] If these types of multifaceted programs prove effective, the most useful role for clinicians may be to support and act as advocates for such programs in their own communities. Environmental, regulatory, or legislative interventions may also prove to be effective in preventing violence. For example, although they do not reduce violent behavior (i.e., threats and fights), metal detectors in schools appear to reduce the prevalence of carrying weapons to school, which would be likely to reduce the morbidity and mortality resulting from any fight that did occur.[37] Again, the most effective role for the clinician might be to sponsor and support interventions that are proven effective in preventing violent injury.

CLINICAL INTERVENTION

There is currently insufficient evidence to recommend for or against clinician counseling to prevent morbidity and mortality from youth violence ("C" recommendation). Adolescent and adult patients should be screened for problem drinking (see Chapter 52). Clinicians may wish to inform patients (and the parents of child and adolescent patients) of the risk to household members associated with the presence of firearms in the home. Clinicians should also be alert for symptoms and signs of drug abuse and dependence (see Chapter 53), the various presentations of family violence (see Chapter 51), and suicidal ideation in persons with established risk factors (see Chapter 50).

In settings where the prevalence of violence is high, clinicians should ask adolescents and young adults about previous violent behavior or victimization, current alcohol and drug use, and the availability of handguns and other firearms. Clinicians should inform those identified as being at high risk for violence about the risks of violent injury associated with easy access to firearms and with intoxication with alcohol or other drugs.

The draft of this chapter was prepared for the U.S. Preventive Services Task Force by Carolyn DiGuiseppi, MD, MPH.

REFERENCES

1. Kochanek KD, Hudson BL. Advance report of final mortality statistics, 1992. Monthly vital statistics report; vol 43, no 6 (suppl). Hyattsville, MD: National Center for Health Statistics, 1995.
2. Centers for Disease Control and Prevention. Trends in years of potential life lost before age 65 among whites and blacks—United States, 1979–1989. MMWR 1992;41:889–891.
3. Centers for Disease Control and Prevention. Years of potential life lost before age 65—United States,1990 and 1991. MMWR 1993;42:251–253.
4. Centers for Disease Control and Prevention. Homicides among 15–19-year-old males—United States, 1963–1991. MMWR 1994;43:725–727.
5. Bureau of Justice Statistics, Department of Justice. Criminal victimization in the United States, 1991. A National Crime Victimization Survey report. Washington, DC: Department of Justice, 1992. (Publication no. NCJ-139563.)
6. Rosenberg ML, Gelles RJ, Holinger PC, et al. Violence: homicide, assault, and suicide. In: Amler RW, Dull HB, eds. Closing the gap: the burden of unnecessary illness. New York: Oxford University Press, 1987:164–178.

7. Federal Bureau of Investigation. Uniform crime reports for the United States, 1992. Washington DC: Government Printing Office, 1993:31–34. (Publication no. 342-498/94321.)

8. Department of Health and Human Services. Report of the Secretary's Task Force on Black and Minority Health. Volume V. Homicide, suicide, and unintentional injuries. Washington DC: Government Printing Office, 1986.

9. Fingerhut LA, Ingram DD, Feldman JJ. Firearm and nonfirearm homicide among persons 15 through 19 years of age. Differences by level of urbanization, United States, 1979 through 1989. JAMA 1992;267:3048–3053.

10. Ropp L, Visintainer P, Uman J, et al. Death in the city: an American childhood tragedy. JAMA 1992; 267:2905–2910.

11. Lauritsen JL, Laub JH, Sampson RJ. Conventional and delinquent activities: implications for the prevention of violent victimization among adolescents. Viol Vict 1992;7:91–109.

12. Smith MD, Brewer VE. A sex-specific analysis of correlates of homicide victimization in United States cities. Viol Vict 1992;7:279–286.

13. Gladstein J, Slater Rusonis EJ, Heald FP. A comparison of inner-city and upper-middle class youths' exposure to violence. J Adolesc Health 1992;13:275–280.

14. Guyer B, Lescohier I, Gallagher S, et al. Intentional injuries among children and adolescents in Massachusetts. N Engl J Med 1989;321:1584–1589.

15. Tardiff K, Marzuk PM, Leon AC, et al. Homicide in New York City: cocaine use and firearms. JAMA 1994;272:43–46.

16. Schwarz DF, Grisso JA, Miles CG, et al. A longitudinal study of injury morbidity in an African-American population. JAMA 1994;271:755–760.

17. DuRant RH, Cadenhead C, Pendergrast RA, et al. Factors associated with the use of violence among urban black adolescents. Am J Public Health 1994;84:612–617.

18. Centers for Disease Control and Prevention. Firearm-related years of potential life lost before age 65 years—United States, 1980–1991. MMWR 1994;43:609–611.

19. Annest JL, Mercy JA, Gibson DR, et al. National estimates of nonfatal firearm-related injuries: beyond the tip of the iceberg. JAMA 1995;273:1749–1754.

20. Kann L, Warren CW, Harris WA, et al. Youth risk behavior surveillance—United States, 1993. MMWR 1995;44(SS-1):1–56.

21. Christoffel KK. Reducing violence—how do we proceed [editorial]? Am J Public Health 1994;84:539–540.

22. Spivak H, Harvey B. The role of the pediatrician in violence prevention. Pediatrics 1994;94(suppl): 577–651.

23. American Psychological Association Commission on Violence and Youth. Violence and youth: psychology's response. Vol 1: summary report. Washington, DC: American Psychological Association, 1993.

24. Sloan JH, Kellermann AL, Reay DT, et al. Handgun regulations, crime, assaults, and homicide: a tale of two cities. N Engl J Med 1988;319:1256–1262.

25. Lester D. Firearm availability and the incidence of suicide and homicide. Acta Psychiatr Belg 1988;88:387–393.

26. Cook PJ. The effect of gun availability on robbery and robbery murder. Policy Stud Rev Annu 1979;3:743–781.

27. Wintemute GJ. Firearms as a cause of death in the United States, 1920–1982. J Trauma 1987;27:532–536.

28. Killias M. International correlations between gun ownership and rates of homicide and suicide. Can Med Assoc J 1993;148:1721–1725.

29. Centerwall BS. Homicide and the prevalence of handguns: Canada and the United States, 1976 to 1980. Am J Epidemiol 1991;134:1245–1260.

30. Kellermann AL, Rivara FP, Rushforth NB, et al. Gun ownership as a risk factor for homicide in the home. N Engl J Med 1993;329:1084–1091.

31. Patterson PJ, Smith LR. Firearms in the home and child safety. Am J Dis Child 1987;141:221–223.

32. Weil DS, Hemenway D. Loaded guns in the home: analysis of a national random survey of gun owners. JAMA 1992;267:3033–3037.

33. Senturia YD, Christoffel KK, Donovan M. Children's household exposure to guns: a pediatric practice-based survey. Pediatrics 1994;93:469–475.

34. Sheley JF, Wright JD. Gun acquisition and possession in selected juvenile samples. In: Research in brief. Washington, DC: Department of Justice, 1993. (Publication no. NCJ 145326.)

35. Kellermann AL, Westphal L, Fischer L, et al. Weapon involvement in home invasion crimes. JAMA 1995;273: 1759–1762.

36. Kellermann AL, Reay DT. Protection or peril? An analysis of firearm-related deaths in the home. N Engl J Med 1986; 314:1557–1560.

37. Centers for Disease Control and Prevention. Violence-related attitudes and behaviors of high school students—New York City, 1992. MMWR 1993;42:773–777.

38. Webster DW, Gainer PS, Champion HR. Weapon carrying among inner-city junior high school students: defensive behavior vs aggressive delinquency. Am J Public Health 1993;83:1604–1608.

39. Callahan CM, Rivara FP. Urban high school youth and handguns. JAMA 1992;267:3038–3047.

40. Callahan CM, Rivara FP, Farrow JA. Youth in detention and handguns. J Adolesc Health 1993;14:350–355.

41. Sheley JF, Brewer VE. Possession and carrying of firearms among suburban youth. Public Health Rep 1995;110: 18–26.

42. Comptroller General of the United States. Report to the Congress. Handgun control: effectiveness and costs. Washington, DC: Government Printing Office, 1978.

43. Loftin C, McDowall D, Wiersema B, et al. Effects of restrictive licensing of handguns on homicide and suicide in the District of Columbia. N Engl J Med 1991;325:1615–1620.

44. Fife D, Abrams WR. Firearms' decreased role in New Jersey homicides after a mandatory sentencing law. J Trauma 1989;29:1548–1551.

45. O'Carroll PW, Loftin C, Waller JB, et al. Preventing homicide: an evaluation of the efficacy of a Detroit gun ordinance. Am J Public Health 1991;81:576–581.

46. Loftin C, McDowall D, Wiersema B. Evaluating effects of changes in gun laws. Am J Prev Med 1993;9 (Suppl 1):39–43.

47. Valois RF, Vincent ML, McKeown RE, et al. Adolescent risk behaviors and the potential for violence: a look at what's coming to campus. J Am Coll Health 1993;41:141–147.

48. Hausman AJ, Spivak H, Roeber JF, et al. Adolescent interpersonal assault injury admissions in an urban municipal hospital. Pediatr Emerg Care 1989;5:275–279.

49. Graham PM, Weingarden SI. Victims of gun shootings. A retrospective study of 36 spinal cord injured adolescents. J Adolesc Health Care 1989;10:534–536.

50. Cotten NU, Resnick J, Browne DC, et al. Aggression and fighting behavior among African-American adolescents: individual and family factors. Am J Public Health 1994;84:618–622.

51. Slaby RG, Guerra NG. Cognitive mediators of aggression in adolescent offenders: 1. Assessment. Dev Psychol 1988; 24:580–588.

52. Forum on youth violence in minority communities: setting the agenda for prevention. Summary of the proceedings, December 10–12, 1990, Atlanta, GA. Public Health Rep 1991;106:225–279.

53. Prothrow-Stith D. Can physicians help curb adolescent violence? Hosp Pract 1992;193–207.

54. Slaby RG, Stringham P. Prevention of peer and community violence: the pediatrician's role. Pediatrics 1994;94:608–616.

55. Abel EL, Zeidenberg P. Age, alcohol and violent death: a postmortem study. J Stud Alcohol 1985;46:228–231.

56. Batten PJ, Hicks LJ, Penn DW. A 28-year (1963–90) study of homicide in Marion County, Oregon. Am J Forensic Med Pathol 1991;12:227–234.

57. Garriott JC. Drug use among homicide victims. Changing patterns. Am J Forensic Med Pathol 1993;14:234–237.

58. Haberman PW, Baden MM. Alcoholism and violent death. Q J Stud Alcohol 1974;35:221–231.

59. Welte JW, Abel EL. Homicide: drinking by the victim. J Stud Alcohol 1989;50:197–201.

60. Goodman RA, Mercy JA, Loya F, et al. Alcohol use and interpersonal violence: alcohol detected in homicide victims. Am J Public Health 1986;76:144–149.

61. Norton RN, Morgan MY. The role of alcohol in mortality and morbidity from interpersonal violence. Alcohol Alcoholism 1989;24:565–576.

62. Shepherd J, Irish M, Scully C, et al. Alcohol consumption among victims of violence and among comparable U.K. populations. Br J Addict 1989;84:1045–1051.

63. Gottlieb P, Gabrielsen G. Alcohol-intoxicated homicides in Copenhagen, 1959–1983. Int J Law Psychiatry 1992;15: 77–87.

64. Virkkunen M. Alcohol as a factor precipitating aggression and conflict behavior leading to homicide. Br J Addict 1974;69: 149–154.

65. Albrektsen SB, Thomsen JL, Aalund O, et al. Injuries due to deliberate violence in areas of Denmark IV. Alcohol intoxication in victims of violence. Forensic Sci Int 1989;41:181–191.

66. Moller-Madsen B, Dalgaard JB, Grymer F, et al. Alcohol involvement in violence. A study from a Danish community. Z Rechtsmed 1986;97:141–146.

67. Busch KG, Zagar R, Hughes JR, et al. Adolescents who kill. J Clin Psychol 1990;46:472–485.

68. Collins JJ, Schlenger WE. Acute and chronic effects of alcohol use on violence. J Stud Alcohol 1988;49:516–521.

69. Leonard KE, Bromet EJ, Parkinson DK, et al. Patterns of alcohol use and physically aggressive behavior in men. J Stud Alcohol 1985;46:279–282.

70. Murdoch D, Pihl RO, Ross D. Alcohol and crimes of violence: present issues. Int J Addict 1990;25:1065–1081.

71. Cherpitel CJ. Alcohol and violence-related injuries: an emergency room study. Addiction 1993;88:79–88.

72. Roslund B, Larson CA. Crimes of violence and alcohol abuse in Sweden. Int J Addict 1979;14:1103–1115.

73. Langevin R, Paitich D, Orchard B, et al. The role of alcohol, drugs, suicide attempts, and situational strains in homicide committed by offenders seen for psychiatric assessment. Acta Psychiatr Scand 1982;66:229–242.

74. Klatsky AL, Armstrong MA. Alcohol use, other traits, and risk of unnatural death: a prospective study. Alcohol Clin Exp Res 1993;17:1156–1162.

75. Hingson R, Merrigan D, Heeren T. Effects of Massachusetts raising its legal drinking age from 18 to 20 on deaths from teenage homicide, suicide, and nontraffic accidents. Pediatr Clin North Am 1985;32:221–232.

76. Jones NE, Pieper CF, Robertson LS. The effect of legal drinking age on fatal injuries of adolescents and young adults. Am J Public Health 1992;82:112–115.

77. Hanzlick R, Gowitt GT. Cocaine metabolite detection in homicide victims. JAMA 1991;265:760–761.

78. Goodman RA, Mercy JA, Rosenberg ML. Drug use and interpersonal violence: barbiturates detected in homicide victims. Am J Epidemiol 1986;124:851–855.

79. Hanzlick R, Koponen M, Floyd V, et al. Homicides of persons aged 18 years—Fulton County, Georgia, 1988–1992. MMWR 1994;43:254–255, 261.

80. Wood NP Jr, Amanfo J, Rodgers D, et al. Intentional injury—homicide as a public health problem. Md Med J 1993;42: 771–773.

81. National Center for Injury Prevention and Control. The prevention of youth violence: a framework for community action. Atlanta: Centers for Disease Control and Prevention, 1993.

82. Webster DW. The unconvincing case for school-based conflict resolution programs for adolescents. Health Aff (Millwood) 1993;12:126–141.

83. Gainer PS, Webster DW, Champion HR. A youth violence prevention program. Description and preliminary evaluation. Arch Surg 1993;128:303–308.

84. Davidson LL, Durkin MS, Kuhn L, et al. The impact of the Safe Kids/Healthy Neighborhoods injury prevention program in Harlem, 1988 through 1991. Am J Public Health 1994;84:580–586.

85. American Academy of Pediatrics. Firearms and adolescents. Pediatrics 1992;89:784–787.

86. American Academy of Pediatrics. Firearm injuries affecting the pediatric population. Pediatrics 1992; 89:788–790.

87. American Academy of Family Physicians. Age charts for periodic health examination. Kansas City, MO: American Academy of Family Physicians, 1994. (Reprint no. 510.)

88. American College of Physicians. Preventing firearm violence: a public health imperative. Ann Intern Med 1995;122: 311–313.

89. Department of Health and Human Services and Department of Justice. Report of the Surgeon General's workshop on violence and public health. Washington, DC: Health Resources and Services Administration, 1986. (Publication no. HRS-D-MC 86-1.)

90. Mason J. Reducing youth violence—the physician's role. JAMA 1992;267:3003.

60. Counseling to Prevent Low Back Pain

RECOMMENDATION

There is insufficient evidence to recommend for or against counseling patients to exercise to prevent low back pain, but recommendations for regular physical activity can be made based on other proven benefits (see
Chapter 55). There is also insufficient evidence to recommend for or
against the routine use of educational interventions, mechanical supports,
or risk factor modification to prevent low back pain (see *Clinical Intervention*).

Burden of Suffering

Low back pain affects 60–80% of U.S. adults at some time during their
lives, and up to 50% have back pain within a given year.[1-8] Back symptoms
are among the 10 leading reasons for patient visits to emergency rooms,
hospital outpatient departments, and physicians' offices.[9-11] Although
symptoms are usually acute and self-limited, low back pain often recurs,[12]
and in 5–10% of patients low back pain becomes chronic.[1-4,13] Back symptoms are the most common cause of disability for persons under age 45.[14]
Treatment is expensive.[2,3,15-18] In 1990, direct medical costs for low back
pain exceeded $24 billion. Total annual costs for back pain increase from
$35 to $56 billion when disability costs are included.[3,8,18]

Many back injuries are occupational in nature. Occupational back injury is clearly related to lifting and repeated activities. Persons in occupations that require repetitive lifting, such as nursing[19] and heavy industry,[20]
are especially at risk. Based on national data, occupational groups with the
highest estimated prevalence of low back pain (10.1–10.5%) include mechanics and repairers of vehicles, engines and heavy equipment; operators
of extractive, mining, and material-moving equipment; and people in construction trades and other construction occupations.[20]

Efficacy of Risk Reduction

Among the most commonly proposed strategies to prevent low back pain
and injury are: (*a*) back flexion, back extension, and general fitness exercises; (*b*) improved back mechanic and ergonomic techniques (i.e., maxi-

mizing the efficient use of human energy in performing work); (*c*) mechanical back supports (back belts or corsets); and (*d*) risk factor modification (such as reducing obesity and smoking).[6,7,21] Clinical strategies for preventing low back pain are aimed at asymptomatic subjects both with and without a history of back pain.[13,22] The pathophysiology of low back pain and the efficacy of prevention strategies do not differ substantially in these two groups, so prevention studies that enrolled subjects with or without prior acute back pain are included in this review. The Task Force does not specifically address occupational interventions to prevent low back pain such as worker selection, changes in workplace design, or the role of the clinician in the workplace. Studies in occupational settings have been included, however, if they might be generalizable to the primary care setting.

Exercise is typically aimed at strengthening back extensors or flexors and increasing back flexibility to reduce injury risk, improving cardiovascular fitness to minimize injury and enhance recovery should injury occur, and improving mood and pain perception to reduce the impact of injury. Observational studies generally support an association between greater fitness or higher levels of physical activity and reduced prevalence of low back pain or injury, but results are less consistent regarding the effect of greater strength or flexibility on low back pain.[23-35]

Five controlled trials have evaluated the prevention of low back pain with exercise compared to no intervention.[36-41] Two of these trials evaluated back-strengthening exercises. In one trial, nurses and aides with and without a history of prior back pain were randomized to receive instructions on exercises for strengthening back extensors (during five half-hour sessions), followed by 13 months of exercise sessions at work (averaging 6 hours per month), or no intervention.[36] Intervention subjects demonstrated greater extensor strength, fewer self-reported days with low back pain, and reduced absenteeism related to low back pain; total absenteeism was not reported. In another hospital-based trial, employees with a history of low back pain during the year before enrollment were randomized to receive (*a*) 45-minute exercise sessions for strengthening back flexors, twice weekly for 3 months at work; (*b*) five 90-minute back education sessions; or (*c*) no intervention. The number of self-reported "painful months" was significantly less for subjects in the exercise group than in the other groups.[37] Total days lost from work were not reported.

Three controlled trials evaluated exercise aimed at increasing cardiovascular fitness. In the first trial, 125 industrial workers with a history of back pain were randomized to receive aerobic exercise sessions once per week at work for 18 months, or no intervention.[38] Withdrawal rates were high: 19 of the 67 controls and 21 of the 58 exercise subjects (including five who withdrew from the exercise group because of an increase in back or neck pain). Over the 18-month period there was a significantly greater decrease in mean number of back pain episodes, and in sick days attributable to back pain, in intervention subjects compared to controls. Total sick days were not reported, however. In a randomized controlled trial enrolling nurses with a history of back pain during the 2 years before enrollment, intervention subjects attended a 5-week program combining 4 hours of aerobic exercise and 4 hours of back education daily.[39] Although study subjects had fewer self-reported back symptoms than controls at 6 months, it is not clear whether this was due to exercise, education, or both. At the 18-month followup, sick days for the intervention group had increased from baseline.[40] In a nonrandomized trial of 45 nursing aides with mild nondebilitating low back pain,[41] 15 subjects attended training to increase aerobic capacity twice weekly for 8 weeks, 14 subjects were taught "short arm" lifting techniques to protect the back, and the remaining subjects served as controls. Following the intervention, subjects in the exercise cohort had significantly improved aerobic capacity, but there was no reduction in duration or frequency of recurrent back episodes compared with controls.

Thus, most of the trials showed a statistically significant benefit from exercise, but the effects were modest and of uncertain duration. The interventions used may not be relevant to the clinical setting since all allocated work time for exercise, thus greatly increasing the likelihood of compliance. In most of the trials, the authors do not specify whether the control groups continued to work while the intervention groups were allowed time during the workday for exercise.[36–39,42] If so, the results may have been biased by the greater exposure time to work conditions associated with back injury in controls compared to the intervention subjects. A common methodologic problem is the lack of precision in specifying whether the goal was to prevent the first episode of low back symptoms, activity limitations, recurrent episodes, work absenteeism, or chronic disability.[43] Finally, the inclusion criteria and clinical outcomes of the studies differ and therefore are difficult to compare. Thus, the evidence regarding the effectiveness of exercise in preventing low back pain is inconclusive.

Orthotic devices such as back supports (corsets or back belts) are frequently used to prevent back pain and injuries.[44] These devices may be prescribed by physicians, but individuals generally obtain them on their own or from employers. Several studies have attempted to evaluate back belts in the occupational setting. In a controlled trial, 642 airline baggage handlers were randomized to one of four groups: back belt only, training only, back belt and training combined, and control.[45] Previously injured workers were included, but the proportion of workers with prior back injury in each group was not reported. Back belts were to be worn only at work. The 1-hour training session included information on back mechanics, proper lifting techniques, and warm-up exercises. At 8-month followup no statistically significant differences in mean rates of work loss were observed between subjects in either the belt only group or the belt and training groups and controls. When all subjects randomized to use a back belt were aggregated and compared to controls, the intervention group showed a trend toward increased frequency of back pain. Results are difficult to interpret, however, because analysis was performed according to intervention received rather than intention to treat, and 58% of subjects assigned to one of the back belt groups who had not yet developed back pain stopped using the supports before the end of the study. In a trial of 90 warehouse workers,[22] one third were randomized to a 1-hour educational intervention emphasizing back biomechanics and were provided with a corset for use during work hours; one third received education only; and one third received no intervention. There were no differences in productivity or injury rates, but subjects in the corset plus education group had a significantly greater decrease in days lost from work compared with controls (2.5-day decrease vs. 0.4-day increase). These differences in outcomes occurred only in the subgroup of previously injured workers, suggesting that prophylactic bracing may only benefit those with a history of back injury. A retrospective cohort study assessed 1,316 workers at an Air Force base where policy mandated use of the belt for all employees with a history of back injury whose position required frequent heavy lifting. Those who wore belts were the intervention group while employees in comparable positions who chose not to wear belts were controls, suggesting likely selection bias. The risk of low back injury was reduced 40% among those using back belts, but this difference was not statistically significant. Costs of injury sustained while wearing a belt, however, were substantially higher than if injured without a belt.[12] Thus evidence is inadequate to show a benefit from back belts, and suggests possible harms. In addition, poor compliance in these and other studies[46] raises the question of whether subjects will routinely use corsets for prevention of back pain.

Epidemiologic evidence suggests that several **modifiable risk factors,** including smoking, obesity, and certain psychological profiles, predispose subjects to develop low back pain.[2,4,6,7,47,48] Risk factors are presumed to exert their influence either by increasing a subject's risk of a precipitating event, or by increasing the chance that such an event will be perceived as painful or disabling. Cross-sectional and prospective studies have consistently shown that smokers have a 1.5–2.5-fold increased risk of back pain compared to nonsmokers.[21,23,24,30,49–57] A biologic basis for this risk is suggested by a recent study of identical twins discordant for smoking, showing that smoking increases degenerative changes of the spine.[58] Prospective and cross-sectional studies have also associated obesity with back pain, although one study did not support this association.[21,23,24,59] The association may be stronger in women.[23] Based on these associations some authors have recommended smoking cessation and, for obese persons, weight loss to prevent back pain,[6,21] but direct evidence to support these recommendations has not been identified. Psychological risk factors, including depression, anxiety, and perceived high occupational stress, have also been associated with the development of low back pain.[23,24,54,60–63] Again, there is no direct evidence that modifying these factors reduces low back pain.

Effectiveness of Counseling

Education is the most common back pain prevention strategy used in the occupational setting and may also be used by clinicians.[44,64,65] Education through "back school" training, including information on back biomechanics, preferred lifting strategies, optimal posture, exercises to prevent back pain, and stress and pain management, has been effective in reducing employment-related injuries and relieving chronic low back pain.[66–70] Such programs are delivered in the workplace, however, and are not necessarily generalizable to education in the clinical setting.[71] Other types of education programs that are potentially relevant to clinicians have also been evaluated. The studies all included patients with and without prior back pain, generally had small sample sizes, and except for one, were conducted in the workplace. As it would be difficult to do a blinded trial on back education, and since patient reports of low back pain are inherently subjective, all the results have a potential for subject bias.

There have been five randomized controlled trials of educational interventions for the prevention of low back pain. Already described above, two of these combined education with exercise interventions, and one combined education with back supports.[22,37,39] In the trial[37] of hospital employees randomized to either exercise, back education, or control groups, both exercise and education groups' knowledge of body mechanics improved. The education group, however, had no reduction of low back pain episodes. In the trial[39] randomizing nurses to either exercise and low back education or to no intervention, intervention subjects had greater improvements in self-reported pain, fatigue, and activities of daily living at 6-month followup; the effects of education, however, could not be separated from those of the exercise intervention. The previously cited randomized trial[22] that evaluated both lumbar supports (corsets) and back education for warehouse workers included a group that received only a 1-hour educational program stressing proper lifting techniques. Those in the educational program had significantly greater knowledge about low back pain than did controls at 6-month followup. Patients with a previous history of injury had lower injury rates and days lost from work after the education compared with controls, while there was no effect on subjects with no history of back injury. In another randomized controlled trial in U.S. postal workers, knowledge about back pain was higher in those attending an educational program, but self-reported frequency of "tired backs" was no different at 2.5-year followup.[72] In the fifth trial, teenagers enrolled in a summer work program were randomized to a 1-hour session providing information about proper lifting techniques and two on-the-job feedback sessions, or to simple orientation sessions. While the intervention subjects were rated as having better body mechanics than controls at 4-week followup, followup data were not available beyond 4 weeks and the incidence of back pain was not measured.[73]

None of six nonrandomized trials and one case-control study that evaluated educational interventions found a statistically significant difference between control and intervention subjects in the incidence or duration of low back injuries, pain episodes, or, in one study, absenteeism.[41,74–79] One of these, conducted on nursing students, did find that students in the intervention group had significantly better patient handling skills when evaluated by nonblinded observers.[75] Nurses observed to have better transfer skills (regardless of study group) while in school had significantly fewer back injuries than did others (2% vs. 24%), but intervention and control groups did not differ in the occurrence of back pain. Thus, educational interventions do increase knowledge and may improve lifting behavior, but there is little evidence that these changes prevent low back pain or injury.

Two studies have evaluated educational interventions for low back pain prevention during pregnancy. In a nonrandomized trial, 85 pregnant women attended two 1-hour sessions in which the causes of back pain, favorable working postures, and lifting strategies were discussed.[80] Ninety pregnant women who enrolled in the clinic after the intervention program or enrolled in a nearby clinic served as controls. Baseline rates of low back pain were similar in both groups. Following the educational program, women in the intervention group had significantly less self-reported "troublesome or severe" backache than controls (32% vs. 54%). The benefit continued until delivery, but subjects were not followed further. In another controlled trial, 407 pregnant women were assigned, based on birthday, to no intervention, to two 45-minute back school classes, or to five individualized 30-minute lessons with the same content as the second group.[81] Overall, the interventions had no significant effect on the incidence or intensity of back pain. In the subgroup of women who had back or posterior pelvic pain, however, both interventions reduced the pain and the individualized lessons reduced sick leave taken and the intensity of pain reported at 8 weeks postpartum. The study has methodologic weaknesses in both analysis and reporting.

There is currently limited evidence that counseling patients to incorporate regular physical activity into their daily routines will have a positive effect on their behavior (see Chapter 55 for details). Establishing the effectiveness of counseling about modifiable risk factors to prevent low back pain also requires further study. Multiple studies have shown that clinician counseling can substantially increase the rate of smoking cessation (see Chapter 54). Similarly, a number of interventions have been proven effective in inducing short-term weight loss (see Chapter 21). There is also effective treatment for diagnosed depression (see Chapter 49). There is little evidence, however, specifically addressing the effectiveness of counseling patients about smoking, obesity, or psychological conditions as it relates to the prevention of low back pain.

Recommendations of Other Groups

The American Academy of Family Physicians recommends "back-conditioning exercises" for persons aged 19–64 years who are at increased risk for low back injury because of past history, body configuration, or certain types of activities.[82] This policy is currently under review. The Agency for Health Care Policy and Research (AHCPR) recommends patient education about low back symptoms and, in occupational settings, back school. AHCPR has also issued recommendations on the management of acute low back problems.[43,83] The American Academy of Orthopaedic Surgeons' "Lift it Safe" program recommends specific lifting techniques to prevent back pain, and exercises to minimize problems with back pain.[84] The National Institute for Occupational Safety and Health (NIOSH) does not recommend the use of back belts to prevent injuries among workers who have never been injured. NIOSH recommends that the most effective means of minimizing the likelihood of back injury in the workplace is to develop and implement a comprehensive ergonomics program.[85,86]

Discussion

With low back pain affecting the majority of adults in the U.S. at some time during their lives, the associated direct and indirect costs make it one of the most expensive ailments in industrialized countries. At present, studies on the prevention of low back pain and its risk factors do not establish a benefit from intervention. Exercise may be mildly protective against back pain, but data are unavailable beyond 18 months. The best results appeared to occur with comprehensive programs that combined exercise training with other educational interventions. Such intensive programs are more typical of work place interventions, but clinicians might expect similar results if resources were available to duplicate the interventions evaluated in published research. Aerobic exercise appears to be at least as effective as exercises aimed at trunk muscles, and can be readily recommended on the basis of other proven benefits (see Chapter 55). The studies on back education offer minimal support for the use of such strategies in low back pain prevention. Although some educational interventions may have a modest effect, the variability of the interventions and the fact that none of the studies was conducted in typical clinical settings make it difficult to recommend a specific intervention that might be effective in practice. With respect to corsets or back belts, the evidence is contradictory and hence insufficient to make any recommendation at this time. Indeed, the largest studies suggested that mechanical supports may increase the risk of low back pain and the cost of injury in some individuals. Finally, no studies have examined the effect of modifying smoking, obesity, or psychological factors on back pain risk.

CLINICAL INTERVENTION

Although there is some evidence that exercise (flexion, extension, aerobic, or fitness) protects against the development of low back pain, the effect is modest and of unknown duration, and the interventions have not been demonstrated in typical clinical settings. Thus, there is insufficient evidence to recommend for or against counseling patients to exercise specifically to prevent low back pain ("C" recommendation). Recommendations for regular physical activity can be made on other grounds, including its proven efficacy in preventing coronary heart disease, hypertension, obesity, and diabetes (see Chapter 55). There is insufficient evidence to recommend for or against educational interventions or the use of mechanical supports in the prevention of low back pain ("C" recommendation). Given some evidence that mechanical supports may increase the risk of low back pain, recommendations can be made against their use except in the context of comprehensive programs where their use can be carefully monitored to avoid injury. There is insufficient evidence to recommend for or against risk factor modification specifically for the prevention of low back pain ("C" recommendation). Screening for obesity (see Chapter 21) and counseling to prevent tobacco use (see Chapter 54) are recommended based on proven benefits unrelated to low back pain.

Worksite screening and job placement practices are beyond the scope of this report (see NIOSH recommendations[85–87]).

Note: See the relevant background paper: Lahad A, Malter AD, Berg AO, et al. The effectiveness of four interventions for the prevention of low back pain. JAMA 1994;272:1286–1291. Copyright 1994, American Medical Association.

The draft of this chapter was prepared for the U.S. Preventive Services Task Force by Ann S. O'Malley, MD, MPH, and Carolyn DiGuiseppi, MD, MPH, based on a background paper prepared by Amnon Lahad, MD, MPH, Alex D. Malter, MD, MPH, Alfred O. Berg, MD, MPH, and Richard A. Deyo, MD, MPH.

REFERENCES

1. Liebenson CS. Pathogenesis of chronic back pain. J Manipulative Physiol Ther 1992;15:299–308.
2. Frymoyer JW. Back pain and sciatica. N Engl J Med 1988;318:291–300.
3. Frymoyer JW. Can low back pain disability be prevented? Bailliere's Clin Rheumatol 1992;6:595–606.
4. Nachemson AL. Prevention of chronic back pain: the orthopaedic challenge for the 80's. Bull Hosp Joint Dis Orthop Inst 1984;44:1–15.
5. McElligott J, Miscovich SJ, Fielding LP. Low back injury in industry: the value of a recovery program. Conn Med 1989;53:711–715.
6. Nordin M, Weiser S, Halpern N. Education: the prevention and treatment of low back disorders. In: Frymoyer JW, ed. The adult spine and practice. New York: Raven Press; 1991:1641–1654.
7. Deyo RA, Loeser JD, Bigos SJ. Herniated lumbar intervertebral disk. Ann Intern Med 1990;112:598–603.
8. Anderson GBJ, Pope MH, Frymoyer JW, et al. Epidemiology and cost. In: Pope MH, Anderson GBJ, Frymoyer JW, et al., eds. Occupational low back pain. St. Louis, MO: Mosby-Year Book, 1991:95–113.
9. McCaig LF. National Hospital Ambulatory Medical Care Survey: 1992 emergency department summary. Advance data from vital and health statistics; no 245. Hyattsville, MD: National Center for Health Statistics, 1994.
10. McCaig LF. Outpatient department summary: National Hospital Ambulatory Medical Care Survey, 1992. Advance data from vital and health statistics; no 248. Hyattsville, MD: National Center for Health Statistics, 1994.
11. Schappert SM. National Ambulatory Medical Care Survey: 1992 summary. Advance data from vital and health statistics; no 253. Hyattsville, MD: National Center for Health Statistics, 1994.
12. Mitchell LV, Lawler FH, Bowen D, et al. Effectiveness and cost-effectiveness of employer-issued back belts in areas of high risk for back injury. J Occup Med 1994;36:90–94.
13. Dwyer AP. Backache and its prevention. Clin Orthop 1987;222:35–43.
14. Cunningham LS, Kelsey JL. Epidemiology of musculoskeletal impairments and associated disability. Am J Public Health 1984;74:574–579.
15. Nachemson A. Work for all; for those with low back pain as well. Clin Orthop Relat Res 1983;179:77–85.
16. Liles DH. Using NIOSH lift guide decreases risk of back injuries. Occup Health Safety 1985;54:57–60.
17. Frymoyer JW, Mooney V. Current concepts review: occupational orthopaedics. J Bone Joint Surg 1986;68:469.
18. Haag AB. Ergonomic standards, guidelines, and strategies for prevention of back injury. Occup Med 1992;7:155–165.
19. Venning PJ, Walter SD, Stitt LW. Personal and job-related factors as determinants of incidence of back injuries among nursing personnel. J Occup Med 1987;29:820–825.
20. Behrens V, Seligman P, Cameron L, et al. The prevalence of back pain, hand discomfort, and dermatitis in the US working population. Am J Public Health 1994;84:1780–1785.
21. Deyo RA, Bass JE. Lifestyle and low-back pain; the influence of smoking and obesity. Spine 1989;14:501–506.
22. Walsh NE, Schwartz RK. The influence of prophylactic orthoses on abdominal strength and low back injury in the workplace. Am J Phys Med Rehabil 1990;69:245–250.
23. Leino PI. Does leisure time physical activity prevent low back disorders? A prospective study of metal industry employees. Spine 1993;18:863–871.
24. Gyntelberg F. One year incidence of low back pain among male residents of Copenhagen aged 40–59. Dan Med Bull 1974;21:30–36.
25. Pope MH, Bevins T, Wilder DG, et al. The relationship between anthropometric, postural, muscular, and mobility characteristics of males ages 18–55. Spine 1985;10:644–648.
26. Cady L, Bischoff DP, O'Connell ER, et al. Strength and fitness and subsequent back injuries in firefighters. J Occup Med 1979;21:269–272.
27. Cady L, Thomas P, Karwasky R. Program for increasing health and physical fitness of firefighters. J Occup Med 1985;27:110–114.
28. Biering-Sorensen F. Physical measurements as risk indicators for low back trouble over a one year period. Spine 1984;9:106–119.
29. Battié M, Bigos S, Fisher L, et al. Isometric lifting strength as a predictor of industrial back pain complaints. Spine 1989;14:851–856.
30. Battié M, Bigos S, Fisher L, et al. A prospective study of the role of cardiovascular risk factors and fitness in industrial back pain complaints. Spine 1989;14:141–147.

31. Battié M, Bigos S, Fisher L, et al. The role of spinal flexibility in back pain complaints within industry, a prospective study. Spine 1990;15:768–773.

32. Leino P, Aro S, Hasan J. Trunk muscle function and low back disorders: a ten-year follow-up study. J Chronic Dis 1987;40:289–296.

33. Troup JDG, Foreman TK, Baxter CE, et al. The perception of back pain and the role of psychophysical tests of lifting capacity. Spine 1987;12:645–657.

34. McNeill T, Warwick D, Andersson G, et al. Trunk strengths in attempted flexion, extension, and lateral bending in healthy subjects and patients with low back disorders. Spine 1980;5:529–538.

35. Nachemson A, Lindh M. Measurement of abdominal and back muscle strength with and without low back pain. Scand J Rehabil Med 1969;1:60–65.

36. Gundewall B, Liljeqvist M, Hansson T. Primary prevention of back symptoms and absence from work. A prospective randomized study among hospital employees. Spine 1993;18:587–594.

37. Donchin M, Woolf O, Kaplan L, et al. Secondary prevention of low-back pain: a clinical trial. Spine 1990;15: 1317–1320.

38. Kellett KM, Kellett DA, Nordholm LA. Effects of an exercise program on sick leave due to low back pain. Phys Ther 1991;4:283–293.

39. Linton SJ, Bradley LA, Jensen I, et al. The secondary prevention of low back pain: a controlled study with follow-up. Pain 1989;36:197–207.

40. Linton SJ, Bradley LA. An 18-month follow-up of a secondary prevention program for back pain: help and hindrance factors related to outcome maintenance. Clin J Pain 1992;8:227–236.

41. Dehlin O, Berg S, Andersson GBJ, et al. Effect of physical training and ergonomic counseling on the psychological perception of work and on the subjective assessment of low back insufficiency. Scand J Rehabil Med 1981;13:1–9.

42. Dehlin O, Berg S, Hedinrud B, et al. Muscle training, psychological perception of work and low back symptoms in nurses aides. Scan J Rehabil Med 1978;10:201–209.

43. Agency for Health Care Policy and Research. Clinical practice guideline, acute low back problems in adults. Washington, DC: Department of Health and Human Services, 1994. (Publication no. 95-0642.)

44. BNA special report. Back injuries: cost, causes, cases & prevention. Washington, DC: The Bureau of National Affairs, Inc., 1988.

45. Reddell CR, Congleton JJ, Huchingson RD, et al. An evaluation of a weightlifting belt and back injury prevention training class for airline baggage handlers. Appl Ergon 1992;23:319–329.

46. Ahlgren SA, Hansen T. The use of lumbosacral corsets prescribed for low back pain. Prosthet Orthot Int 1978;2: 101–104.

47. Andersson GB. Factors important in the genesis and prevention of occupational back pain and disability. J Manipulative Physiol Ther 1992;15:43–46.

48. Heliovaara M. Risk factors for low back pain and sciatica. Ann Med 1989;21:257–264.

49. Boshuizen HC, Verbeek JH, Broersen JP, et al. Do smokers get more back pain? Spine 1993;18:35–40.

50. Frymoyer JW, Pope MH, Clement JH, at el. Risk factors in low back pain; an epidemiologic survey. J Bone Joint Surg 1983;65:213–218.

51. Battié MC, Bigos SJ. Industrial back pain complaints: a broader perspective. Orthop Clin North Am 1991;22:273–282.

52. Bigos SJ, Battié MC, Fisher LD, et al. A prospective evaluation of preemployment screening methods for acute industrial back pain. Spine 1992;17:922–926.

53. Heliovaara M, Makela M, Knekt P, et al. Determinants of sciatica and low-back pain. Spine 1991;16: 608–618.

54. Holmstrom EB, Lindell J, Moritz U. Low back and neck/shoulder pain in construction workers: occupational workload and psychosocial risk factors. Spine 1992;17:663–672.

55. Roncarati A, McMullen W. Correlates of low back pain in a general population sample: a multidisciplinary perspective. J Manipulative Physiol Ther 1988;11:158–164.

56. Cox JM, Trier KK. Exercise and smoking habits in patients with and without low back and leg pain. J Manipulative Physiol Ther 1987;10:239–245.

57. O'Connor FG, Marlowe SS. Low back pain in military basic trainees: a pilot study. Spine 1993;18:1351–1354.

58. Battié MC, Videman T, Gill K, et al. Smoking and lumbar intervertebral disk degeneration: an MRI study of identical twins. Spine 1991;16:1015–1021.

59. Harvey BL. Self-care practices to prevent low back pain. Am Assoc Occup Health Nurs J 1988;36:211–217.

60. Bigos SJ, Battié MC, Spengler DM, et al. A prospective study of work perceptions and psychosocial factors affecting the report of back injury. Spine 1991;16:1–6.
61. Frymoyer JW, Pope MH, Costanza MC, et al. Epidemiologic studies of low-back pain. Spine 1980;5:419–424.
62. Frymoyer JW, Rosen JC, Clements J, et al. Psychologic factors in low-back-pain disability. Clin Orthop 1985;195: 178–184.
63. Pope MH, Rosen JC, Wilder DG, et al. The relation between biomechanical and psychological factors in patients with low-back pain. Spine 1980;5:173–178.
64. Snook SH, White AH. Education and training. In: Pope MH, Frymoyer JW, Andersson G, et al. Occupational low back pain. New York: Praeger Press, 1984:233–244.
65. Fielding JE, Piserchia PU. Frequency of worksite health promotion activities. Am J Public Health 1989;79:6–20.
66. Mattmiller AW. The California back school. Physiotherapy 1980;66:118–122.
67. Schlapbach P. Back school. In: Schlapbach P, Gerber NJ, eds. Physiotherapy: controlled trials and facts. Rheumatology, vol 14. Basel: S. Karger, 1991:25–33.
68. Forssell MZ. The back school. Spine 1981;6:104–106.
69. Linton SJ, Kamwendo K. Low back schools, a critical review. Phys Ther 1987;67:1375–1383.
70. Hall H. The Canadian back education units. Physiotherapy 1980;66:115–117.
71. Graveling RA. The prevention of back pain from manual handling. Ann Occup Hyg 1991;35:427–432.
72. Daltroy LH, Iversen MD, Larson MG, et al. Teaching and social support: effects on knowledge, attitudes, and behaviors to prevent low back injuries in industry. Health Educ Q 1993;20:43–62.
73. McCauley M. The effect of body mechanics instruction on work performance among young workers. Am J Occup Ther 1990;44:402–407.
74. Hellsing AL, Linton SJ, Andershed B, et al. Ergonomic education for nursing students. Int J Nurs Stud 1993;30: 499–510.
75. Videman T, Rauhala H, Asp S, et al. Patient handling skill, back injuries, and back pain: an intervention study in nursing. Spine 1989;14:148–156.
76. Wood DJ. Design and evaluation of a back injury prevention program within a geriatric hospital. Spine 1987;12: 77–82.
77. Feldstein A, Valanis B, Vollmer W, et al. The Back Injury Prevention Project pilot study; assessing the effectiveness of back attack, an injury prevention program among nurses, aides, and orderlies. J Occup Med 1993;35:114–120.
78. Versloot JM, Rozeman A, van Son AM, et al. The cost-effectiveness of a back school program in industry. Spine 1992;17:22–27.
79. Snook SH, Campanelli RA, Hart JW. A study of three preventative approaches to low back injury. J Occup Med 1978;20:478–481.
80. Mantle MJ, Holmes J, Currey HLF. Backache in pregnancy II: Prophylactic influence of back care classes. Rheumat Rehab 1981;20:227–232.
81. Ostgaard HC, Zetherstrom G, Roos-Hansson E, et al. Reduction of back and posterior pelvic pain in pregnancy. Spine 1994;19:894–900.
82. American Academy of Family Physicians. Age charts for periodic health examination. Kansas City, MO: American Academy of Family Physicians, 1994. (Reprint no. 510.)
83. Agency for Health Care Policy and Research. Quick reference guide for clinicians. Acute low back problems in adults: assessment and treatment. Washington, DC: Department of Health and Human Services, 1994. (Publication no. 95-0643.)
84. "Lift it safe!" [brochure] Rosemont, IL: American Academy of Orthopaedic Surgeons.
85. National Institute for Occupational Safety and Health Back Belt Working Group. Workplace use of back belts: review and recommendations. Washington, DC: Government Printing Office, 1994. (Publication no. 550-147/00029.)
86. Waters TR, Putz-Anderson V, Garg A, et al. Revised NIOSH equation for the design and evaluation of manual lifting tasks. Ergonomics 1993;36:749–776.
87. National Institute for Occupational Safety and Health. Back belts: do they prevent injury? Washington, DC: National Institute for Occupational Safety and Health, 1994. (DHHS [NIOSH] Publication no. 94-127.)

61. Counseling to Prevent Dental and Periodontal Disease

RECOMMENDATION

Counseling patients to visit a dental care provider on a regular basis, floss daily, brush their teeth daily with a fluoride-containing toothpaste, and appropriately use fluoride for caries prevention and chemotherapeutic mouth rinses for plaque prevention is recommended based on evidence for risk reduction from these interventions. Educating parents to curb the practice of putting infants and children to bed with a bottle is also recommended based on limited evidence of risk reduction. The effectiveness of clinician counseling to change any of these behaviors has not been adequately evaluated. Appropriate dietary fluoride supplements are recommended for children living in communities with inadequate water fluoridation. While examining the oral cavity, clinicians should be alert for obvious signs of oral disease (see *Clinical Intervention*). Screening for oral cancer is discussed in Chapter 16, and recommendations regarding counseling to promote healthful diets are provided in Chapter 56.

Burden of Suffering

A large proportion of the population of the U.S. suffers from dental caries (tooth decay) and periodontal (gum and bone) disease. Although the prevalence of dental caries among school-aged children has declined in recent years, the most recent national survey (1986–1987) indicates that the average schoolchild has at least one cavity in permanent teeth by age 9, three cavities by age 12, and eight cavities by age 17.[1] About one quarter have five or more decayed, missing, or filled teeth.[1] In 1986–1987, about 50% of children age 5–17 were completely free of decay and of restorations in their permanent teeth.[1] The average adult in the U.S. has 10–17 decayed, missing, or filled permanent teeth.[2]

About half of all adults have gingivitis (gum inflammation), and 80% have experienced some degree of periodontitis (inflammation of the gums leading to destruction of the bone supporting the teeth).[3,4] About 60% of children and adolescents have at least one tooth site with gingival bleeding.[5] Ninety-five percent of elderly persons have periodontitis, with more than one third experiencing moderate to severe periodontal disease (i.e., at least one site with attachment loss of 6 mm or greater).[2] About 22% of American adults over age 45, and over half of adults over age 65, are edentulous.[6] In 1989, dental conditions accounted for 164 million hours of missed work, 51 million hours of missed school, and 41 million restricted activity days in the U.S.[7] Dental expenditures in the U.S. exceeded $30 billion in 1990.[8] Dental and periodontal diseases are more common in persons whose personal behaviors (e.g., tobacco use, alcohol abuse, poor diet), medications, or coexisting medical illnesses (e.g., diabetes mellitus, xerostomia, Sjögren syndrome, human immunodeficiency virus [HIV] infection) increase the risk of oral pathology. Dental caries is also more common among minorities and children whose parents are of low socioeconomic status.[9]

Tooth and gum diseases are part of an overall category of oral health that includes conditions that fall outside the dental focus of this review (e.g., orofacial pain, salivary conditions, congenital anomalies). These include oral conditions that are manifestations of systemic diseases or treatment modalities. With the aging of the population, a growing number of older Americans are experiencing chronic diseases and taking medications that affect their oral health. The exclusion of these conditions from this discussion is not meant to minimize their important effect on other health behaviors (e.g., nutrition) and overall well-being, their importance as a source of morbidity or mortality in the U.S., the role of certain health behaviors (e.g., tobacco use) in causing these conditions, or the potential benefits of early detection by clinicians.[10]

Efficacy of Risk Reduction

Personal oral disease prevention practices can reduce the risk of developing caries and periodontal disease. These measures include regular use of fluoride and some antiplaque and antigingivitis chemical agents, reduced amount and frequency of dietary intake of foods containing refined sugars or adherent carbohydrates, and tooth brushing and flossing. The incidence of caries has been reduced significantly by the fluoridation of community water supplies.[11-16] Although 87% of the U.S. population is served by community water supplies, only 62% of these communities have optimally fluoridated water.[17] In locations where adequate community water fluoridation is not available, the risk of caries can be reduced by providing alternate sources of fluoride.[18-23] These sources include systemic (e.g., school water fluoridation, and fluoride tablets and drops) and topical (e.g., fluoride mouth rinse, professional fluoride treatment) forms. Virtually all toothpastes sold in the U.S. contain fluoride, which has been shown to be effective in reducing the incidence of caries by about 20–40%.[24,25]

The adverse effects of water fluoridation appear to be minimal. Although an increase in the prevalence of dental fluorosis has been observed,[26,27] this trend has been attributed to inappropriate use of fluoride supplements by health professionals and parents.[28,29] Inappropriate use of fluoride supplements and fluoride dentifrices is particularly common among infants and toddlers, who may swallow large amounts of fluoridated toothpaste.[30,31] Most cases are mild and do not affect the appearance of teeth. Observational studies have provided conflicting evidence regarding the association between fluoride ingestion and the incidence of osteoporosis and hip fractures.[32-37]

Nonfluoride chemicals contained in some mouthwashes and gels may also be effective as antiplaque and antigingivitis agents.[38-40] Regular use of some phenolic antiseptic mouthwashes (e.g., Listerine) has been associated with a 28–34% reduction in plaque and gingivitis at 6-month followup.[41-43] Chlorhexidine gluconate rinses, when combined with toothbrushing, have been reported to achieve 50–55% reduction in plaque and a 45% reduction in gingivitis[44-46] but the product can also stain teeth, increase calculus deposition, and produce an unpleasant taste. Dentifrices containing triclosan, when combined with zinc citrate or a copolymer of methoxyethylene and maleic acid, have been associated with a significant reduction in plaque and gingivitis,[47-50] but the products are currently not available in the U.S.

Reduced exposure of the teeth to certain dietary carbohydrates, especially refined sugars and carbohydrates that adhere to the teeth, may lower the risk of developing caries. Studies in the 1950s and 1960s conducted in institutionalized settings suggested that diets including large amounts or frequent consumption of sucrose and other sugary foods were associated with a higher incidence of caries.[51,52] The correlation has been more difficult to demonstrate in more recent studies, in which dietary intake was less carefully controlled, but the data are suggestive that the consumption of sugary foods, especially between meals, is cariogenic.[53-58] Some data from animal studies also support this conclusion. For ethical reasons, definitive studies to prove a causal relationship between diet and carious lesions in humans are unlikely to be performed.

Improper infant feeding practices are another postulated source of caries in young children, especially the cariogenic damage to the maxillary incisors seen in early childhood caries (baby bottle tooth decay). This condition was first attributed to prolonged pooling of liquids around the anterior primary teeth in infants who regularly fall asleep sucking the nipple of a baby bottle containing an acidic or cariogenic beverage (fruit juice, soda, and formula).[59] The etiology of the condition now appears to be multifactorial, and an association between infant feeding practices and early childhood caries is less clear.[60-62] Some evidence suggests that other dietary factors and vertical transmission of certain bacteria from the mother may play an etiologic role.[62a] Education to curb the practice of putting children to bed with a bottle, encouragement of breastfeeding, early restoration and treatment of tooth decay, and optimizing the oral health care of the mother have each been proposed to decrease the risk of early childhood caries, but definitive evidence of effectiveness is lacking.

It is mainly the fluoride contained in toothpastes, rather than tooth-brushing and flossing per se, that reduces tooth decay. It has been known for two decades, however, that brushing and flossing can prevent the development and progression of periodontal disease by removing bacterial plaque deposits.[63-65] Mechanical interdental cleaning (e.g., flossing) and toothbrushing appear to be more effective than toothbrushing alone or antimicrobial mouth rinses in reducing gingivitis.[66,67] Their efficacy, however, depends on the ability of the patient to keep teeth adequately plaque-free, and this necessitates thorough daily tooth brushing and cleaning between teeth with dental floss or other mechanical devices. It is unclear whether home electrical toothbrushes with rotating bristles are more effective than manual brushing in removing plaque and controlling gingivitis.[68-70] These devices may be of greater benefit for persons with physical limitations due to arthritis or other conditions. Due to the difficulty many patients have in adopting and maintaining these habits, personal oral hygiene measures often fail to remove plaque adequately and prevent gingivitis. For this reason, it is also important for patients to receive regular professional dental care.

Different types of professional care are provided by dental specialists, dental hygienists, and dental public health professionals. Among the most important measures performed by dentists and dental hygienists are primary preventive measures, such as prophylactic scaling and root planing of teeth, and secondary preventive maneuvers, such as careful oral and dental examination for the early detection and treatment of dental disease. Other potentially effective preventive interventions offered by dental health professionals include the application of topical fluoride[71,72] and occlusal sealants[73-75] to prevent caries, placement of orthodontic space-maintaining appliances to prevent malocclusion, and the early detection of oral cancer (see Chapter 16) and the oral manifestations of infection with HIV (see also Chapter 28). Experimental studies in the 1970s demonstrated that meticulous and very frequent dental prophylaxis can reduce the incidence of caries in schoolchildren,[76-81] but these studies required an intense program of professional dental care that would not be feasible under typical dental practice conditions in the U.S. Other studies suggest that topical fluoride application may be equally effective with or without dental prophylaxis, making it unclear whether the procedure needs to be restricted to dental practices.[39] Professional care can also delay progression of periodontal disease because the dentist or dental hygienist can remove plaque and calculus from subgingival areas generally not reached by the patient. Professional dental care alone, however, is inadequate to prevent periodontal disease. Failure by the patient to regularly remove plaque deposits between dental visits can lead to extension of supragingival plaque beneath the gum, bacterial recolonization of the gingival crevice, accumulation of calculus, and recurrent periodontitis.[83] Thus, regimens that combine personal oral hygiene with professional prophylaxis are most effective in the prevention of periodontal disease.[84]

Although annual (or more frequent) dental examinations and prophylaxis are often recommended, there is little scientific evidence that this frequency is necessary on a routine basis for the maintenance of oral health in asymptomatic persons. Regular examinations may be necessary to detect and treat disease processes before they threaten the viability of the teeth, gums, and other oral soft tissues; in addition, more frequent visits may be necessary for persons at increased risk by virtue of their age, risk factors (e.g., pregnancy, tobacco and alcohol use), state of periodontal health, rate of accumulation of tartar, personal oral hygiene practices, and medical and dental history (e.g., diabetes mellitus, xerostomia, HIV infection).

Effectiveness of Counseling

Survey data suggest that many patients, especially persons in minority groups or those of low socioeconomic status, lack adequate knowledge about how to prevent oral diseases.[85] There is little information on the effectiveness of physician advice in changing oral hygiene or dietary habits, increasing the optimal use of fluoride supplements, or increasing patient visits to dentists. Studies of patient education involving dentists, dental hygienists, dietitians, physicians, and other providers have reported mixed results in changing personal oral health practices and suffer from numerous design problems.[86–88] It is well known among oral health professionals that patients frequently face difficulties in complying with guidelines for proper tooth brushing and dental flossing without repeated reinforcement. Studies suggest that compliance with oral hygiene instruction is often poor.[89] There is little information regarding the willingness or ability of patients to comply with clinicians' advice to visit their dental care provider on a regular basis. The effectiveness of counseling to promote a healthy diet is discussed in Chapter 56.

In communities with inadequate water fluoridation, primary care physicians are an important source of supplemental fluoride drops or tablets to prevent dental caries in children. There is little information on patient compliance with such prescriptions. Studies have shown, however, that clinicians often fail to prescribe dietary fluoride supplements in accordance with existing guidelines[90] or to determine the fluoride content of the local water supply before doing so.[91]

Recommendations of Other Groups

The Canadian Task Force on the Periodic Health Examination recommends water fluoridation, fluoride supplementation in low-fluoride areas, professional topical fluoride and self-administered fluoride mouth rinses for persons with active decay or specific risk factors, and use of fluoride dentifrices. It found insufficient evidence to recommend for or against toothbrushing and flossing, traditional prophylaxis prior to a topical fluoride application or given at a dental recall visit, and dietary counseling of the general population about cariogenic foods.[92] The American Dental Association (ADA) advises that the frequency of dental examinations be tailored to the individual.[93] The ADA and American Academy of Pediatrics (AAP) have issued new guidelines on the prescription of dietary fluoride supplements for children in areas with inadequate water fluoridation (see below).[94,95] The AAP[96] and other organizations have also issued guidelines on the prevention of early childhood caries (baby bottle tooth decay).

Discussion

Although there is little scientific evidence that clinician counseling can reduce the incidence of dental diseases such as caries and periodontal disease, it is reasonable to provide patients with information about methods to reduce the risk of developing these potentially painful and disfiguring conditions. There is sufficient evidence of benefit to justify efforts by physicians and other health care professionals to encourage frequent tooth brushing, daily dental flossing, appropriate use of fluorides and certain mouth rinses, healthful diet, and periodic visits to the dental care provider. There is, however, little evidence that this form of counseling must be performed frequently, or that annual or semiannual dental checkups are necessary for persons without clinical evidence of dental disease. Although it is likely that decreased or less frequent consumption of foods containing refined sugars or avoiding between-meal sweets will reduce the incidence of dental caries, this has not been demonstrated recently in a controlled prospective study involving humans (see Chapter 56 for information about the effectiveness of other forms of counseling to promote a healthy diet). Finally, clinicians can offer advice regarding effective measures to reduce the risk of developing oral cancer (see Chapter 16), such as discontinuing the use of tobacco products (see Chapter 54) and reducing the consumption of alcoholic beverages (see Chapter 52).

CLINICAL INTERVENTION

Counseling patients to visit a dental care provider on a regular basis is recommended based on evidence for risk reduction from such visits when combined with regular personal oral hygiene ("B" recommendation); the effectiveness of advising patients to visit a dental care provider has not been evaluated ("C" recommendation). There is little evidence regarding the optimal frequency of visits; this recommendation should be made by the patient's dental care provider. Counseling all patients to brush their teeth daily with a fluoride-containing toothpaste and to clean thoroughly between their teeth with dental floss each day is recommended based on the proven efficacy of risk reduction from doing so ("B" recommendation); the effectiveness of clinician counseling to encourage these behaviors has not been adequately evaluated ("C" recommendation). Parents of small children should be encouraged to perform or supervise their children's brushing and to monitor the amount of toothpaste used; wiping the teeth with a piece of gauze or damp cloth is typically recommended for cleaning the teeth of children who are too young to use a toothbrush. Parents of infants and young children should be encouraged to breastfeed (see Chapter 56). Providing advice to parents to put infants and children to bed without a bottle may reduce the risk of baby bottle tooth decay ("B" recommendation). See Chapter 56 for other recommendations regarding counseling to promote a healthy diet.

Clinicians caring for children should ascertain the fluoride concentration of their water supply. For children living in an area with inadequate water fluoridation (<0.6 parts per million [ppm]), the prescription of daily fluoride drops or tablets is recommended ("A" recommendation). According to recently revised guidelines,[94,95] in communities with a water fluoride concentration of less than 0.3 ppm, the recommended dose is 0.25 mg/day for children 6 months to 3 years of age, 0.50 mg/day for children aged 3–6, and 1.0 mg/day for children aged 6–16. In areas with a water fluoride level of 0.3–0.6 ppm, fluoride supplementation is not recommended for children 6 months to 3 years of age. For older children, the recommended dose is 0.25 mg/day for children aged 3–6 and 0.50 mg/day for children aged 6–16. Some groups have issued more conservative recommendations that limit fluoride supplementation to children age 3 and older living in communities with water fluoride concentrations of less than 0.3 ppm.[97]

When examining the oral cavity, clinicians should be alert for obvious signs of untreated tooth decay or mottling, inflamed or cyanotic gingiva, loose teeth, and severe halitosis, and for signs and symptoms of oral cancer or premalignancy in persons who use tobacco or excessive amounts of alcohol (see Chapter 16). All patients should be counseled to avoid the use of tobacco products (see Chapter 54). When examining children, clinicians should be alert for evidence of early childhood caries (baby bottle tooth decay), mismatching of upper and lower dental arches, crowding or malalignment of the teeth, premature loss of primary posterior teeth (baby molars), and obvious mouth breathing. Patients with these or other suspected abnormalities should be referred to appropriate specialists for further evaluation.

The draft update of this chapter was prepared for the U.S. Preventive Services Task Force by Steven H. Woolf, MD, MPH, with contributions from materials prepared for the Canadian Task Force on the Periodic Health Examination by Amid I. Ismail, BDS, MPH, DrPH, Donald W. Lewis, DDS, DDPH, MScD, FRCDC, and Jennifer L. Dingle, MBA.

REFERENCES

1. Public Health Service. Oral health of United States children: the national survey of dental caries in U.S. school children: 1986–1987. National and regional findings. Bethesda: National Institutes of Health, 1989. (NIH Publication no. 89-2247.)
2. National Institute of Dental Research. Oral health of United States adults, the national survey of oral health in U.S. employed adults and seniors: 1985–86. Bethesda: National Institute of Dental Research, 1987. (NIH Publication no. 87-2868.)
3. Beck JD, Lainson PA, Field HM, et al. Risk factors for various levels of periodontal disease and treatment need in Iowa. Community Dent Oral Epidemiol 1984;12:17–22.
4. Oliver RC, Brown LJ, Loe H. An estimate of periodontal treatment needs in the U.S. based on epidemiologic data. J Periodontol 1989;60:371–380.
5. Bhat M. Periodontal health of 14–17-year-old U.S. schoolchildren. J Public Health Dent 1991;51:5–11.
6. National Center for Health Statistics. Dental services and oral health: United States, 1989. Vital and health statistics; series 10 no 183. Hyattsville, MD: National Center for Health Statistics. 1992:4–5. (PHS Publication no. 93-1511.)
7. Gift HC, Reisine ST, Larach DC. The social impact of dental problems and visits. Am J Public Health 1992;82: 1663–1668.
8. Lazenby HC, Letsch SW. National health expenditures, 1989. Health Care Financing Rev 1990;12:1–26.
9. Oral Health Coordinating Committee, Public Health Service. Toward improving the oral health of Americans: an overview of oral health status, resources, and care delivery. Public Health Rep 1993;108:657–672.
10. Gift HC, Redford M. Oral health and the quality of life. Clin Geriatr Med 1992;8:673–683.
11. Newbrun E. Effectiveness of water fluoridation. J Public Health Dent 1989;49(Special Issue):279–289.
12. Lewis DW, Banting DW. Water fluoridation—current effectiveness and dental fluorosis. Community Dent Oral Epidemiol 1994;22:153–158.
13. Stamm JW, Banting DW, Imrey PB. Adult root caries: survey of two similar communities with contrasting natural fluoride water levels. J Am Dent Assoc 1990;120:143–149.
14. Burt BA, Eklund SA. Dentistry, dental practice, and the community, 4th ed. Philadelphia: WB Saunders, 1992: 162–165.
15. Public Health Service. Review of fluoride benefits and risks: report of the ad hoc subcommittee of fluoride of the Committee to Coordinate Environmental and Health Related Programs. Washington, DC: Department of Health and Human Services, 1991.
16. American Dietetic Association. Position of the American Dietetic Association: the impact of fluoride on dental health. J Am Diet Assoc 1994;94:1428–1431.
17. Centers for Disease Control. Fluoridation census, 1992. Washington, DC: Department of Health and Human Services, 1993.
18. Changing patterns of fluoride intake: workshop, Chapel Hill, NC, April 23–25, 1991. J Dent Res 1992;71:1214–1227.

19. Heifetz SB, Meyers RJ, Kingman A. A comparison of the anticaries effectiveness of daily and weekly rinsing with sodium-fluoride: final results after three years. Pediatr Dent 1982;4:300–303.

20. Johnson MF. Comparative efficacy of NaF and SMFP dentifrices in caries prevention: a meta-analytic overview. Caries Res 1993;27:328–336.

21. Driscoll WS, Nowjack-Raymer R, Selwitz RH, et al. A comparison of the caries-preventive effects of fluoride mouthrinsing, fluoride tablets, and both procedures combined: final results after eight years. J Public Health Dent 1992;52:111–116.

22. Nowjack-Raymer RE, Gift HC. Contributing factors to maternal and child oral health. J Public Health Dent 1990;50 370–378.

23. Stephen KW, Kay EJ, Tullis JI. Combined fluoride therapies: a 6-year double-blind school-based preventive dentistry study in Inverness, Scotland. Community Dent Oral Epidemiol 1990;18:244–248.

24. Mellberg JM, Ripa LW. Fluoride dentifrices. In: Mellberg JM, Ripa LW, eds. Fluoride in preventive dentistry: theory and clinical application. Chicago: Quintessence, 1983:215–241.

25. Jensen ME, Kohout FJ. The effect of a fluoridated dentifrice on root and coronal caries in an older adult population. J Am Dent Assoc 1988;117:829–832.

26. Ismail AI, Brodeur JM, Kavanagh M, et al. Prevalence of dental caries and dental fluorosis in students, 11–17 years of age, in fluoridated and non-fluoridated cities in Quebec. Caries Res 1990;24:290–297.

27. Brunelle JA. The prevalence of dental fluorosis in U.S. children, 1987. J Dent Res 1989;68(Special Issue):995.

28. Woolfolk MW, Faja BW, Bagramian RA. Relation of sources of systemic fluoride to prevalence of dental fluorosis. J Public Health Dent 1989;49:78–82.

29. Szpunar SM, Burt BA. Evaluation of appropriate use of dietary fluoride supplements in the US. Community Dent Oral Epidemiol 1992;20:148–154.

30. Nourjah P, Horowitz AM, Wagener DK. Factors associated with the use of fluoride supplements and dentifrice by infants and toddlers. J Public Health Dent 1994;54:47–54.

31. Osuji OO, Leake JL, et al. Risk factors for dental fluorosis in a fluoridated community. J Dent Res 1988;67: 1488–1492.

32. Sowers MFR, Clark MK, Jannausch ML, et al. A prospective study of bone mineral content and fracture in communities with differential fluoride exposure. Am J Epidemiol 1991;133:649–660.

33. Cooper C, Wickham CAC, Barker DJR, et al. Water fluoridation and hip fracture. JAMA 1991;266:513–514.

34. Danielson C, Lyon JL, Egger M, et al. Hip fractures and fluoridation in Utah's elderly population. JAMA 1992;268:746–748.

35. Jacobsen SJ, O'Fallon WM, Melton LJ III. Hip fracture incidence before and after the fluoridation of the public water supply, Rochester, Minnesota. Am J Public Health 1993;83:743–745.

36. Suarez-Almazor ME, Flowerdew G, Saunders LD, et al. The fluoridation of drinking water and hip fracture hospitalization rates in two Canadian communities. Am J Public Health 1993;83:689–693.

37. Gordon SL, Corbin SB. Summary of workshop on drinking water fluoride influence on hip fracture and on bone health. Osteoporosis Int 1992;286:109–117.

38. Brecx M, MacDonald LL, Legary K, Cheang M, Forgay MGE. Long-term effects of Meridol and chlorhexidine mouthrinses on plaque, gingivitis, staining, and bacterial vitality. J Dent Res 1993;72:1194–1197.

39. Olivier M, Brodeur JM, Simard PL. Efficacy of APF treatments without prior toothcleaning targeted to high-risk children. Community Dent Oral Epidemiol 1992;20:38–42.

40. Zimmermann A, Flores-de-Jacoby L, Pan P, Gingivitis, plaque accumulation and plaque composition under long-term use of Meridol. J Clin Periodontol 1993;20:346–351.

41. Lamster IB, Alfano MC, Seiger MC, et al. The effect of Listerine antiseptic on reduction of existing plaque and gingivitis. Clin Prev Dent 1983;5:12.

42. Gordon JM, Lamster IB, Seiger MC. Efficacy of Listerine antiseptic in inhibiting the development of plaque and gingivitis. J Clin Periodontol 1985;12:697–704.

43. DePaola LG, Overholser CD, Meiller TF, et al. Chemotherapeutic inhibition of supergingival dental plaque and gingivitis development. J Clin Periodontol 1989;16:311–315.

44. Lang NP, Hotz P, Graff H, et al. Effect of supervised chlorhexidine mouthrinses in children. J Periodont Res 1982;17: 101–111.

45. Banting D, Bosma M, Bollmer B. Clinical effectiveness of a 0.12% chlorhexidine mouthrinse over two years. J Dent Res 1989;68:1716–1718.

46. Yates R, Jenkins S, Newcombe R, et al. A 6-month home usage trial of a 1% chlorhexidine toothpaste (I). Effects on plaque, gingivitis, calculus and toothstaining. J Clin Periodontol 1993;20:130–138.

47. Svatun B, Saxton CA, Rolla G. Six-month study of the effect of a dentifrice containing zinc citrate and triclosan on plaque, gingival health, and calculus. Scand J Dent Res 1990;98:301–304.

48. Cubells AB, Dalman LB, Petrone ME, et al. The effect of a triclosan/copolymer/fluoride dentifrice on plaque formation and gingivitis: a six-month clinical study. J Clin Dent 1991;2:63–69.

49. Bolden TE, Zambon JJ, Sowinski J, et al. The clinical effect of a dentifrice containing triclosan and a copolymer in a sodium fluoride/silica base on plaque formation and gingivitis: a six-month clinical study. J Clin Dent 1992;3: 125–131.

50. Deasy MJ, Singh SM, Rustogi KN, et al. Effect of a dentifrice containing triclosan and a copolymer on plaque formation and gingivitis. Clin Prev Dent 1991;13:12–19.

51. Gustafsson BE, Quensel CE, Lanke LS, et al. The Vipeholm dental caries study: the effect of different levels of carbohydrate intake on caries activity in 436 individuals observed for 5 years. Acta Odontol Scand 1954;11:232–364.

52. Harris R. Biology of the children of Hopewood House, Bowral, Australia. IV. Observations of dental caries experience extending over five years (1957–1961). J Dent Res 1963;42:1387–1398.

53. Burt RA, Eklund SA, Morgan KJ, et al. The effect of diet on the development of dental caries. Final report, contract DE-22438. Bethesda: National Institute of Dental Research, 1987.

54. Rugg-Gunn AJ, Hackett AF, Appleton DR, et al. Relationship between dietary habits and caries increments assessed over two years in 405 English adolescent schoolchildren. Arch Oral Biol 1984;29:983–992.

55. Burt BA, Eklund SA, Morgan KJ, et al. The effects of sugar intake and frequency of ingestion on dental caries increment in a three-year longitudinal study. J Dent Res 1988;67:1422–1429.

56. Akpata ES, Al-Shammery AR, Saeed HI. Dental caries, sugar consumption and restorative dental care in 12–13-year-old children in Riyadh, Saudi Arabia. Community Dent Oral Epidemiol 1992;20:343–346.

57. Frostell G, Birkhed D, Edwardsson S, et al. Effect of partial substitution of invert sugar for sucrose in combination with Duraphat treatment on caries development in preschool children: the Malmo study. Caries Res 1991;25: 304–310.

58. Holt RD. Foods and drinks at four daily time intervals in a group of young children. Br Dent J 1991;170:137–143.

59. Ripa LW. Nursing caries: a comprehensive review. Pediatr Dent 1988;10:268–282.

60. Serwint JR, Mungo R, Negrete VF, et al. Child-rearing practices and nursing caries. Pediatrics 1993;92: 233–237.

61. Roberts GJ, Cleaton-Jones PE, Fatti LP, et al. Patterns of breast and bottle feeding and their association with dental caries in 1- to 4-year-old South African children. 2. A case control study of children with nursing caries. Community Dent Health 1994;11:38–41.

62. O'Sullivan DM, Tinanoff N. Social and biological factors contributing to caries of the maxillary anterior teeth. Pediatr Dent 1993;15:41–44.

62a. Navia JM. Caries prevention in infants and young children: which etiologic factors should we address? J Public Health Dent 1994;54:195–196.

63. Suomi JD, Greene JC, Vermillion JR, et al. The effect of controlled oral hygiene procedures on the progression of periodontal disease in adults: results after third and final year. J Periodontol 1971;42:152–160.

64. Horowitz AM, Suomi JD, Peterson JK, et al. Effects of supervised daily dental plaque removal by children after 3 years. Community Dent Oral Epidemiol 1980;8:171–176.

65. Lang NP, Cumming BR, Loe H. Toothbrush frequency as it is related to plaque development and gingival health. J Periodontol 1973;44:398–405.

66. Caton JG, Blieden TM, Lowenguth RA, et al. Comparison between mechanical cleaning and an antimicrobial rinse for the treatment and prevention of interdental gingivitis. J Clin Periodontol 1993;20:172–178.

67. Graves RC, Disney JA, Stamm JW. Comparative effectiveness of flossing and brushing in reducing interproximal bleeding. J Periodontol 1989;50:243–247.

68. Barnes CM, Weatherford TW, Menaker L. A comparison of the Braun Oral-B Plaque Remover (D5) electric and a manual toothbrush in affecting gingivitis. J Clin Dent 1993;4:48–51.

69. Stoltze K, Bay L. Comparison of a manual and a new electric toothbrush for controlling plaque and gingivitis. J Clin Periodontol 1994;21:86–90.

70. van der Weijden GA, Timmerman MF, Reijerse E, et al. The long-term effect of an oscillating/rotating electric toothbrush on gingivitis: an 8-month clinical study. J Clin Periodontol 1994;21:139–145.

71. Helfenstein U, Steiner M. Fluoride varnishes (Duraphat): a meta-analysis. Community Dent Oral Epi-

demiol 1994;22:1–5.

72. Ripa LW. A critique of topical fluoride methods (dentifrices, mouthrinses, operator-, and self-applied gels) in an era of decreased caries and increased fluorosis prevalence. J Public Health Dent 1991;51:23–41.

73. Mertz-Fairhurst EJ, Fairhurst CW, Williams JE, et al. A comparative clinical study of two pit and fissure sealants: 7-year results in Augusta, Georgia. J Am Dent Assoc 1984;109:252–255.

74. Llodra JC, Bravo M, Delgado-Rodriguez M, et al. Factors influencing the effectiveness of sealants—a meta-analysis. Community Dent Oral Epidemiol 1993;21:261–268.

75. Weintraub JA. The effectiveness of pit and fissure sealants. J Public Health 1989;49(Special Issue):317–330.

76. Axelsson P, Lindhe J. The effect of a preventive program on dental plaque, gingivitis and caries in school children: results after one and two years. J Clin Periodontol 1974;1:126–138.

77. Axelsson P, Lindhe J. The effect of various plaque control measures on gingivitis and caries in school children. Community Dent Oral Epidemiol 1976;4:232–239.

78. Agerback N, De Paola PF, Brudevold F. Effects of professional toothcleaning every third week on gingivitis and dental caries in children. Community Dent Oral Epidemiol 1978;6:40–41.

79. Ashley FP, Sainsbury RH. The effect of a school-based plaque control programme on caries and gingivitis. Br Dent J 1981;150:41–45.

80. Badersten A, Egelberg J, Koch G. Effect of monthly prophylaxis on caries and gingivitis in schoolchildren. Community Dent Oral Epidemiol 1975;3:1–4.

81. Hamp SE, Lindhe J, Fornell LA, et al. Effect of a field program based on systematic plaque control on caries and gingivitis in schoolchildren after 3 years. Community Dent Oral Epidemiol 1978;6:17–23.

82. *Deleted in proof.*

83. Loe H, Kleinman DV. Dental plaque control measures and oral hygiene practices. Proceedings from a state-of-the-science workshop. Washington, DC: IRL Press, 1986.

84. Axelsson P, Lindhe J. Effect of controlled oral hygiene procedures on caries and periodontal disease in adults: results after six years. J Clin Periodontol 1981;8:239–248.

85. Gift HC, Corbin SB, Nowjack-Raymer RE. Public knowledge of prevention of dental disease. Public Health Rep 1994;109:397–404.

86. Brown LF. Research in dental health education and health promotion: a review of the literature. Health Educ Q 1994;21:83–102.

87. Horowitz AM. Effective oral health education and promotion programs to prevent dental caries. Int Dent J 1982;33:171–181.

88. Hollund U. Effect of a nutrition education program, "learning by teaching," on adolescents' knowledge and beliefs. Community Dent Oral Epidemiol 1990;18:61–65.

89. Weinstein P, Milgrom P, Melnick S, et al. How effective is oral hygiene instruction? Results after 6 and 24 weeks. J Public Health Dent 1989;49:32–38.

90. Kuthy RA, McTigue DJ. Fluoride prescription practices of Ohio physicians. J Public Health Dent 1987;47:172–176.

91. Levy SM, Rozier RG, Bawden JW. Use of systemic fluoride supplements by North Carolina dentists. J Am Dent Assoc 1987;114:347–350.

92. Canadian Task Force on the Periodic Health Examination. Canadian guide to clinical preventive health care. Ottawa: Canada Communication Group, 1994:408–431.

93. American Dental Association. The importance of professional teeth cleaning. Chicago: American Dental Association, 1985.

94. American Academy of Pediatrics. Fluoride supplementation for children: interim policy recommendations. Pediatrics 1995;95:777.

95. New fluoride guidelines proposed. J Am Dent Assoc 1994;125:366.

96. American Academy of Pediatrics policy statement: juice in ready-to-use bottles and nursing bottle caries (RE1422). Elk Grove Village, IL: American Academy of Pediatrics, 1978.

97. Clark DC. Appropriate use of fluorides in the 1990s. J Can Dent Assoc 1993;59:272–279.

62. Counseling to Prevent HIV Infection and Other Sexually Transmitted Diseases

RECOMMENDATION

All adolescent and adult patients should be advised about risk factors for human immunodeficiency virus (HIV) infection and other sexually transmitted diseases (STDs), and counseled appropriately about effective measures to reduce the risk of infection (*see* Clinical Intervention). Counseling should be tailored to the individual risk factors, needs, and abilities of each patient. This recommendation is based on the proven efficacy of risk reduction, although the effectiveness of clinician counseling in the primary care setting is uncertain. Individuals at risk for specific STDs should be offered testing in accordance with recommendations on screening for syphilis, gonorrhea, hepatitis B virus infection, HIV infection, and chlamydial infection (see Chapters 24, 26–29). Injection drug users should be advised about measures to reduce their risk and referred to appropriate treatment facilities (see Chapter 53).

Burden of Suffering

The precise incidence of STDs is not known, but it is estimated that each year there are 12 million new infections in the U.S.[1] This figure includes an estimated 4 million cases of *Chlamydia trachomatis* infection, 800,000 cases of gonorrhea, over 110,000 cases of syphilis, and several million cases of *Trichomonas* vaginitis and nonspecific urethritis. Each year there are 0.5–1 million cases of human papillomavirus (HPV) infection, 200,000–300,000 cases of hepatitis B virus (HBV) infection, 200,000–500,000 cases of genital herpes (HSV), and 40,000–80,000 new infections with HIV.[1-3a] An estimated 1 million Americans are currently infected with HIV, 31 million infected with HSV, 24 million infected with HPV, and over 1 million are chronic HBV carriers.[1] High-risk practices remain common in the U.S.: 13% of men and 5% of women in metropolitan areas report heterosexual activity with two or more partners in the last 12 months without consistent use of condoms.[4] Injection drug use, practiced by 1–1.6 million Americans,[1] is a major cause of new infections with HIV, HBV, and hepatitis C virus[4a] through sharing of needles (see Chapter 53).

The consequences of STDs in infected individuals range from mild urogenital symptoms due to trichomoniasis to the nearly uniformly fatal outcomes from HIV infection (see Chapters 24, 26–30). Left untreated, bacterial STDs can produce painful anogenital symptoms (urethritis, cervicitis, etc.), serious illness requiring hospitalization (e.g., pelvic inflammatory disease [PID]), or life-threatening complications (e.g., tertiary syphilis). Both ulcerative and nonulcerative genital STDs are associated with increased risk of acquiring HIV infection.[5–7] Viral STDs, for which there are no curative treatments at present, may be associated with persistent infection, chronic recurrences (genital herpes and HPV), or potentially fatal sequelae (e.g., fulminant or chronic hepatitis).

Women. Many women are at risk for STDs—14% of sexually active women ages 18–44 had more than one sex partner in the previous year and an additional 12–24% had a partner who had multiple sex partners[8]—and STDs have a disproportionate impact on women. Many STDs are more easily transmitted from men to women or have more severe consequences in women. Gonorrhea and chlamydial infection can result in PID, ectopic pregnancy, or infertility. HPV infection is associated with an increased risk of cervical cancer.[9] Pregnant women can transmit various STDs to their offspring in utero or at delivery with serious or potentially fatal consequences (see Chapters 24, 26–30). Nonetheless, in a recent survey, most women reported limited knowledge about common STDs: fewer than one fourth of those at highest risk—younger women and those with multiple partners—believed they were at risk.[10]

Adolescents and Young Adults. STDs are a particular problem in adolescents and young adults. Men and women under 25 account for two thirds of all cases of chlamydia and gonorrhea,[3] and men and women under 35 account for two thirds of newly reported HIV infections.[11,12] Among 9th to 12th graders surveyed in 1993, more than a third had had intercourse within the previous 3 months; 19% reported having had four or more sex partners.[13] Although condom use has increased among high school students, nearly half of all students did not use condoms at last intercourse.[13]

High-Risk Groups. Individual behavior is the strongest determinant of STD risk, and HIV and STDs are common among persons who exchange sex for money or drugs, injection drug users (IDUs), incarcerated persons, and other persons who have numerous sex partners.[11,12,14,15] Reductions in high-risk sexual behavior since the appearance of AIDS have lowered the incidence of STDs in the gay community,[16] but many younger men who have sex with men continue to be at risk.[15] Individuals in communities where STDs are prevalent are also at higher risk: rates of gonorrhea, syphilis, and HIV infection are substantially higher in blacks and Hispanics than among whites, especially among adolescents and young adults.[3,12]

The economic consequences of STDs remain enormous. The medical costs of treating HIV and AIDS were projected to reach $15 billion in 1995.[17] The estimated direct and indirect costs of treating PID and its sequelae were $4.2 billion in 1990.[1]

Efficacy of Risk Reduction

Sexual Behavior. Avoiding sexual contact or needle sharing with infected partners is the most effective way to prevent infection with HIV and other STDs. Identifying infected sex partners is difficult, however, since many infected persons are unaware that they are infected, few infections are readily apparent to sex partners, and some persons may conceal the fact that they are infected.[18] Sexual contact with high-risk partners (e.g., IDUs, persons with a history of STDs or multiple sex partners, men who have sex with men) is also a strong risk factor for HIV and other STDs, but many men and women are reluctant to discuss their sexual history or drug use with their sex partners. Because accurately assessing risk in individual partners is difficult, maintaining a mutually monogamous relationship and limiting the number of sex partners may be more practical strategies for reducing the risk of STDs. Regardless of sexual orientation, risk increases steadily with increasing number of sex partners (especially casual partners).[19,20]

Certain sexual practices may increase the risk of STDs. Unprotected anal intercourse (especially receptive anal intercourse) is an important risk factor for HIV infection among both homosexual men and female partners of HIV-infected men; other practices that increase rectal trauma may also increase transmission of HIV.[20–22] Oral-genital contact can transmit herpes and gonorrhea, and it may pose a risk for transmitting HIV.[20,23]

Male Condoms. Consistent and appropriate use of latex condoms reduces the risk of many STDs.[24] Condoms have been shown in the laboratory to prevent transmission of chlamydia, HSV,[25] trichomonas, cytomegalovirus, and HIV.[26,27] In epidemiologic studies, persons who use condoms consistently are at decreased risk of gonorrhea, nongonococcal urethritis (ureaplasma or chlamydia), and genital herpes simplex.[28] In Thailand, reported cases of the five major STDs declined 69% after institution of an aggressive program to promote condom use at commercial sex establishments.[29]

Correct and consistent use of latex condoms can also reduce the risk of HIV infection.[20,22,30–32] A meta-analysis of retrospective studies of HIV transmission within heterosexual couples calculated that "regular" condom use reduced transmission from an HIV-infected partner by 69% compared to infrequent users;[33] HIV infection was rare among women who reported always using condoms. In a prospective study following 256 serodiscordant heterosexual couples (i.e., one member HIV-positive) over an average of 20 months, no seroconversions occurred among 124 couples who used condoms for every episode of intercourse, versus 12 among 121 couples who used condoms inconsistently.[7]

Condoms infrequently slip off the penis during intercourse or withdrawal (less than 1% of episodes in one study).[34] Reported rates of condom breakage have ranged from 0.6–2% for vaginal intercourse, and 1–7% for anal intercourse.[28] A substantial proportion of condom breakage or leakage may be attributable to improper handling of condoms or inadequate or improper use of lubricant. When condom skills were studied among more than 3,000 patients at STD clinics, patients correctly performed an average of 3.6 of 6 key steps in placing a condom on a penile model.[35] Use of petroleum- or oil-based lubricants causes degradation of condoms[36] and was an independent risk factor for HIV infection among prostitutes.[37] Up to 60% of homosexual men in one study reported using inappropriate lubricants.[38] Condoms are less protective against infections spread through external genital contact (e.g., HPV),[9] and failure to put on a condom before any genital contact may also account for some infections. Natural membrane condoms may be less effective than latex condoms, due to pores that may allow passage of HIV[28] and other viruses, and due to less uniform quality.[39] Nonetheless, failure to use condoms consistently remains the most important obstacle to condom effectiveness.[40,41] Dissatisfaction with condoms is higher in men than in their female partners and is attributed to reduced sensation, fear of condom breakage, inconvenience, and concern that condom use conveys mistrust of sex partners.[42,43]

Spermicides and Female Barrier Contraceptives. Use of barrier methods such as diaphragm, contraceptive sponge (no longer available in the U.S.), or cervical cap is associated with a 33–70% lower risk of gonorrhea, chlamydia, trichomoniasis, and PID in cross-sectional and case-control studies, compared with women using oral contraceptives or no contraception.[28] Although the physical barrier may provide some protection against cervical infections, much of the protective effect is likely to be due to the spermicides used with these methods. The most common spermicide, nonoxynol-9, exhibits in vitro activity against HSV,[44] HBV, chlamydia,[45] and HIV.[46,47] Clinical trials in sex workers and STD patients have demonstrated reductions of 25–60% in both gonococcal and chlamydial cervical infections with various preparations of nonoxynol-9 (gel, sponge, suppository, or film).[48–52] More consistent use of spermicides was associated with increasing levels of protection but was not as protective as consistent condom use.[28,51]

A female condom, consisting of a polyurethane sheath with flexible rings on each end, has been approved by the Food and Drug Administration (FDA), but clinical experience remains limited.[53] The female condom is impermeable to HIV, cytomegalovirus, and other STD organisms in in vitro testing[54] and is an effective contraceptive when used regularly (see Chapter 63).[55] In studies to date, however, the majority of women did not use the female condom consistently; the cost (estimated $2.25 per unit), inconvenience, and unfamiliar appearance are potential obstacles to widespread acceptance.[56]

The effect of spermicide use on HIV infection has not been consistent in clinical studies.[57] A randomized, placebo-controlled trial of contraceptive sponges among Kenyan prostitutes observed significantly higher rates of vulvitis and genital ulcers among women using the sponge, with no reduction in HIV seroconversion.[48] Given the high prevalence of STDs in this population and the high dose of nonoxynol (1,000 mg/sponge), these findings may not be generalizable to average women using lower doses or different preparations of spermicides.[57] In a cohort study of prostitutes given condoms and lower dose spermicide suppositories, more consistent use of spermicides was associated with substantial reductions in the incidence of HIV, especially among women who used condoms less consistently.[32,58] Nonetheless, spermicides could increase susceptibility to HIV by increasing vaginal irritation or altering vaginal flora, especially if used at high doses.[59] Methods that deliver spermicide high up in the vagina may also be more protective against infections that require a cervical portal of entry (i.e., gonorrhea and chlamydia) than against those that do not (i.e., most viruses, syphilis).[60] Efforts are currently under way to develop a microbicide that is effective against HIV without disrupting vaginal epithelium.[61] Even if spermicides and female barrier methods are less effective than male condoms under optimal conditions, they could provide comparable protection in everyday use if they are used more consistently than male condoms.[62]

Injection Drug Use. The risk of HIV and HBV infection among IDUs is closely related to the number of persons with whom an individual shares injection equipment (needles, syringes, drug preparation materials). Treatment programs that decrease injection drug use reduce the incidence of HIV infection in heroin addicts (see Chapter 53).[63] Drug users can also reduce their risk by avoiding contaminated injection equipment. In a retrospective study of drug users in Bangkok, risk of HIV seroconversion was much lower among those who reported they had stopped sharing injection equipment.[64] A review of needle exchange programs concluded that such programs reduced needle sharing among drug users, without increasing the number of persons injecting drugs or the frequency of drug use.[65,66] Due to difficulties in study design, however, no study has yet demonstrated a reduction in new HIV infections as a direct result of needle exchange programs.[67] Based on changes in reported needle sharing or in HIV contamination of returned needles, modeling studies have estimated that needle exchange programs reduce HIV incidence among IDUs by 33%.[65] Comparisons between cities and countries have demonstrated lower rates of HIV in areas with needle exchange programs and areas where drug behaviors have changed.[68] Where new needles and syringes are not available, disinfecting used equipment with bleach has been recommended,[69] but the effectiveness of this strategy has been questioned.[65,69a] Although bleach sterilizes HIV-contaminated needles in in vitro studies, most IDUs use ineffective procedures to clean needles in actual practice.[65,70]

Effectiveness of Counseling

There have been few controlled studies examining whether or not clinician counseling in the primary care setting is effective in reducing the incidence of STDs.[71] Recent publications, however, have systematically reviewed the evidence that counseling interventions, delivered in a variety of settings, can reduce specific STD risk behaviors.[72–76] The most commonly studied interventions were HIV counseling, with or without antibody testing, in high-risk populations (men who have sex with men, IDUs, or persons with STDs) and condom promotion in at-risk heterosexual populations. Additional evidence is provided by interventions delivered in nonclinical settings, such as school[77] or community programs.[73,74]

Counseling in conjunction with HIV testing is associated with significant reductions in high-risk sexual behavior among homosexual men, but testing may be more important than counseling (see Chapter 28).[72] Behavior change after counseling and testing has been more consistent in seropositive than seronegative patients. Drug users have reduced needle sharing in response to the threat of AIDS,[78] but it has been difficult to demonstrate a benefit of specific counseling interventions in IDUs. A recent review[76] identified only nine studies with appropriate control groups, only two of which found significant, lasting effects on risk behaviors among IDUs.

Counseling to promote condom use has been effective in very high-risk populations.[73] The combination of education and condom distribution increased condom use and produced substantial reductions in HIV and other STDs in studies involving foreign sex workers.[29] Interventions in STD clinics have improved compliance with treatment and follow-up for infected patients[79,80] and increased subsequent use of condoms.[81]

Counseling in the primary care setting has less consistent effects on sexual behavior. Counseling increased the number of patients obtaining or using condoms in some studies[82] and reduced the incidence of STDs in a 1950 study;[83] other recent studies reported no significant effect of counseling.[84,85] Condom promotion appears to be more effective in men than in women.[81,85,86] There are few data on the effect of clinician counseling about other contraceptive methods, but women increased spermicide use after a brief counseling intervention (including vouchers for spermicides) in one study.[87] Whether using female-controlled methods (barriers and spermicide) influences condom use by male partners is also unknown.[88]

The efficacy of 23 school-based programs aimed at reducing sexual risk behaviors was reviewed in 1994.[77] Not all programs had significant effects, but selected programs improved specific outcomes: delaying initiation of intercourse, reducing frequency of intercourse or the number of sex partners, or increasing the use of condoms or other contraceptives. Changes in behavior have generally been modest, however, and the results of school programs are not easily generalized to counseling by clinicians.[89] Nonetheless, concern that promoting condom use in adolescents will lead to increased sexual activity is not supported by data from school-based programs,[77] community interventions,[90] or condom campaigns in other countries.[91]

Important questions remain about the long-term impact of counseling in the primary care setting. Few studies reported data on clinical outcomes (STD incidence), follow-up was often short, and most successful trials enrolled selected populations (e.g., patients with STDs) or employed interventions that may not be feasible in the average primary care practice (e.g., group counseling, role-playing, videotape programs, or multiple educational sessions). Cultural differences between clinician and patient (due to age, ethnicity, or sexual orientation) may also pose an obstacle to effective counseling; culturally tailored interventions may be more effective in certain populations.[92] Finally, an individual's susceptibility to advice about risky behavior varies over time (i.e., "stages of behavior change"[93]). As a result, effective interventions to prevent STDs are likely to require repeated individual messages, follow-up to prevent relapse, community-wide efforts to change norms and attitudes, and screening and treatment of infected individuals.[74,94]

Recommendations of Other Groups

Recommendations for physicians to counsel adolescent and adult patients on measures to prevent STDs (primarily HIV) have been issued by a number of organizations, including the American Medical Association,[95] the American College of Physicians,[96] the American Academy of Pediatrics (AAP),[97] the American Academy of Family Physicians,[98] and the American College of Obstetricians and Gynecologists (ACOG).[99] The AMA Guidelines for Adolescent Preventive Services (GAPS) recommend providing routine advice to all adolescents about responsible sexual behaviors, including abstinence and the use of condoms.[100] ACOG[101] and AAP[102] support encouraging abstinence among adolescents, but both organizations endorse educating sexually active teens about proper condom use and increasing the availability of condoms at sites serving youth. The Canadian Task Force on the Periodic Health Examination concluded there was fair evidence to advise adolescent patients about the correct use of condoms to prevent STDs and pregnancy.[103] Healthy People 2000, a U.S. Public Health Service (PHS) report of national health objectives, endorses efforts to increase age-appropriate counseling on HIV and STD prevention by primary care providers.[104]

The key elements for reducing risk of HIV infection were outlined by the PHS in 1987:[105] abstain from sex or maintain a mutually faithful monogamous sexual relationship with an uninfected partner; abstain from sex with individuals who are not known with certainty to be seronegative and who have not been the sole partner for 6 months prior to or any time after the test; do not practice anal intercourse; do not use unsterilized syringes, needles, or drugs; and always use a condom if there are any doubts about the status of the sex partner. Revised guidelines from the Centers for Disease Control and Prevention (CDC) recommend using all opportunities to reinforce risk reduction messages; tailoring counseling to behaviors, needs, and circumstances of the individual; providing a personalized risk assessment; developing a personalized plan with the patient to reduce risk; and providing appropriate referrals.[106] Detailed instructions for patients on the proper use of condoms have been published by the CDC[24] and the FDA.[39] The CDC recommends that condoms be made more widely available by health care providers in clinics for sexually transmitted diseases, family planning, and drug treatment. A 1993 workshop co-sponsored by several PHS agencies concluded that bleach disinfection was an important way to reduce the risk of HIV transmission for IDUs who do not have the option of using sterile injection equipment; provisional recommendations on the proper use of bleach were described.[107]

Discussion

The ability of primary care clinicians to influence high-risk sexual behaviors and drug use is limited, but there is consistent evidence that American men and women have changed their behavior in response to information about HIV and other STDs, provided through public education and clinical encounters.[16,74,108] Improvements have not been consistent for all behaviors or all populations, however. Those at highest risk (drug users and their partners) may find it difficult to change behavior even when motivated to do so due to poverty, homelessness, addiction, or limited access to condoms or clean needles. Whereas use of condoms has increased in the general population, there is little evidence that heterosexual men and women have reduced the number of sex partners or delayed the onset of sexual activity. A substantial number of young persons have multiple sex partners and few use condoms consistently.[4,13]

Clinicians nonetheless are potentially an important component of the effort to educate patients about HIV and other STDs. Whereas most persons are aware of the effects of HIV infection, few realize the serious consequences of more common STDs such as chlamydia and gonorrhea. Men and women may underestimate their risk of STDs from steady sex partners who use drugs or engage in other high-risk activities. Recent surveys indicate, however, that many physicians do not routinely take a sexual history on all patients, do not ask about specific high-risk practices, and do not offer detailed counseling about methods to reduce risk of HIV or other STDs.[109-111] Clinicians can help promote behavior change by reinforcing educational messages, identifying high-risk behaviors, helping patients plan a feasible strategy to reduce risk, and advising patients about sources of additional information. Clinicians provide an important source of information for high-risk groups (e.g., drug users and commercial sex workers) who otherwise have little access to prevention information. They are also an important source of referrals to various community resources such as drug treatment centers, STD and family planning clinics, and community programs offering free condoms, sterilized drug equipment, and cleaning solutions for needles.

CLINICAL INTERVENTION

All adolescent and adult patients should be advised about risk factors for STDs and counseled appropriately about effective measures to reduce risk of infection ("B" recommendation). This recommendation is based on the proven efficacy of risk reduction, although the effectiveness of clinician counseling in the primary care setting has not been evaluated adequately ("C" recommendation). Counseling should be tailored to the individual risk factors, needs, and abilities of each patient. Assessment of risk should be based on a careful sexual and drug use history and consideration of the local epidemiology of STDs. Sexual history should include questions about number and nature of current and past sex partners (including same-sex partners or partners who have injected drugs), any history of past STD infections, the use of condoms or other barrier protection, and particular high-risk sexual practices such as anal intercourse. Patients at risk of STDs should receive information on their risk and be advised about measures to reduce their risk. Effective measures include abstaining from sex, maintaining a mutually faithful monogamous sexual relationship with a partner known to be uninfected, regular use of latex condoms, and avoiding sexual contact with casual partners and high-risk individuals (e.g., IDUs, commercial sex workers, and persons with numerous sex partners).

Patients who have sex with multiple partners, casual partners, or other persons who may be infected should be advised to use a latex condom at each encounter and to avoid anal intercourse. Condoms need not be recommended to prevent infection in longstanding, mutually monogamous relationships in which neither partner is an injection drug user or is infected with HIV. Patients using condoms should be informed about the importance of using them in accordance with recommended guidelines:[24]

- Handle condoms carefully to avoid damaging with fingernails or sharp objects.
- Use a new condom in good condition for each act of intercourse.
- Place the condom on an erect penis before any intimate contact and unroll completely to the base.
- Leave a space at the tip of the condom and remove air pockets in the space.
- Ensure adequate lubrication during intercourse. Water-based lubricants (e.g., K-Y jelly, spermicidal foam or gel) should be used. Petroleum jelly, mineral oil, hand lotion, baby oil, cold cream, massage oil, and other oil-based lubricants should not be used because they may damage latex condoms.
- Hold condom firmly against base of penis during withdrawal, and withdraw while the penis is still erect so that the condom remains in place.

Women at risk of STDs should be advised of options to reduce their risk in situations when their male partner does not use a condom, including the female condom. Women should be informed that spermicides and female barrier methods (diaphragm or cervical cap) can reduce the risk of gonorrhea and chlamydia but are not likely to be as effective as properly used male condoms, and their effectiveness against HIV and other STDs remains unproven. Pregnant women at risk of STDs should be informed of the potential risks to the fetus of HIV and other sexually transmitted infections (chlamydia, gonorrhea, syphilis, hepatitis B, and herpes) and the importance of being screened for HIV and other STDs during pregnancy.

Advice should be provided as appropriate that using alcohol or drugs can lead to high-risk sexual behavior. Persons who inject drugs should be referred to available drug treatment facilities, warned against sharing drug equipment, and, where possible, referred to sources for uncontaminated injection equipment and condoms. Drug users should be advised of the importance of being tested for HIV, of using condoms regularly with both casual and steady partners, and of following specific steps to reduce the risk of transmitting infection during preparation and injection of drugs (see Chapter 53). All patients at risk for STDs should be offered testing in accordance with recommendations on screening for syphilis, gonorrhea, HIV infection, and chlamydial infection (see Chapters 26–29) and should receive hepatitis B vaccine (see Chapter 66).

The draft update of this chapter was prepared for the U.S. Preventive Services Task Force by David Atkins, MD, MPH, with contributions from materials prepared by William Feldman, MD, FRCPC, Anne Martell, MA, CMC, and Jennifer L. Dingle, MBA, for the Canadian Task Force on the Periodic Health Examination.

REFERENCES

1. Centers for Disease Control and Prevention, Division of STD/HIV Prevention. 1993 annual report. Atlanta: Centers for Disease Control and Prevention, 1994.
2. Division of STD/HIV Prevention. Sexually transmitted disease surveillance, 1993. U.S. Department of Health and Human Services, Public Health Service. Atlanta: Centers for Disease Control and Prevention, December 1994.
3. Centers for Disease Control. HIV prevalence estimates and AIDS case projections for the United States. MMWR 1990;39(RR-16):1–31.
3a. Centers for Disease Control. Hepatitis B virus: a comprehensive strategy for eliminating transmission in the United States through universal childhood vaccination. Recommendations of the Immunization Practices Advisory Committee (ACIP). MMWR 1991;40(RR-13):1–25.
4. Berrios DC, Hearst N, Coates TJ, et al. HIV antibody testing among those at risk for infection. The National AIDS Behavioral Surveys. JAMA 1993;270:1576–1580.
4a. Alter M. Epidemiology of hepatitis C in the West. Semin Liver Dis 1995;15:5–14.
5. Mertens TE, Hayes RJ, Smith PG. Epidemiological methods to study the interaction between HIV infection and other sexually transmitted diseases. AIDS 1990;4:57–65.
6. Laga M, Alary M, Nzila N, et al. Condom promotion, sexually transmitted disease treatment, and declining incidence of HIV-1 infection in female Zairian sex workers. Lancet 1994;344:246–248.
7. de Vincenzi I, for the European Study Group on Heterosexual Transmission of HIV. A longitudinal study of human immunodeficiency virus transmission by heterosexual partners. N Engl J Med 1994;331:341–346.
8. Kost K, Forrest JD. American women's sexual behavior and exposure to risk of sexually transmitted diseases. Fam Plann Perspect 1992;24:244–254.
9. American College of Obstetricians and Gynecologists. Genital human papillomavirus infections. Technical Bulletin no. 193. Washington, DC: American College of Obstetricians and Gynecologists, 1994.
10. Women and sexually transmitted diseases: the dangers of denial. New York: EDK Associates, February 1994.
11. Centers for Disease Control and Prevention. HIV/AIDS surveillance report. Atlanta: Centers for Disease Control and Prevention, 1995;7(1):1–34.
12. National Center for Infectious Diseases, Division of HIV/AIDS. National HIV Serosurveillance Summary—results through 1992. Vol 3. Atlanta: Centers for Disease Control and Prevention, 1993. (Publication no. HIV/NCID/11-93/036.)
13. Centers for Disease Control and Prevention. Trends in sexual risk behavior among high school students—United States, 1990, 1991, and 1993. MMWR 1995;44:124–125, 131–132.
14. Edlin BR, Irwin KL, Faruque S, et al. Intersecting epidemics—crack cocaine use and HIV infection among inner-city young adults. N Engl J Med 1994;331:1422–1427.
15. Holmberg SD. Emerging epidemiologic patterns of HIV in the United States. AIDS Res Hum Retroviruses 1994; 10(Suppl 2):S1.
16. Winkelstein W Jr, Wiley JA, Padian NS, et al. The San Francisco Men's Health Study: continued decline in HIV seroconversion rates among homosexual/bisexual men. Am J Public Health 1988;78:1472–1474.
17. Hellinger FJ. Forecasts of the costs of medical care for persons with HIV: 1992–1995. Inquiry 1992;29:356–365.
18. Marks G, Richardson JL, Maldonado N. Self-disclosure of HIV infection to sexual partners. Am J Public Health 1991;81:1321–1323.
19. Hearst N, Hulley SB. Preventing the heterosexual spread of AIDS: are we giving our patients the best advice? JAMA 1988;259:2428–2432.
20. Detels R, English P, Visscher BR, et al. Seroconversion, sexual activity, and condom use among 2915 seronegative men followed for up to 2 years. J Acquired Immune Defic Syndr 1989;2:77–83.

21. Winkelstein W, Lyman DM, Padian N, et al. Sexual practices and risk of infection by the human immunodeficiency virus—the San Francisco men's health study. JAMA 1987;257:321–325.

22. Lazzarin A, Saracco A, Musicco M, et al. Man-to-woman sexual transmission of the human immuno-deficiency virus. Arch Intern Med 1991;151:2411–2416.

23. Samuel MC, Hessol N, Shiboski S, et al. Factors associated with human immunodeficiency virus sero-conversion in homosexual men in three San Francisco cohort studies, 1984–1989. J Acquired Immune Defic Syndr 1993;6:303–312.

24. Centers for Disease Control and Prevention. Update: barrier protection against HIV infection and other sexually transmitted diseases. MMWR 1993;42:589–591, 597.

25. Conant MA, Spicer DW, Smith CD. Herpes simplex virus transmission: condom studies. Sex Transm Dis 1984;11:94–95.

26. Conant M, Hardy D, Sernatinger J, et al. Condoms prevent transmission of AIDS-associated retrovirus. JAMA 1986;255:1706.

27. Carey RF, Herman WA, Retta SM, et al. Effectiveness of latex condoms as a barrier to human immun-odeficiency virus-sized particles under conditions of simulated use. Sex Transm Dis 1992;19:230–234.

28. Cates W, Stone KM. Family planning, sexually transmitted diseases and contraceptive choice: a literature update—part I. Fam Plann Perspect 1992;24:75–84.

29. Hanenberg RS, Rojanapithayakorn W, Kunasol P, et al. Impact of Thailand's HIV-control programme as indicated by the decline of sexually transmitted diseases. Lancet 1994;344:243–245.

30. Fischl MA, Dickinson GM, Scott GB, et al. Evaluation of heterosexual partners, children, and household contacts of adults with AIDS. JAMA 1987;257:640–644.

31. Mann J, Quinn TC, Piot P, et al. Condom use and HIV infection among prostitutes in Zaire. N Engl J Med 1987;316:345.

32. Zekeng L, Feldblum PJ, Oliver RM, Kapute L. Barrier contraceptive use and HIV infection among high-risk women in Cameroon. AIDS 1993;7:725–731.

33. Weller SC. A meta-analysis of condom effectiveness in reducing sexually transmitted HIV. Soc Sci Med 1993;36:1635–1644.

34. Trussell JE, Warner DL, Hatcher R. Condom performance during vaginal intercourse: comparison of Trojan-Enz and Tactylon condoms. Contraception 1992;45:11–19.

35. Langer LM, Zimmerman RS, Cabral RJ. Perceived versus actual condom skills among patients at sexually transmitted disease clinics. Public Health Rep 1994;109:683–687.

36. Reitmeijer CAM, Judson FN. In vitro testing of condoms for prevention of HIV infection: a review. In: Alexander NJ, Gabelnick HL, Spieler JM, eds. Heterosexual transmission of AIDS. New York: Wiley-Liss, 1989:355–363.

37. European Working Group on HIV Infection in Female Prostitutes. HIV infection in European female sex workers: epidemiologic link with use of petroleum-based lubricants. AIDS 1993;7:401–408.

38. Martin DJ. Inappropriate lubricant use with condoms by homosexual men. Public Health Rep 1992;107:468–473.

39. Food and Drug Administration. Counseling patients about prevention. FDA Drug Bull 1987;Sept: 17–19.

40. Tanfer K, Grady WR, Klepinger DH. Condom use among U.S. men, 1991. Fam Plann Perspect 1993; 25:61–66.

41. Jones EF, Forrest JD. Contraceptive failure rates based on the 1988 NSFG. Fam Plann Perspect 1992;24:12–19.

42. Pleck JH, Sonenstein FL, Ku L. Changes in adolescent males' use of and attitudes towards condoms, 1988–1991. Fam Plann Perspect 1993;25:106–109.

43. Grady WR, Klepinger DH, Billy JOG, Tanfer K. Condom characteristics: the perceptions and preferences of men in the United States. Fam Plann Perspect 1993;25:67–73.

44. Singh B, Postic B, Cutler JC. Virucidal effect of certain chemical contraceptives on type 2 herpes virus. Am J Obstet Gynecol 1976;126:422–425.

45. Benes S, McCormack WM. Inhibition of growth of Chlamydia trachomatis by nonoxynol-9 in vitro. Antimicrob Agents Chemother 1985;27:760–762.

46. Hicks DR, Martin LS, Getchell JP, et al. Inactivation of HTLV-III/LAV-infected culture of normal human lymphocytes by nonoxynol-9 in vitro. Lancet 1985;ii:1422–1423.

47. Polsky B, Berran PA, Gold JWM, et al. In vitro inactivation of HIV-1 by contraceptive sponge containing nonoxynol-9. Lancet 1988;i:1456.

48. Kreiss J, Ngugi E, Holmes K, et al. Efficacy of nonoxynol-9 contraceptive sponge use in preventing heterosexual acquisition of HIV in Nairobi prostitutes. JAMA 1992;268:477–482.

49. Rosenberg MJ, Rojanapithayakorn W, Feldblum PJ, et al. Effect of the contraceptive sponge on chlamydial infection, gonorrhea, and candidiasis: a comparative clinical trial. JAMA 1987;257:2308–2312.

50. Luov WC, Austin H, Alexander WJ, et al. A clinical trial of nonoxynol-9 for preventing gonococcal and chlamydial infections. J Infect Dis 1988;158:518–523.

51. Niruthisard S, Roddy R, Chutivongse S. Use of nonoxynol 9 and reduction in rate of gonococcal and chlamydial cervical infections. Lancet 1992;339:1371–1375.

52. Weir SS, Feldblum PJ, Zekeng L, et al. The use of nonoxynol-9 for protection against cervical gonorrhea. Am J Public Health 1994;84:910–914.

53. Soper DE, Shoupe D, Shangold GA, et al. Prevention of vaginal trichomoniasis by compliant use of the female condom. Sex Transm Dis 1993;20:137–139.

54. Drew WL, Blair M, Miner RC, Conant M. Evaluation of the virus permeability of a new condom for women. Sex Transm Dis 1990;17:110–112.

55. Farr G, Gabelnick H, Sturgen K, et al. Contraceptive efficacy and acceptability of the female condom. Am J Public Health 1994;84:1960–1964.

56. Gollub EL, Stein ZA. Commentary: the new female condom—item 1 on a women's AIDS prevention agenda. Am J Public Health 1993;83:498–500.

57. Lange JMA, Karam M, Piot P. Boost for vaginal microbicides against HIV. Lancet 1993;341:1356.

58. Feldblum PJ, Weir SS. The protective effect of nonoxynol-9 against HIV infection. Am J Public Health 1994;84:1032–1034.

59. Niruthisard S, Roddy RE, Chutivongse S. The effects of frequent nonoxynol-9 use on the vaginal and cervical mucosa. Sex Transm Dis 1991;18:176–179.

60. Stone KM, Peterson HB. Spermicides, HIV, and the vaginal sponge. JAMA 1992;268:520–522.

61. Potts M. The urgent need for a vaginal microbicide in the prevention of HIV transmission. Am J Public Health 1994;84:890–891.

62. Rosenberg MJ, Gollub EL. Commentary: methods women can use that may prevent sexually transmitted disease, including HIV. Am J Public Health 1992;82:1473–1478.

63. Gerstein DR, Harwood HJ, eds. Treating drug problems. Washington, DC: National Academy Press, 1990.

64. Des Jarlais DC, Choopanya K, Vanicheseni S, et al. AIDS risk reduction and reduced HIV seroconversion among injection drug users in Bangkok. Am J Public Health 1994;84:452–455.

65. Normand JL, Vlahov D, Moses LE, eds. Preventing HIV transmission: the role of sterile needles and bleach. Panel on Needle Exchange and Bleach Distribution Programs, National Research Council and Institute of Medicine. Washington, DC: National Academy Press, 1995.

66. Lurie P, ed. The public health impact of needle exchange programs in the United States and abroad: summary, conclusions, and recommendations. San Francisco: University of California, Institute for Health Policy Studies, 1993.

67. Vlahov D, Brookmeyer RS. Editorial: the evaluation of needle exchange programs. Am J Public Health 1994;84: 1889–1891.

68. Washington AE, Kahn JG, Showstack JA, et al. Updated estimates of the impact and cost of HIV prevention in injecting drug users. Final report from the Institute of Health Policy Studies, University of California, San Francisco to Centers for Disease Control and Prevention, Division of STD/HIV Prevention. San Francisco: Institute of Health Policy Studies, University of California, San Francisco, 1992.

69. Centers for Disease Control and Prevention. Use of bleach for disinfection of drug injection equipment. MMWR 1993;42:418–419.

69a. Jones TS, Haverkos HW. HIV, drug-use paraphernalia, and bleach. J Acquired Immune Defic Syndr 1994;7:741–742.

70. Watters JK, Estilo MJ, Clark GL, Lorvick J. Syringe and needle exchange as HIV/AIDS prevention for injection drug users. JAMA 1994;271:115–120.

71. Aral SO, Peterman TA. Defining behavioral methods to prevent sexually transmitted diseases through intervention research. Infect Dis Clin North Am 1993;7:861–873.

72. Higgins DL, Galavotti C, O'Reilly KR, et al. Evidence for the effects of HIV antibody counseling and testing on risk behaviors. JAMA 1991;266:2419–2429.

73. Choi KH, Coates TJ. Prevention of HIV infection. AIDS 1994;8:1371–1389.

74. Holtgrave DR, Qualls NL, Curran JW, et al. An overview of the effectiveness and efficiency of HIV prevention programs. Public Health Rep 1995;110:134–146.

75. Auerbach JD, Wypijewska C, Brodie HKH, eds. Institute of Medicine. AIDS and behavior: an integrated approach. Washington, DC: National Academy Press, 1994.

76. Booth RE, Watters JK. How effective are risk-reduction interventions targeting injecting drug users? AIDS 1994;8:1515–1524.

77. Kirby D, Short L, Collins J, et al. School-based programs to reduce sexual risk behaviors: a review of effectiveness. Public Health Rep 1994;109:339–360.

78. Des Jarlais DC, Friedman SR, Sotheran JL, et al. Continuity and change within an HIV epidemic. JAMA 1994;271:121–127.

79. Solomon MZ, DeJong W. Recent sexually transmitted disease prevention efforts and their implications for AIDS health education. Health Educ Q 1986;13:301–316.

80. Healton CG, Messeri P. The effect of video interventions on improving knowledge and treatment compliance in the sexually transmitted disease setting. Sex Transm Dis 1993;20:70–76.

81. Cohen DA, MacKinnon DP, Dent C, et al. Group counseling at STD clinics to promote use of condoms. Public Health Rep 1992;107:727–731.

82. Rickert VI, Gottlieb AA, Jay MS. Is AIDS education related to condom acquisition? J Clin Pediatr (Phila) 1992;31: 205–210.

83. Vaughn CL, Freiberg AD. A pilot study of the navy's educational program on venereal disease. Am J Syphil 1950;34:476–480.

84. Wenger NS, Greenberg JM, Hilborne LH, et al. Effect of HIV antibody testing and AIDS education on communication about HIV risk and sexual behavior. Ann Intern Med 1992;117:905–911.

85. Rickert VI, Gottlieb A, Jay MS. A comparison of three clinic-based AIDS education programs on female adolescents' knowledge, attitudes and behavior. J Adolesc Health Care 1990;11:298–303.

86. Cohen DA, Dent C, MacKinnon D, et al. Condoms for men, not women. Sex Transm Dis 1992; 19:245–251.

87. Cohen D, Reardon K, Alleyne D. Influencing spermicide use among low-income minority women. J Am Med Women Assoc 1995;50:11–13.

88. Stein Z. HIV prevention: an update on the status of methods that women can use. Am J Public Health 1993;83:1379–1382.

89. Walter HJ, Vaughan RD. AIDS risk reduction among a multiethnic sample of urban high school students. JAMA 1993;270:725–730.

90. Sellers DE, McGraw SA, McKinlay JB. Does the promotion of condoms increase teen sexual activity? Evidence from an HIV prevention program for Latino youth. Am J Public Health 1994;84:1952–1959.

91. Hausser D, Michaud PA. Does a condom-promoting strategy (the Swiss STOP-AIDS Campaign) modify sexual behavior among adolescents? Pediatrics 1994;93:580–585.

92. Kalichman SC, Kelly JA, Hunter TL, et al. Culturally tailored HIV-AIDS risk-reduction messages targeted to African-American urban women: impact on risk sensitization and risk reduction. J Consult Clin Psychol 1993;61:291–295.

93. Prochaska JO, DiClemente CC, Norcross JC. In search of how people change: applications to addictive behaviors. Am Psychol 1992;47:1102–1114.

94. Stryker J, Coates TJ, DeCarlo P, et al. Prevention of HIV infection. Looking back, looking ahead. JAMA 1995;273: 1143–1148.

95. American Medical Association. HIV blood test counseling. Physician guidelines, 2nd ed. Chicago: American Medical Association, 1993.

96. American College of Physicians and Infectious Disease Society of America. Human immunodeficiency virus (HIV) infection. Ann Intern Med 1994;120:310–319.

97. American Academy of Pediatrics, Committee on Adolescence. Sexually transmitted diseases. Pediatrics 1994;94: 568–572.

98. American Academy of Family Physicians. Age charts for periodic health examination. Kansas City, MO: American Academy of Family Physicians, 1994. (Reprint no. 510.)

99. American College of Obstetricians and Gynecologists. Human immunodeficiency virus infection. Technical Bulletin no. 169. Washington, DC: American College of Obstetricians and Gynecologists, 1992.

100. American Medical Association. Guidelines for adolescent preventive services (GAPS): recommendations and rationale. Chicago: American Medical Association, 1994.

101. American College of Obstetricians and Gynecologists. Condom availability for adolescents. Committee Opinion no. 154. Washington, DC: American College of Obstetricians and Gynecologists, 1995.

102. American Academy of Pediatrics. Condom availability for youth. Pediatrics 1995;95:281–285.

103. Canadian Task Force on the Periodic Health Examination. Canadian guide to clinical preventive health care. Ottawa: Canada Communication Group, 1994:540–557.

104. U.S. Department of Health and Human Services. Healthy people 2000: national health promotion and disease prevention objectives. Washington, DC: Public Health Service, 1991:479–510. (Publication no. PHS-91-50212.)

105. Centers for Disease Control. Public Health Service guidelines for counseling and antibody testing to prevent HIV infection and AIDS. MMWR 1987;36:509–515.

106. Centers for Disease Control and Prevention. Technical guidance on HIV counseling. MMWR 1993;42(RR-2):8–17.

107. Centers for Disease Control and Prevention, Center for Substance Abuse Treatment, and the National Institute on Drug Abuse. HIV/AIDS Prevention Bulletin, April 19. Rockville, MD: National Institute on Drug Abuse, 1993.

108. Schoenborn CA, Marsh SL, Hardy AM. AIDS knowledge and attitudes for 1992. Data from the National Health Interview Survey. Advance data no. 243. Hyattsville, MD: National Center for Health Statistics, 1994. (Publication no. DHHS (PHS) 94-1250.)

109. National Center for Health Statistics. Healthy People 2000 review, 1994. Hyattsville, MD: Public Health Service, 1995. (Publication no. DHHS(PHS) 95-1256-1.)

110. Russell NK, Boekeloo BO, Rafi IZ, et al. Unannounced simulated patients observations of physician STD/HIV prevention practices. Am J Prev Med 1992;8:235–240.

111. Centers for Disease Control and Prevention. HIV prevention practices of primary-care physicians— United States, 1992. MMWR 1994;42:988–992.

63. Counseling to Prevent Unintended Pregnancy

RECOMMENDATION

Periodic counseling about effective contraceptive methods is recommended for all women and men at risk for unintended pregnancy (see _Clinical Intervention_). Counseling should be based on information from a careful sexual history and should take into account the individual preferences, abilities, and risks of each patient. Sexually active patients should also receive information on measures to prevent sexually transmitted diseases (see Chapter 62).

Burden of Suffering

Approximately two thirds of all American women are at risk for unintended pregnancy (i.e., they are sexually active but do not want to become pregnant),[1] and a substantial proportion of all pregnancies each year in the U.S. are unintended.[2] In a national survey of over 8,000 women ages 15–44,[a] 57% of all pregnancies were _unintended_, including those that were _unwanted_ (i.e., in women who did not want more children) and those that were _mistimed_ (i.e., in women who did not want children at that time).[3,4] The proportion of pregnancies that are unintended is high in women of all ages: 42% of all pregnancies in women ages 30–34 and 77% in women ages 40–44.[3] Births resulting from unintended and unwanted pregnancies have gradually increased since 1982. Approximately 40% of live births to women ages 15–44 were the result of unintended pregnancies, including 12% due to unwanted pregnancies.[1]

Unintended Teenage Pregnancies. An increasing number of teenagers are at risk for unintended pregnancy. In a 1993 survey, 32% of 9th grade girls, 44% of 9th grade boys, and over two thirds of all high school seniors reported having had sexual intercourse; over half of seniors were sexually active within the previous 3 months.[5] Factors associated with early sexual activity include: lower socioeconomic status; use of tobacco, alcohol, or other drugs; and single-parent households.[6] Approximately 20% of sexu-

---

[a] The 1988 National Survey of Family Growth (NSFG) is the source of the most widely cited statistics on unintended pregnancies and births. Data from the 1995 NSFG are scheduled to be released in 1996.

ally active teenage girls (age 15–19) become pregnant each year in the U.S., and over 80% of teen pregnancies are unintended.[6] Teenagers account for over 1 million pregnancies and over 500,000 births a year in the U.S.[7] Almost 40% of teenage births in 1992 were to mothers age 17 or younger, including 12,000 births in girls under age 15.[8] Although pregnancy rates among sexually active teens declined steadily from 1972 to 1986, pregnancy and birth rates have increased for the entire teen population, due to increasing teenage sexual activity and declining abortion rates.[6,7] The rates of teenage pregnancy and teenage birth (61 births/1,000 women ages 15–19 in 1992)[8] remain substantially higher in the U.S. than in most Western countries.[6]

Adverse Effects of Unintended Pregnancy. A 1995 Institute of Medicine (IOM) report on unintended pregnancy summarized the consequences of unintended pregnancy for both the parents and the child.[2] The most obvious adverse consequence of unintended pregnancies is elective abortion. Roughly half of all unintended pregnancies end in abortion, accounting for most of the 1.5 million abortions performed annually in the U.S.[9,10] Although abortion rates have declined modestly over the past 15 years in the U.S.,[10] they remain higher in the U.S. than in most Western countries.[11]

Separating the effects of unplanned births from other important social and environmental factors (e.g., maternal health, education, and income) is difficult. Adverse social and medical consequences are most consistently observed for teenaged childbearing, most of which is attributable to unintended pregnancy. Teenage mothers are less likely to get or stay married, less likely to complete high school or college, and more likely to require public assistance and live in poverty.[2] Infants born to teenage mothers, especially mothers under age 15, are more likely to suffer from low birth weight, neonatal mortality, and sudden infant death syndrome (SIDS),[2] and they may be at greater risk of child abuse, neglect, and behavioral and educational problems at later ages.[12] Risk factors common in young mothers (poverty, single parenthood, poor nutrition, and inadequate prenatal care) may be more important than young maternal age itself, however.[13] From 1985 to 1990, the public costs of births to teenage mothers (Aid to Families with Dependent Children, Medicaid, etc.) were estimated to be over $120 billion.[14]

The adverse consequences of unintended pregnancy and childbirth are not restricted to teenagers. Women who become pregnant unexpectedly forego the opportunity to receive preconception counseling to improve the health of the fetus.[2] Pregnancies after age 40 are often unintended and are associated with increased risks to both mother and infant. Women with unwanted pregnancies are less likely to receive adequate prenatal care, more likely to smoke or drink, and more likely to have low birth weight babies.[2] Some studies have suggested that developmental problems are more frequent among unwanted children,[15] but other environmental factors are probably important; more than 40% of children resulting from unintended pregnancies in the U.S. are born into single-parent families.[2]

Efficacy of Risk Reduction

Complete sexual abstinence is the only certain form of contraception. Without contraception, an estimated 85% of heterosexual couples who engage in regular intercourse will conceive within 1 year.[16] Available methods to prevent conception vary considerably in their effectiveness, convenience, reversibility, side effects, and cost, and are reviewed in detail in a number of up-to-date references.[16,17]

The effectiveness of contraceptive methods is usually expressed in two ways: the failure rate under "perfect use" (annual pregnancy rates among persons who use the method correctly on every occasion) and under "typical use" (average users in retrospective surveys or clinical trials).[16,18] Because many methods are not used consistently and correctly by the average couple, failure rates with typical use are often considerably higher than with perfect use. Nearly half of all unintended pregnancies occur in women who report using some form of contraception,[3] and inconsistent or incorrect use of contraception is the major cause of such contraception "failures." User knowledge, motivation and ability, cooperation of their partner, the cost, comfort, and ease of use of a particular method, and individual concerns about side effects or safety are all important determinants of compliance with a chosen method of contraception.

Contraceptive hormones include oral contraceptives (combined estrogen/progestin preparations and progestin-only pills), long-acting progestational agents that are injected or implanted, and postcoital preparations.[19] **Combination oral contraceptives** (OCs) are the most popular method of reversible contraception, used by an estimated 10 million American women. The pill is generally taken daily for 21 days, followed by either placebo or no pills for 7 days. The failure rate is about 3% per year with typical use and as low as 0.1% per year when used correctly and consistently.[16] Noncompliance remains the major cause of OC failure, especially in unmarried women. Failure rates calculated from a 1988 survey were 7%; rates were higher among women who were young, unmarried, or poor.[18]

Side effects of OCs, such as breakthrough bleeding, nausea, and breast tenderness, decline over time and have been minimized in recent years by lowering the dose of hormones.[16] Epidemiologic studies demonstrated an association between early OCs and cardiovascular disease (myocardial infarction, stroke, and thromboembolic disorders).[20] This effect was most

742 Section II: Counseling

pronounced in heavy smokers and older women, and has been attributed to thrombotic effects of higher doses of hormones in early formulations.[19,21] Any risks associated with current OCs seem to be minimal.[16,22,23] In several studies conducted after 1985, OC use was associated with an increased risk of occlusive stroke (an extremely rare event in young women),[24-26] but effects on the risk of myocardial infarction have not been consistent.[27,28] For most women (with the possible exception of older smokers), potential risks of OCs are lower than the risks of pregnancy and childbirth.[29] In one U.S. study of newer OCs, there were no cardiovascular deaths in 55,000 patient-years of use.[30] Patient satisfaction is generally higher for OCs (94%) than most other methods.[31]

The net effect of OC use on cancer risk appears to be negligible and may be favorable (see Chapter 64).[32] The lifetime risk of breast cancer is similar in OC users and nonusers, but some studies suggest a modest increase in early breast cancer among long-term users or those beginning OC use at a young age.[33,34] The absolute increase in risk is small, may be due to factors other than OCs (e.g., delayed childbearing), and may not apply to current formulations. A modest increase in cervical cancer has also been reported, but the significance of this association is also controversial.[19] In contrast, OC use is associated with a 40–50% reduction in the risk of ovarian and endometrial cancer (see Chapter 64). Additional noncontraceptive benefits of OCs include lower incidence of menstrual disorders, benign breast disease, uterine fibroids, and clinical pelvic inflammatory disease (PID).[17,35] Extended follow-up (12–20 years) of several large cohorts reported no effect of prolonged OC use on overall or cause-specific mortality.[22,23]

The **progestin-only pill** ("mini-pill") is less effective than combination OCs (failure rate 0.5–4%) and is more likely to cause irregular menses.[16,36] It is a useful alternative for women who are breast-feeding or who have contraindications to estrogen. **Injectable progestins** (depot-medroxyprogesterone acetate [DMPA], i.e., Depo-Provera) and **subdermal progestin implants** (i.e., Norplant) provide long-term contraception without the need for daily compliance. DMPA is administered as intramuscular injections given 4 times a year and has a failure rate of only 0.3%.[16] Subdermal implants can be inserted and removed as an office procedure and provide effective contraception for up to 5 years. Cumulative 5-year pregnancy rates in large case-series were 0.5–1.2%.[37,38] Satisfaction with subdermal implants seems high among selected groups[39,40] but it is not as high as with OCs. Common side effects with progestin-only contraceptives include irregular bleeding (up to 50–70%), headache, and weight gain; cases of stroke and pseudotumor cerebri have been reported among users of Norplant, but no causal association has been established.[41] Removal complications (e.g., broken or imbedded implants) occurred in 5% of patients in 1985–1993.[42] Initial studies reported no significant increase in breast cancer,[43] and a substantial reduction in endometrial cancer,[44] among women using DMPA. DMPA causes modest adverse effects on serum lipids, but the long-term effects on cardiovascular disease are not known for any of the progestin-only contraceptives.

Postcoital administration of estrogen and progestin can reduce subsequent pregnancy if initiated within 72 hours after unprotected intercourse.[45] The best-evaluated regimen consists of two doses of 100 μg ethinyl estradiol and 1 mg levonorgestrel (i.e., two 50 μg combination OC pills), given 12 hours apart. Based on reported failure rates (0.2–7.4%),[46] it is estimated to reduce risk of pregnancy by 75%.[16] Prominent side effects include irregular bleeding, nausea (up to 50%), and vomiting.[45] Alternate regimens using danocrine (Danazol) have fewer side effects but have been less well studied.[47] In two recent trials in Great Britain, mifepristone (RU 486) was as effective as, and better tolerated than, estrogen/progestin regimens for postcoital contraception.[47,48] RU 486 is under study in the U.S. but not yet available.[49] Surveys indicate that knowledge of and use of postcoital contraception remains low among patients and clinicians.[16]

Barrier contraceptive methods include the male and female condom and female barriers used with spermicide. Barrier methods have fewer side effects than hormonal contraception, but average effectiveness is more variable due to inconsistent or incorrect use. When used reliably, latex **condoms** have a 3% failure rate, compared to 12–16% among average users.[16,18] The **female condom** has failure rates comparable to other female barriers: 5% under perfect use and 20% under typical use.[16] Cost ($2.50) and unfamiliar appearance may be obstacles to regular use.[50] Latex condoms (and presumably female condoms) also provide protection against human immunodeficiency virus (HIV) and other sexually transmitted diseases (STDs) (see Chapter 62). Condoms infrequently slip or rupture, but most failure is due to inconsistent or improper use.

Other female barriers include the diaphragm, cervical cap, vaginal sponge, and vaginal film. **Diaphragms** have a failure rate of about 6% when used consistently, and 18–22% under average conditions.[16,18] Among reliable users, failure rates appear higher (10% vs. 3%) in women having more frequent intercourse (≥3 times per week).[16] The **cervical cap** and contraceptive vaginal sponge are as effective as the diaphragm in nulliparous women, but less effective in parous women (failure rates 20–36%).[16] Both can be left in for longer periods than the diaphragm (24 hours). The only American manufacturer of sponges discontinued production in 1995, however.[51] **Spermicides** (foams, creams, jellies) used alone are estimated to have failure rates of 6% when used consistently and

21–25% under typical usage conditions.[16,18] Both barrier methods and spermicides can reduce the risk of infection with gonorrhea and chlamydia, but effects on HIV transmission are uncertain (see Chapter 62).

Intrauterine devices (IUDs) can provide very effective contraception (0.1–0.6% failure rate) for extended periods.[16] Two IUDs are currently available in the U.S.: a copper IUD (Paragard), approved for continued use for up to 8 years, and a progesterone-releasing IUD (Progestasert), which should be replaced annually; approval of a levonorgestrel IUD, which can be left in place for 5 years, is pending in the U.S.[16] Despite adverse publicity in the 1980s that led to the withdrawal of most IUDs from the U.S. market, these newer IUDs have been used widely in other countries and have proven to be safe and reliable.[52] In a study of nearly 23,000 women, the risk of PID was increased only in the first 20 days following IUD insertion, but thereafter remained low (1.6 cases/1,000 years of use);[53] risk was not increased among monogamous women using IUDs. Between 2% and 10% of women will experience expulsion of their IUD in the first year, and up to 15% may require removal due to pain or bleeding. For many women, especially those at low risk of STDs, IUDs offer excellent alternatives to OCs and other methods.

Coitus interruptus (withdrawal) and **periodic abstinence** may be more acceptable alternatives for persons with religious objections to artificial contraception[54] and others who are unwilling or unable to use other methods. It is often difficult to perform these methods correctly. Abstinence during fertile periods can be based on date of last menstrual period (calendar or "rhythm" method) or changes in temperature or cervical mucus (ovulation method). The ovulation method is more effective than the calendar method (1–3% vs. 9% failure rate under perfect use)[16,55] but requires abstinence for about 17 days of each cycle.[17,56,57] Coitus interruptus can fail if withdrawal is not timed properly or if preejaculatory fluid contains sperm. Due to these difficulties, failure rates of withdrawal and periodic abstinence are 18–20% annually in actual practice.[16,18] Effectiveness may be improved by combining these methods with other contraception during the fertile period of the menstrual cycle.

Sterilization is the most common method of contraception in the U.S.[62] and has no proven long-term risks.[16] It differs from other methods in that it is intended to provide permanent contraception. The average failure rate is 0.1–0.2% for male sterilization (vasectomy) and 0.4% for female sterilization (tubal ligation).[16] Between 1% and 2% of vasectomies are accompanied by transient side effects (hematoma, infection, or epididymitis).[16] The complication rate from tubal ligation depends on the type of procedure (e.g., mini-laparotomy, laparoscopy, colpotomy) but is generally less than 1%.[16] Within 2 years of the procedure, up to 3% of American women reported regret over sterilization.[58,59] Fertility can be restored in up to 50% of men after reversal of vasectomy, and up to 70% of women after reversal of tubal ligation.[16] Sterilization does not protect against sexually transmitted infections, but tubal ligation is associated with lower risk of PID and ovarian cancer.[60,61]

Effectiveness of Counseling

Many adolescents and adults could potentially benefit from counseling about how to prevent unintended pregnancy. In a 1990 survey, 12% of sexually active women ages 15–44, and 22% of sexually active teens, reported not practicing any form of contraception.[62] Contraception use at first premarital intercourse remains lower than at any other stage in life: 29% of all teens and more than half of women under age 17 report using no contraception at first intercourse.[63] Many more persons use contraception but fail to use it consistently or correctly. Nearly half of all unintended pregnancies occur in women using a contraceptive method. Among teenagers, the most common reasons given by teenagers for not using contraception at last intercourse were "Didn't expect to have sex" and "Just didn't think pregnancy would occur."[64] In one study of college students fitted for a diaphragm, only 57% reported using it with each coitus.[65]

Information on the effectiveness of counseling by primary care clinicians in altering sexual practices or improving the use of contraception remains limited, however. What evidence does exist comes primarily from studies of interventions delivered in other settings (classrooms, school clinics, family planning clinics) or targeted to AIDS-related behaviors rather than unintended pregnancy. The 1995 IOM report identified 23 pregnancy prevention programs that had been adequately evaluated, most of which targeted high-risk adolescents.[2] These programs employed a variety of interventions: community- and school-based education about sexuality, life skills, and contraception; individual counseling through school or hospital clinics; and provision of contraceptive services. Most evaluations were based on change in self-reported sexual activity and contraceptive use rather than actual rates of unintended pregnancy. There were several major conclusions of the IOM review: only 13 of 23 programs were even somewhat effective in changing behavior, and magnitude of effect was often small; evidence of the effectiveness of abstinence-only programs was inconclusive; education programs that provided information on both abstinence and contraceptive use had generally favorable effects, without promoting early sexual activity or frequency of intercourse; and only a few programs included measures to ensure access to contraception.

One of the most effective programs combined a school curriculum with free contraceptive services through a school-linked clinic.[66] Another community-based program that included contraceptive services demonstrated early success in preventing adolescent pregnancy,[67] but not in later years after contraceptive services were dropped.[68] Evaluations of other school-based clinics suggest no clear effect on teenage birth rates,[64,69,70] but most pregnancies occurred before students had used the clinic or discussed birth control.[64]

Kirby et al.[71] reviewed the effects of 23 school programs providing sex and HIV education (including some reviewed in the IOM report). They noted isolated positive effects of some programs on use of contraception at first intercourse, but less effect on contraception use among sexually experienced teens. As in the IOM report, they found no evidence that education about sexuality or instruction about contraception led to earlier or more frequent sexual activity among teenagers. All effective programs went well beyond simply providing factual information about contraception and sexuality; most sought to reinforce specific norms about sexual behavior and to develop skills to help teens resist sexual pressures.

A variety of HIV prevention programs have employed individual or group counseling in a clinic setting (see Chapter 62). A number of these demonstrated an increase in condom use after counseling men, but interventions emphasized STD prevention rather than contraception. A randomized trial of reproductive health counseling of young men age 15–18 did not increase overall use of contraception or use of condoms.[72]

Access to family planning clinics appears to help prevent unintended adolescent pregnancy. Teenagers who attend family planning clinics were more likely to use oral contraceptives and less likely to engage in unprotected sexual intercourse;[73] adolescents living in communities with subsidized family planning services were less likely to become pregnant in one analysis.[74] Clinic attenders are self-selected, however, and many of the effects of counseling are short-lived. In one study, less than one half of all adolescents attending a family planning clinic were compliant with contraception after 1 year.[75] Attempts to improve compliance through family counseling, telephone follow-up, or contingency planning have met with limited success.[76,77]

There are obvious limitations in generalizing from such programs to routine office counseling by clinicians. Furthermore, little is known about interventions to improve contraception in nonadolescent women and men.[2] At the same time, the potential to improve counseling practices in the primary care setting is apparent. A minority of primary care providers—from 18% of pediatricians to 53% of nurse practitioners—routinely ask their female patients about family planning needs.[78] Surveys document that many adolescents and adults are misinformed about the risks of unintended pregnancy, the benefits and risks of particular contraceptive methods, and the proper use of contraception.[2] Misperceptions about risks of contraception (especially OCs and IUDs) are important reasons why women delay seeking contraceptive services, use contraceptives inconsistently, or prematurely discontinue their use.

The effectiveness of counseling depends on the age, maturity, sex, and experience of the patient, as well as on the level of training and counseling skills of the provider.[79] Selection of an appropriate method of birth control must take into consideration the personal preferences, religious beliefs, and abilities of the patient, and the nature of their relationship with their partner(s). As documented in the IOM report, physician training in family planning is highly variable and often limited.[2] Many clinicians are reluctant to prescribe contraceptives for adolescents without parental consent,[80] although most states explicitly or implicitly permit minors to consent[b] to contraceptive services without parental approval.[81] Informing parents may discourage adolescents from seeking needed assistance and conflict with the duty to protect the well-being of the patient and the confidentiality of the doctor-patient relationship.[82] Concern that a physician will inform parents is commonly cited by adolescents as a reason for choosing family planning clinics over private physicians to obtain contraception.[83] Of the estimated 5 million teenaged women at risk for unintended pregnancy in the U.S., however, only 1.2 million receive services at publicly funded family planning clinics.[84]

Recommendations of Other Groups

Numerous organizations recommend counseling sexually active adolescents and adults about unintended pregnancy. The American Academy of Family Physicians,[85] the AMA Guidelines for Adolescent Preventive Services (GAPS),[86] the American Academy of Pediatrics (AAP)[87], the American College of Obstetricians and Gynecologists (ACOG),[88] the Society for Adolescent Medicine,[89] the Canadian Task Force on the Periodic Health Examination,[90] and Bright Futures[94] each recommends that clinicians counsel all adolescents about preventing unintended pregnancy (including the role of abstinence) and provide effective contraception for all sexually active patients. These groups also encourage physicians to protect the confidentiality of the doctor-adolescent relationship within the confines of local legal requirements regarding parental consent. Healthy People 2000, a U.S. Public Health Service report of national health objectives, endorses efforts to increase sexual abstinence among adolescents and increase the proportion of primary care providers offering age-appropriate family planing counseling.[91] Updated family planning information from the World Health Organization was released in 1995.[92]

Discussion

Unintended pregnancy remains a critical problem in the U.S. Although the consequences of unintended pregnancy are most pronounced in

---

[b] Some states permit minor consent on the basis of age (age 14 or 16) or if referred by doctor, family planning agency or school.

young, unmarried women, the problem affects women and men through-out the reproductive period of their lives. Multiple factors are involved in unintended pregnancy, including personal and societal attitudes toward sex, contraception, and pregnancy. Postponing early sexual activity among teens and increasing the consistent use of effective contraception continue to be elusive goals for parents, clinicians, and educators alike. Nonetheless, a variety of evidence indicates that a combination of patient education and access to effective contraception can reduce unintended pregnancy. Although their ability to influence patient sexual behavior may be limited, clinicians can offer information about contraceptive options and prescribe effective and appropriate contraception. The public health benefits of better contraceptive practices would be enormous: reducing the proportion of women not using contraception by half could prevent as many as one third of all unintended pregnancies and 500,000 abortions per year.[93]

There is no ideal contraceptive method for all patients. The choice of an appropriate method must consider each patient's motivation and ability to use a particular method, their individual preferences (and partner's preferences), cost and safety factors, and their relationship with their sexual partner(s). Women bear the largest burden from unintended pregnancy, and methods under female control (hormonal contraception, IUDs, and female barriers) appear to be used more regularly than those requiring male cooperation (condoms, coitus interruptus, periodic abstinence). On the other hand, female methods (with the possible exception of the female condom) do not offer reliable protection against transmission of HIV or other STDs, which are important threats to many individuals. The importance of measures to reduce the risk of STDs (abstinence, maintaining monogamous relationships, avoiding sex with high-risk persons, and using condoms consistently) need to be emphasized along with the importance of effective contraception. Clinicians need to remain alert to factors that may contribute to noncompliance (anxiety, cost, discomfort, embarrassment, etc.).

The effectiveness of counseling depends in part on the clinician's sensitivity to the personal concerns and privacy of the patient. These issues are especially important when addressing issues of sexuality with adolescents, who may have conflicted feelings about sexuality or childbearing, limited information about fertility and contraception, and unrealistic perceptions of the risks of unprotected sex. Clinicians can encourage abstinence as the safest choice, provide support for individuals choosing to postpone sexual activity, and prescribe effective contraceptive methods for young persons who continue to be at risk. The low rate of contraception at first intercourse indicates that discussion of sexuality and contraception should begin before adolescents become sexually active.

CLINICAL INTERVENTION

Periodic counseling about effective contraceptive methods is recommended for all women and men at risk for unintended pregnancy ("B" recommendation). Counseling should be based on information from a careful history that includes direct questions about sexual activity, current and past use of contraception, level of concern about pregnancy, and past history of unintended pregnancies. Counseling should take into account the individual preferences, concerns, abilities, and risks of each patient and his or her partner, including risk of STDs (see Chapter 62). Counseling should include a discussion of the risk associated with the patient's current contraceptive practice and, when indicated, available alternatives for more effective contraception. Clinicians should inform adolescent patients that abstinence is the most effective way to prevent unintended pregnancy and STDs, although the effectiveness of abstinence counseling has not been established.

Clear instructions should be provided for the proper use of recommended contraceptive techniques. Hormonal contraceptives, barrier methods used with spermicides, and IUDs should be recommended as the most effective reversible means of preventing pregnancy in sexually active persons. Sexual abstinence, the maintenance of a mutually faithful monogamous sexual relationship, and consistent use of condoms should be emphasized as important measures to reduce the risk of STDs (see Chapter 62). Clinicians should monitor satisfaction and compliance of patients with any chosen form of contraception.

Empathy, confidentiality, and a nonjudgmental, supportive attitude are especially important when discussing issues of sexuality with adolescents. Clinicians should involve young pubertal patients (and their parents, where appropriate) in early, open discussion of sexual development and effective methods to prevent unintended pregnancy and STDs. Clinicians should explore attitudes and expectations of adolescents and other patients who are not currently involved in a sexual relationship to anticipate future need for contraception, and inform them how to obtain information and contraception if they plan to begin engaging in sexual intercourse. Preferably, adolescents should be examined without their parent(s) present. Clinicians providing birth control for minors should take into consideration both the confidentiality of the doctor-patient relationship as well as local legal restrictions when deciding whether to notify parents before prescribing contraception. The optimal frequency of counseling to prevent unintended pregnancy is unknown and is left to clinical discretion.

The draft update of this chapter was prepared for the U.S. Preventive Services Task Force by David Atkins, MD, MPH, with contributions from materials prepared by

William Feldman, MD, FRCPC, Anne Martell, MA, CMC, and Jennifer L. Dingle, MBA, for the Canadian Task Force on the Periodic Health Examination.

REFERENCES

1. Forrest JD, Singh S. The sexual and reproductive behavior of American women, 1982–1988. Fam Plann Perspect 1990;22:206–214.
2. Committee on Unintended Pregnancy, Institute of Medicine. The best intentions: unintended pregnancy and the well-being of children and families. Brown SS, Eisenberg L, eds. Washington DC: National Academy Press, 1995.
3. Forrest JD. Epidemiology of unintended pregnancy and contraceptive use. Am J Obstet Gynecol 1994; 170(Suppl 2):1485–1489.
4. Piccinino LJ. Unintended pregnancy and childbearing. In: Wilcox LS, Marks JS, eds. From data to action: CDC's public health surveillance for women, infants, and children. Washington, DC: U.S. Department of Health and Human Services, 1994:73–82.
5. Centers for Disease Control and Prevention. Youth Risk Behavior Surveillance—United States, 1993. MMWR 1995; 44(SS-1):1–56.
6. Alan Guttmacher Institute. Sex and America's teenagers. New York: Alan Guttmacher Institute, 1994.
7. Ventura SJ, Taffel SM, Mosher WD, et al. Trends in pregnancies and pregnancy rates: estimates for the United States, 1980–92. Monthly vital statistics report; vol 43 no 11 (suppl). Hyattsville, MD: National Center for Health Statistics, 1995.
8. Ventura SJ, Martin JA, Taffel SM, et al. Advance report of final natality statistics, 1992. Monthly vital statistics report; vol 43 no 5 (suppl). Hyattsville, MD: National Center for Health Statistics, 1994.
9. Koonin LM, Smith JC, Ramick M. Abortion surveillance—United States, 1991. In: CDC Surveillance Summaries, May 1995. MMWR 1995;44(SS-2):23–53.
10. Henshaw SK, Van Vort J. Abortion services in the United States, 1991 and 1992. Fam Plann Perspect 1994;26: 100–106, 112.
11. Henshaw SK. Induced abortion: a world review, 1990. Fam Plann Perspect 1990;22:76–89.
12. Furstenberg FF Jr, Brooks-Gunn J, Morgan SP. Adolescent mothers and their children in later life. Fam Plann Perspect 1987;19:142–51.
13. National Institute of Child Health and Human Development. Summary of a conference. Outcomes of early childbearing: an appraisal of recent evidence. Bethesda: National Institute of Child Health and Development, May 1992.
14. Center for Population Options. Teenage pregnancy and too-early childbearing: public costs, personal consequences. 6th ed. Washington, DC: Center for Population Options, 1992.
15. Myhrman A. Family relation and social competence of children unwanted at birth: a follow-up study at the age of 16. Acta Psychiatr Scand 1988;77:181–187.
16. Hatcher RA, Guest F, Stewart F, et al. Contraceptive technology. 16th rev ed. New York: Irvington, 1994.
17. Speroff L, Darney P. A clinical guide for contraception. Baltimore: Williams & Wilkins, 1992.
18. Jones EF, Forrest JD. Contraceptive failure rates based on the 1988 NSFG. Fam Plann Perspect 1992;24:12–19.
19. Baird DT, Glasier AF. Hormonal contraception. N Engl J Med 1993;328:1543–1549.
20. Stampfer MJ, Willett WC, Colditz GA, et al. Past use of oral contraceptives and cardiovascular disease: a meta-analysis in the context of the Nurses' Health Study. Am J Obstet Gynecol 1990;163:285–291.
21. DaVanzo J, Parnell AM, Foege WH. Health consequences of contraceptive use and reproductive patterns. Summary of a report from the U.S. National Research Council. JAMA 1991;265:2692–2696.
22. Vessey MP, Villard-Mackintosh I, McPherson K, et al. Mortality among oral contraceptive users: 20 years follow up of women in a cohort study. BMJ 1989;299:1487–1491.
23. Colditz GA for the Nurses' Health Study Research Group. Oral contraceptive use and mortality during 12 years of follow-up: the Nurses' Health Study. Ann Intern Med 1994;120:821–826.
24. Thorogood M, Mann J, Vessey M. Fatal stroke and use of oral contraceptives: findings from a case-control study. Am J Epidemiol 1992;136:35–45.
25. Hannaford PC, Croft PR, Kay CR. Oral contraception and stroke. Evidence from the Royal College of General Practitioners' oral contraception study. Stroke 1994;25:935–942.
26. Lidegard O. Oral contraception and risk of cerebral thromboembolic attack: results of a case-control study. BMJ 1993;306:956–963.

27. Rosenberg L, Palmer JR, Lesko S, et al. Oral contraceptive use and the risk of myocardial infarction. Am J Epidemiol 1990;131:1009–1016.

28. Thorogood M, Mann J, Murphy M, et al. Is oral contraceptive use still associated with an increased risk of fatal myocardial infarction? Report of a case-control study. Br J Obstet Gynaecol 1991;98:1245–1253.

29. Kost K, Forrest JD, Harlap S. Comparing the health risks and benefits of contraceptive choices. Fam Plann Perspect 1991;23:54–61.

30. Porter JB, Hershel J, Walker AM. Mortality among oral contraceptive users. Obstet Gynecol 1987;70:29–32.

31. Forrest JD, Fordyce RR. Women's contraceptive attitudes and use in 1992. Fam Plann Perspect 1993;25:175–179.

32. Schlesselman JJ. Net effect of oral contraceptive use on the risk of cancer in women in the United States. Obstet Gynecol 1995;85:793–801.

33. Malone KE, Daling JR, Weiss NS. Oral contraceptives in relation to breast cancer. Epidemiol Rev 1993;15:80–97.

34. Romieu I, Berlin JA, Colditz G. Oral contraceptives and breast cancer: review and meta-analysis. Cancer 1990;66: 2253–2263.

35. Harlap S, Kost K, Forrest JD, eds. Preventing pregnancy, protecting health: a new look at birth control choices in the United States. New York: Alan Guttmacher Institute, 1991.

36. Chi I. The safety and efficacy issues of progestin-only oral contraceptives—an epidemiologic perspective. Contraception 1993;47:1–21.

37. Xiao BL, Gu SJ, Wang SL, et al. Norplant and the levonorgestrel IUD in Chinese family planning programs. Ann Med 1993;25:161–163.

38. Su-Juan G, Ming Kun D, Ling-De Z, et al. A 5-year evaluation of NORPLANT contraceptive implants in China. Obstet Gynecol 1994;83:673–678.

39. Polaneczky M, Slap G, Forke C, et al. The use of levonorgestrel implants (Norplant) for contraception in adolescent mothers. N Engl J Med 1994;331:1201–1206.

40. Berenson AB, Wiemann CM. Patient satisfaction and side effects with levonorgestrel implant (Norplant) use in adolescents 18 years or younger. Pediatrics 1993;92:257–260.

41. Wysowski DK, Green L. Serious adverse events in Norplant users reported to the Food and Drug Administration's MedWatch spontaneous reporting system. Obstet Gynecol 1995;85:538–542.

42. Dunson TR, Amatya RN, Krueger SL. Complications and risk factors associated with the removal of Norplant implants. Obstet Gynecol 1995;85:543–548.

43. World Health Organization. Depot-medroxyprogesterone acetate (DMPA) and cancer: memorandum from a WHO meeting. Bull WHO 1993;71:669–676.

44. Kaunitz AM. Long-acting injectable contraception with DMPA. Am J Obstet Gynecol 1994;170:1543–1549.

45. Trussell J, Stewart F, Hatcher RA. Emergency contraceptive pills: a simple proposal to reduce unintended pregnancies. Fam Plann Perspect 1992;24:269–273.

46. Fasoli M, Parazzini F, Cecchetti G, et al. Post-coital contraception: an overview of published studies. Contraception 1989;39:459–468. [Erratum, Contraception 1989;39:699].

47. Webb A, Russell J, Elstein M. Comparison of Yuzpe regimen, danazol, and mifepristone (RU 486) in postcoital contraception. BMJ 1992;305:927–931.

48. Glasier A, Thong KJ, Dewar M, et al. Mifepristone (RU 486) compared with high-dose estrogen and progestogen for emergency postcoital contraception. N Engl J Med 1992;327:1041–1044.

49. The contraception report. Warren Township, NJ: Emron, Inc., 1994. Vol V, no. 3, p. 14.

50. Farr G, Gabelnick H, Sturgen K, et al. Contraceptive efficacy and acceptability of the female condom. Am J Public Health 1994;84:1960–1964.

51. Choice of contraceptives. Med Lett Drugs Ther 1995;37:9–12.

52. Diagnostic and therapeutic technology assessment. Intrauterine devices. JAMA 1989;261:2127–2130.

53. Farley TMM, Rosenberg MJ, Rowe PJ, et al. Intrauterine devices and pelvic inflammatory disease: an international perspective. Lancet 1992;339:785–788.

54. Notzer N, Levran D, Mashiach S, et al. Effect of religiosity on sex attitudes, experience and contraception among university students. J Sex Marital Ther 1984;10:57–62.

55. Trussell J, Grummer-Strawn L. Contraceptive failure of the ovulation method of periodic abstinence. Fam Plann Perspect 1990;22:65–75.

56. World Health Organization. A prospective multicenter trial of the ovulation method of natural family planning. IV. The outcome of pregnancy. Fertil Steril 1984;41:593–598.

57. Klaus H, Goebel JM, Muraski B, et al. Use-effectiveness and client satisfaction in six centers teaching the Billings ovulation method. Contraception 1979;19:613–629.

58. Grubb G, Refoser H, Layde PM, et al. Regret after decision to have a tubal sterilization. Fertil Steril 1985;44: 248–253.

59. Wilcox LS, Chu SY, Peterson HB, et al. Characteristics of women who considered or obtained tubal reanastomosis: results from a prospective study of tubal sterilization. Obstet Gynecol 1990;75:661–665.

60. Phillips AJ, D'Ablaing G. Acute salpingitis subsequent to tubal ligation. Obstet Gynecol 1986;67:55S–58S.

61. Hankinson SE, Hunter DJ, Colditz GA, et al. Tubal ligation, hysterectomy, and risk of ovarian cancer: a prospective study. JAMA 1993;270:2813–2818.

62. Peterson LS. Contraceptive use in the United States, 1982–90. Advance data from vital and health statistics; no. 260. Hyattsville, MD: National Center for Health Statistics, 1995.

63. Mosher WD, McNally JW. Contraceptive use at first pre-marital intercourse: United States, 1965–1988. Fam Plann Perspect 1991;23:108–116.

64. Kirby D, Waszak C, Ziegler J. Six school-based clinics: their reproductive health services and impact on sexual behavior. Fam Plann Perspect 1991;23:6–16.

65. Loucks A. A comparison of satisfaction with types of diaphragms among women in a college population. J Obstet Gynecol Neonatal Nurs 1989;18:194–200.

66. Zabin LS, Hirsch MB, Smith EA, et al. Evaluation of a pregnancy prevention program for urban teenagers. Fam Plann Perspect 1986;18:119–26.

67. Vincent ML, Clearie AR, Schluchter MD. Reducing adolescent pregnancy through school and community-based education. JAMA 1987;257:3382–3386.

68. Koo HP, Dunteman GH, George G, et al. Reducing adolescent pregnancy through a school- and community-based intervention: Denmark, South Carolina, revisited. Fam Plann Perspect 1994;26:206–211, 217.

69. Edwards L, Steinman M, Arnold K, et al. Adolescent pregnancy services in high school clinics. Fam Plann Perspect 1980;12:6–14.

70. Kirby D, Resnick MD, Downes B, et al. The effects of school based health clinics in St. Paul on schoolwide birthrates. Fam Plann Perspect 1993;25:12–16.

71. Kirby D, Short L, Collins J, et al. School-based programs to reduce sexual risk behaviors: a review of effectiveness. Public Health Rep 1994;109:339–360.

72. Danielson R, Marcy S, Plunkett A, et al. Reproductive health counseling for young men: what does it do? Fam Plann Perspect 1990;22:115–121.

73. Forrest JD, Hermalin A, Henshaw SK. The impact of family planning clinic programs on adolescent pregnancy. Fam Plann Perspect 1981;13:109–116.

74. Moore KA, Caldwell SB. The effect of government policies on out-of-wedlock sex and pregnancy. Fam Plann Perspect 1977;9:164–169.

75. Emans SJ, Grace E, Woods E, et al. Adolescents' compliance with the use of oral contraceptives. JAMA 1987;257: 3377–3381.

76. Herceg-Baron R, Furstenberg FF Jr, Shea J, et al. Supporting teenagers' use of contraceptives: a comparison of clinic services. Fam Plann Perspect 1986;18:61–66.

77. Namerow PB, Weatherby N, Williams-Kaye J. The effectiveness of contingency-planning counseling. Fam Plann Perspect 1989;21:115–119.

78. National Center for Health Statistics. Healthy People 2000 review, 1994. Hyattsville, MD: U.S. Public Health Service, 1995. (Publication no. PHS-95-1256-1).

79. Nathanson CA, Becker MH. The influence of client-provider relationships on teenage women's subsequent use of contraception. Am J Public Health 1985;75:33–38.

80. Orr M. Private physicians and the provision of contraceptives to adolescents. Fam Plann Perspect 1984;16:83–86.

81. Donovan P. Our daughter's decisions: the conflict in state law on abortion and other issues. New York: Alan Guttmacher Institute, 1992.

82. Committee on Education in Family Life, American College of Obstetricians and Gynecologists. The management of sexual crises in the minor female. Washington, DC: American College of Obstetricians and Gynecologists, 1982.

83. Chamie M, Eisman S, Forrest JD, et al. Factors affecting adolescents' use of family planning clinics. Fam Plann Perspect 1982;14:126–139.

84. Smith JC, Franchino B, Henneberry JF. Surveillance of family planning services at Title X clinics and characteristics of women receiving these services, 1991. In: CDC surveillance summaries, May 5, 1995. MMWR 1995;44(SS-2):1–21.

85. American Academy of Family Physicians. Age charts for periodic health examination. Kansas City, MO: American Academy of Family Physicians, 1994. (Reprint no. 510.)

86. American Medical Association. Guidelines for adolescent preventive services (GAPS): recommendations and rationale. Chicago: American Medical Association, 1994.

87. American Academy of Pediatrics. Contraception and adolescents. Pediatrics 1990;86:134–138.

88. American College of Obstetricians and Gynecologists. The adolescent obstetric-gynecologic patient. Technical Bulletin no. 145. Washington, DC: American College of Obstetricians and Gynecologists, 1990.

89. Society for Adolescent Medicine. Position papers on reproductive health care for adolescents. J Adolesc Health Care 1983;4:208–210.

90. Canadian Task Force on the Periodic Health Examination. Canadian guide to clinical preventive health care. Ottawa: Canada Communication Group, 1994:540–547.

91. U.S. Department of Health and Human Services. Healthy People 2000: national health promotion and disease prevention objectives. Washington, DC: Public Health Service, 1991:185–205. (Publication no. PHS-91-50212.)

92. World Health Organization Special Programme of Research, Development and Research Training in Human Reproduction. Annual technical report—1994. Geneva: WHO, 1995. (WHO/HRP/ATR/94/95.)

93. Mosher W. Fertility and family planning in the United States: insights from the National Survey of Family Growth. Fam Plann Perspect 1988;20:207–217.

94. Green M, ed. Bright Futures: guidelines for health supervision of infants, children, and adolescents. Arlington VA: National Center for Education in Maternal and Child Health, 1994.

64. Counseling to Prevent Gynecologic Cancers

RECOMMENDATION

There is insufficient evidence to recommend for or against routine counseling of women about measures for the primary prevention of gynecologic cancers. Clinicians counseling women about contraceptive practices should include information on the potential benefits of oral contraceptives, barrier contraceptives, and tubal sterilization with respect to specific gynecologic cancers (see Chapter 63). Clinicians should also promote other practices (maintaining desirable body weight, smoking cessation, and safe sex practices) that may reduce the incidence of certain gynecologic cancers and have other proven health benefits (see Chapters 21, 54, and 62).

Burden of Suffering

Gynecologic malignancies are an important cause of morbidity and mortality in women.[1] Ovarian cancer is the fourth most common cause of death from cancer among women of all ages in the U.S.[2] Estimates for 1995 anticipated that there would be 15,800 new cases and 4,800 deaths from cervical cancer, 32,500 new cases and 5,900 deaths from endometrial cancer, and 26,600 new cases and 14,500 deaths from ovarian cancer.[2] Although Papanicolaou (Pap) smear screening has helped reduce mortality from cervical cancer (see Chapter 9), there are no screening strategies that have been proved effective in reducing mortality from endometrial or ovarian cancer (see Chapter 14).

Even when cancers are detected early, the treatment of invasive cervical cancer, endometrial cancer, and ovarian cancer involves surgery and often additional radiation therapy or chemotherapy. Despite aggressive treatment, 5-year survival of women with ovarian cancer is only about 40%.[2] In addition to the costs and morbidity from treatment, the loss of reproductive function and ovarian function can have important psychological and physical consequences in premenopausal women. Compared to early detection and treatment, primary preventive strategies offer the potential to reduce both mortality and morbidity from gynecologic cancers.[3]

Efficacy of Risk Reduction

Cervical Cancer. Certain sexual behaviors are consistently associated with an increased risk for cervical cancer. Women who became sexually active at an early age and women with a high lifetime number of sex partners have a significantly increased risk of cervical cancer.[4] Use of barrier contraception (diaphragm and condoms) and spermicides (foam or contraceptive jelly) is associated with lower risk of invasive cervical cancer. Of 11 case-control studies[5–15] and one cohort study[16] examining this issue, 10 reported that at least one of these methods of contraception was associated with a significantly lower risk of cervical cancer. This protective effect persisted after controlling for the potential influence of age at first intercourse, cytology screening history, and smoking.[11,13,16] Substantial reductions in risk of invasive cervical cancer were observed among both condom users (odds ratios [OR] = 0.4–0.8, i.e., 20–60% reduction in risk)[11] and diaphragm users (OR = 0.2–0.7).[5,16] A longer duration of use was associated with greater protection.[11] In one study, barrier contraceptives reduced risk only among women with multiple sex partners.[13] Spermicides afforded protection comparable to physical barriers in three studies;[12–14] proving an independent effect of spermicides is difficult since they are often used in conjunction with other barrier methods.

The apparent protective effect of avoiding high-risk sexual activity and using barrier contraceptives or spermicides is presumably mediated through reducing the incidence of sexually transmitted diseases (STDs). Human papillomavirus (HPV) appears to be an important factor in the etiology of cervical cancers:[1,4,17] women with HPV infection have a 10-fold higher risk of developing invasive cervical cancer.[18] Direct evidence that spermicides or barrier contraception prevents HPV infection is limited, however.[19] Despite in vitro activity against many sexually transmitted viruses and bacteria, nonoxynol-9 did not inhibit papillomaviruses in one recent study.[20]

Smoking is also associated with an increased risk of invasive cervical cancer.[17,21–23] Recent case-control studies report a 2-fold increased risk among smokers versus nonsmokers; risk remained significantly elevated after controlling for other risk factors.[13,24–26] Most studies suggest a dose-response relationship between risk and cigarette use. Ex-smokers have a risk below that of current smokers, but higher than in nonsmokers.[13,25–27]

Some dietary factors, such as high levels of vitamin C, have also been associated with reduced risk of cervical cancer.[28,29] Two case-control studies have reported significantly lower risk (30–50% lower) in women with the highest versus lowest vitamin C intake.[30,31] The relationship of dietary folate, vitamin E, and dietary carotenoids to invasive cervical cancer is unclear.[4,29,32] Attributing a protective effect to any specific dietary component is problematic, however, due to the possible influence of other dietary constituents or lifestyle factors.[29,33] The mechanisms by which dietary factors might protect against cervical neoplasia remain speculative, but include antioxidant effects or enhancement of the immune system.[30]

Long-term use (>5 years) of oral contraceptives (OCs) has been associated with an increased risk of invasive cervical cancer,[17,34,35] which remains elevated after controlling for sexual history and cytologic screening.[36–38] Two large collaborative case-control studies[36,38] and a large cohort study in the United Kingdom[39] each reported increased risks of cervical cancer among women who have ever used OCs (OR = 1.2–1.8). A meta-analysis of 18 methodologically sound epidemiologic studies[40] reported an increased risk for invasive cancer among OC users (OR = 1.21, 95% confidence interval [CI], 1.1 to 1.4), with increasing risk with longer durations of use. Although a causal association between OC use and cervical cancer is biologically plausible (OCs cause endocervical hyperplasia), it is difficult to exclude the effect of other risk factors among long-term OC users (e.g., multiple sex partners or low use of barrier contraceptives).[17,41]

Endometrial Cancer. Childbearing seems to protect against endometrial cancer,[42] and the use of combination oral contraceptives is consistently associated with a lower risk of endometrial cancer. Of 13 case-control studies,[38,43–54] and three cohort studies,[39,55,56] all but two indicated a protective effect of oral contraceptive use (OR = 0.1–0.6).[1] In the largest study, the Cancer and Steroid Hormone (CASH) study which involved 433 cases and 3191 controls, women who had used combination OCs for at least 1 year had an age-adjusted OR of endometrial cancer of 0.6 (95% CI, 0.3 to 0.9).[51] The protective effect began after 1 year of use and lasted up to 15 years after discontinuing the pills, but it was most evident in nulliparous women. Two of three cohort studies have reported similar protective effects.[39,51,56] The Royal College of General Practitioners study from the United Kingdom followed 47,000 women and found an 80% reduction in risk (RR = 0.2; 95% CI, 0.0 to 0.7) among OC users.[39]

In the CASH study, lower risk was seen with a variety of different combination OCs (OR = 0.2–0.7).[51] In one report, high-dose estrogen/low-dose progestin pills were less effective (OR = 1.1; 95% CI, 0.1 to 10.0) than low-dose estrogen/high-dose progestin pills (OR = 0.0; 95% CI, 0.0 to 1.1),[57] but the importance of formulation remains controversial.[58] Other unresolved questions include the duration of protection, since most endometrial cancer occurs after age 60, and the effects of past OC use in women taking postmenopausal hormone therapy.[58] Use of unopposed estrogen after the menopause is associated with an increased risk of endometrial cancer, but the risk is reduced or eliminated by regimens combining estrogen with progestins (see Chapter 68).[59]

Overweight women have an increased risk of endometrial cancer.[17] Nineteen reports, using varying definitions of overweight, observed relative risks ranging from 1.0–20.3 for overweight women.[42,54,60] Most RRs were above 2, and body mass was significantly correlated with cancer risk. In contrast with several other diseases, the total amount of adiposity may be more important than its distribution (i.e., waist-hip ratio) in the development of endometrial cancer.[61]

The protective effects of OCs and of normal weight may reflect the adverse effects on the endometrium of unopposed estrogen stimulation.[62] Obesity is associated with increased anovulation, increasing levels of circulating estrogens, and lower progesterone levels, due to conversion of androstenedione into estrone (an estrogen) by adipose tissue.[17] OCs containing progestins reduce the period of unopposed estrogen stimulation of the endometrium.

Ovarian Cancer. Childbearing reduces the risk of ovarian cancer,[63] and use of oral contraceptives may have a similar effect. Of 20 case-control studies[38,49,64–81] of the association between OC use and ovarian cancer, all but two found a lower risk among users of OCs.[79,80] Three cohort studies, one from the U.S.[55] and two from the U.K.,[39,82] all reported substantial protective effects of oral contraceptives (RR = 0.4, 0.6, and 0.3, respectively). In a 1992 meta-analysis of these studies, the pooled risk of ovarian cancer was 30–40% lower in OC users in case-control studies, and 60% lower in cohort studies (RR = 0.4; 95% CI, 0.3 to 0.8).[83] In the CASH study, with 546 cases and 4,228 controls,[64] a protective effect was evident after as little as 3–6 months of pill use, persisted for at least 15 years after discontinuation, increased with duration of use (80% reduction after 10 or more years), and was evident for each of 11 commonly used formulations.

Breastfeeding also appears to lower a woman's risk of ovarian cancer.[44,64,69,79,84–86] In an analysis of 12 case-control studies, women who had breast fed an infant had a 20% lower risk of ovarian cancer (OR = 0.8; 95% CI, 0.7 to 1.0) than parous women who had never breastfed;[63] each month of breastfeeding was associated with a 1% reduction in overall risk. Childbearing, OC use, and breastfeeding may reduce the risk of malignant transformation by prolonging periods of anovulation or suppressing gonadotropin levels.

Tubal sterilization is associated with a lower risk of ovarian cancer in a number of case-control studies (OR = 0.2–0.9).[63,78,80,86–89] A recent, large cohort study of nearly 78,000 premenopausal nurses demonstrated a substantial reduction in subsequent ovarian cancer among women who had tubal ligation (RR = 0.3; 95% CI, 0.2 to 0.6).[90] A meta-analysis of published studies estimated that tubal sterilization reduced risk by 40% (RR = 0.6; 95% CI, 0.4 to 0.9).[90] This protective effect may be due to isolation of the ovaries from carcinogens imported from the external environment.[91,92] Hysterectomy, which has a simiar effect, is associated with a somewhat smaller reduction in ovarian cancer (RR = 0.6–0.7).[63,88,90]

Recent trends in the U.S. and U.K. are consistent with a protective effect of OCs on endometrial and ovarian cancer.[62,93,94] In women under 50 (those with greatest exposure to combination OCs) incidence of endometrial cancer fell 28% between 1973 and 1986 in the U.S., and incidence of ovarian cancer declined 20%, similar to changes predicted based on a protective effect of OCs.[62,95] Interpreting temporal trends is complicated by changes in other risk factors (e.g., parity, estrogen use) and in screening practices, however.

Effectiveness of Counseling

There are no data to determine whether counseling women specifically about primary prevention of gynecologic cancers influences their choice of contraception or their attention to other risk factors (sexual practices, weight control, diet, or smoking). Women and men choosing a particular method of contraception may regard other considerations—costs, effectiveness, convenience, and protection against STDs—as more important than long-term effects on gynecologic cancers, which account for less than 10% of all cancer deaths in women. Some women may place a higher value on reducing their risk of cancer, however, or have risk factors that place them at higher risk for specific cancers. These important noncontraceptive benefits of modern OCs are often not mentioned when the risks and benefits of these agents are discussed. A recent survey of female employees, students, and faculty at a large university revealed that 80% did not know that use of OCs protects against ovarian cancer.[96]

There is only limited evidence that clinical counseling can reduce the high-risk sexual behaviors in young women that put them at future risk for cervical cancer (see Chapter 62). Early sexual activity and multiple sex partners remain common among young men and women. Counseling men is more effective than counseling women in increasing regular use of condoms.[97] Although methods under female control (diaphragms, spermicides and female condom) may also be protective, they remain less popular, especially among high-risk populations.[98]

Discussion

A large body of evidence suggests that specific measures can reduce the risk of cervical, ovarian, or endometrial cancer. Although this evidence comes from epidemiologic studies rather than from controlled trials, various considerations support the conclusion that certain interventions have a protective effect against cancer:[99] the observed associations are strong, consistent in multiple studies, biologically plausible, dose-dependent, and not explained by differences in other risk factors. Evidence of a protective effect of OCs on endometrial and ovarian cancer is compelling and stronger than that for adverse effects of OCs on cervical cancer. Furthermore, ovarian and endometrial cancers together account for four times as many deaths as cervical cancer, which can often be prevented by effective screening. Tubal sterilization, hysterectomy, and breastfeeding also appear to reduce risk of ovarian cancer, but evidence is more limited. Other measures (breastfeeding, avoiding smoking, obesity, and high-risk sexual activity) also appear to reduce the risk of specific gynecologic cancers, and there are other compelling reasons to promote these measures routinely for all patients. In contrast, the evidence is not yet sufficient to recommend specific diets to reduce the risk of cervical cancer. More information may come from ongoing chemoprevention trials of vitamin supplementation.[100]

Women selecting contraception need to consider not only the convenience and effectiveness of a given method, but other important noncontraceptive risks and benefits as well (see Chapter 63).[101,102] The favorable effects of OCs on endometrial and ovarian cancer are more consistent yet less widely appreciated than some of the possible risks of OCs, such as cardiovascular disease or breast cancer. Despite the relative safety of oral contraceptives, however, it is not clear that the potential benefits with respect to ovarian and endometrial cancer would justify the expense, inconvenience, and possible risks of OC use in women who do not otherwise need contraception. One study estimated that treating 100,000 women with OCs for 8 years might prevent 193 cases of ovarian cancer and 197 cases of endometrial cancer;[103] net benefit, however, would be negligible if OCs increase the risk of cervical or breast cancer. Nonetheless, for women with specific concerns about gynecologic cancers, information about effective measures that they can take to reduce their risk of cervical, ovarian, or endometrial cancer may be particularly useful.

CLINICAL INTERVENTION

There is insufficient evidence to recommend for or against routine counseling of female patients about measures to reduce the risk of cervical, ovarian, and endometrial cancer ("C" recommendation). Clinicians counseling women about contraceptive practices should include information about the potential benefits of specific methods with respect to gynecologic cancers (see Chapter 63). These potential benefits include reduced risks of ovarian and endometrial cancer in women using OCs, cervical cancer in women who use barrier contraception and spermicides, and ovarian cancer after tubal sterilization. All women should be counseled about effective means to prevent STDs (see Chapter 62) and about the benefits of

breastfeeding (see Chapter 56), avoiding obesity (see Chapter 21), and avoiding tobacco use (see Chapter 54).

Note: See background paper: Grimes DA, Economy KE. Primary prevention of gynecologic malignancies. Am J Obstet Gynecol 1995;172:227–235.

The draft of this chapter was prepared for the U.S. Preventive Services Task Force by David Grimes, MD, and David Atkins, MD, MPH, based on a background paper by David Grimes, MD, and Katherine E. Economy, MD.

REFERENCES

1. Grimes DA, Economy KE. Primary prevention of gynecologic malignancies. Am J Obstet Gynecol 1995;172: 227–235.
2. Wingo PA, Tong T, Bolden S. Cancer statistics, 1995. CA Cancer J Clin 1995;45:8–30.
3. Last JM, ed. Scope and methods of prevention. In: Maxcy-Rosenau public health and preventive medicine. 11th ed. New York: Appleton-Century-Crofts, 1980:3–8.
4. Brinton LA. Epidemiology of cervical cancer—overview. In: Munoz N, Bosch FX, Shah KV, Meheus A, eds. The epidemiology of cervical cancer and human papillomavirus. Lyon, France: IARC, 1992:3–23.
5. Parazzini F, Negri E, La Vecchia C, Fedele L. Barrier methods of contraception and the risk of cervical neoplasia. Contraception 1989;40:519–530.
6. Boyd JT, Doll R. A study of the aetiology of carcinoma of the cervix uteri. Br J Cancer 1964;18:419–434.
7. Aitken-Swan J, Baird D. Cancer of the uterine cervix in Aberdeenshire. Etiological aspects. Br J Cancer 1966;20: 642–659.
8. Martin CE. Epidemiology of cancer of the cervix. II. Marital and coital factors in cervical cancer. Am J Public Health 1967;57:803–814.
9. Boyce JG, Lu T, Nelson JH, Fruchter RG. Oral contraceptives and cervical carcinoma. Am J Obstet Gynecol 1977;128:761–766.
10. Fasal E, Simmons ME, Kampert JB. Factors associated with high and low risk of cervical neoplasia. J Natl Cancer Inst 1981;66:631–636.
11. Peters RK, Thomas D, Hagan DG, et al. Risk factors for invasive cervical cancer among Latinas and non-Latinas in Los Angeles County. J Natl Cancer Inst 1986;77:1063–1077.
12. Celentano DD, Klassen AC, Weisman CS, Rosenshein NB. The role of contraceptive use in cervical cancer: the Maryland cervical cancer case-control study. Am J Epidemiol 1987;126:592–604.
13. Slattery ML, Overall JC Jr, Abbott TM, et al. Sexual activity, contraception, genital infections, and cervical cancer: support for a sexually transmitted disease hypothesis. Am J Epidemiol 1989;130:248–258.
14. Hildesheim A, Brinton LA, Malin K, et al. Barrier and spermicidal contraceptive methods and risk of invasive cervical cancer. Epidemiology 1990;1:266–272.
15. Brinton LA, Reeves WC, Brenes MM, et al. Oral contraceptive use and risk of invasive cervical cancer. Int J Epidemiol 1990;19:4–11.
16. Wright NH, Vessey MP, Kenward B, et al. Neoplasia and dysplasia of the cervix uteri and contraception: a possible protective effect of the diaphragm. Br J Cancer 1978;38:273–279.
17. Daly MB, Bookman MA, Lerman CE. Female reproductive tract: cervix, endometrium, ovary. In: Greenwald P, Kramer BS, Weed DL, eds. Cancer prevention and control. New York: Marcel Dekker, 1995.
18. Schiffman MH. Recent progress in defining the epidemiology of human papillomavirus infection and cervical neoplasia. J Natl Cancer Inst 1992;84:394–398.
19. Cates W, Stone KM. Family planning, sexually transmitted diseases and contraceptive choice: a literature update—Part I. Fam Plann Perspect 1992;24:75–84.
20. Hermonat PL, Daniel RW, Shah KV. The spermicide nonoxynol-9 does not inactivate papillomavirus. Sex Transm Dis 1992;19:203–205.
21. Winkelstein W Jr. Smoking and cervical cancer—current status: a review. Am J Epidemiol 1990;131:945–957.
22. Baron JA, Byers T, Greenberg ER, et al. Cigarette smoking in women with cancers of the breast and reproductive organs. J Natl Cancer Inst 1986;77:677–680.

23. Slattery ML, Robison LM, Schuman KL, et al. Cigarette smoking and exposure to passive smoking are risk factors for cervical cancer. JAMA 1989;261:1594–1598.

24. La Vecchia C, Franceschi S, Decarli A, et al. Cigarette smoking and the risk of cervical neoplasia. Am J Epidemiol 1986;123:22–29.

25. Brisson J, Roy M, Fortier M, et al. Condyloma and intraepithelial neoplasia of the uterine cervix: a case-control study. Am J Epidemiol 1988;128:337–342.

26. Brinton LA, Schairer C, Haenszel W, et al. Cigarette smoking and invasive cervical cancer. JAMA 1986;255: 3265–3269.

27. Mayberry RM. Cigarette smoking, herpes simplex virus type 2 infection, and cervical abnormalities. Am J Public Health 1985;75:676–678.

28. Block G, Patterson B, Subar A. Fruit, vegetables, and cancer prevention: a review of the epidemiological evidence. Nutr Cancer 1992;18:1–29.

29. Potischman N. Nutritional epidemiology of cervical neoplasia. J Nutr 1993;123:424–429.

30. Herrero R, Potischman N, Brinton LA, et al. A case-control study of nutrient status and invasive cervical cancer. I. Dietary indicators. Am J Epidemiol 1991;134:1335–1346.

31. Verreault R, Chu J, Mandelson M, Shy K. A case-control study of diet and invasive cervical cancer. Int J Cancer 1989;43:1050–1054.

32. Schneider A, Shah K. The role of vitamins in the etiology of cervical neoplasia: an epidemiological review. Arch Gynecol Obstet 1989;246:1–13.

33. Brock KE, Berry G, Mock PA, et al. Nutrients in diet and plasma and risk of in situ cervical cancer. J Natl Cancer Inst 1988;80:580–585.

34. Hannaford PC. Cervical cancer and methods of contraception. Adv Contracept 1991;7:317–324.

35. Brinton LA. Oral contraceptives and cervical neoplasia. Contraception 1991;43:581–595.

36. Brinton LA, Huggins GR, Lehman HF, et al. Long-term use of oral contraceptives and risk of invasive cervical cancer. Int J Cancer 1986;38:339–344.

37. Parazzini F, La Vecchia C, Negri E, Maggi R. Oral contraceptive use and invasive cervical cancer. Int J Epidemiol 1990;19:259–263.

38. Thomas DB. The WHO collaborative study of neoplasia and steroid contraceptives: the influence of combined oral contraceptives on risk of neoplasms in developing and developed countries. Contraception 1991;43:695–710.

39. Beral V, Hannaford P, Kay C. Oral contraceptive use and malignancies of the genital tract. Results from the Royal College of General Practitioners' oral contraception study. Lancet 1988;ii:1331–1335.

40. Delgado-Rodriguez M, Sillero-Arenas M, Martin-Moreno JM, et al. Oral contraceptives and cancer of the cervix uteri. A meta-analysis. Acta Obstet Gynecol Scand 1992;71:368–376.

41. WHO Scientific Group. Oral contraceptives and neoplasia. WHO Technical Report series, no. 817. Geneva: World Health Organization, 1992.

42. Parazzini F, La Vecchia C, Bocciolone L, Franceschi S. The epidemiology of endometrial cancer. Gynecol Oncol 1991;41:1–16.

43. Horwitz RI, Feinstein AR. Case-control study of oral contraceptive pills and endometrial cancer. Ann Intern Med 1979;91:226–227.

44. Weiss NS, Sayvetz TA. Incidence of endometrial cancer in relation to the use of oral contraceptives. N Engl J Med 1980;302:551–554.

45. Kaufman DW, Shapiro S, Slone D, et al. Decreased risk of endometrial cancer among oral contraceptive users. N Engl J Med 1980;303:1045–1047.

46. Kelsey JL, LiVolsi VA, Holford TR, et al. A case-control study of cancer of the endometrium. Am J Epidemiol 1982;116:333–342.

47. Hulka BS, Chambless LE, Kaufman DG, et al. Protection against endometrial carcinoma by combination-product oral contraceptives. JAMA 1982;247:475–477.

48. Henderson BE, Casagrande JT, Pike MC, et al. The epidemiology of endometrial cancer in young women. Br J Cancer 1983;47:749–756.

49. La Vecchia C, Decarli A, Fasoli M, et al. Oral contraceptives and cancers of the breast and of the female genital tract. Interim results from a case-control study. Br J Cancer 1986;54:311–317.

50. Pettersson B, Adami HO, Bergstrom R, Johansson EDB. Menstruation span - a time-limited risk factor for endometrial carcinoma. Acta Obstet Gynecol Scand 1986;65:247–255.

51. The Cancer and Steroid Hormone Study of the Centers for Disease Control and the National Institute of Child Health and Human Development. Combination oral contraceptive use and the risk of endometrial cancer. JAMA 1987;257: 796–800.

52. Koumantaki Y, Tzonou A, Koumantakis E, et al. A case-control study of cancer of the endometrium in Athens. Int J Cancer 1989;43:795–799.
53. Brinton LA, Hoover RN, and the Endometrial Cancer Collaborative Group. Estrogen replacement therapy and endometrial cancer risk: unresolved issues. Obstet Gynecol 1993;81:265–271.
54. Jick SS, Walker AM, Jick H. Oral contraceptives and endometrial cancer. Obstet Gynecol 1993;82:931–935.
55. Ramcharan S, Pellegrin FA, Ray R, Hsu J-P. The Walnut Creek contraceptive drug study: a prospective study of the side effects of oral contraceptives, vol 3. Bethesda: National Institute of Child Health and Human Development,1981.
56. Trapido EJ. A prospective cohort study of oral contraceptives and cancer of the endometrium. Int J Epidemiol 1983;12:297–300.
57. Rosenblatt KA, Thomas DB, and the WHO Collaborative Study of Neoplasia and Steroid Contraceptives. Hormonal content of combined oral contraceptives in relation to the reduced risk of endometrial carcinoma. Int J Cancer 1991;49:870–874.
58. Schlesselman JJ. Oral contraceptives and neoplasia of the uterine corpus. Contraception 1991;43: 557–579.
59. Grady D, Rubin SM, Petitti DB, et al. Hormone therapy to prevent disease and prolong life in postmenopausal women. Ann Intern Med 1992;117:1016–1037.
60. Sturgeon SR, Brinton LA, Berman ML, et al. Past and present physical activity and endometrial cancer risk. Br J Cancer 1993;68:584–589.
61. Folsom AR, Kaye SA, Potter JD, Prineas RJ. Association of incident carcinoma of the endometrium with body weight and fat distribution in older women: early findings of the Iowa Women's Health Study. Cancer Res 1989;49: 6828–6831.
62. Henderson BE, Ross RK, Pike MC. Hormonal chemoprevention of cancer in women. Science 1993; 259:633–638.
63. Whittemore AS, Harris R, Itnyre J, and the Collaborative Ovarian Cancer Group. Characteristics relating to ovarian cancer risk: collaborative analysis of 12 U.S. case-control studies. II. Invasive epithelial ovarian cancers in white women. Am J Epidemiol 1992;136:1184–1203.
64. The Cancer and Steroid Hormone Study of the Centers for Disease Control and the National Institute of Child Health and Human Development. The reduction in risk of ovarian cancer associated with oral-contraceptive use. N Engl J Med 1987;316:650–655.
65. Newhouse ML, Pearson RM, Fullerton JM, et al. A case- control study of carcinoma of the ovary. Br J Prev Soc Med 1977;31:148–153.
66. Casagrande JT, Louie EW, Pike MC, et al. "Incessant ovulation" and ovarian cancer. Lancet 1979; 2:170–173.
67. Annegers JF, Strom H, Decker DG, et al. Ovarian cancer: incidence and case-control study. Cancer 1979;43:723–729.
68. McGowan L, Parent L, Lednar W, Norris HJ. The woman at risk for developing ovarian cancer. Gynecol Oncol 1979;7:325–344.
69. Hildreth NG, Kelsey JL, LiVolsi VA, et al. An epidemiologic study of epithelial carcinoma of the ovary. Am J Epidemiol 1981;114:398–405.
70. Willett WC, Bain C, Hennekens CH, et al. Oral contraceptives and risk of ovarian cancer. Cancer 1981;48:1684–1687.
71. Weiss NS, Lyon JL, Liff JM, et al. Incidence of ovarian cancer in relation to the use of oral contraceptives. Int J Cancer 1981;28:669–671.
72. Rosenberg L, Shapiro S, Slone D, et al. Epithelial ovarian cancer and combination oral contraceptives. JAMA 1982;247:3210–3212.
73. Franceschi S, La Vecchia C, Helmrich SP, et al. Risk factors for epithelial ovarian cancer in Italy. Am J Epidemiol 1982;115:714–719.
74. Cramer DW, Hutchison GB, Welch WR, et al. Factors affecting the association of oral contraceptives and ovarian cancer. N Engl J Med 1982;307:1047–1051.
75. Tzonou A, Day NE, Trichopoulos D, et al. The epidemiology of ovarian cancer in Greece: a case-control study. Eur J Cancer Clin Oncol 1984;20:1045–1052.
76. Wu ML, Whittemore AS, Paffenbarger RS, et al. Personal and environmental characteristics related to epithelial ovarian cancer. I. Reproductive and menstrual events and oral contraceptive use. Am J Epidemiol 1988;128: 1216–1227.

77. Harlow BL, Weiss NS, Roth GJ, et al. Case-control study of borderline ovarian tumors: reproductive history and exposure to exogenous female hormones. Cancer Res 1988;48:5849–5852.

78. Booth M, Beral V, Smith P. Risk factors for ovarian cancer: a case-control study. Br J Cancer 1989;60:592–598.

79. Hartge P, Schiffman MH, Hoover R, et al. A case-control study of epithelial ovarian cancer. Am J Obstet Gynecol 1989;161:10–16.

80. Shu XO, Brinton LA, Gao YT, Yuan JM. Population-based case-control study of ovarian cancer in Shanghai. Cancer Res 1989;49:3670–3674.

81. Parazzini F, La Vecchia C, Negri E, et al. Oral contraceptive use and the risk of ovarian cancer: an Italian case-control study. Eur J Cancer 1991;27:594–598.

82. Vessey M, Metcalfe A, Wells C, et al. Ovarian neoplasms, functional ovarian cysts, and oral contraceptives. BMJ 1987;294:1518–1520.

83. Hankinson SE, Colditz GA, Hunter DJ, et al. A quantitative assessment of oral contraceptive use and risk of ovarian cancer. Obstet Gynecol 1992;80:708–714.

84. Cramer DW, Hutchison GB, Welch WR, et al. Determinants of ovarian cancer risk. I. Reproductive experiences and family history. J Natl Cancer Inst 1983;71:711–716.

85. Nasca PC, Greenwald P, Chorost S, et al. An epidemiologic case-control study of ovarian cancer and reproductive factors. Am J Epidemiol 1984;119:705–713.

86. Whittemore AS, Wu ML, Paffenbarger RS Jr, et al. Personal and environmental characteristics related to epithelial ovarian cancer. II. Exposures to talcum powder, tobacco, alcohol, and coffee. Am J Epidemiol 1988;128:1228–1240.

87. Mori M, Harabuchi I, Miyake H, et al. Reproductive, genetic, and dietary factors for ovarian cancer. Am J Epidemiol 1988;128:771–777.

88. Irwin KL, Weiss NS, Lee NC, Peterson HB. Tubal sterilization, hysterectomy, and the subsequent occurrence of epithelial ovarian cancer. Am J Epidemiol 1991;134:362–369.

89. Koch M, Jenkins H, Gaedke H. Risk factors of ovarian cancer of epithelial origin: a case control study. Cancer Detect Prev 1988;13:131–136.

90. Hankinson SE, Hunter DJ, Colditz GA, et al. Tubal ligation, hysterectomy, and risk of ovarian cancer: a prospective study. JAMA 1993;270:2813–2818.

91. Grimes DA. Primary prevention of ovarian cancer. JAMA 1993;270:2855–2856.

92. Egli GE, Newton MD. The transport of carbon particles in the human female reproductive tract. Fertil Steril 1961;12:151–155.

93. Villard L, Murphy M. Endometrial cancer trends in England and Wales: a possible protective effect of oral contraception. Int J Epidemiol 1990;19:255–258.

94. Villard-Mackintosh L, Vessey MP, Jones L. The effects of oral contraceptives and parity on ovarian cancer trends in women under 55 years of age. Br J Obstet Gynaecol 1989;96:783–788.

95. Ries LAG, Miller BA, Hankey RF, et al, eds. SEER Cancer Statistic Review, 1973–1991: tables and graphs. Bethesda: National Cancer Institute, 1994.

96. Peipert J, Gutmann J. Oral contraceptive risk assessment: a survey of 247 educated women. Obstet Gynecol 1993;82:112–117.

97. Cohen DA, Dent C, MacKinnon D, Hahn G. Condoms for men, not women. Sex Transm Dis 1992;19:245–251.

98. Peterson LS. Contraceptive use in the United States, 1982–90. Advance data from vital and health statistics; no. 260. Hyattsville, MD: National Center for Health Statistics, 1995.

99. Hill AB. Principles of medical statistics. 9th ed. London: Lancet, 1971:313.

100. Greenwald P, Kelloff G, Burch-Whitman C, et al. Chemoprevention. CA Cancer J Clin 1995;45:31–49.

101. Vessey MP. The Jephcott Lecture, 1989. An overview of the benefits and risks of combined oral contraceptives. In: Mann RD, ed. Oral contraceptives and breast cancer. Carnforth, England: Parthenon Publishing Group, 1990:121–135.

102. Hatcher RA, Guest F, Stewart F, et al. Contraceptive technology. 16th rev ed. New York: Irvington, 1994.

103. Schlesselman JJ. Net effect of oral contraceptive use on the risk of cancer in women in the United States. Obstet Gynecol 1995;85:793–801.

IMMUNIZATIONS AND CHEMOPROPHYLAXIS

65. Childhood Immunizations

RECOMMENDATION

All children without established contraindications should receive diphtheria-tetanus-pertussis (DTP), oral poliovirus (OPV), measles-mumps-rubella (MMR), conjugate Haemophilus influenzae type b, hepatitis B, and varicella vaccines, in accordance with recommended schedules (see *Clinical Intervention*). Hepatitis A vaccine is recommended for children and adolescents at high risk for hepatitis A virus (HAV) infection. Pneumococcal vaccine and annual influenza vaccine are recommended for children and adolescents at high risk (see Clinical Intervention and Chapter 66). See Chapter 67 for recommendations on postexposure prophylaxis against selected infectious diseases, and Chapter 25 for recommendations regarding the Bacille Calmette-Guérin (BCG) vaccine.

Burden of Suffering

A number of infectious diseases are preventable through routine childhood immunizations. Largely as a result of widespread childhood vaccination over the past several decades, diphtheria, pertussis, tetanus, poliomyelitis, measles, mumps, rubella, and congenital rubella syndrome have become remarkably less common in the U.S. than in prevaccination years, and the numbers of cases reported are at or near the lowest levels ever.[1] Comparisons of the total numbers of reported cases in the U.S. in 1994 and in the years preceding vaccination reveal an impressive decrease in reported cases of diphtheria (from 9,493 [1948] to 2 cases), tetanus (from 601 [1948] to 51 cases), paralytic poliomyelitis (from 18,308 [1954] to 0 cases due to endemic wild virus), measles (from 481,530 [1962] to 963 cases), mumps (from 152,209 [1968] to 1,537 cases), rubella (from 57,686 [1969] to 227 cases), and congenital rubella syndrome (from 77 [1970] to 7 cases).[2,2a] Before the introduction of poliovirus vaccine in 1955, polio occurred in epidemic waves of increasing magnitude, reaching a peak incidence of more than 20,000 paralytic cases in 1952.[3] The last outbreak, in 1979, totaled only 10 paralytic cases. Although the number of pertussis cases has also declined markedly since the prevaccination years (from 74,715 [1948] to 4,617 cases), long-term trends suggest an overall increase in the reported incidence of pertussis since 1976, rising from 0.5/100,000 to 2.6/100,000 in 1993 and 1.8/100,000 in 1994.[4,4a] Many of these cases occurred in unvaccinated or inadequately vaccinated infants and children.

Newer childhood vaccines include *H. influenzae* type b (Hib), hepatitis B, hepatitis A, and varicella vaccines. Systemic illness from Hib disease, including meningitis, pneumonia, arthritis, and epiglottitis, previously occurred before age 5 in about 1 of every 200 children born in the U.S.[5] The highest rates of Hib disease in the U.S. have been reported in Alaska Native and certain Native American populations. The incidence of invasive Hib disease in children <5 years old declined by an estimated 95% (from 41 to 2/100,000) between 1987, when the first Hib vaccine was licensed, and 1994.[6,6a]

Children less than 5 years old account for only 1% of reported cases of hepatitis B and 1–3% of the 200,000 to 300,000 hepatitis B virus (HBV) infections estimated to occur annually in the U.S., but 20–30% of chronic infections.[7] The likelihood of developing chronic infection has been estimated to be 80–90% in perinatally infected neonates, decreasing to 25% for those infected at age 5, and to <10% for infected adults.[8] Chronic infection can lead to severe complications including chronic active hepatitis, cirrhosis, and hepatocellular carcinoma.[9–11]

Nearly 27,000 cases of hepatitis A were reported in the U.S. in 1994 (10.3/100,000),[2a] although the actual number of cases is estimated to be several times higher.[9] Children aged 5–14 years have the highest rate of reported hepatitis A (about 15 cases per 100,000 in 1993).[2] About half of reported cases of hepatitis in the U.S. are attributable to hepatitis A.[9] High-risk groups include travelers to countries with intermediate or high hepatitis A endemicity,[12] some religious communities, and Alaska Native, Pacific Islander, and Native American populations; persons institutionalized for custodial care may also have an increased risk. Day care centers may be an important source of epidemic HAV infection.[13]

Because chickenpox, caused by infection with varicella-zoster virus (VZV), infects nearly everyone by adulthood, its annual incidence approximates the birth cohort (4 million in 1993).[14,15] At least 90% of cases occur in children less than 15 years old.[14] Most adults are immune.[16] Although generally mild in healthy children, chickenpox often results in missed school days for the child, missed work days for their parents, and visits to health care providers, and it occasionally leads to serious complications (e.g., encephalitis, pneumonia, bacterial superinfection), hospitalizations, and, rarely, death.[14,17–20] Complication rates per case of varicella and case-fatality rates are substantially higher for older adolescents and adults than for children.[14,17] Infants are also at high risk of complications.

Efficacy of Vaccines

DTP Vaccine. The efficacy of the DTP vaccine is established on the basis of clinical studies and decades of experience with universal childhood immunization.[21-24] Substantial declines in diphtheria, tetanus, and pertussis disease followed the introduction of whole-cell pertussis vaccine combined with diphtheria and tetanus toxoids in the late 1940s.[24,25] The diphtheria and tetanus toxoids are generally safe and are most commonly associated with self-limited local reactions,[26] although case reports have described allergic or Arthus-like reactions and peripheral neuropathy following frequent tetanus boosters. Anaphylaxis occurs in rare instances.[27-29]

Increased attention has focused in recent years on the efficacy and safety of the pertussis component of the vaccine.[30-32] In a national surveillance study of households with laboratory-confirmed pertussis, the efficacy of currently used whole-cell pertussis vaccines in fully vaccinated (three or more doses) children 1 through 4 years of age was estimated to be 59–89% for prolonged cough, 78% for typical paroxysmal cough, and 96–97% for severe clinical illness.[22] In another national surveillance study, vaccine efficacy in preventing pertussis, defined as either any culture-proven cough illness or typical pertussis illness, was 64% for three doses and 82% for four or more doses.[4a] The whole-cell preparation commonly produces local redness, swelling, and pain, and systemic events such as fever, fretfulness, and protracted, inconsolable crying.[33] DTP has also been associated with more serious adverse events such as febrile seizures in about 57/100,000 doses and hypotonic/hyporesponsive episodes in 3.5–291/100,000 doses.[33] The risk of seizures may be higher in certain children, such as those with a personal or family history of seizures.[34,35] Limited follow-up of such cases, however, suggests that most, if not all, are associated with benign outcomes.[36,37] The National Childhood Encephalopathy Study (NCES), a large British case-control study, reported that pertussis-containing vaccines were associated with more severe neurologic illnesses at a rate of 6.8 per million doses (95% CI, 2.1–15.9 per million), including acute encephalopathy in 2.7 (0–10.5) per million doses.[38] A 10-year follow-up study reported an association between death or permanent neurologic dysfunction and DTP vaccine only among children who had developed a serious acute neurologic illness within 7 days of receiving DTP.[39] The NCES has been criticized for possible bias and error in case ascertainment and other methodologic problems.[33] Detailed analysis of this and other controlled and uncontrolled observational studies led the Institute of Medicine to conclude that evidence was consistent with (but did not establish) a causal relationship between DTP vaccine and acute encephalopathy, with a range of excess risk between 0 and 10.5 per million doses,[33] and between DTP and chronic neurologic dysfunction in those rare children who experienced a serious acute neurologic illness within 7 days after receiving DTP.[40] The incidence of serious neurologic disorders following DTP administration is substantially less than that following pertussis disease.[38] Nevertheless, the high rate of adverse local and mild systemic reactions, as well as the possibility of rare adverse neurologic sequelae, has stimulated interest in development of less reactogenic vaccines.[41]

Acellular forms of pertussis vaccine induce fewer local and systemic side effects than does the whole cell vaccine when administered to infants and children up to 6 years old.[42–48] In a randomized placebo-controlled trial of 3,801 Swedish children aged 5–11 months, the efficacy of two acellular pertussis vaccines was 79–80% in preventing severe culture-proven pertussis and 54–69% for preventing culture-proven cases with any cough.[49–51] Four-year follow-up indicates persistent efficacy ranging from 69% to 95%, depending on case definition.[52] Household exposure studies in Japan have reported efficacy >90% against typical pertussis among children receiving acellular vaccines at age ≥2 years.[53–55a] In a prospective institutional exposure study, children vaccinated with acellular pertussis-component DTP (DTaP) beginning at a median age of 5 months (range, 3–26) were significantly less likely to develop typical pertussis symptoms compared with unvaccinated children.[56] None of these studies directly compared the acellular vaccine to the whole-cell vaccine. Immunogenicity appears comparable to the whole cell vaccine for the antigens present in the acellular vaccines.[44,57] Preliminary results from two European randomized, double-blind trials indicate that DTaP at 2, 4, and 6 months of age was at least as efficacious as DTP with significantly fewer side effects; DTaP is likely to be licensed for use in infancy in the near future (personal communication, John R. La Montagne, PhD, National Institutes of Health (NIH), Bethesda, Aug. 15, 1995). DTaP is currently licensed in the U.S. for use in children ≥15 months of age as the fourth and/or fifth doses of the recommended DTP series.[58,59]

OPV Vaccine. Three doses of live oral poliovirus (OPV) vaccine offers protection against all three poliovirus types in 95–100% of children. As a result, disease caused by indigenous wild poliovirus has been eliminated in the U.S.[60] An estimated 1 out of every 2.5 million vaccine doses results in paralytic poliomyelitis, however, and all cases of endemic paralytic poliomyelitis in the U.S. since 1980 (about eight cases per year) have been associated with the vaccine.[60] The vaccine has also resulted in several cases of fatal vaccine-strain poliovirus infections, primarily in immunocompromised patients.[29] The licensing of enhanced-potency inactivated poliovirus vaccine (IPV), which has no documented serious adverse effects and appears to have comparable immunogenicity,[61,62] has led some to propose replacment of the live vaccine with this product.[63] IPV may be less effective, however, in limiting transmission of wild poliovirus among susceptible members of the population.[64] OPV has few significant adverse effects other than the risk of paralytic poliomyelitis.[29] The rare occurrence of Guillain-Barré syndrome (GBS) was associated with a one-time OPV mass vaccination program in controlled studies in Finland, where IPV had been used routinely.[29] A retrospective epidemiologic survey of GBS in southern California, however, found no correlation between the usual age of OPV immunization and the incidence of GBS.[65] Because it requires injection, IPV is associated with greater discomfort and possibly greater administrative costs than is OPV. Combining IPV with other infant vaccines[66,67] would alleviate this problem.

MMR Vaccine. A single dose of MMR is highly protective against measles, mumps, and rubella and its widespread use has resulted in substantial declines in the incidence of all three diseases.[2,68] It is generally associated with only mild adverse effects in healthy individuals.[68,69] MMR vaccine rarely causes thrombocytopenia (2.5–3.3/100,000 vaccinated persons), urticaria (0.6/100,000), and anaphylaxis (estimated at 0.1–5/100,000).[29,70] Several deaths from vaccine-strain viral infection have been reported, all in severely immunocompromised children; none has been reported in children infected with human immunodeficiency virus (HIV).[29] The efficacy and adverse effects of rubella vaccine are described in detail in Chapter 32.

Despite the efficacy and safety of the vaccine, measles remains an important public health problem in the U.S. due to failure to immunize and to immunization failure. Between 1989 and 1994, 27–64% of measles cases occurred among unvaccinated but vaccine-eligible persons and 19–22% among persons who had received one vaccine after 12 months of age (immunization failure).[71–72a] Most immunization failures appear to occur in children who fail to respond to the vaccine (primary immunization failure), an estimated 5% of children immunized after 15 months of age.[73,74] In the past, the rate of primary immunization failure has been higher among children vaccinated before 15 months of age, presumably because maternal antibody interfered with response.[75] More recent studies indicate excellent serologic response and similar clinical efficacy in children vaccinated at 12–14 months, perhaps because maternal antibody levels achieved in a vaccinated cohort of mothers decline earlier than levels achieved by natural infection.[76–82] Antibody response remains lower than when the vaccine is given at 15 months, however. Current evidence indicates that revaccination of primary immunization failures results in seroconversion rates comparable to that of never vaccinated persons[83] and prevents measles outbreaks.[84]

Although some evidence suggests that waning immunity (secondary immunization failure) may also be a factor in immunization failure,[85–91] seropositivity rates generally remain high at least 10–15 years following vaccination,[92–94] anamnestic antibody responses occur in vaccinated persons who apparently lack antibody,[83,93] and cohorts of known seroconverters followed through time in Great Britain and Japan have shown little evidence of increasing disease incidence with time since immunization.[93] In 27-year follow-up of a British vaccine trial, there was no significant decline in vaccine efficacy with time (although the number of cases was quite small).[95]

Because of immunization failures, a two-dose vaccination protocol against measles appears necessary to eliminate transmission of this highly communicable disease.[88,96–98] Indirect evidence in support of a two-dose regimen comes from studies showing that attack rates during outbreaks are lower among populations of individuals who have had two doses of vaccine,[82,88–91,99] and from the rarity of reported measles cases among persons who had received two doses of vaccine.[72,72a] In Finland, a two-dose vaccination program administered at 14–18 months and at 6 years (with >95% coverage), along with "catch-up" vaccination for children 11–13 years and for individuals at occupational risk, has essentially eliminated indigenous measles, mumps, and rubella.[70] Adverse reactions to a second dose of vaccine seem to be no more common than to the first.

Hib Vaccine. The efficacy of a capsular polysaccharide (polyribosyl-ribitol phosphate [PRP]) vaccine in preventing infection with Hib in children over age 2 was first demonstrated in Finland in 1984.[100] Newer vaccines with substantially improved immunogenicity were subsequently developed by covalently conjugating PRP with protein antigens and were licensed for use in children 15–18 months of age in the late 1980s. Postlicensure studies have indicated vaccine efficacy of 74–88% for children 18–59 months of age.[101–103] Licensure of Hib conjugate vaccines for infants under 6 months of age followed demonstration of 93% efficacy of two doses of PRP-OMP conjugate vaccine in a randomized trial, and 100% efficacy of three doses of Hib oligosaccharide conjugate (HbOC) in a quasi-randomized trial.[104–106] A postlicensure case-control study reported protective efficacies of 71%, 89%, and 94% after one, two, and three doses, respectively, of HbOC.[107] Although U.S. controlled trials of a third vaccine (PRP-T) were terminated after the licensure of other Hib conjugate vaccines for use in infancy, no cases of invasive Hib disease were reported among more than 6,200 vaccine recipients at the time of termination,[108] and protective efficacy has been reported from a British trial in which infants were given this vaccine at 2, 3, and 4 months,[109] and from a Finnish immunization program using historical controls.[110] A combined DTP-HbOC vaccine and use of PRP-T vaccine reconstituted with DTP (from a single manufacturer) have been licensed based on immunogenicity similar to that of the individual vaccines, although no clinical efficacy information is available.[111,112] These combined vaccines allow a reduced number of injections when both vaccines are indicated. Other combination vaccines are currently being evaluated.[113] Declines in antibody levels occur with all vaccines after administration of the primary series, but booster vaccination at ≥12 months of age elicits a good antibody response.[114–116] Surveillance in a number of different populations indicates a 55–95% decline in the incidence of Hib disease with widespread use of Hib conjugate vaccines.[6,117–122] A substantial decline in the incidence of Hib disease among unvaccinated children[120] and in persons ≥5 years[6] may be due to reduced carriage and transmission of the bacteria from vaccinated children.[123,124] In randomized controlled trials, serial combinations of different vaccines (PRP-OMP, HbOC, or PRP-T) were as safe and at least as immunogenic as single conjugate vaccine series, supporting the interchangeability of these vaccines.[125–127] Adverse effects of the Hib vaccine are generally mild (local tenderness, redness and swelling, irritability, fever, malaise, etc.).[128]

Hepatitis B Vaccine. In the U.S., infants born to hepatitis B surface antigen-positive (HBsAg+) mothers are at high risk of becoming infected with HBV, but most other infants have little risk of infection before adolescence. Controlled trials,[129–135a] cohort studies,[136,137] and a time series study,[138] have demonstrated that hepatitis B vaccine given alone to infants of HBsAg+ mothers is 62–92% effective (depending on dosage, interval, vaccine, and maternal antigen status) in preventing the development of the HBV chronic carrier state during the first 1–5 years of life. The protective efficacy of vaccine combined with hepatitis B immune globulin (HBIG) is somewhat higher (85–95%) than for vaccine alone in these infants (see Chapter 24).

Because universal vaccination of low-risk infants has only been introduced recently in the U.S., its ability to protect these infants later in life must be inferred from studies in other populations. From controlled trials[139–141] and time series studies[142–147] conducted in populations where horizontal HBV transmission is common, universal vaccination of infants, children, and/or adolescents with a three- or four-dose regimen is estimated to be >84% effective in preventing HBV infection and >80% effective in preventing the development of chronic HBV carriage. Mass vaccination of children in New Zealand[142] and infants in Taiwan,[148] American Samoa,[149] and Alaska Native communities[150] has led to substantial reductions in acute HBV events and the prevalence of chronic infection in both vaccinated and unvaccinated populations. Controlled trials and time series indicate protection against HBV infection and chronic carriage lasting from 3 to as long as 11–12 years in vaccinated infants, children, and adolescents, despite declines in antibody levels.[130,142,143, 146,151–155] Breakthrough infections appear to be associated more with low initial antibody response than with declining antibody levels.[139,146,156] The recombinant vaccines currently in use in the U.S. induce antibody responses and short-term (up to 5 years) efficacy in children similar to those of the plasma-derived vaccine.[131,133,138,142,147,157–163] Mild reactions—including local soreness and induration, low-grade fever, irritability, and poor feeding—are reported by the parents of up to 13% of vaccinated children and 4–7%

of vaccinated infants.[161,162,164] There have been several case reports of nonfatal anaphylaxis from recombinant hepatitis B vaccine.[29]

Hepatitis A Vaccine. Inactivated hepatitis A vaccine, delivered in two doses 1 month apart, protected against hepatitis A for at least 1 year in a double-blind randomized controlled trial in more than 30,000 Thai children aged 1–16 years.[165] Protective efficacy was 94% at 12 months, and 100% at 17.5 months after a booster dose at 12 months. After the trial ended, all controls received two doses of the vaccine and were followed for an additional 10 months. The subsequent attack rate was 6 cases per 100,000, compared to 114 cases per 100,000 in this control group during the same interval while the trial was ongoing, and to 52–101 cases per 100,000 in historical controls. In a smaller U.S. trial of healthy children aged 2–16 years, a single dose of a different inactivated vaccine was 100% efficacious (lower bound 87%) in preventing hepatitis A at mean 103-day follow-up.[166] In other high-risk populations, seroconversion rates of 82–95% after one dose and 100% after two to three doses of inactivated hepatitis A vaccine have been reported in children ranging in age from 1 to 15 years.[167–169] Although the duration of clinical immunity has not been established, protective levels of antibody have been shown to persist at least four years after administration of three doses of vaccine.[170–173] Estimates derived from models of antibody decline after vaccination predict that protective levels of antibody could last for at least 20 years.[170] Vaccine efficacy is low in the first week after vaccination, rising to 77–90% at 2 weeks and 90–100% at 3–4 weeks.[166,174–176,179] To provide immediate protection for those at high risk of exposure (e.g., travelers to endemic areas), administration of immune globulin (IG) with the first vaccine dose may be necessary. Although several studies have reported lower mean antibody titers when the vaccine is administered concomitantly with IG, vaccine seroconversion rates appear to be comparable.[177,179] In direct comparisons with IG, traditionally used as preexposure prophylaxis against hepatitis A for high-risk persons such as international travelers (see Chapter 67), the vaccine led to higher and longer-lasting antibody titers.[178–184] The reported 94–100% protective efficacy of hepatitis A vaccine is higher than that reported for IG (80–90%) (see Chapter 67), but the clinical efficacies of the two interventions have not been directly compared in clinical trials.

Adverse effects of the vaccine, including mild local reactions (pain, tenderness, redness, and swelling) and minor systemic symptoms such as fever, headache, and malaise, occur in 10–30% of recipients, and are more common after the second and third doses.[165–167,169] Serious allergic reactions, without long-term consequences, have been reported rarely in temporal association with hepatitis A vaccination.[12]

Varicella Vaccine. The efficacy of a live attenuated Oka strain varicella-zoster vaccine was 98% in preventing chickenpox through two varicella seasons in a randomized, double-blind, placebo-controlled trial in healthy children and adolescents aged 1–14 years.[185,186] Other studies in children and adolescents have compared the attack rate after household or other close exposure to that of historical controls and estimated vaccine efficacy at 86–98%.[186–190] Breakthrough infections occur at a rate of about 1–2% per year, but illness is attenuated, with fewer lesions and a reduced incidence of fever compared to natural infections.[186,191,192] Protective efficacy and antibody levels have been shown to persist for at least 7–10 years.[186,193] In a 17–20-year follow-up study, only 2 of 96 adults who received vaccine in childhood (age 10 months to 13 years) developed breakthrough infections (both mild cases), despite 100 documented episodes of contact with persons infected with VZV.[194] Antibody levels were higher than those observed 10 years earlier. It is unclear what effect immune boosting caused by reinfection with wild-type VZV had on the level or duration of protection against disease.

The vaccine has been less well studied in older adolescents and adults than in children. Adolescents ≥13 years and adults have a poorer immune response to the varicella vaccine, and two doses are required to achieve optimal seroconversion rates.[187,190,195] A hospital and household exposure study, conducted in health care workers and parents of young children, reported a protective efficacy of only 50%, but all breakthrough infections were mild.[196]

Adverse effects of the vaccine have included injection site reactions and, less commonly, varicella-like rashes and fever.[185,187,190] Experience with substantially greater numbers of vaccine recipients would be required to rule out rare, serious adverse reactions. Mild herpes zoster has been reported in several healthy children after varicella vaccine, but it appears to occur at a reduced rate compared to that associated with natural varicella,[197] as has been demonstrated for vaccinated children with leukemia.[198,199] Herpes zoster has been reported in one adult recipient of the vaccine.[200] The most important potential adverse consequence of universal preschool varicella vaccination is a shift of the age distribution of cases into adulthood, when the disease is more severe.[14,17] Such a shift would occur if immunity from childhood vaccination wanes in adulthood, or if a large number of older children enter adolescence and adulthood without having been vaccinated and without having acquired natural immunity to VZV because of reduced circulation of wild virus. An age-structured theoretical transmission model suggests, however, that over a plausible range of values for vaccine efficacy, duration of immunity, and levels of coverage, routine immunization of preschool children would greatly reduce the number of primary varicella cases and would therefore reduce overall morbidity (as measured by hospitalizations) despite a shift in the age distribution of cases.[201] This model also suggests that "catch-up" immunization of 12-year-olds for the first 11 years of the vaccination program would reduce the likelihood that a large pool of susceptible adolescents and adults would be created by universal preschool vaccination.

Recommendations of Other Groups

Recommendations on the administration of childhood vaccines are issued regularly by the Advisory Committee on Immunization Practices (ACIP),[202,203] the American Academy of Pediatrics (AAP),[13] and the American Academy of Family Physicians (AAFP).[204] These three groups, working with federal agencies, have approved a unified childhood immunization schedule.[205] The recommendations for the vaccines in the synthesized schedule are generally similar to those recommended by the Task Force (see *Clinical Intervention*), except: giving a second dose of MMR at either age 4–6 or 11–12 years is considered equally acceptable in this schedule, whereas the Task Force recommends 4–6 years as the preferred age (see Discussion); and routine hepatitis B vaccine was recommended only in infancy in the unified schedule, whereas the Task Force also recommends its routine use in all children and adolescents not previously immunized. ACIP and AAP have subsequently revised their recommendations for hepatitis B vaccine to include all children aged 11–12 years who have not previously been vaccinated; ACIP also recommends vaccinating unimmunized children under 11 years who are Pacific Islanders or who reside in households of first-generation immigrants from countries with high or intermediate HBV endemicity.[206,216] ACIP and AAP recommend one dose of varicella vaccine for all healthy children age 12 months to the 13th birthday who have not been previously immunized and who lack a reliable history of varicella, with a target age of 12–18 months for routine vaccination; two doses of vaccine 4–8 weeks apart are recommended for susceptible adolescents aged ≥13 years.[207,207a] AAP recommends optional serologic testing in healthy adolescents older than 18 years who lack a history of varicella.[207] Recommendations for the use of varicella vaccine are being developed by AAFP and other organizations. The Food and Drug Administration has approved inactivated hepatitis A vaccine for use in selected groups including travelers, military personnel, and laboratory workers.[208] Recommendations for the use of hepatitis A vaccine in children are being developed by ACIP, AAP, AAFP, and other groups. ACIP has issued recommendations for the use of inactivated hepatitis A vaccine for susceptible persons aged ≥2 years traveling to or working in countries with intermediate or high HAV endemicity.[208a]

Discussion

All of the vaccines licensed for routine use in children have been proved efficacious in controlled studies or multiple time series. Those that have been in widespread use for some years (diphtheria, pertussis, tetanus, polio, measles, mumps, rubella, Hib) have already demonstrated a dramatic effect on the incidence of childhood disease. In the case of polio, more than a decade has passed since the last documented transmission of wild poliovirus in the U.S., and more recently poliomyelitis has been eradicated in the entire Western hemisphere.[209] Global eradication efforts are now concentrated on interrupting transmission in Asia and sub-Saharan Africa. All cases of endemic paralytic poliomyelitis in the U.S. are now caused by vaccine-strain poliovirus infections, indicating that there may be a benefit from replacing OPV with enhanced-potency IPV. The use of combination vaccines that include IPV may reduce the costs and adverse effects associated with adding another injection to the infant vaccine schedule. Such combination vaccines are not yet available in the U.S.

Whether universal hepatitis B and varicella vaccination will lead to benefits similar to those attributable to previously approved vaccines is unknown. Their appropriateness for routine use in healthy children is a policy decision that must take into account other issues in addition to vaccine efficacy, including cost-effectiveness, available resources, and competing priorities. Routine infant vaccination against hepatitis B in the U.S. has been recommended primarily as a way to prevent HBV infection in adolescents and adults, but this benefit has not yet been documented. Universal vaccination in early adolescence (e.g., age 11–12) would be effective in preventing adolescent HBV infection, but it would not prevent transmission in early childhood, when the risk of developing chronic carriage is highest and which continued to occur in the U.S. despite selective vaccination of infants born to HBsAg+ mothers. One cost-effectiveness analysis reported an incremental cost of universal newborn vaccination relative to screening pregnant women and selective vaccination of high-risk newborns to be $30,347 per discounted life-year gained, which is comparable to that of other health care strategies commonly used in North America, such as treatment for mild hypertension.[210] Another cost-effectiveness analysis[211] reported that screening all pregnant women and giving vaccine plus HBIG to neonates of HBsAg+ mothers (as currently recommended in Chapter 24), combined with universal vaccination of children at age 10 with a booster at age 20, was more cost-effective than universal vaccination of newborns (with boosters at age 10 and 20) or universal vaccination of adolescents at age 10 (with a booster at age 20) without screening in pregnancy. This analysis did not account, however, for the consequences of horizontal transmission and consequent chronic infection during childhood. A cost-effectiveness analysis has evaluated prevaccination testing for hepatitis B in adolescents or preadolescents; this strategy was not effective in terms of cost or rate of completed vaccination unless the seroprevalence of antibodies to HBsAg was at least 40% (also see Chapter 24).[211a]

For varicella vaccine, there are few data regarding protective efficacy beyond about 10 years after vaccination. The likely change in VZV epidemiology as a result of universal childhood immunization, i.e., that chickenpox would occur primarily in adulthood when it tends to be more severe, remains an important concern. While the previously cited model[201] found that the overall effect of universal preschool vaccination would be beneficial, longer experience will be necessary to demonstrate this. Cost effectiveness analysis suggests that routine vaccination for preschool-age children results in cost savings when the analysis includes both direct medical costs and indirect costs (i.e., current work-loss of parents and of infected adults, and future work-loss of those who die or who are permanently disabled from encephalitis).[212] Vaccination before age 13 is preferable because two doses 4–8 weeks apart are required to achieve optimal seroconversion rates when the vaccine is given after age 12. The use of combined vaccines (e.g., MMRV,[213,214] which is not currently available in the U.S.) would reduce the number of injections needed, reducing the adverse effects associated with multiple needlesticks and potentially reducing costs. Vaccinating all adolescents and adults with a negative or uncertain history of chickenpox is likely to be more effective in preventing chickenpox than serologic testing followed by immunization of test-negative adolescents and adults, because with the latter strategy, loss to follow-up and false-positive test results will reduce the proportion protected. Serologic testing prior to vaccination may be more cost-effective, however, because many adolescents and most adults with negative or uncertain histories of chickenpox are in fact immune, and because the need for two doses to be given at two separate visits increases the costs of vaccination.[215]

Recommendations have been made to give a second MMR dose at either 4–6 years or 11–12 years.[205] Giving the second dose at 4–6 years has two apparent advantages: primary immunization failures are corrected sooner and the health care and school systems are poised to capture the most individuals for immunization at the time of school entry. The advantage of a dose at 11–12 years is that it should have a more immediate impact on outbreaks involving middle, junior high, and high schools, and colleges. Studies directly comparing different two-dose schedules are under way. The weight of the currently available evidence would not appear to favor delaying the second dose into late childhood with the intent of preventing secondary immunization failure. Efforts should be made, however, to vaccinate all children aged 11–12 years who have not previously received a second dose of MMR.

CLINICAL INTERVENTION

All children without established contraindications should receive diphtheria-tetanus-pertussis (DTP), oral poliovirus (OPV), measles-mumps-rubella

(MMR), conjugate *H. influenzae* type b (Hib), hepatitis B, and varicella vaccines ("A" recommendation).

The recommended childhood immunization schedule includes *DTP vaccine* at ages 2 months, 4 months, and 6 months; DTP at 12–18 months or DTaP at 15–18 months; and DTP or DTaP between ages 4 and 6 years, just prior to school entry. A combined tetanus-diphtheria (Td) booster should be administered at age 11–12 years (14–16 years is an acceptable alternative) and periodically in adulthood (see Chapter 66). *OPV vaccine* is recommended at ages 2 months, 4 months, 6–18 months, and 4–6 years.

MMR vaccine should be administered at age 12–15 months and again at 4–6 years of age; 11–12 years is an acceptable alternative for the second dose. Giving the first dose at 15 months may be preferable when compliance with a visit at this age is assured, because efficacy and immunogenicity are slightly higher than at 12 months. Children over 6 years of age who present for care and have not yet received two doses of measles vaccine should be vaccinated with MMR, with the goal that all children will have had two doses of measles or MMR vaccine by 11–12 years of age.

Hib conjugate vaccine should be given at 2, 4, and 6 months (HbOC or PRP-T) or 2 and 4 months (PRP-OMP), with a booster dose at 12–15 months of age using any of the conjugate vaccines. While giving a single conjugate Hib vaccine for the primary series is preferred because of proven clinical efficacy, there is good evidence for the safety and immunogenicity of heterogenous Hib conjugate vaccine series. Therefore, immunization at the recommended intervals (2, 4, 6, and 12–15 months) should not be delayed by efforts to determine the type of vaccine previously received. When this information is unavailable, any of the conjugate vaccines approved for use in infants may be given to complete the series. Licensed combined vaccines (e.g., DTP-HbOC [Tetrammune®]*) may be substituted for the relevant individual vaccines in cases where both vaccines would normally be given in order to reduce the total number of injections given.

Hepatitis B vaccine is recommended for all infants, and for all children and adolescents not previously immunized, particularly those in high-risk populations (see Chapters 24 and 66). For infants, the first dose is recommended at 0–2 months (preferably prior to hospital discharge), the second dose 1–2 months after the first, and the third dose at 6–18 months (preferably at least 4 months after the second dose). Giving hepatitis B vaccine at 0, 1, 2, and 12 months of age is also acceptable. After infancy, the vaccine schedule is at the current visit and 1 and 6 months latter. Clinicians may wish to inform parents that booster doses may be required in the future to maintain immunity through adolescence and adulthood.

---

*Use of trade names is for identification only and does not imply endorsement by the Public Health Service or the U.S. Department of Health and Human Services.

Varicella vaccine, administered subcutaneously in one 0.5-mL dose, is recommended for routine use in healthy children 12–18 months of age, and in children under age 13 with no reliable history of varicella infection or previous immunization. Clinicians should inform parents that varicella disease in adulthood is associated with increased risk of serious complications, the duration of immunity provided by varicella vaccine has not been established, and booster doses of the vaccine may be required to maintain protection throughout adulthood. Two doses of vaccine delivered 4–8 weeks apart are recommended for healthy adolescents ≥13 years of age with no reliable history of varicella infection or previous vaccination. Given the relatively high prevalence of immunity in adolescents with no history of chickenpox and the results of cost-effectiveness analysis, clinicians may wish to offer serologic testing for varicella susceptibility to history-negative adolescents ≥13 years who are likely to comply with return visits.

Clinicians may wish to conduct an assessment of immunization status for all children at age 11–12, in particular to determine whether the patient needs Td, MMR, varicella, or hepatitis B vaccines. Clinicians are referred to published guidelines for details on vaccine contraindications, instructions for immunizing children with medical disorders (including human immunodeficiency virus infection), and modified protocols recommended during community outbreaks or epidemics or for children with delayed immunization.[13,202]

Hepatitis A vaccine is recommended for all high-risk children aged ≥2 years and all high-risk adolescents ("A" recommendation). High-risk groups include persons living in, traveling to, or working in areas where the disease is endemic and periodic outbreaks occur (e.g., countries with high or intermediate endemicity, Alaska Native, Pacific Islander, and Native American communities, certain religious communities) (see Chapter 66 for additional high-risk groups and recommendations for adult immunization). Hepatitis A vaccination may also be considered for institutionalized persons (e.g., those living in chronic care facilities). Where tracking or identification of high-risk patients is not practical or cost-effective, universal vaccination may be a reasonable policy given the minimal adverse consequences of the vaccine. At this writing, the only licensed hepatitis A vaccine is Havrix® (SmithKline Beecham Pharmaceuticals).* Three doses (360 ELISA units/dose), administered intramuscularly, are recommended for persons aged 2–18 years; the second and third doses are given 1 and 6–12 months after the first dose. The need for periodic booster doses has not been established. For persons requiring immediate protection against hepatitis A (e.g., travelers to high-risk areas who have not previously been vaccinated), IG (0.02 mL/kg) should be given simultaneously with the first

---

*Use of trade names is for identification only and does not imply endorsement by the Public Health Service or the U.S. Department of Health and Human Services.

dose of hepatitis A vaccine, although the clinical efficacy of this approach has not been established. IG can also be recommended as an efficacious intervention for short-term ($\leq$5–6 months) preexposure prophylaxis against hepatitis A (see Chapter 67). While some evidence suggests that the vaccine may be more efficacious than IG, the clinical efficacies of the two regimens have not been directly compared in clinical trials. Other factors to consider in choosing between the two interventions are patient preference, the likely frequency and duration of exposure, the need for immediate protection, and cost.

Annual *influenza vaccine* is recommended for adolescents and children $\geq$6 months of age who are residents of chronic care facilities or have chronic cardiopulmonary disorders, metabolic diseases (including diabetes mellitus), hemoglobinopathies, immunosuppression, or renal dysfunction ("B" recommendation) (see Chapter 66 for the review of evidence regarding influenza vaccine). Split-virus vaccine is recommended for children $\leq$12 years; the recommended vaccine dose is 0.25 mL for children 6–35 months of age and 0.5 mL for children $\geq$3 years of age.[13] Amantadine and rimantadine prophylaxis against influenza A is discussed in Chapter 66.

Pneumococcal vaccine is recommended for immunocompetent adolescents and children ($\geq$2 years of age) with chronic cardiac or pulmonary disease, diabetes mellitus, and anatomic asplenia (excluding sickle cell disease), and those living in special environments or social settings with an identified increased risk of pneumococcal disease (e.g., certain Native American and Alaska Native populations) ("B" recommendation) (see Chapter 66 for the review of evidence regarding pneumococcal vaccine). Routine revaccination is not recommended, but it may be appropriate to consider periodic revaccination in immunocompetent individuals at highest risk for morbidity and mortality from pneumococcal disease (e.g., those with severe chronic disease) who were vaccinated more than 5 years previously. There is insufficient evidence to recommend for or against pneumococcal vaccine as an efficacious vaccine for immunocompromised children $\geq$2 years of age, but recommendations for vaccinating these persons may be made on other grounds, including high incidence and mortality rates of pneumococcal disease and minimal adverse effects from vaccine ("C" recommendation). Examples of immunocompromised conditions associated with high risk for pneumococcal disease include acquired or congenital immunodeficiency (including HIV infection), sickle cell disease, nephrotic syndrome, chronic renal failure, metastatic or hematologic malignancy, and other conditions associated with immunosuppression, such as organ transplant. It may be appropriate to consider periodic revaccination in these patients, who are likely to have poor initial antibody response and rapid decline of antibodies after vaccination.

See Chapter 25 (screening for tuberculous infection) for recommendations regarding the BCG vaccine. Recommendations on postexposure prophylaxis against selected infectious diseases, including tetanus, hepatitis A, hepatitis B, and Hib, are given in Chapter 67.

The draft update of this chapter was prepared for the U.S. Preventive Services Task Force by Carolyn DiGuiseppi, MD, MPH, based in part on background papers on measles and Hib vaccines prepared by Modena Wilson, MD, MPH, and Donald Robinson, MD, MPH.

REFERENCES

1. Centers for Disease Control and Prevention. Reported vaccine-preventable disease—United States, 1993, and the Childhood Immunization Initiative. MMWR 1994;43:57–60.
2. Centers for Disease Control and Prevention. Summary of notifiable diseases, United States, 1993. MMWR 1994;42:1–73.
2a. Centers for Disease Control and Prevention. Final 1994 reports of notifiable diseases. MMWR 1995;44:537–543.
3. Langmuir AD. Inactivated virus vaccines: protective efficacy. In: International Poliomyelitis Congress. Poliomyelitis. Philadelphia: JB Lippincott, 1961:240–256.
4. Davis SF, Strebel PM, Cochi SL, et al. Pertussis surveillance—United States, 1989–1991. MMWR 1992;41(SS-8):11–19.
4a. Centers for Disease Control and Prevention. Pertussis—United States, January 1992–June 1995. MMWR 1995;44:525–529.
5. Cochi SL, Broome CV, Hightower AW. Immunization of children with *Haemophilus influenzae* type b vaccine: a cost-effectiveness model of strategy assessment. JAMA 1985;253:521–529.
6. Centers for Disease Control and Prevention. Progress toward elimination of *Haemophilus influenzae* type b disease among infants and children—United States, 1987–1993. MMWR 1994;43:144–148.
6a. Centers for Disease Control and Prevention. Progress toward elimination of *Haemophilus influenzae* type b disease among infants and children—United States, 1993–1994. MMWR 1995;44:545–550.
7. Margolis HS, Alter MJ, Hadler SC. Hepatitis B: evolving epidemiology and implications for control. Semin Liver Dis 1991;11:84–92.
8. Edmunds WJ, Medley GF, Nokes DJ, et al. The influence of age on the development of the hepatitis B carrier states. Proc R Soc Lond 1993;253:197–201.
9. Advisory Committee on Immunization Practices (ACIP). Protection against viral hepatitis. MMWR 1990;39:1–26.
10. Sakuma K, Takhara T, Okuda K, et al. Prognosis of hepatitis B virus surface antigen carriers in relation to routine liver function tests: a prospective study. Gastroenterology 1982;83:114–117.
11. Lo KJ, Tong MJ, Chien MC, et al. The natural course of hepatitis B surface antigen-positive chronic active hepatitis in Taiwan. J Infect Dis 1982;146:205–210.
12. Steffen R, Kane MA, Shapiro CN, et al. Epidemiology and prevention of hepatitis A in travelers. JAMA 1994;272:885–889.
13. American Academy of Pediatrics. 1994 Red Book: report of the Committee on Infectious Diseases. 23rd ed. Elk Grove Village, IL: American Academy of Pediatrics, 1994.
14. Preblud SR. Varicella: complications and costs. Pediatrics 1986;78(suppl):728–735.
15. National Center for Health Statistics. Annual summary of births, marriages, divorces, and deaths: United States, 1993. Monthly vital statistics report; vol 42, no 13. Hyattsville, MD: Public Health Service, 1994.
16. Kelly PW, Petruccelli BP, Stehr-Green P, et al. The susceptibility of young adult Americans to vaccine-preventable infections: a national serosurvey of US Army recruits. JAMA 1991;266:2724–2729.
17. Guess HA, Broughton DD, Melton LJ III, et al. Chickenpox hospitalizations among residents of Olmsted County, Minnesota, 1962 through 1981. Am J Dis Child 1984;138:1055–1057.
18. Sullivan-Bolyai JZ, Yin EK, Cox P, et al. Impact of chickenpox on households of healthy children. Pediatr Infect Dis J 1987;6:33–35.
19. Jackson MA, Burry VF, Olson LC. Complications of varicella requiring hospitalization in previously healthy children. Pediatr Infect Dis J 1992;11:441–445.

20. Fleisher G, Henry W, McSorley M, et al. Life-threatening complications of varicella. Am J Dis Child 1981;135:896–899.
21. Edsall G. Specific prophylaxis of tetanus. JAMA 1959;171:417–427.
22. Onorato IM, Wassilak SG, Meade B. Efficacy of whole-cell pertussis vaccine in preschool children in the United States. JAMA 1992;267:2745–2749.
23. Fine PEM, Clarkson JA. Reflections on the efficacy of pertussis vaccines. Rev Infect Dis 1987;9:866–883.
24. Centers for Disease Control. Diphtheria, tetanus, and pertussis: recommendations for vaccine use and other preventive measures: recommendations of the Immunization Practices Advisory Committee (ACIP). MMWR 1991;40(RR-10):1–28.
25. Mortimer EA, Jones PK. An evaluation of pertussis vaccine. Rev Infect Dis 1979;1:927–932.
26. Cody CL, Baraff LJ, Cherry JD, et al. Nature and rates of adverse reactions associated with DTP and DT immunizations in infants and children. Pediatrics 1981;68:650–660.
27. Reinstein L. Peripheral neuropathy after multiple tetanus toxoid boosters. Arch Phys Med Rehabil 1982;63:332–334.
28. Edsall G, Elliot MW, Peebles TG, et al. Excessive use of tetanus toxoid boosters. JAMA 1967;202:111–113.
29. Institute of Medicine. Adverse events associated with childhood vaccines: evidence bearing on causality. Washington, DC: National Academy Press, 1994.
30. Hinman AR, Koplan JP. Pertussis and pertussis vaccine: reanalysis of benefits, risks, and costs. JAMA 1984;251:3109–3113.
31. Hinman AR, Koplan JP. Pertussis and pertussis vaccine: further analysis of benefits, risks and costs. Dev Biol Stand 1985;61:429–437.
32. Miller DL, Alderslade R, Ross EM. Whooping cough and whooping cough vaccine: the risks and benefits debate. Epidemiol Rev 1982;4:1–24.
33. Institute of Medicine. Adverse effects of pertussis and rubella vaccines. Washington, DC: National Academy Press, 1991.
34. Stetler HC, Orenstein WA, Bart KJ, et al. History of convulsions and use of pertussis vaccine. J Pediatr 1985;107:175–179.
35. Livengood JR, Mullen JR, White JW, et al. Family history of convulsions and use of pertussis vaccine. J Pediatr 1989;115:527–531.
36. Baraff LJ, Shields WD, Beckwith L, et al. Infants and children with convulsions and hypotonic-hyporesponsive episodes following diphtheria-tetanus-pertussis immunization: follow-up evaluation. Pediatrics 1988;81:789–794.
37. Centers for Disease Control. Adverse events following immunization. MMWR 1985;34:43–47.
38. Miller D, Wadsworth J, Diamond J, et al. Pertussis vaccine and whooping cough as risk factors in acute neurological illness and death in young children. Dev Biol Stand 1985;61:389–394.
39. Miller D, Madge N, Diamond J, et al. Pertussis immunisation and serious acute neurological illnesses in children. BMJ 1993;307:1171–1176.
40. Institute of Medicine. DPT vaccine and chronic nervous system dysfunction: a new analysis. Washington, DC: National Academy Press, 1994.
41. Shapiro ED. Pertussis vaccines: seeking a better mousetrap [editorial]. JAMA 1992;267:2788–2790.
42. Morgan CM, Blumberg DA, Cherry JD, et al. Comparison of acellular and whole-cell pertussis-component DTP vaccines: a multicenter double-blind study in 4- to 6-year-old children. Am J Dis Child 1990;144:41–45.
43. Blumberg DA, Mink CM, Cherry JD, et al. Comparison of an acellular pertussis-component diphtheria-tetanus-pertussis (DTP) vaccine with a whole-cell pertussis-component DTP vaccine in 17- to 24-month-old children, with measurement of 69-kilodalton outer membrane protein antibody. J Pediatr 1990;117:46–51.
44. Blumberg DA, Mink CM, Cherry JK, et al. Comparison of acellular and whole-cell pertussis-component diphtheria-tetanus-pertussis vaccines in infants. J Pediatr 1991;119:194–204.
45. Englund JA, Decker MD, Edwards KM, et al. Acellular and whole-cell pertussis vaccines as booster doses: a multicenter study. Pediatrics 1994;93:37–43.
46. Bernstein HH, Rothstein EP, Pichichero ME, et al. Clinical reactions and immunogenicity of the BIKEN acellular diphtheria and tetanus toxoids and pertussis vaccine in 4- through 6-year-old US children. Am J Dis Child 1992;146:556–559.
47. Bernstein HH, Rothstein EP, Pennridge Pediatric Association, et al. Comparison of a three-component acellular pertussis vaccine with a whole-cell pertussis vaccine in 15- through 20-month-old infants. Pediatrics 1994;93:656–659.

48. Blennow M, Granstrom M, Jatmaa E, et al. Primary immunization of infants with an acellular pertussis vaccine in a double-blind randomized clinical trial. Pediatrics 1988;82:293–299.

49. Ad Hoc Group for the Study of Pertussis Vaccines. Placebo-controlled trial of two acellular pertussis vaccines in Sweden—protective efficacy and adverse events. Lancet 1988;1:955–960.

50. Storsaeter J, Hallander H, Farrington CP, et al. Secondary analyses of the efficacy of two acellular pertussis vaccines in a Swedish phase III trial. Vaccine 1990;8:457–461.

51. Blackwelder WC, Storsaeter J, Olin P, et al. Acellular pertussis vaccine: efficacy and evaluation of clinical case definitions. Am J Dis Child 1991;145:1285–1289.

52. Olin P, Storsaeter J. The efficacy of acellular pertussis vaccine [letter]. JAMA 1989;261:560.

53. Aoyama T, Murase Y, Kato M, et al. Efficacy and immunogenicity of acellular pertussis vaccine by manufacturer and patient age. Am J Dis Child 1989;143:655–659.

54. Kato T, Goshima T, Nakajima N, et al. Protection against pertussis by acellular pertussis vaccines (Takeda, Japan): household contact studies in Kawasaki City, Japan. Acta Paediatr Jpn 1989;31:698–701.

55. Mortimer EA, Kimura M, Cherry JD, et al. Protective efficacy of the Takeda acellular pertussis vaccine combined with diphtheria and tetanus toxoids following household exposure of Japanese children. Am J Dis Child 1990;144:899–904.

55a. Isomura S. Clinical studies on efficacy and safety of an acellular pertussis vaccine in Aichi Prefecture, Japan. Dev Biol Stand 1991;73:37–42.

56. Aoyama T, Iwata T, Iwai H, et al. Efficacy of acellular pertussis vaccine in young infants. J Infect Dis 1993;167:483–486.

57. Kimura M, Kuno-Sakai H, Sato Y, et al. A comparative trial of the reactogenicity and immunogenicity of Takeda acellular pertussis vaccine combined with tetanus and diphtheria toxoids: outcome in 3- to 8-month-old infants, 9- to 23-month-old infants and children, and 24- to 30-month-old children. Am J Dis Child 1991;145:734–741.

58. Centers for Disease Control. Pertussis vaccination: acellular pertussis vaccine for reinforcing and booster use—supplementary ACIP statement. Recommendations of the Immunization Practices Advisory Committee (ACIP). MMWR 1992;41(RR-1):1–10.

59. Centers for Disease Control. Pertussis vaccination: acellular pertussis vaccine for the fourth and fifth doses of the DTP series; update to supplementary ACIP statement. Recommendations of the Advisory Committee on Immunization Practices (ACIP). MMWR 1992;41(RR-15):1–5.

60. Prevots DR, Sutter RW, Strebel PM, et al. Completeness of reporting for paralytic poliomyelitis, United States, 1980 through 1991. Arch Pediatr Adolesc Med 1994;148:479–485.

61. McBean AM, Thomas MI, Johnson RH, et al. A comparison of the serological responses to oral and injectable trivalent poliovirus vaccine. Rev Infect Dis 1984;6:S552–S555.

62. Centers for Disease Control. Poliomyelitis prevention: enhanced-potency inactivated poliomyelitis vaccine—supplementary statement. MMWR 1987;36:795–798.

63. Institute of Medicine. An evaluation of poliomyelitis vaccine policy options. Washington, DC: National Academy Press, 1988.

64. Hinman AR, Koplan JP, Orenstein WA, et al. Live or inactivated poliomyelitis vaccine: an analysis of benefits and risks. Am J Public Health 1988;78:291–295.

65. Rantala H, Cherry JD, Shields WD, et al. Epidemiology of Guillain-Barré syndrome in children: relationship of oral polio vaccine administration to occurrence. J Pediatr 1994;124:220–223.

66. Dagan R, Botujansky C, Watemberg N, et al. Safety and immunogenicity in young infants of Haemophilus b-tetanus protein conjugate vaccine, mixed in the same syringe with diphtheria-tetanus-pertussis-enhanced inactivated poliovirus vaccine. Pediatr Infect Dis J 1994;13:356–361.

67. Gold R, Scheifele D, Barreto L, et al. Safety and immunogenicity of Haemophilus influenzae vaccine (tetanus toxoid conjugate) administered concurrently or combined with diphtheria and tetanus toxoids, pertussis vaccine and inactivated poliomyelitis vaccine to healthy infants at two, four and six months of age. Pediatr Infect Dis J 1994;13:348–355.

68. Centers for Disease Control. Measles prevention. MMWR 1987;36:409–418, 423–425.

69. Fescharek R, Quast U, Maass G, et al. Measles-mumps vaccination in the FRG: an empirical analysis after 14 years of use. II. Tolerability and analysis of spontaneously reported side effects. Vaccine 1990;8:446–456.

70. Peltola H, Heinonen OP, Valle M, et al. The elimination of indigenous measles, mumps, and rubella from Finland by a 12-year, two-dose vaccination program. N Engl J Med 1994;331:1397–1402.

71. Gindler JS, Atkinson WL, Markowitz LE, et al. Epidemiology of measles in the United States in 1989 and 1990. Pediatr Infect Dis 1992;11:841–846.

72. Centers for Disease Control and Prevention. Measles—United States, first 26 weeks, 1993. MMWR 1993;42:813–816.

72a. Centers for Disease Control and Prevention. Measles—United States, 1994. MMWR 1995;44:486–487, 493–494.

73. Markowitz LE, Orenstein WA. Measles vaccine. Pediatr Clin North Am 1990;37:603–625.

74. Fescharek R, Quast U, Maass G, et al. Measles-mumps vaccination in the FRG: an empirical analysis after 14 years of use. I. Efficacy and analysis of vaccine failures. Vaccine 1990;8:333–336.

75. Orenstein WA, Markowitz LE, Preblud SR, et al. The appropriate age for measles vaccination in the United States. Dev Biol Stand 1986;65:13–21.

76. Lennon JL, Black FL. Maternally-derived measles immunity in sera of vaccine-protected mothers. J Pediatr 1986;108:671–676.

77. Yeager AS, Harvey B, Crosson FJ, et al. Need for measles revaccination in adolescents: correlation with birth date prior to 1972. J Pediatr 1983;102:191–194.

78. Johnson CE, Nalin DR, Chui LW, et al. Measles vaccine immunogenicity in 6- versus 15-month-old infants born to mothers in the measles vaccine era. Pediatrics 1994;93:939–944.

79. Makino S, Sasaki K, Nakayama T, et al. A new combined trivalent live measles (AIK-C strain), mumps (Hoshino strain), and rubella (Takahashi strain) vaccine. Am J Dis Child 1990;144:905–910.

80. Kakakios AM, Burgess MA, Bransby RD, et al. Optimal age for measles and mumps vaccination in Australia. Med J Aust 1990;152:472–474.

81. Robertson CM, Bennett VJ, Jefferson N, et al. Serological evaluation of a measles, mumps, and rubella vaccine. Arch Dis Child 1988;63:612–616.

82. Yuan L. Measles outbreak in 31 schools: risk factors for vaccine failure and evaluation of a selective revaccination strategy. Can Med Assoc J 1994;150:1093–1098.

83. Orenstein WA, Albrecht P, Herrmann KL, et al. The plaque-neutralization test as a measure of prior exposure to measles virus. J Infect Dis 1987;155:146–149.

84. Crawford GE, Gremillion DH. Epidemic measles and rubella in air force recruits: impact of immunization. J Infect Dis 1981;144:403–410.

85. Krugman S, Giles JP, Friedman H, et al. Studies on immunity to measles. J Pediatr 1965;66:471–488.

86. Krugman S. Further-attenuated measles vaccine: characteristics and use. Rev Infect Dis 1983;5:477–481.

87. Mathias RG, Meekison WG, Arcand TA, et al. The role of secondary vaccine failures in measles outbreaks. Am J Public Health 1989;79:475–478.

88. Davis RM, Whitman ED, Orenstein WA, et al. A persistent outbreak of measles despite appropriate prevention and control measures. Am J Epidemiol 1987;126:438–449.

89. Hutchins SS, Markowitz LE, Mead P, et al. A school-based measles outbreak: The effect of a selective revaccination policy and risk factors for vaccine failure. Am J Epidemiol 1990;132:157–168.

90. Nkowane BM, Bart SW, Orenstein WA, et al. Measles outbreak in a vaccinated school population: epidemiology, chains of transmission and the role of vaccine failures. Am J Public Health 1987;77:434–438.

91. Shasby DM, Shope TC, Downs H, et al. Epidemic measles in a highly vaccinated population. N Engl J Med 1977; 296:585–589.

92. Krugman S. Present status of measles and rubella immunization in the United States: a medical progress report. J Pediatr 1977;90:1–12.

93. Markowitz LE, Preblud SR, Fine PEM, Orenstein WA. Duration of live measles vaccine-induced immunity. Pediatr Infect Dis J 1990;9:101–110.

94. Dai B, Chen Z, Lui Q, et al. Duration of immunity following immunization with live measles vaccine: 15 years of observation in Zhejiang province, China. Bull WHO 1991;69:415–423.

95. Ramsay MEB, Moffatt D, O'Connor M. Measles vaccine: a 27-year follow-up. Epidemiol Infect 1994;409–412.

96. Chen RT, Goldbaum GM, Wassilak SGF, et al. An explosive point-source measles outbreak in a highly vaccinated population. Am J Epidemiol 1989;129:173–182.

97. Edmonson MB, Addiss DG, McPherson JT, et al. Mild measles and secondary vaccine failure during a sustained outbreak in a highly vaccinated population. JAMA 1990;263:2467–2471.

98. Markowitz LE, Preblud SR, Orenstein WA, et al. Patterns of transmission in measles outbreaks in the United States, 1985–1986. N Engl J Med 1989;320:75–81.

99. Hersh BS, Markowitz LE, Hoffman RE, et al. A measles outbreak at a college with a prematriculation immunization requirement. Am J Public Health 1991;81:360–364.

100. Peltola H, Kayhty H, Virtanen M, et al. Prevention of *Haemophilus influenzae* type b bacteremic infection with the capsular polysaccharide vaccine. N Engl J Med 1984;310:1561–1566.

101. Wenger JD, Pierce R, Deaver KA, et al. Efficacy of *Haemophilus influenzae* type b polysaccharide-diphtheria toxoid conjugate vaccine in US children aged 18–59 months. Lancet 1991;338:395–398.

102. Greenberg DP, Vadheim CM, Bordenave N, et al. Protective efficacy of *Haemophilus influenzae* type b polysaccharide and conjugate vaccines in children 18 months of age and older. JAMA 1991;265:987–992.

103. Loughlin AM, Marchant CD, Lett S, et al. Efficacy of *Haemophilus influenzae* type b vaccines in Massachusetts children 18–59 months of age. Pediatr Infect Dis J 1992;11:374–379.

104. Black SB, Shinefield HR, Fireman B, et al. Efficacy in infancy of oligosaccharide conjugate *Haemophilus influenzae* type b (HbOC) vaccine in a United States population of 61,080 children. Pediatr Infect Dis J 1991;10:97–104.

105. Black SB, Shinefield HR, Lampert D, et al. Safety and immunogenicity of oligosaccharide conjugate *Haemophilus influenza* type b (HbOC) vaccine in infancy. Pediatr Infect Dis J 1991;10:92–96.

106. Santosham M, Wolff M, Reid R, et al. The efficacy in Navajo infants of a conjugate vaccine consisting of *Haemophilus influenzae* type b polysaccharide and *Neisseria meningitides* outer-membrane protein complex. N Engl J Med 1991;324:1767–1772.

107. Vadheim CM, Greenberg DP, Eriksen E, et al. Protection provided by *Haemophilus influenzae* type b conjugate vaccines in Los Angeles County: a case-control study. Pediatr Infect Dis J 1994;13:274–280.

108. Vadheim CM, Greenberg DP, Partridge S, et al. Effectiveness and safety of an *Haemophilus influenzae* type b conjugate vaccine (PRP-T) in young infants. Pediatrics 1993;92:272–279.

109. Booy R, Moxon ER, Macfarlane JA, et al. Efficacy of *Haemophilus influenzae* type b conjugate vaccine in Oxford region. Lancet 1992;340:847.

110. Fritzell B, Plotkin S. Efficacy and safety of a *Haemophilus influenzae* type b capsular polysaccharide-tetanus protein conjugate vaccine. J Pediatr 1992;212:355–362.

111. Centers for Disease Control and Prevention. Food and Drug Administration approval of use of *Haemophilus influenzae* type b conjugate vaccine reconstituted with diphtheria-tetanus-pertussis vaccine for infants and children. MMWR 1993;42:964–965.

112. Paradiso PR, Hogerman DA, Madore DV, et al. Safety and immunogenicity of a combined diphtheria, tetanus, pertussis and *Haemophilus influenzae* type b vaccine in young infants. Pediatrics 1993; 827–832.

113. Centers for Disease Control and Prevention. Recommendations for use of *Haemophilus influenzae* b conjugate vaccines and a combined diphtheria, tetanus, pertussis, and *Haemophilus influenzae* b vaccine. Recommendations of the Advisory Committee on Immunization Practices (ACIP). MMWR 1993;42(RR-13):1–15.

114. Kayhty H, Eskola J, Peltola H, et al. High antibody response to booster doses of either *Haemophilus influenzae* capsular polysaccharide or conjugate vaccine after primary immunization with conjugate vaccines. J Infect Dis 1992;165(Suppl 1):S165–S166.

115. Decker MD, Edwards KM, Bradley R, et al. Responses of children to booster immunization with their primary conjugate *Haemophilus influenzae* type b vaccine or with polyribosylribitol phosphate conjugated with diphtheria toxoid. J Pediatr 1993;122:410–413.

116. Granoff DM, Holmes SJ, Osterholm MT, et al. Induction of immunologic memory in infants primed with *Haemophilus influenzae* type b conjugate vaccines. J Infect Dis 1993;168:663–671.

117. Black SB, Shinefield HR, and the Kaiser Permanente Pediatric Vaccine Study Group. Immunization with oligosaccharide conjugate *Haemophilus influenzae* type b (HbOC) vaccine on a large health maintenance organization population: extended follow-up and impact on *Haemophilus influenzae* disease epidemiology. Pediatr Infect Dis J 1992;11:610–613.

118. Adams WG, Deaver KA, Cochi SL, et al. Decline of childhood *Haemophilus influenzae* type b (Hib) disease in the Hib vaccine era. JAMA 1993;269:221–226.

119. Broadhurst LE, Erickson RL, Kelley PW. Decreases in invasive *Haemophilus influenzae* diseases in US army children, 1984 through 1991. JAMA 1993;269:227–231.

120. Murphy TV, White KE, Pastor P, et al. Declining incidence of *Haemophilus influenzae* type b disease since introduction of vaccination. JAMA 1993;269:246–248.

121. Vadheim CM, Greenberg DP, Eriksen E, et al. Eradication of *Haemophilus influenzae* type b disease in southern California. Kaiser-UCLA Vaccine Study Group. Arch Pediatr Adolesc Med 1994;148:51–56.

122. Loughlin AM, Marchant CD, Lett SM. The changing epidemiology of invasive bacterial infections in Massachusetts children, 1984 through 1991. Am J Public Health 1995;85:392–394.

123. Barbour ML, Mayon-White RT, Coles C, et al. The impact of conjugate vaccine on carriage of *Haemophilus influenzae* type b. J Infect Dis 1995;171:93–98.

124. Murphy TV, Pastor P, Medley F, et al. Decreased *Haemophilus* colonization in children vaccinated with *Haemophilus influenzae* type b conjugate vaccine. J Pediatr 1993;122:517–523.

125. Greenberg DP, Lieberman JM, Marcy SM, et al. Enhanced antibody responses in infants given different sequences of heterogeneous *Haemophilus influenzae* type b conjugate vaccines. J Pediatr 1995;126:206–211.

126. Daum RS, Milewski WM, Ballanco GA. Interchangeability of *H. influenzae* type B vaccines for the primary series ("mix and match")—a preliminary analysis [Abstract 976]. Pediatr Res 1993;33:166A.

127. Anderson EL, Decker MD, Englund JA, et al. Interchangeability of conjugated *Haemophilus influenzae* type b vaccines in infants. JAMA 1995;273:849–853.

128. Decker MD, Edwards KM, Bradley R, et al. Comparative trial in infants of four conjugate *Haemophilus influenzae* type b vaccines. J Pediatr 1992;120:184–189.

129. Ip HMH, Wong VCW, Lelie PN, et al. Hepatitis B infection in infants after neonatal immunization. Acta Paediatr Jpn 1989;31:654–658.

130. Zhu QR, Duan SC, Xu HF. A six-year survey of immunogenicity and efficacy of hepatitis B vaccine in infants born to HBsAg carriers. Chin Med J 1992;105:194–198.

131. Halliday ML, Kang LY, Rankin JG, et al. An efficacy trial of a mammalian cell-derived recombinant DNA hepatitis B vaccine in infants born to mothers positive for HBsAg, in Shanghai, China. Int J Epidemiol 1992;21:564–573.

132. Theppisai U, Thanuntaseth C, Chiewsilp P, et al. Long-term immunoprophylaxis of hepatitis B surface antigen carrier in infants born to hepatitis B surface antigen positive mothers using plasma derived vaccine. Asia-Oceania J Obstet Gynaecol 1989;15:111–115.

133. Assateerawatt A, Tanphaichitr VS, Suvatte V, et al. Immunogenicity and protective efficacy of low dose recombinant DNA hepatitis B vaccine in normal and high-risk neonates. Asian Pac J Allergy Immunol 1991;9:89–93.

134. Sehgal A, Gupta I, Sehgal R, et al. Hepatitis B vaccine alone or in combination with anti-HBS immunoglobulin in the perinatal prophylaxis of babies born to HBsAg carrier mothers. Acta Virol 1992;36:359–366.

135. Lo KJ, Tsai YT, Lee SD, et al. Immunoprophylaxis of infection with hepatitis B virus in infants born to hepatitis B surface antigen-positive carrier mothers. J Infect Dis 1985;152:817–822.

135a. Xu ZY, Duan SC, Margolis HS, et al. Long-term efficacy of active postexposure immunization of infants for prevention of hepatitis B virus infection. J Infect Dis 1995;171:54–60.

136. Hsu HM, Chen DS, Chuang CH, et al. Efficacy of a mass hepatitis B vaccination program in Taiwan. Studies on 3464 infants of hepatitis B surface antigen-carrier mothers. JAMA 1988;260:2231–2235.

137. Assateerawatt A, Tanphaichitr VS, Suvatte V, et al. Immunogenicity and efficacy of a recombinant DNA hepatitis B vaccine, GenHevac B Pasteur in high risk neonates, school children and healthy adults. Asian Pac J Allergy Immunol 1993;11:85–91.

138. Poovorawan Y, Sanpavat S, Pongpunlert W, et al. Protective efficacy of a recombinant DNA hepatitis B vaccine in neonates of HBe antigen-positive mothers. JAMA 1989;261:3278–3281.

139. Coursaget P, Yvonnet B, Chotard J, et al. Seven-year study of hepatitis B vaccine efficacy in infants from an endemic area (Senegal). Lancet 1986;1143–1145.

140. Sun ZT, Zhu Y, Stjernsward J, et al. Design and compliance of HBV vaccination trial on newborns to prevent hepatocellular carcinoma and 5-year results of its pilot study. Cancer Detect Prev 1991;15:313–318.

141. Hayashi J, Kashiwagi S, Nomura H, et al. The control of hepatitis B virus infection with vaccine in Japanese nursery schools. Am J Epidemiol 1987;126:474–479.

142. Milne A, Krugman S, Waldon JA, et al. Hepatitis B vaccination in children: five year booster study. NZ Med J 1992;105:336–338.

143. Whittle HC, Maine N, Pilkington J, et al. Long-term efficacy of continuing hepatitis B vaccination in infancy in two Gambian villages. Lancet 1995;345:1089–1092.

144. Fortuin M, Chotard J, Jack AD, et al. Efficacy of hepatitis B vaccine in the Gambian expanded programme on immunisation. Lancet 1993;341:1129–1131.

145. Craxi A, Vinci M, Almasio P, et al. Hepatitis B vaccination of relatives of hepatitis B virus DNA positive carriers: an experience with plasma-derived vaccine. Eur J Epidemiol 1989;5:65–69.

146. Wainwright RB, McMahon BJ, Bulkow LR, et al. Protection provided by hepatitis B vaccine in a Yupik Eskimo population. Arch Intern Med 1991;151:1634–1636.

147. Moulia-Pelat J-P, Spiegel A, Martin PMV, et al. A 5-year immunization field trial against hepatitis B using a Chinese hamster ovary cell recombinant vaccine in French Polynesian newborns: results at 3 years. Vaccine 1994;12:499–503.

148. Tsen YJ, Chang MH, Hsu HY, et al. Seroprevalence of hepatitis B virus infection in children in Taipei, 1989: five years after a mass hepatitis B vaccination program. J Med Virol 1991;34:96–99.

149. Mahoney FJ, Woodruff BA, Erben JJ, et al. Effect of a hepatitis B vaccination program on the prevalence of hepatitis B virus infection. J Infect Dis 1993;167:203–207.

150. McMahon BJ, Rhoades ER, Heyward WL, et al. A comprehensive programme to reduce the incidence of hepatitis B virus infection and its sequelae in Alaskan Natives. Lancet 1989;ii:1134–1136.

151. Pongpipat D, Suvatte V, Assateerawatt A. Efficacy of hepatitis B virus (HBV) vaccine in long term prevention of HBV infection. Asian Pac J Allergy Immunol 1988;6:19–22.

152. Lo KJ, Lee SD, Tsai YT, et al. Long-term immunogenicity and efficacy of hepatitis B vaccine in infants born to HBeAg-positive HBsAg-carrier mothers. Hepatology 1988;8:1647–1650.

153. Hwang L-Y, Lee C-Y, Beasley RP. Five-year follow-up of HBV vaccination with plasma-derived vaccine in neonates: evaluation of immunogenicity and efficacy against perinatal transmission. In: Hollinger FB, Lemon SM, et al, eds. Viral hepatitis and liver disease. Baltimore: Williams & Wilkins, 1990:759–761.

154. Lieming D, Mintai Z, Yinfu W, et al. A 9-year follow-up study of the immunogenicity and long-term efficacy of plasma-derived hepatitis B vaccine in high-risk Chinese neonates. Clin Infect Dis 1993;17:475–479.

155. Coursaget P, Leboulleux D, Soumare M, et al. Twelve-year follow-up study of hepatitis B immunization of Senegalese infants. J Hepatol 1994;21:250–254.

156. Whittle HC, Inskip H, Hall AJ, et al. Vaccination against hepatitis B and protection against chronic viral carriage in The Gambia. Lancet 1991;337:747–750.

157. West DJ. Clinical experience with hepatitis B vaccines. Am J Infect Control 1989;17:172–180.

158. Panda SK, Ramesh R, Rao KVS, et al. Comparative evaluation of the immunogenicity of yeast-derived (recombinant) and plasma-derived hepatitis B vaccine in infants. J Med Virol 1991;35:297–302.

159. Hayashi J, Kashiwagi S, Kajiyama W, et al. Comparison of results of recombinant and plasma-derived hepatitis B vaccines in Japanese nursery-school children. J Infect 1988;17:49–55.

160. Halliday ML, Rankin JG, Bristow NJ, et al. A randomized double-blind clinical trial of a mammalian cell-derived recombinant DNA hepatitis B vaccine compared with a plasma-derived vaccine. Arch Intern Med 1990;150:1195–1200.

161. Gunn TR, Bosley A, Woodfield DG. The safety and immunogenicity of a recombinant hepatitis B vaccine in neonates. NZ Med J 1989;102:1–3.

162. Tan KL, Oon CJ, Goh KT, et al. Immunogenicity and safety of low doses of recombinant yeast-derived hepatitis B vaccine. Acta Paediatr Scand 1990;79:593–598.

163. Goh KT, Tan KL, Kong KH, et al. Comparison of the immune response of four different dosages of a yeast-recombinant hepatitis B vaccine in Singapore children: a four-year follow-up study. Bull WHO 1992;70:233–239.

164. Andre FE. Overview of a 5-year clinical experience with a yeast-derived hepatitis B vaccine. Vaccine 1990;8:S74–S78.

165. Innis BL, Snitbhan R, Hunasol P, et al. Protection against hepatitis A by an inactivated vaccine. JAMA 1994;271:1328–1334.

166. Werzberger A, Mensch B, Kuter B, et al. A controlled trial of a formalin-inactivated hepatitis A vaccine in healthy children. N Engl J Med 1992;327:453–457.

167. Riedemann S, Reinhardt G, Frosner GG, et al. Placebo-controlled efficacy study of hepatitis A vaccine in Valdivia, Chile. Vaccine 1992:10(Suppl 1):S152–S155.

168. Newcomber W, Rivin B, Reid R, et al. Immunogenicity, safety and tolerability of varying doses and regimens of inactivated hepatitis A virus vaccine in Navajo children. Pediatr Infect Dis J 1994;13:640–642.

169. Horng Y-C, Chang M-H, Lee C-Y, et al. Safety and immunogenicity of hepatitis A vaccine in healthy children. Pediatr Infect Dis J 1993;12:359–362.

170. Van Damme P, Thoelen S, Cramm M, et al. Inactivated hepatitis A vaccine: reactogenicity, immunogenicity and long-term antibody persistence. J Med Virol 1994;44:446–451.

171. Tilzey AJ, Palmer SJ, Barrow S, et al. Clinical trial with inactivated hepatitis A vaccine and recommendations for its use [published erratum BMJ 1992;304:1352]. BMJ 1992;304:1272–1276.

172. Ellerbeck EF, Lewis JA, Nalin D, et al. Safety profile and immunogenicity of an inactivated vaccine derived from an attenuated strain of hepatitis A. Vaccine 1992;10:668–672.

173. Clemens R, Safary A, Hepburn A, et al. Clinical experience with an inactivated hepatitis A vaccine. J Infect Dis 1995;171(Suppl 1):S44–S49.

174. Briem H, Safary A. Immunogenicity and safety in adults of hepatitis A virus vaccine administered as a single dose with a booster 6 months later. J Med Virol 1994;44:443–445.

175. Van Damme P, Mathei C, Thoelen S, et al. Single dose inactivated hepatitis A vaccine: rationale and clinical assessment of the safety and immunogenicity. J Med Virol 1994;44:435–441.
176. Jilg W, Bittner R, Bock HL, et al. Vaccination against hepatitis A: comparison of different short-term immunization schedules. Vaccine 1992;10(Suppl 1):S126–S128.
177. Wagner G, Lavanchy D, Darioli R, et al. Simultaneous active and passive immunization against hepatitis A studied in a population of travelers. Vaccine 1993;11:1027–1032.
178. Shouval D, Ashur Y, Adler R, et al. Safety, tolerability, and immunogenicity of an inactivated hepatitis A vaccine: effects of single and booster injections, and comparison to administration of immune globulin. J Hepatol 1993;18(Suppl 2):S32–S37.
179. Leentvaar-Kuijpers A, Coutinho RA, Brulein V, et al. Simultaneous passive and active immunization against hepatitis A. Vaccine 1992;10(Suppl 1):S138–S141.
180. Fujiyama S, Odoh K, Kuramoto I, et al. Current seroepidemiological status of hepatitis A with a comparison of antibody titers from infection and vaccination. J Hepatol 1994;21:641–645.
181. Fujiyama S, Iino S, Odoh K, et al. Time course of hepatitis A virus antibody titer after active and passive immunization. Hepatology 1992;15:983–988.
182. Iino S, Fujiyama S, Horiuchi K, et al. Clinical trial of a lyophilized inactivated hepatitis A candidate vaccine in healthy adult volunteers. Vaccine 1992;10:323–328.
183. Wiedermann G, Ambrosch F, Kollaritsch H, et al. Safety and immunogenicity of an inactivated hepatitis A candidate vaccine in healthy adult volunteers. Vaccine 1990;8:581–584.
184. Green MS, Cohen D, Lerman Y, et al. Depression of the immune response to an inactivated hepatitis A vaccine administered concomitantly with immune globulin. J Infect Dis 1993;168:740–743.
185. Weibel RE, Neff BJ, Kuter BJ, et al. Live attenuated varicella virus vaccine. Efficacy trial in healthy children. N Engl J Med 1984;310:1409–1415.
186. Kuter BJ, Weibel RE, Guess HA, et al. Oka/Merck varicella vaccine in healthy children: final report of a 2-year efficacy study and 7-year follow-up studies. Vaccine 1991;9:643–647.
187. White CJ, Kuter BJ, Hildebrand CS, et al. Varicella vaccine (VARIVAX) in healthy children and adolescents: results from clinical trials, 1987 to 1989. Pediatrics 1991;87:604–610.
188. Arbeter AM, Starr SE, Preblud SR, et al. Varicella vaccine trials in healthy children: a summary of comparative and follow-up studies. Am J Dis Child 1984;138:434–438.
189. Johnson CE, Shurin PA, Fattlar D, et al. Live attenuated varicella vaccine in healthy 12- to 24-month-old children. Pediatrics 1988;81:512–518.
190. Arbeter AM, Starr SE, Plotkin SA. Varicella vaccine studies in healthy children and adults. Pediatrics 1986;78(suppl):748–756.
191. Watson BM, Piercy SA, Plotkin SA, et al. Modified chickenpox in children immunized with the Oka/Merck varicella vaccine. Pediatrics 1993;91:17–22.
192. White CJ, Kuter BJ, Ngai A, et al. Modified cases of chickenpox after varicella vaccination: correlation of protection with antibody response. Pediatr Infect Dis J 1992;11:19–23.
193. Asano Y, Nagai T, Miyata T, et al. Long-term protective immunity of recipients of the OKA strain of live varicella vaccine. Pediatrics 1985;75:667–671.
194. Asano Y, Suga S, Yoshikawa T, et al. Experience and reason: twenty-year follow-up of protective immunity of the Oka strain live varicella vaccine. Pediatrics 1994;94:524–526.
195. Nader S, Bergen R, Sharp M, et al. Age-related differences in cell-mediated immunity to varicella-zoster virus among children and adults immunized with live attenuated varicella vaccine. J Infect Dis 1995;171:13–17.
196. Gershon AA, Steinberg SP, LaRussa P, et al. Immunization of healthy adults with live attenuated varicella vaccine. J Infect Dis 1988;158:132–137.
197. Plotkin SA, Starr SE, Connor K, et al. Zoster in normal children after varicella vaccine [letter]. J Infect Dis 1989;159:1000–1001.
198. Brunell PA, Taylor-Wiedeman J, Geiser CF, et al. Risk of herpes zoster in children with leukemia: varicella vaccine compared with history of chickenpox. Pediatrics 1986;77:53–56.
199. Hardy I, Gershon AA, Steinberg SP, et al. The incidence of zoster after immunization with live attenuated varicella vaccine. N Engl J Med 1991;325:1545–1550.
200. Hammerschlag MR, Gershon AA, Steinberg SP, et al. Herpes zoster in an adult recipient of live attenuated varicella vaccine. J Infect Dis 1989;160:535–537.
201. Halloran ME, Cochi SL, Lieu TA, et al. Theoretical epidemiologic and morbidity effects of routine varicella immunization of preschool children in the United States. Am J Epidemiol 1994;140:81–104.

202. Centers for Disease Control and Prevention. General recommendations on immunization: recommendations of the Advisory Committee on Immunization Practices (ACIP). MMWR 1994;43(RR-1):1–38.

203. Centers for Disease Control and Prevention. Standards for pediatric immunization practices. Recommended by the National Vaccine Advisory Committee. MMWR 1993;42(RR-5):1–10.

204. American Academy of Family Physicians. Age charts for periodic health examination. Kansas City, MO: American Academy of Family Physicians, 1994. (Reprint no. 510.)

205. Advisory Committee on Immunization Practices, American Academy of Pediatrics, American Academy of Family Physicians, and the National Immunization Program, Centers for Disease Control and Prevention. Recommended childhood immunization schedule—United States, January 1995. MMWR 1995;43:959–960.

206. Centers for Disease Control and Prevention. Update: recommendations to prevent hepatitis B virus transmission—United States. MMWR 1995;44:574–575.

207. American Academy of Pediatrics. Recommendations for the use of live attenuated varicella vaccine. Pediatrics 1995;95:791–796.

207a. Centers for Disease Control and Prevention. Varicella prevention: recommendations of the Advisory Committee on Immunization Practices (ACIP). MMWR 1996 (in press).

208. Food and Drug Administration. FDA licenses hepatitis A vaccine. FDA Talk Paper 1995;Feb 22:T95-11.

208a. Advisory Committee on Immunization Practices. Licensure of inactivated hepatitis A vaccine and recomendations for use among international travelers. MMWR 1995;44:559–560.

209. Centers for Disease Control and Prevention. Certification of poliomyelitis eradication—the Americas, 1994. MMWR 1994;43:720–722.

210. Krahn M, Detsky AS. Should Canada and the United States universally vaccinate infants against hepatitis B? A cost-effectiveness analysis. Med Decis Making 1993;13:4–20.

211. Bloom BS, Hillman AL, Fendrick AM, et al. A reappraisal of hepatitis B virus vaccination strategies using cost-effectiveness analysis. Ann Intern Med 1993;118:298–306.

211a. Kwan-Gett TS, Whitaker RC, Kemper KJ. A cost-effectiveness analysis of prevaccination testing for hepatitis B in adolescents and preadolescents. Arch Pediatr Adolesc Med 1994;148:915–920.

212. Lieu TA, Cochi SL, Black SB, et al. Cost-effectiveness of a routine varicella vaccination program for US children. JAMA 1994;271:375–381.

213. Brunell PA, Novelli VM, Lipton SV, et al. Combined vaccine against measles, mumps, rubella, and varicella. Pediatrics 1988;81:779–784.

214. Englund JA, Suarez CS, Kelly J, et al. Placebo-controlled trial of varicella vaccine given with or after measles-mumps-rubella vaccine. J Pediatr 1989;114:37–44.

215. Lieu TA, Finkler LJ, Sorel ME, et al. Cost-effectiveness of varicella serotesting versus presumptive vaccination of school-age children and adolescents. Pediatrics 1995;95:632–638.

216. American Academy of Pediatrics. Recommended ages for administration of currently licensed childhood vaccines—August 1995. AAP News, August 1995.

66. Adult Immunizations—
Including Chemoprophylaxis Against Influenza A

RECOMMENDATION

Annual influenza vaccine is recommended for all persons aged 65 and older and persons in selected high-risk groups (see *Clinical Intervention*). Pneumococcal vaccine is recommended for all immunocompetent individuals who are age 65 years and older or otherwise at increased risk for pneumococcal disease (see Clinical Intervention). There is insufficient evidence to recommend for or against pneumococcal vaccine for high-risk immunocompromised individuals, but recommendations for vaccinating these persons may be made on other grounds. The series of combined tetanus-diphtheria toxoids (Td) should be completed for adults who have not received the primary series, and all adults should receive periodic Td boosters. Vaccination against measles and mumps should be provided to all adults born after 1956 who lack evidence of immunity. A second measles vaccination is recommended for adolescents and young adults in settings where such individuals congregate (e.g., high schools and colleges). See Chapter 32 for recommendations for rubella vaccine. Hepatitis B vaccine is recommended for all young adults not previously immunized and for all persons at high risk for infection (see Clinical Intervention). Hepatitis A vaccine is recommended for persons at high risk for hepatitis A virus (HAV) infection (see *Clinical Intervention*). Varicella vaccine is recommended for susceptible adults (see also Chapter 65). See Chapter 25 for recommendations regarding the Bacille Calmette-Guérin (BCG) vaccine. Recommendations for postexposure prophylaxis against selected infectious diseases are in Chapter 67; see also Chapter 24, Screening for Hepatitis B Virus Infection.

INFLUENZA

Burden of Suffering

Influenza, which frequently causes incapacitating malaise for several days, is responsible for significant morbidity and decreased productivity during epidemics. Twenty thousand or more excess deaths have been reported during each of 10 different epidemics from 1972–1973 to 1990–1991; more than 40,000 excess deaths occurred in each of three of these epidemics.[1] During severe pandemics (e.g., 1957 and 1968), there are often high attack rates across all age groups, and mortality usually is markedly increased. Elderly persons and persons of all ages with certain chronic medical disorders (see *Clinical Intervention*) are at increased risk for complications from influenza infections. More than 90% of the deaths attributed to pneumonia and influenza in these epidemics occurred among persons aged 65 and older.[1] Influenza has been estimated to cause a yearly average of 4.1–4.4 million excess respiratory illnesses and 16.6–17.9 million excess bed and restricted activity days in persons over 20 years of age.[2] Excess rates of hospitalization have also been documented for children with influenza who have chronic conditions such as severe asthma, cystic fibrosis, and diabetes.[3]

Efficacy of Vaccine

Inactivated (killed-virus) influenza vaccine containing antigens identical or similar to currently circulating influenza A and B viruses has been shown in controlled trials to be 70–80% effective in preventing influenza illness or reducing severity of influenza illness in healthy children, adolescents, and adults under age 65.[4–8] The vaccine has also been reported to reduce clinical symptoms in health care workers,[9] which may translate into a reduction in transmission to high-risk patients.

Only one randomized placebo-controlled trial has studied vaccine efficacy in high-risk persons for whom the vaccine is generally recommended. This trial enrolled 1,838 persons aged 60 years and older, three fourths of whom had no risk factors other than age.[10] During the influenza season, the vaccine significantly reduced the proportion with influenza-like illness (from 3% to 2%) and with serologically diagnosed infections (from 9% to 4%). In stratified analyses, protective efficacy was similar in healthy older adults and those with chronic disease but was reduced in subjects ≥70 years of age. In a poorly reported randomized controlled trial comparing different types and dosages of influenza vaccine in elderly persons living in the community,[11] one of the vaccines reduced clinical illness rates by 50–70% compared with other vaccine types and dosages. Illness rates were also substantially reduced compared to an unvaccinated cohort not enrolled in the trial. In a large serial cohort study of community-dwelling elderly persons, influenza vaccination reduced hospitalization rates by 48–57% for pneumonia and influenza and by 27–39% for all acute and chronic respiratory conditions, after adjustment for covariates.[12] Case-control studies in persons who are 65 years or older have reported that during epidemic periods when there was a good antigenic match between vaccine and virus, influenza vaccination prevented 31–45% of hospitalizations for pneumonia and influenza[13–15] and 43–49% of deaths due to all respiratory conditions.[13] In a separate analysis using vital statistics data, influenza vaccination reduced total mortality by 27–30% among individuals aged 45 years or older.[13]

Adequately designed and performed observational studies conducted during influenza outbreaks also generally support the efficacy of influenza vaccine in preventing illness, hospitalization, and mortality in the institutionalized elderly population and in community-dwelling elderly persons with high-risk chronic conditions, although efficacy estimates vary widely (e.g., 24–58% efficacy against pneumonia).[16–22] Vaccination of nursing home residents also may prevent institutional outbreaks.[23] Randomized controlled trials in nursing homes have suggested that greater protection may be offered by other, as yet unlicensed, vaccine formulations or combinations (e.g., diphtheria toxoid conjugate vaccine or addition of live intranasal vaccine).[24,25] Data are more limited for younger high-risk persons. One cohort study in children with moderate to severe asthma demonstrated 49% vaccine efficacy against clinical illness despite a poor antigenic match with the epidemic influenza A virus, but no effect was seen on hospitalizations or asthma attack rates or severity.[26]

Because of frequent seasonal variation in the hemagglutinin and neuraminidase antigens of circulating viruses ("antigenic drift"), it is necessary to administer the vaccine annually each fall, prior to the epidemic season. This schedule allows the annually reformulated influenza vaccine to include antigens detected from recent global viral surveillance, which are likely to be circulating during the subsequent season. Although allergic reactions have been described, principally in patients with hypersensitivity to eggs, serious adverse effects from influenza vaccine are quite uncommon.[1] Randomized placebo-controlled trials of influenza vaccine have reported no difference in systemic reactions, but mild local side effects were more common after vaccine and occurred in up to 20% of patients.[27,28]

Amantadine and rimantadine are 70–90% effective in preventing illness caused by outbreaks of naturally occurring strains of influenza A viruses when used prophylactically in healthy community-living or institutionalized persons.[29–34] Several trials have shown much lower protection rates,[35,36] however, possibly due to late initiation of chemoprophylaxis or inadequate compliance. No controlled trials of these medications have been conducted in nursing home populations, but observational studies support the efficacy of chemoprophylaxis as an adjunct to vaccination during influenza A outbreaks in these institutions.[21,37,38] Neither drug is effective as prophylaxis against influenza A for household members of simultaneously treated index cases,[39,40] although amantadine has been proven efficacious in preventing influenza A disease when the index case is not treated.[41] Transmission of resistant viruses from treated patients may reduce the efficacy of chemoprophylaxis in household or institutional contacts.[22,39] Neither drug prevents influenza B infection, so they are appropriate only in presumed influenza A epidemics.

Amantadine and rimantadine produce transient insomnia, anxiety, nausea, dizziness, and impaired concentration in 5–25% of patients.[42–47] The risk of adverse central nervous system effects has been shown to be significantly lower with rimantadine.[33] Adverse effects occur more frequently and with greater severity in older persons and have been associated with increased risk of falls.[48,49] Toxic levels resulting from reduced drug clearance have been identified in elderly persons.[42,49]

PNEUMOCOCCAL DISEASE

Burden of Suffering

Pneumococcal disease is a significant cause of morbidity and mortality in the U.S. Although pneumococcal infection is not a reportable disease, population-based surveillance studies have reported annual invasive pneumococcal disease rates of at least 15–19/100,000 population and pneumococcal meningitis rates of 0.3–1.2/100,000.[50–54] Significantly higher incidence rates are reported for persons less than 5 years of age or over age 65; blacks, Native Americans, and Alaska Natives; nursing home residents; alcoholics; and those with underlying chronic medical or immunodeficient conditions.[50–57] Pneumococcal disease accounts for about 15% of severe community-acquired pneumonia, which has a case-fatality rate (proportion of cases resulting in death) of 9–26%.[58–63] Pneumococcal bacteremia and meningitis are also associated with high case-fatality rates.[50–54,63,64] The highest case-fatality rates from invasive pneumococcal infection occur in elderly persons (30–43%) and patients with co-morbid conditions (25–27%), and the lowest occur in healthy children (0–3%).[50–53,63] In recent years, drug-resistant strains of *Streptococcus pneumoniae* have emerged; recent estimates suggest that in some locales 15% or more of pneumococcal isolates are drug resistant.[50,65,65a] The emergence of drug-resistant strains underscores the importance of preventing pneumococcal disease by vaccination.

Efficacy of Vaccine

The 14-valent polysaccharide pneumococcal vaccine, which was licensed in 1977, was replaced in 1983 by a 23-valent polysaccharide vaccine.[66] The latter contains purified capsular materials from 88% of the strains of *S. pneumoniae* causing bacteremic pneumococcal disease reported in the U.S.[67] In randomized controlled trials, 4- to 13-valent pneumococcal vaccines were 76–92% efficacious in preventing pneumococcal pneumonia in healthy young adult populations living in epidemic conditions.[68–70] A 14-valent vaccine was also efficacious in reducing respiratory mortality in a population from a developing country.[71] The efficacy of pneumococcal vaccine in the general U.S. population has not been determined with certainty. Controlled trials in the U.S. involving low-risk middle-aged and older adults failed to demonstrate protective efficacy,[72] although the relatively low incidence of pneumococcal infection in healthy U.S. adults makes efficacy difficult to establish in a prospective clinical trial. A meta-analysis combining the most recent trials (follow-up periods of 16–36 months) in low-risk populations in the U.S. and elsewhere reported significant reductions in definitive and presumptive pneumococcal pneumonia with vaccination.[73] Vaccinated individuals had 11 fewer episodes of definitive pneumococcal pneumonia and 25 fewer episodes of presumptive pneumococcal pneumonia per 1,000 subjects. Results were similar for definitive and presumptive pneumonia due to vaccine types only. Small reductions in mortality were not statistically significant.

Trials in relatively healthy institutionalized elderly (≥50–55 years of age) have demonstrated significant reductions in the incidence of pneumonia, and in mortality in one study, with 3- and 14-valent vaccines, although these trials were limited by flaws in design and conduct.[74,75] Other trials of 14- to 17-valent vaccines in high-risk populations, all adequately designed and conducted, have been unable to detect significant reductions in pneumococcal or all-cause pneumonia or mortality.[76–79] A meta-analysis combining five trials in high-risk populations also reported no effects of vaccine on pneumococcal pneumonia, all-cause pneumonia, or mortality.[73] The sample sizes were much smaller than for the analyses in low-risk populations, but effect estimates for most outcomes did not suggest important benefits.

One possible explanation for the lack of vaccine efficacy in trials in high-risk populations is that the trials may have included subsets of individuals for whom the vaccine has little benefit. Case-control studies and indirect cohort studies (comparing the distribution of pneumococcal serotypes in the blood of vaccinated and unvaccinated persons) have been much more feasible to perform than controlled trials, although such observational studies may be more prone to bias. These studies support the protective value of pneumococcal vaccine in immunocompetent recipients, with vaccine efficacy estimates of 60–75% reported but not in severely or relatively immunocompromised individuals, including those with alcoholism, chronic renal failure, immunoglobulin deficiency, nephrotic syndrome, sickle cell disease, multiple myeloma, metastatic or hematologic malignancies, or systemic lupus erythematosus.[80–86] For some of these disorders, efficacy point estimates suggest a benefit, but confidence intervals are wide and include the possibility of no benefit. Additional research is needed to obtain more definitive data on the efficacy of pneumococcal vaccine and to develop vaccines that have better efficacy in both immunocompetent and immunocompromised individuals, as well as in high-risk children under 2 years of age.

The total duration of antibody protection from pneumococcal vaccination is unknown; elevated titers appear to persist in adults for at least 5 years after immunization, but in some persons, they may fall to prevaccination levels within 10 years.[66] A case-control study reported a statistically significant decline in protective efficacy with increasing time since vaccination (e.g., from 88% within 3 years to 75% if ≥5 years since vaccination in persons aged 55–64).[81] On the other hand, an indirect cohort study reported that clinical efficacy persisted at least 7–10 years.[84]

There is little evidence of serious adverse effects from this vaccine, although erythema, induration, or pain at the injection site occur in about one third to one half of patients. Fever, myalgia, and severe reactions occur in no more than 1% of patients.[66,72] Most evidence indicates little difference in adverse reactions to revaccination compared to initial vaccination.[66]

TETANUS AND DIPHTHERIA

Burden of Suffering

Largely as a result of routine immunization, tetanus and diphtheria have become uncommon diseases in the U.S.: 51 cases of tetanus (0.02/100,000) and 2 cases of diphtheria were reported in 1994.[86a] In 1948, before tetanus and diphtheria toxoids were widely introduced, there were over 600 cases of tetanus and about 9,500 cases of diphtheria in the U.S.[87] The prevalence of immunity to tetanus in the U.S. population, as measured by serum antibodies, declines with age beginning at age 40 and is only 28% among persons ages 70 or older.[88] Adults ages 50 and older account for the majority of cases of tetanus.[87,88] Tetanus remains a serious infection, with death occurring in 19–24% of cases.[88,89] Reports may underrepresent tetanus mortality by as much as 60%.[90] The tetanus case-fatality rate increases with age and is 26% for persons ages 70 and older.[88] The case-fatality rate is also high in neonates, indicating the need to adequately immunize women of childbearing age against tetanus. Diphtheria is a potentially severe illness, with a case-fatality rate of 5–10% in unvaccinated individuals. The disease is rare in the U.S., but large outbreaks have occurred in other developed countries despite relatively high rates of childhood immunization.[91–94]

Efficacy of Vaccine

The efficacy of the tetanus and diphtheria toxoids is established on the basis of clinical studies and decades of experience with universal childhood immunization.[95,96] A primary series of three doses of Td, followed by a booster dose, is highly effective in producing protective antibody titers lasting as long as 15–25 years and results in anamnestic responses with booster immunization as much as 20–30 years later.[97–104] In Sweden, a five-dose regimen (primary series plus boosters at age 8–10 and 18 years) resulted in greater than 90% of subjects having protective tetanus antitoxin levels at age 50 years, slightly fewer than at age 30.[105] Tetanus is unlikely in Americans who have received a primary vaccination series,[89,90,106] although clinical immunity may wane somewhat after 10–20 years.[89] Td often produces mild local inflammation, occasionally Arthus-type reactions and peripheral neuropathy (following frequent boosters), and rarely, anaphylaxis.[107–110]

MEASLES, MUMPS, AND RUBELLA

Burden of Suffering

Measles, a childhood illness, was reported in 232 (0.1/100,000) American adults (aged 20 or older) in 1994, a substantial decline from the recent peak of 6,210 cases (3.9/100,000) reported in 1990.[87,111] Adults accounted for nearly one fourth of all cases with known age reported in 1994.[111] About one third of adult infections occur among persons ages 20–24,[87] often in places where young adults congregate, such as schools or college campuses.[111] Hospitalization for measles and complications such as pneumonia and encephalitis are more common in adults than in school-aged children. Mumps infection was reported in 319 persons ≥20 years of age in 1993 (0.2/100,000), accounting for 20% of reported cases with known age.[87] Mumps outbreaks continue to occur periodically in schools and similar settings; in several recent outbreaks, most of those infected had previously been vaccinated against mumps.[111a] Rubella infection is discussed in Chapter 32.

Efficacy of Vaccine

A single dose of measles vaccine is 95% effective in producing long-term immunity.[112,113] Seropositivity rates remain high at least 10–15 years following vaccination,[114,115] and cohorts of known seroconverters have shown little evidence of increasing disease incidence with time since immunization.[115] Adult infections occur primarily in persons who have not been naturally infected or appropriately vaccinated in the past,[111] as well as those who were vaccinated before age 15 months.[116,117] Persons born before 1957 are likely to have been naturally infected and need not be considered susceptible.[118] Based on the age distribution and location of recent measles outbreaks,[111,117] revaccination of young adults in settings such as colleges and the workplace is likely to be most effective in reducing incidence in adults. Measles outbreaks are less common at colleges where two doses of vaccine are required prior to matriculation.[119] When outbreaks do occur in these settings, attack rates are lower among persons who have had two doses of vaccine.[117,120,122–124] Measles has been virtually eliminated among military recruits by revaccinating those whose screening sera suggest they are susceptible despite a history of vaccination.[125]

Since the introduction of mumps vaccine in the United States in 1967, there has been a 99% decline in the incidence of mumps, supporting the efficacy of this vaccine.[111a] The incidence of mumps in adults declined 50% between 1988–1990 and 1991–1993.[111a] Recommendations issued in 1989 for a two-dose measles vaccination schedule, with MMR recommended as the preferred vaccine, may have contributed to this recent decline. The age distribution and location of recent mumps outbreaks also suggests that revaccinating young adults in settings such as schools and colleges may be effective in reducing the incidence in adults. As with measles, persons born before 1957 can generally be considered immune to mumps and need not be vaccinated. Rubella screening and immunization are discussed in Chapter 32.

Adverse effects of measles or combined measles-mumps-rubella (MMR) vaccine in adults are usually mild and self-limited.[118,126] Administration of MMR vaccine is not associated with adverse effects in persons already immune to these diseases, and thus the combined MMR vaccine is preferable to individual vaccines such as measles vaccine, since many recipients may be susceptible to more than one of the three diseases MMR prevents.

HEPATITIS B

Burden of Suffering

An estimated 200,000–300,000 persons become infected with hepatitis B virus (HBV) in the U.S. each year and more than 10,000 require hospitalization.[127,128,188] The risk of developing a chronic HBV infection (i.e., carrier state) after acute infection is about 6–10% in adults.[127,130,131] Some 1–1.25 million persons in the U.S. are chronic HBV carriers.[188] About one quarter of carriers develop chronic active hepatitis, which can progress to cirrhosis; carriers are also at risk for developing hepatocellular carcinoma.[128,132,133] Some 5,000 hepatitis B-related deaths occur each year as a result of cirrhosis and liver cancer.[128] Persons with acute or chronic HBV infection are also at risk for infection with hepatitis delta virus (HDV), which can itself cause acute, possibly fulminant, hepatitis or chronic hepatitis that may progress to cirrhosis.[128] Since HDV cannot be transmitted in the absence of HBV infection, measures to prevent HBV infection will also prevent the complications of HDV infection.

Efficacy of Vaccine

Plasma-derived hepatitis B vaccine, which became available in 1982, has 85–95% protective efficacy when administered in three intramuscular doses to immunocompetent patients.[134–138] Controlled trials and time series in adult responders to plasma-derived vaccine indicate persistent protection against clinical HBV infection and chronic carriage lasting at least 7–9 years despite declines in protective antibody levels.[139–141,147] The recombinant vaccines licensed in 1986 and currently in use in the U.S. induce antibody responses and short-term efficacy (up to 5 years) similar to those of the plasma-derived vaccine.[142–145] Information on longer-term efficacy is not yet available for recombinant vaccines. The possible need for booster doses after longer intervals will be assessed as additional data become available.

Compared to healthy young persons, older adults, overweight persons, smokers, chronic hemodialysis patients, injection drug users, and human immunodeficiency virus (HIV)-infected patients are significantly less likely to have an adequate antibody response to the vaccine; those who do respond have a more rapid decline in antibody levels.[142,146–155] A repeat vaccination series in persons who fail to respond to the first series results in moderate antibody response in up to 50%.[156] Injection into the buttocks has been associated with a suboptimal immune response, and therefore the deltoid muscle is the preferred injection site.[128,146] Local soreness at the injection site is a common side effect.[145] There have been several case reports of nonfatal anaphylaxis from recombinant hepatitis B vaccine.[157]

HEPATITIS A

Burden of Suffering

Almost 27,000 cases of hepatitis A were reported in the U.S. in 1994 (10.3/100,000),[86a] although the actual number of cases is estimated to be several times higher.[128] Adults aged 20–39 years account for 43% of reported cases.[87] About half of reported hepatitis cases in the U.S. are attributable to hepatitis A.[128] The case-fatality rate and clinical severity of hepatitis A increase with increasing age.[128,158] Groups at high risk for hepatitis A include certain Alaska Native, Pacific Islander, and Native American populations, institutionalized persons and workers in these institutions, men who have sex with men, users of injection or street drugs (depending on local epidemiology), certain laboratory workers, some religious communities, and travelers to countries where hepatitis A has intermediate or high endemicity.[128,159,160] For susceptible travelers visiting developing countries, the incidence rate of hepatitis A has been estimated at 300 cases per 100,000 persons per month and the mortality rate at 3 deaths per 100,000 per month.[160]

Efficacy of Vaccine

Inactivated hepatitis A vaccine, now licensed in the U.S., has been proven efficacious against hepatitis A in randomized controlled trials in children (see Chapter 65).[161,162] Although trials evaluating clinical outcomes have not been performed in adults, hepatitis A vaccine produces seroconversion rates of 90–100% after one dose and 99–100% after two doses in healthy adult volunteers, including Alaska Natives.[163–169] The duration of immunity has not been established, but in adults, protective levels of antibody have been shown to persist at least 4 years after administration of three doses of vaccine.[164,168,170,170a] Estimates from models of antibody decline after vaccination predict that protective levels could last at least 20 years.[164] Vaccine efficacy is low in the first week after vaccination, rising to 77–90% at 2 weeks and 90–100% at 3–4 weeks.[162,165,171,172,176]

To provide immediate protection for those at high risk of exposure (e.g., travelers to endemic areas), giving immune globulin (IG) with the first vaccine dose may be necessary (see Chapter 67). Although several studies have reported lower mean antibody titers when the vaccine is administered concomitantly with IG, vaccine seroconversion rates appear to be comparable.[173,176,181] Seroconversion rates do not appear to be adversely affected when hepatitis A vaccine is given with hepatitis B vaccine.[174]

In direct comparisons with IG, traditionally used as preexposure prophylaxis against hepatitis A for high-risk persons (see Chapter 67), the vaccine led to higher and longer-lasting antibody titers.[175–181] The reported protective efficacy of hepatitis A vaccine is higher than that reported for IG (see Chapters 65 and 67), but the clinical efficacies of the two interventions have not been directly compared.

Adverse effects of the vaccine, including mild local reactions (pain, tenderness, redness, and swelling) and minor systemic symptoms such as fever, headache, and malaise, occur in 10–30% of recipients and are more common after the second and third doses.[161,162,169,170,182,183] Serious allergic reactions without long-term consequences have been reported rarely in temporal association with hepatitis A vaccine.[160]

Recommendations of Other Groups

Guidelines on adolescent and adult immunizations have been published by the American College of Physicians (ACP) and the Infectious Diseases Society of America (IDSA),[184] the American Academy of Family Physicians,[185] the American Academy of Pediatrics,[3] the Canadian Task Force on the Periodic Health Examination,[186] the American College of Obstetricians and Gynecologists (ACOG),[186a] and the Advisory Committee on Immunization Practices (ACIP).[187] ACIP has also issued specific recommendations on the use of Td;[96] pneumococcal,[66] influenza,[1] hepatitis B,[128,170a,188] rubella,[189] measles,[118] varicella,[189a] and hepatitis A[189b] vaccines; and the use of vaccines in persons with altered immunocompetence.[190] ACOG has issued detailed guidelines on the use of vaccines during pregnancy.[191]

A few of these recommendations differ from those made in this chapter. The Canadian Task Force recommends against pneumococcal vaccine in immunocompromised individuals and found insufficient evidence to recommend for or against routine pneumococcal vaccination for healthy community-living elderly persons.[186] ACP[184] recommends that a single Td booster at age 50 for those who have completed the full five-dose pediatric series is an equally acceptable alternative strategy to decennial Td boosters.[96] ACIP and AAP recommend catch-up immunization with hepatitis B vaccine for adolescents aged 11–12 who have not been vaccinated previously, but they do not recommend routine hepatitis B vaccination for low-risk persons over 12 years, primarily because of cost and implementation considerations.[3,188,188a] ACIP recommends two doses of live measles vaccine or evidence of measles immunity for two groups in addition to those entering schools or colleges: persons who travel abroad and medical personnel at the time they begin employment.[118] ACOG recommends routine influenza vaccine beginning at age 55 rather than 65 and hepatitis B vaccine only for high-risk groups.[186a]

Antiviral chemoprophylaxis against influenza A, using either rimantadine hydrochloride or amantadine hydrochloride, has been recommended by the ACP, IDSA, and ACIP for high-risk persons and their caretakers who cannot be or have very recently been vaccinated (i.e., within 2 weeks for adults; within 2 weeks of the second dose for children), immunodeficient individuals as a supplement to vaccine, and residents and unvaccinated staff during outbreaks in institutions.[184,192]

Discussion

Most adults have not been immunized in accordance with existing immunization guidelines.[193] Perceptions that adult vaccine-preventable infections are not important health problems and that available vaccines are not safe and efficacious[193] can be readily refuted by the evidence already described. The cost of vaccines is another possible barrier to widespread immunization, but studies have shown that the prevention of morbidity and mortality from infectious diseases makes immunization cost-effective. For example, analyses of routine influenza and pneumococcal vaccination of persons aged 65 and older suggest that their cost-effectiveness is comparable to that of other widely recommended preventive services such as mammography or screening for hypertension.[12,15,194,195] Hepatitis B vaccination of high-risk groups (those with HBV incidence >5%), with or without prior screening for susceptibility, has been shown to be cost-effective, even cost-saving in some analyses.[196–198]

Cost-effectiveness analysis may also provide guidance on appropriate vaccination strategies. Vaccination of high-risk newborns and adults against hepatitis B has been ineffective in eliminating the disease. One cost-effectiveness analysis reported that vaccinating all adolescents against hepatitis B, in addition to the current strategy of screening pregnant women and vaccinating high-risk newborns, would cost only $3,695 per year of life saved.[198] While Td booster vaccination every 10 years is efficacious in preventing disease, antibody studies suggest that an interval of 15–30 years between boosters is likely to be adequate, especially given the small absolute risk of either disease in the U.S. A recent cost-effectiveness analysis reported that a decennial-booster strategy added a 2-minute survival advantage compared with a single booster at age 65 years, at a cost of $281,748 per year of additional life saved,[199] although potential costs related to diphtheria were not incorporated into the analysis.[200]

Compared to IG, hepatitis A vaccine appears to have greater and longer-lasting efficacy against infection with fewer adverse effects, but it is unclear whether the benefits outweigh the costs of the vaccine. One cost-effectiveness analysis reported that for all age groups, use of IG for post-exposure prophylaxis or for preexposure short-term (≤6 months) prophylaxis is less expensive than vaccination.[201] Testing for hepatitis A antibodies in groups with a high prevalence of immunity (e.g., frequent travelers, military personnel, older persons) reduces vaccination costs, however. An analysis for British soldiers calculated a more favorable cost-benefit ratio for the vaccine than for IG if there were at least two exposures to areas endemic for hepatitis A in 4 years.[202]

CLINICAL INTERVENTION

Influenza vaccine should be administered annually to all persons ages 65 and older and to persons 6 months of age or older who are residents of chronic care facilities or suffer from chronic cardiopulmonary disorders, metabolic diseases (including diabetes mellitus), hemoglobinopathies, immunosuppression, or renal dysfunction ("B" recommendation). Influenza vaccine is also recommended for health care providers for high-risk patients ("B" recommendation). In persons at high risk for influenza A (e.g., during institutional outbreaks), *amantadine* or *rimantadine prophylaxis* (200 mg/day orally) may be started at the time of vaccination and continued for 2 weeks ("B" recommendation). A lower dose (≤100 mg/day) of amanta-

dine is recommended for persons with reduced creatinine clearance and those 65 years of age and older. A reduced dosage (100 mg/day) of rimantadine is indicated for those with reduced renal or hepatic function and for elderly nursing home residents and may also be necessary in healthy persons 65 years and older who experience side effects. Amantadine and rimantadine are most useful as short-term prophylaxis for high-risk persons who have not yet received the vaccine or are vaccinated after influenza A activity in the community has already begun; when the vaccine may be ineffective due to major antigenic changes in the virus; for unimmunized persons who provide care for high-risk persons; to supplement protection provided by vaccine in persons who are expected to have a poor antibody response; and for high-risk persons in whom the vaccine is contraindicated (i.e., those with anaphylactic hypersensitivity to egg protein). If vaccine is contraindicated, amantadine or rimantadine should be started at the beginning of the influenza season and continued daily for the duration of influenza activity in the community.

Pneumococcal vaccine is recommended for all immunocompetent individuals who are aged 65 years and older or otherwise at increased risk for pneumococcal disease ("B" recommendation). High-risk groups include institutionalized persons ≥50 years of age, persons ≥2 years of age with certain medical conditions, including chronic cardiac or pulmonary disease, diabetes mellitus, and anatomic asplenia (excluding sickle cell disease), and persons ≥2 years of age who live in special environments or social settings with an identified increased risk of pneumococcal disease (e.g., certain Native American and Alaska Native populations). Routine revaccination is not recommended, but it may be appropriate to consider revaccination in immunocompetent individuals at highest risk for morbidity and mortality from pneumococcal disease (e.g., persons ≥75 years of age or with severe chronic disease) who were vaccinated more than 5 years previously. Revaccination with the 23-valent vaccine may be appropriate for high-risk persons who previously received the 14-valent vaccine. There is insufficient evidence to recommend for or against pneumococcal vaccine as an efficacious vaccine for immunocompromised individuals, but recommendations for vaccinating these persons may be made on other grounds, including high incidence and case-fatality rates of pneumococcal disease and minimal adverse effects from the vaccine ("C" recommendation). Immunocompromised conditions associated with high risk for pneumococcal disease include alcoholism, cirrhosis, chronic renal failure, ne-phrotic syndrome, sickle cell disease, multiple myeloma, metastatic or hematologic malignancy, acquired or congenital immunodeficiency (including HIV infection), and other conditions associated with immunosuppression, such as organ transplant. It may be appropriate to consider periodic revaccination in these high-risk immunocompromised patients, who are likely to have poor initial antibody response and rapid decline of antibodies after vaccination.

The *Td vaccine series* should be completed for patients who have not received the primary series, and all adults should receive periodic Td boosters ("A" recommendation). For persons not previously immunized, the recommended schedule for the primary Td series is 0, 2, and 8–14 months. The optimal interval for booster doses is not established. The standard regimen is to provide a Td booster at least once every 10 years, but in the U.S., intervals of 15–30 years between boosters are likely to be adequate in persons who received a complete five-dose series in childhood (see Chapter 65). For international travelers, an interval of 10 years between boosters is recommended.

MMR vaccine should be administered to all persons born after 1956 who lack evidence of immunity to measles (receipt of live vaccine on or after the first birthday, laboratory evidence of immunity, or a history of physician-diagnosed measles) ("A" recommendation). A second measles vaccination is recommended for adolescents and young adults in settings where such individuals congregate (e.g., high schools, technical schools, and colleges), if they have not previously received a second dose (see Chapter 65) ("B" recommendation). The combined MMR vaccine is preferable to monovalent measles vaccine, since many recipients may also be susceptible to mumps or rubella due to inadequate vaccination or primary vaccine failure. Susceptible individuals should be vaccinated against mumps ("B" recommendation). Administration of the MMR or measles vaccine during pregnancy is not recommended. See Chapter 32 for recommendations on rubella screening and vaccination.

Hepatitis B vaccine is recommended for all young adults not previously immunized ("A" recommendation). Hepatitis B vaccine is also recommended for susceptible adults in high-risk groups, including men who have sex with men, injection drug users and their sex partners, persons who have a history of sexual activity with multiple partners in the previous 6 months or have recently acquired another sexually transmitted disease, international travelers to countries where HBV is of high or intermediate endemicity, recipients of certain blood products (including hemodialysis patients), and persons in health-related jobs with frequent exposure to blood or blood products ("A" recommendation). The recommended regimen for the recombinant hepatitis B vaccine is to administer 10 or 20 μg (depending on vaccine product) intramuscularly in the deltoid muscle at the current visit and at 1 and 6 months later. Clinicians should consider testing antibody response to the vaccine in individuals at very high risk from hepatitis B who are likely to have an inadequate antibody response (i.e., chronic renal dialysis patients, injection drug users, HIV-infected patients). Recommendations on screening for HBV infection and prevention of perinatal transmission are in Chapter 24. Recommendations for persons with possible percutaneous or sexual exposure to individuals infected with hepatitis B virus are in Chapter 67.

Hepatitis A vaccine is recommended for all high-risk adults ("B" recommendation). High-risk groups include persons living in, traveling to, or working in areas where the disease is endemic and periodic hepatitis A outbreaks occur (e.g., Alaska Native, Pacific Islander, and Native American communities, certain religious communities, countries with high or intermediate endemicity), men who have sex with men, users of injection or street drugs (depending on local epidemiology), military personnel, and certain hospital and laboratory workers. Hepatitis A vaccine may also be considered for institutionalized persons (e.g., in prisons and institutions for the developmentally disabled) and workers in these institutions and in day care centers. Where tracking or identification of high-risk patients is not practical or cost-effective, universal vaccination may be a reasonable policy given the minimal adverse consequences of the vaccine. At this writing, the only licensed hepatitis A vaccine is Havrix® (SmithKline Beecham Pharmaceuticals).* Two doses (1,440 ELISA units/dose) at 0 and 6–12 months are recommended for persons over age 18 years. The need for periodic booster doses of the vaccine has not been established. For persons requiring immediate protection against hepatitis A (e.g., travelers to high-risk areas who have not previously been vaccinated), clinicians may wish to consider giving IG simultaneously with the first dose of hepatitis A vaccine, although the clinical efficacy of this approach has not been established. IG can also be recommended as an efficacious intervention for short-term (≤5–6 months) preexposure prophylaxis against hepatitis A (see Chapter 67). While some evidence suggests that the vaccine may be more efficacious than IG, the clinical efficacies of these two interventions have not been directly compared. Other factors to consider in choosing between these two interventions include patient preference, the likely duration of exposure, the need for immediate vs. long-term protection, and cost.

Two doses of *varicella vaccine* delivered 4–8 weeks apart are recommended for healthy adults with no history of varicella infection or previous vaccination ("B" recommendation) (see Chapter 65 for the review of evidence regarding varicella vaccine). Vaccination efforts should be targeted to susceptible health care workers and family contacts of immunocompromised individuals, and may also be targeted to susceptible adults who live or work in environments with a high likelihood of varicella transmission (e.g., day care centers, residential institutions, colleges, military bases). Given the high prevalence of immunity in adults with no history of

---

*Use of trademarks is for identification only and does not imply endorsement by the Public Health Service or the U.S. Department of Health and Human Services.

chickenpox and the results of cost-effectiveness analysis (see Chapter 65), clinicians may wish to offer serologic testing for varicella susceptibility to history-negative adults who are likely to comply with return visits.

See Chapter 25 for recommendations regarding the Bacille Calmette-Guérin (BCG) vaccine. Recommendations on postexposure prophylaxis against selected infectious diseases, including tetanus, hepatitis A, and hepatitis B, are given in Chapter 67.

The draft update of this chapter was prepared for the U.S. Preventive Services Task Force by Carolyn DiGuiseppi, MD, MPH, based in part on background papers prepared for the U.S. Preventive Services Task Force by Modena Wilson, MD, MPH, and Donald Robinson, MD, MPH (measles vaccine), and for the Canadian Task Force on the Periodic Health Examination by Elaine Wang, MD, CM, FRCPC (pneumococcal vaccine).

REFERENCES

1. Centers for Disease Control and Prevention. Prevention and control of influenza: recommendations of the Advisory Committee on Immunization Practices (ACIP). MMWR 1995;44(RR-3):1–22.
2. Sullivan KM, Monto AS, Longini IM Jr. Estimates of the US health impact of influenza. Am J Public Health 1993;83:1712–1716.
3. American Academy of Pediatrics. In: Peter G, ed. 1994 Red Book: report of the Committee on Infectious Diseases. 23rd ed. Elk Grove Village, IL: American Academy of Pediatrics, 1994.
4. Meiklejohn G. Effectiveness of monovalent influenza A-prime vaccine during the 1957 influenza A-prime epidemic. Am J Hyg 1958;67:237–249.
5. Hoskins TW, Davies JR, Allchin A, et al. Controlled trial of inactivated influenza vaccine containing the A/Hong Kong strain during an outbreak of influenza due to the A/England/42/72 strain. Lancet 1973;ii:116–120.
6. Hammond ML, Ferris AA, Faine S, et al. Effective protection against influenza after vaccination with subunit vaccine. Med J Aust 1978;1:301–303.
7. Edmondson WP Jr, Rothenberg R, White PW, et al. A comparison of subcutaneous, nasal, and combined influenza vaccination. II. Protection against natural challenge. Am J Epidemiol 1971;93:480–486.
8. Edwards KM, Dupont WD, Westrich MK, et al. A randomized controlled trial of cold-adapted and inactivated vaccines for the prevention of influenza A disease. J Infect Dis 1994;169:68–76.
9. Weingarten S, Staniloff H, Ault M, et al. Do hospital employees benefit from the influenza vaccine? A placebo-controlled clinical trial. J Gen Intern Med 1988;3:32–37.
10. Govaert TME, Thijs CTMCN, Masurel N, et al. The efficacy of influenza vaccination in elderly individuals: a randomized double-blind placebo-controlled trial. JAMA 1994;272:1661–1665.
11. Schoenbaum SC, Mostow SR, Dowdle WR, et al. Studies with inactivated influenza vaccines purified by zonal centrifugation. 2. Efficacy. Bull WHO 1969;41:531–535.
12. Nichol KL, Margolis KL, Wuorenma J, et al. The efficacy and cost effectiveness of vaccination against influenza among elderly persons living in the community. N Engl J Med 1994;331:778–784.
13. Fedson DS, Wajda A, Nicol JP, et al. Clinical effectiveness of influenza vaccination in Manitoba[published erratum in JAMA 1994;271:1578]. JAMA 1993;270:1956–1961.
14. Foster DA, Talsma A, Furumoto-Dawson A, et al. Influenza vaccine effectiveness in preventing hospitalization for pneumonia in the elderly. Am J Epidemiol 1992;136:296–307.
15. Centers for Disease Control and Prevention. Final results: Medicare influenza vaccine demonstration—selected states, 1988–1992. MMWR 1993;42:601–604.
16. Barker WH, Mullooly JP. Influenza vaccination of elderly persons: reduction in pneumonia and influenza hospitalizations and deaths. JAMA 1980;244:2547–2549.

17. Saah AJ, Neufeld R, Rodstein M, et al. Influenza vaccine and pneumonia mortality in a nursing home population. Arch Intern Med 1986;146:2353–2357.

18. Horman JT, Stetler HC, Israel E, et al. An outbreak of influenza A in a nursing home. Am J Public Health 1986;76: 501–504.

19. Gross PA, Quinnan GV, Rodstein M, et al. Association of influenza immunization with reduction in mortality in an elderly population. A prospective study. Arch Intern Med 1988;148:562–565.

20. Patriarca PA, Weber JA, Parker RA, et al. Efficacy of influenza vaccine in nursing homes: reduction in illness and complications during an influenza A (H3N2) epidemic. JAMA 1985;253:1136–1139.

21. Arden NH, Patriarca PA, Fasano MB, et al. The roles of vaccination and amantadine prophylaxis in controlling an outbreak of influenza A (H3N2) in a nursing home. Arch Intern Med 1988;148:865–868.

22. Mast EE, Harmon MW, Gravenstein S, et al. Emergence and possible transmission of amantadine-resistant viruses during nursing home outbreaks of influenza A (H3N2). Am J Epidemiol 1991;134:988–997.

23. Patriarca PA, Weber JA, Parker RA, et al. Risk factors for outbreaks of influenza in nursing homes. A case-control study. Am J Epidemiol 1986;124:114–119.

24. Gravenstein S, Drinka P, Duthie EH, et al. Efficacy of an influenza hemagglutinin-diphtheria toxoid conjugate vaccine in elderly nursing home subjects during an influenza outbreak. J Am Geriatr Soc 1994;42:245–251.

25. Treanor JJ, Mattison HR, Dammed G, et al. Protective efficacy of combined live intranasal and inactivated influenza A virus vaccines in the elderly. Ann Intern Med 1992;117:625–633.

26. Sugaya N, Nerome K, Ishida M, et al. Efficacy of inactivated vaccine in preventing antigenically drifted influenza type A and well-matched type B. JAMA 1994;272:1122–1126.

27. Govaert TME, Dinant GJ, Aretz K, et al. Adverse reactions to influenza vaccine in elderly people: randomised double blind placebo controlled trial. BMJ 1993;307:988–990.

28. Margolis KL, Nichol KL, Poland GA, et al. Frequency of adverse reactions to influenza vaccine in the elderly: a randomized, placebo-controlled trial. JAMA 1990;264:1139–1141.

29. Oker-Blom N, Houi T, Leinikki P, et al. Protection of man from natural infection with influenza Hong Kong virus by amantadine: a controlled study. BMJ 1970;3:676–678.

30. Finklea JF, Hennessy AV, Davenport FM. A field trial of amantadine prophylaxis in naturally-occurring acute respiratory illness. Am J Epidemiol 1967;85:403–412.

31. Wendel HA, Snyder MT, Pell S. Trial of amantadine in epidemic influenza. Clin Pharmacol Ther 1966;7:38–43.

32. Dolin R, Reichman RC, Madore HP, et al. A controlled trial of amantadine and rimantadine in the prophylaxis of influenza A infection. N Engl J Med 1982;307:580–584.

33. Monto AS, Gunn RA, Bandyk MG, et al. Prevention of Russian influenza by amantadine. JAMA 1979;241: 1003–1007.

34. Nafta I, Turcanu AG, Braun I, et al. Administration of amantadine for the prevention of Hong Kong influenza. Bull WHO 1970;42:423–427.

35. Pettersson RF, Hellstrom P-E, Penttinen K, et al. Evaluation of amantadine in the prophylaxis of influenza A (H1N1) virus infection: a controlled field trial among young adults and high-risk patients. J Infect Dis 1980;142:377–383.

36. Mate J, Simon M, Juvancz I, et al. Prophylactic use of amantadine during Hong Kong influenza epidemic. Acta Microbiol Acad Sci Hung 1970;17:285–296.

37. Atkinson WL, Arden NH, Patriarca PA, et al. Amantadine prophylaxis during an institutional outbreak of Type A (H1N1) influenza. Arch Intern Med 1986;146:1751–1756.

38. Peters NL, Oboler S, Hair C, et al. Treatment of an influenza A outbreak in a teaching nursing home: effectiveness of a protocol for prevention and control. J Am Geriatr Soc 1989;37:210–218.

39. Hayden FG, Belshe RB, Clover RD, et al. Emergence and apparent transmission of rimantadine-resistant influenza A virus in families. N Engl J Med 1989;321:1696–1702.

40. Galbraith AW, Oxford JS, Schild GC, et al. Study of l-adamantanamine hydrochloride used prophylactically during the Hong Kong influenza epidemic in the family environment. Bull WHO 1969;41:677–682.

41. Galbraith AW, Oxford JS, Schild GC, et al. Protective effect of l-adamantanamine hydrochloride on influenza A2 infections in the family environment: a controlled double-blind study. Lancet 1969; 2:1026–1028.

42. Patriarca PA, Kater NA, Kendal AP, et al. Safety of prolonged administration of rimantadine hydrochloride in the prophylaxis of influenza A virus infections in nursing homes. Antimicrob Agents Chemother 1984;26:101–103.

43. Bryson YJ, Monahan C, Pollack M, et al. A prospective double-blind study of side effects associated with the administration of amantadine for influenza A virus prophylaxis. J Infect Dis 1980;141:543–547.

44. Soo W. Adverse effects of rimantadine: summary from clinical trials. J Respir Dis 1989;10:S26–31.

45. Brady MT, Sears SD, Clements ML, et al. Safety and efficacy of low-dose rimantadine for prophylaxis. J Respir Dis 1989;10:S32–37.

46. Bernstein JM, Betts RF, Demmler RW, et al. Safety and tolerance of rimantadine in elderly patients. J Respir Dis 1989;10:S38–41.

47. Reuman PD, Bernstein DI, Keefer MC, et al. Efficacy and safety of low dosage amantadine hydrochloride as prophylaxis for influenza A. Antiviral Res 1989;11:27–40.

48. Stange KC, Little DW, Blatnik B. Adverse reactions to amantadine prophylaxis of influenza in a retirement home. J Am Geriatr Soc 1991;33:700–705.

49. Degelau J, Somani S, Cooper SL, et al. Occurrence of adverse effects and high amantadine concentrations with influenza amantadine in the nursing home. J Am Geriatr Soc 1990;38:428–432.

50. Haglund LA, Istre GR, Pickett DA, et al. Invasive pneumococcal disease in Central Oklahoma: emergence of high-level penicillin resistance and multiple antibiotic resistance. J Infect Dis 1993;168:1532–1536.

51. Wenger JD, Hightower AW, Facklam RR, et al. Bacterial meningitis in the United States, 1986: report of a multistate surveillance study. J Infect Dis 1990;162:1316–1323.

52. Breiman RF, Spika JS, Navarro VJ, et al. Pneumococcal bacteremia in Charleston County, South Carolina. A decade later. Arch Intern Med 1990;150:1401–1405.

53. Bennett NM, Buffington J, LaForce FM. Pneumococcal bacteremia in Monroe County, New York. Am J Public Health 1992;82:1513–1516.

54. Schlech WF III, Ward JI, Band JD, et al. Bacterial meningitis in the United States, 1978 through 1981. The National Bacterial Meningitis Surveillance Study. JAMA 1985;253:1749–1754.

55. Davidson M, Schraer C, Parkinson A, et al. Invasive pneumococcal disease in an Alaska Native population, 1980 through 1986. JAMA 1989;261:715–718.

56. Cortese MM, Wolff M, Almeido-Hill J, et al. High incidence rates of invasive pneumococcal disease in the White Mountain Apache population. Arch Intern Med 1992;152:2277–2282.

57. Sims RV, Boyko EJ, Maislin G, et al. The role of age in susceptibility to pneumococcal infections. Age Ageing 1992;21:357–361.

58. Fine MJ, Orloff JJ, Arisumi D, et al. Prognosis of patients hospitalized with community-acquired pneumonia. Am J Med 1990;88:1N–8N.

59. Fang G-D, Fine M, Orloff J, et al. New and emerging etiologies for community-acquired pneumonia with implications for therapy. A prospective multicenter study of 359 cases. Medicine 1990;69:307–316.

60. Torres A, Serra-Batlles J, Ferrer A, et al. Severe community-acquired pneumonia: epidemiology and prognostic factors. Am Rev Respir Dis 1991;144:312–318.

61. Ortqvist A, Kalin M, Julander I, et al. Deaths in bacteremic pneumococcal pneumonia. A comparison of two populations—Huntington, WVa, and Stockholm, Sweden. Chest 1993;103:710–716.

62. Fine MJ, Smith MA, Carson CA, et al. A meta-analysis of prognostic studies in patients with community-acquired pneumonia [abstract]. Clin Res 1993;41:518A.

63. Jette LP, Lamothe F, and the Pneumococcus Study Group. Surveillance of invasive Streptococcus pneumoniae infection in Quebec, Canada, from 1984 to 1986: serotype distribution, antimicrobial susceptibility, and clinical characteristics. J Clin Microbiol 1989;27:1–5.

64. Plouffe JF, Moore SK, Davis R, et al. Serotypes of Streptococcus pneumoniae blood culture isolates from adults in Franklin County, Ohio. J Clin Microbiol 1994;32:1606–1607.

65. Breiman RF, Butler JC, Tenover FC, et al. Emergence of drug-resistant pneumococcal infections in the United States. JAMA 1994;271:1831–1835.

65a. Hofmann J, Cetron MS, Farley MM, et al. The prevalence of drug-resistant Streptococcus pneumoniae in Atlanta. N Engl J Med 1995;333:481–486.

66. Centers for Disease Control. Pneumococcal polysaccharide vaccine: recommendations of the Immunization Practices Advisory Committee (ACIP). MMWR 1989;38:64–68, 73–76.

67. Spika JS, Fedson DS, Facklam RR. Pneumococcal vaccination. Controversies and opportunities. Infect Dis Clin North Am 1990;4:11–27.

68. MacLeod CM, Hodges RG, Heidelberger M, et al. Prevention of pneumococcal pneumonia by immunization with specific capsular polysaccharides. J Exp Med 1945:82:445–465.

69. Smit P, Oberholzer D, Hayden-Smith S, et al. Protective efficacy of pneumococcal polysaccharide vaccines. JAMA 1977;238:2613–2616.

70. Austrian R, Douglas RM, Schiffman G, et al. Prevention of pneumococcal pneumonia by vaccination. Trans Assoc Am Phys 1976;89:184–194.

71. Riley ID, Tarr PI, Andrews M, et al. Immunisation with a polyvalent pneumococcal vaccine: reduction of adult respiratory mortality in a New Guinea Highlands community. Lancet 1977;1:1338–1341.

72. Austrian R. Surveillance of pneumococcal infection for field trials of polyvalent pneumococcal vaccines. Report DAB-VDP-12-84. Bethesda: National Institutes of Health, 1980.

73. Fine MJ, Smith MA, Carson CA, et al. Efficacy of pneumococcal vaccination in adults: a meta-analysis of randomized controlled trials. Arch Intern Med 1994;154:2666–2677.

74. Kaufman P. Pneumonia in old age. Active immunization against pneumonia with pneumococcus polysaccharide: results of a six year study. Arch Intern Med 1947;79:518–531.

75. Gaillat J, Zmirous D, Mallaret MR, et al. Essai clinique du vaccin antipneumococcique chez des personnes agées vivant en institution. Rev Epidemiol Santé Publique 1985;33:437–444.

76. Klastersky J, Mommen P, Cantraine F, et al. Placebo controlled pneumococcal immunization in patients with bronchogenic carcinoma. Eur J Cancer Clin Oncol 1986;22:807–813.

77. Simberkoff MS, Cross AP, Al-Ibrahim M, et al. Efficacy of pneumococcal vaccine in high-risk patients: results of a Veterans Administration Cooperative Study. N Engl J Med 1986;315:1318–1327.

78. Davis AL, Aranda CP, Schiffman G, et al. Pneumococcal infection and immunologic response to pneumococcal vaccine in chronic obstructive pulmonary disease: a pilot study. Chest 1987;92:204–212.

79. Leech JA, Gervais A, Ruben FL. Efficacy of pneumococcal vaccine in severe chronic obstructive pulmonary disease. Can Med Assoc J 1987;136:361–365.

80. Shapiro ED, Clemens JD. A controlled evaluation of the protective efficacy of pneumococcal vaccine for patients at high risk of serious pneumococcal infections. Ann Intern Med 1984;101:325–330.

81. Shapiro ED, Berg AT, Austrian R, et al. The protective efficacy of polyvalent pneumococcal polysaccharide vaccine. N Engl J Med 1991;325:1453–1460.

82. Bolan G, Broome CV, Facklam RR, et al. Pneumococcal vaccine efficacy in selected populations in the United States. Ann Intern Med 1986;104:1–6.

83. Sims RV, Steinmann WC, McConville JH, et al. The clinical effectiveness of pneumococcal vaccine in the elderly. Ann Intern Med 1988;108:653–657.

84. Butler JC, Breiman RF, Campbell JF, et al. Pneumococcal polysaccharide vaccine efficacy. An evaluation of current recommendations. JAMA 1993;270:1826–1831.

85. Forrester HL, Jahnigen DW, LaForce FM. Inefficacy of pneumococcal vaccine in a high-risk population. Am J Med 1987;83:425–430.

86. Ammann AJ, Addiego J, Wara DW, et al. Polyvalent pneumococcal-polysaccharide immunization of patients with sickle-cell anemia and patients with splenectomy. N Engl J Med 1977;297:897–900.

86a. Centers for Disease Control and Prevention. Final 1994 reports of notifiable diseases. MMWR 1995;44:537–543.

87. Centers for Disease Control and Prevention. Summary of notifiable diseases, United States, 1993. MMWR 1994;42:1–73.

88. Gergen PJ, McQuillan GM, Kiely M, et al. A population-based serologic survey of immunity to tetanus in the United States. N Engl J Med 1995;332:761–766.

89. Centers for Disease Control. Tetanus surveillance—United States, 1989–1990. MMWR 1992;41(SS-8):1–9.

90. Sutter RW, Cochi SL, Brink EW, et al. Assessment of vital statistics and surveillance data for monitoring tetanus mortality, United States, 1979–1984. Am J Epidemiol 1990;131:132–142.

91. Bjorkholm B, Bottiger M, Christenson B, et al. Antitoxin antibody levels and the outcome of illness during an outbreak of diphtheria among alcoholics. Scand J Infect Dis 1986;18:235–239.

92. Rappuoli R, Perugini M, Falsen E. Molecular epidemiology of the 1984–1986 outbreak of diphtheria in Sweden. N Engl J Med 1988;318:12–14.

93. Youwang Y, Jianming D, Yong X, et al. Epidemiological features of an outbreak of diphtheria and its control with diphtheria toxoid immunization. Int J Epidemiol 1992;21:807–811.

94. Centers for Disease Control and Prevention. Diphtheria epidemic—New Independent States of the former Soviet Union, 1990–1994. MMWR 1995;44:177–181.

95. Edsall G. Specific prophylaxis of tetanus. JAMA 1959;171:417–427.

96. Centers for Disease Control. Diphtheria, tetanus, and pertussis: recommendations for vaccine use and other preventive measures. Recommendations of the Immunization Practices Advisory Committee (ACIP). MMWR 1991;40(RR-10):1–28.

97. Simonsen O, Bentzon MW, Kjeldsen K, et al. Evaluation of vaccination requirements to secure continuous antitoxin immunity to tetanus. Vaccine 1987;5:115–122.

98. Simonsen O, Badsberg JH, Kjeldsen K, et al. The fall-off in serum concentrations of tetanus antitoxin after primary and booster vaccination. Acta Pathol Microbiol Scand 1986;94:77–82.

99. Simonsen O, Kjeldsen K, Heron I. Immunity against tetanus and effect of revaccination 25–30 years after primary vaccination. Lancet 1984;2:1240–1242.

100. Bottiger M, Pettersson G. Vaccine immunity to diphtheria: a 20-year follow-up study. Scand J Infect Dis 1992;753–758.

101. Gottlieb S, McLaughlin FX, Levine L, et al. Long term immunity to tetanus: a statistical evaluation and its clinical implications. Am J Public Health 1964;54:961–971.

102. McCarroll JR, Abrahams I, Skudder PA. Antibody response to tetanus toxoid 15 years after initial immunization. Am J Public Health 1962;52:1669–1675.

103. Trinca JC. Active immunization against tetanus: the need for a single all-purpose toxoid. Med J Aust 1965;2:116–120.

104. Trinca JC. Antibody response to successive booster doses of tetanus toxoid in adults. Infect Immun 1974;10:1–5.

105. Christenson B, Bottiger M. Epidemiology and immunity to tetanus in Sweden. Scand J Infect Dis 1987;19:429–435.

106. Wassilak SG, Walter AO. Tetanus. In: Plotkin SA, Mortimer EA, eds. Vaccines. Philadelphia: WB Saunders, 1988:45–73.

107. Reinstein L. Peripheral neuropathy after multiple tetanus toxoid boosters. Arch Phys Med Rehabil 1982;63:332–334.

108. Edsall G, Elliot MW, Peebles TG, et al. Excessive use of tetanus toxoid boosters. JAMA 1967; 202:111–113.

109. Hagen-Coenen J, Drinka PJ, Siewert M. Tetanus-diphtheria vaccinations in a veterans nursing home. J Am Geriatr Soc 1992;40:513–514.

110. Stratton KR, Johnson Howe C, Johnston RB Jr. Adverse events associated with childhood vaccines other than pertussis and rubella. JAMA 1994;271:1602–1605.

111. Centers for Disease Control and Prevention. Measles—United States, 1994. MMWR 1995;44:486–487, 493–494.

111a. Van Loon FPL, Holmes SJ, Sirotkin BI, et al. Mumps surveillance—United States, 1988–1993. In: CDC surveillance summaries, Aug 11, 1995. MMWR 1995;44(SS-3):1–14.

112. Markowitz E, Preblud SR, Katz SL. Measles vaccine. In: Plotkin SA, Mortimer EA, ed. Vaccines. 2nd ed. Philadelphia: WB Saunders, 1994.

113. Markowitz LE, Orenstein WA. Measles vaccine. Pediatr Clin North Am 1990;37:603–625.

114. Krugman S. Present status of measles and rubella immunization in the United States: a medical progress report. J Pediatr 1977;90:1–12.

115. Markowitz LE, Preblud SR, Fine PEM, et al. Duration of live measles vaccine-induced immunity. Pediatr Infect Dis J 1990;9:101–110.

116. Orenstein WA, Markowitz LE, Preblud SR, et al. The appropriate age for measles vaccination in the United States. Dev Biol Stand 1986;65:13–21.

117. Hersh BS, Markowitz LE, Hoffman RE, et al. A measles outbreak at a college with a prematriculation immunization requirement. Am J Public Health 1991;81:360–364.

118. Centers for Disease Control. Measles prevention: recommendations of the Immunization Practices Advisory Committee (ACIP). MMWR 1989;38(Suppl 9):1–18.

119. Baughman AL, Williams WW, Atkinson WL, et al. The impact of college prematriculation immunization requirements on risk for measles outbreaks. JAMA 1994;272:1127–1132.

120. Davis RM, Whitman ED, Orenstein WA, et al. A persistent outbreak of measles despite appropriate prevention and control measures. Am J Epidemiol 1987;126:438–449.

121. *Deleted in proof.*

122. Hutchins SS, Markowitz LE, Mead P, et al. A school-based measles outbreak: the effect of a selective revaccination policy and risk factors for vaccine failure. Am J Epidemiol 1990;132:157–168.

123. Nkowane BM, Bart SW, Orenstein WA, et al. Measles outbreak in a vaccinated school population: epidemiology, chains of transmission and the role of vaccine failures. Am J Public Health 1987;77:434–438.

124. Shasby DM, Shope TC, Downs H, et al. Epidemic measles in a highly vaccinated population. N Engl J Med 1977;296:585–589.

125. Crawford GE, Gremillion DH. Epidemic measles and rubella in air force recruits: impact of immunization. J Infect Dis 1981;144:403–410.

126. Chen RT, Moses JM, Markowitz LE, et al. Adverse events following measles-mumps-rubella and measles vaccinations in college students. Vaccine 1991;9:297–299.

127. Margolis HS, Alter MJ, Hadler SC. Hepatitis B: evolving epidemiology and implications for control. Semin Liver Dis 1991;11:84–92.

128. Advisory Committee on Immunization Practices (ACIP). Protection against viral hepatitis. MMWR 1990;39:1–26.

129. *Deleted in proof.*

130. McMahon BJ, Alward WL, Hall DB, et al. Acute hepatitis B virus infection: relation of age to the clinical expression of disease and subsequent development of the carrier state. J Infect Dis 1985;151:599–603.

131. Edmunds WJ, Medley GF, Nokes DJ, et al. The influence of age on the development of the hepatitis B carrier state. Proc R Soc Lond B Biol Sci 1993;253:197–201.

132. Sakuma K, Takahara T, Okuda K, et al. Prognosis of hepatitis B virus surface antigen carriers in relation to routine liver function tests: a prospective study. Gastroenterology 1982;83:114–117.

133. Lo KJ, Tong MJ, Chen MC, et al. The natural course of hepatitis B surface antigen-positive chronic active hepatitis in Taiwan. J Infect Dis 1982;146:205–210.

134. Szmuness W, Stevens CE, Harley EJ, et al. Hepatitis B vaccine: demonstration of efficacy in a controlled clinical trial in a high-risk population in the United States. N Engl J Med 1980;303:833–841.

135. Szmuness W, Stevens CE, Zang EA, et al. A controlled clinical trial of the efficacy of hepatitis B vaccine (Heptavax B): a final report. Hepatology 1981;1:377–385.

136. Francis DP, Hadler SC, Thompson SE, et al. The prevention of hepatitis B with vaccine: report of the Centers for Disease Control multi-center efficacy trial among homosexual men. Ann Intern Med 182;97:362–366.

137. Krugman S. The newly licensed hepatitis B vaccine. JAMA 1982;247:2012–2015.

138. Crosnier J, Jungers P, Courouce AM, et al. Randomised placebo-controlled trial of hepatitis B surface antigen vaccine in French haemodialysis units: I, medical staff. Lancet 1981;i:455–459.

139. Courouce AM, Laplanche A, Benhamou E, et al. Long-term efficacy of hepatitis B vaccination in healthy adults. In: Hollinger FB, Lemon SM, Margolis HF, eds. Viral hepatitis and liver disease. Baltimore: Williams & Wilkins, 1988:1002–1005.

140. Pongpipat D, Suvatte V, Assateerawatt A. Efficacy of hepatitis B virus (HBV) vaccine in long term prevention of HBV infection. Asian Pac J Allergy Immunol 1988;6:19–22.

141. Tabor E, Cairns J, Gerety RJ, et al. Nine-year follow-up study of a plasma-derived hepatitis B vaccine in a rural African setting. J Med Virol 1993;40:204–209.

142. Halliday ML, Rankin JG, Bristow NJ, et al. A randomized double-blind clinical trial of a mammalian cell-derived recombinant DNA hepatitis B vaccine compared with a plasma-derived vaccine. Arch Intern Med 1990;150:1195–1200.

143. Andre FE. Summary of safety and efficacy data on a yeast-derived hepatitis B vaccine. Am J Med 1989;87: 14S–20S.

144. Van Damme P, Vranckx R, Safary A, et al. Protective efficacy of a recombinant deoxyribonucleic acid hepatitis B vaccine in institutionalized mentally handicapped clients. Am J Med 1989;87:26S–29S.

145. Andre FE. Overview of a 5-year clinical experience with a yeast-derived hepatitis B vaccine. Vaccine 1990;8(suppl):S74–S78.

146. Shaw FE Jr, Guess HA, Roets JM, et al. Effect of anatomic injection site, age, and smoking on the immune response to hepatitis B vaccination. Vaccine 1989;7:425–430.

147. Wainwright RB, McMahon BJ, Bulkow LR, et al. Protection provided by hepatitis B vaccine in a Yupik Eskimo population. Arch Intern Med 1991;151:1634–1636.

148. Roome AJ, Walsh SJ, Cartter M, et al. Hepatitis B vaccine responsiveness in Connecticut public safety personnel. JAMA 1993;270:2931–2934.

149. Wood RC, MacDonald KL, White KE, et al. Risk factors for lack of detectable antibody following hepatitis B vaccination of Minnesota health care workers. JAMA 1993;270:2935–2939.

150. Crosnier J, Jungers P, Courouce AM, et al. Randomised placebo-controlled trial of hepatitis B surface antigen vaccine in French haemodialysis units: II, haemodialysis patients. Lancet 1981;i:797–800.

151. Stevens CE, Alter HJ, Taylor PE, et al. Hepatitis B vaccine in patients receiving hemodialysis: immunogenicity and efficacy. N Engl J Med 1984;311:496–501.

152. Buti M, Viladomiu L, Jardi R, et al. Long-term immunogenicity and efficacy of hepatitis B vaccine in hemodialysis patients. Am J Nephrol 1992;12:144–147.

153. Collier AC, Corey L, Murphy VL, et al. Antibody to human immunodeficiency virus (HIV) and suboptimal response to hepatitis B vaccination. Ann Intern Med 1988;109:101–105.

154. Rodrigo JM, Serra MA, Aparisi L, et al. Immune response to hepatitis B vaccine in parenteral drug abusers. Vaccine 1992;10:798–801.

155. Rumi MG, Colombo M, Romeo R, et al. Suboptimal response to hepatitis B vaccine in drug users. Arch Intern Med 1991;151:574–578.

156. Hadler SC, Francis DP, Maynard JE, et al. Long-term immunogenicity and efficacy of hepatitis B vaccine in homosexual men. N Engl J Med 1986;315:209–214.

157. Institute of Medicine. Adverse events associated with childhood vaccines: evidence bearing on causality. Washington, DC: National Academy Press, 1994.

158. Forbes A, Williams R. Increasing age—an important adverse prognostic factor in hepatitis A virus infection. J R Coll Phys Lond 1988;22:237–239.

159. Centers for Disease Control. Hepatitis A among homosexual men—United States, Canada, and Australia. MMWR 1992;41:155, 161–164.

160. Steffen R, Kane MA, Shapiro CN, et al. Epidemiology and prevention of hepatitis A in travelers. JAMA 1994;272:885–889.

161. Innis BL, Snitbhan R, Hunasol P, et al. Protection against hepatitis A by an inactivated vaccine. JAMA 1994;271:1328–1334.

162. Werzberger A, Mensch B, Kuter B, et al. A controlled trial of a formalin-inactivated hepatitis A vaccine in healthy children. N Engl J Med 1992;327:453–457.

163. McMahon BJ, Williams J, Bulkow L, et al. Immunogenicity of an inactivated hepatitis A vaccine in Alaska Native children and Native and non-Native adults. J Infect Dis 1995;171:676–679.

164. Van Damme P, Thoelen S, Cramm M, et al. Inactivated hepatitis A vaccine: reactogenicity, immunogenicity and long-term antibody persistence. J Med Virol 1994;44:446–451.

165. Briem H, Safary A. Immunogenicity and safety in adults of hepatitis A virus vaccine administered as a single dose with a booster 6 months later. J Med Virol 1994;44:443–445.

166. Westblom TU, Gudipati S, DeRousse C, et al. Safety and immunogenicity of an inactivated hepatitis A vaccine: effect of dose and vaccination schedule. J Infect Dis 1994;169:996–1001.

167. Kallinowski B, Gmelin K, Kommerell B, et al. Immunogenicity, reactogenicity and consistency of a new, inactivated hepatitis A vaccine—a randomized multicentre study with three consecutive vaccine lots. Vaccine 1992;10:500–501.

168. Tilzey AJ, Palmer SJ, Barrow S, et al. Clinical trial with inactivated hepatitis A vaccine and recommendations for its use [published erratum BMJ 1992;304:1352]. BMJ 1992;304:1272–1276.

169. Clemens R, Safary A, Hepburn A, et al. Clinical experience with an inactivated hepatitis A vaccine. J Infect Dis 1995;171(Suppl 1):S44–S49.

170. Ellerbeck EF, Lewis JA, Nalin D, et al. Safety profile and immunogenicity of an inactivated vaccine derived from an attenuated strain of hepatitis A. Vaccine 1992;10:668–672.

170a. Centers for Disease Control and Prevention. Update: recommendations to prevent hepatitis B virus transmission—United States. MMWR 1995;44:574–575.

171. Van Damme P, Mathei C, Thoelen S, et al. Single dose inactivated hepatitis A vaccine: rationale and clinical assessment of the safety and immunogenicity. J Med Virol 1994;44:435–441.

172. Jilg W, Bittner R, Bock HL, et al. Vaccination against hepatitis A: comparison of different short-term immunization schedules. Vaccine 1992;10(Suppl 1):S126–S128.

173. Wagner G, Lavanchy D, Darioli R, et al. Simultaneous active and passive immunization against hepatitis A studied in a population of travelers. Vaccine 1993;11:1027–1032.

174. Ambrosch F, Andre FE, Delem A, et al. Simultaneous vaccination against hepatitis A and B: results of a controlled study. Vaccine 1992;10(Suppl 1):S142–S145.

175. Shouval D, Ashur Y, Adler R, et al. Safety, tolerability, and immunogenicity of an inactivated hepatitis A vaccine: effects of single and booster injections, and comparison to administration of immune globulin. J Hepatol 1993; 18(Suppl 2):S32–S37.

176. Leentvaar-Kuijpers A, Coutinho RA, Brulein V, et al. Simultaneous passive and active immunization against hepatitis A. Vaccine 1992;10(Suppl 1):S138–S141.

177. Fujiyama S, Odoh K, Kuramoto I, et al. Current seroepidemiological status of hepatitis A with a comparison of antibody titers from infection and vaccination. J Hepatol 1994;21:641–645.

178. Fujiyama S, Iino S, Odoh K, et al. Time course of hepatitis A virus antibody titer after active and passive immunization. Hepatology 1992;15:983–988.

179. Iino S, Fujiyama S, Horiuchi K, et al. Clinical trial of a lyophilized inactivated hepatitis A candidate vaccine in healthy adult volunteers. Vaccine 1992;10:323–328.

180. Wiedermann G, Ambrosch F, Kollaritsch H, et al. Safety and immunogenicity of an inactivated hepatitis A candidate vaccine in healthy adult volunteers. Vaccine 1990;8:581–584.

181. Green MS, Cohen D, Lerman Y, et al. Depression of the immune response to an inactivated hepatitis A vaccine administered concomitantly with immune globulin. J Infect Dis 1993;168:740–743.

182. Riedemann S, Reinhardt G, Frosner GG, et al. Placebo-controlled efficacy study of hepatitis A vaccine in Valdivia, Chile. Vaccine 1992:10(Suppl 1):S152–S155.

183. Horng Y-C, Chang M-H, Lee C-Y, et al. Safety and immunogenicity of hepatitis A vaccine in healthy children. Pediatr Infect Dis J 1993;12:359–362.

184. American College of Physicians Task Force on Adult Immunization and Infectious Diseases Society of America. Guide for adult immunization. 3rd ed. Philadelphia: American College of Physicians, 1994.

185. American Academy of Family Physicians. Age charts for periodic health examination. Kansas City, MO: American Academy of Family Physicians, 1994. (Reprint no. 510.)

186. Canadian Task Force on the Periodic Health Examination. Canadian guide to clinical preventive health care. Ottawa: Canada Communication Group, 1994: 386–395, 744–751.

186a. American College of Obstetricians and Gynecologists. The obstetrician-gynecologist and primary-preventive care. Washington, DC: American College of Obstetricians and Gynecologists, 1993.

187. Centers for Disease Control. Update on adult immunization: recommendations of the Immunization Practices Advisory Committee (ACIP). MMWR 1991;40(RR-12):1–94.

188. Centers for Disease Control. Hepatitis B virus: a comprehensive strategy for eliminating transmission in the United States through universal childhood vaccination. Recommendations of the Immunization Practices Advisory Committee (ACIP). MMWR 1991;40(RR-13):1–25.

189. Centers for Disease Control. Rubella prevention: recommendations of the Immunization Practices Advisory Committee (ACIP). MMWR 1990;39(RR-15):1–18.

189a. Centers for Disease Control and Prevention. Varicella prevention: recommendations of the Advisory Committee on Immunization Practices (ACIP). MMWR 1996 (in press).

189b. Advisory Committee on Immunization Practices. Licensure of inactivated hepatitis A vaccine and recommendations for use among international travelers. MMWR 1995;44:559–560.

190. Centers for Disease Control and Prevention. Recommendations of the Advisory Committee on Immunization Practices (ACIP): use of vaccines and immune globulins in persons with altered immunocompetence. MMWR 1993;42(RR-4):1–18.

191. American College of Obstetricians and Gynecologists. Immunization during pregnancy. Technical Bulletin no. 160. Washington, DC: American College of Obstetricians and Gynecologists, 1991.

192. Centers for Disease Control and Prevention. Prevention and control of influenza: part II, antiviral agents: recommendations of the Advisory Committee on Immunization Practices (ACIP). MMWR 1994;43(RR-15):1–10.

193. Fedson DS. Adult immunization: summary of the National Vaccine Advisory Committee Report. JAMA 1994;272:1133–1137.

194. Sisk JE, Riegelman RK. Cost effectiveness of vaccination against pneumococcal pneumonia: an update. Ann Intern Med 1986;104:79–86.

195. Mullooly JP, Bennett MD, Hornbrook MC, et al. Influenza vaccination programs for elderly persons: cost-effectiveness in a health maintenance organization. Ann Intern Med 1994;121:947–952.

196. Jonsson B. Cost-benefit analysis of hepatitis B vaccination. Postgrad Med J 1987;63(Suppl 2):27–32.

197. Mulley AG, Silverstein MD, Dienstag JL. Indications for use of hepatitis B vaccine, based on cost-effectiveness analysis. N Engl J Med 1982;307:644–652.

198. Bloom BS, Hillman AL, Fendrick AM, et al. A reappraisal of hepatitis B virus vaccination strategies using cost-effectiveness analysis. Ann Intern Med 1993;118:298–306.

199. Balestra DJ, Littenberg B. Should adult tetanus immunization be given as a single vaccination at age 65? A cost-effectiveness analysis. J Gen Intern Med 1993;8:405–412.
200. Sutter RW, Strikas RA, Hadler SC. Tetanus immunization: concerns about the elderly and about diphtheria reemergence [letter]. J Gen Intern Med 1994;9:117–118.
201. Bryan JP, Nelson M. Testing for antibody to hepatitis A to decrease the cost of hepatitis A prophylaxis with immune globulin or hepatitis A vaccines. Arch Intern Med 1994;154:663–668.
202. Jefferson TO, Behrens RH, Demicheli V. Should British soldiers be vaccinated against hepatitis A? An economic analysis. Vaccine 1994;12:1379–1383.

67. Postexposure Prophylaxis for Selected Infectious Diseases

RECOMMENDATION

Postexposure prophylaxis should be provided to selected persons with exposure or possible exposure to Haemophilus influenzae type b, hepatitis A, hepatitis B, meningococcal, rabies, or tetanus pathogens (see *Clinical Intervention*). See Chap-ter 66 for recommendations on postexposure prophylaxis against influenza A.

HAEMOPHILUS INFLUENZAE TYPE B DISEASE

Burden of Suffering

The incidence of invasive *H. influenzae* type b (Hib) disease (e.g., meningitis, epiglottitis, septic arthritis) has decreased dramatically in recent years, most likely due to the immunization of infants and young children with effective vaccines, with 1,174 cases reported in 1994.[1] The incidence of invasive Hib disease among children less than 5 years of age decreased from 41/100,000 in 1987 to fewer than 2/100,000 in 1994.[2] Most cases occur during infancy,[3,4] but many children remain susceptible to infection until age 4–5 years. Young children are at especially increased risk if they are exposed to infected persons at home or in day care.[3,5–7] Most secondary cases of Hib disease in household contacts occur within 1–2 weeks of the primary case.[5]

Efficacy of Prophylaxis

Rifampin prophylaxis can reduce the risk of secondary infection in persons exposed to Hib. A randomized controlled clinical trial and an uncontrolled trial have shown that a 4-day antibiotic regimen can reduce both the rate of asymptomatic carriage of Hib and the incidence of secondary infection in household and day care contacts of infected persons.[8,9] Postexposure prophylaxis for Hib may prove unnecessary eventually, given widespread childhood immunization with the Hib conjugate vaccine (see Chapter 65). In addition to protecting the vaccinated child against Hib infection, conjugate vaccine appears to decrease Hib pharyngeal colonization,[10,11] which would also reduce Hib transmission to unvaccinated children.

HEPATITIS A AND B

Burden of Suffering

Epidemics caused by hepatitis A virus (HAV) remain a major public health problem, with 26,796 cases reported in 1994 in the U.S.[1] HAV is transmitted through the fecal-oral route, and the most frequent source of infection is household or sexual contact with a person who has hepatitis A. Day care centers have become an important source of epidemic HAV infection.[12] In the U.S. each year, hepatitis B virus (HBV) causes an estimated 200,000 to 300,000 acute infections and 4,000–5,000 deaths from chronic liver disease and hepatocellular carcinoma.[13] More than 1 million Americans have chronic HBV infection. HBV may be transmitted by perinatal (see Chapter 24), percutaneous, sexual, or mucosal exposure.[14]

Efficacy of Prophylaxis

Since the 1940s, passive immunization with immune globulin (IG), administered within 2 weeks of exposure, has been shown to be an effective means of preventing or markedly attenuating clinical hepatitis A in persons exposed to HAV.[15] Studies in household contacts have shown that IG can reduce the incidence of clinical hepatitis A by 80–90%.[16] The earlier that IG is given after exposure the more likely it is that protection will result.[16] Adverse effects of IG include local symptoms and, less commonly, systemic symptoms such as headache, chills, and nausea.[12] Serious adverse effects with IG have been rare.[13] There is no evidence of transmission of HBV, human immunodeficiency virus, or other viruses in the U.S. by IG prepared for intramuscular injection.[13] Hepatitis C transmission has been reported with intravenous administration of an immune globulin product.[16a]

Immunogenic inactivated hepatitis A vaccines, recently licensed in the U.S., have been shown to be highly protective against hepatitis A (see Chapters 65 and 66).[17,18] Because an adequate immune response does not develop for 1–2 weeks after vaccine administration,[17,19–22] the vaccine alone is likely to be inadequate for postexposure prophylaxis. Vaccine may be given simultaneously with IG for individuals with both immediate and continued risk of hepatitis A. Although studies have reported lower mean antibody titers when the vaccine is administered concomitantly with IG, vaccine seroconversion rates appear to be adequate.[20,23,24]

Administration of hepatitis B immune globulin (HBIG) promptly after exposure and 1 month later has a combined efficacy of about 75% in protecting susceptible persons with perinatal, percutaneous, sexual, or mucosal exposure to HBV.[25–28] Hepatitis B vaccine is highly immunogenic and efficacious and can be used to provide both preexposure and postexposure protection (see Chapters 24, 65, and 66).[29] Two recombinant DNA hepatitis B vaccines are currently licensed in the U.S. and, in recommended dosages, provide similar seroconversion rates. Combined active-passive immunization has the advantage of providing both immediate and long-term protection.[30] For infants born to mothers who are infected with HBV, the combination of HBIG given at birth and hepatitis B vaccine given at birth and ages 1 and 6 months is 85–90% effective in preventing perinatal HBV transmission (see Chapter 24).[31-34] Regimens involving a vaccine series alone have shown 70–85% efficacy in preventing perinatal transmission (see Chapters 24 and 65).

MENINGOCOCCAL INFECTION
Burden of Suffering

Infection with *Neisseria meningitidis* serotypes A, B, C, X, Y, Z, 29-E, and W-135 can lead to meningitis and fulminant septicemia. Meningococcal infections occur sporadically, with 2,886 cases reported in the U.S. in 1994.[1] The estimated incidence during 1989–1991 in the U.S. was 1/100,000 persons annually.[35] The potential exists for epidemic meningococcal disease.

Efficacy of Prophylaxis

Both chemoprophylaxis and vaccination are available for postexposure prophylaxis against meningococcal infection, although vaccines are not routinely recommended for postexposure prophylaxis. Rifampin prophylaxis in contacts of patients with meningococcal infection can reduce the rate of meningococcal colonization, thereby reducing the risk of secondary infection.[36-38] Rifampin dosage schedules effective in eliminating meningococci in adults have included 600 mg taken once daily for 4 days or twice daily for 2 days.[36-40] One study has shown that a single intramuscular dose of ceftriaxone is at least as effective as oral rifampin in eliminating pharyngeal carriage in family contacts;[39] its efficacy has only been confirmed for serogroup A strains.

Due to the relatively long interval (as long as 14–30 days) that can occur between primary and secondary cases,[41,42] meningococcal vaccines also may be efficacious for postexposure prophylaxis against serogroups contained in the vaccine.[43] A quadrivalent vaccine effective against meningococcal serogroups A, C, Y, and W-135,[12,44] is available in the U.S. and has been effective in interrupting epidemic disease in other developed countries.[45,46] The serogroup A component is immunogenic in children ≥3 months of age,[47] but children less than 2 years of age do not always respond to the vaccine's other components. The current vaccine does not provide adequate long-term protection. A satisfactory vaccine to prevent group B meningococcal disease has yet to be developed. One vaccine against group B meningococcus was estimated to be 74% effective in children aged 4–6 years but was not proven effective in younger children.[48] Conjugate meningococcal vaccines, which may be more immunogenic, are currently being evaluated.[49,50] The serogroup specificity of currently available meningococcal vaccines requires that the infecting organism be properly characterized.

RABIES

Burden of Suffering

In the absence of adequate prophylaxis, persons infected with rabies almost always die from rabies encephalitis.[51] Human rabies is an uncommon disease in the U.S., with only 33 cases diagnosed from 1977 to 1994, 15 of which were associated with exposure to dogs outside the country or at the U.S.-Mexican border.[52] Bat-associated rabies virus has been associated with at least 10 cases.[52] Wild animals now constitute the largest source of human infection acquired in the U.S. A recent outbreak among raccoons in the northeastern states has been responsible for a large increase in the incidence of animal rabies, although no human transmission has been reported.[53] In the U.S., squirrels, chipmunks, and other rodents have not been implicated in any human cases.[51] More than 18,000 persons receive postexposure prophylaxis yearly for rabies.[54] Another 10,000 persons at increased risk receive preexposure prophylaxis.

Efficacy of Prophylaxis

Currently recommended postexposure prophylaxis consists of wound cleansing, human rabies immune globulin (HRIG) administered at the site of the bite and into the gluteal muscle, and a vaccination series administered into the deltoid muscle. Two vaccine preparations, human diploid cell vaccine (HDCV) and rabies vaccine, adsorbed (RVA) are available in the U.S. No vaccine failure has been reported in the U.S. in anyone who received postexposure prophylaxis using the current regimen.[55] Field experience has shown that this regimen provides adequate virus-neutralizing antibody titers.[56–59] Studies from developing countries have reported adequate antibody titers and clinical efficacy with varied dosages, schedules, and routes of administration of potent rabies vaccines (HDCV and others).[55,60–62b] Deviations from current recommendations, including gluteal HDCV administration, inadequate wound cleansing, and incorrect use of HRIG, may have been responsible for 13 rabies cases that occurred after administration of postexposure prophylaxis in other countries.[63–66] Two cohort studies have shown that gluteal, as opposed to deltoid, administration of HDCV results in lower antibody titers.[67,68] Reported adverse effects of HDCV include systemic allergic reactions[69] and, rarely, Guillain-Barré-like illnesses.[70–72]

Preexposure rabies vaccination is recommended for persons at high risk of rabies exposure. A three-dose series of HDCV (1.0 mL intramuscularly [IM] or 0.1 mL intradermally) or RVA (1.0 mL IM), given in the deltoid region on days 0, 7, and 21 or 28, provides an antibody response in virtually all individuals, lasting at least 2 years.[73–76] Recent studies have reported a continuous decline in antibody levels over time.[77,78] A two-dose booster is therefore recommended after an exposure. One rabies case has been reported following preexposure rabies vaccination;[79] this patient did not receive the recommended two-dose booster following exposure. Immune complex hypersensitivity develops in 6% of persons given a HDCV booster dose after the initial series.[69,80,81] A recent randomized clinical trial reports that purified HDCV used for boosters causes fewer severe and urticarial reactions.[82]

TETANUS

Burden of Suffering

Largely as a result of childhood immunization, tetanus has become uncommon in the U.S., with only 51 cases reported in 1994.[1] Tetanus remains a serious disease with 24% of recent cases resulting in death. Reports may underrepresent tetanus mortality by as much as 60%.[83] Most persons with tetanus had not received a primary immunization series.[84] Seventy-eight percent of cases followed an acute injury, half of which were puncture wounds. At least half of cases of tetanus and deaths from tetanus occur in persons over the age of 60.[1,84] In the third National Health and Nutrition Examination Survey (NHANES III), the prevalence of immunity to tetanus declined with increasing age beginning at age 40.[85] More than 80% of persons aged 6–39 years, but only 28% of persons 70 years and older, had protective antibody levels.

Efficacy of Prophylaxis

The use of equine tetanus immune globulin (TIG) resulted in a dramatic decline in the incidence of clinical tetanus during World War I.[86,87] Numerous animal trials[88,89] and an uncontrolled experiment involving two humans[90] established the protective serum antitoxin level at 0.01 unit/mL, although there have been several case reports of clinical tetanus despite higher serum antitoxin levels.[91–93] In unimmunized individuals, the combination of 250 units human TIG and 0.5 mL adsorbed tetanus toxoid provides a serum antitoxin level of 0.01 unit/mL immediately that lasts beyond 4 weeks.[94–98] Individuals who have completed a primary vaccination series (three doses and one booster) have serum antitoxin levels of ≥0.01 unit/mL for at least 20 years.[99–101] Booster immunization results in a vigorous anamnestic response after periods as long as 20–30 years following a three-dose primary vaccination series;[100,101] recent data suggest, however, that some individuals who receive their first booster 17–20 years after a primary vaccination series may not develop protective antitoxin levels immediately.[102] There is animal evidence to suggest that protection begins before a rise in antitoxin is detected.[103] Furthermore, tetanus is unlikely in persons who have received a primary vaccination series at any time.[83,104] Serious adverse effects of tetanus toxoid are rare, although several case reports and a case series have described allergic or Arthus-like reactions and peripheral neuropathy following frequent boosters.[105,106]

Recommendations of Other Groups

The Advisory Committee on Immunization Practices,[13,54,55,74,107–109] the American Academy of Pediatrics,[12] and the American College of Physicians[110] have issued recommendations on postexposure prophylaxis for Hib disease, hepatitis A and B, meningococcal infection, rabies, and tetanus that are similar to those described below. The American College of Obstetricians and Gynecologists has issued detailed guidelines on the use of vaccines during pregnancy.[111]

CLINICAL INTERVENTION

Postexposure prophylaxis is recommended for selected persons with exposure or possible exposure to *H. influenzae* type b, hepatitis A, hepatitis B, meningococcal, rabies, or tetanus pathogens ("A" recommendation). Details are given below.

H. influenzae Type b Disease. **Oral rifampin prophylaxis should be prescribed promptly for patients with Hib disease and for all their household contacts regardless of age, if at least one of the contacts is a child less than 4 years of age who has not been fully vaccinated with a licensed Hib conjugate vaccine. Experts define a household contact as a person residing with the index patient or a nonresident who spent 4 hours or more with the index patient for at least 5 of the 7 days preceding the day of hospital admission of the index patient.[12] The dosage of rifampin for children and adults is 20 mg/kg (maximum 600 mg) as a single daily dose for 4 days. The dose for infants younger than 1 month of age has not been established, but experts recommend reducing the dose to 10 mg/kg/day.[12] Published guidelines also recommend postexposure prophylaxis for all day care attendees and staff, regardless of vaccination status, when 2 or more cases have occurred within 60 days and unvaccinated or incompletely vaccinated children attend.[12] When a single case has occurred in a day care center, rifampin prophylaxis should be given to all attendees and staff** only if unvaccinated or incompletely vaccinated children less than 2 years of age are present in the center for at least 25 hours per week.[12] Day care contacts of children with Hib disease should receive rifampin prophylaxis using the same regimen as for household contacts. All children who are less than 5 years of age and who are unvaccinated or incompletely vaccinated should be brought up to date by administration of the recommended doses of a licensed Hib conjugate vaccine (see Chapter 65).

Hepatitis A. Immune globulin should be administered at a dose of 0.02 mL/kg IM as soon as possible within 2 weeks of exposure to sexual and close household contacts of persons with hepatitis A, staff and children at day care centers where a hepatitis A case is recognized, staff and patients at custodial institutions where HAV transmission is documented, and food handlers at food service establishments where a food handler is diagnosed with hepatitis A. Detailed published protocols are available.[12,13,110] Hepatitis A vaccine is recommended for persons ≥2 years of age who are at high risk for infection (see Chapters 65 and 66).

Hepatitis B. The use of HBIG and hepatitis B vaccine is recommended to prevent HBV infection in the following circumstances: birth of an infant to a hepatitis B surface antigen (HBsAg)-positive mother (see Chapter 24), percutaneous or permucosal exposure to HBsAg-positive blood, sexual exposure to an HBsAg-positive person, and household exposure of an infant less than 1 year of age to a primary caregiver who has acute HBV infection. For needlesticks and other percutaneous exposures, and for sexual exposures, the precise protocol for postexposure prophylaxis against hepatitis B depends on the nature of the exposure, the availability from the source of exposure of blood for testing, the HBsAg status of the source, and the hepatitis B vaccination and vaccine-response status of the exposed person. Detailed guidelines are available.[12,13] See Chapter 24 for detailed recommendations on prenatal screening and perinatal postexposure prophylaxis against HBV infection, and Chapters 65 and 66 for recommendations regarding routine use of hepatitis B vaccine in children and adults.

Meningococcal Infection. Oral rifampin prophylaxis is indicated for household or day care contacts of persons with meningococcal infection, as well as for those with direct exposure to oral secretions (e.g., kissing) of an index patient. The dose is 600 mg for adults, 10 mg/kg for children 1–12 years of age, and 5 mg/kg for infants 3 months to 1 year of age, given twice daily for 2 days (for a total of four doses). Rifampin is contraindicated during pregnancy. There is currently insufficient evidence to recommend for or against the use of ceftriaxone for routine meningococcal prophylaxis ("C" recommendation). Ceftriaxone at a dose of 250 mg IM for adults and 125 mg IM for children is efficacious for eliminating meningococcal carriage of serogroup A strains of meningococcus. In outbreaks caused by serogroup A strains, the use of meningococcal vaccine is recommended in addition to antibiotic prophylaxis for all persons ≥3 months of age. In outbreaks caused by serogroup C, Y, and W-135 strains, vaccination is recommended for persons ≥2 years of age.[12]

Rabies. Postexposure prophylaxis against rabies should be instituted if a possible exposure to rabies has occurred. Criteria for making this assessment, which include the type of animal (e.g., carnivorous wild animals, bats), the circumstances of the attack (e.g., unprovoked attack), and the type of exposure (e.g., bite), are available in published guidelines[55,110] and from local health departments. HRIG is given at a dose of 20 IU/kg; half of the dose is infiltrated around the wound, and the remainder is given intramuscularly at another site. The upper outer gluteal region of the buttocks is preferred because of the large volume administered. HDCV or RVA is administered in the deltoid muscle in five 1.0 mL injections on days 0, 3, 7, 14, and 28. Persons who were immunized before the incident require only two 1.0 mL doses of vaccine on days 0 and 3, and do not require HRIG. Preexposure prophylaxis with three injections (1.0 mL IM or 0.1 mL intradermally) of vaccine (days 0, 7, and 21 or 28) is recommended for those at high risk of contact with rabies virus, including rabies laboratory workers, veterinarians, animal handlers, and persons planning to spend more than 1 month in countries where rabies is endemic. Persons with frequent exposure should have their antibody level checked every 6 months and receive booster injections if antibody titers are below protective levels. Published guidelines suggest more frequent testing for certain continuously exposed laboratory workers.[55,110]

Tetanus. All individuals who have not completed a primary vaccination series of at least three doses and who present with wounds should receive 0.5 mL IM adsorbed tetanus toxoid. Diphtheria and tetanus toxoids and whole-cell or acellular pertussis vaccine adsorbed (DTP or DTaP, respectively) or diphtheria and tetanus toxoids adsorbed (DT) (as appropriate) for patients less than 7 years old and tetanus and diphtheria toxoids adsorbed (Td) for patients ≥7 years old, are preferred so that adequate levels of diphtheria and pertussis immunity are maintained (see Chapters 65 and 66). For a wound that is serious and/or contaminated (e.g., with dirt, feces), the incompletely vaccinated patient should receive both vaccine and human TIG (250 units IM at a separate site). Although there is inadequate evidence on which to make a recommendation for or against TIG prophylaxis for clean, minor wounds in inadequately immunized persons, experts recommend against the routine use of human TIG.[12,109,110] For individuals presenting with a wound who have completed a primary vaccination series of at least three doses, tetanus toxoid is recommended if more than 10 years have elapsed since the last dose or if only three doses of fluid toxoid (which was used prior to the availability of adsorbed toxoid) were received. There is insufficient evidence to document increased risk after a shorter interval for major or contaminated wounds, but expert opinion supports vaccination when more than 5 years have elapsed.[12,109,110] Human TIG is not recommended for persons who have completed a primary vaccination series. All wounds should be properly cleaned and debrided.

Influenza. See Chapter 66 for recommendations regarding the use of amantadine and rimantadine to protect against influenza A.

The draft update of this chapter was prepared for the U.S. Preventive Services Task Force by Robert Reid, MD, MPH, Carolyn DiGuiseppi, MD, MPH, Cameron Grant, MBChB, and Modena Wilson, MD, MPH.

REFERENCES

1. Centers for Disease Control and Prevention. Final 1994 reports of notifiable diseases. MMWR 1995;44:537–543.
2. Centers for Disease Control. Progress toward elimination of *Haemophilus influenzae* type b disease among infants and children—United States, 1993–1994. MMWR 1995;44:545–550.
3. Redmond SR, Pichichero ME. *Haemophilus influenzae* type b disease: an epidemiologic study with special reference to day-care centers. JAMA 1984;252:2581–2584.
4. Casto DT, Edwards DL. Preventing *Haemophilus influenzae* type b disease. Clin Pharmacol 1985;4:637–648.
5. Ward JI, Fraser DW, Baraff LJ, et al. *Haemophilus influenzae* meningitis: a national study of secondary spread in household contacts. N Engl J Med 1979;301:122–126.
6. Fleming DW, Leibenhaut MH, Albanes D, et al. Secondary *Haemophilus influenzae* type b in day-care facilities: risk factors and prevention. JAMA 1985;254:509–514.
7. Makintubee S, Istre GR, Ward JI. Transmission of invasive *Haemophilus influenzae* type b disease in day care settings. J Pediatr 1987;111:180–186.
8. Band JD, Fraser DW, Ajello G. Prevention of *Haemophilus influenzae* type b disease. JAMA 1984;251: 2381–2386.
9. Granoff DM, Gilsdorf J, Gessert C, et al. *Haemophilus influenzae* type B disease in a day care center: eradication of carrier state by rifampin. Pediatrics 1979;63:397–401.
10. Murphy TV, Pastor P, Medley F, et al. Decreased *Haemophilus* colonization in children vaccinated with *Haemophilus influenzae* type b conjugate vaccine. J Pediatr 1993;122:517–523.
11. Barbour ML, Mayon-White RT, Coles C, et al. The impact of conjugate vaccine on carriage of *Haemophilus influenzae* type b. J Infect Dis 1995;171:93–98.
12. American Academy of Pediatrics. 1994 Red Book: report of the Committee on Infectious Diseases. 23rd ed. Elk Grove, IL: American Academy of Pediatrics, 1994.
13. Immunization Practices Advisory Committee. Protection against viral hepatitis. MMWR 1990;39(RR-2):1–26.
14. Gerberding JL. Management of occupational exposures to blood-borne viruses. N Engl J Med 1995;332:444–451.
15. Hollinger FB, Glombicki AP. Hepatitis A virus. In: Mandell GL, Douglas RG, Bennett JE, eds. Principles and practice of infectious diseases. 3rd ed. New York: Churchill Livingstone, 1990:1383–1399.
16. Mosley JW, Reisler DM, Brachott D, et al. Comparison of two lots of immune serum globulin for prophylaxis of infectious hepatitis. Am J Epidemiol 1968;87:539–550.
16a. Bresee JS, Mast E, Alter MJ, et al. Hepatitis C associated with intravenous immunoglobulin administration [abstr]. Presented at the 44th Annual Epidemic Intelligence Service Conference, Atlanta, GA, March 27–31, 1995.

17. Werzberger A, Mensch B, Kuter B, et al. A controlled trial of a formalin-inactivated hepatitis A vaccine in healthy children. N Engl J Med 1992;327:453–457.

18. Innis BL, Snitbhan R, Kunasol P, et al. Protection against hepatitis A by an inactivated vaccine. JAMA 1994;271:1328–1334.

19. Briem H, Safary A. Immunogenicity and safety in adults of hepatitis A virus vaccine administered as a single dose with a booster 6 months later. J Med Virol 1994;44:443–445.

20. Leentvaar-Kuijpers A, Coutinho RA, Brulein V, et al. Simultaneous passive and active immunization against hepatitis A. Vaccine 1992;10(Suppl 1):S138–S141.

21. Van Damme P, Mathei C, Thoelen S, et al. Single dose inactivated hepatitis A vaccine: rationale and clinical assessment of the safety and immunogenicity. J Med Virol 1994;44:435–441.

22. Jilg W, Bittner R, Bock HL, et al. Vaccination against hepatitis A: comparison of different short-term immunization schedules. Vaccine 1992;10(Suppl 1):S126–S128.

23. Green MS, Cohen D, Lerman Y, et al. Depression of the immune response to an inactivated hepatitis A vaccine administered concomitantly with imune globulin. J Infect Dis 1993;168:740–743.

24. Wagner G, Lavanchy D, Darioli R, et al. Simultaneous active and passive immunization against hepatitis A studied in a population of travelers. Vaccine 1993;11:1027–1032.

25. Maynard JE. Passive immunization against hepatitis B: a review of recent studies and comment on current aspects of control. Am J Epidemiol 1978;107:77–86.

26. Hoofnagle JH, Seeff LB, Bales ZB, et al. Passive-active immunity from hepatitis B immune globulin: reanalysis of a Veterans Administrative cooperative study of needle stick hepatitis, the Veterans Administration Cooperative Study Group. Ann Intern Med 1979;91:813–818.

27. Perrillo RP, Campbell CR, Strang S, et al. Immune globulin and hepatitis B immune globulin: prophylactic measures for intimate contacts exposed to acute type B hepatitis. Arch Intern Med 1984;144:81–85.

28. Beasley RP, Hwang LY, Stevens CE, et al. Efficacy of hepatitis B immune globulin for prevention of perinatal transmission of the hepatitis B carrier state: final report of a randomized double-blind, placebo-controlled trial. Hepatology 1983;3:135–141.

29. Centers for Disease Control. Hepatitis B virus: a comprehensive strategy for eliminating transmission in the United States through universal childhood vaccination. Recommendations of the Immunization Practices Advisory Committee (ACIP). MMWR 1991;40(RR-13):1–25.

30. Palmovic D. Prevention of hepatitis B infection in health care workers after accidental exposure. J Infect 1987;15:221–224.

31. Stevens CE, Taylor PE, Tong MJ, et al. Yeast-recombinant hepatitis B vaccine: efficacy with hepatitis B immune globulin in prevention of perinatal hepatitis B virus transmission. JAMA 1987;257:2612–2616.

32. Beasley RP, Hwang LY, Lee GC, et al. Prevention of perinatally transmitted hepatitis B virus infections with hepatitis immune globulin and hepatitis B vaccine. Lancet 1983;2:1099–1102.

33. Wong VC, Ip HM, Reesink HW, et al. Prevention of HBsAg carrier state in newborn infants of mothers who are chronic carriers of HBsAg and HBeAg by administration of hepatitis-B vaccine and hepatitis-B immunoglobulin: double-blind randomised, placebo-controlled study. Lancet 1984;1:921–926.

34. Stevens CE, Toy PT, Tong MJ, et al. Perinatal hepatitis B transmission in the United States: prevention by passive-active immunization. JAMA 1985;253:1740–1745.

35. Jackson LA, Wenger JD, Meningococcal Disease Study Group. Laboratory-based surveillance for meningococcal disease in selected areas, United States—1989–1991. MMWR 1993;42(SS-2):21–30.

36. Kaiser AB, Hennekens CH, Saslaw MS, et al. Seroepidemiology and chemoprophylaxis of disease due to sulfonamide resistant *Neisseria meningitidis* in a civilian population. J Infect Dis 1974;130:217–224.

37. Munford RS, Sussuarana de Vasconcelos ZJ, Phillips CJ, et al. Eradication of carriage of *Neisseria meningitidis* in families: a study in Brazil. J Infect Dis 1974;129:644–649.

38. Guttler RB, Counts GW, Avent CK, et al. Effect of rifampin and minocycline on meningococcal carrier rates. J Infect Dis 1971;124:199–205.

39. Schwartz B, Al-Tobaiqi A, Al-Ruwais A, et al. Comparative efficacy of ceftriaxone and rifampin in eradicating pharyngeal carriage of group A *Neisseria meningitidis*. Lancet 1988;1:1239–1242.

40. Deal WB, Sanders E. Efficacy of rifampin in treatment of meningococcal carriers. N Engl J Med 1969;281:641–645.

41. Munford RS, Taunay AE, Morais JS, et al. Spread of meningococcal infection within households. Lancet 1974;1:1275–1278.

42. Meningococcal Disease Surveillance Group. Meningococcal disease: secondary attack rate and chemoprophylaxis in the United States, 1974. JAMA 1976;235:261–265.

43. Greenwood BM, Hassan-King M, Whittle HC. Prevention of secondary cases of meningococcal disease in household contacts by vaccination. BMJ 1978;2:1317–1318.

44. Jones DM. Meningococcal vaccines [editorial]. J Med Microbiol 1993;38:77–78.

45. Lennon D, Gellin B, Hood D, et al. Successful intervention in a group A meningococcal outbreak in Auckland, New Zealand. Pediatr Infect Dis J 1992;11:617–623.

46. Biselli R, Fattorossi A, Matricardi PM, et al. Dramatic reduction of meningococcal meningitis among military recruits in Italy after introduction of specific vaccination. Vaccine 1993;11:578–581.

47. Peltola H, Makela HP, Kayhty H, et al. Clinical efficacy of meningococcal group A capsular polysaccharide vaccine in children three months to five years of age. N Engl J Med 1977;297:686–691.

48. de Moraes JC, Perkins BA, Camargo MC, et al. Protective efficacy of a serogroup B meningococcal vaccine in Sao Paulo, Brazil. Lancet 1992;340:1074–1078.

49. Twumasi PA Jr, Kumah S, Leach A, et al. A trial of a group A plus group C meningococcal polysaccharide-protein conjugate vaccine in African infants. J Infect Dis 1995;171:632–638.

50. Bjune G, Nokleby H, Hareide B. Clinical trials using a new Norwegian vaccine against disease caused by group B meningococci. Tidsskr Nor Laegeforen 1990;110:614–617.

51. Fishbein DB, Robinson LE. Rabies. N Engl J Med 1993;329:1632–1638.

52. Centers for Disease Control and Prevention. Human rabies—Alabama, Tennessee, and Texas, 1994. MMWR 1995;44:269–272.

53. Centers for Disease Control and Prevention. Raccoon rabies epizootic—United States, 1993. MMWR 1994;43: 269–273.

54. Centers for Disease Control. Update on adult immunizations: recommendations of the Immunization Practices Advisory Committee. MMWR 1991;40(RR-12):36–39.

55. Centers for Disease Control. Rabies prevention—United States, 1991: recommendations of the Immunization Practices Advisory Committee. MMWR 1991;40(RR-3):1–19.

56. Berlin BS, Mitchell JR, Burgoyne GH, et al. Rhesus diploid vaccine (adsorbed), a new rabies vaccine: II. results of clinical studies simulating prophylactic therapy for rabies exposure. JAMA 1983;249:2663–2665.

57. Helmick CG, Johnstone C, Sumner J, et al. A clinical study of Merieux human rabies immune globulin. J Biol Stand 1982;10:357–367.

58. Anderson LJ, Sikes RK, Langkop CW, et al. Postexposure trial of a human diploid cell strain rabies vaccine. J Infect Dis 1980;142:133–138.

59. Bahmanyar M, Fayaz A, Nour-Salehi S, et al. Successful protection of humans exposed to rabies infection: post exposure treatment with the new human diploid cell rabies vaccine and antirabies serum. JAMA 1976;236:2751–2754.

60. Chutivongse S, Wilde H, Supich C, et al. Postexposure prophylaxis for rabies with antiserum and intradermal vaccination. Lancet 1990;2:896–898.

61. Warrell MJ, Nicholson KG, Warrell DA, et al. Economical multiple-site intradermal immunization with human diploid cell strain vaccine is effective for post exposure rabies prophylaxis. Lancet 1985;1: 1059–1062.

62. Vodopija I, Sureau P, Smerdel S, et al. Interaction of rabies vaccine with human rabies immunoglobulin and reliability of the 2-1-1 schedule application for postexposure treatment. Vaccine 1988; 6:283–286.

62a. Suntharasamai P, Warrell MJ, Warrell DA, et al. New purified vero cell vaccine prevents rabies in patients bitten by rabid animals. Lancet 1986;2:129–131.

62b. Sehgal S, Bhattacharya D, Bhardwaj M. Clinical evaluation of purified vero-cell rabies vaccine in patients bitten by rabid animals in India. J Commun Dis 1994;26:139–146.

63. Shill M, Baynes RD, Miller SD. Fatal rabies encephalitis despite appropriate post-exposure prophylaxis: a case report. N Engl J Med 1987;316:1257–1258.

64. Wilde H, Choomkasien O, Hemachudka T, et al. Failure of rabies postexposure treatment in Thailand. Vaccine 1989;7:49–52.

65. Centers for Disease Control. Human rabies despite treatment with rabies immune globulin and human diploid cell vaccine—Thailand. MMWR 1987;36:759–760, 765.

66. Review: rabies vaccine failures. Lancet 1988;1:917–918.

67. Reid-Sanden FL, Fishbein DB, Stevens CA, et al. Administration of rabies vaccine in the gluteal area: a continuing problem [letter]. Arch Intern Med 1991;151:821.

68. Fishbein DB, Sawyer LA, Reid-Sanden FL. Administration of human diploid-cell vaccine in the gluteal area [letter]. N Engl J Med 1988;318:214–215.

69. Centers for Disease Control. Systemic allergic reactions following immunization with human diploid cell rabies vaccine. MMWR 1984;33:185–187.

70. Bernard KW, Smith PW, Kader FJ, et al. Neuroparalytic illness and human diploid cell rabies vaccine. JAMA 1982;248:3136–3138.

71. Boe E, Nyland H. Guillain-Barré syndrome after vaccination with human diploid cell rabies vaccine Scand J Infect Dis 1980;12:231–232.

72. Knittel T, Ramadori G, Mayet WJ. Guillain-Barré syndrome and human diploid cell rabies vaccine [letter]. Lancet 1989;1:1334–1335.

73. Turner GS, Nicholson KG, Tyrrell DA, et al. Evaluation of a human diploid cell strain rabies vaccine: final report of a three year study of pre-exposure immunization. J Hyg (Lond) 1982;89:101–110.

74. Immunization Practices Advisory Committee. Rabies prevention: supplemental statement on the pre-exposure use of human diploid cell vaccine by the intradermal route. MMWR 1986;35:767–769.

75. Rosanoff E, Tint H. Responses to human diploid cell rabies vaccine: neutralizing antibody responses of vaccinees receiving booster doses of human diploid cell rabies vaccine. Am J Epidemiol 1979;110:322–327.

76. Bernard KW, Mallonee J, Wright JC, et al. Preexposure immunization with intradermal human diploid cell rabies vaccine: risks and benefits of primary and booster vaccination. JAMA 1987;257:1059–1063.

77. Berlin BS. Rabies vaccine adsorbed: neutralizing antibody titers after three-dose pre-exposure vaccination. Am J Public Health 1990;80:476–478.

78. Briggs DJ, Schwenke JR. Longevity of rabies antibody titre in recipients of human diploid cell rabies vaccine. Vaccine 1992;10:125–129.

79. Centers for Disease Control. Human rabies—Kenya. MMWR 1983;32:494–495.

80. Dreesen DW, Bernard KW, Parker RA, et al. Immune complex disease in 23 persons following a booster dose of rabies human diploid cell vaccine. Vaccine 1986;4:45–49.

81. Fishbein DB, Yenne KM, Dreesen DW, et al. Risk factors for systemic hypersensitivity reactions after booster vaccinations with human diploid cell rabies vaccine: a nationwide prospective study. Vaccine 1993;11:1390–1394.

82. Fishbein DB, Dreesen DW, Holmes DF, et al. Human diploid rabies vaccine purified by zonal centrifugation: a controlled study of antibody response and side effects following primary and booster pre-exposure immunizations. Vaccine 1989;7:437–442.

83. Sutter RW, Cochi SL, Brink EW, Sirotkin BI. Assessment of vital statistics and surveillance data for monitoring tetanus mortality, United States, 1979–1984. Am J Epidemiol 1990;131:132–142.

84. Centers for Disease Control. Tetanus surveillance—United States, 1989–1990. MMWR 1992;41(SS-8):1–9.

85. Gergen PJ, McQuillan GM, Kiely M, et al. A population-based serologic survey of immunity to tetanus in the United States. N Engl J Med 1995;332:761–766.

86. Sachs A. Modern views on the prevention of tetanus in wounded. Proc R Soc Med 1952;45:641–652.

87. Bruce D. Tetanus: analysis of 1458 cases which occurred in home military hospitals during the years 1914–1918. J Hyg (Lond) 1920;19:1–32.

88. Edsall G. Specific prophylaxis of tetanus. JAMA 1959;171:417–427.

89. Looney JM, Edsall G, Ipsen J, et al. Persistence of antitoxin levels after tetanus-toxoid inoculation in adults and effect of a booster dose after various intervals. N Engl J Med 1956;254:6–12.

90. Wolters KL, Dehmel H. Abschliessende Untersuchungen uber die Tetanusprophylaxe durch aktive Immunisierung. Z Hyg Infektionskr 1942;124:326–332.

91. Passen EL, Andersen BR. Clinical tetanus despite a 'protective' level of toxin-neutralizing antibody. JAMA 1986;255:1171–1173.

92. Berger SA, Cherubin CE, Nelson S, Levine L. Tetanus despite preexisting antitetanus antibodies. JAMA 1978;240:769–770.

93. Goulon M, Girard O, Grosbuis S, et al. Les anticorps antitétaniques: titrage avant séro-anatoxinothérapie chez 64 tétaniques. Press Med 1972;1:3049–3050.

94. Levine L, McComb JA, Dwyer RC, et al. Active-passive tetanus immunization: choice of toxoid, dose of tetanus immune globulin and timing of injections. N Engl J Med 1966;274:186–190.

95. Rubbo SD, Suri JC. Combined active-passive immunization against tetanus with human immune globulin. Med J Aust 1965;2:109–113.

96. McComb JA, Dwyer RC. Passive-active immunization with tetanus immune globulin (human). N Engl J Med 1963; 268:857–862.

97. Tasman A, Huygen FJ. Immunization against tetanus of patients given injections of antitetanus serum. Bull WHO 1962;26:397–407.

98. Smolens J, Vogt AB, Crawford MN, et al. The persistence in the human circulation of horse and human tetanus antitoxin. J Pediatr 1961;59:899–902.

99. Simonsen O, Bentzon MW, Kjeldsen K, et al. Evaluation of vaccination requirements to secure continuous antitoxin immunity to tetanus. Vaccine 1987;5:115–122.

100. Simonsen O, Badsberg JH, Kjeldsen K, et al. The fall-off in serum concentrations of tetanus antitoxin after primary and booster vaccination. Acta Pathol Microbiol Scand 1986;94:77–82.

101. Simonsen O, Kjeldsen K, Heron I. Immunity against tetanus and effect of revaccination 25–30 years after primary vaccination. Lancet 1984;2:1240–1242.

102. Simonsen O, Klærke M, Jensen JE, et al. Revaccination against tetanus 17–20 years after primary vaccination: kinetics of antibody response. J Trauma 1987;27:1358–1361.

103. Ipsen J. Changes in immunity and antitoxin level immediately after secondary stimulus with tetanus toxoid in rabbits. J Immunol 1961;86:50–55.

104. Wassilak SG, Walter AO. Tetanus. In: Plotkin SA, Mortimer EA, eds. Vaccines. Philadelphia: WB Saunders, 1988:45–73.

105. Reinstein L. Peripheral neuropathy after multiple tetanus toxoid boosters. Arch Phys Med Rehabil 1982;63:332–334.

106. Edsall G, Elliot MW, Peebles TG, et al. Excessive use of tetanus toxoid boosters. JAMA 1967; 202:111–113.

107. Immunization Practices Advisory Committee. Update: prevention of *Haemophilus influenzae* type b disease. MMWR 1986;35:170–180.

108. Immunization Practices Advisory Committee. Meningococcal vaccines. MMWR 1985;34:255–259.

109. Immunization Practices Advisory Committee. Diphtheria, tetanus and pertussis; recommendations for vaccine use and other preventive measures. MMWR 1991;40(RR-10):1–2, 20–25.

110. American College of Physicians Task Force on Adult Immunization and Infectious Diseases Society of America. Guide for adult immunization. 3rd ed. Philadelphia: American College of Physicians, 1994.

111. American College of Obstetricians and Gynecologists. Immunization during pregnancy. Technical Bulletin no. 160. Washington, DC: American College of Obstetricians and Gynecologists, 1991.

68. Postmenopausal Hormone Prophylaxis

RECOMMENDATION

Counseling all perimenopausal and postmenopausal women about the potential benefits and risks of hormone prophylaxis is recommended. There is insufficient evidence to recommend for or against hormone therapy for all postmenopausal women. Women should participate fully in the decision-making process, and individual decisions should be based on patient risk factors for disease, clear understanding of the probable benefits and risks of hormone therapy, and patient preferences (*see* Clinical Intervention).

Burden of Suffering

The median age of menopause in American women is 51 years (range 41–59),[1,2] but ovarian production of estrogen and progestin begins to decline years before the complete cessation of menses. Lower levels of circulating estrogen contribute to accelerated bone loss, vulvovaginal atrophy, changes in urethral mucosa and vaginal flora[3] and substantial rises in total and low-density lipoprotein cholesterol (LDL-C) that occur during the perimenopausal and postmenopausal period.[4,5] Hormonal changes produce vasomotor symptoms ("hot flashes") in 50–85% of women by the time of menopause.[1,2,6,7] Hot flashes may be severe in 20% of women, may contribute to sleep disturbances and somatic symptoms, and are present 4 years after menopause in 20% of women.[1,7] Urogenital symptoms (dyspareunia, dysuria, incontinence, and urinary tract infections) are also common in postmenopausal women: up to 45% of women complain of vaginal dryness after menopause,[8] and 10–15% of women over age 60 have frequent urinary tract infections.[9]

The average life expectancy of an American woman reaching menopause is approximately 30 years. Many of the most important causes of morbidity in older women (cardiovascular disease, osteoporosis, and various cancers) appear to be influenced by female hormones. Cardiovascular disease is the leading cause of morbidity and mortality in postmenopausal women: nearly half will develop coronary heart disease (CHD) in their lifetime, 30% will die from CHD (more than 230,000 women per year), and 20% will have a stroke.[10–12] An estimated 1.3 million osteoporosis-related fractures occur each year in the U.S., nearly all in postmenopausal women.[13] A 50-year-old white woman is estimated to have a 16% chance of eventually suffering a hip fracture and a 32% risk of vertebral fracture.[11] In comparison, the lifetime probability of developing endometrial cancer and breast cancer is only 2.6% and 10%, respectively, and the chance of dying from these cancers is only 0.3% and 3%.[12]

Efficacy of Chemoprophylaxis

Controlled trials of the effects of hormone therapy on clinical endpoints are difficult because of the large numbers of subjects and long follow-up required. The recently launched Women's Health Initiative, a multicenter randomized trial with 25,000 women assigned to placebo, estrogen alone (for women with prior hysterectomy only), or combined estrogen-progestin therapy, should provide important new evidence, but results will not be reported for 8–12 years.[14] Additional information may come from secondary prevention trials examining the benefits of hormone therapy in women with CHD or cerebrovascular disease. Numerous cross-sectional, case-control, and cohort studies, however, suggest that postmenopausal estrogen therapy has important effects on a number of major clinical outcomes.[12]

Osteoporotic Fractures. There is good evidence from retrospective studies and clinical trials that oral or parenteral estrogen can reduce the rate of bone loss and improve bone mineral density in postmenopausal women.[15] In epidemiologic studies[16–20] and nonrandomized clinical trials,[21] use of postmenopausal estrogen was associated with a decreased rate of fractures of the hip, forearm and spine. An overview of 11 studies estimated that risk of hip fracture was reduced 25% among women who had used estrogens;[12] greater benefit has been observed with current use (vs. past use), long-term use (>5 years), and therapy begun close to menopause. Since accelerated bone loss resumes when estrogen is discontinued, hormones may be needed indefinitely to provide maximal protection after age 75, when risk of fracture is highest.[22] One model predicted that fracture risk in women ages 75–85 would be reduced 73% in women who took estrogen continuously after menopause, 57–69% in women who began therapy at age 65, and only 23% in women who began therapy at menopause but stopped at age 65.[23] Several studies have reported that past estrogen use provides minimal or no protection to women over age 75 in terms of bone density[24] or reduced risk of hip fracture.[20,25,26]

Coronary Heart Disease and Lipids. Numerous studies have demonstrated significantly lower risks of fatal and nonfatal CHD among postmenopausal women taking estrogen.[12,27] Overviews of these studies have estimated a

37–44% reduction in risk of CHD among ever-users of estrogen.[12,28] In the Nurses' Health Study, one of the largest and best-designed studies, the beneficial effect was most evident in current users of estrogen (relative risk (RR) of major CHD = 0.56) and diminished in former users (RR = 0.83); benefit of estrogen did not increase with long-term use.[29] Studies of women undergoing angiography report less severe coronary stenosis among women taking estrogen,[28,30,31] and one follow-up study of women with angiographically confirmed coronary disease reported reduced mortality in those who had taken estrogen.[32] Generalizing from angiographic studies is problematic, since they do not examine a representative sample of hormone users and non-users.

Whether age or other risk factors modify the cardiac benefits of estrogen is uncertain.[28] Some studies reported a reduced benefit of estrogen (or even increased risk) in smokers,[33,34] while others reported comparable or greater benefits in smokers compared to nonsmokers.[29] Similarly, some studies reported that protective effects of estrogen were lower among older women (over age 60),[29,33] but others observed protective effects of estrogen independent of age[35] and in cohorts of elderly women.[28,36]

The beneficial effects of estrogen on serum lipids are believed to be responsible for some but not all of the observed reduction in the risk of CHD.[35–37] In short-term studies, oral estrogen therapy lowers LDL-C 14–20% and raises high-density lipoprotein cholesterol (HDL-C) 15–20%, but it also raises serum triglycerides 24–38%.[38,39] These effects are mediated through first-pass effects of oral estrogen on hepatic cholesterol metabolism; transdermal and vaginal estrogens, which circumvent this first-pass effect, have less effect on serum lipids.[38] Beneficial effects of estrogen on vascular tone[40,41] or lipid oxidation[42] represent additional mechanisms by which estrogen therapy may reduce cardiovascular risk, independent of effects on serum lipid levels.

Whether or not combined estrogen-progestin therapy has similar effects on CHD remains a matter of considerable debate.[12] The use of progestins attenuates the beneficial effects of estrogen on HDL-C, but effects depend on dose, duration, and type of progestin.[39] The effects of four different hormone regimens on cardiovascular risk factors were examined in the 3-year "PEPI" trial,[43] which randomized 875 women to: placebo; unopposed conjugated equine estrogen (CEE) 0.625 mg daily; daily CEE (0.625 mg) plus cyclic medroxyprogesterone acetate (MPA) (10 mg/day for 12 days each month); daily CEE (0.625 mg) plus daily MPA (2.5 mg); or daily CEE (0.625 mg) plus cyclic micronized progesterone (MP) (200 mg/day for 12 days each month).[43] Compared to placebo, all hormone regimens decreased LDL-C (7–10%), decreased fibrinogen (1–11%), and increased triglycerides (6–7%), without significant effects on blood pressure or insulin responsiveness. Increases in HDL-C were significantly greater with unopposed estrogen or estrogen with cyclic MP (+9–11%) than with regimens using MPA (+4%).

These results suggest that MPA, the most commonly prescribed progestin in the U.S.,[44] may attenuate the cardiac benefits of estrogen therapy, but the importance of this physiologic effect remains controversial.[12] In a large cross-sectional survey, women taking estrogen and progestins (largely MPA) had lipid levels comparable to women taking unopposed estrogen.[45] In two recent observational studies, estrogen/progestin therapy and unopposed estrogen each were associated with significant and comparable reductions in risk of CHD compared to women who did not use hormones.[46,47] The effects of progestins on other estrogen-sensitive endpoints (vascular tone, lipid oxidation) have not yet been clearly defined.[45,48]

Cerebrovascular Disease. Studies to date have not demonstrated a consistent association between postmenopausal hormone use and cerebrovascular disease.[12] Individual studies have demonstrated significant increases (primarily in smokers)[33] or decreases[49,50] in stroke risk among women who report ever having used estrogen. A pooled estimate of risk from 15 studies calculated that there was no significant effect of estrogen use on risk of stroke among ever-users versus never-users.[12] The failure to distinguish between ischemic and hemorrhagic strokes is a limitation of most studies, since risk factors are distinct for each stroke type. In the Nurses' Health Study, there was no significant effect of current use or past use of estrogen on risk of any stroke, ischemic stroke, or hemorrhagic stroke.[29] This finding is consistent with the observation that serum lipids are weaker risk factors for stroke than for heart disease.[51,52] There are few data on the effects of progestins on stroke. A Swedish cohort study reported significantly lower risk of stroke among women taking combination therapy (and among women taking unopposed estrogen) than in the general population, but it could not adjust for differences in other stroke risk factors.[53]

Other Potential Benefits of Hormone Therapy. Estrogen taken orally, transdermally, or vaginally is effective in relieving vulvovaginal atrophy and urogenital symptoms.[3,7] These benefits may help improve sexual function, but independent effects of estrogen on libido or sexual responsiveness have not been clearly demonstrated.[3] Vaginal estrogen cream reduced recurrence of urinary tract infections in a randomized trial in older women.[54] The effects of estrogen on mood and cognitive function have been inconsistent.[3] In a small randomized trial among women without menopausal symptoms, estrogen significantly improved depression scores but not scores on several other psychological indices.[55] There was no evidence of an effect of past or current estrogen therapy on cognitive function in a large cross-sectional study in a retirement community.[56] Two case-control studies reported a reduced risk of Alzheimer's disease (AD) among women who were currently using estrogen[57] or had previously used estrogen,[58] but a third study found no association between estrogen therapy and AD.[59]

Potential Risks of Hormone Therapy: Endometrial Cancer. Prolonged use of unopposed estrogens increases the risk of endometrial hyperplasia and endometrial cancer.[60–62] Risk appears elevated at all doses and increases with dose and duration of therapy. A recent meta-analysis of 37 observational studies reported that risk was increased almost 6-fold among women who used estrogen for 5–10 years, and more than 9-fold with use for more than 10 years.[60] Although association was strongest for early stage, noninvasive tumors that have a good prognosis, the risks for invasive cancer (RR = 3.8; 95% confidence interval [CI], 2.9 to 5.1) and for endometrial cancer death (RR = 2.7; 95% CI, 0.9 to 8.0) were also increased among women who had used estrogen.

Both continuous and cyclic regimens of progestins prevent estrogen-induced endometrial hyperplasia.[43,63] In the PEPI trial, incidence of adenomatous or atypical hyperplasia was similar among women taking various combination therapies or placebo (0–2%), compared to 34% among women on unopposed estrogen.[43] Several observational studies and a small trial reported that women taking estrogen with cyclic MPA had a lower risk of endometrial cancer than did women who never took hormones, but several more recent case-control studies observed nonsignificant 2-fold increases in endometrial cancer.[60] One study reported increased risk only when progestins were taken for fewer than 10 days each month.[64] There are few data on cancer risk with other progestin regimens (i.e., daily). For women who do not tolerate daily or monthly progestins, regular endometrial surveillance (annual endometrial biopsy) or less frequent progestin cycles (e.g., every 3 months) have been proposed as alternative ways to reduce risks of estrogen; neither of these methods has been adequately assessed for its ability to prevent endometrial cancer, however.

Breast Cancer. Endogenous estrogen appears to be important in the etiology of breast cancer, but the effect of exogenous estrogens on breast cancer risk remains uncertain.[65,66] More than 40 observational studies, and 6 meta-analyses of individual studies, have examined the association between postmenopausal estrogen therapy and the risk of breast cancer, with varying results.[12,67–71] Although cancer risk was not increased among women who had ever used postmenopausal estrogens, several overviews reported a modest but significant increase in risk among women who were currently using estrogen (RR = 1.2–1.4)[70,71] or had used estrogen for long periods (RR = 1.2–1.3 for durations >10–15 years).[12,69–71] These findings were affirmed in a 1995 report from the Nurses' Health Study, with over

725,000 person-years of follow-up: risk of breast cancer was increased only among current, long-term users (>5 years) of hormones and increased with age. Compared to women who had never taken hormones, breast cancer incidence among current long-term users of hormones was increased 50%.[72] Risk was not increased among past users of hormones, however, even those who took hormones for long periods. There was no clear effect of dose of estrogen on risk in most studies.

A number of studies reported that women who develop breast cancer during estrogen therapy have earlier disease at diagnosis,[73–76] lower rates of metastasis,[75] and longer survival with breast cancer,[74,77,78] compared to women with cancer who had never used estrogen. These findings suggest that some of the apparent increase in cancer incidence among women taking estrogens may be due to earlier diagnosis (i.e., "surveillance bias")[79,80] or effects of estrogen on well-differentiated cancers with better prognosis.[75,76] The effect of hormones on breast cancer mortality is not consistent. There was no association between past or current estrogen use and death from breast cancer in the Nurses Health Study,[72] in long term follow-up of a smaller British cohort,[81] or in 12-year follow-up of 23,000 Swedish women prescribed hormones.[82] Among a subgroup of current long-term users in the Nurses' Health Study, however, breast cancer mortality was increased (RR = 1.45, 95% CI, 1.01 to 2.09).[72] The lack of risk attributable to past hormone use may indicate that hormones promote growth of existing cancers rather than cause new cancers.[77]

There is little evidence that adding progestins to estrogen therapy influences the risk of breast cancer. An early study that reported protective effects of progestins[83] has been largely discounted due to methodologic flaws. In more recent studies, the risks associated with combination therapy are comparable to those observed for estrogen alone.[84–86] Estrogen-progestin therapy was associated with modest but significant increases in risk in three large cohort studies with long-term follow-up (RR =1.2–1.6)[72,76,87] but no increase in a recent community-based case-control study.[87a] In the only long-term controlled trial of hormone therapy, 84 pairs of institutionalized women were randomized to 2.5 mg/day conjugated estrogen plus cyclic MPA, or placebo for 10 years. After an additional 12 years of follow-up, none of 116 women who had ever received hormone therapy (during trial or follow-up) developed breast cancer, compared to 6 of 52 controls who never received therapy (p < 0.01).[88] The select nature of the participants precludes generalizing these results to the average perimenopausal woman.

Thrombosis, Gallbladder Disease, Glucose Tolerance, and Other Side Effects. High-dose estrogen has been associated with alterations in clotting factors and an increased risk of thrombosis in studies of early contraceptives and in a trial of estrogen therapy in men with CHD.[48] There is no clear evidence of an increased risk of clinical thrombosis in women taking postmenopausal estrogens, however.[12,89] High-dose CEE (2.5–5 mg daily) doubled the incidence of gallbladder disease in a trial in men[90] and in a small trial in postmenopausal women.[91] Several larger observational studies report a similar 2–3-fold increased risk of gallstone disease or cholecystectomy among women taking postmenopausal estrogen;[92,93] this effect was not consistently seen in smaller studies.[94,95] Transdermal estrogens, which avoid first-pass effects on the liver, may have less effect on thrombosis and gallbladder disease. In the PEPI trial, neither estrogen nor estrogen/progestin therapy had a significant effect on mean systolic blood pressure or glucose tolerance, and all hormone regimens lowered fibrinogen levels.[43]

Estrogen and progestin each can cause unpleasant side effects. Progestin is a more common cause of bothersome side effects, including bloating, headache, irritability, and depression; the most prominent effect of estrogen is breast tenderness. Many of these side effects subside with continued treatment or can be relieved by adjusting dose or timing of administration. Women who have not had a hysterectomy will experience resumption of menses while taking cyclic progestins. Up to 40% of women on continuous progestins will experience erratic and unpredictable bleeding within the first 6 months, but 75–95% have amenorrhea after 12 months.[3,7,96]

Limitations of Epidemiologic Evidence. There are some important limitations in the ability to predict the benefits and risks of long-term hormone therapy from currently available studies: the average duration of hormone use in most studies was relatively short (several years), most long-term users of hormones had specific indications for estrogen therapy (e.g., early menopause, surgical menopause, persistent symptoms, or osteoporosis), and few women had used long-term progestin or regimens other than cyclic MPA.[44] In many studies, differences between hormone users and never-users may have independently influenced the risk of specific diseases or death. Compared to never-users, women who take estrogen are: thinner, better educated, and of higher income; more likely to exercise and drink alcohol; more likely to have had a surgical menopause and less likely to have a family history of breast cancer; in more frequent contact with physicians; and, by definition, compliant with medical therapy.[45,50,97–99] Although "selection bias" (i.e., the greater tendency for low-risk, healthy women to take hormones) may exaggerate the protective effects of estrogen on CHD, it is unlikely to account for the large and consistent effects seen in multiple studies. Confounding, selection bias, and surveillance bias are of greater concern when the observed associations are weak and inconsistent (i.e., breast cancer). The net effect of these different biases is difficult to predict, and they could plausibly have increased *or* decreased the risk of breast cancer among hormone users in observational studies.

Risk-Benefit Analyses. Several analyses have estimated the net benefit of prolonged hormone therapy for the average postmenopausal woman.[12,100–102] Because CHD is much more common than breast cancer after the menopause,[11] both estrogen and estrogen-progestin therapy are predicted to prolong life expectancy for most women even if the risk of breast cancer is increased up to 50%.[101,102] Predicted benefits exceed those of most other preventive interventions in older women[101] and are particularly large for women at increased risk of CHD (>2-year average increase in life expectancy).[12,101] For women at high risk of breast cancer and low risk of CHD, effects may be small or even adverse, depending on the influence of progestins on these outcomes. These predictions assume that the effects of estrogen are independent of age, race, or underlying risk factors, but data on the effects of long-term hormone use are limited for some important groups of women: women over age 70, black women, and women who are obese. Cost-effectiveness of therapy is highly sensitive to costs of medication and follow-up visits. In a British study, combined estrogen-progestin therapy was predicted to cost roughly $10,000 per quality-adjusted life-year gained, assuming an annual cost of less than $150 for medications and follow-up.[100] A 1995 report of the Office of Technology Assessment estimated that unopposed estrogen would cost up to $25,000 per year of life gained, and that therapy begun at age 65 might be even more cost-effective.[114,115]

Effectiveness of Counseling

Few studies have examined the effectiveness of physician counseling of asymptomatic postmenopausal women to use estrogen. Long-term compliance with estrogen therapy may be limited by side effects, concerns about cancer risk, or inconvenience of taking daily medication.[103] In one study, up to 20–30% of women never had their prescriptions for estrogen filled; of those who began therapy, 20% discontinued the drug within 9 months.[104] The strongest determinants of use in one survey were a clear physician recommendation and knowledge that estrogen deficiency was a risk factor for osteoporosis.[105] Women who have documented low bone density appear more likely to take hormone therapy,[106] but up to 40% of those with low bone density in one study did not comply with recommendations to take hormone therapy.[107] Studies have demonstrated that targeted education and screening for osteoporosis or heart disease prevention can increase the proportion of women remaining on hormone therapy to over 80%.[107,108]

In women without a hysterectomy, breakthrough bleeding or withdrawal bleeding are important reasons for noncompliance;[103,109] more than half of such women assigned to unopposed estrogen in the PEPI study changed or stopped therapy.[43] Continuous combination therapy, which usually causes amenorrhea, or less frequent progestin cycles (e.g., every 3 months) may improve patient satisfaction. In the PEPI trial, however, compliance did not differ between continuous and cyclic estrogen/progestin regimens.[43]

Recommendations of Other Groups

The American College of Obstetricians and Gynecologists,[110] the American Academy of Family Physicians,[111] the Canadian Task Force on the Periodic Health Examination,[112] and the American College of Physicians (ACP)[113] recommend that physicians counsel all postmenopausal women about the risks and benefits of estrogen replacement and make decisions regarding therapy on an individual basis. The ACP concluded that women with a hysterectomy and those at increased risk of coronary disease are likely to benefit from therapy, but that risks may outweigh benefits among women at increased risk of breast cancer. A 1984 National Institutes of Health consensus conference on osteoporosis recommended that estrogen therapy after menopause should be considered in high-risk women who have no medical contraindications and who are willing to adhere to a program of careful follow-up.[13]

Discussion

Estrogen therapy after the menopause relieves vasomotor and urogenital symptoms, produces clinically important improvements in bone density and blood lipids, and is associated with significant reductions in the risk of heart disease and fracture. Ongoing clinical trials can be expected to provide more reliable estimates of the magnitude of these benefits. Nonetheless, the strength and consistency of the results of observational studies strongly suggest that estrogen therapy can substantially reduce morbidity and mortality from coronary disease and osteoporosis in older women. Although models suggest a net benefit of hormone use in most postmenopausal woman, important questions remain about the appropriate duration of treatment, the benefits and risks in older women (over age 65) and non-white women, the net effect of adding progestins, and interactions with other risk factors. Recommendations about hormone therapy are best made on an individual basis, weighing probable benefits against the costs, inconvenience, and possible adverse effects of estrogen and progestin.

Whether current postmenopausal hormone regimens increase the risk of breast cancer remains uncertain. Although there is little evidence of harm from short-term use of postmenopausal estrogen, overviews suggest that continued, long-term use of hormones may increase the risk of breast cancer in older women. The reported association is biologically plausible and could alter the balance of risks and benefits for some patients, but it has not been consistent in all studies. Moreover, the absolute increase in breast cancer mortality from hormone therapy (if any exists) is likely to be small: a 30–40% increase in mortality would increase the lifetime risk of dying of breast cancer by only 1% (i.e., from 3% to 4%). Regular mammography may further reduce any risk, but patients will have to make their own decisions regarding possible risks vs. potential benefits of therapy.

Despite many areas of uncertainty, clinicians play an essential role in helping women decide whether or not to begin hormone therapy. Clinicians can elicit symptoms related to estrogen deficiency (e.g., vasomotor or urogenital symptoms), assess other potential indications (major risk factors for osteoporosis or heart disease) or contraindications (prior breast cancer, liver diseases, or estrogen-related complications) for estrogen therapy, and explain the probable benefits and risks of prolonged therapy. Although direct evidence is not available, the asymptomatic women most likely to benefit from estrogen therapy include those with early or surgical menopause, those with other cardiac risk factors (especially adverse lipid profile; see Chapter 2), and women at high risk of osteoporosis or fracture (women who are thin, smoke, or have a family history of fracture).

The balance of benefits and risks of estrogen therapy in women at increased risk of breast cancer is not known. Since the risk of cardiovascular disease is much higher than the risk of breast cancer for most postmenopausal women, benefits may outweigh any harms even in women with a family history of breast cancer. Fear of breast cancer is particularly high in these women, however, and many may be reluctant to do anything that might increase risk. Patients should also understand that current estimates are based on available (often incomplete) knowledge and may change with new information. Because many of the benefits of estrogen may require continuing therapy indefinitely, clinicians should clarify the reasons for recommending hormone therapy and periodically assess patient concerns about side effects or risks of treatment.

CLINICAL INTERVENTION

Clinicians should counsel all women around the time of menopause about the possible benefits and risks of postmenopausal hormone therapy and the available treatment options ("B" recommendation). Counseling should include asking about presence and severity of menopausal symptoms (hot flashes, urogenital symptoms), as well as assessing risk factors for heart disease, osteoporosis, and breast cancer. Women should be advised of the probable benefits of hormone therapy on menopausal symptoms, myocardial infarction, and fracture; the increased risks of endometrial cancer with unopposed estrogen; and a possible increased risk of breast cancer.

Each woman should consider the relative importance of these benefits and risks, the possible side effects of treatment, and her willingness to take medication for an indefinite period.

Women considering estrogen therapy should be counseled about the available estrogen and progestin preparations and routes of administration. The minimum effective dose of estrogen is 0.625 mg conjugated estrogen or the equivalent once a day. For women who have not had a hysterectomy, progestin therapy or regular endometrial surveillance is recommended to reduce risk of endometrial cancer. The most common progestin regimens include a continuous regimen of daily administration of 2.5 mg medroxyprogesterone acetate (MPA) or equivalent, or a cyclic regimen of 5–10 mg MPA daily for 10–14 days each month. Transdermal estrogen preparations are effective in relieving menopausal symptoms and preventing osteoporosis, but they have less effect on lipids and are of undetermined benefit against heart disease.

All women should receive information about potential alternatives to hormones for treating menopausal symptoms (e.g., vaginal lubricants for dyspareunia, etc.), for preventing osteoporosis (see Chapter 46) and for reducing their risk of heart disease, including screening for high cholesterol (see Chapter 2) and hypertension (see Chapter 3) and counseling to prevent tobacco use and promote physical activity and healthy diet (see Chapters 54–56).

See also relevant background paper: Grady D, Rubin SM, Petitti DB, et al. Hormone therapy to prevent disease and prolong life in postmenopausal women. Ann Intern Med 1992;117:1016–1037.

The draft update of this chapter was prepared for the U.S. Preventive Services Task Force by David Atkins, MD, MPH, and Robert B. Wallace, MD, MSc, based in part on material prepared for the American College of Physicians by Deborah Grady, MD, MPH, Susan M. Rubin, MPH, Diana B. Petitti, MD, MPH, Cary S. Fox, MS, Dennis Black, PhD, Bruce Ettinger, MD, Virginia L. Ernster, PhD, and Steven R. Cummings, MD.

REFERENCES

1. McKinlay SM, Brambilla DJ, Posner JG. The normal menopause transition. Maturitas 1992;14:103–115.
2. Barbo DM. The physiology of the menopause. Med Clin North Am 1987;71:11–39.
3. Greendale GA, Judd HL. The menopause: health implications and clinical management. J Am Geriatr Soc 1993;41:426–436.
4. Kannel WB. Metabolic risk factors for coronary heart disease in women: perspectives from the Framingham Study. Am Heart J 1987;114:413–419.
5. van Beresteijn ECH, Korevaar JC, Huijbregts PCW, et al. Perimenopausal increase in serum cholesterol: a 10-year longitudinal study. Am J Epidemiol 1993;137:4:383–393.
6. Oldenhave A, Jaszman LJB, Haspels AA, et al. Impact of climacteric on well-being. Am J Obstet Gynecol 1993;168:772–780.
7. Belchetz PE. Hormonal treatment of postmenopausal women. N Engl J Med 1994;1062–1071.

8. Oldenhave A, Netelenbos C. Pathogenesis of climacteric complaints: ready for the change? Lancet 1994;343:649–653.

9. Romano JM, Kaye D. UTI in the elderly: common yet atypical. Geriatrics 1981;36:113–115.

10. Kuhn FE, Rackley CE. Coronary artery disease in women: risk factors, evaluation, treatment and prevention. Arch Intern Med 1993;153:2626–2636.

11. Cummings SR, Black DM, Rubin SM. Lifetime risks of hip, Colles' or vertebral fracture and coronary heart disease among white postmenopausal women. Arch Intern Med 1989;149:2445–2448.

12. Grady D, Rubin SM, Petitti DB, et al. Hormone therapy to prevent disease and prolong life in postmenopausal women. Ann Intern Med 1992;117:1016–1037.

13. Consensus conference: osteoporosis. JAMA 1984;252:799–802.

14. Rossouw JE, Finnegan LP, Harlan WR, et al. The evolution of the Women's Health Initiative: perspectives from the NIH. J Am Med Wom Assoc 1995;50:50–55.

15. Johnston CC, Melton LJ Lindsay R, et al. Clinical indications for bone mass measurements: a report from the Scientific Advisory Board of the National Osteoporosis Foundation. J Bone Min Res 1989;4 (Suppl 2):1–28.

16. Weiss NS, Ure CL, Ballard JH, et al. Decreased risk of fractures of the hip and lower forearm with postmenopausal use of estrogen. N Engl J Med 1980;303:1195–1198.

17. Hutchinson TA, Polansky SM, Feinstein AR. Post-menopausal oestrogens protect against fractures of hip and distal radius: a case-control study. Lancet 1979;2:705–709.

18. Paganini-Hill A, Ross RK, Gerkins VR, et al. Menopausal estrogen therapy and hip fractures. Ann Intern Med 1981;95:28–31.

19. Ettinger B, Genant HK, Cann CE. Long-term estrogen replacement therapy prevents bone loss and fractures. Ann Intern Med 1985;102:319–324.

20. Kiel DP, Felson DT, Anderson JJ, et al. Hip fracture and the use of estrogens in postmenopausal women: the Framingham Study. N Engl J Med 1987;317:1169–1174.

21. Lindsay R, Hart DM, Forrest C, et al. Prevention of spinal osteoporosis in oophorectomized women. Lancet 1980;2:1151–1154.

22. Ettinger B, Grady D. The waning effect of postmenopausal estrogen therapy on osteoporosis. N Engl J Med 1993;329:1192–1193.

23. Ettinger B, Grady D. Maximizing the benefit of estrogen therapy for prevention of osteoporosis. Menopause 1994;1:19–24.

24. Felson DT, Zhang Y, Hannan MT, et al. The effect of postmenopausal estrogen therapy on bone-density in elderly women. N Engl J Med 1993;329:1141–1146.

25. Paganini-Hill A, Chao AA, Ross RK, et al. Exercise and other factors in the prevention of fracture: the Leisure World study. Epidemiology 1991;2:16–25.

26. Cauley JA, Seeley DG, Ensrud K, et al. Estrogen replacement therapy and fractures in older women. Ann Intern Med 1995;122:9–16.

27. Barrett-Connor E, Bush TL. Estrogen and coronary heart disease in women. JAMA 1991;265:1861–1867.

28. Stampfer MJ, Colditz GA. Estrogen replacement and coronary heart disease: a quantitative assessment of the epidemiologic evidence. Prev Med 1991;20:47–63.

29. Stampfer MJ, Colditz GA, Willett WC, et al. Postmenopausal estrogen therapy and cardiovascular disease. Ten year follow-up from the Nurses' Health Study. N Engl J Med 1991;325:756–762.

30. Sullivan JM, Vander Zwagg R, Lemp GF, et al. Postmenopausal estrogen use and coronary atherosclerosis. Ann Intern Med 1988;108:358–363.

31. Hong MK, Romm PA, Reagan K, et al. Effects of estrogen replacement therapy on serum lipid values and angiographically defined coronary artery disease in postmenopausal women. Am J Cardiol 1992;69:176–178.

32. Sullivan JM, Vander Zwaag R, Hughes JP, et al. Estrogen replacement and coronary artery disease: effect on survival in post-menopausal women. Arch Intern Med 1990;150:2557–2562.

33. Wilson PW, Garrison RJ, Castelli WP. Postmenopausal estrogen use, cigarette smoking, and cardiovascular morbidity in women over 50. The Framingham Study. N Engl J Med 1985;313:1038–1043.

34. Mann RD, Lis Y, Chukwujindu J. A study of the association between hormone replacement therapy, smoking and the occurrence of myocardial infarction in women. J Clin Epidemiol 1994;47:307–312.

35. Bush TL, Barrett-Connor E, Cowan LD, et al. Cardiovascular mortality and noncontraceptive use of estrogen in women: results from the Lipid Research Clinics Program follow-up study. Circulation 1987;75:1102–1109

36. Henderson BE, Paganini-Hill A, Ross RK. Estrogen replacement therapy and protection from acute myocardial infarction. Am J Obstet Gynecol 1988;159:312–317.

37. Grodstein F, Stampfer M. The epidemiology of coronary heart disease and estrogen replacement therapy in postmenopausal women. In: Manson J, ed. Progress in cardiovascular diseases. Philadelphia: WB Saunders, 1996 (in press).

38. Walsh BW, Schiff I, Rosner B, et al. Effects of postmenopausal estrogen replacement on the concentrations and metabolism of plasma lipoproteins. N Engl J Med 1991;325:1196–1204.

39. Lobo RA. Clinical review 27: effects of hormonal replacement on lipids and lipoproteins in postmenopausal women. J Clin Endocrinol Metab 1991;73:925–930.

40. Rosano GMC, Sarrel PM, Poole-Wilson PA, et al. Beneficial effect of estrogen on exercise-induced myocardial ischemia in women with coronary artery disease. Lancet 1993;342:133–136.

41. Gilligan DM, Quyyumi AA, Cannon RO, et al. Effects of physiological levels of estrogen on coronary vasomotor function in postmenopausal women. Circulation 1994;89:2545–2551.

42. Sack MN, Rader DJ, Cannon RO. Estrogen and inhibition of oxidation of low-density lipoproteins in postmenopausal women. Lancet 1994;343:269–270.

43. The Postmenopausal Estrogen/Progestin Interventions (PEPI) Trial. Effects of estrogen or estrogen/progestin regimens on heart disease risk factors in postmenopausal women. JAMA 1995;273:199–208.

44. Wysowski DK, Golden L, Burke L. Use of menopausal estrogens and medroxyprogesterone in the United States, 1982–1992. Obstet Gynecol 1995;85:6–10.

45. Nabulsi AA, Folsom AR, White A, et al. Association of hormone-replacement therapy with various cardiovascular risk factors in postmenopausal women. N Engl J Med 1993;328:1069–1075.

46. Psaty BM, Heckbert SR, Atkins D, et al. The risk of myocardial infarction associated with the combined use of estrogens and progestins in postmenopausal women. Arch Intern Med 1994;154:1333–1339.

47. Falkeborn M, Persson I, Adami HO, et al. The risk of acute myocardial infarction after oestrogen and oestrogen-progestogen replacement. Br J Obstet Gynaecol 1992;99:821–828.

48. Psaty BM, Heckbert SR, Atkins D, et al. A review of the association of estrogens and progestins with cardiovascular disease in postmenopausal women. Arch Intern Med 1993;153:1421–1427.

49. Henderson BE, Paganini-Hill A, Ross RK. Decreased mortality in users of estrogen replacement therapy. Arch Intern Med 1991;151:75–78.

50. Finucane FF, Madans JH, Bush TL, et al. Decreased risk of stroke among postmenopausal hormone users. Results from a national cohort. Arch Intern Med 1993;153:73–79.

51. Atkins D, Psaty BM, Koepsell TD, et al. Cholesterol reduction and the risk for stroke in men. A meta-analysis of randomized, controlled trials. Ann Intern Med 1993;119:136–145.

52. Dyken ML, Wolf PA, Barnett HJ, et al. Risk factors for stroke. A statement for physicians by the Subcommittee on Risk Factors and Stroke of the Stroke Council. Stroke 1984;15:1105–1111.

53. Falkeborn M, Persson I, Terent A, et al. Hormone replacement therapy and the risk of stroke. Followup of a population-based cohort in Sweden. Arch Intern Med 1993;153:1201–1209.

54. Raz R, Stamm WE. A controlled trial of intravaginal estriol in postmenopausal women with recurrent urinary tract infections. N Engl J Med 1993;329:752–756.

55. Ditkoff EC, Crary WC, Cristo M. Estrogen improves psychological function in asymptomatic postmenopausal women. Obstet Gynecol 1991;78:991–996.

56. Barrett-Connor E, Kritz-Silverstein D. Estrogen replacement therapy and cognitive function in older women. JAMA 1993;269:2637–2641.

57. Henderson VW, Paganini-Hill A, Emanuel CK, et al. Estrogen replacement therapy in older women. Comparisons between Alzheimer's disease cases and nondemented control subjects. Arch Neurol 1994;51:896–900.

58. Paganini-Hill A, Henderson VW. Estrogen deficiency and risk of Alzheimer's disease in women. Am J Epidemiol 1994;140:256–261.

59. Brenner DE, Kukull WA, Stergachis A, et al. Postmenopausal estrogen replacement therapy and the risk of Alzheimer's disease: a population-based case-control study. Am J Epidemiol 1994;140:262–267.

60. Grady D, Gebretsadik T, Kerlikowske K, et al. Hormone replacement therapy and endometrial cancer risk: a meta-analysis. Obstet Gynecol 1995;85:304–313.

61. Brinton LA, Hoover RN, and the Endometrial Cancer Collaborative Group. Estrogen replacement therapy and endometrial cancer risk: unresolved issues. Obstet Gynecol 1993;81:265–271.

62. Shapiro S, Kelly JP, Rosenberg L, et al. Risk of localized and widespread endometrial cancer in relation to recent and discontinued use of conjugated estrogens. N Engl J Med 1985;313:969–972.

63. Williams DB, Moley KH. Progestin replacement in the menopause: effects on the endometrium and serum lipids. Curr Opin Obstet Gynecol 1994;6:284–292.
64. Voigt L, Weiss N, Chu J, et al. Progestogen supplementation of exogenous oestrogens and risk of endometrial cancer. Lancet 1991;338:274–277.
65. Key TJA, Pike MC. The role of oestrogens and progestogens in the epidemiology and prevention of breast cancer. Eur J Cancer Clin Oncol 1988;24:29–43.
66. Kelsey JL, Gammon MD. Epidemiology of breast cancer. Epidemiol Rev 1990;12:228–240.
67. Armstrong BK. Oestrogen therapy after the menopause—boon or bane. Med J Aust 1988;148: 213–214.
68. Dupont WD, Page DL. Menopausal estrogen replacement therapy and breast cancer. Arch Intern Med 1991;151:67–72.
69. Steinberg KK, Thacker SB, Smith J, et al. A meta-analysis of the effect of estrogen replacement therapy on the risk of breast cancer. JAMA 1991;265:1985–1990.
70. Sillero-Arenas M, Delgado-Rodriguez M, Rodrigues-Cateras R, et al. Menopausal hormone replacement therapy and breast cancer: a meta-analysis. Obstet Gynecol 1992;79:286–294.
71. Colditz GA, Egan KM, Stampfer MJ. Hormone replacement therapy and risk of breast cancer: results from epidemiologic studies. Obstet Gynecol 1993;168:1473–1480.
72. Colditz GA, Hankinson SE, Hunter DJ, et al. The use of estrogens and progestins and the risk of breast cancer in postmenopausal women. N Engl J Med 1995;332:1589–1593.
73. Brinton LA, Hoover R, Fraumeni JF. Menopausal oestrogens and breast cancer risk: an expanded case-control study. Br J Cancer 1986;54:825–832.
74. Strickland DM, Gambrell RD, Butzin CA, et al. The relationship between breast cancer survival and prior postmenopausal estrogen use. Obstet Gynecol 1992;80:400–404.
75. Bonnier P, Romain S, Giacalone PL, et al. Clinical and biologic prognostic factors in breast cancer diagnosed during postmenopausal hormone replacement therapy. Obstet Gynecol 1995;85:11–17.
76. Schairer C, Byrne C, Keyl PM, et al. Menopausal estrogen and estrogen-progestin therapy and risk of breast cancer (United States). Cancer Causes Control 1994;5:491–500.
77. Colditz GA, Stampfer MJ, Willett WC, et al. Type of postmenopausal hormone use and risk of breast cancer: 12-year follow-up from the Nurses Health Study. Cancer Causes Control 1992;3:433–439.
78. Bergkvist L, Adami HO, Persson I, et al. Prognosis after breast cancer diagnosis in women exposed to estrogen and estrogen-progestogen replacement therapy. Am J Epidemiol 1989;130:221–228.
79. Henrich JB. The postmenopausal estrogen/breast cancer controversy. JAMA 1992;268:1900–1902.
80. Brinton LA, Schairer C. Estrogen replacement therapy and breast cancer risk. Epidemiol Rev 1993;15: 66–79.
81. Hunt K, Vessey M, McPherson K. Mortality in a cohort of long-term users of hormone replacement therapy: an updated analysis. Br J Obstet Gynaecol 1990;97:1080–1086.
82. Yuen J, Persson I, Bergkvist L, et al. Hormone replacement therapy and breast cancer in Swedish women: results after adjustment for "healthy drug-user" effect. Cancer Causes Control 1993;4:369–374.
83. Gambrell RD Jr, Maier RC, Sanders BI. Decreased incidence of breast cancer in post-menopausal estrogen-progestogen users. Obstet Gynecol 1983;62:435–443.
84. Bergkvist L, Adami HO, Persson I, et al. The risk of breast cancer after estrogen and estrogen-progestin replacement. N Engl J Med 1989;321:293–297.
85. Kaufman DW, Palmer JR, Mouzon J, et al. Estrogen replacement therapy and the risk of breast cancer: results from the case-control surveillance study. Am J Epidemiol 1991;134:1375–1385.
86. Yang CP, Daling JR, Band PR, et al. Non-contraceptive hormone use and risk of breast cancer. Cancer Causes Control 1992;3:475–479.
87. Persson I, Yuen J, Bergkvist L, et al. Combined oestrogen-progestogen replacement and breast cancer risk. Lancet 1992;340:1044.
87a. Stanford JL, Weiss NS, Voigt LF, et al. Combined estrogen and progestin hormone replacement therapy in relation to risk of breast cancer in middle-aged women. JAMA 1995;274:137–142.
88. Nachtigall MJ, Smilen SW, Nachtigall RD, et al. Incidence of breast cancer in a 22-year study of women receiving estrogen-progestin replacement therapy. Obstet Gynecol 1992;80:827–830.
89. Devor M, Barrett-Connor E, Renvall M, et al. Estrogen replacement therapy and the risk of venous thrombosis. Am J Med 1992;92:275–282.
90. The Coronary Drug Project Research Group. Gallbladder disease as a side effect of drugs influencing lipid metabolism: experience in the Coronary Drug Project. N Engl J Med 1977;296:1185–1190.

91. Nachtigall LE, Nachtigall RH, Nachtigall RD, et al. Estrogen replacement therapy II: a prospective study in relationship to carcinoma and cardiovascular and metabolic problems. Obstet Gynecol 1979;54:74–79.
92. Grodstein F, Colditz G, Stampfer MJ. Postmenopausal hormone use and cholecystectomy in a large prospective study. Obstet Gynecol 1994;83:5–11.
93. LaVecchia C, Negri E, D'Avanzo B, et al. Oral contraceptives and non-contraceptive estrogens in the risk of gallstone disease requiring surgery. J Epidemiol Community Health 1992;46:234–236.
94. Scragg RKR, McMichael AJ, Seamark RF. Oral contraceptives, pregnancy and endogenous estrogen in gallstone disease—a case-control study. BMJ 1984;288:1795–1799.
95. Kakar F, Weiss NS, Strite SA. Non-contraceptive estrogen use and the risk of gallstone disease in women. Am J Public Health 1988;78:564–566.
96. Udoff L, Langenberg P, Adashi EY. Combined continuous hormone replacement therapy: a critical review. Obstet Gynecol 1995;86:306–316.
97. Barrett-Connor E. Post-menopausal estrogen and prevention bias. Ann Intern Med 1991;115:455–456.
98. Petitti DB. Coronary heart disease and estrogen replacement therapy: can compliance bias explain the results of observational studies? Ann Epidemiol 1994;4:115–118.
99. Cauley JA, Cummings SR, Black DM, et al. Prevalence and determinants of estrogen replacement therapy in elderly women. Am J Obstet Gynecol 1990;163:1438–1444.
100. Daly E, Roche M, Barlow D, et al. HRT: an analysis of benefits, risks, and costs. Br Med Bull 1992;48:368–400.
101. Zubialde JP, Lawler F, Clemenson N. Estimated gains in life expectancy with use of postmenopausal estrogen therapy: a decision analysis. J Fam Pract 1993;36:271–280.
102. Gorsky RD, Koplan JP, Peterson HB, et al. Relative risks and benefits of long-term estrogen replacement therapy: a decision analysis. Obstet Gynecol 1994;83:161–166.
103. Wren BG, Brown L. Compliance with hormonal replacement therapy. Maturitas 1991;13:17–21.
104. Ravnikar VA. Compliance with hormone therapy. Am J Obstet Gynecol 1987;156:1332–1334.
105. Ferguson KJ, Hoegh C, Johnson S. Estrogen replacement therapy—a survey of women's knowledge and attitudes. Arch Intern Med 1989;149:133–136.
106. Rubin SM, Cummings SR. Results of bone densitometry affect women's decisions about taking measures to prevent fractures. Ann Intern Med 1992;116:990–995.
107. Ryan PJ, Harrison R, Blake GM. Compliance with hormone replacement therapy (HRT) after screening for postmenopausal osteoporosis. Br J Obstet Gynaecol 1992;99:325–328.
108. Coope J, Marsh J. Can we improve compliance with long-term HRT? Maturitas 1992;15:151–158.
109. Hahn RG. Compliance considerations with estrogen replacement: withdrawal bleeding and other factors. Am J Obstet Gynecol 1989;161:1854–1858.
110. American College of Obstetricians and Gynecologists. Hormone replacement therapy. Technical Bulletin no. 166. Washington, DC: American College of Obstetricians and Gynecologists, 1992.
111. American Academy of Family Physicians. Age charts for periodic health examination. Kansas City, MO: American Academy of Family Physicians, 1994. (Reprint no. 510.)
112. Canadian Task Force on the Periodic Health Examination. Canadian guide to clinical preventive health care. Ottawa: Canada Communication Group, 1994:620–631.
113. American College of Physicians. Guidelines for counselling postmenopausal women about preventive hormone therapy. Ann Intern Med 1992;117:1038–1041.
114. U.S. Congress, Office of Technology Assessment. Effectiveness and costs of osteoporosis screening and hormone replacement therapy, vol. I: cost-effectiveness analysis. Washington, DC:U.S. Government Printing Office, 1995. (Publication no. OTA-BP-H-160.)
115. U.S. Congress, Office of Technology Assessment. Effectiveness and costs of osteoporosis screening and hormone replacement therapy, vol. II: evidence on benefits, risks, and costs. Washington, DC:U.S. Government Printing Office, 1995. (Publication no. OTA-BP-H-144.)

69. Aspirin Prophylaxis for the Primary Prevention of Myocardial Infarction

RECOMMENDATION

There is insufficient evidence to recommend for or against routine aspirin prophylaxis for the primary prevention of myocardial infarction (MI) in asymptomatic persons. Although aspirin reduces the risk of MI in men ages 40–84, its use is associated with important adverse effects, and the balance of benefits and harms is uncertain. If aspirin prophylaxis is considered, clinicians and patients should discuss potential benefits and risks for the individual before beginning its use (see *Clinical Intervention*).

Burden of Suffering

Cardiovascular diseases are the leading causes of death in the U.S., with a mortality rate in 1993 of 366.3/100,000 population.[1] There are approximately 1.5 million myocardial infarctions (MIs) annually and nearly 500,000 deaths from ischemic heart disease.[1,2] Each year, about 150,000 Americans die from stroke.[1,2] The cost to the U.S. of medical care and lost productivity due to cardiovascular diseases was estimated at $117.4 billion in 1990.[2] MI and sudden death often occur without warning in persons with no history of angina pectoris or other cardiovascular symptoms. The principal risk factors for coronary heart disease are smoking, high blood pressure, elevated serum cholesterol, obesity, diabetes mellitus, physical inactivity, increased age, male sex, and a family history of premature coronary artery disease. Postmenopausal hormone replacement is associated with reduced risk of coronary heart disease in women (see Chapter 68).

Efficacy of Chemoprophylaxis

Two randomized controlled trials, one each in the U.S. and Great Britain, have examined the efficacy of aspirin in the primary prevention of MI in healthy middle-aged and older men. In the American trial, more than 22,000 asymptomatic male physicians received either 325 mg aspirin or placebo every other day.[3–5] Physicians ages 40 to 84 years were enrolled, although few subjects were older than 75 years. The study was terminated prematurely, after 60.2 months of follow-up, when a statistically significant 44% reduction in the incidence of total (fatal plus nonfatal) MIs was noted in the group receiving aspirin. This represents an absolute risk reduction of less than two events per thousand individuals per year. In subgroup analyses, this beneficial effect occurred only in individuals age 50 years and older, although the absolute number of MIs occurring in those under the age of 50 was very small. Total cardiovascular mortality was equal between the two groups (81 in the aspirin group vs. 83 in the placebo group).

The British trial, with a smaller sample size (5139 male physicians 80 years of age) and a higher dose of aspirin (500 mg daily), found no significant change in incidence of MI (1% increase) or total cardiovascular mortality (6% reduction) in the treated group.[6] Although the apparent absence of an effect on these outcomes may have been due to lack of efficacy, the British trial may have failed to demonstrate a significant effect due to inadequate sample size or other differences in study design (e.g., high dropout rate, higher dose, no placebo).[7]

In the American physician trial, an increase in sudden death was noted in the aspirin group (22 vs. 12) which offset the reduction in fatal MI, leading to similar rates of total cardiovascular mortality. Both the American and British trials observed an increase in the incidence of stroke among persons taking aspirin, which in the American trial was due primarily to an increase in hemorrhagic stroke.[4] However, none of these differences was statistically significant.[4,6] In addition to possible increases in risk of hemorrhagic stroke and sudden death, other side effects of aspirin therapy must be considered in evaluating its long-term safety. Aspirin can produce unpleasant gastrointestinal symptoms such as stomach pain, heartburn, nausea, and constipation, as well as gastrointestinal blood loss, gastritis, and peptic ulcer disease.[8] The likelihood of these side effects in otherwise healthy persons is directly related to the dose of aspirin.[9] In the British trial, in which the dose was 500 mg daily, 20% of the doctors taking aspirin had to discontinue the drug due to dyspepsia or constipation, 3.6% experienced bleeding or bruising, and 2.2% had gastrointestinal blood loss.[6] In the American trial, in which the dose was 325 mg every other day, there was less than a 1% difference in gastrointestinal complaints between the aspirin and placebo groups. Although the transfusion rate was statistically significantly higher in the aspirin group, only one case (which was unconfirmed) of fatal gastrointestinal hemorrhage was reported in this group in 5 years of treatment.[4] Similarly, a large secondary prevention trial also reported little difference in epigastric discomfort, decreased hemoglobin concentration, or occult blood in stool in persons receiving 325 mg/day.[10]

There are no randomized controlled trials that assess the role of aspirin prophylaxis in the primary prevention of cardiovascular disease in women, although one such study is currently being conducted among 40,000 U.S. female health professionals over the age of 45.[11] A 1991 prospective cohort study[12] followed 87,678 women (registered nurses) for 6 years to examine the association between self-selected aspirin use and risk of a first MI. After controlling for risk factors, they found a statistically significant association between taking one to six aspirins a week and a 25% reduction in first (nonfatal plus fatal) MI. The association was seen at all ages, but was strongest in women age 50 and older. No benefit was seen for those using 7–14 or 15 or more aspirins per week. Aspirin usage did not affect the rate of hemorrhagic stroke. There was a nonsignificant reduction in total cardiovascular and all-cause mortality in the aspirin group. The association between aspirin prophylaxis and reduction in first MI was accentuated in women who currently smoked, had a history of hypertension, or had an elevated serum cholesterol level.

The success of aspirin prophylaxis in persons who have documented disease (secondary prevention) is felt by some to support the practice of prescribing aspirin in asymptomatic, high-risk persons. Several secondary prevention trials have shown that daily aspirin ingestion can lower the risk of subsequent nonfatal ischemic strokes, nonfatal MI, and total cardiovascular mortality in persons at increased risk for thrombotic cardiovascular events (those with unstable angina, previous MI, transient ischemic attacks, prior ischemic stroke, and after coronary artery bypass graft surgery and thrombolysis).[10,13–17] Three meta-analyses extend the populations for whom aspirin is beneficial for secondary prevention to include women, the elderly, hypertensives, and diabetics.[18–20] Aspirin has also been shown to reduce mortality in acute evolving MI.[14]

The use of aspirin to prevent stroke has also been proposed for persons without neurologic symptoms who are at increased risk for thromboembolic events, including those with carotid bruits (see Chapter 4), valvular heart disease, and atrial fibrillation.[21,28] Some evidence supports the use of aspirin in nonrheumatic atrial fibrillation,[22–26] but convincing data to support its efficacy in persons with valvular heart disease or carotid bruits are lacking. There have been no randomized trials designed to evaluate the role of aspirin in the primary prevention of stroke.

A review of 25 secondary prevention trials with a total of 29,000 patients[27] found little difference in outcome in dosages ranging from 300 to 1500 mg/day, suggesting that lower-dose therapy is as effective as higher dose regimens in reducing cardiovascular risks while reducing the risk of side effects. It is possible that high-dose therapy may even have less platelet-inhibitory effect than low-dose therapy, because of inhibition of vessel wall synthesis of prostacyclin along with platelet production of thromboxane A_2.

Effectiveness of Counseling

There is little information on whether asymptomatic patients will comply with physician advice to take aspirin for an extended period of time. Aspirin is the most consumed drug in the U.S., with an estimated 20–30 billion tablets ingested each year,[10] but most patients use aspirin to relieve pain, fever, or other symptoms. It is not known whether healthy individuals would be able or willing to comply with a lifelong daily (or alternate day) regimen, especially if it produces unpleasant side effects. As noted above, over the course of 6 years, 20% of the doctors participating in the British trial were forced to discontinue a daily 500 mg aspirin regimen because of dyspepsia or constipation. In the American study, 33,223 male physicians were initially willing to participate, but after an 18 week run-in period one third of them (11,152) were excluded prior to randomization because of poor compliance, the development of an exclusion criterion or side effects, or an unwillingness to continue participation. Compliance by physicians may not accurately predict compliance in the general population.

Recommendations of Other Groups

The American Heart Association has recently stated that the use of aspirin seems prudent in middle-aged and older men whose risks of a first MI are sufficiently high to warrant the possible adverse effects of long-term use of the drug.[28] They emphasize that the decision to use aspirin should be made on an individual basis, that aspirin prophylaxis is only an adjunct to coronary heart disease risk factor management, and that efforts should first be directed at modifying primary risk factors for heart disease and stroke, assessing potential contraindications to aspirin, and counseling patients about potential side effects and symptoms requiring medical attention.[29]

The Canadian Task Force on The Periodic Health Examination states that there is no clear evidence that routine use of aspirin in asymptomatic men leads to a reduction in all-cause mortality, cardiovascular disease, or MI (when sudden deaths are taken into account). They concluded that the evidence was not strong enough to support a recommendation for or against routine aspirin therapy for the primary prevention of cardiovascular disease in asymptomatic men and women. The Canadian Task Force recommended that the decision whether to prescribe aspirin should be made on an individual basis after the benefits of decreased risk of ischemic cardiovascular events have been balanced against the potential risks associated with prolonged aspirin use.[30]

The American Academy of Family Physicians recommends that physicians discuss aspirin prophylaxis with men who have risk factors for MI (e.g., high blood cholesterol, smoking, diabetes mellitus, family history of early-onset coronary artery disease) and who lack a history of gastrointestinal or other bleeding problems and other risk factors for bleeding or cerebral hemorrhage.[31] This policy is currently under review.

Discussion

Data from a large trial have provided evidence that low-dose aspirin therapy can reduce the risk of MI in asymptomatic men.[4] However, it is important to note that these benefits were demonstrated in a select population: male doctors between the ages of 40 and 84, in exceptionally good health, who were prescreened to eliminate persons unable to tolerate aspirin. In addition, there was no benefit in total cardiovascular mortality, because the reduction in the rate of acute fatal MI was offset by an increased rate of sudden death. No study to date, however, has had sufficient power to adequately evaluate the effectiveness of low-dose aspirin in reducing total cardiovascular mortality. Some patients might judge the reduced risk of nonfatal MI inadequate to justify the increased complication rates associated with aspirin prophylaxis. In both the U.S. and British studies, significant complications including duodenal ulcers and gastrointestinal bleeding were noted in the aspirin group. Moreover, in both trials, strokes were more common in men taking aspirin. Although the differences were not statistically significant, the consistency of the findings suggests that further study of the relationship between aspirin therapy and cerebral hemorrhage is warranted. Some have suggested that hypertensive patients, a population at increased risk for both coronary artery and cerebrovascular disease, may be more likely to experience hemorrhagic stroke while taking this drug.[10,32]

CLINICAL INTERVENTION

There is insufficient evidence to determine whether the proven benefits of routine aspirin prophylaxis given for the primary prevention of MI in asymptomatic men ages 40 to 84 years outweigh the proven harms, and thus the U.S. Preventive Services Task Force does not recommend for or against its use ("C" recommendation). In men with other risk factors for coronary heart disease who lack contraindications to aspirin use (including allergy to aspirin, history of uncontrolled hypertension, liver or kidney disease, diabetic retinopathy, peptic ulcer or other gastrointestinal disease, bleeding problems, or other risk factors for bleeding or cerebral hemorrhage), the benefits may outweigh the harms. In asymptomatic men without risk factors for coronary heart disease or with relative contraindications to aspirin use, the harms may outweigh the benefits. If aspirin therapy is considered, physicians and patients should understand the potential benefits and risks of aspirin therapy before beginning treatment. At the present time, data are insufficient to support or oppose the

use of aspirin prophylaxis for the prevention of MI in women ("C" recommendation). All patients should be encouraged to focus their efforts on modifying primary risk factors for cardiovascular disease such as smoking (Chapter 54), elevated cholesterol (Chapters 2 and 56), and hypertension (Chapter 3).

The draft update of this chapter was prepared for the U.S. Preventive Services Task Force by Peter W. Pendergrass, MD, MPH, and Carolyn DiGuiseppi, MD, MPH.

REFERENCES

1. National Center for Health Statistics. Annual summary of births, marriages, divorces, and deaths: United States, 1993. Monthly vital statistics report; vol 42 no 13. Hyattsville, MD: Public Health Service, 1994.
2. American Heart Association. 1993 heart and stroke fact statistics. Dallas, TX: American Heart Association, 1993.
3. The Steering Committee of the Physicians' Health Study Research Group. Preliminary report: findings from the aspirin component of the ongoing Physicians' Health Study. N Engl J Med 1988;318:262–264.
4. The Steering Committee of the Physicians' Health Study Research Group. Final report on the aspirin component of the ongoing Physicians' Health Study. N Engl J Med 1989;321:129–135.
5. Manson JE, Buring JE, Satterfield S, et al. Baseline characteristics of participants in the Physicians' Health Study: a randomized trial of aspirin and beta-carotene in U.S. physicians. Am J Prev Med 1991;7:150–154.
6. Peto R, Gray R, Collins R, et al. Randomised trial of prophylactic daily aspirin in British male doctors. BMJ 1988;296:313–316.
7. Hennekens CH, Peto R, Hutchison GB, et al. An overview of the British and American aspirin studies. N Engl J Med 1988;318:923–924.
8. Fuster V, Cohen M, Chesebro JH. Usefulness of aspirin for coronary artery disease. Am J Cardiol 1988;61:637–640.
9. UK-TIA Study Group. United Kingdom transient ischemic attack (UK-TIA) aspirin trial interim results. BMJ 1988;296: 316–320.
10. Lewis HD, Davis JW, Archibald DG, et al. Protective effects of aspirin against acute myocardial infarction and death in men with unstable angina: results of a Veterans Administration cooperative study. N Engl J Med 1983;309:396–403.
11. Buring JE, Hennekens CH. The Women's Health Study: summary of the study design. J Myocardial Ischemia 1992;4: 27–29.
12. Manson JE, Stampfer MJ, Colditz GA, et al. A prospective study of aspirin use and primary prevention of cardiovascular disease in women. JAMA 1991;266:521–527.
13. ISIS-2 (Second International Study of Infarct Survival) Collaborative Group. Randomized trial of intravenous streptokinase, oral aspirin, both or neither among 17,187 cases of suspected acute myocardial infarction: ISIS-2. Lancet 1988;2:349–360.
14. Wallentin LC. Aspirin (75 mg/day) after an episode of unstable coronary artery disease: long-term effects on the risk for myocardial infarction, occurrence of severe angina and the need for revascularization. J Am Coll Cardiol 1991;18:1587–1593.
15. The Salt Collaborative Group. Swedish aspirin low-dose trial (SALT) of 75 mg aspirin as secondary prophylaxis after cerebrovascular ischemic events. Lancet 1991;338:1345–1349.
16. The Dutch TIA Trial Study Group. A comparison of two doses of aspirin (30 mg vs 283 mg a day) in patients after a transient ischemic attack or minor ischemic stroke. N Engl J Med 1991;325:1261–1266.
17. Nyman I, Larsson H, Wallentin L. Prevention of serious cardiac events by low-dose aspirin in patients with silent myocardial ischemia. Lancet 1992;340:497–501.
18. Antiplatelet Trialists' Collaboration. Collaborative overview of randomised trials of antiplatelet therapy—I: prevention of death, myocardial infarction, and stroke by prolonged antiplatelet therapy in various categories of patients. BMJ 1994;308:81–106.

19. Antiplatelet Trialists' Collaboration. Collaborative overview of randomised trials of antiplatelet therapy—II: maintenance of vascular graft or arterial patency by antiplatelet therapy. BMJ 1994;308:159–168.
20. Antiplatelet Trialists' Collaboration. Collaborative overview of randomised trials of antiplatelet therapy—III: reduction in venous thrombosis and pulmonary embolism by antiplatelet prophylaxis among surgical and medical patients. BMJ 1994;308:235–246.
21. Foster JW, Hart RG. Antithrombotic therapy for cerebrovascular disease: prevention and treatment of stroke. Postgrad Med 1986;80:199–206.
22. Stroke Prevention in Atrial Fibrillation Investigators. Predictors of thromboembolism in atrial fibrillation study: final report. Circulation 1991;84:527–539.
23. Peterson P, Boyson G, Godtredsen J, et al. Placebo-controlled, randomized trial of warfarin and aspirin for prevention of thromboembolic complications in chronic atrial fibrillation. Lancet 1989;1:175–179.
24. Veterans Affairs Stroke Prevention in Nonrheumatic Atrial Fibrillation Investigators. Warfarin in the prevention of stroke associated with nonrheumatic atrial fibrillation. N Engl J Med 1992;327:1406–1412.
25. The Boston Area Anticoagulation Trial for Atrial Fibrillation Investigators. The effect of low-dose warfarin on the risk of stroke in patients with nonrheumatic atrial fibrillation. N Engl J Med 1990;323:1505–1511.
26. Connolly SJ, Laupacis A, Gent M, et al. Canadian atrial fibrillation anticoagulation (CAFA) study. J Am Coll Cardiol 1991;18:349–355.
27. Anti-Platelet Trialists' Collaboration. Secondary prevention of vascular disease by prolonged antiplatelet treatment. BMJ 1988;296:320–331.
28. Fuster V, Dyken ML, Vokonas PS, et al. Aspirin as a therapeutic agent in cardiovascular disease. Circulation 1993;87: 659–675.
29. American Heart Association. Physicians' Health Study report on aspirin. Circulation 1988;77:1447A.
30. Canadian Task Force on the Periodic Health Examination. Canadian guide to clinical preventive health care. Ottawa: Canada Communication Group, 1994:680–691.
31. American Academy of Family Physicians. Age charts for periodic health examination. Kansas City, MO: American Academy of Family Physicians, 1994. (Reprint no. 510.)
32. Shapiro S. The Physicians' Health Study: aspirin for the primary prevention of myocardial infarction [letter]. N Engl J Med 1988;318:924.

70. Aspirin Prophylaxis in Pregnancy

RECOMMENDATION

There is insufficient evidence to recommend for or against the routine use of aspirin to prevent preeclampsia or intrauterine growth retardation in pregnant women, including those at high risk (see *Clinical Intervention*).

Burden of Suffering

Pregnancy-associated hypertension/preeclampsia/eclampsia syndrome (see Chapter 37 for definitions) is the second leading cause of maternal death in the U.S.[1,2] In 1992, over 112,000 pregnant women (28.5/1,000 live births) developed pregnancy-associated hypertension, of whom approximately 13% were classified as severe.[3] Maternal complications associated with preeclampsia include abruptio placentae, acute renal failure, cerebral hemorrhage, disseminated intravascular coagulation, pulmonary edema, circulatory collapse, eclampsia, and death.[4] Preeclampsia also increases the rate of cesarean delivery and prolongs the duration of hospitalization.[3,5] Neonatal complications include low birth weight (due to preterm delivery and/or intrauterine growth retardation), preterm delivery, hypoxia, and perinatal death.[6] Risk factors for preeclampsia include age (<20 or ≥40 years), Native American race, family history, nulliparity, twin gestation, chronic hypertension, diabetes, collagen vascular disease, and a previous history of pregnancy-associated hypertension or preeclampsia.[3,7,8]

Efficacy of Chemoprophylaxis

Preeclampsia may be due to endothelial dysfunction caused by the systemic effects of decreased placental blood flow.[8] Compared to women with normal pregnancies, women with preeclampsia have a relative excess of thromboxane A_2 (a platelet-derived vasoconstrictor and platelet aggregation promoter) compared to prostacyclin (an endothelial cell-derived vasodilator and platelet aggregation inhibitor).[9–11] The correction of the thromboxane A_2 to prostacyclin ratio caused by aspirin may help prevent the development of preeclampsia and its complications.[12]

A number of randomized controlled trials have evaluated the potential benefit of prophylactic aspirin in preventing preeclampsia. Two studies[13,14] were performed in routine obstetric patients. Hauth[13] et al. randomized 604 nulliparous women under the age of 28 years to 60 mg aspirin or placebo daily from 24 weeks' gestation until delivery. Compared with the placebo group, the group receiving aspirin experienced a statistically significant reduction in total and severe preeclampsia and in levels of thromboxane B_2, a metabolite of thromboxane A_2. No statistically significant differences emerged in the rates of neonatal complications (including low birth weight, prematurity, and fetal death), maternal complications, or cesarean deliveries. Sibai[14] et al. studied 3,135 nulliparous women. These women received either 60 mg aspirin (n = 1,485) or placebo (n = 1,500) daily from <26 weeks' gestation to delivery. The treated group had a 26% reduction in the incidence of preeclampsia compared with the placebo group (4.6% vs. 6.3%, p = 0.05). Women who received aspirin had a significant increase in the risk of abruptio placentae: 0.7% vs. 0.1% (p = 0.01). This outcome was not defined before the trial, however; its definition was not standardized nor was the diagnosis confirmed by external review. There were no other significant differences in maternal or fetal outcomes.

In the largest trial to date, the CLASP Collaborative Group[15] randomized 9,364 women to either 60 mg aspirin or placebo daily. Women were eligible for entry into the study for prophylactic (n = 8,021) or therapeutic (n = 1,343) treatment if they were between 12 and 32 weeks' gestation and either had signs or symptoms of preeclampsia or intrauterine growth retardation (IUGR) or were considered by the physician to be at high risk for preeclampsia or IUGR (based on a history of preeclampsia or IUGR in a previous pregnancy, chronic hypertension, renal disease, maternal age, family history, or multiple gestation). This study found a significant, small reduction in preterm deliveries in the aspirin group (12% reduction among high-risk asymptomatic women), but no difference in the incidence of preeclampsia or IUGR. An increase in transfusion rates was noted in the aspirin group; it was not associated with the occurrence or severity of postpartum hemorrhage, however, nor were there significant differences in abruptio placentae or other antepartum bleeding. No other maternal or fetal complications were noted. This trial may have failed to show an effect of aspirin on preeclampsia because of the variability and subjectivity of entry criteria (which were based on the responsible clinician's rating of risk), and the use of a more conservative statistical analysis ($\alpha = 0.01$ and two-tailed test of significance).

Three smaller trials[16–18] also examined the use of aspirin in women at increased risk of preeclampsia. These studies identified women at increased risk on the basis of results of various screening tests, including the "rollover" test,[16] wave form ultrasound,[17] and angiotensin test.[18] Intervention began between 24 and 32 weeks, and the dose of aspirin ranged from

60 to 100 mg/day. Each study found a statistically significant reduction in preeclampsia in the aspirin-treated group, but no significant differences in fetal or maternal complications. The cesarean delivery rate was significantly lower in the aspirin group in two of the studies.[17,18]

Three other randomized controlled trials enrolled women with risk factors for preeclampsia, including nulliparity, multiple gestations, chronic hypertension, and previous pregnancy with preeclampsia, IUGR, or fetal death.[19–21] All three studies showed a significant reduction in preeclampsia in the aspirin group. Two additional trials, from Finland[22] and Italy,[23] found no significant reduction in pregnancy-associated hypertension in the aspirin-treated group. These study populations included women who had pregnancy-associated hypertension or preeclampsia in the current pregnancy as well as asymptomatic high-risk women, however, which may have masked a benefit.

Three trials, two randomized[15,24] and one nonrandomized,[25] tested the efficacy of low-dose aspirin in the prevention of IUGR in asymptomatic high-risk women. The CLASP trial[15] (see above) of women at increased risk of IUGR found no difference in incidence of IUGR between those who were randomized to receive aspirin prophylaxis compared to placebo. In the other randomized controlled trial,[24] pregnant women with a history of poor outcomes (including IUGR) in two earlier pregnancies were randomized to receive either aspirin 150 mg/day or a placebo, beginning at 15 to 18 weeks' gestation. Those given aspirin had significantly heavier babies (mean 225 g higher; $p = 0.03$), and the proportion weighing less than the 10th percentile was decreased from 26% to 13% in the treated group ($p < 0.02$). The nonrandomized trial also found a significant reduction in IUGR in the aspirin group. Two other randomized controlled trials cited above found no difference in IUGR incidence with aspirin prophylaxis, but the inclusion of both symptomatic and asymptomatic high-risk women may have concealed an effect.[22,23]

The safety of aspirin prophylaxis in pregnancy must be carefully considered. While there have been sporadic reports of congenital heart defects associated with aspirin use in the first trimester of pregnancy, no causal link between aspirin and birth defects has been established.[26] Preterm closure of the ductus arteriosus has also been reported. High-dose aspirin consumption close to delivery can result in maternal and fetal clotting abnormalities such as increased maternal bleeding and neonatal intracranial hemorrhage.[12,27] Maternal effects were seen with doses of 1,500–2,500 mg/day, and neonatal effects with doses of 325–1,500 mg/day. Bleeding problems have not generally been reported at low doses (60–150 mg/day),[28–30] although most trials were too small to detect rare adverse effects. The two largest trials each found a significantly increased risk of bleeding: abruptio placentae in one trial[14] and an increased risk of postpartum maternal transfusion in the other.[15] A meta-analysis of 11 randomized controlled trials of low-dose aspirin prophylaxis in pregnancy did not find an association, however, between aspirin and either abruptio placentae or perinatal mortality.[31]

Effectiveness of Counseling

Little information on compliance with daily aspirin prophylaxis during pregnancy is available. In one trial, 315 of 919 women failed a 2-week run-in period due to poor compliance with either visits or medication.[13] In another trial, 35 of 39 women recruited for a placebo-controlled study of low-dose aspirin therapy in the prevention of preeclampsia refused participation.[32] Reasons for refusal included fear that aspirin would harm the fetus or the pregnant woman, the belief that pregnant women should not participate in experimental studies of drugs, and the belief that women should avoid medications during pregnancy.

Recommendations of Other Groups

No organization currently recommends routine aspirin prophylaxis in pregnancy for the prevention of preeclampsia or intrauterine growth retardation.

Discussion

Numerous randomized controlled trials among both low-risk and high-risk pregnant women indicate that aspirin prophylaxis reduces the incidence and severity of preeclampsia. Nevertheless, no consistent reductions in other fetal or maternal complications have been seen. Although the CLASP trial found a significant reduction in preterm delivery, most trials to date have had insufficient power to identify clinically important differences in rates of prematurity, respiratory distress syndrome, and perinatal death. A meta-analysis of controlled trials reported no significant effect of aspirin on perinatal mortality.[31] In addition, the largest trial in healthy low-risk women[14] found a significant increase in the risk of abruptio placentae, a potentially life-threatening complication for both the fetus and the woman, while the CLASP trial[15] reported an increased risk of maternal transfusion postpartum. Hence, the net health impact of routine aspirin prophylaxis remains uncertain. While aspirin appears to reduce the incidence of preeclampsia, it is unknown whether it improves other, perhaps more important, fetal and maternal outcomes. Preeclampsia may be only one manifestation of a broader underlying pathophysiologic defect. Complications commonly attributed to preeclampsia may be due to the underlying pathology and not to preeclampsia per se. If so, prevention of preeclampsia may not translate into an overall clinical benefit.

One randomized trial found a beneficial effect of aspirin on birth weight among women at increased risk for delivering an infant with IUGR. While statistically significant, this effect may have little clinical impact due to problems with the definition of "growth retardation." This study did not differentiate constitutionally small infants with progressive intrauterine growth from infants with faulty growth patterns. In addition, other randomized trials in asymptomatic and symptomatic women have not reported significant effects on IUGR. Further studies are warranted to confirm any benefit, to determine the optimal gestational ages for administration, and to find the lowest effective dose of aspirin.

CLINICAL INTERVENTION

There is insufficient evidence to recommend for or against routine aspirin prophylaxis in pregnancy for the prevention of either preeclampsia ("C" recommendation) or intrauterine growth retardation ("C" recommendation). Clinicians may wish to inform patients at high risk of preeclampsia that aspirin prophylaxis has been shown to decrease this risk, but such patients should also be informed that aspirin has not been proven to improve overall fetal or maternal outcomes, that one large trial raised the possibility of an increased risk of abruptio placentae, and that aspirin can have additional unpleasant and occasionally serious side effects.

The draft of this chapter was prepared for the U.S. Preventive Services Task Force by Peter W. Pendergrass, MD, MPH, and Carolyn DiGuiseppi, MD, MPH.

REFERENCES
1. Kaunitz AM, Hughes JM, Grimes DA, et al. Causes of maternal mortality in the United States. Obstet Gynecol 1985;65:605–612.
2. Rochat RW, Koonin LM, Atrash HK, et al. Maternal mortality in the United States: report from the maternal mortality collaborative. Obstet Gynecol 1988;72:91–97.
3. Ventura SJ, Martin JA, Taffel SM, et al. Advance report of final natality statistics, 1992. Monthly vital statistics report; vol 43 no 5 (suppl). Hyattsville, MD: National Center for Health Statistics, 1994.
4. Saftlas AF, Olson DR, Franks AL, et al. Epidemiology of preeclampsia and eclampsia in the United States, 1979–1986. Am J Obstet Gynecol 1988;95:644–653.
5. Redman CWG, Robert JM. Management of pre-eclampsia. Lancet 1993;341:1451–1454.
6. Page EW, Christianson R. The impact of mean arterial pressure in the middle trimester upon the outcome of pregnancy. Am J Obstet Gynecol 1976;125:740–746.
7. Cooper DW, Hill JA, Chesley LC, et al. Genetic control of susceptibility to eclampsia and miscarriage. Br J Obstet Gynaecol 1988;95:644–653.
8. Roberts JM, Redman CW. Pre-eclampsia: more than pregnancy-induced hypertension. Lancet 1993;341:1447–1451.
9. Friedman SA. Preeclampsia: a review of the role of prostaglandins. Obstet Gynecol 1988;71:122–137.
10. Noort WA, Keirse MJNC. Prostacyclin versus thromboxane metabolite excretion: changes in pregnancy and labor. Eur J Obstet & Gynecol Reprod Biol 1990;35:15–21.
11. Walsh SW. Preeclampsia: an imbalance in placental prostacyclin and thromboxane production. Am J Obstet Gynecol 1985;152:335–340.
12. Schiff E, Mashiach S. The use of low dose aspirin in pregnancy. Am J Reprod Immunol 1992;28:153–156.
13. Hauth JC, Goldenberg RL, Parker CR, et al. Low-dose aspirin therapy to prevent preeclampsia. Am J Obstet Gynecol 1993;168:1083–1093.

14. Sibai B, Caritis S, Phillips E, et al. Prevention of preeclampsia with low-dose aspirin in healthy, nulliparous pregnant women. N Engl J Med 1993;329:1213–1218.

15. CLASP (Collaborative Low-dose Aspirin Study in Pregnancy) Collaborative Group. CLASP: a randomised trial of low-dose aspirin for the prevention and treatment of pre-eclampsia among 9364 pregnant women. Lancet 1994;343:619–629.

16. Schrocksnadel H, Sitte B, Alge A, et al. Low-dose aspirin in primigravidae with positive roll-over test. Gynecol Obstet Invest 1992;34:146–150.

17. McParland P, Pearce JM, Chamberlain GVP. Doppler ultrasound and aspirin in recognition and prevention of pregnancy-induced hypertension. Lancet 1990;335:1552–1555.

18. Wallenburg HCS, Dekker GA, Markovitz JW, et al. Low-dose aspirin prevents pregnancy-induced hypertension and pre-eclampsia in angiotensin-sensitive primigravidae. Lancet 1986;1:1–3.

19. Schiff E, Peleg E, Goldenberg M, et al. The use of aspirin to prevent pregnancy-induced hypertension and lower the ratio of thromboxane A_2 to prostacyclin in relatively high risk pregnancies. N Engl J Med 1989;321:351–356.

20. Beaufils M, Donsimoni R, Uzan S, et al. Prevention of pre-eclampsia by early antiplatelet therapy. Lancet 1985;1:840–842.

21. Benigni A, Gregorini G, Frusca T, et al. Effect of low-dose aspirin on fetal and maternal generation of thromboxane by platelets in women at risk for pregnancy-induced hypertension. N Engl J Med 1989;321:357–362.

22. Vinikka L, Hartikainen-Sorri AL, Lumme R, et al. Low dose aspirin in hypertensive pregnant women: effect on pregnancy outcome and prostacyclin-thromboxane balance in mother and newborn. Br J Obstet Gynaecol 1993;100: 809–815.

23. Italian Study of Aspirin in Pregnancy. Low-dose aspirin in prevention and treatment of intrauterine growth retardation and pregnancy-induced hypertension. Lancet 1993;341:396–400.

24. Uzan S, Beaufils M, Breart G, et al. Prevention of fetal growth retardation with low-dose aspirin: findings of the EPREDA trial. Lancet 1991;337:1427–1431.

25. Wallenburg HCS, Rotmans N. Prevention of recurrent idiopathic fetal growth retardation by low-dose aspirin and dipyridamole. Am J Obstet Gynecol 1987;157:1230–1235.

26. Hertz-Picciotto I, Hopenhayn-Rich C, Golub M, et al. The risk and benefits of taking aspirin during pregnancy. Epidemiol Rev 1990;12:108–148.

27. Stuart MJ, Gross SJ, Elrad H, et al. Effects of acetylsalicylic acid ingestion on maternal and neonatal hemostasis. N Engl J Med 1982;307:909–912.

28. Valcamonico A, Foschini M, Soregaroli M, et al. Low dose aspirin in pregnancy: a clinical and biochemical study of effects on the newborn. J Perinat Med 1993;21:235–240.

29. Benigni A, Gregorini G, Frusca T, et al. Effects of low dose aspirin on fetal and maternal generation of thromboxane by platelets in women at risk for pregnancy induced hypertension. N Engl J Med 1989;321:357–362.

30. Sibai BM, Mirro R, Chesney C, et al. Low dose aspirin in pregnancy. Obstet Gynecol 1989;74:551–556.

31. Hauth JC, Goldenberg RL, Parker CR Jr, et al. Low-dose aspirin: lack of association with an increase in abruptio placentae or perinatal mortality. Obstet Gynecol 1995;85:1055–1058.

32. Hutton JD, Wilkinson AM, Neale J. Poor participation of nulliparous women in a low dose aspirin study to prevent preeclampsia. NZ Med J 1990;103:511–512.

APPENDICES

Task Force Ratings

The tables of ratings on the following pages were developed for the U.S. Preventive Services Task Force using the methodology adapted from the Canadian Task Force on the Periodic Health Examination[a] and described in Chapter ii. For this edition of the *Guide*, the Task Force developed ratings for all of the topics examined.

The Task Force graded the *strength of recommendations* for or against preventive interventions as follows.

Strength of Recommendations

A: There is good evidence to support the recommendation that the condition be specifically considered in a periodic health examination.

B: There is fair evidence to support the recommendation that the condition be specifically considered in a periodic health examination.

C: There is insufficient evidence to recommend for or against the inclusion of the condition in a periodic health examination, but recommendations may be made on other grounds.

D: There is fair evidence to support the recommendation that the condition be excluded from consideration in a periodic health examination.

E: There is good evidence to support the recommendation that the condition be excluded from consideration in a periodic health examination.

Determination of the quality of evidence (i.e., "good," "fair," "insufficient") in the strength of recommendations was based on a systematic consideration of three criteria: the burden of suffering from the target condition, the characteristics of the intervention, and the effectiveness of the intervention as demonstrated in published clinical research. Effectiveness of the intervention received special emphasis. In reviewing clinical studies, the Task Force used strict criteria for selecting admissible evidence and placed emphasis on the quality of study designs. In grading the *quality of evidence*, the Task Force gave greater weight to those study designs that, for methodologic reasons, are less subject to bias and inferential error. The following rating system was used.

---

[a] Canadian Task Force on the Periodic Health Examination. The periodic health examination. Can Med Assoc J 1979;121:1193–1254.

Quality of Evidence

I: Evidence obtained from at least one properly randomized controlled trial.

II-1: Evidence obtained from well-designed controlled trials without randomization.

II-2: Evidence obtained from well-designed cohort or case-control analytic studies, preferably from more than one center or research group.

II-3: Evidence obtained from multiple time series with or without the intervention. Dramatic results in uncontrolled experiments (such as the results of the introduction of penicillin treatment in the 1940s) could also be regarded as this type of evidence.

III: Opinions of respected authorities, based on clinical experience; descriptive studies and case reports; or reports of expert committees.

Well-designed and well-conducted meta-analyses were also considered, and were graded according to the quality of the studies on which the analyses were based (e.g., Grade I if the meta-analysis pooled properly randomized controlled trials).

An exact correlation does not exist between the strength of the recommendation and the level of evidence, i.e., Level I evidence did not necessarily lead to an "A" grade, nor did an "A" grade require Level I evidence. For example, there may have been evidence of good quality that did not prove that an intervention is effective (e.g., mammography in women under age 50, which received a "C" recommendation). On the other hand, an "A" recommendation was given to screening for cervical cancer with Papanicolaou testing, based on burden of suffering and Level II evidence supporting the effectiveness of the intervention. For many preventive services, there is insufficient evidence to determine whether or not routine intervention will improve clinical outcomes ("C" recommendation). A variety of different circumstances can result in a "C" recommendation: available studies are not adequate to determine effectiveness (e.g., insufficient statistical power, unrepresentative populations, lack of clinically important endpoints, or other important design flaws); high-quality studies have produced conflicting results; evidence of significant benefits is offset by evidence of important harms from intervention; or studies of effectiveness have not been conducted. As a result, lack of evidence of effectiveness does not constitute evidence of ineffectiveness. Chapter ii provides further information about the methodology used to develop the body of this report.

Table 1.
Screening for Asymptomatic Coronary Artery Disease

Intervention	Level of Evidence	Strength of Recommendation
Routine resting, ambulatory, or exercise electrocardiography in middle-aged or older persons	II-2	C
Routine resting electrocardiography in healthy children, adolescents, or young adults, including those undergoing pre-participation sports physicals	III	D

Table 2.
Screening for High Blood Cholesterol and Other Lipid Abnormalities

Intervention	Level of Evidence	Strength of Recommendation
Routine measurement of total serum or blood cholesterol		
Men aged 35–65 yr	I, II-2	B
Women aged 45–65 yr	II-2	B
Persons aged > 65 yr	II-2	C
Children, adolescents, young adults	II-2	C
Routine measurement of HDL-C	II-2, III	C
Routine measurement of triglycerides	II-2	C

Table 3.
Screening for Hypertension

Intervention	Level of Evidence	Strength of Recommendation
Periodic blood pressure measurement in persons aged ≥ 21 yr	I	A
Measurement of blood pressure in children and adolescents during office visits	II-2, II-3, III	B

Table 4.
Screening for Asymptomatic Carotid Artery Stenosis

Intervention	Level of Evidence	Strength of Recommendation
Routine carotid ultrasound or auscultation for carotid bruits in older persons	I, II-2	C

Table 5.
Screening for Peripheral Arterial Disease

Intervention	Level of Evidence	Strength of Recommendation
Routine history-taking for classic claudication, palpation of peripheral pulses, ultrasound, or other noninvasive tests in older persons	III	D

Table 6.
Screening for Abdominal Aortic Aneurysm

Intervention	Level of Evidence	Strength of Recommendation
Routine abdominal palpation	II-2	C
Routine abdominal ultrasound	II-2	C

Table 7.
Screening for Breast Cancer

Intervention	Level of Evidence	Strength of Recommendation
Routine mammogram every 1-2 yr with or without annual clinical breast exam		
Women aged 40–49 yr	I	C
50–69 yr	I, II-2	A
70–74 yr	I, II-3	C
≥ 75 yr	III	C
Annual clinical breast exam without periodic mammograms		
Women aged 40–49 yr	III	C
50–59 yr	I	C
≥ 60 yr	III	C
Routine breast self-exam	I, II-2, III	C

Table 8.
Screening for Colorectal Cancer

Intervention	Level of Evidence	Strength of Recommendation
Annual fecal occult blood testing of persons aged 50 yr and older	I, II-1, II-2	B
Routine sigmoidoscopy in persons aged 50 yr and older	II-2, II-3	B
Routine digital rectal exam	III	C
Routine barium enema	III	C
Routine colonoscopy	III	C

Table 9.
Screening for Cervical Cancer

Intervention	Level of Evidence	Strength of Recommendation
Regular Pap testing in women who are or have been sexually active and who have a cervix	II-2, II-3	A
Discontinuation of regular Pap testing in women aged >65 yr	III	C
Routine cervicography or colposcopy	III	C
Routine testing for HPV infection	III	C

Table 10.
Screening for Prostate Cancer

Intervention	Level of Evidence	Strength of Recommendation
Routine digital rectal exam	II-2	D
Routine prostate-specific antigen or other serum tumor markers	I, II-2, III	D
Routine transrectal ultrasound	II-2, III	D

Table 11.
Screening for Lung Cancer

Intervention	Level of Evidence	Strength of Recommendation
Routine chest x-ray or sputum cytology	I, II-1, II-2	D

Table 12.
Screening for Skin Cancer—Including Counseling to Prevent Skin Cancer

Intervention	Level of Evidence	Strength of Recommendation
Screening		
Total body skin exam by primary care clinicians	II-3, III	C
Periodic skin self-exam	II-3, III	C
Primary Prevention		
Sun avoidance or use of protective clothing by high-risk* persons	II-2	B
Routine use of sunscreens	I, II-2	C
Clinician counseling to increase the use of sun protection measures	III	C

*See relevant chapter for definition of high risk.

Table 13.
Screening for Testicular Cancer

Intervention	Level of Evidence	Strength of Recommendation
Routine self-exam or physician exam of the testes in men	III	C

Table 14.
Screening for Ovarian Cancer

Intervention	Level of Evidence	Strength of Recommendation
Routine pelvic exam, ultrasound, or serum tumor markers		
General female population	II-3, III	D
High-risk* women	III	C

Table 15.
Screening for Pancreatic Cancer

Intervention	Level of Evidence	Strength of Recommendation
Routine abdominal palpation, ultrasound, or serum tumor markers	III	D

Table 16.
Screening for Oral Cancer

Intervention	Level of Evidence	Strength of Recommendation
Routine oral exam by primary care clinicians	III	C

Table 17.
Screening for Bladder Cancer

Intervention	Level of Evidence	Strength of Recommendation
Routine urine dipstick or microscopy	II-2, III	D
Routine urine cytology	III	D

*See relevant chapter for definition of high risk.

Table 18.
Screening for Thyroid Cancer

Intervention	Level of Evidence	Strength of Recommendation
Routine neck palpation or ultrasound		
General population	II-2, III	D
High-risk* adults or children	III	C

Table 19.
Screening for Diabetes Mellitus

Intervention	Level of Evidence	Strength of Recommendation
Non-insulin-dependent		
Routine measurement of plasma glucose, glycosylated hemoglobin, or urine glucose	II-2	C
Gestational		
Routine oral 1-hr glucose challenge test, glycosolated hemoglobin, fasting or random plasma glucose, or urine glucose	I, II-2	C
Insulin-dependent		
Routine measurement of serum auto-antibodies in the general population	III	D

Table 20.
Screening for Thyroid Disease

Intervention	Level of Evidence	Strength of Recommendation
Routine thyroid function tests		
General population	III	D
High-risk* persons	I, II-3	C

Table 21.
Screening for Obesity

Intervention	Level of Evidence	Strength of Recommendation
Periodic height and weight measurements	I, II-2, II-3	B
Routine determination of the waist/hip ratio	II-2	C

*See relevant chapter for definition of high risk.

Table 22.
Screening for Iron Deficiency Anemia—Including Iron Prophylaxis

Intervention	Level of Evidence	Strength of Recommendation
Screening		
Routine hemoglobin/hematocrit		
Pregnant women at first prenatal visit	II-1, II-2	B
High-risk* infants	I	B
High-risk* children	I	C
General population	I, II-1, II-2	C
Repeat hemoglobin/hematocrit in pregnant women or high-risk* infants not anemic at initial testing	III	C
Primary Prevention		
Breastfeeding and use of iron-enriched formula or food for all infants and toddlers	I, II-1, II-2, II-3	B
Routine use of iron supplements		
Healthy pregnant women	I, II-1, II-2	C
Healthy infants	I, III	C

Table 23.
Screening for Elevated Lead Levels in Childhood and Pregnancy

Intervention	Level of Evidence	Strength of Recommendation
Screening		
Routine blood lead measurement		
High-risk* children	II-1, II-2, II-3	B
Pregnant women	III	C
Primary Prevention		
Routinely counseling families to control lead dust by repeated household cleaning, or to optimize caloric, iron, and calcium intake specifically to reduce lead absorption	II-2, III	C

Table 24.
Screening for Hepatitis B Virus Infection

Intervention	Level of Evidence	Strength of Recommendation
Routine measurement of HBsAg		
Pregnant women	I, II-1, II-2, II-3	A
High-risk* persons (to assess eligibility for vaccination)	III	C
General population	III	D

*See relevant chapter for definition of high risk.

Table 25.
Screening for Tuberculous Infection—Including BCG Immunization

Intervention	Level of Evidence	Strength of Recommendation
Tuberculin skin testing of high-risk* persons	I	A
BCG vaccination of selected high-risk* infants and children	I, II-2	B

Table 26.
Screening for Syphilis

Intervention	Level of Evidence	Strength of Recommendation
Routine serologic testing		
High-risk* persons	II-3	A
Pregnant women	II-3	A

Table 27.
Screening for Gonorrhea—Including Ocular Prophylaxis in Newborns

Intervention	Level of Evidence	Strength of Recommendation
Screening		
Routine gonorrhea culture or nonculture screening test		
High-risk* women	II-2, III	B
High-risk* pregnant women	II-2	B
Other pregnant women	III	C
High-risk* men	II-3, III	C
General population	III	D
Primary Prevention of Gonococcal Ophthalmia Neonatorum		
Routine ophthalmic antibiotic in newborns	II-3, III	A

Table 28.
Screening for Human Immunodeficiency Virus Infection

Intervention	Level of Evidence	Strength of Recommendation
Enzyme immunoassay, with confirmatory test for positive results		
High-risk* adolescents and adults	I, II-2	A
High-risk* pregnant women	I, II-2	A
High-risk* infants	II-2	B
Low-risk pregnant women, adolescents, and adults	III	C

*See relevant chapter for definition of high risk.

Table 29.
Screening for Chlamydial Infection—Including Ocular Prophylaxis in Newborns

Intervention	Level of Evidence	Strength of Recommendation
Screening		
Routine culture or nonculture screening test		
Sexually active female adolescents and other high-risk* women	I, II-2, III	B
High-risk* pregnant women	II-2	B
Other pregnant women	III	C
High-risk* men	II-3, III	C
General population	III	D
Primary Prevention of Chlamydial Ophthalmia Neonatorum		
Routine ophthalmic antibiotic in newborns	I, II-2, III	C

Table 30.
Screening for Genital Herpes Simplex

Intervention	Level of Evidence	Strength of Recommendation
Screening		
Routine viral culture, serology, or other tests		
General population	II-3, III	D
Pregnant women	II-2, II-3, III	D
Examination of pregnant women in labor for signs of active genital HSV lesions	II-2, III	C
Primary Prevention of Neonatal Herpes Infection		
Routine use of systemic acyclovir in pregnant women with recurrent herpes	III	C
Counseling uninfected women with infected partners to use condoms or abstain from intercourse during pregnancy	III	C

Table 31.
Screening for Asymptomatic Bacteriuria

Intervention	Level of Evidence	Strength of Recommendation
Routine urine culture in pregnant women at 12-16 weeks' gestation	I	A
Routine urine dipstick for leukocyte esterase/nitrites		
Pregnant women	II-2	D
Diabetic women	III	C
Noninstitutionalized elderly women	I, II-1, II-2	C
Institutionalized elders	I	E
School-aged girls	I	E
Other persons	I, II-2, III	D
Routine urine microscopy	II-2	D

*See relevant chapter for definition of high risk.

Table 32.
Screening for Rubella—Including Immunization of Adolescents and Adults

Intervention	Level of Evidence	Strength of Recommendation
Routine rubella serology or vaccination history		
Women of childbearing age (including pregnant women)	II-2, II-3, III	B
Young men in high-risk* settings	II-3, III	C
Other men and postmenopausal women	III	D
Routine rubella vaccination without screening		
Children	I, II-1, II-2, II-3	A
Nonpregnant women of childbearing age	II-2, III	B
Young men in high-risk* settings	II-2, III	C
Other men and postmenopausal women	III	D

Table 33.
Screening for Visual Impairment

Intervention	Level of Evidence	Strength of Recommendation
Routine testing for amblyopia and strabismus in preschool children	II-1, II-2	B
Routine Snellen acuity testing in elderly persons	II-3	B
Routine ophthalmoscopy by primary care clinicians in elderly persons	III	C
Routine vision screening in other children, adolescents, and adults	III	C

Table 34.
Screening for Glaucoma

Intervention	Level of Evidence	Strength of Recommendation
Routine tonometry	I, II-2, III	C
Routine ophthalmoscopy by primary care clinicians	III	C

*See relevant chapter for definition of high risk.

Table 35.
Screening for Hearing Impairment

Intervention	Level of Evidence	Strength of Recommendation
Periodically questioning older adults about their hearing	I, III	B
Routine audiometric testing in older adults	I, III	C
Routine hearing testing in adolescents and working-age adults[1]	III	C
Routine evoked otoacoustic emission testing or auditory brainstem response in newborns	II-2, III	C
Routine hearing testing in children aged >3 yr	II-2	D

[1]Screening of workers for noise-induced hearing loss should be performed in the context of existing worksite programs and occupational medicine guidelines.

Table 36.
Screening Ultrasonography in Pregnancy

Intervention	Level of Evidence	Strength of Recommendation
Routine midtrimester ultrasound in pregnant women	I	C
Routine third-trimester ultrasound in pregnant women	I	D

Table 37.
Screening for Preeclampsia

Intervention	Level of Evidence	Strength of Recommendation
Periodic blood pressure measurement during pregnancy, as part of routine prenatal care	II-3, III	B

Table 38.
Screening for D (Rh) Incompatibility

Intervention	Level of Evidence	Strength of Recommendation
Routine D (Rh) blood typing and antibody testing of pregnant women at the first visit	I, II-1, II-3	A
Repeat antibody testing of all unsensitized D-negative pregnant women at 24-28 weeks' gestation	II-1	B
Routine administration of D immuno-globulin to unsensitized D-negative women		
Postpartum	I, II-1	A
At 24-28 weeks' gestation	II-1	B
After amniocentesis or induced abortion	II-1, II-3	B
After CVS, other high-risk* obstetric procedures or complications	I, III	C

Table 39.
Intrapartum Electronic Fetal Monitoring

Intervention	Level of Evidence	Strength of Recommendation
Routine intrapartum electronic fetal monitoring		
Low-risk pregnancies	I	D
High-risk* pregnancies	I	C

Table 40.
Home Uterine Activity Monitoring

Intervention	Level of Evidence	Strength of Recommendation
Home uterine activity monitoring		
Normal risk pregnancies	III	D
High-risk* pregnancies	I, II-2	C

*See relevant chapter for definition of high risk.

Table 41.
Screening for Down Syndrome

Intervention	Level of Evidence	Strength of Recommendation
Offering amniocentesis or CVS to high-risk* pregnant women	II-2	B
Offering maternal serum multiple-marker testing to all pregnant women	II-2	B
Offering maternal serum individual marker testing to pregnant women	II-2	C
Offering midtrimester ultrasound to pregnant women	II-2, III	C

Table 42.
Screening for Neural Tube Defects—Including Folate Prophylaxis

Intervention	Level of Evidence	Strength of Recommendation
Screening		
Offering maternal serum a-fetoprotein measurement to all pregnant women	II-2	B
Offering midtrimester ultrasound to all pregnant women	I, II-2, III	C
Primary Prevention		
Periconceptional folic acid 4.0 mg daily for women with previous affected pregnancy	I	A
Daily multivitamin or multivitamin/ multimineral containing 0.4–0.8 mg folic acid for women planning pregnancy	I, II-2	A
Daily multivitamin containing 0.4 mg folic acid for women capable of pregnancy	II-2	B
Dietary folate intake of 0.4 mg/day for women capable of pregnancy	II-2	C

Table 43.
Screening for Hemoglobinopathies

Intervention	Level of Evidence	Strength of Recommendation
Testing for hemoglobinopathies in newborns	I, II-2	A
Offering testing for hemoglobinopathies with counseling		
Pregnant women at first prenatal visit	II-2, II-3, III	B
High-risk* adolescents and young adults	II-1, III	C

*See relevant chapter for definition of high risk.

Table 44.
Screening for Phenylketonuria

Intervention	Level of Evidence	Strength of Recommendation
Routine measurement of phenylalanine level on dried-blood spot specimens in newborns	II-3	A
Routine measurement of blood phenylalanine level in pregnant women	II-2, III	C

Table 45.
Screening for Congenital Hypothyroidism

Intervention	Level of Evidence	Strength of Recommendation
Routine measurement of T_4 and/or TSH on dried-blood spot specimens in newborns	II-3	A

Table 46.
Screening for Postmenopausal Osteoporosis

Intervention	Level of Evidence	Strength of Recommendation
Routine bone densitometry in postmenopausal women	II-2, III	C

Table 47.
Screening for Adolescent Idiopathic Scoliosis

Intervention	Level of Evidence	Strength of Recommendation
Routine forward-bending test, visual inspection of the back, inclinometer, or other tests in adolescents	II-3, III	C

Table 48.
Screening for Dementia

Intervention	Level of Evidence	Strength of Recommendation
Routine use of standardized screening tests in elderly persons	III	C

Table 49.
Screening for Depression

Intervention	Level of Evidence	Strength of Recommendation
Routine use of standardized screening tests in primary care patients	I, II-1	C

Table 50.
Screening for Suicide Risk

Intervention	Level of Evidence	Strength of Recommendation
Screening		
Routine use by primary care clinicians of direct questions or standardized screening tests in the general population	I, II-2, II-3	C
Primary Prevention		
Training primary care clinicians to recognize and treat affective disorders	II-3	B

Table 51.
Screening for Family Violence

Intervention	Level of Evidence	Strength of Recommendation
Routine standardized interview or physical exam to detect child abuse	III	C
Routine standardized interview to detect elder abuse	III	C
Routine standardized questionnaire to detect domestic violence	II-3, III	C

Table 52.
Screening for Problem Drinking

Intervention	Level of Evidence	Strength of Recommendation
Routine interview or standardized questionnaire to detect problem drinking		
Adolescents and adults	I, II-2	B
Pregnant women	II-2	B

Table 53.
Screening for Drug Abuse

Intervention	Level of Evidence	Strength of Recommendation
Routine screening with standardized questionnaires or biologic assays	III	C

Table 54.
Counseling to Prevent Tobacco Use

Intervention	Level of Evidence	Strength of Recommendation
Efficacy of Risk Reduction		
Avoidance or cessation of tobacco use to reduce the risk of cancer, cardiovascular and respiratory diseases, adverse pregnancy and neonatal outcomes, and effects of passive smoking	II-2	A
Effectiveness of Counseling and Other Clinical Interventions		
Clinician counseling of all patients, including pregnant women, who use tobacco to reduce or stop use	I	A
Nicotine patches or gum as an adjunct to counseling	I	A
Clonidine as an adjunct to counseling	I	C
Clinician counseling of school-aged children and adolescents to avoid tobacco use	III[1]	C

[1]Controlled trials have demonstrated the ability of school-based intervention programs to delay the initiation of tobacco use in children and adolescents.

Table 55.
Counseling to Promote Physical Activity

Intervention	Level of Evidence	Strength of Recommendation
Efficacy of Risk Reduction		
Regular physical activity to prevent coronary heart disease, hypertension, obesity, and other diseases	II-2	A
Effectiveness of Counseling		
Counseling patients to incorporate regular physical activity into their daily routines	I, II-2	C

Table 56.
Counseling to Promote a Healthy Diet

Intervention	Level of Evidence	Strength of Recommendation
Efficacy of Risk Reduction in the General Population		
Limiting intake of dietary fat (especially saturated fat)	I, II-2, II-3	A
Limiting intake of dietary cholesterol	II-2	B
Emphasizing fruits, vegetables and grain products containing fiber	II-2, II-3	B
Maintaining caloric balance through diet and exercise	II-2	B
Maintaining adequate intake of dietary calcium in women	I, II-1, II-2, II-3	B
Reducing intake of dietary sodium	II-3	C
Increasing intake of dietary iron	II-2, II-3, III	C
Increasing intake of beta-carotene and other antioxidants	II-2, II-3	C
Breastfeeding infants	I, II-2	A
Effectiveness of Counseling		
Counseling to change dietary habits		
Specially trained educators	I[1]	B
Primary care clinicians	III	C

[1]These trials generally involved specially trained educators such as dieticians delivering intensive interventions (e.g., multiple sessions, tailored materials) to selected patients with known risk factors.

Table 57.
Counseling to Prevent Motor Vehicle Injuries

Intervention	Level of Evidence	Strength of Recommendation
Efficacy of Risk Reduction		
Child safety seats, lap/shoulder belts, and motorcycle helmets	II-2, II-3	A
Avoidance of driving while impaired by alcohol or other drugs	II-2, II-3	A
Driver- and passenger-side air bags	II-2	A
Alteration of pedestrian behavior	II-1, II-2, II-3	C
Effectiveness of Counseling		
Counseling parents to have their children use car safety seats or seat belts as appropriate for age	I, II-1, II-2	B
Counseling adolescent and adult patients to use lap/shoulder belts	II-1, II-3	B
Counseling patients to use motorcycle helmets	III	C
Counseling problem drinkers to reduce their alcohol consumption (see Ch. 52)	I	B
Counseling patients to avoid driving while impaired by alcohol or other drugs	III	C
Counseling patients and parents of child patients on safe pedestrian behavior	III	C

Table 58.
Counseling to Prevent Household and Recreational Injuries

Intervention	Level of Evidence	Strength of Recommendation
Efficacy of Risk Reduction		
Fires and Burns		
Properly installed/tested smoke detectors	II-2	B
Smoking cessation (see Ch. 54)	II-2	A
Flame-retardant sleepwear for children	II-3	A
Hot water heaters set to <120–130° F	II-3	A
Drowning		
Four-foot, four-sided isolation fences with self-latching gates	II-2	B
Cardiopulmonary resuscitation (CPR) training	II-2, III	B
Poisonings		
Child-proof containers for medications	II-3	A
Limitation of number of tablets packaged	II-3	A
Poison-warning stickers designed for children (e.g., "Mr. Yuk" stickers)	II-1	D
Bicycling and ATV Injuries		
Approved bicycle and ATV helmets	II-2, II-3	A
Avoidance of bicycling near traffic	II-2, III	B
ATVs with smaller engines and 4 wheels	II-2	B
Training in safe bicycling behavior	I, III	C
Alcohol-Related Injuries		
Avoidance of swimming, boating, bicycling, hunting, or smoking while intoxicated	II-2	B
Falls in Children		
Window guards in high-risk* buildings	II-3	A
Falls in Elderly Persons		
Exercise, especially balance training	I, II-1, II-2	B
Home-based multifactorial fall prevention interventions in high-risk* elders	I, II-2	B
External hip protectors in institutionalized elderly persons	II-1	C
Other Injury Prevention Measures		
(see Ch. 58 for details)	III	C
Effectiveness of Counseling		
Counseling parents of young children on measures to reduce injury risk	I, II-1, II-2, II-3	B
Counseling adolescents and adults on measures to reduce injury risk	I, III	C
Counseling problem drinkers to reduce alcohol consumption (see Ch. 52)	I	B
Counseling elderly patients to address risk factors for falls	I	C

*See relevant chapter for definition of high risk.

Table 59.
Counseling to Prevent Youth Violence

Intervention	Level of Evidence	Strength of Recommendation
Efficacy of Risk Reduction		
Removal or safe storage of firearms in the home	II-2, II-3, III	B
Acquisition of interpersonal - problem solving skills	II-2, III	C
Reduction of heavy or problem drinking	II-2, II-3, III	B
Reduction of illicit drug use or drug trafficking	II-2, III	C
Effectiveness of Counseling		
Counseling problem drinkers to reduce alcohol consumption (see Ch. 52)	I	B
Counseling on measures to reduce violence risk	III	C

Table 60.
Counseling to Prevent Low Back Pain

Intervention	Level of Evidence	Strength of Recommendation
Efficacy of Risk Reduction		
Exercise to strengthen back or abdominal muscles or to improve overall fitness	I, II-1, II-2	C
Corsets/back belts	I, II-2	C
Modification of risk factors (smoking, obesity, psychological factors)	II-2, III	C
Effectiveness of Counseling		
Back pain prevention education		
Workplace	I, II-1, II-2	C
Pregnant women	II-1	C
Primary care patients	III	C

Table 61.

Counseling to Prevent Dental and Periodontal Disease

Intervention	Level of Evidence	Strength of Recommendation
Efficacy of Risk Reduction		
Regular visits to dental care provider (for services such as professionally applied topical fluorides, sealants)	I	B
Toothbrushing with fluoride-containing toothpaste	I, III	B
Dental flossing	II-1	B
Avoidance of putting infants and children to bed with a bottle	II-2, III	B
Reduced and less frequent intake of sugary foods	II-2	C
Fluoride supplementation of persons aged ≤16 yr, in areas with inadequate water fluoridation	II-1	A
Effectiveness of Counseling		
Counseling patients (parents) to follow measures to reduce their (their children's) risk of oral disease	II-2, II-3	C

Table 62.

Counseling to Prevent HIV Infection and Other Sexually Transmitted Diseases

Intervention	Level of Evidence	Strength of Recommendation
Efficacy of Risk Reduction		
Sexual abstinence or maintenance of mutually faithful monogamous sexual relationship	II-2	A
Regular use of condoms	II-2, II-3	A
Regular use of female barrier contraceptives and spermicides	I[1], II-2	B
Avoidance of contaminated injection equipment	II-2	A
Effectiveness of Counseling		
Counseling by primary care clinicians to reduce high-risk* sexual behavior or injection drug use	I, II-2	C

[1]Benefit demonstrated for gonorrhea and chlamydia, but effects on HIV infection uncertain.

*See relevant chapter for definition of high risk.

Table 63.
Counseling to Prevent Unintended Pregnancy

Intervention	Level of Evidence	Strength of Recommendation
	Efficacy of Risk Reduction	
Sexual abstinence or regular use of contraceptives	II-2	A
	Effectiveness of Counseling	
Clinician counseling to improve the effective use of contraceptives	II-3	B
Clinician counseling to promote sexual abstinence among adolescents	III	C

Table 64.
Counseling to Prevent Gynecologic Cancers

Intervention	Level of Evidence	Strength of Recommendation
	Efficacy of Risk Reduction	
Oral contraceptives to prevent ovarian and endometrial cancer	II-2	B
Avoidance of high-risk* sexual activity, use of barrier contraceptives and spermicides to prevent cervical cancer	II-2	A
Tubal sterilization to prevent ovarian cancer	II-2	B
	Effectiveness of Counseling	
Counseling about measures to reduce risk of gynecologic cancers	III	C

*See relevant chapter for definition of high risk.

Table 65.
Childhood Immunizations[1]

Intervention	Level of Evidence	Strength of Recommendation
Routine Childhood Immunizations		
Diphtheria ⎫		
Pertussis		
Tetanus		
Poliomyelitis ⎬	I, II-3	A
Measles		
Rubella		
Mumps ⎭		
H. influenzae type b conjugate	I, II-1, II-2, II-3	A
Hepatitis B	I, II-2, II-3	A
Varicella	I, II-3	A
Immunizations for High-Risk Children*		
Hepatitis A (age ≥2 yr)	I, II-3	A
Influenza (age ≥6 mo) (see Ch. 66)	II-2	B
Pneumococcus (age ≥2 yr) (see Ch. 66)		
Immunocompetent	I, II-2	B
Immunocompromised	I, II-2	C
Healthy persons living in epidemic conditions	I	A
Chemoprophylaxis Against Influenza A		
Amantadine/rimantadine - for high risk* children (see Ch. 66)	I	B

[1]See Ch. 25 for recommendations on the use of BCG vaccine against tuberculosis.

*See relevant chapter for definition of high risk.

Table 66.
Adult Immunizations—Including Chemoprophylaxis Against Influenza A

Intervention	Level of Evidence	Strength of Recommendation
Routine Adult Immunizations		
Influenza (age ≥65 yr)	I, II-2	B
Pneumococcus (age ≥65 yr)	II-2	B
Tetanus-diphtheria	I, II-3	A
Hepatitis B (young adults)	I, II-3	A
Immunizations for High-Risk Adults*		
Influenza	II-2	B
Pneumococcus		
Immunocompetent	I, II-2	B
Immunocompromised	I, II-2	C
Healthy young adults living in epidemic conditions	I	A
Hepatitis B	I, II-3	A
Hepatitis A	I	B
Measles-mumps-rubella	I	A
Measles-mumps-rubella (second dose)	II-2, II-3	B
Varicella (see Ch. 65)	I, II-3	B
Chemoprophylaxis Against Influenza A		
Amantadine/rimantadine for high-risk* adults	I	B

Table 67.
Postexposure Prophylaxis for Selected Infectious Diseases

Disease	Intervention	Level of Evidence	Strength of Recommendation
H. influenzae type b	Rifampin	I, II-3	A
Hepatitis A	Immune globulin	II-1	A
Hepatitis B	Immune globulin/vaccine	I	A
N. meningitidis	Rifampin	I, II-1	A
	Vaccine[1]	I, II-1, II-3	A
	Ceftriaxone	I	C[2]
Rabies	Immune globulin/ postexposure vaccine	I, II-3	A
	Preexposure vaccine in high-risk* persons	II-1	A
Tetanus	Vaccine/immune globulin	II-1, II-2, II-3	A

[1]Persons ≥3 mo in serogroup A outbreaks; persons ≥2 yr in serogroup C, Y, and W135 outbreaks.

[2]The efficacy of ceftriaxone in eliminating pharyngeal carriage of meningococcus has been confirmed only for serogroup A strains.

*See relevant chapter for definition of high risk.

Table 68.
Postmenopausal Hormone Prophylaxis

Intervention	Level of Evidence	Strength of Recommendation
Routinely counseling peri- and postmenopausal women about the risks and benefits[1] of hormone prophylaxis	I, II-2	B

[1]Hormone prophylaxis reduces the risk of osteoporosis and coronary heart disease, but may increase the risk of endometrial and breast cancer.

Table 69.
Aspirin Prophylaxis for the Primary Prevention of Myocardial Infarction

Intervention	Level of Evidence	Strength of Recommendation
Routine aspirin prophylaxis		
Middle-aged or older men	I	C
Middle-aged women	II-2	C

Table 70.
Aspirin Prophylaxis in Pregnancy

Intervention	Level of Evidence	Strength of Recommendation
Routine aspirin prophylaxis to prevent preeclampsia		
Pregnant women	I	C
High-risk* pregnant women	I	C
Routine aspirin prophylaxis to prevent intrauterine growth retardation in high-risk* pregnant women	I, II-1	C

*See relevant chapter for definition of high risk.

Reviewers

Listed below are nearly 700 Federal and non-Federal experts who reviewed Task Force draft background papers, chapters, and recommendations during their various stages of preparation. Many of these reviews were arranged by the liaisons to the Task Force (listed in the Acknowledgments) from primary care specialty societies, including the American Academy of Family Physicians (AAFP), American Academy of Pediatrics (AAP), American College of Obstetricians and Gynecologists, and American College of Physicians, and from Public Health Service (PHS) agencies, and by other professional organizations. We gratefully acknowledge the contribution of many other unnamed reviewers who provided helpful comments through various PHS agencies, professional societies, and voluntary organizations. Staff from the Food and Drug Administration (FDA) also reviewed draft chapters, background papers, and recommendations for the Task Force. Their review of these documents does not necessarily imply FDA approval of specific products for the indications described in the Task Force recommendations.

It should be emphasized that while reviewer comments and suggestions were of substantial assistance and are gratefully acknowledged, the Task Force is solely responsible for the final recommendations. Service as a reviewer does not necessarily reflect endorsement of any or all of the Task Force recommendations.

Rhoda Abrams, M.B.A.
Health Resources and Services
    Administration
Bethesda, MD

Harold P. Adams, Jr., M.D.
University of Iowa
Iowa City, IA

M.J. Adams, M.D.
Centers for Disease Control and
    Prevention
Atlanta, GA

Nancy E. Adler, Ph.D.
University of California at San Francisco
San Francisco, CA

David A. Ahlquist, M.D.
Mayo Clinic
Rochester, MN

Dennis J. Ahnen, M.D., F.A.C.G.
University of Colorado
Denver, CO

Beth Alexander, M.D., M.S.
Michigan State University/AAFP
East Lansing, MI

John Allen, Ph.D.
National Institutes of Health
Rockville, MD

Michael Allerton, M.S.
Kaiser Permanente Medical Care Program
Oakland, CA

Elaine J. Alpert, M.D., M.P.H.
Boston University
Boston, MA

Miriam J. Alter, Ph.D.
Centers for Disease Control and
    Prevention
Atlanta, GA

Tom Anan, M.D.
Providence Hospital/AAFP
Novi, MI

Robert Anda, M.D.
Centers for Disease Control and
    Prevention
Atlanta, GA

Jay R. Anderson, D.M.D., M.H.S.A.
Health Resources and Services
    Administration
Bethesda, MD

Reubin Andres, M.D.
National Institutes of Health
Baltimore, MD

James C. Anthony, Ph.D.
The Johns Hopkins University
Baltimore, MD

Richard Atkinson, M.D.
University of Wisconsin at Madison
Madison, WI

N. Burton Attico, M.D., M.P.H.
Indian Health Service
Phoenix, AZ

Thomas F. Babor, Ph.D.
University of Connecticut
Farmington, CT

Ronald Bachman, M.D.
Kaiser Permanente Medical Care Program
Oakland, CA

Christine Bachrach, Ph.D.
National Institutes of Health
Bethesda, MD

Shirley Bagley
National Institutes of Health
Bethesda, MD

David R. Baines, M.D., F.A.A.F.P.
American Academy of Family Physicians
St. Maries, ID

Ray Baker, M.D.
Ray Baker, M.D., Inc.
White Rock, British Columbia

Susan S. Baker, M.D., Ph.D.
Medical University of South Carolina
Charleston, SC

Albert Barrocas, M.D.
Pendleton Memorial Methodist Hospital
New Orleans, LA

Michael J. Barry, M.D.
Massachusetts General Hospital
Boston, MA

Joel L. Bass, M.D.
MetroWest Medical Center
Framingham, MA

David M. Baughan, M.D.
University of California at San
  Diego/AAFP
La Jolla, CA

David D. Bayse, Ph.D.
Centers for Disease Control and
  Prevention
Atlanta, GA

Roberta K. Beach, M.D.
Westside Health Center/AAP
Denver, CO

John W. Beasley, M.D.
University of Wisconsin at Madison/AAFP
Madison, WI

Marie-Dominique Beaulieu, M.D.,
M.Sc., F.C.F.P.
University of Montreal
Montreal, Quebec

David V. Becker, M.D.
New York Hospital-Cornell Medical Center
New York, NY

Myron L. Belfer, M.D.
Substance Abuse and Mental Health
  Services Administration
Rockville, MD

David Bellinger, M.D.
Children's Hospital Medical Center
Boston, MA

Beryl Benacerraf, M.D.
Diagnostic Ultrasound Associates, P.C.
Boston, MA

Birgitte H. Bendixen, M.D., Ph.D.
University of Iowa
Iowa City, IA

Heinz Berendes, M.D.
National Institutes of Health
Rockville, MD

Cynthia J. Berg, M.D., M.P.H.
Centers for Disease Control and
  Prevention
Atlanta, GA

Alan L. Berman, Ph.D.
Washington Psychological Center
Washington, DC

S. Thomas Bigos, M.D.
Maine Medical Center
Portland, ME

William F. Bina, III, M.D., M.P.H.
Family Practice Residency Program/AAFP
Macon, GA

Sue Binder, M.D.
Centers for Disease Control and
  Prevention
Atlanta, GA

George L. Blackburn, M.D., Ph.D.
New England Deaconess Hospital
Boston, MA

Steven Blair, P.E.D.
Cooper Institute for Aerobics Research
Dallas, TX

David A. Blandino, M.D.
Shadyside Hospital/AAFP
Pittsburgh, PA

C. Richard Boland, M.D.
University of Michigan
Ann Arbor, MI

John H. Bond, M.D.
University of Minnesota
Minneapolis, MN

Emily A. Boohaker, M.D.
Georgetown University
Washington, DC

John W. Boslego, M.D.
Walter Reed Army Institute of Research
Washington, DC

G. Stephen Bowen, M.D., M.P.H.
Health Resources and Services
  Administration
Rockville, MD

John M. Bowman, M.D.
Rh Laboratory
Winnipeg, Manitoba

William E. Boyle, Jr., M.D.
Dartmouth-Hitchcock Medical
    Center/AAP
Lebanon, NH

Katharine Bradley, M.D., M.P.H.
Department of Veterans Affairs
Seattle, WA

William E. Brady, M.P.H.
Centers for Disease Control and
    Prevention
Atlanta, GA

Frederick L. Brancati, M.D., M.H.S.
The Johns Hopkins University
Baltimore, MD

J. Timothy Bricker, M.D.
Texas Children's Hospital
Houston, TX

Peter A. Briss, M.D.
Centers for Disease Control and
    Prevention
Atlanta, GA

John W. Britt, R.N., M.P.H.
Harborview Injury Prevention & Research
    Center
Seattle, WA

Robert Brodell, M.D.
American Academy of Pediatrics
Cumberland, MD

Yvonne Bronner, Sc.D., R.D., L.D.
The Johns Hopkins University
Baltimore, MD

Neil Brooks, M.D.
Rockville Family Physicians, P.C./AAFP
Rockville, CT

W. Blair Brooks, M.D.
Dartmouth-Hitchcock Medical Center
Lebanon, NH

Zane A. Brown, M.D.
University of Washington
Seattle, WA

Kendall J. Bryant, Ph.D.
National Institutes of Health
Rockville, MD

Bill Bukoski, M.D.
National Institutes of Health
Bethesda, MD

Lisa M. Bundara, M.P.H.
National Institutes of Health
Bethesda, MD

William P. Bunnell, M.D.
Loma Linda University
Loma Linda, CA

Virginia B. Burggraf, M.S.N., R.N.
American Nurses Association
Washington, DC

Julie E. Buring, Sc.D.
Brigham and Women's Hospital
Boston, MA

Mary Ann Burkman, M.P.H., R.D.
Dairy Council of California
San Ramon, CA

Randall W. Burt, M.D.
University of Utah
Salt Lake City, UT

Benjamin T. Burton, Ph.D.
National Institutes of Health
Bethesda, MD

Jamie Calabrese, M.D.
Mercy Hospital of Pittsburgh/AAP
Pittsburgh, PA

Mariel Caldwell, M.P.H., M.S., R.D.
American Dietetic Association
Chicago, IL

C. Wayne Callaway, M.D.
George Washington University
Washington, DC

John L. Cameron, M.D.
The Johns Hopkins University
Baltimore, MD

Joseph Caprioli, M.D.
American Academy of Ophthalmology
San Francisco, CA

C. Eugene Carlton, M.D.
American Urological Association, Inc.
Baltimore, MD

David F. Carpenter, Ph.D.
Illinois Department of Public Health
Springfield, IL

Joseph S. Carra
U.S. Environmental Protection Agency
Washington, DC

H. Ballentine Carter, M.D.
James Buchanan Brady Urological
   Institute
Baltimore, MD

Carl J. Caspersen, Ph.D., M.P.H.
Centers for Disease Control and
   Prevention
Atlanta, GA

Kenneth G. Castro, M.D.
Centers for Disease Control and
   Prevention
Atlanta, GA

Willard Cates, Jr., M.D., M.P.H.
Centers for Disease Control and
   Prevention
Atlanta, GA

Ralph R. Cavalieri, M.D.
Department of Veterans Affairs Medical
   Center
San Francisco, CA

Arturo Cazares, M.D., M.P.H.
National Institutes of Health
Bethesda, MD

David L. Chadwick, M.D.
Children's Hospital Health Center/AAP
San Diego, CA

Evan Charney, M.D.
University of Massachusetts
Worcester, MA

Vivian Chen, Sc.D., M.S.W.
Health Resources and Services
   Administration
Rockville, MD

Robert T. Chen, M.D.
Centers for Disease Control and
   Prevention
Atlanta, GA

Ronni Chernoff, Ph.D., R.D.
University of Arkansas
Little Rock, AR

Francis D. Chesley, M.D.
Agency for Health Care Policy and
   Research
Rockville, MD

Emily Chew, M.D.
National Institutes of Health
Bethesda, MD

James E. Childs, Sc.D.
Centers for Disease Control and
   Prevention
Atlanta, GA

J. Julian Chisolm, Jr., M.D.
The Johns Hopkins University
Baltimore, MD

Gerald W. Chodak, M.D.
The University of Chicago
Chicago, IL

*Terence L. Chorba, M.D., M.P.H.,
   M.P.A.*
Centers for Disease Control and
   Prevention
Atlanta, GA

*Katherine Kaufer Christoffel, M.D.,
   M.P.H.*
The Children's Memorial Hospital
Chicago, IL

Carolyn Clancy, M.D.
Agency for Health Care Policy and
   Research
Rockville, MD

Ellen W. Clayton, M.D.
Vanderbilt University/AAP
Nashville, TN

James I. Cleeman, M.D.
National Institutes of Health
Bethesda, MD

John D. Clemens, M.D.
National Institutes of Health
Bethesda, MD

Janet C. Cleveland, M.S.
Centers for Disease Control and
    Prevention
Atlanta, GA

Nathaniel Cobb, M.D.
Indian Health Service
Albuquerque, NM

Cecil H. Coggins, M.D.
Massachusetts General Hospital
Boston, MA

Peter F. Cohn, M.D.
State University of New York at Stony
    Brook
Stony Brook, NY

George C. Coleman, M.D.
Medical College of Virginia/AAFP
Richmond, VA

George Cooney, Ph.D.
Macquarie University
Sydney, New South Wales, Australia

James Cooper, M.D.
Agency for Health Care Policy and
    Research
Rockville, MD

Judith A. Cooper, Ph.D.
National Institutes of Health
Rockville, MD

Jose F. Cordero, M.D., M.P.H.
Centers for Disease Control and
    Prevention
Atlanta, GA

Lawrence Corey, M.D.
University of Washington
Seattle, WA

E. Jane Costello, Ph.D.
Duke University
Durham, NC

Edward O. Cox, M.D.
American Academy of Pediatrics
Grand Rapids, MI

James Cox, M.D.
Navajo Area Indian Health Service
Gallup, NM

Janet Cragan, M.D.
Centers for Disease Control and
    Prevention
Atlanta, GA

Thomas C. Croft
Health Resources and Services
    Administration
Rockville, MD

Linda S. Crossett, R.D.H., B.S.
Centers for Disease Control and
    Prevention
Atlanta, GA

George Cunningham, M.D., M.P.H.
California State Department of Health
Berkeley, CA

Linda L. Dahlberg, M.A., Ph.D.
Centers for Disease Control and
    Prevention
Atlanta, GA

Peter R. Dallman, M.D. (ret.)
University of California at San Francisco
San Francisco, CA

Thomas W. Davidson, M.D.
Omaha Family Medicine/AAFP
Omaha, NE

Dana Davis, M.Ed.
American School Health Association
Kent, OH

Michael P. Davis, M.A.
National Institutes of Health
Bethesda, MD

Lauren DeAlleaume, M.D.
St. Joseph's Medical Center/AAFP
Yonkers, NY

Felix F. de la Cruz, M.D.
National Institutes of Health
Bethesda, MD

Margo A. Denke, M.D.
University of Texas
Dallas, TX

Robert Dershewitz, M.D.
Harvard Community Health Plan
Braintree, MA

Paul Dick, M.D.C.M., F.R.C.P.C.
University of Toronto
Toronto, Ontario

Charlotte Dickinson, Ph.D.
Centers for Disease Control and
 Prevention
Atlanta, GA

Robert A. Dickson, M.A., Ch.M.
University of Leeds
Leeds, United Kingdom

Allen Dietrich, M.D.
Dartmouth Medical School
Hanover, NH

Kim N. Dietrich, Ph.D.
University of Cincinnati
Cincinnati, OH

Susan E. Dietz, R.N., M.S.
Centers for Disease Control and
 Prevention
Atlanta, GA

William Dietz, M.D., Ph.D.
New England Medical Center
Boston, MA

Robin DiMatteo, Ph.D.
University of California at Riverside
Riverside, CA

Jennifer L. Dingle, M.B.A.
Dalhousie University
Halifax, Nova Scotia

Richard C. Dobyns, M.D., M.S.P.H.
University of Iowa/AAFP
Iowa City, IA

Theodore C. Doege, M.D., M.S.
American Medical Association
Chicago, IL

Karen Donato, M.S., R.D.
National Institutes of Health
Bethesda, MD

Samuel W. Dooley, Jr., M.D.
Centers for Disease Control and
 Prevention
Atlanta, GA

Louise Doss-Martin, M.A., A.C.S.W.
Health Resources and Services
 Administration
Bethesda, MD

Marion P. Downs, M.A., D.H.S.
University of Colorado
Denver, CO

Joseph S. Drage, M.D.
National Institutes of Health
Bethesda, MD

D. Peter Drotman, M.D., M.P.H.
Centers for Disease Control and
 Prevention
Atlanta, GA

Philippe Duclos, D.V.M., Ph.D.
Laboratory Center for Disease Control
Ottawa, Ontario

Ann C. Duerr, Ph.D., M.D.
Centers for Disease Control and
 Prevention
Atlanta, GA

Johanna Dwyer, D.Sc., R.D.
Frances Stern Nutrition Center
Boston, MA

Donald D. Dyson, M.D.
Kaiser Permanente Medical Center
Santa Clara, CA

James R. Eckman, M.D.
Emory University
Atlanta, GA

David M. Eddy, M.D., Ph.D.
Kaiser Permanente Medical Care Program
Pasadena, CA

Kathryn M. Edwards, M.D.
Vanderbilt University
Nashville, TN

Theodore C. Eickhoff, M.D.
University of Colorado
Denver, CO

Tedd V. Ellerbrock, M.D., F.A.C.O.G.
Centers for Disease Control and
 Prevention
Atlanta, GA

John B. Emans, M.D.
Children's Orthopaedic Surgery
　　Foundation
Boston, MA

Michael M. Engelgau, M.D.
Centers for Disease Control and
　　Prevention
Atlanta, GA

Daniel R. Erickson, M.D.
American Academy of Family Physicians
Horicon, WI

J. David Erickson, D.D.S., Ph.D.
Centers for Disease Control and
　　Prevention
Atlanta, GA

Martin Erlichman, M.D.
Agency for Health Care Policy and
　　Research
Rockville, MD

Claire B. Ernhart, Ph.D.
Case Western Reserve University
Cleveland, OH

Judith Ernst, D.M.Sc., R.D.
Indiana University
Indianapolis, IN

E. Harvey Estes, Jr., M.D.
North Carolina Medical Society
　　Foundation, Inc.
Raleigh, NC

Bruce Ettinger, M.D.
Kaiser Permanente Medical Care Program
Oakland, CA

Ruth A. Etzel, M.D.
American Academy of Pediatrics
Chamblee, GA

Geoffrey Evans, M.D.
Health Resources and Services
　　Administration
Rockville, MD

Kenneth L. Evans, M.D.
American Academy of Family Physicians
Edmond, OK

Bruce Lee Evatt, M.D.
Centers for Disease Control and
　　Prevention
Atlanta, GA

W. Douglas Everett, M.D., M.P.H.
American Academy of Family Physicians
Huntsville, AL

Bernard G. Ewigman, M.D.
University of Missouri at Columbia
Columbia, MO

Harmon J. Eyre, M.D.
American Cancer Society
Atlanta, GA

Henry Falk, M.D., M.P.H.
Centers for Disease Control and
　　Prevention
Atlanta, GA

Donna Falvo, Ph.D.
Family Practice Center/AAFP
Carbondale, IL

David F. Fardon, M.D.
Knoxville Orthopedic Clinic
Knoxville, TN

Denise J. Fedele, D.M.D., M.S.
Department of Veterans Affairs
Perry Point, MD

**John W. Feightner, M.D., M.Sc.,
　　F.C.F.P.**
McMaster University
Hamilton, Ontario

Bruce B. Feinberg, M.D.
Brigham and Women's Hospital
Boston, MA

Bernadine Feldman, Ph.D.
Agency for Health Care Policy and
　　Research
Rockville, MD

William Feldman, M.D., F.R.C.P.C.
Hospital for Sick Children
Toronto, Ontario

Jonathan E. Fielding, M.D., M.P.H.
University of California at Los Angeles
Santa Monica, CA

Walter M. Fierson, M.D., P.C.
American Academy of Pediatrics
Elk Grove Village, IL

David H. Filipi, M.D.
HMO Nebraska/AAFP
Omaha, NE

Michael J. Fine, M.D., M.P.H.
University of Pittsburgh
Pittsburgh, PA

Michael C. Fiore, M.D., M.P.H.
University of Wisconsin at Madison
Madison, WI

Kenneth D. Fisher, Ph.D.
Federation of American Societies for
  Experimental Biology
Bethesda, MD

Arthur C. Fleischer, M.D.
Vanderbilt University
Nashville, TN

David Fleischer, M.D.
American Society for Gastrointestinal
  Endoscopy
Washington, DC

Alan R. Fleischman, M.D.
The New York Academy of Medicine/AAP
New York, NY

Michael F. Fleming, M.D., M.P.H.
University of Wisconsin at Madison
Madison, WI

Food and Nutrition Board
National Academy of Sciences
Washington, DC

Jacqueline Darroch Forrest, Ph.D.
The Alan Guttmacher Institute
New York, NY

Willis R. Foster, M.D.
National Institutes of Health
Bethesda, MD

Steven Fox, M.D., M.P.H.
Agency for Health Care Policy and
  Research
Rockville, MD

**John W. Frank, M.D., C.C.F.P., M.S.,
  F.R.C.P.C.**
Ontario Workers' Compensation Institute
Toronto, Ontario

C. James Frankish, Ph.D.
Institute of Health Promotion Research
Vancouver, British Columbia

Adele L. Franks, M.D.
Centers for Disease Control and
  Prevention
Atlanta, GA

Linda French, M.D.
Oakwood Hospital/AAFP
Dearborn, MI

Gary D. Friedman, M.D.
Kaiser Permanente Medical Care Program
Oakland, CA

Victor F. Froelicher, M.D.
Stanford University
Palo Alto, CA

Paul G. Fuller, Jr., M.D.
American Academy of Pediatrics
Rome, NY

Robinson Fulwood, M.S.P.H.
National Institutes of Health
Bethesda, MD

Barbara Gaffield, M.S., R.D.
Children's Hospital
Oakland, CA

Eduardo Gaitan, M.D., F.A.C.P.
Department of Veterans Affairs Medical
  Center
Jackson, MS

Theodore G. Ganiats, M.D.
University of California at San
  Diego/AAFP
La Jolla, CA

Alan Michael Garber, M.D., Ph.D.
Department of Veterans Affairs
Palo Alto, CA

A. Isabel Garcia, D.D.S., M.P.H.
Agency for Health Care Policy and
  Research
Rockville, MD

Pierce Gardner, M.D.
State University of New York at Stony
  Brook
Stony Brook, NY

Robert J. Garrison, Ph.D.
National Institutes of Health
Bethesda, MD

Marilyn H. Gaston, M.D.
Health Resources and Services
  Administration
Rockville, MD

James R. Gavin, III, M.D., Ph.D.
American Diabetes Association
Alexandria, VA

David W. Gelfand, M.D.
Wake Forest University
Winston-Salem, NC

Melvin D. Gerald, M.D., M.P.H.
Gerald Family Care Associates/AAFP
Washington, DC

A. Russell Gerber, M.D.
Centers for Disease Control and
  Prevention
Atlanta, GA

Marianne Gerson, M.D.
Kaiser Permanente Medical Care Program
Vallejo, CA

Helen Gift, Ph.D.
National Institutes of Health
Bethesda, MD

Wayne H. Giles, M.D., M.S.
Centers for Disease Control and
  Prevention
Atlanta, GA

Gary A. Giovino, Ph.D.
Centers for Disease Control and
  Prevention
Atlanta, GA

Fred S. Girton, M.D.
Family Health Center/AAFP
Macon, GA

*Cindy Quinton Gladstone, M.H.Sc.,
  M.D., F.R.C.P.C.*
University of Toronto
Toronto, Ontario

John Gohagan, Ph.D.
National Institutes of Health
Rockville, MD

Dorothy Gohdes, M.D.
Indian Health Service
Albuquerque, NM

Michael Goldberg, M.D.
New England Medical Center/AAP
Boston, MA

*Richard B. Goldbloom, O.C., M.D.,
  F.R.C.P.C.*
Dalhousie University
Halifax, Nova Scotia

Robert L. Goldenberg, M.D.
University of Alabama at Birmingham
Birmingham, AL

Lee Goldman, M.D.
University of California at San Francisco
San Francisco, CA

Sherwin Goldman, M.D.
Mayo Clinic
Rochester, MN

Ronald H. Goldschmidt, M.D.
San Francisco General Hospital/AAFP
San Francisco, CA

Junius J. Gonzales, M.D.
Georgetown University
Washington, DC

Nancy P. Gordon, Sc.D.
Kaiser Permanente Medical Care Program
Oakland, CA

Barbara Gosink, M.D.
University of California at San Diego
San Diego, CA

Madelyn S. Gould, Ph.D., M.P.H.
Columbia University
New York, NY

Laura B. Gowen
National Scoliosis Foundation
Watertown, MA

Deborah Grady, M.D., M.P.H.
University of California at San Francisco
San Francisco, CA

Philippe Grandjean, M.D., Ph.D.
Odense Universitet
Miljemedicin, Denmark

Dan M. Granoff, M.D.
American Academy of Pediatrics
Berkeley, CA

Gilman D. Grave, M.D.
National Institutes of Health
Bethesda, MD

Joseph H. Graziano, Ph.D.
Columbia University
New York, NY

Beverly B. Green, M.D., M.P.H.
Group Health Cooperative of Puget
  Sound
Bainbridge Island, WA

Clarice A. Green, M.D., M.S.
Centers for Disease Control and
  Prevention
Atlanta, GA

John L. Green, M.D.
American Academy of Pediatrics
Rochester, NY

Lawrence W. Green, Dr.P.H.
University of British Columbia
Vancouver, British Columbia

Lee Green, M.D., M.P.H.
University of Michigan/AAFP
Ann Arbor, MI

John C. Greene, D.M.D., M.P.H. (ret.)
University of California at San Francisco
  School of Dentistry
San Rafael, CA

Michael F. Greene, M.D.
Brigham and Women's Hospital
Boston, MA

Donald E. Greydanus, M.D.
Michigan State University/AAP
Kalamazoo, MI

Marie R. Griffin, M.D.
Vanderbilt University
Nashville, TN

Don Gromisch, M.D.
American Academy of Pediatrics
Elk Grove Village, IL

George A. Gross, D.O., M.P.H. (ret.)
Michigan State University College of
  Osteopathic Medicine
East Lansing, MI

Peter A. Gross, M.D.
Hackensack Medical Center
Hackensack, NJ

Robert D. Gross, M.D.
Children's Eye Specialists/AAP
Fort Worth, TX

Ronald L. Gross, M.D.
Baylor College of Medicine
Houston, TX

Erica P. Gunderson, M.S., M.P.H., R.D.
American Dietetic Association
Larkspur, CA

Gordon Guyatt, M.D.
McMaster University
Hamilton, Ontario

Julian Haber, M.D.
American Academy of Pediatrics
Fort Worth, TX

James E. Haddow, M.D.
Foundation for Blood Research
Scarborough, ME

Stephen C. Hadler, M.D.
Centers for Disease Control and
  Prevention
Atlanta, GA

Evan Hadley, M.D.
National Institutes of Health
Bethesda, MD

Caroline Breese Hall, M.D.
University of Rochester Medical
   Center/AAP
Rochester, NY

Neal Halsey, M.D.
The Johns Hopkins University
Baltimore, MD

Edward N. Hanley, Jr., M.D.
American Academy of Orthopaedic
   Surgeons
Rosemont, IL

W.B. Hanley, M.D.
Hospital for Sick Children
Toronto, Ontario

W. Harry Hannon, Ph.D.
Centers for Disease Control and
   Prevention
Atlanta, GA

Toni J. Hanson, M.D.
Mayo Clinic
Rochester, MN

Jeffrey Harris, M.D., M.P.H.
Centers for Disease Control and
   Prevention
Atlanta, GA

Birt Harvey, M.D.
Packard Children's Hospital
Palo Alto, CA

Richard A. Hatch, O.D.
Indian Health Service
Gallup, NM

Barton F. Haynes, M.D.
Duke University
Durham, NC

R. Brian Haynes, M.D., Ph.D.,
   F.R.C.P.C.
McMaster University
Hamilton, Ontario

Denise Haynie, Ph.D.
National Institutes of Health
Bethesda, MD

Gregory W. Heath, D.Sc., M.P.H.
Centers for Disease Control and
   Prevention
Atlanta, GA

Susan C. Hellerstein, M.D., M.P.H.
Beth Israel Hospital
Boston, MA

Charles G. Helmick, III, M.D.
Centers for Disease Control and
   Prevention
Atlanta, GA

Elina Hemminki, M.D., Ph.D.
National Research and Development
   Centre for Welfare and Health
Helsinki, Finland

William R. Hendee, Ph.D.
Medical College of Wisconsin
Milwaukee, WI

Eric Henley, M.D.
Indian Health Service
Albuquerque, NM

Charles H. Hennekens, M.D., Dr.P.H.
Brigham and Women's Hospital
Boston, MA

Carol Herbert, M.D.
Institute of Health Promotion Research
Vancouver, British Columbia

James W. Herbert, M.D.
American Academy of Pediatrics
San Angelo, TX

Moses Herrera, M.D.
Medical Center Physicians, P.A./AAFP
Nampa, ID

Lisa J. Herrinton, Ph.D.
Kaiser Permanente Medical Care Program
Oakland, CA

Jerome M. Hershman, M.D.
American Thyroid Association
Los Angeles, CA

Stephen P. Heyse, M.D., M.P.H.
National Institutes of Health
Bethesda, MD

Robert A. Hiatt, M.D., Ph.D.
Kaiser Permanente Medical Care Program
Oakland, CA

Ronald J. Hicks, M.D.
University of Oklahoma Health Sciences
    Center/AAFP
Oklahoma City, OK

Gerry B. Hill, M.D., Ch.B., M.Sc.
Laboratory Centre for Disease Control
Tunney's Pasture, Ottawa

Washington C. Hill, M.D.
Sarasota Memorial Hospital
Sarasota, FL

E. Susan Hodgson, M.D.
Rutgers University/AAP
Somerset, NJ

C.C. Hoekstra, Ph.D.
Child Audiological Center, University
    Hospital
Nijmegen, Netherlands

Joe Hollowell, M.D.
Centers for Disease Control and
    Prevention
Atlanta, GA

King K. Holmes, M.D., Ph.D.
University of Washington
Seattle, WA

David Holtgrave, Ph.D.
Centers for Disease Control and
    Prevention
Atlanta, GA

Neil A. Holtzman, M.D., M.P.H.
The Johns Hopkins University
Baltimore, MD

Charles Homer, M.D.
Children's Hospital/AAP
Boston, MA

Steven Hotta, M.D., Ph.D.
Agency for Health Care Policy and
    Research
Rockville, MD

Jan Howard, Ph.D.
National Institutes of Health
Rockville, MD

Van Hubbard, M.D.
National Institutes of Health
Bethesda, MD

William J. Hueston, M.D.
Eau Claire Family Practice/AAFP
Eau Claire, WI

Stephen B. Hulley, M.D., M.P.H.
University of California at San Francisco
San Francisco, CA

Corinne G. Husten, M.D., M.P.H.
Centers for Disease Control and
    Prevention
Atlanta, GA

Vince L. Hutchins, M.D.
National Center for Education in MCH
Arlington, VA

Jay D. Iams, M.D.
Ohio State University Hospital
Columbus, OH

Debbie M. Jackson, M.A.
Health Resources and Services
    Administration
Rockville, MD

Laird G. Jackson, M.D.
Thomas Jefferson University
Philadelphia, PA

Richard J. Jackson, M.D., M.P.H.
Centers for Disease Control and
    Prevention
Atlanta, GA

Ian Jacobs, M.D., M.R.C.O.G.
Cambridge University Teaching Hospitals
    Trust
Cambridge, England

Richard F. Jacobs, M.D.
Arkansas Children's Hospital/AAP
Little Rock, AR

A.D. Jacobson, M.D.
American Academy of Pediatrics
Phoenix, AZ

Robert M. Jacobson, M.D.
Mayo Clinic
Rochester, MN

Mary A. Jansen, Ph.D.
Substance Abuse and Mental Health
   Administration
Rockville, MD

Carole Jenny, M.D.
The Children's Hospital/AAP
Denver, CO

James Jerger, Ph.D.
Journal of the American Academy of
   Audiology
Houston, TX

Patrick Johannes, P.H.A.
Indian Health Service
Albuquerque, NM

Barry L. Johnson, Ph.D.
Centers for Disease Control and
   Prevention
Atlanta, GA

Denise Johnson, M.S.
Centers for Disease Control and
   Prevention
Atlanta, GA

Joy L. Johnson, Ph.D., R.N.
University of British Columbia
Vancouver, British Columbia

Robert E. Johnson, M.D., M.P.H.
Centers for Disease Control and
   Prevention
Atlanta, GA

A. Patrick Jonas, M.D.
Ohio State University/AAFP
Columbus, OH

Donna S. Jones, M.D., M.P.H.
Centers for Disease Control and
   Prevention
Atlanta, GA

Wanda K. Jones, Dr.P.H.
Centers for Disease Control and
   Prevention
Atlanta, GA

Douglas E. Jorenby, Ph.D.
University of Wisconsin at Madison
Madison, WI

Elaina R. Jurecki, M.S., R.D.
Kaiser Permanente Medical Care Program
Oakland, CA

Norman M. Kaplan, M.D.
University of Texas Southwestern Medical
   Center
Dallas, TX

William Kassler, M.D., M.P.H.
Centers for Disease Control and
   Prevention
Atlanta, GA

Wayne J. Katon, M.D.
University of Washington
Seattle, WA

Samuel L. Katz, M.D.
Duke University
Durham, NC

Steven C. Kaufman, M.D., M.S.
National Institutes of Health
Bethesda, MD

Joseph W. Kelaghan, M.D.
National Institutes of Health
Bethesda, MD

Arthur L. Kellermann, M.D., M.P.H.
Emory Center for Injury Control
Atlanta, GA

Kathi J. Kemper, M.D., M.P.H.
Harborview Medical Center/AAP
Seattle, WA

Karla Kerlikowske, M.D.
University of California at San Francisco
San Francisco, CA

Muin J. Khoury, M.D., Ph.D.
Centers for Disease Control and
   Prevention
Atlanta, GA

Edwin M. Kilbourne, M.D.
Centers for Disease Control and
   Prevention
Atlanta, GA

Gail King, M.D., M.P.H.
Centers for Disease Control and
    Prevention
Atlanta, GA

Howard A. King, M.D.
Children's Hospital and Medical Center
Seattle, WA

Douglas Kirby, Ph.D.
ETR Associates
Santa Cruz, CA

Barbara Klein, M.D., M.P.H.
University of Wisconsin at Madison
Madison, WI

**Robert N. Kleinstein, O.D., M.P.H.,
    Ph.D.**
University of Alabama at Birmingham
Birmingham, AL

William J. Klish, M.D.
Texas Children's Hospital/AAP
Houston, TX

Ruth N. Knollmueller, Ph.D., R.N.
American Nurses Association
Hamden, CT

Richard Koch, M.D.
Children's Hospital Los Angeles
Los Angeles, CA

Howard K. Koh, M.D., F.A.C.P.
Boston University
Boston, MA

Steve Kohl, M.D.
San Francisco General Hospital/AAP
San Francisco, CA

Ann M. Koontz, Dr.P.H.
Health Resources and Services
    Administration
Rockville, MD

Daniel B. Kopans, M.D., F.A.C.R.
Massachusetts General Hospital
Boston, MA

Lorrin M. Koran, M.D.
Stanford University
Stanford, CA

Doreen Koretz, Ph.D.
National Institutes of Health
Bethesda, MD

Thomas E. Kottke, M.D.
Mayo Clinic
Rochester, MN

Barnett S. Kramer, M.D., M.P.H.
National Institutes of Health
Bethesda, MD

Norman A. Krasnegor, Ph.D.
National Institutes of Health
Bethesda, MD

Robert Kreisberg, M.D.
University of Alabama at Birmingham
Birmingham, AL

David B. Krier, M.D., M.S.P.H.
American Academy of Family Physicians
St. Paul, OR

Richard D. Krugman, M.D.
University of Colorado/AAP
Denver, CO

Saul Krugman, M.D.
New York University
New York, NY

Laura Kruse, M.D.
Health Resources and Services
    Administration
Rockville, MD

Lewis H. Kuller, M.D., Dr.P.H.
University of Pittsburgh
Pittsburgh, PA

Stephen La Franchi, M.D.
Oregon Health Sciences University/AAP
Portland, OR

F. Marc LaForce, M.D.
The Genesee Hospital
Rochester, NY

Kathleen A. Lamping, M.D.
EENT Associates, Inc.
South Euclid, OH

Sandra A. Larsen, Ph.D.
Centers for Disease Control and
   Prevention
Atlanta, GA

Eric B. Larson, M.D., M.P.H.
University of Washington
Seattle, WA

Reva C. Lawrence, M.P.H.
National Institutes of Health
Bethesda, MD

Nancy C. Lee, M.D.
Centers for Disease Control and
   Prevention
Atlanta, GA

R. Dee Legako, M.D.
Canyon Park Family Physicians/AAFP
Edmond, OK

Rudolph L. Leibel, M.D.
Rockefeller University
New York, NY

Richard A. Lemen, Ph.D.
Centers for Disease Control and
   Prevention
Atlanta, GA

Claude Lenfant, M.D.
National Institutes of Health
Bethesda, MD

M. Cristina Leske, M.D., Ph.D.
State University of New York at Stony
   Brook
Stony Brook, NY

Carl M. Leventhal, M.D.
National Institutes of Health
Bethesda, MD

Gary I. Levine, M.D.
Southwest Georgia Family Practice
   Residency/AAFP
Albany, GA

Harvey L. Levy, M.D.
Children's Hospital
Boston, MA

**Donald W. Lewis, D.D.S., D.D.P.H.,
   M.Sc.D., F.R.C.D.**
University of Toronto
Toronto, Ontario

Tracy Lieu, M.D., M.P.H.
Kaiser Permanente Medical Care Program
Oakland, CA

Irwin Light, M.D.
University of Cincinnati
Cincinnati, OH

Elmer S. Lightner, M.D.
University of Arizona/AAP
Phoenix, AZ

Jane S. Lin-Fu, M.D.
Health Resources and Services
   Administration
Rockville, MD

Robert Lindsay, M.B.Ch.B., Ph.D.
Helen Hayes Hospital
West Haverstraw, NY

Mack Lipkin, Jr., M.D.
New York University
New York, NY

Scott M. Lippman, M.D.
University of Texas
Houston, TX

John R. Livengood, M.D.
Centers for Disease Control and
   Prevention
Atlanta, GA

Alexander G. Logan, M.D., F.R.C.P.C.
Mount Sinai Hospital
Toronto, Ontario

Everett Logue, Ph.D.
Family Practice Clinical Research
   Center/AAFP
Akron, OH

Jacob Lohr, M.D.
University of North Carolina
Chapel Hill, NC

Douglas G. Long, M.D.
American Academy of Family Physicians
East Boothbay, ME

John E. Lonstein, M.D.
Minnesota Spine Center
Minneapolis, MN

Carolyn C. Lopez, M.D.
Rush Prudential Health Plans/AAFP
Chicago, IL

Fred Lorey, Ph.D.
California State Department of Health
Berkeley, CA

Betsy Lozoff, M.D., M.S.
University of Michigan
Ann Arbor, MI

Russell V. Luepker, M.D.
University of Minnesota
Minneapolis, MN

Sheila A. Lukehart, Ph.D.
University of Washington
Seattle, WA

James Lustig, M.D.
Denver General Hospital/AAP
Denver, CO

David A. Luthy, M.D.
Swedish Medical Center
Seattle, WA

Jerry M. Lyle, M.D.
Indian Health Service
Rockville, MD

Henry T. Lynch, M.D.
Creighton University
Omaha, NE

Noni E. MacDonald, M.D., F.R.C.P.C.
Children's Hospital of Eastern
    Ontario/AAP
Ottawa, Ontario

Michael I. MacEntee, Ph.D., L.D.S.(I),
    F.R.C.D.C.
University of British Columbia
Vancouver, British Columbia

Abe Macher, M.D.
Health Resources and Services
    Administration
Rockville, MD

Harriet L. MacMillan, M.D., F.R.C.P.C.
Chedoke-McMaster Hospitals/McMaster
    University
Hamilton, Ontario

Kathryn R. Mahaffey, Ph.D.
U.S. Environmental Protection Agency
Cincinnati, OH

Frank J. Mahoney, M.D
Centers for Disease Control and
    Prevention
Atlanta, GA

Louis Emmet Mahoney, M.D., Dr.P.H.
Health Resources and Services
    Administration
Rockville, MD

Lois A. Maiman, Ph.D.
National Institutes of Health
Bethesda, MD

Jack S. Mandel, Ph.D., M.P.H.
University of Minnesota
Minneapolis, MN

Marc Manley, M.D., M.P.H.
National Institutes of Health
Bethesda, MD

R. Jerry Mann, M.D.
University of Arkansas/AAFP
Little Rock, AR

Edgar K. Marcuse, M.D., M.P.H.
Children's Hospital & Medical Center
Seattle, WA

Harold S. Margolis, M.D.
Centers for Disease Control and
    Prevention
Atlanta, GA

Donald W. Marianos, D.D.S., M.P.H.
Centers for Disease Control and
    Prevention
Atlanta, GA

Lauri Markowitz, M.D.
Centers for Disease Control and
    Prevention
Atlanta, GA

Morri Markowitz, M.D.
Montefiore Medical Center
Bronx, NY

James S. Marks, M.D.
Centers for Disease Control and
    Prevention
Atlanta, GA

Susan Marks, R.N., M.S.N.
Kaiser Permanente Medical Care Program
Oakland, CA

R.G. Mathias, M.D., F.R.C.P.C.
University of British Columbia
Vancouver, British Columbia

Tim McAfee, M.D., M.P.H.
Group Health Cooperative of Puget
    Sound
Seattle, WA

Elizabeth McAnarney, M.D.
University of Rochester Medical
    Center/AAP
Rochester, NY

Jerome McAndrews, D.C.
American Chiropractic Association
Arlington, VA

Patrick E. McBride, M.D., M.P.H.
University of Wisconsin at Madison
Madison, WI

Harrison C. McCandless, M.D.
American Academy of Family Physicians
Torrance, CA

Wayne McCormick, M.D.
University of Washington
Seattle, WA

George McCoy, Ph.D.
Indian Health Service
Rockville, MD

Judith McFarlane, Dr.P.H.
Texas Woman's University
Houston, TX

Joan A. McGowan, Ph.D.
National Institutes of Health
Bethesda, MD

Pamela McInnes, D.D.S., M.Sc.
National Institutes of Health
Bethesda, MD

Pamela M. McMahon, Ph.D.
Centers for Disease Control and
    Prevention
Atlanta, GA

Lynn McQueen, M.S., M.P.H.
Agency for Health Care Policy and
    Research
Rockville, MD

Robert Mecklenburg, D.D.S., M.P.H.
National Institutes of Health
Bethesda, MD

Jack H. Medalie, M.D., M.P.H.
Case Western Reserve University
Cleveland, OH

L.J. Melton, III, M.D.
Mayo Clinic
Rochester, MN

James A. Mercy, Ph.D.
Centers for Disease Control and
    Prevention
Atlanta, GA

Gerald B. Merenstein, M.D.
The Children's Hospital/AAP
Denver, CO

Gregory J. Mertz, M.D.
University of New Mexico
Albuquerque, NM

Edward M. Messing, M.D., F.A.C.S.
University of Wisconsin at Madison
Madison, WI

Curtis Mettlin, Ph.D.
Roswell Park Cancer Institute
Buffalo, NY

Angela D. Mickalide, Ph.D.
National SAFE KIDS Campaign
Washington, DC

Wm. Phillip Mickelson, M.D., M.A.
Health Canada
Ottawa, Ontario

Anthony B. Miller, M.B., F.R.C.P.C.
University of Toronto
Toronto, Ontario

Bess I. Miller, M.D., M.Sc.
Centers for Disease Control and
    Prevention
Atlanta, GA

Daniel S. Miller, M.D., M.P.H.
Centers for Disease Control and
    Prevention
Atlanta, GA

Stephen C. Miller, O.D.
American Optometric Association
St. Louis, MO

Connie Mobley, Ph.D., R.D., L.D.
University of Texas at San Antonio
San Antonio, TX

Alison A. Moore, M.D., M.P.H.
University of California at Los Angeles
Los Angeles, CA

Barbara Moore, M.D.
National Institutes of Health
Bethesda, MD

Prof. Michael R. Moore
National Research Centre for
    Environmental Toxicology
Brisbane, Queensland, Australia

Dale C. Moquist, M.D.
American Academy of Family Physicians
Kansas City, MO

John S. Moran, M.D.
Centers for Disease Control and
    Prevention
Atlanta, GA

Bruce Z. Morgenstern, M.D.
Mayo Clinic
Rochester, MN

Gregory Morosco, Ph.D.
National Institutes of Health
Bethesda, MD

John C. Morris, M.D.
Mayo Clinic
Rochester, MN

Brenda J. Morrison, Ph.D.
University of British Columbia
Vancouver, British Columbia

John C. Morrison, M.D.
University of Mississippi Medical Center
Jackson, MS

Raymond T. Morrissy, M.D.
Children's Orthopaedics of Atlanta
Atlanta, GA

James A. Mortimer, Ph.D.
University of Minnesota
Minneapolis, MN

Eve K. Moscicki, Sc.D., M.P.H.
National Institutes of Health
Rockville, MD

Susan M. Mou, M.D.
University of Missouri
Kansas City, MO

Jean-Marie Moutquin, M.D.
Hopital Saint-François d'Assise
Quebec, Quebec

Julie Graves Moy, M.D., M.P.H.
Baylor College of Medicine/AAFP
Houston, TX

Joseph Mulinare, M.D., M.S.P.H.
Centers for Disease Control and
    Prevention
Atlanta, GA

George E. Murphy, M.D.
Washington University in St. Louis
St. Louis, MO

Alf L. Nachemson, M.D., Ph.D.
Health Care Excellence
Washington, DC

Donald C. Nagel, M.D.
American Academy of Family Physicians
Black Mountain, NC

National Association of School Nurses
Scarborough, ME

Marion Nestle, Ph.D., M.P.H.
New York University
New York, NY

Susan Newcomer, Ph.D.
National Institutes of Health
Rockville, MD

Thomas B. Newman, M.D., M.P.H.
University of California at San Francisco
San Francisco, CA

Vicky Newman, M.S., R.D.
Wellstart International/American Dietetic
  Association
San Diego, CA

Sheila A. Newton, Ph.D.
National Institutes of Health
Bethesda, MD

Theresa A. Nicklas, Dr.P.H., L.D.N.
Tulane University
New Orleans, LA

Lindsay E. Nicolle, M.D.
University of Manitoba
Winnipeg, Manitoba

Richard Niska, M.D., F.A.C.E.P.
Health Resources and Services
  Administration
Rockville, MD

Audrey H. Nora, M.D., M.P.H.
Health Resources and Services
  Administration
Rockville, MD

J.W. Norris, M.D., F.R.C.P.C.
University of Toronto
North York, Ontario

Charles North, M.D.
Indian Health Service
Albuquerque, NM

Jerry L. Northern, Ph.D.
University of Colorado
Denver, CO

Ruth Nowjack-Raymer, R.D.H., M.P.H.
National Institutes of Health
Bethesda, MD

Lennarth Nysbrom, B.A.
Umea University Hospital
Umea, Sweden

Denis M. O'Day, M.D., F.A.C.S.
American Academy of Ophthalmology
San Francisco, CA

Godfrey P. Oakley, Jr., M.D.
Centers for Disease Control and
  Prevention
Atlanta, GA

Joseph Oesterling, M.D.
University of Michigan
Ann Arbor, MI

James G. Olson, Ph.D.
Centers for Disease Control and
  Prevention
Atlanta, GA

Thomas C. Olsen, M.D.
St. Joseph Mercy Community Health Care
  System/AAP
Pontiac, MI

Walter Orenstein, M.D.
Centers for Disease Control and
  Prevention
Atlanta, GA

Fred C. Osher, M.D.
Agency for Health Care Policy and
  Research
Rockville, MD

Frank A. Oski, M.D.
The Johns Hopkins University
Baltimore, MD

Gary L. Oxman, M.D., M.P.H.
Multnomah County Health Department
Portland, OR

Pasquale J. Palumbo, M.D.
Mayo Clinic
Scottsdale, AZ

Robert Pantell, M.D.
University of California at San Francisco/
  AAP
San Francisco, CA

Michael D. Parkinson, M.D., M.P.H.
Health Resources and Services
  Administration
Rockville, MD

**Patrick J. Parsons, Ph.D., C.Chem.,
F.R.S.C.**
State of New York Department of Health
Albany, NY

Christopher Patterson, M.D., F.R.C.P.C.
Chedoke-McMaster Hospitals
Hamilton, Ontario

Kay C. Pearson, R.Ph., M.P.H.
Agency for Health Care Policy and
    Research
Rockville, MD

Jeffrey F. Peipert, M.D., M.P.H.
Women and Infants'
Providence, RI

Thomas A. Peterman, M.D., M.Sc.
Centers for Disease Control and
    Prevention
Atlanta, GA

Kenneth Petersen, M.D.
Indian Health Service
Anchorage, AK

Herbert B. Peterson, M.D.
Centers for Disease Control and
    Prevention
Atlanta, GA

William R. Phillips, M.D., M.P.H.
University of Washington/AAFP
Seattle, WA

Gregory A. Poland, M.D., F.A.C.P.
Mayo Clinic
Rochester, MN

Ronald L. Poland, M.D., F.A.A.P.
Pennsylvania State College of Medicine
    Children's Hospital
Hershey, PA

Malcolm H. Pope, M.D.
University of Iowa
Iowa City, IA

Barry Portnoy, Ph.D.
National Institutes of Health
Bethesda, MD

Barbara Millen Posner, Dr.P.H., R.D.
Boston University
Boston, MA

Lloyd B. Potter, Ph.D., M.P.H.
Centers for Disease Control and Prevention
Atlanta, GA

Jerilynn Prior, M.D., F.R.C.P.C.
University of British Columbia
Vancouver, British Columbia

Charles G. Prober, M.D.
Stanford University
Palo Alto, CA

Bruce Psaty, M.D., Ph.D.
University of Washington
Seattle, WA

Robert F. Purtell, Jr., M.D.
American Academy of Family Physicians
Milwaukee, WI

Michelle A. Puryear, M.D., Ph.D.
Health Resources and Services
    Administration
Rockville, MD

John T. Queenan, M.D.
Georgetown University
Washington, DC

N. Regina Rabinovich, M.D., M.P.H.
National Institutes of Health
Bethesda, MD

James A. Raczek, M.D.
Eastern Maine Medical Center/AAFP
Bangor, ME

Juan Ramos, Ph.D.
National Institutes of Health
Bethesda, MD

Peter Rappo, M.D.
American Academy of Pediatrics
West Bridgewater, MA

Pamela A. Ratner, R.N.
University of Alberta
Vancouver, British Columbia

Elizabeth Raymond, M.D., M.P.H.
Family Health International
Research Triangle Park, NC

**Barbara K. Redman, Ph.D., R.N.,
    F.A.A.N.**
The Johns Hopkins University
Baltimore, MD

Joan Reede, M.D., M.P.H.
Harvard University/AAP
Boston, MA

Paul J. Reiss, M.D.
Vermont Academy of Family
   Physicians/AAFP
Willston, VT

John T. Repke, M.D.
Brigham and Women's Hospital
Boston, MA

Ken Resnicow, Ph.D.
Emory University
Atlanta, GA

Sheldon M. Retchin, M.D., M.S.P.H.
Medical College of Virginia
Richmond, VA

George G. Rhoads, M.D., M.P.H.
The Environmental and Occupational
   Health Sciences Institute
Piscataway, NJ

Darrell S. Rigel, M.D.
New York University
New York, NY

B. Lawrence Riggs, M.D.
Mayo Clinic
Rochester, MN

Frederick P. Rivara, M.D., M.P.H.
Harborview Medical Center
Seattle, WA

Milisa K Rizer, M.D., M.P.H.
University of Texas at San Antonio/AAFP
San Antonio, TX

Helen Elizabeth Roberts, M.D.
Centers for Disease Control and
   Prevention
Atlanta, GA

Richard Roberts, M.D., J.D.
University of Wisconsin at Madison/AAFP
Madison, WI

William O. Robertson, M.D.
Washington Poison Center
Seattle, WA

Lee N. Robins, Ph.D.
Washington University
St. Louis, MO

Edward J. Roccella, Ph.D.
National Institutes of Health
Bethesda, MD

Roger B. Rodrigue, M.D., M.P.H.
Medical Center of Delaware/AAFP
Wilmington, DE

Martha Rogers, M.D.
Centers for Disease Control and
   Prevention
Atlanta, GA

Michael Rosenberg, M.D., M.P.H.
Health Decisions, Inc.
Chapel Hill, NC

Zeda F. Rosenberg, Sc.D.
National Institutes of Health
Bethesda, MD

Lisa S. Rosenblum, M.D., M.P.H.
Centers for Disease Control and Prevention
Atlanta, GA

*Edward C. Rosenow III, M.D., F.C.C.P.,
   F.A.C.P.*
Mayo Clinic
Rochester, MN

Anthony L. Rosner, Ph.D.
Foundation for Chiropractic Education
   and Research
Arlington, VA

Douglas S. Ross, M.D.
Massachusetts General Hospital
Boston, MA

Louise B. Russell, Ph.D.
Rutgers University
New Brunswick, NJ

Marcia Russell, Ph.D.
Research Institutes on Addictions
Buffalo, NY

Mark S. Ruttum, M.D.
Medical College of Wisconsin
Milwaukee, WI

*Benjamin P. Sachs, M.B., B.S.,
   D.P.H. (C)*
Beth Israel Hospital
Boston, MA

Henrietta Sachs, M.D. (ret.)
Glencoe, IL

Bertha H. Safford, M.D.
American Academy of Family Physicians
Ferndale, WA

Marcel Salive, M.D., M.P.H.
National Institutes of Health
Bethesda, MD

Daniel H. Saltzman, M.D.
Brigham and Women's Hospital
Boston, MA

Linda E. Saltzman, Ph.D.
Centers for Disease Control and
  Prevention
Atlanta, GA

Neil H. Sampson, M.P.H., M.G.A.
Health Resources and Services
  Administration
Rockville, MD

Jean E. Sanders, M.D.
Fred Hutchinson Cancer Research
  Center/AAP
Seattle, WA

M. Olwen Sanderson, M.D.
American Academy of Family Physicians
Portland, OR

Mathuram Santosham, M.D.
The Johns Hopkins University
Baltimore, MD

Clark T. Sawin, M.D.
Department of Veterans Affairs Medical
  Center
Boston, MA

Robert Sayers, M.D.
American Academy of Pediatrics
Ocean Springs, MS

Charles A. Schable, M.S.
Centers for Disease Control and
  Prevention
Atlanta, GA

Lawrence Schachner, M.D.
American Academy of Pediatrics
Miami, FL

Catherine Schaefer, Ph.D.
Kaiser Permanente Medical Care Program
Oakland, CA

William Schaffner, M.D.
Vanderbilt University
Nashville, TN

James J. Schlesselman, Ph.D.
University of Pittsburgh
Pittsburgh, PA

Candace M. Schlife, M.P.H.
Indian Health Service
Albuquerque, NM

Edgar J. Schoen, M.D.
Kaiser Permanente Medical Care Program
Oakland, CA

Herbert C. Schulberg, Ph.D.
University of Pittsburgh
Pittsburgh, PA

Manuel Schydlower, M.D.
William Beaumont Army Medical
  Center/AAP
El Paso, TX

*Carol Jack Scott, M.D., M.S.Ed.,
  F.A.C.E.P.*
University of Maryland/The Medical
  Education Group, Inc.
Baltimore, MD

Gwendolyn B. Scott, M.D.
University of Miami/AAP
Miami, FL

F. Douglas Scutchfield, M.D.
San Diego State University
San Diego, CA

Margretta R. Seashore, M.D.
Yale University/AAP
New Haven, CT

Joe Selby, M.D., M.P.H.
Kaiser Permanente Medical Care Program
Oakland, CA

Mary C. Sengstock, Ph.D., C.C.S.
Wayne State University
Detroit, MI

F.J. Service, M.D., Ph.D.
Mayo Clinic
Rochester, MN

David Shaffer, M.D.
Columbia University
New York, NY

Barbara Shannon, Ph.D.
Pennsylvania State University
University Park, PA

Craig N. Shapiro, M.D.
Centers for Disease Control and
  Prevention
Atlanta, GA

Henry R. Shinefield, M.D.
Kaiser Permanente Medical Care Program
Oakland, CA

Hugh M. Shingleton, M.D.
American Cancer Society
Atlanta, GA

Barbara M. Shulman
The Scoliosis Association, Inc.
Raleigh, NC

Baha M. Sibai, M.D.
University of Tennessee at Memphis
Memphis, TN

Ellen K. Silbergeld, M.D.
University of Maryland at Baltimore
Baltimore, MD

Denise G. Simons-Morton, M.D., Ph.D.
National Institutes of Health
Bethesda, MD

Peter A. Singer, M.D.
University of Southern California
Los Angeles, CA

David A. Sleet, Ph.D.
Centers for Disease Control and
  Prevention
Atlanta, GA

Jean Slutsky, P.A., M.S.P.H.
Agency for Health Care Policy and
  Research
Rockville, MD

Clark B. Smith, M.D.
University of Tennessee at
  Memphis/AAFP
Memphis, TN

Richard J. Smith, III
Indian Health Service
Rockville, MD

Suzanne M. Smith, M.D., M.P.H.
Centers for Disease Control and
  Prevention
Atlanta, GA

Linda Snetselaar, Ph.D., R.D., L.D.
University of Iowa
Iowa City, IA

David B. Snyder, R.P.H., D.D.S.
Health Resources and Services
  Administration
Rockville, MD

Alfred Sommer, M.D., M.H.S.
The Johns Hopkins University
Baltimore, MD

Edward J. Sondik, Ph.D.
National Institutes of Health
Bethesda, MD

Stephen J. Spann, M.D.
University of Texas at Galveston/AAFP
Galveston, TX

Marjorie A. Speers, Ph.D.
Centers for Disease Control and
  Prevention
Atlanta, GA

Carole A. Spencer, Ph.D., M.T.
University of Southern California
Los Angeles, CA

Sachiko T. St. Jeor, Ph.D., R.D.
University of Nevada
Reno, NV

Michael E. St. Louis, M.D.
Centers for Disease Control and
  Prevention
Atlanta, GA

Walter E. Stamm, M.D.
University of Washington
Seattle, WA

Meir Stampfer, M.D., Dr.P.H.
Harvard University
Boston, MA

Robert J. Stanley, M.D.
American College of Radiology
Reston, VA

Jeffrey R. Starke, M.D.
Texas Children's Hospital/AAP
Houston, TX

Pamela E. Starke-Reed, Ph.D., H.S.A., B.A.P.
National Institutes of Health
Bethesda, MD

Jeffrey A. Stearns, M.D.
University of Illinois at Rockford/AAFP
Rockton, IL

Russell W. Steele, M.D.
Louisiana State University/AAP
New Orleans, LA

Bruce C. Steffens, M.D.
American Academy of Family Physicians
Moline, IL

Martin T. Stein, M.D.
University of California at San Diego/AAP
La Jolla, CA

Zena Stein, M.A., M.B., B.Ch.
New York State Psychiatric Institute
New York, NY

William M. Steinberg, M.D.
George Washington University
Washington, DC

Thomas Stephens, Ph.D.
Thomas Stephens & Associates
Manotick, Ontario

Barbara Sternfeld, Ph.D.
Kaiser Permanente Medical Care Program
Oakland, CA

Gene R. Sterritt, D.D.S., M.P.H.
Centers for Disease Control and Prevention
Atlanta, GA

David Stoff, Ph.D.
National Institutes of Health
Rockville, MD

Lisa B. Stollman, M.A., R.D.
American Dietetic Association
North Port, NY

David Stone, Ph.D.
Institute for Urban Health
Boston, MA

Katherine M. Stone, M.D.
Centers for Disease Control and
    Prevention
Atlanta, GA

Mary Story, Ph.D., R.D.
University of Minnesota
Minneapolis, MN

D. Eugene Strandness, Jr., M.D.
University of Washington
Seattle, WA

Victor Strasburger, M.D.
American Academy of Pediatrics
Elk Grove Village, IL

Karen F. Strauss, M.S., R.D.
Indian Health Service
Rockville, MD

Raymond A. Strikas, M.D.
Centers for Disease Control and
    Prevention
Atlanta, GA

Albert J. Stunkard, M.D.
University of Pennsylvania
Philadelphia, PA

Roger F. Suchyta, M.D.
American Academy of Pediatrics
Elk Grove Village, IL

Christina M. Surawicz, M.D., F.A.C.G.
American College of Gastroenterology
Arlington, VA

Roland W. Sutter, M.D., M.P.H.
Centers for Disease Control and
    Prevention
Atlanta, GA

Judith Swan, M.H.S.
National Institutes of Health
Bethesda, MD

Jack T. Swanson, M.D.
McFarland Clinic/AAP
Ames, IA

Zachary Taylor, M.D., M.S.
Centers for Disease Control and
  Prevention
Atlanta, GA

Bruce D. Tempest, M.D., F.A.C.P.
Indian Health Service
Gallup, NM

Milton Tenenbein, M.D.
Children's Hospital/AAP
Winnipeg, Manitoba

Stephen B. Thacker, M.D., M.Sc.
Centers for Disease Control and
  Prevention
Atlanta, GA

Robert S. Thompson, M.D.
Group Health Cooperative of Puget
  Sound
Seattle, WA

Robert H. Threlkel, M.D.
American Academy of Pediatrics
Jacksonville, FL

James M. Tielsch, Ph.D.
The Johns Hopkins University
Baltimore, MD

Donald D. Timmerman, M.D.
Elmcrest Psychiatric Institute/AAFP
Portland, CT

Mary E. Tinetti, M.D.
Yale University
New Haven, CT

Tokos Medical Corporation
Cambridge, MA

Riva Touger-Decker, Ph.D., R.D.
University of Medicine and Dentistry of
  New Jersey
Newark, NJ

Frederick Trowbridge, M.D.
Centers for Disease Control and
  Prevention
Chamblee, GA

Cyndee Trower, M.D.
Health Resources and Services
  Administration
Rockville, MD

Myra Tucker, B.S.N., M.P.H.
Centers for Disease Control and
  Prevention
Atlanta, GA

James R. Ullom
Agency for Health Care Policy and
  Research
Rockville, MD

Ronald O. Valdiserri, M.D., M.P.H.
Centers for Disease Control and Prevention
Atlanta, GA

Peter C. Van Dyck, M.D., M.P.H.
Health Resources and Services
  Administration
Rockville, MD

Theodore B. Van Itallie, M.D.
St. Luke's-Roosevelt Hospital Center
New York, NY

Lester Van Middlesworth, Ph.D, M.D.
University of Tennessee/Memphis
Memphis, TN

Gert J. Vanderwilt, Ph.D.
Katholieke Universiteit Nijmegen
Nijmegen, Netherlands

Maria E. Vegega, Ph.D.
National Highway Traffic Safety
  Administration
Washington, DC

M. Elsa Villarino, M.D., M.P.H.
Centers for Disease Control and
  Prevention
Atlanta, GA

Frank Vinicor, M.D., M.P.H.
Centers for Disease Control and
  Prevention
Atlanta, GA

Carey Vinson, M.D., M.P.M.
Forbes Regional Hospital/AAFP
Monroeville, PA

Donna L. Vogel, Ph.D.
National Institutes of Health
Bethesda, MD

H. Bruce Vogt, M.D.
University of South Dakota
Sioux Falls, SD

William C. Wadland, M.D., M.S.
Michigan State University/AAFP
East Lansing, MI

Bailus Walker, Jr., Ph.D., M.P.H.
Alliance to End Childhood Lead
  Poisoning
Washington, DC

Elinor Walker
Agency for Health Care Policy and
  Research
Rockville, MD

Michael D. Walker, M.D.
National Institutes of Health
Bethesda, MD

Eric Wall, M.D., M.P.H.
Oregon Health Sciences University/AAFP
Portland, OR

Mark E. Wallace, M.D., M.P.H.
North Colorado Family Medicine/AAFP
Greeley, CO

Sharon L. Walmsley, M.D., F.R.C.P.C.
University of Toronto
Toronto, Ontario

Patrick C. Walsh, M.D.
The Johns Hopkins Hospital
Baltimore, MD

**Elaine E.L. Wang, M.D. C.M., M.Sc.
F.R.C.P.C.**
Hospital for Sick Children
Toronto, Ontario

Wendy Warren, M.D.
American Academy of Family Physicians
Klamath Falls, OR

Reginald L. Washington, M.D.
American Academy of Pediatrics
Denver, CO

Judith H. Wasserheit, M.D.
Centers for Disease Control and
  Prevention
Atlanta, GA

Thomas R. Waters, Ph.D.
Centers for Disease Control and
  Prevention
Cincinnati, OH

Alan G. Waxman, M.D., M.P.H.
Indian Health Service
Gallup, NM

Daniel W. Webster, Sc.D., M.P.H.
The Johns Hopkins University
Baltimore, MD

Robert Weibel, M.D.
Health Resources and Services
  Administration
Rockville, MD

Milton C. Weinstein, Ph.D.
Harvard University
Boston, MA

Stuart L. Weinstein, M.D.
University of Iowa
Iowa City, IA

Noel S. Weiss, M.D., Dr.P.H.
University of Washington
Seattle, WA

Michael Weitzman, M.D.
Rochester General Hospital
Rochester, NY

Jay D. Wenger, M.D.
Centers for Disease Control and
  Prevention
Atlanta, GA

Martha M. Werler, Sc.D.
Boston University
Brookline, MA

David J. West, Ph.D., M.P.H.
Merck Research Laboratories
West Point, PA

David W. Wetter, Ph.D.
University of Wisconsin at Madison
Madison, WI

Judith Whalen, M.P.A.
National Institutes of Health
Bethesda, MD

Melinda E. Wharton, M.D., M.P.H.
Centers for Disease Control and
    Prevention
Atlanta, GA

Jane White, Ph.D., R.D.
University of Tennessee at Knoxville
Knoxville, TN

John C. Whitener, O.D., M.P.H.
American Optometric Association
Alexandria, VA

William L. Whittington, M.D.
Centers for Disease Control and
    Prevention
Atlanta, GA

David O. Wiebers, M.D.
Mayo Clinic
Rochester, MN

William H. Wiese, M.D., M.P.H.
University of New Mexico
Albuquerque, NM

Lynne S. Wilcox, M.D., M.P.H.
Centers for Disease Control and
    Prevention
Atlanta, GA

Allan J. Wilke, M.D.
Family Practice Center/AAFP
St. Cloud, MN

Stephen D. Williams, M.D.
Indiana University Cancer Center
Indianapolis, IN

Walter W. Williams, M.D., M.P.H.
Centers for Disease Control and
    Prevention
Atlanta, GA

David F. Williamson, Ph.D., M.S.
Centers for Disease Control and
    Prevention
Atlanta, GA

Sidney J. Winawer, M.D.
Memorial Sloan-Kettering Cancer Center
New York, NY

Phyllis A. Wingo, Ph.D., M.S.
Centers for Disease Control and
    Prevention
Atlanta, GA

Peter D. Wood, D.Sc., Ph.D., F.A.C.S.M.
Stanford University
Palo Alto, CA

Steffie Woolhandler, M.D.
Harvard University
Cambridge, MA

Catherine E. Woteki, Ph.D., R.D.
The White House, Office of Science
    Technology Policy
Washington, DC

David Wright, M.D.
American Academy of Family Physicians
Austin, TX

Ray Yip, M.D.
Centers for Disease Control and
    Prevention
Atlanta, GA

Jonathan M. Zenilman, M.D.
The Johns Hopkins University
Baltimore, MD

Gerhard Zielhuis, Ph.D.
Katholieke Universiteit Nijmegen
Nijmegen, Netherlands

*Richard Kent Zimmerman, M.D.,
M.P.H.*
University of Pittsburgh/AAFP
Pittsburgh, PA

Barry Zuckerman, M.D.
Boston University
Boston, MA

Index

Mean arterial pressure, preeclampsia, Ch 37

Mean cell volume, iron deficiency and, Ch 22

Mean corpuscular volume, thalassemia screening, Ch 43

Measles, childhood immunization. *See* Measles-mumps-rubella vaccine

Measles-mumps-rubella vaccine
adolescent immunization, Ch 32, Ch 65, Ch 66
adult immunization, Ch 66
in childhood, Ch 32, Ch 65

Mechanical suffocation, prevention counseling, Ch 58

Medroxyprogesterone acetate, postmenopausal hormone prophylaxis, Ch 68

Melanoma, malignant, Ch 12

Meningococcal infection, postexposure prophylaxis, Ch 67

Meningomyelocele, Ch 42

Menopause. *See* Postmenopause period

Menstruation
hemoglobin levels and, Ch 22
microscopic hematuria and, Ch 17

Mental health disorders. *See also* Depression, Suicide
exercise benefits, Ch 55
recognition and treatment, Ch 49, Ch 50

Mental retardation
congenital hypothyroidism, Ch 45
Down syndrome, Ch 41
infant phenylketonuria, Ch 44
intrapartum electronic fetal monitoring and, Ch 39

Mental status, dementia screening, Ch 48

Metabolic disorders. *See also* Diabetes mellitus; Obesity; Thyroid disease
dementia and, Ch 48

Methodology, preventive service evaluation, Ch ii

MHA-TP (microhemagglutination assay for antibodies to *Treponema pallidum*), Ch 26

Michigan Alcoholism Screening Test, Ch 52

Microhemagglutination assay for antibodies to *Treponema pallidum*, Ch 26

Military personnel
hepatitis A vaccine, Ch 66
HIV infection screening, Ch 28
rubella screening and vaccination, Ch 32

Mini-Mental State Examination, dementia screening, Ch 48

"Mini-pill," for contraception, Ch 63

MMR vaccine. *See* Measles-mumps-rubella vaccine

Modified Clinical Technique, visual impairment screening, Ch 33

Moire topography, adolescent idiopathic scoliosis screening, Ch 47

Moles, skin cancer and, Ch 12

Mono-Vacc multiple puncture test, Ch 25

Morbidity/mortality. *See individual conditions*

Motor vehicle injuries, Ch 57
dementia and, Ch 48
motorcycle injuries, Ch 57
visual impairment in elderly, and, Ch 33

MRI. *See* Magnetic resonance imaging

Multiple gestations
maternal serum α-fetoprotein, Ch 42
preeclampsia/eclampsia, Ch 37
ultrasonographic detection, Ch 36

Multiple-marker screening. *See* Serum markers, maternal

Multiple puncture tests, tuberculous infection screening, Ch 25

Multivitamins, neural tube defect prophylaxis, Ch 42

Mycobacterium avium complex (MAC), rifabutin prophylaxis, Ch 28

Mycobacterium tuberculosis. *See* Tuberculous infection

Myocardial infarction. *See also* Coronary heart disease
aspirin prophylaxis for, Ch 69
carotid artery stenosis and, Ch 4

Myopia, glaucoma and, Ch 34

Negative predictive value, screening test accuracy, Ch ii

Neisseria gonorrhoeae. *See* Gonorrhea

Neisseria meningitidis infection, postexposure prophylaxis, Ch 67

Neoplastic diseases. *See specific cancer sites*

Neural tube defects, Ch 42

Nevi, skin cancer and, Ch 12

Newborns. *See also* Infants; Perinatal morbidity/mortality
asymptomatic bacteriuria, Ch 31
breast feeding, Ch 56
chlamydial infection, Ch 29. *See also* Ophthalmia neonatorum
congenital rubella syndrome, Ch 32
genital herpes simplex, Ch 30
gonorrhea. *See also* Ophthalmia neonatorum
hearing impairment, Ch 35
hemoglobinopathies, Ch 43

Guide to Clinical Preventive Services, 3rd Edition, 2000–2002

Report of the U.S. Preventive Services Task Force

The *U.S. Preventive Services Task Force* (USPSTF) was convened by the Public Health Service to rigorously evaluate clinical research in order to assess the merits of preventive measures, including screening tests, counseling, immunizations, and chemoprophylaxis.

The 3rd Edition of the *Guide to Clinical Preventive Services* updates some recommendations from the 2nd Edition and evaluates additional new topics. Recommendations from the Third Task Force are being released incrementally, as they become available.

Third U.S. Preventive Services Task Force

Contents

Introducing the Third U.S. Preventive Services Task Force

Alfred O. Berg, MD, MPH, Janet D. Allan, PhD, RN, CS

Providing preventive services to apparently healthy individuals in clinical settings is such a ubiquitous part of primary care practice that it is easy to forget that the concept is less than 100 years old. The idea that clinicians had anything useful to offer healthy people was a product of the 1930s and 1940s, during an era of rapid advances in public health and progress in the pathophysiologic view of disease. Claims that patients could benefit from "periodic health examinations" were initially met with skepticism on the part of most medical practitioners. But the skeptics were quickly converted, so that by the 1950s and 1960s the proliferation of screening tests and primary preventive advice was far advanced in routine clinical practice. Many clinical conditions for which diagnostic tests were available became targets for inclusion in periodic examinations, at one extreme resulting in programs of excess in which healthy individuals of means might be admitted to hospital to undergo a battery of screening and diagnostic testing over several days.

Despite the quick and general acceptance of screening as a component of routine clinical practice, a few advocates for studies to test directly the efficacy of screening tests and other preventive interventions raised concerns about the lack of evidence that interventions truly improved clinical outcomes. These concerns became organized during the 1970s when critical scientific reviews were first published by individuals and expert groups. Since the 1980s, both the Canadian Task Force on Preventive Health Care and the United States Preventive Services Task Force (Task Force) have provided evidence-based scientific reviews of preventive health services for

From the Department of Family Medicine, University of Washington School of Medicine (Berg), Seattle, Washington; and the School of Nursing, University of Texas Health Science Center (Allan), San Antonio, Texas

Dr. Berg is Chair and Dr. Allan is Vice-Chair of the U.S. Preventive Services Task Force.

Address correspondence to: Alfred O. Berg, MD, MPH, Chair, USPSTF, Professor and Chair, Department of Family Medicine, University of Washington School of Medicine, 1959 Northeast Pacific Avenue, Box 356390, Seattle, Washington 98195. E-mail: Aberg@u.washington.edu.

Reprints are available from the AHRQ Web site at www.ahrq.gov/ clinic/uspstfix.htm, through the National Guideline Clearinghouse (www.guideline.gov), or in print through the AHRQ Publications Clearinghouse (1-800-358-9295).

use in primary care clinical settings, including screening tests, counseling, and chemoprevention. The first Task Force *Guide to Clinical Preventive Services*[1] was published in 1989. The second Task Force *Guide to Clinical Preventive Services*[2] was published in 1996 and served as the basis for the 1998 *Clinicians Handbook of Preventive Services*[3] and the Put Prevention Into Practice national implementation program.

This supplement to the *American Journal of Preventive Medicine* (*AJPM*) introduces the methods and products of the third Task Force. The first background article[4] reviews the philosophy and history of Task Force work, placing our new efforts in historical perspective, discussing challenges faced by the Task Force, and previewing several of the contributions to be made. The second background article[5] summarizes the methods used by the Task Force, its extraordinary length appropriately reflecting the importance we place on public accountability and transparency of the methods used to reach our conclusions. Despite its length, the article cannot fully describe all the details; these will be presented in more depth in each of the Systematic Evidence Reviews that will be published on the AHRQ Web site and in print. The third background article[6] covers one of the significant new additions to the scope of work of the third Task Force: economic evaluation. For the first time, when evaluating preventive interventions, we are attempting to answer not only the question "Does it work?" (the scientific assessment of efficacy), but, for selected conditions, "Is it worth it?" (the assessment of economic benefits and costs).

Following the background articles are four pairs of recommendation and rationale statements (produced principally by Task Force members and staff)[7–10] and evidence summaries (produced principally by the Evidence- based Practice Centers at the Oregon Health Sciences University and Research Triangle Institute–University of North Carolina).[11–14] These recommendation and rationale statements, evidence summaries, and the Systematic Evidence Reviews are available at the U.S. Preventive Services Task Force Web site (www. ahrq.gov/clinic/uspstfix.htm). We also hope to see many of the recommendation and rationale statements published in a variety of peer-reviewed and continuing education journals to reach a broad range of health professionals. The Systematic Evidence Reviews will be used to generate individual papers in the peer-reviewed literature highlighting key meta-analyses, modeling projects, and other work conducted as part of the review process used by the Task Force.

Finally, several commentators[15–17] provide advice on how to use the information provided in this supplement. We believe the readers of *AJPM*, most of whom share our interest, concern, and passion for preventive health care, will appreciate the articles in this "launch" of the work of the third Task Force.

REFERENCES

1. U.S. Preventive Services Task Force. Guide to Clinical Preventive Services, 1st ed. Washington, DC: Office of Disease Prevention and Health Promotion, 1989.
2. U.S. Preventive Services Task Force. Guide to Clinical Preventive Services, 2nd ed. Washington, DC: Office of Disease Prevention and Health Promotion, U.S. Government Printing Office, 1996.
3. U.S. Preventive Services Task Force Put Prevention Into Practice. Clinician's Handbook of Preventive Services, 2nd ed. (Available from the Agency for Healthcare Research and Quality, Pub. No. APPIP 98–0025). Washington, DC: Office of Disease Prevention and Health Promotion, 1996.
4. Woolf SH, Atkins D. The evolving role of prevention in health care: contributions of the U.S. Preventive Services Task Force. Am J Prev Med 2001;20(suppl 3):13–20.
5. Harris RP, Helfand M, Woolf SH, et al., for the Methods Work Group, third U.S. Preventive Services Task Force. Current methods of the U.S. Preventive Services Task Force: a review of the process. Am J Prev Med 2001;20(suppl 3):21–35.
6. Saha S, Hoerger TJ, Pignone MP, Teutsch SM, Helfand M, Mandelblatt JS for the Cost Work Group of the third U.S. Preventive Services Task Force. The art and science of incorporating cost effectiveness into evidence-based recommendations for clinical preventive services. Am J Prev Med 2001; 20(suppl 3):36–43.
7. U.S. Preventive Services Task Force. Screening for skin cancer: recommendations and rationale. Am J Prev Med 2001;20(suppl 3):44–6.
8. U.S. Preventive Services Task Force. Screening for bacterial vaginosis in pregnancy: recommendations and rationale. Am J Prev Med 2001;20(suppl 3):59–61.
9. U.S. Preventive Services Task Force. Screening adults for lipid disorders: recommendations and rationale. Am J Prev Med 2001;20(suppl 3):73–6.
10. U.S. Preventive Services Task Force. Screening for chlamydial infection: recommendations and rationale. Am J Prev Med 2001;20(suppl 3):90–4.
11. Helfand M, Mahon SM, Eden KB, Frame PS, Orleans CT. Screening for skin cancer. Am J Prev Med 2001;20(suppl 3):47–58.
12. Guise J-M, Mahon SM, Aickin M, Helfand M, Peipert JF, Westhoff C. Screening for bacterial vaginosis in pregnancy. Am J Prev Med 2001; 20(suppl 3):62–72.
13. Pignone MP, Phillips CJ, Atkins D, Teutsch SM, Mulrow CD, Lohr KN. Screening and treating adults for lipid disorders. Am J Prev Med 2001; 20(suppl 3):77–89.
14. Nelson HD, Helfand M. Screening for chlamydial infection. Am J Prev Med 2001;20(suppl 3):95–107.
15. Feightner JW, Lawrence RS. Evidence-based prevention and international collaboration. Am J Prev Med 2001;20(suppl 3):5–6.
16. Calonge N. New USPSTF Guidelines: integrating into clinical practice. Am J Prev Med 2001;20 (suppl 3):7–9.
17. Russell LB. The methodologic partnership of effectiveness reviews and cost-effectiveness analysis. Am J Prev Med 2001;20(suppl 3):10–2.

Background

Evaluating Primary Care Behavioral Counseling Interventions: An Evidence-based Approach

By Evelyn P. Whitlock, M.D., M.P.H.[a], C. Tracy Orleans, Ph.D.[b],
Nola Pender, R.N., Ph.D., FAAN[c], Janet Allan, R.N., Ph.D., C.S.[d]

ABSTRACT

Risky behaviors are a leading cause of preventable morbidity and mortality, yet behavioral counseling interventions to address them are underutilized in health care settings. Research on such interventions has grown steadily, but the systematic review of this research is complicated by wide variations in the organization, content, and delivery of behavioral interventions and the lack of a consistent language and framework to describe these differences. The Counseling and Behavioral Interventions Work Group of the U.S. Preventive Services Task Force (USPSTF) was convened to address adapting existing USPSTF methods to issues and challenges raised by behavioral counseling intervention topical reviews.

The systematic review of behavioral counseling interventions seeks to establish whether such interventions addressing individual behaviors improve health outcomes. Few studies directly address this question, so evidence addressing whether changing individual behavior improves health outcomes and whether behavioral counseling interventions in clinical settings help people change those behaviors must be linked. To illustrate this process, we present two separate analytic frameworks derived from screening topic tools that we developed to guide USPSTF behavioral topic reviews.

No simple empirically validated model captures the broad range of intervention components across risk behaviors, but the Five A's construct—assess, advise, agree, assist, and arrange—adapted from tobacco cessation interventions in clinical care provides a workable framework to report behavioral counseling intervention review findings. We illustrate the use of this framework with general findings from recent behavioral counseling intervention studies.

Introduction

In 1998, the Agency for Healthcare Research and Quality (AHRQ) reconvened the U.S. Preventive Services Task Force (USPSTF) to update its recommendations for clinical preventive services. This Task Force represents primary care disciplines (nursing, pediatrics, family practice, internal medicine, and obstetrics/gynecology), preventive medicine, and behavioral medicine. Two evidence-based practice centers (EPCs)—Oregon Health & Science University and RTI/University of North Carolina—were contracted to prepare systematic evidence reviews that the USPSTF uses in developing its recommendations for preventive care.

Although the USPSTF evidence-based methods are widely applicable throughout medicine, to date they have been used primarily to assess services such as preventive screening, rather than those requiring behavioral counseling.[1,2] The current USPSTF recognized a two-fold need:

1. To expand its evidence-based approach to better assess behavioral counseling interventions.
2. To formulate practical communication strategies for describing services that are effective in changing behavior.

The Counseling and Behavioral Interventions Work Group of the USPSTF adapted the USPSTF generic screening analytic framework, which guides systematic reviews, to address behavioral topics more specifically, and it has promoted a consistent organizational construct for describing behavioral counseling interventions. Clinicians are referred to current products of the USPSTF (1-800-358-9295) for systematic evidence reviews of specific behavioral counseling topics and related USPSTF evidence-based recommendations and clinical considerations beyond the scope of this paper.

This paper has three purposes:

1. To promote a broader appreciation of the importance of behavioral counseling interventions in clinical care and the context for their delivery.
2. To describe the generic analytic frameworks developed to guide the systematic review of behavioral counseling topics for the current USPSTF.
3. To detail the practical organizational construct (the Five A's) adopted by the USPSTF to describe intervention research more consistently in order to foster its application in clinical settings.

Background

Healthy People 2010[3] sets two major goals for the United States:

1. To increase quality and years of healthy life.

2. To eliminate health disparities among different segments of the population.

The next decade offers unprecedented opportunities for health care systems and providers to address these goals by promoting healthy lifestyles among the diverse populations they serve and by adopting policies that will institutionalize preventive services.

Changing the health behaviors of Americans has the greatest potential of any current approach for decreasing morbidity and mortality and for improving the quality of life across diverse populations.[4] In their landmark paper, McGinnis and Foege[5] linked 50 percent of the mortality in the United States from the 10 leading causes of death to lifestyle-related behaviors such as tobacco use, poor dietary habits and inactivity, alcohol misuse, illicit drug use, and risky sexual practices. These behaviors remain problematic in today's society despite having been previously targeted for improvement.[6] Thus, the U.S. Department of Health and Human Services has designated five lifestyle factors as Healthy People 2010[3] health indicators by which to track progress in improving the health of the nation over the next decade (Table 1; Text Version). Improving health behaviors is an important approach to health disparities, because those who are economically and/or socially disadvantaged, including those in low-income ethnic/racial minority groups, disproportionately bear the prevalence of risky health behaviors and the burden of preventable morbidity and mortality.[7]

The unabated impact of health-damaging behaviors among Americans makes it imperative that health care providers and health care systems seriously consider these behavioral issues and accept the challenge of routinely providing quality behavioral counseling interventions where proven effective. The 1996 edition of the *Guide to Clinical Preventive Services* by the USPSTF concluded: "Effective interventions that address personal health practices ... [for] ... primary prevention ... hold greater promise for improving overall health than many secondary preventive measures, such as routine screening for early disease. Therefore, clinician counseling that leads to improved personal health practices may be more valuable than conventional clinical activities, such as diagnostic testing."[1]

Nevertheless, rates of behavioral counseling intervention by pediatricians, nurse practitioners, obstetrician-gynecologists, internists, and family physicians for the priority behaviors discussed above still fall far below national targets.[3,8,9] In fact, gaps in the delivery of clinical preventive services are greater for behavioral counseling than for screening or chemoprevention.[10] This stems in part from the relative paucity of good research evidence to support the behavioral counseling intervention recommendations in the 1996 *Guide to Clinical Preventive Services*.[1]

The quality and quantity of good research evidence for the effectiveness of behavioral counseling interventions are increasing. Brief interventions integrated into routine primary care can effectively address the most common and important risk behaviors.[11-22] The strongest evidence for the efficacy of primary care behavior-change interventions comes from tobacco cessation research[11,12,14,15,19] and, to a lesser extent, problem drinking.[11,16-19,21,22] Accumulating evidence also shows the effectiveness of similar interventions for other behaviors.[11,19,20]

These interventions often provide more than brief clinician advice. Effective interventions typically involve behavioral counseling techniques and use of other resources to assist patients in undertaking advised behavior changes.[12,19] For example, intervention adjuncts to brief clinician advice may involve a broader set of health care team members (e.g., nurses, other office staff, health educators, and pharmacists), a number of complementary communication channels (e.g., telephone counseling,[22,23] video or computer-assisted interventions,[24-26] self-help guides,[27] and tailored mailings[28]), and multiple contacts with the patient.[12,14,19,29]

Rationale for Behavioral Counseling Interventions in Clinical Care

Health care providers and their staff play a unique and important role in motivating and assisting patients' healthy behavior changes. Patients report that primary care clinicians are expected sources of preventive health information and recommendations for patients.[30] For instance, in a recent survey, the vast majority (92 percent to 98 percent) of adult members of health maintenance organizations (HMO) indicated that they expected advice and help from the health care system in key behaviors, such as diet, exercise, and substance use.[31] Similarly, health care providers generally accept[32] and value their role in motivating health promotion and disease prevention.[33,34]

Health care systems are natural settings for interventions to improve health behaviors for many individuals because repeated contacts typically occur over a number of years. Interventions to help patients change unhealthy behaviors, like treatments for patients with chronic disease, often require repetition for modest effects over time. Continuity of care offers opportunities to sustain individual motivation, assess progress, provide feedback, and adjust behavior change plans.[35]

In fact, most clinicians have multiple opportunities to intervene with patients on matters related to health behavior change: patients younger than 15 years average 2.4 visits per person annually to office-based physicians, and those 15 years of age and older average 1.6 to 6.3 visits per year, with visit frequency increasing with age.[36] Moreover, 93 percent of children and youth and 84 percent of adults 18 years of age and older have a specific source of ongoing health care.[3] Not surprisingly, people with a usual source of health care are more likely than those without to receive a variety of clinical preventive services.[3]

The health care setting is not the only setting for approaches to support healthy behaviors. The Guide to Community Preventive Services features evidence-based recommendations from the Task Force on Community Preventive Services for population-based interventions. Those recommendations include policy or environmental changes or individual and group interventions outside the clinical setting intended to change risky behaviors; reduce specific diseases, injuries and impairments; and address environmental and ecosystem challenges.[37] These preventive policies and approaches complement the individually focused interventions that the USPSTF addresses.

Objectives and Scope of Behavioral Counseling Interventions

Behavioral counseling interventions in clinical care are those activities delivered by primary care clinicians and related health care staff to assist patients in adopting, changing, or maintaining behaviors proven to affect health outcomes and health status. Common health-promoting behaviors include smoking cessation, healthy diet, regular physical activity, appropriate alcohol use, and responsible use of contraceptives.

Behavioral counseling interventions occur all or in part during routine primary care and may involve both visit-based and outside intervention components. For instance, assessment of behavioral health risks may occur at the time of enrollment in a health plan or at the time of a clinical visit. Behavioral counseling may take place in routine primary care visits and/or through telephone contacts or personalized mailings of self-help guides or materials. Referral to more intensive clinics in the community also may be included. While the USPSTF primarily evaluates interventions that involve clinicians as part of routine primary care, USPSTF liaisons assigned to a particular behavioral topic define the scope of clinical intervention approaches reviewed for any given topic, such as problem drinking or physical activity.

Behavioral counseling interventions differ from screening interventions in several important ways that affect the ease and likelihood of their being delivered. Behavioral counseling interventions address complex behaviors that are integral to daily living; they vary in intensity and scope from patient to patient; they require repeated action by both patient and clinicians, modified over time, to achieve health improvement; and they are strongly influenced by multiple contexts (family, peers, worksite, school, and community).

Further, "counseling" is a broadly used but imprecise term that covers a wide array of preventive and therapeutic activities, from mental health or marital therapy to the provision of health education and behavior change support. Thus, we have chosen to use the term "behavioral counseling interventions" to describe the range of personal counseling and related behavior-change interventions that are effectively employed in primary care to help patients change health-related behaviors. As with its use in other contexts, "counseling" here denotes a cooperative mode of work demanding active participation from both patient and clinician that aims to facilitate the patient's independent initiative and ability to cope.[38] Engaging patients actively in the self-management practices needed to change and maintain healthy behaviors is a central component of effective behavioral counseling interventions.

Theories and Models of Behavior Change

Behavior change theories and models from the social and behavioral sciences explain the biological, cognitive, behavioral, and psychosocial/environmental determinants of health-related behaviors. Thus, they also define interventions to produce changes in knowledge, attitudes, motivations, self-confidence, skills, and social supports required for behavior change and maintenance.[39] The application of relevant theoretical models to behavioral counseling interventions is an important contribution to strengthening health research in this area.[40]

A literature review of 1,174 articles evaluating health behavior, education, and promotion interventions published between 1992 and 1994 found that 44.8 percent of these were explicitly theory based.[41] Six theories and models addressing determinants of health-behavior change at the intrapersonal, interpersonal, and environmental levels (Table 2; Text Version) and two cross-theoretical key constructs/theories were most commonly cited in this research. Promising, if not substantial, empirical evidence supports the validity of all eight theories in predicting or changing health behavior.[41] In addition to those listed in Table 2, self-efficacy and social network/support were the other two most commonly cited constructs in the current literature. Self-efficacy is an individual's level of confidence in his or her own skills and persistence to accomplish a desired goal and predicts future behavior across a wide variety of lifestyle risk factors.[42] Social networks are a person-centered web of social relationships.[43] These relationships provide social support that can assist the individual through "stress-buffering" and other mechanisms.[43]

These theories focus on diverse, interacting levels of influence on an individual's behavior. On the intrapersonal level, multiple internal factors influence an individual's behavioral choices and actions, and there is considerable variability in these factors among individuals with the same objective health behavior. For example, in the stages-of-change/transtheoretical model (Table 2; Text Version), behavioral change is thought of as an ongoing process with multiple stages that often includes relapse and recycling into renewed efforts to change.[44] On the interpersonal level, individual behavioral choices occur in a context that includes the influence of social and environmental conditions in the family and larger community.[41,45]

Behavioral influences operate within a broadly conceptualized ecological paradigm emphasizing that a dynamic interaction between functional levels—intrapersonal, interpersonal, and the physical environment—continues over an individual's lifetime, and that age, gender, race, ethnicity, and socioeconomic status play a critical role in health and health decisions.[40,46] Similarly, the Institute of Medicine[47] recently concluded that "interventions must recognize that people live in social, political, and economic systems that shape behaviors and access to the resources they need to maintain good health."

According to another recent Institute of Medicine report,[40] there is an emerging consensus that social and behavioral research and intervention efforts should be based on this broader ecologic model that incorporates and relates focused approaches across levels. Thus, omission of any key dimension in research or practice reduces the likelihood of successfully addressing problem behaviors, such as smoking.[48] More than a brief overview of theories and models is beyond the scope of this paper and can be found elsewhere.[39–46]

Although these theoretical constructs are unfamiliar to many clinicians, they can help practitioners conceptualize the complex context in which individual behavioral choice occurs and the variability among patients in their receptivity to behavioral counseling interventions at any one time. These insights can clarify barriers, opportunities, and the relative intensity of intervention needed to successfully address behavior change for a given individual.

Generally, less-intensive outside support and intervention are needed for individuals with more change-predisposing attributes than for those with fewer such attributes[48,49] (Table 3). Scarce resources can be focused on strengthening an individual's factors favoring change and targeting the most intensive support to people with the fewest pre-disposing attributes. Theoretical perspectives also make clear the complementary role played by policies and practices in settings outside health care in promoting healthy behaviors across society.

The Clinician-Patient Relationship

As our understanding of behavioral counseling interventions has become more sophisticated, interventions have evolved beyond the limits of one-on-one interactions between a clinician and a patient. However, the use of additional resources within and outside the primary care setting to support the clinician by no means undermines the importance of the clinician-patient relationship in promoting behavior change. Effective clinician communication is important for a variety of patient outcomes.[50,51] Clinician advice to change lifestyle habits is associated with increased efforts to change[52,53] and is effective in encouraging smoking cessation,[11,12,14,15] reducing problem drinking,[11,16] and modifying some activity- and diet-associated cardiovascular risk factors.[11,20] Clinician advice is also associated with increased satisfaction with medical care.[30,54,55] Such advice has been suggested to "prime" patients, especially women, to attend to and act on subsequent educational information.[56] In a recent cross-sectional study among members of a managed care organization,[57] receipt of professional advice to change was associated with a higher readiness to change smoking, physical activity, and diet behaviors. Preliminary data also suggest that advice from one's health care provider based on personal health status is a very strong external cue to health-promoting action.[58]

The clinician employing an empathetic "partnership" approach avoids engendering resistance to behavior change advice.[59] Such an approach emphasizes the patient's role in interpreting advice and explores, rather than prescribes, how best to proceed. According to a Toronto consensus conference on doctor-patient communication,[60] "effective communication between doctor and patient is a central function that cannot be delegated."

The Potential Impact of Health Behavior-Change Programs in Clinical Care

Appreciating behavioral counseling interventions requires a true population-based medicine perspective (i.e., intervening with individuals, but recognizing that the health benefits may not be as clinically visible individually as they are clinically meaningful when considered for the whole). Individually, brief behavioral counseling interventions that are feasible in health care settings often have only modest behavior change impacts. For example, only 5 percent to 15 percent of those receiving an intervention make clinically significant changes, such as quitting smoking[12] or reducing heavy drinking.[11] Even at a population level, overall risk factors typically change only 1 percent to 20 percent.[16,17,19,20,22,61] However, these "modest" impacts translate to significant benefits to the health of the population (and to multiple individuals) when systematically applied to a large proportion of those in need.[48,62–65] This opportunity for substantial public health benefit comes about only when behavior change interventions are applied broadly to entire populations of patients. Given this, population-based behavioral interventions generally offer a range of intervention options including motivational strategies designed for people not ready to change.[64]

Impact of Health Behavior Change Programs

Highly efficacious, intensive group tobacco cessation approaches[12,48,64,66] have typically been perceived as producing higher quit rates than primary care behavioral counseling interventions. Group approaches produce quit rates of 30 percent to 40 percent but reach only a small proportion of highly motivated smokers volunteering for treatment (roughly 3 percent to 5 percent of all smokers). Thus, their potential impact on the prevalence of smoking (Impact = Participation Rate x Efficacy) is substantially less than systematically delivered primary care interventions, which can feasibly reach the 70 percent of smokers who visit their clinicians each year and result in 5 percent to 10 percent overall quit rates.

Applying a similar public health approach, modest effective clinical interventions addressing problem drinking[21,22,62] and dietary change[61] are projected to have significant population impact when broadly delivered.

Practical Approaches to Overcome Barriers to Behavioral and Counseling Interventions

Numerous barriers to preventive service delivery continue to exist in present-day health care settings, most of which are still organized mainly around symptom-driven, acute illness care.[67,68] These barriers include:

- A focus on more medically urgent issues.
- Lack of time.
- Inadequate clinician training, self-confidence, or reimbursement.
- Low patient demand.
- Lack of supportive resources.[3,69]

Further, feedback to clinicians about results of preventive care is largely non-existent or can even be negative.[69] For example, clinicians or their staffs may never "hear" about the patients who followed through on a referral or made positive lifestyle changes, but may encounter complaints about repeated advice to quit smoking, even when voiced by only a few.

Unfortunately, most of these challenges are exacerbated for health behavior-change interventions. Thus, risk assessment and behavioral counseling interventions are delivered even less frequently than screenings.[8] Moreover, although clinicians increasingly agree that most health-promoting behaviors are important to patients' health,[32] they report skepticism about patients' willingness to change these behaviors and about their own ability to intervene successfully in these areas.[70,71] Clinicians often lack the knowledge, skills, and support systems to quickly and easily provide a range of different behavioral counseling interventions, particularly in the limited time available.[69,72,73] These barriers provide an important rationale for proposing a consistent overall approach (such as the Five A's) for describing behavioral counseling interventions across the range of topics in clinical care.

Evaluations of continuing medical education efforts show that programs based on the principles of adult learning that build clinician skills using interactive, sequential learning opportunities in settings such as workshops, small groups, and individual training sessions appear to have the greatest influence on clinician practices and patient outcomes.[74] Even relatively brief physician training along these lines (2 to 3 hours) can improve the delivery of clinical preventive services.[75,76]

However, clinician training may be efficacious only in the presence of an office-support program that assists clinicians in carrying out behavioral counseling interventions and incorporating them into routine care.[77,78] As Solberg et al[79] noted, "Without such systems, delivery of preventive services must depend on the memory, motivation, and time of individual clinicians." Fortunately, we also have a better understanding of the organized office or health-plan processes that support the systematic and consistent delivery of clinical preventive services. These systems typically consist of:

1. Preventive services guidelines.
2. Basic support processes that identify and activate those who need a service, summarize needed services on the patient chart, and remind the clinician during a visit.
3. Prevention resources to provide in-clinic and after-clinic counseling, support, and followup.[80]

A recent randomized controlled trial[81] reported that, compared with control practices, community family practices demonstrated significantly increased clinical preventive services delivery 1 year after receiving practice-tailored systems support for preventive service delivery. Delivery of behavioral counseling interventions was particularly improved. The Put Prevention Into Practice (PPIP) program, sponsored by AHRQ, has a variety of materials to help make these services an integral part of primary care. PPIP has developed tools to assist clinicians in determining which clinical preventive services patients should receive, and it produces guides and materials for service delivery in a variety of settings.[82] PPIP also provides resources for patients to guide health maintenance decisions and to keep track of their preventive care.

Ongoing innovations in the design and delivery of behavioral counseling interventions can also address barriers, improve patient access, and increase treatment effectiveness. Clinicians' efforts are enhanced when the entire health care team takes appropriate and complementary roles in delivering efficacious interventions.[29,83,84] For example, health educators and nurse case managers who contact and support smokers between visits[85] extend intervention opportunities beyond the initial primary care visit. Coordination with resources outside the clinical setting, such as programs and services through voluntary agencies and other community resources, can help patients conveniently access needed supports after they leave the visit.[67] This integration may increase health care system efficiency and impact by creating congruence between clinical interventions and the broader community.[86]

Expanding communication technologies allow both passive and interactive use[25] of telephones, videos, CD-ROMs, the Internet, and other computer-assisted venues to enhance and personalize behavioral intervention content[28,87] and to prolong contact with the patient, while reducing the services that must be directly provided by clinical staff.[67] Such computer-based print, telephone, and video communications have boosted treatment outcomes over standard "one-size-fits-all" interventions in several behavioral areas (e.g., smoking cessation and diet modification), with greatest benefits sometimes seen in low-income populations.[88–90] Although some of these technologies are relatively new and still under evaluation, advances in information and communication technologies hold great promise for enhancing intervention efficiency by automating assessment, education, and patient contacts, especially for ongoing followup and support. Taken together, these ongoing innovations offer opportunities to address key barriers to behavioral counseling interventions in clinical settings.

The Agency for Healthcare Research and Quality and the U.S. Preventive Services Task Force

Public Support for Translating Evidence into Prevention Practice and Policy

John M. Eisenberg, MD, MBA, Douglas B. Kamerow, MD, MPH

In the 12 years since the release of its first report in 1989, the U.S. Preventive Services Task Force(Task Force/USPSTF) has become widely regarded as a premier source of information on the effectiveness of a broad range of clinical preventive services. The work of the Task Force is an important example of a successful public–private partnership to help translate research advances into better preventive care.

The Agency for Healthcare Research and Quality (AHRQ), as required by its reauthorization in 2000, has assumed responsibility for supporting the USPSTF as part of the Agency's mission to enhance the quality, appropriateness, and effectiveness of health care services. From the initial inception of the USPSTF under the auspices of the U.S. Public Health Service Office of Disease Prevention and Health Promotion, federal support has been critical to ensuring both the quality of USPSTF products and the broad participation of relevant professional groups and government agencies. AHRQ's current support of the Task Force typifies the Agency's strategy of improving health care by assuring that decision-makers have access to the evidence they need to draw conclusions about the most effective and efficient screening, diagnostic, and therapeutic choices. AHRQ's support

From the Agency for Healthcare Research and Quality and the U.S. Public Health Service, Rockville, Maryland

Address correspondence to: Douglas B. Kamerow, MD, MPH, Director, Center for Practice and Technology Assessment, AHRQ, and Assistant Surgeon General, U.S. Public Health Service, Agency for Healthcare Research and Quality, 6010 Executive Boulevard, Rockville, MD 20852. E-mail: dkamerow@ahrq.gov.

Reprints are available from the AHRQ Web site at www.ahrq.gov/clinic/uspstfix.htm, through the National Guideline Clearinghouse (www.guideline.gov), or in print through the AHRQ Publications Clearinghouse (1-800-358-9295).

of the Task Force also provides opportunities for public and private partners to translate the evidence that is generated from research into recommendations, clinical practice guidelines, continuing education, and quality assurance or improvement measures.

The first four recommendations[1-8] contained in this supplement to the *American Journal of Preventive Medicine* are based on systematic reviews of the evidence about the effectiveness of screening for skin cancer, bacterial vaginosis during pregnancy, lipid disorders in adults, and chlamydia. These reviews were conducted by two AHRQ-supported Evidence-based Practice Centers (EPCs) and involved consideration of hundreds of research articles and the input of a broad array of federal and private peer reviewers. At the same time, the independence of the USPSTF has ensured that its recommendations are based on an impartial assessment of existing evidence, not the positions of any particular Federal agency or interest group. This approach to improving clinical prevention complements the community-based prevention emphasis of the Centers for Disease Control and Prevention (CDC).

Support of the USPSTF falls within a larger commitment by AHRQ to promote evidence-based health care. It is fitting that the USPSTF, which helped propel the early movement of evidence-based medicine in the United States, is now benefiting from the advances and insights of a growing international network of scholars who are expert in systematic reviews, practice guidelines, and implementation research. Among this network are investigators at 12 AHRQ-supported EPCs, who produce systematic reviews on important questions concerning medical technologies and/or treatment or diagnostic strategies, and who work with private partners interested in developing guidelines, quality improvement tools, and other interventions to improve care.

Some of the information on outcomes and effectiveness emanates from the Patient Outcomes Research Teams (PORTs) that AHRQ supported in the 1990s. AHRQ also supports the on-line National Guideline Clearinghouse (www.guideline.gov), which allows online access to a wide array of evidence-based guidelines on a variety of health care topics. The USPSTF recommendations and the guidelines based on them have been the foundation for performance measures that are used to judge quality, such as those designed and used by oversight organizations such as the National Committee for Quality Assurance (NCQA), Peer Review Organizations (PROs), and the Joint Commission for the Accreditation of Healthcare Organizations (JCAHO). AHRQ's compendium of performance measures, called CONQUEST, provides evidence-based tools for quality assurance and quality improvement; some are based on the conclusions of the USPSTF, making them more accessible to purchasers, institutions, clinicians, and patients.

But just supporting research that can serve as the foundation for recommendations, guidelines, performance measures, and educational programs will not necessarily result in improved quality of care. A decade of AHRQ-supported research has highlighted the challenges of translating evidence into practice. The Put Prevention Into Practice initiative (www.ahrq.gov/clinic/prevenix.htm), sponsored by AHRQ, is developing different tools and products to help translate the USPSTF recommendations for the broad array of audiences (clinicians, educators, policymakers, payers, and patients) who directly and indirectly influence the quality of preventive care. Other ongoing research sponsored or conducted by AHRQ is examining several additional quality-improvement opportunities, such as interventions to improve the delivery of clinical preventive services in different settings; health outcomes, cost-effectiveness, and quality measurement for individual preventive services; changes in payment mechanisms and the organization or delivery of preventive services; and the increasing role of patients in decisions about preventive care.

The work of the USPSTF has helped to establish the importance of including prevention in primary health care, ensuring insurance coverage for effective preventive services, and holding providers and healthcare systems accountable for delivering effective care. Its findings have also highlighted the opportunities for improving delivery of effective services, reducing use of ineffective services, and narrowing gaps between the preventive care of different populations. Equally important, the Task Force has identified an agenda for research on clinical preventive services that is a key component of research on health care quality.

REFERENCES

1. U.S. Preventive Services Task Force. Screening for skin cancer: recommendations and rationale. Am J Prev Med 2001;20(suppl 3):44–6.
2. Helfand M, Mahon SM, Eden KB, Frame PS, Orleans CT. Screening for skin cancer. Am J Prev Med 2001;20(suppl 3):47–58.
3. U.S. Preventive Services Task Force. Screening for bacterial vaginosis in pregnancy: USPSTF recommendations and rationale. Am J Prev Med 2001;20(suppl 3):59–61.
4. Guise J-M, Mahon SM, Aickin M, Helfand M, Peipert JF, Westhoff C. Screening for bacterial vaginosis in pregnancy. Am J Prev Med 2001; 20(suppl 3):62–72.
5. U.S. Preventive Services Task Force. Screening adults for lipid disorders: recommendations and rationale. Am J Prev Med 2001;20(suppl 3):73–6.
6. Pignone MP, Phillips CJ, Atkins D, Teutsch SM, Mulrow CD, Lohr KN. Screening and treating adults for lipid disorders. Am J Prev Med 2001; 20(suppl 3):77–89.
7. U.S. Preventive Services Task Force. Screening for chlamydial infection: recommendations and rationale. Am J Prev Med 2001;20(suppl 3):90–4.
8. Nelson HD, Helfand M. Screening for chlamydial infection. Am J Prev Med 2001;20(suppl 3):95–107.

The Evolving Role of Prevention in Health Care

Contributions of the U.S. Preventive Services Task Force

Steven H. Woolf, MD, MPH, David Atkins, MD, MPH

Many of the leading causes of death and disability in the United States can be prevented.[1] *Primary prevention* can prevent or arrest the disease process in its earliest stages by promoting healthier lifestyles or immunizing against infectious disease. *Secondary prevention*, by detecting and treating asymptomatic risk factors or early asymptomatic disease, can substantially reduce subsequent morbidity or mortality. The clinician plays a pivotal role in both primary and secondary prevention. Health professionals deliver vaccinations, screen for modifiable risk factors such as high blood pressure and high cholesterol, counsel patients about smoking and other behavioral risk factors, provide screening tests for early detection of cancer and other chronic conditions, and advise patients about the benefits and risks of preventive therapies such as postmenopausal hormone replacement therapy.

The health care landscape has changed dramatically in the 17 years since the U.S. Preventive Services Task Force (USPSTF/Task Force) was first established in 1984 to provide advice about prevention for health professionals. Prevention has become an integral component of primary health care.[2] Delivery of clinical preventive services such as immunizations, mammograms, and cholesterol screening has risen steadily over the past two decades.[3] Roughly 90% of employers now include well-child visits, childhood immunizations, screening tests, and adult physical examinations among covered health benefits, compared to less than half that did so in 1988.[4] Interest in prevention has grown significantly among the public, cli-

From Virginia Commonwealth University, Medical College of Virginia (Woolf), Fairfax, Virginia; and Center for Practice and Technology Assessment, Agency for Healthcare Research and Quality (Atkins), Rockville, Maryland

Address correspondence to: Steven H. Woolf, MD, MPH, Virginia Commonwealth University, Medical College of Virginia, 3712 Charles Stewart Drive, Fairfax, VA 22033. E-mail: shwoolf@aol.com.

Reprints are available from the AHRQ Web site at www.ahrq.gov/clinic/uspstfix.htm, through the National Guideline Clearinghouse (www.guideline.gov), or in print through the AHRQ Clearinghouse (1-800-358-9295).

nicians, educators, employers, and policymakers.[5] Furthermore, health plans and individual clinicians are increasingly being held accountable for the quality of the preventive care they provide to their patients.[6]

Substantial gaps in the delivery of effective preventive care in the United States remain, however, because clinicians continue to face many of the same barriers that originally spurred the formation of the first USPSTF.[7] Identifying effective interventions can be difficult in prevention, where prospective controlled trials are often difficult to conduct. Conflicting recommendations from different organizations, further exacerbated by the advocacy positions of some groups, leave many clinicians uncertain about what to do. Clinicians facing increasing time pressures in practice may question the value of some routine preventive interventions, as may employers and other payers struggling with accelerating health care costs. Although more prevention information is reaching the public, the messages conveyed are often inconsistent and increasingly colored by commercial self-interest. Clinicians may feel compelled to provide unproven or ineffective services because patients demand them or they fear being sued, but patients may find that insurance coverage for individual preventive services, especially new technologies, is inconsistent.[4,7]

The importance of clarifying what we know and do not know about the effectiveness of specific preventive services is as important in 2001 as it was in 1984. But the experience of the USPSTF illustrates that understanding effectiveness is only one step on a path to improving preventive health care. In this article, we briefly review the history of the USPSTF from its inception in 1984, reflect on the impact of the Task Force on both preventive care policy and practice and its influence on the contemporary movement of practice guidelines and evidence-based health care in general, and comment on future challenges to the work of the USPSTF and other efforts to promote the implementation of effective preventive health care.

Historical Background: The Journey of the U.S. Preventive Services Task Force

Although major groups had advocated annual physical examinations for decades[8] and promoted routine screening tests such as blood and urine chemistry panels, chest radiographs, and electrocardiograms, a comprehensive review of the scientific evidence to support specific preventive services was lacking in the early 1980s. Doubts grew as critical review articles focused attention on the absence of data for many commonly delivered services.[9] In 1979, the Canadian Task Force on the Periodic Health Examination published its first report,[10] a seminal work using systematic rules of evidence to support the strength of recommendations for a wide variety of preventive services.

In 1984, the U.S. Public Health Service, part of the U.S. Department of Health and Human Services, established the USPSTF to extend the approach of the Canadian Task Force to address a comprehensive set of clinical preventive services. The USPSTF was charged with systematically reviewing the scientific evidence for individual clinical preventive services and making recommendations for practitioners about what services should be routinely offered. The 20-member panel of nonfederal experts included 14 physicians and a dentist, nurse, health services researcher, health educator, economist, and sociologist. In contrast to many other disease-specific guideline panels,[11] the Task Force consisted of generalists with expertise in research methodology and prevention, allowing it to address a wide range of topics. Broad expertise also lessened the potential for conflict of interest on a given issue. Following publication of a series of journal articles on individual services, the USPSTF released the *Guide to Clinical Preventive Services*[12] in 1989. The *Guide* reviewed the evidence for 169 screening tests, counseling interventions, immunizations, and chemopreventive regimens, grading the recommendations on a 5-level (A to E) scale to reflect the quality of the supporting evidence, for age groups ranging from infancy to old age.

The release of the *Guide* had effects both on preventive medicine and on the nascent discipline of evidence- based medicine. The *Guide* represented the first attempt to assess a broad set of services using a consistent approach and with an emphasis on the perspective of the primary care clinician. It provided a single reference to which clinicians and policymakers could turn for the evidence for specific preventive services. The conclusions that the available evidence did not support some services ardently advocated by other medical groups drew heated criticism, but helped establish the credibility of the USPSTF among more skeptical audiences. Casting a spotlight on deficiencies in the evidence also focused attention on the gaps in knowledge and helped guide an agenda for future research needed to establish effectiveness.

The services for which the USPSTF did find compelling evidence— and which typically had wide support from other groups—formed the nucleus of a core set of preventive services advocated by skeptics and enthusiasts alike. This enabled the boundaries of "mainstream" preventive medicine to take form, something that had not occurred before, which in turn became a strategic tool in leveraging policymakers, insurers, and employers to provide a package of well-supported preventive services to large population groups.

The release of the *Guide* accelerated a growing movement to replace traditional "expert consensus" methods for developing clinical recommendations with a systematic and explicit process for reviewing evidence and of linking clinical practice recommendations directly to the quality of the science.[13] Early contributors to this movement included David Eddy[14] and the Evidence-based Medicine Working Group.[15] The strict approach taken by the Task Force drew praise and criticism for eschewing expert opinion as a basis for making recommendations and for taking a neutral position when evidence was lacking. The systems for rating evidence and grading recommendations popularized by the Canadian and U.S. Task Forces were joined by similar schemes used by other groups.[16] The USPSTF formed close collaborations with other groups committed to evidence-based policy, such as the American College of Physicians[17] and American Academy of Family Physicians, staking out similar positions in polarized debates with advocacy organizations using the older opinion-based methods.

Although the USPSTF was disbanded in 1989 with the release of the *Guide*, the need to keep pace with the rapid growth in scientific evidence led to convening a second panel in 1990. The second USPSTF was smaller, with only ten members, eight of whom were primary care physicians. It refined the previous group's methods for reviewing evidence and making recommendations, and expanded the scope of topics. It adopted policies for disclosure of conflicts arising from financial interests, funding sources, or other affiliations. The work of the second USPSTF was marked by strengthened ties with both federal and nongovernmental partners, including primary care subspecialty societies. The work of the second USPSTF culminated in the publication of the second edition of the *Guide*[18] in 1996, which covered over 200 interventions in 70 areas.

The Changing Climate of Prevention

By the time the second edition of the *Guide* appeared, the environment for preventive medicine and evidence based medicine had changed dramatically. Managed care organizations, which had emerged as a dominant paradigm for delivering and paying for health care, included preventive care among basic covered services more commonly than had traditional fee-for-service insurance.[4,19,20] At the same time, the heightened competition spurred by managed care brought increased attention to costs and value. Although clinicians were the primary intended audience for the *Guide*, it soon became clear that the recommendations had an even greater impact on practice by reaching a wider audience of purchasers, health plans, and policymakers, who valued the objective approach to the evidence. The *Guide* was frequently cited by health plans and systems of care in defending their health 14 American Journal of Preventive Medicine, Volume 20, Number 3S maintenance programs and benefits packages, and its recommendations informed many of the Health Plan Employer Data and Information Set (HEDIS)[6] quality measures developed by the National Committee on Quality Assurance for evaluating health plan performance.

These developments occurred against a backdrop of greater interest in health promotion and healthy lifestyles on the part of the American public. Public education campaigns and commercial advertising had spurred interest in low-fat diets, exercise, and weight management. The emergence of new screening technologies and the promotion of specific tests by celebrities and national organizations made patient requests for screening a common occurrence in clinicians' offices. With the advent of the Internet and other information technologies, many patients grew more knowledgeable about options for preventive care and newly released guidelines. Access to information was accompanied by a greater sense of empowerment among patients, including a desire to be more informed consumers and to take a more active role in making health care choices. Health plans, in turn, recognized that including comprehensive health promotion and disease prevention was a valuable marketing tool for attracting patients.

The attention the *Guide* brought to clinical preventive services also highlighted the importance of health promotion and disease prevention efforts outside of the clinician's office. For some health problems (e.g., teenage smoking), the potential impact of the individual clinician was much smaller than that of other community- based interventions. In 1996, the U.S. Centers for Disease Control and Prevention impaneled the Task Force on Community Preventive Services, modeled on the USPSTF, to create the *Guide to Community Preventive Services*, to address a broad range of interventions targeting communities and health care systems rather than individual patients. Recommendations in the *Community Guide* are targeted at persons involved in planning, funding, and implementing population-based services at the state and local levels. The first products of the *Community Guide* effort, including a systematic review of interventions to increase vaccination coverage in children and adults, were published in a January 2000 supplement to the *American Journal of Preventive Medicine*.[21]

Continuing Evolution of Guidelines and Evidence-Based Health Care

By 1996, the enthusiasm for clinical practice guidelines and for evidence-based medicine had been tempered by a realization of their attendant practical and political challenges.[22] At its inception, the U.S. Congress authorized the Agency for Health Care Policy and Research (AHCPR; renamed the Agency for Healthcare Research and Quality [AHRQ] in 1999) to develop practice guidelines as part of its twin goals of improving quality and reducing unnecessary costs. By 1995, however, controversies sparked by several guidelines led to a re-examination of the appropriate role of AHCPR in developing clinical practice policies. At the same time, specialty societies and professional organizations that had reorganized and invested in the early 1990s to establish their own practice guideline programs soon found their efforts eclipsed by guidelines developed by commercial vendors and sold to health plans and hospital systems with the promise of lower health care costs and lengths of stay. Moreover, as experience with evidence-based guidelines grew, observers gained a more mature appreciation of their limitations: a recognition that the critical appraisal of evidence involved more than assigning letter codes; that evidence was lacking for much of medicine; that waiting for better data from controlled trials was often unrealistic or unethical; and that evidence-based guidelines and policies, however well-intentioned, could cause unintended harm to patients, health professionals, and the health care system at large.[23]

Notwithstanding these difficulties, the evidence based perspective gained its footing in health care. Entire journals, and sections of other major journals, are now devoted to the critical appraisal of individual studies, and articles and websites detail the methods for conducting such reviews. Systematic reviews following an explicit methodology[24] and meta-analyses of multiple studies, popularized by the Cochrane Collaboration's *Cochrane Library*,[25,26] appear regularly in most medical journals and offer a more rigorous alternative to the traditional review paper reflecting the opinions of a single expert. Evidence-based guidelines, founded on systematic reviews, are produced throughout the world[23] and the AHRQ National Guideline Clearinghouse (www.guideline. gov), established in 1998, provides access to a steadily growing number of guidelines (over 500 as of October 2000). Software tools to facilitate evidence-based decision making at the bedside are increasingly popular.[27] Policymakers, payers, and legislators are becoming increasingly aware that evidence-based health policy is a tool for quality improvement and for confronting the unrelenting rise in the costs of health care.

The Current USPSTF

It is in this context that a third USPSTF was convened in 1998 to update the recommendations of the second Task Force. Following the release of the second edition of the *Guide*, responsibility for the work of the USPSTF and the related Put Prevention Into Practice[28] initiative (www.ahrq.gov/clinic/prevenix.htm) were transferred to AHRQ as part of its commitment to supporting evidence-based practice. Thirteen Task Force members (including four returning members) were selected from a pool of over 70 individuals nominated by national organizations and experts (see Table 1). Recognizing the need for a broader interdisciplinary approach, the new USPSTF added two nurses, an expert in behavioral medicine, and several experts in cost effectiveness.

Changes are also apparent in the organization of the scientific support to the USPSTF process. Congressional reauthorization of AHRQ in 1999

Table 1. U.S. Preventive Services Task Force and staff (1998–2002)

U.S. PREVENTIVE SERVICES TASK FORCE	

U.S. PREVENTIVE SERVICES TASK FORCE

Afred O. Berg, MD, MPH (chair)
Department of Family Medicine
Univ. of Washington School of
  Medicine
Seattle, Washington

Janet D. Allan, PhD, RN (vice-chair)
School of Nursing
Univ. of Texas Health Science Center
  at San Antonio
San Antonio, Texas

Paul S. Frame, MD
Tri-County Family Medicine
Cohocton, New York

Charles J. Homer, MD, MPH
National Initiative for Children's
  Healthcare Quality
Institute for Healthcare Improvement
Boston, Massachusetts

Tracy A. Lieu, MD, MPH
Dept. of Ambulatory Care and
  Prevention
Harvard Pilgrim Health Care and
  Harvard Medical School
Boston, Massachusetts

Cynthia D. Mulrow, MD, MSc
Dept. of Medicine
University of Texas, San Antonio
Audie L. Murphy Memorial Veterans
  Hospital
San Antonio, Texas

Carole Tracy Orleans, PhD
Robert Wood Johnson Foundation
Princeton New Jersey

Jeffrey F. Peipert, MD, MPH
Department of Obstetrics and
  Gynecology
Women & Infants Hospital of Rhode
  Island
Providence, Rhode Island

Nola J. Pender, PhD, RN, FAAN
School of Nursing
University of Michigan
Ann Arbor, Michigan

Harold C. Sox, Jr, MD
Department of Medicine
Dartmouth-Hitchcock Medical Center
Lebanon, New Hampshire

Steven M. Teutsch, MD, MPH
Merck & Co., Inc.
West Point, Pennsylvania

Carolyn Westhoff, MD, MSc
Department of Obstetrics and
  Gynecology
Columbia University
New York, New York

Steven H. Woolf, MD, MPH
Department of Family Practice
Medical College of Virginia
Virginia Commonwealth University
Fairfax, Virginia

**AGENCY FOR HEALTHCARE
RESEARCH AND QUALITY**

David Atkins, MD, MPH
Scientific and Technical Editor,
  USPSTF

Dana Best, MD, MPH
Assistant Scientific and Technical
  Editor, USPSTF

Randie A. Siegel, MS
Director, Office of Print and Electronic
  Publishing

Eve N. Shapiro
Managing Editor, USPSTF (under
  contract to AHRQ)

Barbara Gordon
Program Analyst, USPSTF

Antoinette P. Wrighton
Assistant Managing Editor, USPSTF
  (under contract to AHRQ)

Table 1. U.S. Preventive Services Task Force and staff (1998–2002) (cont.)

OREGON HEALTH SCIENCES UNIVERSITY
EVIDENCED-BASED PRACTICE CENTER

Mark Helfand, MD, MS
Director, OHSU Clinical Prevention
    Center
Director, OHSU Evidence-based
    Practice Center

Kathryn Pyle Krages, AMLS, MA
Project Manager, OHSU Clinical
    Prevention Center

Benjamin KS Chan, MS

Petronella Davies, MS

Karen B. Eden, PhD

Jeanne-Marie Guise, MD, MPH

Linda L. Humphrey, MD, MPH

Susan Mahon, MPH

Gary Miranda, MA

Heidi D. Nelson, MD, MPH

Margaret M. Nygren, MA

Evelyn P. Whitlock, MD, MPH

Susan Wingenfeld

RESEARCH TRIANGLE INSTITUTE
(RTI)/UNIVERSITY OF NORTH CAROLINA
AT CHAPEL HILL (UNC) EVIDENCEBASED
PRACTICE CENTER

RTI:

Kathleen N. Lohr, PhD
Co-Director, Evidence-based Practice
    Center
Co-Director, RTI-UNC Clinical
    Prevention Center

Sonya Sutton, BSPH
Project Manager, RTI-UNC Clinical
    Prevention Center

Linda Lux, MPA

Sheila White

UNC:

Russell P. Harris, MD, MPH
Co-Director, RTI-UNC Clinical
    Prevention Center

Timothy S. Carey, MD, MPH
Co-Director, RTI-UNC Evidence-based
    Practice Center

Mark Dowell, BA

Anne Jackman, MSW

Carol Krasnov

Michael P. Pignone, MD, MPH

Lynn Whitener, DrPH, MSLS

made federal support for the USPSTF explicit. It also redirected AHRQ from sponsoring guideline development to supporting the production of evidence syntheses for use by outside partners such as professional societies, who could in turn develop guidelines and policies more appropriate for their settings and populations. To this end, AHRQ established a network of 12 Evidence-based Practice Centers (EPCs) in universities and private research organizations with expertise in research synthesis and systematic review. Two of these centers (Oregon Health Sciences University and a collaboration between the Research Triangle Institute and the University of North Carolina at Chapel Hill) provide ongoing support for the USPSTF. Research staff members consult with the USPSTF, conduct systematic reviews, and produce detailed technical reports summarizing the evidence of effectiveness of specific interventions. These reports, which undergo outside review and revision, serve as the foundation for briefer summaries of evidence and for the USPSTF to formulate its recommendations. The centers and their sponsor focus on the science, leaving the formulation of policy and practice recommendations to the independent USPSTF.

Accordingly, the USPSTF process produces three types of documents: a detailed systematic evidence review, written largely by EPC staff with input from the USPSTF; a shorter summary of the evidence, suitable for publication in journals and on the Internet; and a "recommendation and rationale" statement authored by the USPSTF, containing the clinical conclusions derived by the Task Force. These recommendations represent the independent positions of the USPSTF and do not reflect the policies of its sponsor (AHRQ) or the U.S. Public Health Service. Included in this issue of the *Journal* are the first products resulting from this program. An EPC-authored summary of the evidence and a USPSTF-authored recommendation statement appear for each of the four preventive services discussed in this issue (screening for lipid disorders, bacterial vaginosis in pregnancy, chlamydial infection, and skin cancer). The full details of the technical reports are available online (www.ahrq.gov/clinic/prevenix.htm).

This new model of collaboration among the USPSTF, AHRQ, and the academic EPCs offers new opportunities and challenges. The resources provided by the independent, AHRQ-supported centers allow for more detailed reviews than were possible with a small internal staff. Similarly, separating the processes of reviewing evidence and developing recommendations helps ensure that the assessment of the evidence is insulated from policy or political considerations. Clarifying the independence of the USPSTF, and explaining situations in which the conclusions of the USPSTF diverge from that of other federal agencies, will remain ongoing challenges.

Despite its independence, the USPSTF continues to benefit from close relationships with federal health agencies and primary care professional

Table 2. Liaison organizations to USPSTF

Private organizations
American Academy of Family Physicians
American Academy of Pediatrics
American Academy of Physicians Assistants
Americal College of Obstetricians and Gynecologists
American College of Physicians/American Society of Internal Medicine
American College of Preventive Medicine
Canadian Task Force on Preventive Health Care

Federal organizations
Centers for Disease Control and Prevention
National Institutes of Health
Veterans Administration
Health Care Financing Administration
Indian Health Service
Health Resources Services Administration
United States Navy, Bureau of Medicine and Surgery
United States Air Force, Medical Operations Agency
United States Army, Center for Health Promotion and Preventive Medicine

organizations, which regularly attend Task Force meetings and provide peer review of draft documents (see Table 2). These collaborations help to ensure that the evidence that serves as the basis of USPSTF recommendations is complete and accurate, that USPSTF recommendations are clear and credible to practitioners and policymakers, and that consensus is achieved when the position is supported by evidence. In addition, representatives of the USPSTF, Canadian Task Force on Preventive Health Care, and the *Community Guide* Task Force routinely attend each other's meetings and contribute to methods and manuscripts.

Implementation: The Final Frontier of Preventive Medicine

The experiences of the first and second USPSTF, as well as that of other evidence-based guideline efforts, have highlighted the importance of identifying effective ways to implement clinical recommendations. Practice guidelines are relatively weak tools for changing clinical practice when used in isolation.[29,30] To effect change, guidelines must be coupled with strategies to improve their acceptance and feasibility. Such strategies include enlisting the support of local opinion leaders, using reminder systems for clinicians and patients,[31] adopting standing orders, and audit and feedback of information to clinicians about their compliance with recommended practice.[30]

In the case of preventive services guidelines, implementation needs to go beyond traditional dissemination and promotion efforts to recognize the added patient and clinician barriers that affect preventive care. These include clinicians' ambivalence about whether preventive medicine is part of their job, the psychological and practical challenges that patients face in changing behaviors, lack of access to health care or of insurance coverage for preventive services for some patients, competing pressures within the context of shorter office visits, and the lack of organized systems in most practices to ensure the delivery of recommended preventive care.[32,33]

Failure to deal adequately with these challenges is a likely explanation for continuing gaps between USPSTF recommendations and clinical practice. Studies suggest that primary care physicians have variable but generally low awareness of and compliance with USPSTF guidelines.[34-36] USPSTF recommendations have also had less influence on prevention-related legislation and policy than the highly visible efforts of advocacy groups.[37] Under the Balanced Budget Act of 1997, Congress added several preventive services under Medicare, but only one of these (colorectal cancer screening) was recommended for routine use by the Task Force.[38] Similarly, a recent survey of state legislation regarding cancer screening[39] shows many more examples of state-mandated coverage of prostate cancer screening (not recommended by the USPSTF) than of colorectal cancer screening. A recent Institute of Medicine report acknowledged these issues when it recommended a more objective and systematic approach to expanding Medicare coverage of preventive services recommended by the USPSTF.[38] While the USPSTF and AHRQ will work to make their products more relevant to policymakers, these examples also illustrate that factors other than scientific evidence continue to shape policies in both the public and private sectors.

Neither the resources nor the composition of the USPSTF equip it to address these numerous implementation challenges, but a number of related efforts seek to increase the impact of future USPSTF reports. The USPSTF convened representatives from the various audiences for the *Guide*—clinicians, consumers, and policymakers from health plans, national organizations and Congressional staff—about how to modify the content and format of its products to address their needs. With funding from the Robert Wood Johnson Foundation, the USPSTF and *Community Guide* Task Force conducted an audience analysis to further explore implementation needs. The Put Prevention Into Practice[28,40] initiative at AHRQ has developed office tools such as patient booklets, posters, handheld patient mini-records, and a new implementation guide for state health departments.[41]

Dissemination strategies have also changed dramatically in this age of electronic information. While recognizing the continuing value of journals and other print formats for dissemination, AHRQ will make all USPSTF products available through its website (www.ahrq.gov). The combination of electronic access and extensive material in the public domain should make it easier for a broad audience of users to access USPSTF materials and adapt them for their local needs. Online access to USPSTF products also opens up new possibilities for the appearance of the third edition of the *Guide to Clinical Preventive Services*. Freed from having to serve as the primary repository for all USPSTF work, the next *Guide* may be much slimmer than the almost 1000 pages of the second edition.

National efforts such as the USPSTF face inherent limitations in trying to influence practice in individual physicians' offices. To be successful, approaches for implementing prevention have to be tailored to the local level and deal with the specific barriers at a given site, typically requiring the redesign of systems of care. Such a systems approach to prevention has had notable success in established staff-model health maintenance organizations, by addressing organization of care, emphasizing a philosophy of prevention, and altering the training and incentives for clinicians.[42] Staff-model plans also benefit from integrated information systems that can track the use of needed services and generate automatic reminders aimed at patients and clinicians, some of the most consistently successful interventions.[31,43] Information systems remain a major challenge for individual clinicians' offices, however, as well as for looser affiliations of practices in network-model managed care and independent practice associations, where data on patient visits, referrals and test results are not always centralized.

Future Challenges

The USPSTF faces continuing challenges in its attempts to distill evidence and produce clinical recommendations (see the accompanying paper on USPSTF methods in this issue).[44] Increasing explicitness of USPSTF methods cannot completely remove the subjective element involved in making recommendations based on inferences from imperfect evidence on complex issues. Nonetheless, the USPSTF continues to adhere to the general principle that it is appropriate to set a high standard of evidence for preventive care. Premature promotion of services that may be ineffective not only wastes time and money, but could also harm healthy patients, divert attention from more important issues, and undermine efforts to determine what really works.

Over time, the principal question of interest to the USPSTF in the past—Does the preventive service 18 American Journal of Preventive Medicine, Volume 20, Number 3S work?—has matured into more sophisticated questions about the magnitude of benefit, the trade-off between benefits and harms, and the influence of individual preferences on those trade-offs. The Task Force is developing principles for incorporating "shared decision making" into recommendations involving important trade-offs (e.g., tamoxifen to prevent breast cancer, which carries potential benefits and risks), as discussed below. As detailed in the accompanying article about methods, setting the threshold for what constitutes good evidence remains a formidable challenge.

There are inevitable tensions in translating conclusions about the evidence into recommendations that may be widely applied by clinicians in a variety of settings. One approach is simply to describe the quality of the supporting evidence for specific outcomes, leaving it to others to translate that into recommendations appropriate to their practices. This approach recognizes that decision-makers—whether clinicians, legislators, payers, or patients—confront different constraints and priorities in their individual settings. Conversely, blanket recommendations offer clearer guidance but impose the value judgments of the committee and give little account to other determinants of appropriateness (expert opinion, prior experience, standards of care, costs, resources, patient expectations, available services, insurance coverage, medical-legal liability, and ethics). Feedback from a variety of users has clearly indicated a desire for explicit recommendations from the USPSTF, but the group will continue to struggle with its dual duties to describe the evidence and advise on practice policy.

An important challenge is what position to take for the many services reviewed by the USPSTF when available evidence is inadequate to assess the net benefits or harms. Some say the USPSTF should take a neutral position and offer no advice until better evidence becomes available. Others say it should be more permissive, offering such services as "clinical options," especially if the potential harms or costs are minimal. Doing so recognizes that science is only one consideration in judging appropriateness and that clinicians cannot always await better data to make a decision. Some argue the opposite: In an era in which preventive services of proven benefit are not delivered because of limited time and resources, the USPSTF should actively recommend against use of interventions that have not been adequately studied.

For a growing number of preventive services, available data are sufficiently robust to quantify the magnitude of benefits and harms for specific population groups, but this precision gives rise to difficult ethical questions about trade-offs.[45] If a preventive service poses potential benefits and harms, some would recommend that the USPSTF avoid making any generic recommendations and instead uniformly advocate shared decision making, in which the clinician reviews the trade-offs with patients and helps them decide for themselves based on personal preferences. This approach, however, may be impractical and ethically unnecessary except for "close calls" in which judgments about whether benefits outweigh harms fluctuate dramatically based on personal preferences. Even in those cases, a large proportion of patients expects the clinician to give advice.[46] Perhaps the USPSTF has a duty to proffer what that advice should be.

When the original USPSTF was established in 1984, it received explicit instructions not to consider the economic costs of preventive services. Recommending against an effective service because of its cost was considered unpalatable, econometric methods were immature, and controversy over costs could distract attention from more fundamental questions of effectiveness. Although modern methods of cost-effectiveness analysis still need refinement, it is now much more acceptable (in theory, at least) to consider costs in health policy. Here too, however, the role of the USPSTF continues to evolve. At present, the Task Force is reviewing published cost-effectiveness studies and subjecting them to critical appraisal according to accepted criteria, but there is interest in conducting its own analyses when published data fail to address questions of interest. Furthermore, questions of when and how the USPSTF might alter recommendations based on cost effectiveness are not resolved. If economic considerations will influence recommendations, what threshold of cost effectiveness or cost utility is considered acceptable? These issues are explored more fully in the accompanying article on cost effectiveness in this issue.[47]

Finally, for the services the USPSTF does recommend, it is clear that clinicians, health care systems, and payers cannot implement everything at once. For priorities to be set in an evidence-based manner, the USPSTF sees the need for providing users with quantitative information about the relative benefits to individuals and populations. This would require converting the outcomes of preventive services to a common metric, such as quality-adjusted life-years, so that interventions that reduce morbidity or mortality can be compared on a level playing field. Although the USPSTF has decided to include outcomes tables in its reviews with the primary data on which such calculations would be based, views differ on whether it should undertake the additional role of ranking the relative priority of preventive services. The Partnership for Prevention convened a panel to develop methods for prioritizing services. The rankings of the services recommended in 1996 by the second USPSTF are expected to be published in 2001.[48]

The approach the USPSTF is currently taking in dealing with these issues is addressed more fully in the articles that follow. The details of this process, however, flow from fundamental philosophical choices about the roles and responsibilities outlined above, which will remain matters of discussion, debate, and learning for years. As the USPSTF makes adjustments in its sense of purpose to better serve the needs of patients and providers, its methods and procedures can be expected to develop accordingly.

REFERENCES

1. McGinnis JM, Foege WH. Actual causes of death in the United States. JAMA 1993;270:2207–12.
2. Starfield B. Primary care: balancing health needs, services, and technology. New York: Oxford University Press, 1998.
3. National Center for Health Statistics. Healthy People 2000 review, 1998–99. Hyattsville, MD: U.S. Public Health Service, 1999.
4. Partnership for Prevention. Results from the William M. Mercer survey of employer-sponsored health plans. Washington, DC: Partnership for Prevention, 1999.
5. Partnership for Prevention. Recommendations to the Congressional Prevention Coalition: nine high-impact actions Congress can take to protect and promote the nation's health. Washington, DC: Partnership for Prevention, 2000.
6. National Committee for Quality Assurance. HEDIS 2000: The Health Plan Employer Data and Information Set. Volume 1: Narrative—What's in it and why it matters. Washington, DC: National Committee for Quality Assurance, 2000.
7. U.S. Department of Health and Human Services. Healthy People 2010, 2nd ed. Understanding and improving health and objectives for improving health. 2 vols. Washington, DC: Government Printing Office, Nov 2000.
8. Han PK. Historical changes in the objectives of the periodic health examination. Ann Intern Med 1997;127:910–7.
9. Frame PS, Carlson SJ. A critical review of periodic health screening using specific screening criteria. J Fam Practice 1975:2:283–9.
10. Canadian Task Force on the Periodic Health Examination. The periodic health examination. Can Med Assoc J 1979;121:1194–254.
11. American Cancer Society. Summary of current guidelines for the cancerrelated checkup: recommendations. New York: American Cancer Society: 1988.
12. U.S. Preventive Services Task Force. Guide to clinical preventive services: an assessment of the effectiveness of 169 interventions. Baltimore: Williams & Wilkins, 1989.
13. Woolf SH. Practice guidelines: a new reality in medicine. I. Recent developments. Arch Intern Med 1990;150:1811–8.
14. Eddy DM. A manual for assessing health practices and designing practice policies: the explicit approach. Philadelphia: American College of Physicians, 1992.
15. Evidence-Based Medicine Working Group. Evidence-based medicine: a new approach to the practice and teaching of medicine. JAMA 1992;268: 2420–5.
16. Sackett DL. Rules of evidence and clinical recommendations on the use of antithrombotic agents. Arch Intern Med 1986:146:464–5.
17. Eddy DM. Common screening tests. Philadelphia: American College of Physicians, 1991.
18. U.S. Preventive Services Task Force. Guide to clinical preventive services, 2nd ed. Washington, DC: Office of Disease Prevention and Health Promotion, U.S. Government Printing Office, 1996.
19. Schauffler HH, Chapman SA. Health promotion and managed care: surveys of California's health plans and population. Am J Prev Med 1998;14:161–7.
20. Stafford RS, Saglam D, Causino N, et al. Trends in adult visits to primary care physicians in the United States. Arch Fam Med 1999;8:26–32.
21. Task Force on Community Preventive Services. Introducing the Guide to Clinical Preventive Services: methods, first recommendations and expert commentary. Am J Prev Med 2000;18(suppl 1):1–142.
22. Institute of Medicine, Committee on Methods for Setting Priorities for Guideline Development. Setting priorities for clinical practice guidelines. Washington, DC: National Academy Press, 1995.
23. Woolf SH, Grol R, Hutchinson A, Eccles M, Grimshaw J. Potential benefits, limitations, and harms of clinical guidelines. BMJ 1999;318:527–30.
24. Mulrow CD, Cook DJ, Davidoff F. Systematic reviews: critical links in the great chain of evidence. Ann Intern Med 1997;126:389–91.
25. Bero L, Rennie D. The Cochrane Collaboration: preparing, maintaining, and disseminating systematic reviews of the effects of health care. JAMA 1995;274:1935–8.
26. Cochrane Library. Available at: http://hiru.mcmaster.ca/cochrane/cochrane/ cdsr.htm. Accessed 12 October 2000.
27. Ebell M, Rovner D. Information in the palm of your hand. J Fam Pract 2000;49(3):243–51.

28. U.S. Preventive Services Task Force. Put Prevention Into Practice. Clinician's handbook of preventive services, 2nd ed. (Available from the Agency for Healthcare Research & Quality. Pub. No. APPIP 98-0025.) Washington, DC: Office of Disease Prevention and Health Promotion, 1998.

29. Davis DA, Thomson MA, Oxman AD, Haynes RB. Evidence for the effectiveness of CME: a review of 50 randomized controlled trials. JAMA 1992;268:1111–7.

30. Bero LA, Grilli R, Grimshaw JM, et al. Closing the gap between research and practice: an overview of systematic reviews of interventions to promote the implementation of research findings. BMJ 1998;317:465–8.

31. Balas EA, Weingarten S, Garb CT, Blumenthal D, Boren SA, Brown GD. Improving preventive care by prompting physicians. Arch Intern Med 2000;160:301–8.

32. Solberg LI, Kottke TE, Brekke ML, et al. The case of the missing clinical preventive services systems. Effective Clin Pract 1998;1:33–8.

33. Kottke TE, Solberg LI, Brekke ML, Magnan S, Amundson GM. Clinician satisfaction with a preventive services implementation trial: the IMPROVE project. Am J Prev Med 2000;18:219–24.

34. Ewing GB, Selassie AW, Lopez CH, McCutcheon EP. Self-report of delivery of clinical preventive services by U.S. physicians: comparing specialty, gender, age, setting of practice, and area of practice. Am J Prev Med 1999;17:62–72.

35. Christakis DA, Rivara FP. Pediatricians' awareness of and attitudes about four clinical practice guidelines. Pediatrics 1998;101:825–30.

36. Weingarten S, Stone E, Hayward R, et al. The adoption of preventive care practice guidelines by primary care clinicians: do actions match intentions? J Gen Intern Med 1995;10:138–44.

37. Merenstein D, Rabinowitz H, Louis DZ. Health care plan decisions regarding preventive services. Arch Fam Med 1999;8:354–6.

38. Institute of Medicine. Extending Medicare coverage for preventive and other services. Washington, DC: National Academy of Sciences, 2000.

39. Rathore SS, McGreevey JD III, Schulman KA, Atkins D. Mandated coverage for cancer-screening services: whose guidelines do states follow? Am J Prev Med 2000;19:71–8.

40. Agency for Healthcare Research and Quality (AHRQ). Put Prevention Into Practice. Staying healthy at 501. Pub. No. AHRQ00-0002. Rockville, MD: Agency for Healthcare Research and Quality, 2000.

41. Agency for Healthcare Research and Quality (AHRQ). Put Prevention Into Practice. A step-by-step guide to delivering clinical preventive services. Rockville, MD: Agency for Healthcare Research and Quality. In press.

42. Thompson RS, Taplin SH, McAfee TA, et al. Primary and secondary prevention services in clinical practice: twenty years' experience in development, implementation, and evaluation. JAMA 1995;273:1130–5.

43. Briss PA, Rodewald LE, Hinman AR, et al. Reviews of evidence regarding interventions to improve vaccination coverage in children, adolescents, and adults. Am J Prev Med 2000;18(suppl 1):97–140.

44. Harris RP, Helfand M, Woolf SH, et al. Current methods of the U.S. Preventive Services Task Force: a review of the process. Am J Prev Med 2001;20(suppl 3):21–35.

45. Pauker SG, Kassirer JP. Contentious screening decisions: does the choice matter? N Engl J Med 1997;336:1243–4.

46. Frosch DL, Kaplan RM. Shared decision making in clinical medicine: past research and future directions. Am J Prev Med 1999;17:285–94.

47. Saha S, Hoerger TJ, Pignone M, Teutsch SM, Helfand M, Mandelblatt JS. The art and science of incorporating cost effectiveness into evidence-based recommendations for clinical preventive services. Am J Prev Med 2001; 20(suppl 3):36–43.

48. Coffield AB, Maciosek MV, McGinnis JM, et al. Priorities among recommended clinical preventive services. Am J Prev Med 2001. In press.

Current Methods of the U.S. Preventive Services Task Force

Russell P. Harris, MD, MPH, Mark Helfand, MD, MS,
Steven H. Woolf, MD, MPH, Kathleen N. Lohr, PhD,
Cynthia D. Mulrow, MD, MSc, Steven M. Teutsch, MD, MPH,
David Atkins, MD, MPH for the Methods Work Group,
Third U.S. Preventive Services Task Force

ABSTRACT

The U.S. Preventive Services Task Force (USPSTF/Task Force) represents one of several efforts to take a more evidence-based approach to the development of clinical practice guidelines. As methods have matured for assembling and reviewing evidence and for translating evidence into guidelines, so too have the methods of the USPSTF. This paper summarizes the

From the School of Medicine and Cecil G. Sheps Center for Health Services Research, University of North Carolina at Chapel Hill (Harris), North Carolina; Division of Medical Informatics and Outcomes Research, and Evidence-based Practice Center, Oregon Health Sciences University and Portland Veterans Affairs Medical Center (Helfand), Portland, Oregon; Department of Family Practice, Medical College of Virginia, Virginia Commonwealth University (Woolf), Fairfax, Virginia; Research Triangle Institute, Research Triangle Park, and University of North Carolina at Chapel Hill, Program on Health Outcomes and School of Public Health (Lohr), North Carolina; Department of Medicine, University of Texas Health Science Center (Mulrow), San Antonio, Texas; Outcomes Research and Management, Merck & Co., Inc. (Teutsch), West Point, Pennsylvania; Center for Practice and Technology Assessment, Agency for Healthcare Research and Quality (Atkins), Rockville, Maryland

Other members of the Methods Work Group include: Alfred O. Berg, MD, MPH, University of Washington School of Medicine; Karen B. Eden, PhD, Oregon Health Sciences University; John Feightner, MD, MSc, FCFP, University of Western Ontario–Parkwood Published by Elsevier Science Inc. PII S0749-3797(01)00261-6 Hospital; Susan Mahon, MPH, Oregon Health Sciences University; and Michael Pignone, MD, MPH, University of North Carolina School of Medicine.

Address correspondence to: Russell P. Harris, MD, MPH, Cecil G. Sheps Center for Health Services Research, CB# 7590, 725 Airport Rd., The University of North Carolina at Chapel Hill, Chapel Hill, NC 27599-7590. E-mail: rharris@med.unc.edu.

Reprints are available from the AHRQ Web site at www.ahrq.gov/clinic/uspstfix.htm, through the National Guideline Clearinghouse (www.guideline.gov), or in print through the AHRQ Publications Clearinghouse (1-800-358-9295).

current methods of the third USPSTF, supported by the Agency for Healthcare Research and Quality (AHRQ) and two of the AHRQ Evidence-based Practice Centers (EPCs).

The Task Force limits the topics it reviews to those conditions that cause a large burden of suffering to society and that also have available a potentially effective preventive service.It focuses its reviews on the questions and evidence most critical to making a recommendation.It uses analytic frameworks to specify the linkages and key questions connecting the preventive service with health outcomes. These linkages, together with explicit inclusion criteria, guide the literature searches for admissible evidence.

Once assembled, admissible evidence is reviewed at three strata: (1) the individual study,(2) the body of evidence concerning a single linkage in the analytic framework, and (3) the body of evidence concerning the entire preventive service. For each stratum, the Task Force uses explicit criteria as general guidelines to assign one of three grades of evidence:good, fair, or poor. Good or fair quality evidence for the entire preventive service must include studies of sufficient design and quality to provide an unbroken chain of evidence-supported linkages, generalizable to the general primary care population, that connect the preventive service with health outcomes. Poor evidence contains a formidable break in the evidence chain such that the connection between the preventive service and health outcomes is uncertain.

For services supported by overall good or fair evidence, the Task Force uses outcome stables to help categorize the magnitude of benefits, harms, and net benefit from implementation of the preventive service into one of four categories: substantial, moderate,small, or zero/negative.

The Task Force uses its assessment of the evidence and magnitude of net benefit to make a recommendation, coded as a letter: from A (strongly recommended) to D (recommend against). It gives an I recommendation in situations in which the evidence is insufficient to determine net benefit.

The third Task Force and the EPCs will continue to examine a variety of methodologic issues and document work group progress in future communications.

Medical Subject Headings (MeSH): MEDLINE, preventive health services, evidence-based medicines, methods, practice guidelines (Am J Prev Med 2001;20(3S):21–35)

Introduction

The U.S. Preventive Services Task Force (Task Force/USPSTF)represents one of several efforts by governments and national organizations to take a more evidence-based approach to the development of clinical practice guidelines. Guidelines developed by an evidence-based approach tend to be based on conclusions supported more by scientific evidence than by expert opinion.[1] Efforts are made to link the strength of recommendations to the quality of evidence;to make that linkage transparent and explicit,and to ensure that the review of evidence is comprehensive, objective, and attentive to quality.[2]

Methods for reviewing the evidence have matured over the years as groups have gained experience in developing evidence-based guidelines. Systematic searches of multiple bibliographic research databases help ensure thorough and unbiased identification of the relevant literature. Predetermined selection criteria minimize bias and improve the efficiency of reviewing that literature. Quality criteria developed by methodologists guide judgments of weaknesses and strengths of individual research studies. Frameworks and models explicitly define methods for rating and integrating multiple pieces of heterogeneous evidence.[3]

Methods for linking evidence and recommendations have also matured.[4] Initially the recommendations of the USPSTF and other evidence-based groups were strongly correlated with the research design of the most important studies. An A recommendation, for example, usually meant that use of the preventive service was supported by a randomized controlled trial (RCT).[5,6] Guideline developers now understand the need to consider the evidence as a whole, including the trade-offs among benefits, harms, and costs and the net benefit relative to other health care needs for optimal resource allocation.[7]

In the case of prevention, moreover, special scientific and policy considerations apply in reviewing evidence and setting policy. Preventive services require a distinctive logic in considering, for example, the incremental benefit of early detection or the ability of counselors to motivate behavior change. Because the populations affected by preventive care recommendations are often large and have no recognized symptoms or signs of the target condition, harms incurred by even a small percentage can affect a large number of people. Thus, the potential for doing greater harm than good must betaken seriously.

In the context of these methodologic advances and with an awareness of the many unresolved issues for which sound methods are lacking, the third Task Force formed a methods subcommittee (Methods Work Group). It comprises members of the Task Force, representatives of the Canadian Task Force on Preventive Health Care, staff of the two Evidence-based Practice Centers (EPCs) that support the Task Force, and staff of the Agency for Healthcare Research and Quality (AHRQ). The mission of the Work Group is to revisit methods used by previous U.S. Preventive Services Task Forces, to develop more sophisticated methods to be used in current work, and to understand better the theoretical considerations for problems that lack easy answers.

The discussions of this group and subsequent discussions by the entire Task Force have led to several modifications of Task Force methods and identified areas that need further examination. This article describes the methods in current use by the third USPSTF. As the Task Force identifies better ways to do its work, the Methods Work Group will explore additional revisions and refinements to its methods.

We discuss these changes in the sequence of steps of recommendation development: scope and selection of topics, review of the evidence, assessing the magnitude of net benefit, extrapolation and generalization, translating evidence into recommendations, drafting there port, and external review.

Scope and Selection of Topics

Scope

In defining its scope of interest, the Task Force must consider types of services, populations of patients and providers, and sites for which its recommendations are intended. Clarifying these definitions has both methodologic and practical importance. Resource limitations make it impossible for the Task Force to review evidence for all services that prevent disease; the project must, therefore, set boundaries.

The third Task Force has retained the previous policy of focusing on screening tests, counseling interventions, immunizations, and chemo prevention delivered to persons without recognized symptoms or signs of the target condition.

As in the past, this Task Force decided not to make recommendations concerning services to prevent complications in patients with established disease (e.g., coronary artery disease and diabetes). It does, however, make recommendations for preventing morbidity or mortality from a second condition among those who have a different established disease.

The Task Force does make recommendations for people at different levels of risk for a condition. Many people in the general population have one or more risk factors for the Task Force's target conditions. Because the balance between benefits and harms sometimes differs between people at higher risk and those at lower risk, Task Force recommendations may vary across these different groups.

Although the Task Force does not conduct Systematic searches of evidence for services to prevent complications in people with established disease, it may cite such studies when they are relevant for people without established disease. Often, compelling evidence that screening tests and treatments can reduce morbidity and mortality comes from patients with extant disease rather than from asymptomatic populations. For example, the review of lipid screening in this supplement [8] would be incomplete if it did not discuss studies of the efficacy of statins in patients with coronary artery disease.

The populations for whom Task Force recommendations are intended include patients seen in traditional primary care or other clinical settings (e.g., dieticians' offices, cardiologists' offices, emergency departments, hospitals, school-based clinics, urgent care facilities,student health clinics, family planning clinics, nursing homes, and homes). As before, the third Task Force has excluded consideration of preventive services outside the clinical setting (e.g., nonclinic-based programs at schools, worksites, and shopping centers), reserving this analysis to the work of the Centers for Disease Control and Prevention's (CDC) *Guide to Community Preventive Services*[9] effort. For selected topics, however,the Task Force may examine evidence from community-based settings to evaluate the effectiveness of interventions conducted in the clinical arena.

Selection of Topics

In the second edition of the Guide to Clinical Preventive Services,[6] the Task Force reviewed 70 preventive care topics, including more than 100 actual services. These had been selected on the basis of the burden of suffering to society or individuals and the potential effectiveness of one or more preventive interventions. The Task Force briefly considered using an explicit grading process for ranking the priority of topics, an exercise that was undertaken by the second Task Force with disappointing results, and for this reason the current Task Force did not pursue it.

Instead, the third Task Force started with the topics reviewed in the second *Guide to Clinical Preventive Services.*[6] From the 70 topics, the EPCs, AHRQ, and Task Force leaders identified 55 likely to have new evidence or continued controversy. For these 55 topics, the EPCs undertook limited literature searches and prepared brief summaries of the new evidence, current controversies, and critical issues. The EPCs prepared similar summaries of 15 new topics suggested by previous Task Force members, the public, outside experts, federal agencies, and health care organizations. AHRQ and the EPCs also invited about 60 private health and consumer groups and federal agencies to rate the need to update old chapters and to nominate new topics.

Based on this information, the USPSTF ranked the priority of topics at its first meeting in November 1998. It initially assigned 12 topics to the two EPCs (six to each EPC) for review and has subsequently added more topics in a phased schedule (Table 1).

The responsible EPC assigns a lead author and a variable number of additional local personnel to each topic. The Task Force assigns two or three of its own members ("Task Force liaisons") to collaborate on the

Table 1. Topics completed or under review by the third U.S. Preventive
Services Task Force

Evidence-based Practice Center	
Research Triangle Institute– University of North Carolina	**Oregon Health Sciences University**
Updates	**Updates**
Screening for and treating adults for lipid disorders	Screening for breast cancer
Screening for type 2 diabetes mellitus	Counseling to prevent skin cancer
Counseling in the clinical setting to prevent	Screening for family violence
unintended pregnancy	Screening for problem drinking
Counseling to promote a healthy diet	Screening for skin cancerCounseling to prevent youth violence
Screening for visual impairment in children aged 0 to 5 years	Postmenopausal hormone chemoprevention
Screening for depression	Screening for chlamydial infection
Screening for cervical cancer	Universal newborn hearing screening
Screening for prostate cancer	Screening for lung cancer
Screening for colorectal cancer	Screening for ovarian cancer
Aspirin chemoprevention for the primary prevention	Screening for iron deficiency anemia
of cardiovascular events	Screening for neural tube defects
Screening for hypertension	Screening for asymptomatic carotid artery stenosis
Screening for gestational diabetes	Screening for Down syndrome
Screening for asymptomatic coronary artery disease	Screening for osteoporosis
Screening for dementia	Counseling to promote physical activity
Screening for obesity	
Screening for suicide risk	**New**
Counseling to prevent dental and periodontal disease	Screening for bacterial vaginosis in pregnancy
	Counseling to promote breastfeeding
New	Vitamin supplementation to prevent cancer and
Chemoprevention of breast cancer	cardiovascular disease
Screening for developmental delay	

review. The local EPC group and the Task Force liaisons constitute the "topic team" for each review. the EPCs make certain that all topic team personnel are trained in Task Force methods and the content area of the review.

Review of the Evidence

Intensity

Current methods for conducting systematic reviews emphasize a comprehensive literature search and evaluation and detailed documentation of methods and findings.[10] An advantage of this approach is that it avoids the tendency of some guideline panels to cite evidence selectively in support of their recommendations. This approach also enables others outside the process to understand, judge, and replicate the interpretation of the evidence. The disadvantage of this approach is that it produces long, detailed reports of interest to a minority of readers and of limited value to busy clinicians. The process is also resource intensive and requires months of work and considerable expenditures for literature searches and staff. Despite the disadvantages, many evidence-based groups use this approach when reviewing evidence.

For a group such as the Task Force and its EPCs,which must examine multiple topics at once, limited resources and time require compromises in the intensity of reviews. Full-scale systematic reviews for every topic considered are not possible. One strategy for striking a balance, already noted, is topic prioritization. Another strategy, initiated by the second Task Force, is to focus the review on the questions and evidence most critical to making a recommendation.

Setting the Focus for Admissible Evidence

Analytic framework. The second Task Force introduced diagrams, called "causal pathways," to map out the specific linkages in the evidence that must be present for a preventive service to be considered effective. The third Task Force retained these diagrams,renaming them "analytic frameworks." The analytic framework (Figures 1 and 2) uses a graphical format to make explicit the populations, preventive services, diagnostic or therapeutic interventions, and intermediate and health outcomes to be considered in the review. It demonstrates the chain of logic that evidence must support to link the preventive service to improved health outcomes.[11-13]

In the analytic framework, the arrows ("linkages"), labeled with a preventive service or a treatment, represent the questions that evidence must answer; dotted lines represent associations; rectangles represent the intermediate outcomes (rounded corners) or the health states (square corners)

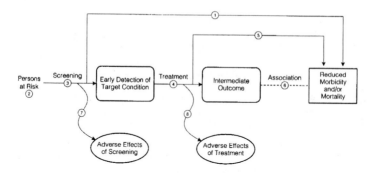

Figure 1. Generic analytic framework for screening topics. Numbers refer to key questions as follows: (1) Is there direct evidence that screening reduces morbidity and/or mortality? (2) What is the prevalence of disease in the target group? Can a high-risk group be reliably identified? (3) Can the screening test accurately detect the target condition? (a) What are the sensitivity and specificity of the test? (b) Is there significant variation between examiners in how the test is performed? (c) In actual screening programs, how much earlier are patients identified and treated? (4) Does treatment reduce the incidence of the intermediate outcome? (a) Does treatment work under ideal, clinical trial conditions? (b) How do the efficacy and effectiveness of treatments compare in community settings? (5) Does treatment improve health outcomes for people diagnosed clinically? (a) How similar are people diagnosed clinically to those diagnosed by screening? (b) Are there reasons to expect people diagnosed by screening to have even better health outcomes than those diagnosed clinically? (6) Is the intermediate outcome reliably associated with reduced morbidity and/or mortality? (7) Does screening result in adverse effects? (a) Is the test acceptable to patients? (b) What are the potential harms, and how often do they occur? (8) Does treatment result in adverse effects?

by which those linkages are measured. Figure 1 illustrates the analytic framework for a screening service, in which a population at risk (left side of the figure) undergoes a screening test to identify early-stage disease. A generic analytic framework for a counseling topic is given in Figure 2.

In Figure 1, an "overarching" linkage (arrow 1) above the primary framework represents evidence that directly links screening to changes in health outcomes. For example, an RCT of chlamydia screening established a direct, causal connection between screening and reduction in a pelvic inflammatory disease.[14] That is, a single body of evidence establishes the connection between the preventive service (screening) and health outcomes.

When direct evidence is lacking or is of insufficient quality to be convincing, the Task Force relies on a chain of linkages to assess the effectiveness of a service. In Figure 1, these linkages correspond to key questions about the accuracy of screening tests (arrow 3), the efficacy of treatment (arrow 4 or arrow 5 for intermediate or health outcomes, respectively), and the association between intermediate measures and health outcomes (dotted line 6). Intermediate outcomes (e.g.,changes in serum lipid levels or

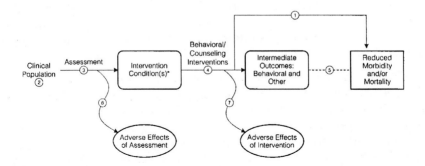

Figure 2. Generic analytic framework for counseling interventions. Numbers refer to key questions as follows: (1) Is there direct evidence that behavioral/counseling interventions reduce disease morbidity and/or mortality? (2) What is the prevalence of risky behavior(s) in the target group? Are there distinct patient groups for whom different intervention strategies apply? (3) Are there effective, feasible, and reliable assessment tools to identify those in need of interventions? (4) Does the behavioral/counseling intervention result in change in intermediate behavioral or other outcomes? (a) What are the essential elements of efficacious interventions? (b) Are there differences in efficacy in important patient subgroups? (c) How do intervention efficacy and effectiveness compare? (5) Does the behavior change lead to reduced morbidity and/or mortality? Do other intermediate outcomes related to the behavior change lead to decreased morbidity and/or mortality? (6) Is assessment for the behavioral/counseling intervention acceptable to patients? Does it result in adverse effects? (7) Is the behavioral/counseling intervention acceptable to patients? Does it result in adverse effects?

*An intervention condition is a distinct group identified through the assessment process that receives a different intervention. Evidence for each of the intervention conditions may be reviewed separately.

eradication of chlamydia infection as measured by a DNA probe) are often used in studies as indicators of efficacy; health outcomes are measures that a patient can feel or experience, including death, quality of life, pain, and function. Curved arrows below the primary framework (arrows 7 and 8 in Figure 1) indicate adverse events or harms (ovals). Each arrow in the analytic framework relates to one or more "key questions" that specify the evidence required to establish the linkage (see the legends for Figures 1 and 2). These questions help organize the literature searches, the results of the review, and the writing of reports.

As can be seen in Figures 1 and 2, the framework supporting a service is considered indirect if two or more bodies of evidence are required to assess the effectiveness of the service. For example, no controlled studies provide direct evidence that screening for skin cancer lowers mortality.[15] To infer benefit, one must piece together evidence about the accuracy of the screening test, how much earlier screening detects skin cancer or its precursors than would be the case without screening, the existence of effective treatment, whether treatment at an earlier stage improves health outcomes, and the existence and magnitude of associated harms. These criteria are similar to those outlined by the World Health Organization[16] and by Frame and Carlson.[17]

Admissible evidence. The third Task Force focuses its reviews primarily on the evidence most likely to influence are commendations. For example, it maintains the tradition of giving greater weight to evidence that preventive services influence health outcomes rather than intermediate outcomes. Although some intermediate outcomes (e.g., advanced-stage breast or colon cancer) are so closely associated with health outcomes that they are logical surrogates, many others (e.g.,physiological changes or histopathologic findings) are less convincing because their reliability in predicting adverse health outcomes has weaker scientific support.[18,19] Accordingly, the topic teams often do not fully review studies that do not address outcomes of interest.

The topic team determines the bibliographic databases to be searched and the specific inclusion and exclusion criteria (i.e., admissible evidence) for the literature on each key question. Such criteria typically include study design, population studied, year of study,outcomes assessed, and length of follow-up. Topic teams specify criteria on a topic-by-topic basis rather than adhering to generic criteria. If high-quality evidence is available, the topic teams may exclude lower quality studies. Conversely, if higher-quality evidence is lacking, the teams may examine lower-quality evidence. In general, the topic teams exclude non-English language references.

The second Task Force reviewed studies published through 1995. Thus, literature searches to update these topics usually extend from 1994 to the present, although new or refocused key questions may extend the search to older literature. For new topics, all searches begin with 1966 unless topic-specific reasons limit the search to a shorter time span or require an examination of even older literature. If a search finds a well-performed systematic review that directly addresses the literature on a key question through a given date, the topic team may use this review to capture the literature for those dates. The team can then restrict its own search to dates not covered by the existing systematic review.

The topic team documents these strategies for sharpening focus—the analytic framework, key questions,and criteria for admissible evidence—in an initial work plan. This work plan is presented to the Task Force at its first meeting after the topic has been assigned, allowing the Task Force the opportunity to modify the direction and scope of the review, as needed.

Literature Search and Abstraction

All searches involve at least the MEDLINE English language database and the Cochrane Collaboration Library, using appropriate search terms to

Table 2. Hierarchy of research design

I	Evidence obtained from at least one properly randomized controlled trial.
II–1	Evidence obtained from well-designed controlled trials without randomization.
II–2	Evidence obtained from well-designed cohort or casecontrol analytic studies, preferably from more than one center or research group.
II–3	Evidence obtained from multiple time series with or without the intervention. Dramatic results in uncontrolled experiments (such as the results of the introduction of penicillin treatment in the 1940s) could also be regarded as this type of evidence.
III	Opinions of respected authorities, based on clinical experience, descriptive studies and case reports, or reports of expert committees.

retrieve studies that meet the previously established inclusion and exclusion criteria. The search also includes other data bases when indicated by the topic. The topic teams supplement these searches with references from reviews, current articles, and suggestions from experts in the field. Two members of the topic team (typically EPC staff) review abstracts of all articles. If either reviewer believes that the abstract meets the inclusion criteria, the EPC retrieves the full text of the article. The eligibility criteria are reapplied by one reviewer who, if the article is included, abstracts information about the patient population, study design, interventions (where appropriate), quality indicators, and findings.

Evaluating evidence: rethinking quality. The Methods Work Group, recognizing the central role that evaluating the quality of the evidence plays in the process of making evidence-based guidelines, focused much effort on this issue and decided to refine the process used by the previous Task Force. Specifically, the third Task Force adopted three important changes to the process: adding a rating of internal validity to the study design criterion for judging individual studies, explicitly assessing evidence at three different strata, and separating the magnitude of effect from the assessment of quality.

Evaluating quality at three strata: Stratum 1, the individual study. For some years, the standard approach to evaluating the quality of individual studies was based on a hierarchical grading system of research design in which RCTs received the highest score (Table 2). The maturation of critical appraisal techniques has drawn attention to the limitations of this approach, which gives inadequate consideration to how well the study was conducted, a dimension known as internal validity.[20] A well-designed cohort study may be more compelling than an inadequately powered or poorly conducted RCT.[21,22]

To accompany the standard categorization of research design, the third Task Force added a three category rating of the internal validity of each study: "good," "fair," and "poor." To distinguish among good, fair, and poor, the Task Force modified criteria developed by others[23-26] to create a set of operational parameters for evaluating the internal validity of five different study designs: systematic reviews, case-control studies, RCTs, cohort studies, and diagnostic accuracy studies (Table 3). These criteria are used not as rigid rules but as guidelines; exceptions are made with adequate justification. In general, a good study meets all criteria for that study design; a fair study does not meet all criteria but is judged to have no fatal flaw that invalidates its results; and a poor study contains a fatal flaw.

Thus, the topic team assigns each study two separate ratings: one for study design and one for internal validity. A well-performed RCT, for example, would receive a rating of I-good, whereas a fair cohort study would be rated II-2-fair. In many cases, narrative text is needed to explain the rating of internal validity for the study, especially for those studies that play a pivotal role in the analytic framework. When the quality of an individual study is the subject of significant disagreement,the entire Task Force may be asked to rate the study and the final rating is applied after debate and discussion.

Even well-designed and well-conducted studies may not supply the evidence needed if the studies examine a highly selected population of little relevance to the general population seen in primary care. Thus, external validity—the extent to which the studies reviewed are generalizable to the population of interest—is considered on a par with internal validity. Deciding whether generalizing in specific situation is appropriate is based on explicit principles developed by the Task Force (see Extrapolation and Generalization section).

Evaluating quality at three strata: Stratum 2, the linkage. The quality of evidence in a single study constitutes only one stratum in analyzing the quality of evidence for a preventive service. One might also consider two additional levels of assessment: the quality of the body of evidence for each linkage (key question) in an analytic framework, and the overall quality of the body or bodies of evidence for a preventive service, including all linkages in the analytic framework (Table 4).

In assessing quality at the second level, the body of evidence supporting a given linkage in the analytic framework, the Task Force recognizes three important criteria. The first two follow directly from criteria for the first stratum. Internal validity (including research design) and external validity (generalizability) remain important, but at this level they are considered in the aggregate for all relevant studies (Table 4).

The third criterion for evaluating the quality of the body of evidence concerning the linkage in an analytic framework is consistency and coher-

Table 3. Criteria for grading the internal validity of individual studies

Study design	Criteria
Systematic reviews	• Comprehensiveness of sources/search strategy used • Standard appraisal of included studies • Validity of conclusions • Recency and relevance
Case–control studies	• Accurate ascertainment of cases • Nonbiased selection of cases/controls with exclusion criteria applied equally to both • Response rate • Diagnostic testing procedures applied equally to each group • Appropriate attention to potential confounding variables

Randomized controlled trials (RCTs) and cohort studies	• Initial assembly of comparable groups:
	    For RCTs: adequate randomization, including concealment and whether potential confounders were distributed equally among groups
	    For cohort studies: consideration of potential confounders with either restriction or measurement for adjustment in the analysis; consideration of inception cohorts
	• Maintenance of comparable groups (includes attrition, crossovers, adherence, contamination)
	• Important differential loss to follow-up or overall high loss to follow-up
	• Measurements: equal, reliable, and valid (includes masking of outcome assessment)
	• Clear definition of interventions
	• All important outcomes considered
	• Analysis: adjustment for potential confounders for cohort studies, or intention-totreat analysis for RCTs

Diagnostic accuracy studies	• Screening test relevant, available for primary care, adequately described • Study uses a credible reference standard, performed regardless of test results • Reference standard interpreted independently of screening test • Handles indeterminate results in a reasonable manner • Spectrum of patients included in study • Sample size • Administration of reliable screening test

Table 4. Evaluating the quality of evidence at three strata

Level of evidence	Criteria for judging quality
1. Individual study	• Internal validity[a] • External validity[b]
2. Linkage in the analytic framework	• Aggregate internal validity[a] • Aggregate external validity[b] • Coherence/consistency
3. Entire preventive service	• Quality of the evidence from Stratum 2 for each linkage in the analytic framework • Degree to which there is a complete chain of linkages supported by adequate evidence to connect the preventive service to health outcomes • Degree to which the complete chain of linkages "fit" together[c] • Degree to which the evidence connecting the preventive service and health outcomes is "direct"[d]

[a] Internal validity is the degree to which the study(ies) provides valid evidence for the population and setting in which it was conducted.

[b] External validity is the extent to which the evidence is relevant and generalizable to the population and conditions of typical primary care practice.

[c] "Fit" refers to the degree to which the linkages refer to the same population and conditions. For example, if studies of a screening linkage identify people who are different from those involved in studies of the treatment linkage, the linkages are not supported by evidence that "fits" together.

[d] "Directness" of evidence is inversely proportional to the number of bodies of evidence required to make the connection between the preventive service and health outcomes. Evidence is direct when a single body of evidence makes the connection, and more indirect if two or more bodies of evidence are required.

ence. Coherence means that a body of evidence makes sense, that is, that the evidence fits together in an understandable model of the situation. The Task Force does not necessarily require consistency, recognizing that studies may produce different results in different populations, and heterogeneity of this sort may still be coherent with the hypothesized model of how interventions relate to outcomes. Consistent results of several studies across different populations and study designs do, however, contribute to coherence.

A topic team considers these three criteria—aggregate internal validity, aggregate external validity, and coherence/consistency—in evaluating the quality of the body of evidence concerning the linkage in ananalytic framework (Table 4). It assigns good, fair, or poor ratings to each of these three factors. In making these judgments, the Task Force has no simple formula but rather considers all the evidence, giving greater weight to studies of higher quality. Topic teams write brief explanatory narratives to provide the rationale for their ratings.

Evaluating quality at three strata: Stratum 3, the entire preventive service. The third level of assessing quality considers the evidence for the entire preventive service.Previous Task Forces used the hierarchical rating of research design (Table 2) to describe the best evidence for a preventive service. The evidence for a preventive service would receive a II-2 code, for example, if the best evidence consisted of a controlled cohort study. As noted above, the current USPSTF has added to this grading of research design an assessment of how well the study was conducted.

Even with this addition, however, examination of the analytic framework shows the difficulty in using this rating scheme alone to judge the quality of the evidence for an entire preventive service. The quality of the evidence may depend on which linkage it is examining. For example, the evidence for smoking cessation counseling could be described as grade I-good evidence(because well-performed RCTs have shown that counseling and nicotine replacement therapy reduce smoking rates) or as grade II-2-good evidence (because only cohort studies have shown that stopping smoking improves health). The more precise conceptualization is that smoking cessation counseling consists of multiple components, as reflected in the linkages for its analytic framework (e.g., Figure 2) and that different levels of evidence support each linkage.

The third Task Force adopted an approach that systematically examines the evidence for each linkage, and all linkages together, in the analytic framework. The underlying issue is whether the evidence is adequate to determine the existence and magnitude of acausal connection between the preventive service (on the left side of the analytic framework) and health outcomes (on the right side of the analytic framework). Rather than applying formal rules for determining the overall quality of evidence, the Task Force adopted a set of general criteria that it considers when making this judgment (Table 4). These criteria are as follows:

- Quality of the evidence from Stratum 2 for each linkage in the analytic framework;
- Degree to which a complete chain of linkages supported by adequate evidence connects the preventive service to health outcomes;
- Degree to which the linkages fit together; and
- Degree to which the evidence connecting the preventive service and health outcomes is direct.

As noted earlier, the directness of evidence is inversely proportional to the number of linkages (bodies of evidence) that must be pieced together to infer that a preventive service has an impact on health. The evidence is most direct if a single body of evidence,corresponding to the overarching linkage in the analytic framework, provides adequate evidence concerning the existence and magnitude of health effects resulting from the use of the preventive service. the evidence is indirect if, instead of having overarching evidence, one must rely on two or more bodies of evidence corresponding to linkages in the analytic framework to make an adequate connection between the use of the preventive service and health.

Based on these considerations, the Task Force grades the overall quality of the evidence using the same tripartite scheme (good, fair, and poor) applied to other levels of evidence. The Task Force decided against a formal system for assigning these grades. Instead, it makes its reasoning explicit in an explanatory narrative in the recommendation statement, providing the overall assessment of the quality of the evidence and the rationale behind this assessment.

In general, good overall evidence includes a high quality direct linkage between the preventive service and health outcomes. Fair evidence is typically indirect but it is adequate to complete a chain of linkages across the analytic framework from the preventive service to health outcomes. The evidence is inadequate to make this connection unless the linkages fit together in a meaningful way. For example, in some situations screening may detect people who are different from those involved in studies of treatment efficacy. In this case, the screening and treatment linkages do not fit together. Poor evidence has a formidable break in the evidence chain such that information is inadequate to connect the preventive service and health outcomes.

To make its reasoning explicit, the Task Force includes an explanatory narrative about its overall rating of the evidence in the recommendation statement.

Separating magnitude of effect from quality. When reviewers consider the quality of evidence, they often confound quality of evidence with magnitude of effect. Evidence for an intervention is sometimes described as good if it shows a dramatic effect on outcomes. Strictly speaking, whether a study provides accurate information should be independent of its findings. The magnitude of observed benefits and/or harms from a service, although of critical importance to decisions about whether it should be recommended, is a separate issue from the quality of the data. The Task Force examines magnitude (or effect size) separately from the quality of evidence, but it merges both issues in making its recommendations (see discussion in "Assessing Magnitude of Net Benefit" section).

Assessing Magnitude of Net Benefit

When the overall quality of the evidence is judged to be good or fair, the Task Force proceeds to consider the magnitude of net benefit to be expected from implementation of the preventive service. Determining net benefit requires assessing both the magnitude of benefits and the magnitude of harms and weighing the two. When the evidence is considered to be poor, the Task Force has no scientific basis for making conjectures about magnitude.

The Task Force classifies benefits, harms, and net benefits on a 4-point scale: "substantial," "moderate,""small," and "zero/negative." It has adopted no standardized metric (such as number needed to screen,number needed to treat, number of lives extended, years of life saved, and/or quality-adjusted life years) for comparing net benefit across preventive services. Ideally, a quantitative definition for such terms as substantial or moderate benefit would make these categorizations more defensible, less arbitrary, and more useful to policymakers in ranking the relative priority of preventive services. Unfortunately, the Task Force has not yet solved the methodologic challenges to deriving such a metric.

Although the Task Force has decided against a rigid formula for defining these terms, it has developed a conceptual framework and a process for making these distinctions. In assessing the magnitude of benefits and harms, the Task Force uses a modification of the statistical concept of the confidence interval. The magnitude of effect in individual studies is given by a point estimate surrounded by a confidence interval. Point estimates and confidence intervals often vary among studies of the same question, sometimes considerably. The Task Force examines all relevant studies to construct a general, conceptual "confidence interval" of the range of effect-size values consistent with the literature. It considers the upper and lower bounds of this confidence interval in assessing the magnitude of benefits and harms.

Assessing Magnitude of Benefits

The Task Force thinks of benefit from both population and individual perspectives. For the benefit to be considered substantial, the service must have

- at least a small relative impact on a frequent condition with a substantial population burden, or
- a large impact on an infrequent condition that poses a significant burden at the individual patient level.

For example, counseling for tobacco cessation produces a change in behavior in only a small proportion of patients,[27] but the societal implications are sizable because of the large number of tobacco users in the population and the burden of illness and death that is averted if even a small percentage of people stop smoking. Conversely, phenylketonuria is a grave condition that affects a very small proportion of the population, but neonatal screening markedly reduces morbidity and mortality from the disease.[6] Although the target conditions in these examples differ considerably in prevalence, the Task Force views both preventive services as having a substantial magnitude of benefit."Outcomes tables" (similar to "balance sheets"[28]) are the Task Force's standard resource for estimating the magnitude of benefit.[28,29] These tables, prepared by the topic teams for use at Task Force meetings, compare the condition-specific outcomes expected for a hypothetical primary care population with and without use of the preventive service. These comparisons may be extended to consider only people of specified age or risk groups or other aspects of implementation. Thus, outcomes tables allow the Task Force to examine directly how the preventive service affects benefits for various groups.

One important problem with outcomes tables is that the evidence typically differs across table cells. For some services and some groups, the frequency of the outcome may be clear, but for others one can calculate the frequency of the outcome only by making broad assumptions, some with greater scientific support than others. Thus, outcomes tables must provide information about both the frequency of outcomes and how certain we are about that information.

Assessing Magnitude of Harms

The Task Force considers all types of potential harms of a service, both direct harms of the service itself (e.g., those from a screening test or preventive medication) and indirect harms that may be downstream consequences of the initial intervention (e.g., invasive follow-up tests or harms of treatments). The Task Force considers potential medical, psychological, and nonhealth harms (e.g., effects on insurability).

All analytic frameworks include linkages concerning the potential harms of preventive services, and all topic teams search for evidence about these harms. The Task Force strives to give equal weight to benefits and harms in its assessment of net benefit, but the amount of evidence about benefits is usually greater. Few studies provide useful information on adverse outcomes. Thus, the Task Force often finds itself trying to estimate harms based on little evidence. Methods of making this estimation are lacking, but the Task Force continues to discuss ways to frame the range of reasonable estimates of harm for each preventive service.

When evidence on harms is available, the topic teams assess its quality in a manner like that for benefits and include adverse events in the outcomes tables. When few harms data are available, the Task Force does not assume that harms are small or nonexistent. It recognizes a responsibility to consider which harms are likely and to judge their potential frequency and the severity that might ensue from implementing the service.[30] It uses whatever evidence exists to construct a general confidence interval on the 4-point scale (e.g., substantial, moderate, small, and zero/negative) described above.

Assessing Net Benefits: Weighing Benefits and Harms

Value judgments are involved in using the information in an outcomes table to rate either benefits or harms on the Task Force's 4-point scale. Value judgments are also needed to weigh benefits against harms to arrive at a rating of net benefit.

The need to invoke value judgments is most obvious when the Task Force must weigh benefits and harms of different types against each other in coming to a collective assessment of net benefits. For example, although breast cancer screening for certain age groups may reduce deaths from breast cancer,[31] it also increases the number of women who must experience the anxiety of a work-up for a false-positive mammogram.[32] Determining which of the four categories of net benefit to assign to this service depends greatly on the value one places on each outcome.

In making its determinations of net benefit, the Task Force strives to consider what it believes are the general values of most people. It does this with greater confidence for certain outcomes (e.g., death) about which there is little disagreement about undesirability, but it recognizes that the degree of risk people are willing to accept to avert other outcomes (e.g., cataracts) can vary considerably.[33] When the Task Force perceives that preferences among individuals vary greatly, and that these variations are sufficient to make the average trade-off of benefits and harms a "close call," then it will often assign a C recommendation (see below). This recommendation indicates that the decision is likely to be sensitive to individual patients' preferences.

Extrapolation and Generalization

As noted in the "Review of the Evidence" section, the Task Force regularly faces the issue of generalization in determining the quality of evidence. The Task Force makes recommendations intended for the general primary care situation; for this purpose, high-quality evidence is evidence that is relevant and valid for this setting. When studies examine different situations and settings, the issue of generalization arises.

Likewise, the magnitude of the effect of interest to the Task Force is that resulting from implementation in the primary care setting. Calculations based on extrapolation are usually required to estimate the likely magnitude of effect for the primary care situation.

Some degree of extrapolation and generalization is invariably required to use evidence in the research literature to make guidelines for the primary care situation. For some services, the evidence may provide high-quality information about the efficacy of a preventive service in the hands of experts for a specific subpopulation. For others, evidence about efficacy often comes from studies of symptomatic patients who are more severely ill than patients who would be discovered by screening. Even when good randomized trials of therapeutic efficacy in asymptomatic patients exist (e.g., therapy of lipid disorders), female, elderly, and younger patients may be under represented, and eligibility criteria might exclude patients with characteristics that are typical of a general primary care population. Other commonly encountered issues are whether the efficiency of screening in one practice setting can be replicated in other settings and whether efficacy persists or diminishes beyond the length of time usually covered by available studies.

In the absence of good evidence, to what extent can one use reasoned judgments based on assumptions with varying degrees of scientific support to draw conclusions about the potential benefits and harms of a preventive service? The Task Force developed a policy for determining the conditions under which extrapolation and generalization are reasonable. These conditions include:

- biologic plausibility;
- similarities of the populations studied and primary care patients (in terms of risk factor profile, demographics, ethnicity, gender, clinical presentation, and similar factors);
- similarities of the test or intervention studied to those that would be routinely available or feasible in typical practice; and
- clinical or social environmental circumstances in the studies that could modify the results from those expected in a primary care setting.

Judgments about extrapolation and generalization, because they are often matters of policy and subjective judgment rather than hard science, are made by the Task Force and not the EPCs.

Translating Evidence into Recommendations

General Principles

Making recommendations for clinical practice involves considerations that extend beyond scientific evidence. Direct scientific evidence is of pre-eminent interest, but such issues as cost effectiveness, resource prioritization, logistical factors, ethical and legal concerns, and patient and societal expectations should also be considered.

Historically, the Task Force has taken a conservative, evidence-based approach to this process, making recommendations that reflect primarily the state of the evidence and refraining from making recommendations when they cannot be supported by evidence. This is done with the understanding that clinicians and policymakers must still consider additional factors in making their own decisions.[34] The Task Force sees its purpose as providing users with information about the extent to which recommendations are supported by evidence, allowing them to make more informed decisions about implementation.

Another important issue in making recommendations is the amount and quality of evidence required. As evidence is rarely adequate to provide decision makers with completely valid information about all important outcomes for the population of interest, those creating guidelines must consider how far they are willing to generalize from imperfect evidence. As noted in the Extrapolation and Generalization section, the Task Force believes that such generalizations can be made under defined conditions.

The general principles the Task Force follows in making recommendations are outlined in Table 5. Most of these principles have been discussed in other parts of this paper. They involve both the factors considered by the Task Force in making recommendations (e.g., the most salient types of evidence, feasibility, harms, economic costs, and its target population) and the way in which it considers these factors (e.g., the place of subjectivity, the importance of the population perspective, and the extent to which the evidence connects the service with positive net benefits for patients).

Codes and Wording of Statements

As in the past, the Task Force assigns letter codes to its recommendations and uses standardized phrasing for each category of recommendations (Table 6), but the details have changed from previous versions. The original five-letter scheme, which included an E recommendation category that was rarely used,[6] has been replaced with a four-letter scheme that allows only one classification for recommendations *against* routinely providing a preventive service (D).

Previous definitions for letter codes focused on whether the evidence supported "including the preventive service in the periodic health examination." Current thinking is that preventive services should also be delivered in other contexts, such as illness visits. The new wording thus focuses on whether the service should be "routinely provided."

In the past, the Task Force assigned a C code to recommendations with "insufficient evidence to make a recommendation." Previous Task Forces used this code for a wide assortment of circumstances and thus assigned it to a large proportion of the preventive services they reviewed. Evidence could be insufficient because no studies existed, available studies were of

Table 5. Principles for making recommendations

- Task Force recommendations are evidence based: They require scientific evidence that persons who receive the preventive service experience better health outcomes than those who do not and that the benefits are large enough to outweigh the harms.

  The Task Force emphasizes evidence that directly links the preventive service with health outcomes. Indirect evidence may be sufficient if it supports the principal links in the analytic framework.

  Although the Task Force acknowledges that subjective judgments do enter into the evaluation of evidence and the weighing of benefits and harms, its recommendations are not based largely on opinion.

  The Task Force is explicit about the scientific rationale for its recommendations.

- The outcomes that matter most in weighing the evidence and making recommendations are health benefits and harms.

  In considering potential benefits, the Task Force focuses on absolute reductions in the risk of outcomes that people can feel or care about.

  In considering potential harms, the Task Force examines harms of all types, including physical, psychological, and nonmedical harms that may occur sooner or later as a result of the preventive service.

  Where possible, the Task Force considers the feasibility of future widespread implementation of the preventive service in making recommendations.

  The Task Force generally takes a population perspective in weighing the magnitude of benefits against the magnitude of harms. In some situations, it may recommend a service with a large potential benefit for a small proportion of the population.

  In assessing net benefits, the Task Force subjectively estimates the population's value for each benefit and harm. When the Task Force judges that the perceived balance of benefits and harms is likely to vary substantially within the population, it may abandon general recommendations and suggest shared decision making at the individual level.

- Where possible, the Task Force considers the total economic costs that result from providing a preventive service, both to individuals and to society, in making recommendations, but costs are not the first priority.

  When the Task Force recommends against a preventive service for economic reasons, it states so explicitly.

- The Task Force does not modify its recommendations to accommodate concerns about insurance coverage of preventive services, medicolegal liability, or legislation, but users of the recommendations may need to do so.

- Recommendations apply only to asymptomatic persons or those with unrecognized signs or symptoms of the target condition for which the preventive service is intended. They also apply only to preventive services initiated in the clinical setting.

Table 6. Standard recommendation language

Recommendation	Language[a]
A	The USPSTF strongly recommends that clinicians routinely provide [the service] to eligible patients. (The USPSTF found good evidence that [the service] improves important health outcomes and concludes that benefits substantially outweigh harms.)
B	The USPSTF recommends that clinicians routinely provide [the service] to eligible patients. (The USPSTF found at least fair evidence that [the service] improves important health outcomes and concludes that benefits outweigh harms.)
C	The USPSTF makes no recommendation for or against routine provision of [the service]. (The USPSTF found at least fair evidence that [the service] can improve health outcomes but concludes that the balance of the benefits and harms is too close to justify a general recommendation.)
D	The USPSTF recommends against routinely providing [the service] to asymptomatic patients. (The USPSTF found at least fair evidence that [the service] is ineffective or that harms outweigh benefits.)
I	The USPSTF concludes that the evidence is insufficient to recommend for or against routinely providing [the service]. (Evidence that [the service] is effective is lacking, of poor quality, or conflicting and the balance of benefits and harms cannot be determined.)

[a]All statements specify the population for which the recommendation is intended and are followed by a rationale statement providing information about the overall grade of evidence and the net benefit from implementing the service. USPSTF, U.S. Preventive Services Task Force.

poor quality, studies were of reasonable quality but conflicting, or results were consistent but the magnitude of net benefit was small.

The C recommendation, because of its location in the hierarchical ranking of recommendation grades, implies that the service is less worthy of implementation than services that receive an A or a B recommendation. The current Task Force believes that such pejorative conclusions should be applied only when the evidence provides a basis for inferring that the magnitude of net benefit is smaller than for interventions that merit higher ratings. In other instances, in which evidence is of poor quality or conflicting, the possibility of substantial benefit (or substantial harm) cannot be excluded on scientific grounds and thus the Task Force can make no evidence-based judgments about the service.

Table 7. Recommendation grid

Quality of evidence	Net benefit			
	Substantial	**Moderate**	**Small**	**Zero/negative**
Good	A	B	C	D
Fair	B	B	C	D
Poor = I				

To address these cases, the Task Force has created a new recommendation category, the I recommendation (insufficient evidence). It has also intentionally chosen a letter distant from the A–D hierarchy to signal its reluctance to pass judgment about the effectiveness of the interventions that receive this rating. The Task Force gives an I recommendation when studies are lacking or of poor quality or when they produce conflicting results that do not permit conclusions about likely benefits and harms.

For the A–D recommendations, the Task Force has adopted a more formalized process for translating the evidence into group judgments about how strongly to recommend the intervention than had been applied in the past. In earlier years, the simplistic notion was that services supported by RCTs always received A recommendations. The new approach recognizes that the importance of providing the preventive service depends not only on the quality of the evidence but also on the magnitude of net benefit to patients or populations. In an effort to ensure that both dimensions— quality and magnitude—are addressed systematically in assigning letter codes, the Task Force now uses a recommendation grid (Table 7) that makes the process more explicit.

As shown, code A indicates that the quality of evidence is good and the magnitude of net benefits is substantial: The Task Force "strongly recommends" that these services be routinely provided (Table 6). The B code indicates that the Task Force has found that either the quality of the evidence or the magnitude of net benefits (or both) is less than would be needed to warrant an A. Primary care providers should not necessarily give higher priority to A over B services. Setting priorities for offering, providing, or reimbursing these services should include consideration of time and resource requirements, which are beyond the scope of the Task Force's review. Other groups have undertaken this important work.[35]

The C code indicates that the quality of evidence is either good or fair but that the magnitude of net benefits, as judged in the subjective process outlined above, is too small to make a general recommendation. In these cases, the Task Force "makes no recommendation for or against routinely providing the service." Clinicians and policymakers may choose to offer the service for other reasons—such as considerations other than scientific evidence or because benefits for individual patients are expected to exceed those observed in studies—but the Task Force rating is meant to advise them that existing evidence does not document substantial net benefit for the average patient.

The D code indicates that the evidence is good or fair but that net benefit is probably either zero or negative. In these situations, the Task Force recommends against routine use of the service.

When the evidence is poor, the Task Force cannot distinguish between substantial or moderate net benefits on the one hand and small or zero/negative net benefits on the other. In these cases, the Task Force uses code I to indicate that it cannot make a recommendation for or against routinely providing the service. Because extant evidence cannot yet clarify whether the net benefits of the service are large or small (or negative), this rating advises clinicians and policymakers that determination of whether to provide these services routinely cannot be based on evidence; such decisions must be based on factors other than science.

Drafting the Report

In its earliest days, background papers and recommendations of the Task Force were written by individual panel members assigned to those topics. In later years, they were written by staff with close oversight by the Task Force. In time a sharp demarcation has evolved between descriptions of the evidence and recommendations.

Thus, for the third Task Force, topic teams led by EPC staff write systematic evidence reviews. These reviews define the strengths and limits of the evidence but stop short of making recommendations.

Systematic evidence reviews typically include the full version (available from AHRQ and accessible on its website, www.ahrq.gov) and a shorter summary such as those published in this issue. As a work product prepared under contract for AHRQ, the systematic evidence reviews must be approved by the agency before public release. The reviews remain pure descriptions of the science; because they are published separately, groups other than the Task Force can use them to formulate their own guidelines and recommendations.

The summary reviews are typically coupled with a "recommendation and rationale" document, written by the Task Force, which contains recommendations and their supporting rationales. Recommendations, which cross the line from science into policy, are based on formal voting procedures that include explicit rules for determining the views of the majority.

The Task Force has an explicit policy concerning conflict of interest. All members and EPC staff disclose at each meeting if they have an important financial, organizational, or intellectual conflict for each topic being discussed. Task Force members and EPC staff with conflicts can participate in discussions about evidence, but members abstain from voting on recommendations about the topic in question.

Recommendations are independent of the government. They neither require clearance from nor represent the policy of AHRQ or the U.S. Public Health Service, although efforts are made to consult with relevant agencies to reduce unnecessary discrepancies among guidelines.

The Task Force chair or liaisons on the topic team generally compose the first draft of the recommendation and rationale statement, which the full panel then reviews and edits. These statements have the general structure of the chapters in previous editions of the *Guide to Clinical Preventive Services*.6 Specifically, they include a recommendation statement and code, a rationale statement, and a brief discussion of clinical interventions. The clinical intervention section is meant to provide more specific information and guidance to clinicians about the service, sometimes discussing factors beyond the quality of the evidence and the magnitude of net benefit that must be considered with implementation.

External Review

Before the Task Force makes its final determinations about recommendations on a given preventive service, the EPC and AHRQ send a draft systematic evidence review to four to six external experts and to federal agencies and professional and disease-based health organizations with interests in the topic. They ask the experts to examine the review critically for accuracy and completeness and to respond to a series of specific questions about the document. After assembling these external review comments and documenting the proposed response to key comments, the topic team presents this information to the Task Force in memo form. In this way, the Task Force can consider these external comments and a final version of the systematic review before it votes on its final recommendations about the service.

Conclusion

Methods for making evidence-based practice policies are evolving. At one extreme, guidelines panels could insist on direct evidence or point to any information gaps to justify a negative recommendation for almost any service. Such an approach would result in positive recommendations only for services that had a very narrow confidence interval for net benefit, but many effective services would not be recommended. At the other extreme, guideline groups that accept incomplete data and allow easy extrapolation make many positive recommendations, but they have less certainty that the services they recommend actually produce more benefit than harm.

In avoiding these extremes, the Task Force has wrestled with several gaps in existing methodology for assessing the quality of evidence, for integrating bodies of evidence, and for translating evidence into guidelines. It continues to address several knotty questions: Can criteria for the internal validity of studies be consistently applied across preventive services? How reliable are such criteria in identifying studies with misleading results? How much weight should be given to various degrees of information gaps, particularly those concerning potential harms and generalizations from research studies to everyday practice? Should the Task Force modify any of these methods when dealing with counseling services?

More methodologic research is warranted in several key areas. Principal among these are efforts to determine the best factors to consider in using evidence based principles to guide judgments about the magnitude of benefits and harms when the available evidence is fair in quality and when gaps exist in the framework supporting effectiveness. These and other challenges will make the methods of the Task Force, like those of other evidence-based guideline programs, a work in progress for many years.

This paper was developed by the Research Triangle Institute-University of North Carolina at Chapel Hill (RTI-UNC) and the Oregon Health Sciences University (OHSU) Evidence-Based Practice Centers under contracts from the Agency for Healthcare Research and Quality (contract nos. 290-97-0011 and 290-97-0018, respectively). We acknowledge the assistance of Jacqueline Besteman, JD, MA, EPC Program Officer; the AHRQ staff working with the third Task Force; and the staffs of the EPCs at RTI-UNC and at OHSU for their many hours of work in support of this effort. We also acknowledge the assistance of the Counseling and Behavioral Issues Work Group of the Task Force, Evelyn Whitlock, MD, MPH, convenor. Finally, we also acknowledge the major contribution of the entire third U.S. Preventive Services Task Force for its support and intellectual stimulation.

The authors of this article are responsible for its contents, including any clinical or treatment recommendations. No statement in this article should be construed as an official position of the Agency for Healthcare Research and Quality or the U.S. Department of Health and Human Services.

REFERENCES

1. Field MJ, Lohr KN, eds. Guidelines for clinical practice: from development to use. Washington, DC: National Academy Press, 1992 (for Institute of Medicine).
2. Woolf SH, George JN. Evidence-based medicine: interpreting studies and setting policy. Hematol Oncol Clin N Amer 2000;14:761–84.
3. Mulrow CD, Cook D, eds. Systematic reviews: synthesis of best evidence for health care decisions. Philadelphia: American College of Physicians, 1998. 34 American Journal of Preventive Medicine, Volume 20, Number 3S
4. Cook D, Giacomini M. The trials and tribulations of clinical practice guidelines. JAMA 1999;281:1950–1.
5. Lawrence RS, Mickalide AD, Kamerow DB, Woolf SH. Report of the U.S. Preventive Services Task Force. JAMA 1990;263:436–7.
6. U.S. Preventive Services Task Force. Guide to clinical preventive services: report of the U.S. Preventive Services Task Force, 2nd ed., Washington, DC: Office of Disease Prevention and Health Promotion, U.S. Government Printing Office, 1996.
7. Eddy DM. Clinical decision making: from theory to practice. A collection of essays from JAMA. Boston: Jones and Bartlett Publishers, 1995.

8. Pignone MP, Phillips CJ, Atkins D, Teutsch SM, Mulrow CD, Lohr KN. Screening and treating adults for lipids disorders. Am J Prev Med 2001; 20(suppl 3):77–89.

9. Briss PA, Zaza S, Pappaioanou M, et al. Developing an evidence-based guide to community preventive services: methods. Am J Prev Med 2000; 18(suppl 1):35–43.

10. Meade MO, Richardson WS. Selecting and appraising studies for a systematic review. In: Mulrow CD, Cook D, eds. Systematic reviews: synthesis of best evidence for health care decisions. Philadelphia: American College of Physicians, 1998:81–90.

11. Woolf SH, DiGuiseppi CG, Atkins D, Kamerow DB. Developing evidence based clinical practice guidelines: lessons learned by the U.S. Preventive Services Task Force. Ann Rev Public Health 1996;17:511–38.

12. Battista RN, Fletcher SW. Making recommendations on preventive practices: methodological issues. Am J Prev Med 1988;4(suppl 4):53–67.

13. Mulrow C, Langhorne P, Grimshaw J. Integrating heterogeneous pieces of evidence in systematic reviews. In: Mulrow CD, Cook D, eds. Systematic reviews: synthesis of best evidence for health care decisions. Philadelphia: American College of Physicians, 1998:103–12.

14. Nelson HD, Helfand M. Screening for chlamydial infection. Am J Prev Med 2001;20(suppl 3):95–107.

15. Helfand M, Mahon SM, Eden KB, Frame PS, Orleans CT. Screening for skin cancer. Am J Prev Med 2001;20(suppl 3):47–58.

16. Wilson JMG, Junger G. Principles and practice of screening for disease. Geneva: World Health Organization, 1968 (Public Health Papers No. 34). 17. Frame PS, Carlson SJ. A critical review of periodic health screening using specific screening criteria. J Fam Pract 1975;2:29–36, 123–9, 189–94, 283–9.

18. Bucher HC, Guyatt GH, Cook DJ, Holbrook A, McAlister FA. Users' guides to the medical literature. XIX. Applying clinical trial results. A. How to use an article measuring the effect of an intervention on surrogate end points. JAMA 1999;282:771–8.

19. Gøtzsche PC, Liberati A, Torri V, Rossetti L. Beware of surrogate outcome measures. Int J Tech Assess Health Care 1996;12:238–46.

20. Lohr KN, Carey TS. Assessing "best evidence": issues in grading the quality of studies for systematic reviews. J Qual Improv 1999;25:470–9.

21. Hornberger J, Wrone E. When to base clinical policies on observational versus randomized trial data. Ann Intern Med 1997;127:697–703.

22. Feinstein AR, Horwitz RI. Problems in the "evidence" of "evidence-based medicine." Am J Med 1997;103:529–35.

23. Oxman AD, Cook DJ, Guyatt GH, Evidence-Based Medicine Working Group. Users' guides to the medical literature: how to use an overview. JAMA 1994;272:1367–71.

24. Mulrow CD, Linn WD, Gaul MK, Pugh JA. Assessing quality of a diagnostic test evaluation. J Gen Intern Med 1989; 4:288–295.

25. Guyatt GH, Sackett DL, Cook DJ, Evidence-Based Medicine Working Group. Users' guides to the medical literature. I. How to use an article about therapy or prevention. A. Are the results of the study valid? JAMA 1993;270:2598–601.

26. Laupacis A, Wells G, Richardson WS, Tugwell P, Evidence-Based Medicine Working Group. Users' guides to the medical literature V. How to use an article about prognosis. JAMA 1994;272:234–7.

27. Russell MA, Wilson C, Taylor C, Baker CD. Effect of general practitioners' advice against smoking. BMJ 1979;2:231–5.

28. Eddy DM. Comparing benefits and harms: the balance sheet. JAMA 1990;263:2493, 2498, 2501.

29. Braddick M, Stuart M, Hrachovec J. The use of balance sheets in developing clinical guidelines. J Am Board Fam Pract 1999;12:48–54.

30. Ewart RM. Primum non nocere and the quality of evidence: rethinking the ethics of screening. J Am Board Fam Pract 2000;13:188–96.

31. Fletcher SW, Black W, Harris R, Rimer B, Shapiro S. Report of the International Workshop on Screening for Breast Cancer. J Natl Cancer Inst 1993;85:644–56.

32. Elmore JG, Barton MB, Moceri VM, Polk S, Arena PJ, Fletcher SW. Ten-year risk of false positive screening mammograms and clinical breast examinations. N Engl J Med 1998;338:1089–96.

33. Nease RF Jr, Kneeland T, O'Connor GT, et al. Variation in patient utilities for outcomes of the management of chronic stable angina: implications for clinical practice guidelines. JAMA 1995;273:1185–90.

34. Woolf SH, Dickey LL. Differing perspectives on preventive care guidelines: a new look at the mammography controversy. Am J Prev Med 1999;17: 260–8.

35. Coffield AB, Maciosek MV, McGinnis JM, et al. Priorities among recommended clinical preventive services. Am J Prev Med 2001. In press.

The Art and Science of Incorporating Cost Effectiveness into Evidence-Based Recommendations for Clinical Preventive Services

Somnath Saha, MD, MPH, Thomas J. Hoerger, PhD,
Michael P. Pignone, MD, MPH, Steven M. Teutsch, MD, MPH,
Mark Helfand, MD, MS, Jeanne S. Mandelblatt, MD, MPH, for the Cost
Work Group of the Third U.S. Preventive Services Task Force

ABSTRACT

As medical technology continues to expand and the cost of using all effective clinical services exceeds available resources, decisions about health care delivery may increasingly rely on assessing the cost-effectiveness of medical services. Cost-effectiveness is particularly relevant for decisions about how to implement preventive services, because these decisions typically represent major investments in the future health of large populations.

From the Evidence-Based Practice Center (Saha, Helfand) and Division of Medical Informatics and Outcomes Research (Helfand), Oregon Health Sciences University; Section of General Internal Medicine, Portland Veterans Affairs Medical Center (Saha, Helfand), Portland, Oregon; Evidence-based Practice Center, Research Triangle Institute and University of North Carolina (Hoerger, Pignone), and Center for Economics Research, Research Triangle Institute (Hoerger), Research Triangle Park; Department of Internal Medicine, University of North Carolina at Chapel Hill (Pignone), North Carolina; Merck & Co., Inc. (Teutsch), West Point, Pennsylvania; Departments of Oncology and Medicine, Georgetown University Medical Center (Mandelblatt), Washington, DC

Address correspondence to: Somnath Saha, MD, MPH, Portland VA Medical Center (P3MED), 3710 SW US Veterans Hospital Rd., Portland, OR 97207. E-mail: sahas@ohsu.edu

Reprints are available from the AHRQ Web site at www.ahrq.gov/clinic/uspstfix.htm, through the National Guideline Clearinghouse (www.guideline.gov), or in print through the AHRQ Publications Clearinghouse at (1-800-358-9295).

Other members of the Cost Work Group of the third U.S. Preventive Services Task Force include: David Atkins, MD, MPH, Agency for Healthcare Research and Quality, Rockville, Maryland; Alfred O. Berg, MD, MPH, University of Washington, Seattle, Washington; Tracy A. Lieu, MD, MPH, Harvard Community Health Plan, Boston, Massachusetts; Cynthia D. Mulrow, MD, MSc, University of Texas Health Science Center, San Antonio, Texas; Harold C. Sox, Jr, Dartmouth-Hitchcock Medical Center, Lebanon, New Hampshire; and Carolyn Westhoff, MD, MSc, Columbia University, New York, New York.

As such, decisions regarding the implementation of preventive services frequently involve, implicitly if not explicitly, consideration of costs. Cost-effectiveness analysis summarizes the expected benefits, harms, and costs of alternative strategies to improve health and has become an important tool for explicitly incorporating economic considerations into clinical decision making. Acknowledging the usefulness of this tool, the third U.S. Preventive Services Task Force (USPSTF) has initiated a process for systematically reviewing cost-effectiveness analyses as an aid in making recommendations about clinical preventive services. In this paper, we provide an overview and examples of roles for using cost-effectiveness analyses to inform preventive services recommendations, discuss limitations of cost-effectiveness data in shaping evidence-based preventive health care policies, outline the USPSTF approach to using cost-effectiveness analyses, and discuss the methods the USPSTF is developing to assess the quality and results of cost-effectiveness studies. While this paper focuses on clinical preventive services (i.e., screening, counseling, immunizations, and chemo-prevention), the framework we have developed should be broadly portable to other health care services.

Medical Subject Headings (MeSH): economic models, costs and cost analysis, cost-benefit analysis, methods, MEDLINE, preventive health services, evidence-based medicine, practice guidelines (Am J Prev Med 2001; 20(3S):36–43)

Introduction

At the close of the twentieth century, health care costs in the United States continued to rise steadily, accounting for 13.5% of the gross domestic product in 1998,[1] and debate on health care funding for the aging American population intensified. In this environment, preventive services often compete with one another and with diagnostic- and treatmentoriented care for increasingly constrained resources.[2] While preventive services are often believed to save costs, delivery of most preventive services, with few exceptions (e.g., some immunizations), incurs net costs.[3]

Cost-effectiveness analyses (CEAs) summarize the expected benefits, harms, and costs of adopting and translating a clinical recommendation into practice.[4] The results of a CEA are typically presented as a ratio of the net costs to the net health outcomes of alternative intervention strategies, illustrated in the formula:

$$(C_1 - C_2)/(O_1 - O_2),$$

where C represents costs associated with an intervention, O represents outcomes, and 1 and 2 refer to alternative interventions. Costs associated with an intervention include the costs of the intervention itself plus those induced by the intervention (e.g., the costs of treating side effects), minus the costs averted because of the intervention (i.e., the costs of care for the prevented disease).

Outcomes in CEAs may be measured in different ways. Frequently, they are measured as life-years saved (LYS). While this measure accounts for how an intervention strategy affects mortality, it does not reflect the quality of life associated with different health outcomes. To capture the effect that intervention strategies have on both loss of and quality of life, the number of years with an illness or injury can be multiplied by a value weight from 0 (death) to 1 (full health) to generate quality-adjusted life-years (QALYs).[5] CEAs that use QALYs in the denominator of their cost-effectiveness ratios are often referred to as cost-utility analyses (CUAs), because they incorporate people's preferences, or utilities, for different states of health, illness, and injury. In our discussion, we treat CUAs as a subset of CEAs.

Economic analyses other than CEAs, such as costminimization analyses and cost-benefit analyses (CBAs), also provide information about the potential value of health services. CEAs differ from most of these types of analysis in that they describe how different strategies for allocating resources affect health outcomes.[4] For the third U.S. Preventive Services Task Force (USPSTF), this focus on health outcomes reflects an essential element of the approach to reviewing evidence. CBAs also incorporate health outcomes, but convert outcomes into dollars. Because assigning dollar values to health outcomes is controversial and not frequently used in U.S. health policy, the USPSTF has chosen to focus primarily on CEAs.

By quantifying the immediate and downstream benefits, harms, and costs of interventions, CEA demonstrates the trade-offs involved in choosing among different intervention strategies to effect desired health outcomes. As such, CEAs may provide valuable information for those designing or implementing policies about preventive services. In this paper, we discuss uses of CEA to guide policies related to clinical preventive services, some of the limitations in using CEA to inform recommendations for services, and the approach and methods the USPSTF is developing to systematically review CEAs and incorporate cost-effectiveness data into its process for developing recommendations for the forthcoming third edition of the *Guide to Clinical Preventive Services* (the *Guide*), slated for publication in 2003.

Potential Uses of CEA in Informing Preventive Service Recommendations

Evidence-based recommendations are increasingly used to help determine which preventive and other services to include in clinical practice, public health programs, and benefits packages.[6,7] Most of these recommendations

Table 1. Uses of cost effectiveness analysis in informing evidence-based recommendations for preventive services

(1) Quantifying the differences between two or more effective services for the same condition
(2) Illustrating the impact of delivering a given intervention at different intervals, different ages, or to different risk groups
(3) Evaluating the potential role of new technologies
(4) Identifying key conditions that must be met to achieve the intended benefit of an intervention
(5) Incorporating preferences for intervention outcomes
(6) Developing a ranking of services in order of their costs and expected benefits[a]

[a]The current U.S. Preventive Services Task Force will not use cost effectiveness analyses for this purpose.

have not systematically incorporated evidence related to cost-effectiveness. CEAs, however, can be used in several ways to inform and extend clinical service recommendations (Table 1).

One of the most important and common uses of CEA is to examine the costs and health benefits associated with alternative interventions to achieve a given health outcome. For instance, effective screening strategies for colorectal cancer include fecal occult blood testing (FOBT),[8] sigmoidoscopy,[9] and possibly barium enema and colonoscopy.[10] More effective screening strategies often cost more than less effective strategies. Depending on available resources, some might screen initially with FOBT, which provides moderate effectiveness at relatively low cost, while others might choose colonoscopy, which is more costly but may also be more effective.[11-14] CEA makes explicit the trade-offs involved in these decisions.

CEAs can also help in selecting the most efficient application of effective interventions, such as the intervals between screening tests,[15,16] the ages for starting or stopping a service,[17] or the population subgroup likely to benefit most from a service.[18] Early detection of cervical neoplasia provides a pertinent example. In a CEA of cervical cancer screening, Eddy[15,16] demonstrated that Pap testing every 3 years saved 97% of the lives that would be saved using annual screening and reduced costs by 67%. These results prompted several leading professional groups to issue a joint statement changing their recommendations to include triennial screening as a valid option.[16] Other CEAs have noted that screening women aged ≥65 who have had limited prior testing or are at high risk for cervical cancer can save both health care dollars and lives.[19] In contrast, screening low-risk women with a history of regular screening before age 65 increases the cost-effectiveness ratio more than tenfold over results for all women.[20] These results suggest that recommendations for screening older women for cervical cancer should be stratified according to risk of disease and prior screening history.

CEAs can also be used to evaluate new technologies related to prevention. For example, tests for mutations in the BRCA1 and BRCA2 genes, which confer high lifetime risks of developing breast and ovarian cancer,[21] can identify high-risk individuals, who can then be counseled about intensive surveillance for early disease detection or prophylactic surgery.[22,23] It is not clear, however, how such tests should be used in general practice. In this situation, one can model the costs and health consequences of using BRCA testing in different populations and calculate the marginal cost and effectiveness. For example, one could conduct a CEA to compare the cost effectiveness of screening all women versus screening only those with a strong family history of breast cancer. The results of such an analysis could help set policies about who should receive genetic testing and counseling.

CEAs can also help determine how factors that are not typically considered in clinical trials of intervention efficacy might influence the "real-world" effectiveness of a preventive service. For instance, there is evidence that doxycycline and azithromycin are equally efficacious in eradicating genital chlamydia infection in women.[24] It might seem reasonable to recommend doxycycline as the antibiotic of choice, since it is less expensive than azithromycin. However, when one considers that azithromycin is given as a single dose and is therefore associated with higher rates of adherence than doxycycline, azithromycin may in some settings improve outcomes compared with doxycycline and therefore be the more cost-effective choice.[25]

CEAs—more specifically, CUAs—can also be used to make explicit the impact of the target population's preferences for different health outcomes. By using QALYs as an outcome measure, CUAs account for the fact that most people prefer some states of health and illness to others. These preferences may need to be considered in deciding whether or not to implement a given preventive service. For instance, clinical trials typically report the effectiveness of tamoxifen in reducing overall morbidity and mortality as a balance between the benefits and harms of the drug, but fail to account for the different values that women place on various outcomes (e.g., breast cancer and endometrial cancer). In a CUA, the net effectiveness of the intervention is modeled as a weighted sum of benefits and harms, where the weights reflect women's preferences among these potential outcomes. Such information may be useful in establishing policies for large populations.

Finally, if CEAs are conducted in a standardized manner using the same units for measuring outcomes, preventive services can be ranked in a "league table," a listing of interventions in order of their costs of saving a year of life or QALY.[26-28] In a setting of limited resources, these methods for prioritizing services could be used as a guide in providing services for a population to maximize overall health for a given investment. Overall, CEAs are a dynamic tool for developing and adapting effective preventive service interventions to obtain the best value for the greatest number of individuals at risk for poor health outcomes. However, they also have shortcomings. In the following section, we present a summary of limitations associated with using CEAs to inform evidence-based recommendations.

Limits of Using CEAs to Inform Preventive Service Recommendations

Prior USPSTFs and other groups have chosen not to incorporate cost effectiveness into their recommendations for several reasons, including a historical lack of standardized, high-quality CEAs; a paucity of CEAs for many preventive services; the questionable validity of QALYs in capturing preferences; a lack of transparency in the complex models used in many analyses; and concerns about the ethics and politics of rationing.

Until the last decade, there were few efforts in the United States to standardize the conduct of CEAs. As a result, many published analyses would not meet current criteria for high-quality CEA research.[29] Lack of standardization has made it difficult to compare studies about a specific preventive service or across different interventions.[30,31] In addition, for many services there has been a paucity of cost-effectiveness data, and for some services there are no economic evaluations at all.

Expanded use of QALYs as an outcome measure may improve the comparability of CEAs. Current use of QALYs, however, is limited by the shortcomings of existing preference measures, many of which are unvalidated and narrow in focus, not fully capturing the multifaceted nature of personal preference. QALYs as a measure are also not intuitively understood by most clinicians, policymakers, or patients. Moreover, results from a CEA using preferences of the general population to generate QALYs may not always be helpful to clinicians in their offices caring for individual patients with specific values that may differ from the average.

Using CEAs in making health decisions has also raised ethical concerns. CEAs typically assume that a year of life saved or a QALY for an infant is equal to that for a 70-year-old, or that a gain of 1 year for one person is the same as a gain of a tenth of a year for ten people. These assumptions could be considered the least biased and a protection against discriminating against any group, but they may also inadequately reflect societal and individual values.[32-33]

Other ethical concerns relate to the use of CEA to ration health care services. Implicit in the use of CEAs in developing clinical recommendations is that societal health care resources are limited. In some industrialized countries this assumption, and the rationing of health care services, are made explicit. In the United States, CEAs have only rarely been used explicitly to set recommendations about services or funding levels. In the best-known case, the Oregon Health Services Commission ranked health care services according to their cost effectiveness, in order to expand health care coverage among low-income populations within the constrained Medicaid budget.[34] This approach was abandoned in the face of public criticism; many observers argued that rationing is not ethical, and that individuals should have access to all effective interventions.[35,36] Patients and health professionals alike expressed concern about the prospect of potentially valuable services being withheld to save money. In Oregon, cost effectiveness was ultimately used as one of several considerations in setting Medicaid-covered services. The Oregon experience illustrates that ranking services by their cost-effectiveness ratios may be a useful but not likely sufficient process for developing clinical service priorities. Most observers recognize that while CEAs are an important decision-making tool, they are not the only tool, and that many other factors, including ethical implications, public perceptions, and political and operational feasibility, need to be considered when prioritizing health care spending.

The perspective of a CEA—whose costs and benefits are considered in the analysis—is also important. A CEA using the societal perspective ideally incorporates an intervention's impact, in terms of costs and outcomes, on all members of society. If, however, an analysis is conducted from the perspective of a specific organization, such as a managed care provider, other costs (e.g., out-of-pocket patient costs and caregiver time) that are not relevant from the provider's perspective are not considered.[30] Such an analysis may be useful only to a select group of decision-makers. Moreover, because studies from varying perspectives assess different sets of costs and outcomes, they are not directly comparable. The Panel on Cost-Effectiveness in Health and Medicine4 has recommended that all CEAs include the societal perspective. One limitation of this approach, however, is that the societal perspective may not reflect the specific concerns of some parties interested in using CEAs, such as individual practitioners, patients, or health care organizations. Another limitation is that enumerating all of the costs society experiences is often more difficult than quantifying those experienced by a specific entity, such as a health care system.

For these and other reasons, the USPSTF has, in the past, not used CEAs to inform its recommendations. Over the past several years, however, the quantity and quality of CEAs have increased substantially.[29] Theoretical refinement, methodologic advances, and the development of standards for reporting and conducting CEAs have improved their usefulness as decision-making tools. Moreover, as the cost of health care delivery has continued to rise, policymakers have found it increasingly difficult to decide about implementing clinical services solely on evidence of effectiveness, without consideration of costs. The third USPSTF has therefore decided to incorporate information from CEAs into its process for developing recommendations. While CEAs may never be able to address all of the complex issues involved in deciding how to allocate health care resources, their ability to quantify the trade-offs involved in choosing among different alternatives to improve health make them a valuable source of information in deciding which clinical preventive services to select and implement.

The USPSTF Approach

The USPSTF will conduct systematic reviews of CEAs to inform its recommendation process. These reviews will not replace the USPSTF's harms-benefits analyses and will not be conducted for every topic, but rather where relevant questions about cost effectiveness exist. Most of these questions will address the trade-offs between two or more effective strategies for achieving a given health outcome; the cost effectiveness of applying an intervention at varying intervals or to different target populations or risk groups; and the impact of factors such as adherence that may affect the costs and effectiveness of a given intervention. Examples of questions for which a CEA review might be initiated include the following: What is the cost-effectiveness of screening average-risk adults aged 20 to 30 for dyslipidemia? What is the comparative cost effectiveness of universal versus selective screening for chlamydial infection among women aged <25? What is the impact of varying levels of adherence on the cost effectiveness of colorectal cancer screening using sigmoidoscopy versus colonoscopy?

The USPSTF has set specific requirements for the use of CEAs in its recommendation process. First, there should be reasonable evidence that the intervention in question is effective. When definitive proof of effectiveness is difficult to achieve, the USPSTF may consider information from CEAs that make reasonable assumptions about the intervention's likely effectiveness. In general, however, the USPSTF will initiate a CEA review only for services where evidence of effectiveness exists.

Second, the USPSTF will use only economic analyses assessing the costs associated with achieving health outcomes. The results of studies that examine only intermediate measures, such as those reporting costs per patient screened or costs per case detected, are less interpretable in that the value of what is achieved for the costs accrued is less clear. These studies will therefore not be included in USPSTF CEA reviews.

Third, the USPSTF will focus primarily on CEAs that are conducted from the societal perspective. It will also give highest priority to studies in which valuations of outcomes, or QALYs, are derived from the perspective of general, rather than selected, populations.[4] In this manner, consistent with the USPSTF perspective, CEAs used in making decisions should reflect the public interest, and not be biased by any group that stands to gain or lose by the implementation of a particular preventive service.[26] Many CEAs include most but not all relevant costs accrued by society. Costs such as time and resources expended by patients and caregivers are frequently omitted. Such studies may nonetheless provide valuable information and will be considered. When reviewing these studies, the USPSTF will consider how including the relevant societal costs might have affected the studies' results.

Finally, the USPSTF will not create league tables to rank preventive services in order of cost effectiveness. Although the USPSTF strives to provide as much information as possible to guide decision-makers in their use of preventive services, a preliminary review of the cost effectiveness literature for several preventive services revealed that the quality and comparability of CEAs across services were not sufficient to allow direct comparisons and rankings. As standardization of methods and comparability of CEAs across preventive, diagnostic, and therapeutic services improves, future *Guides* may include league tables to allow for prioritizing services based on costs and expected benefits. In the meantime, *Partnership for Prevention*, a national nonprofit organization, has developed methods to estimate the relative value of services recommended by the second USPSTF to guide decision-makers in prioritizing effective preventive services.[37]

To sum up, CEAs are valuable decision-making tools that, when properly applied, can help maximize efficiency and appropriateness in health care delivery. The USPSTF recognizes that CEAs have limitations and that their use in informing health policies is controversial. It also recognizes, however, that users of the third *Guide*, if not provided with information from CEAs, are still likely to use economic analyses, potentially in an unsystematic way. The USPSTF will therefore attempt to provide unbiased summaries of cost-effectiveness data where relevant, based on a systematic approach to, and critical appraisal of, the literature. In circumstances where information on cost-effectiveness is unavailable but is felt to be vital to the shaping of a recommendation, the USPSTF may conduct an original CEA.

Methods to Review CEAs to Inform Recommendations for Preventive Services

Conceptual Approach

Systematically reviewing CEAs shares much in common with the process for reviewing studies of intervention effectiveness.[38] The goal in both cases is to identify the best available evidence regarding a specific question and to critically review and synthesize that evidence in order to answer the question in an evidence-based way. However, reviewing CEAs is also fundamentally different from reviewing effectiveness studies. For example, in a systematic review of the effectiveness of a single intervention, the effect sizes from several clinical trials, which represent unique samples of data gathered in a similar fashion, might be pooled in order to obtain a more accurate estimate of the intervention's effectiveness. It is difficult, however, to combine the results of several CEAs into a single cost-effectiveness ratio, because they often do not involve primary data collection and are frequently based on assumptions and models that vary in a way that may make combining results from multiple studies difficult or conceptually unsound. In addition, while the USPSTF's systematic reviews of intervention effectiveness involve developing an analytic framework of the various components of effectiveness and critically appraising the literature related to each component separately,[38] CEAs typically use decision analytic modeling to include all the components of such a framework in a single study.

Why then, conduct a systematic review of CEAs rather than identify a single study that addresses the question at hand? CEAs vary widely in their methods and assumptions. Because of this variation, systematically reviewing CEAs provides several benefits. First, because CEAs draw on a variety of cost and effectiveness data sources to develop input parameters, a systematic review can identify which analyses use the best available evidence for key inputs and are therefore the most evidence based. Second, because the credibility of CEAs rests on their quality, a critical review of CEAs and a rating of the quality of each allow for identifying the most methodologically rigorous studies. Third, a comprehensive review can identify the studies that best address the question being asked. Fourth, comparatively assessing CEAs can help to identify variables and methods that significantly influence the estimated benefits and cost effectiveness of an intervention. For instance, some CEAs might assume no harms from a given intervention, while others might assume that the intervention has significant harms. Comparing these studies side by side may provide insight into how the assumption or lack of assumption of harm affects the estimated benefit of the intervention. While some assumptions are varied within a single study using sensitivity analysis, most CEAs provide a limited number of sensitivity analyses. Thus, systematically reviewing CEAs may help identify, through a side-by-side comparison that amounts to a "virtual sensitivity analysis," the impact of different assumptions on the benefits of a given intervention. Finally, the more high-quality, independently conducted CEAs there are for a given intervention, the more convincing the evidence.

Developing the Instrument and Process for Abstracting Data

To systematically review CEAs, we first developed a tool for abstracting relevant information from individual studies in a standardized way. Through

---

Table 2. Sample quality rating items for cost effectiveness analyses

Framing

    Are the interventions and populations compared appropriate?   .

    Is the study conducted from the societal perspective?

    Is the time horizon clinically appropriate and relevant to the study question?

Effects

    Are all important drivers of effectiveness included?

    Are key harms included?

    Is the best available evidence used to estimate effectiveness?

    Are long-term outcomes used?

    Do effect measures capture preferences or utilities?

Costs

    Are all appropriate downstream medical costs included?

    Are charges converted to costs appropriately?

    Are the best available data used to estimate costs?

Results

    Are incremental cost-effectiveness ratios presented?

    Are appropriate sensitivity analyses performed?

---

a literature search and consultation with experts, we located several existing abstraction tools[28,39] and quality-rating criteria.[4,40,41] We drew on the strengths of each of these instruments to develop a novel abstraction tool that met the needs and objectives of the USPSTF. The tool is largely adapted from the CEA abstraction instruments developed by the Task Force on Community Preventive Services[39] and the Harvard Center for Risk Analysis.[29]

    The USPSTF CEA abstraction instrument, which we are currently piloting, was designed to (1) ensure that the CEAs being reviewed are applicable to the question posed, (2) assess the studies' methodological rigor, (3) ascertain that their models contain the appropriate components of effectiveness, (4) examine the degree to which they use the best available evidence of effectiveness, (5) evaluate the validity and impact of their assumptions, and (6) assess the type and quality of cost information used. Our criteria for rating methodological quality are based on recommendations of the Panel on Cost-Effectiveness in Health and Medicine.[4] Sample quality rating items are listed in Table 2. Because simple counts of criteria fulfilled do not differentiate studies of varying quality with great precision, these criteria will not be used to generate quality scores but rather as a guide in categorizing study quality as high, fair, or poor.

    Our reviews will focus mainly on high-quality studies. When few or no high-quality studies exist for a given question, we will also consider studies rated fair. Poorquality studies will not be considered. Our objective is to present the best evidence currently available while appropriately identify-

---

Table 3. U.S. Preventive Services Task Force process for conducting a
systematic review of cost-effectiveness analyses

---

(1) Define the question to be addressed.
(2) Comprehensively search relevant literature databases.
(3) Screen abstracts for inclusion.
(4) Review reference lists and call experts to identify studies not captured by the
     literature search.
(5) Abstract relevant studies.
(6) Compare the impact of varying assumptions and resolve differential results
     across studies through consensus.
(7) Synthesize and present results in evidence tables.

---

ing study limitations, because policymakers are sometimes required to
make decisions without having perfect information.

Process for Reviewing Studies

The process for systematically reviewing CEAs is similar to that for reviewing studies of effectiveness (Table 3). As with any systematic review, before
reviewing the evidence, one must define the question at hand. USPSTF
"topic teams"[38] reviewing the evidence for the effectiveness of preventive
services within specific clinical topics (e.g., screening for hypertension) are
asked to identify relevant questions related to the cost effectiveness of services within each topic (Table 1).

Once the question is identified, a comprehensive search for appropriate CEAs is conducted. Searches may be limited by year (e.g., after 1990),
based on when relevant technologies came into use. Abstracts identified by
the search are screened for inclusion using three items: (1) Does the study
address the identified question? (2) Is the study an original CEA? (3) Does
the study report results using an appropriate outcome metric (e.g., LYS,
QALY, or cases of illness averted)?. If no CEAs exist for a specific question,
we consider reviewing other types of economic analyses, such as CBAs.

Studies meeting inclusion criteria are abstracted by at least two reviewers. To determine whether the best available evidence was used in each
study, whether included assumptions are reasonable, and whether each
study appropriately addresses the question at hand, the CEA review team
for each question includes a member of the topic team reviewing the effectiveness evidence for that topic.[38] The data used in the CEA are compared
with the evidence derived from the systematic review of effectiveness conducted by the topic team, which serves as the "gold standard" for whether
the best available evidence was used.

After abstracting studies, reviewers discuss how studies differ in their assumptions, how varying assumptions affect study results, and how different studies may arrive at different conclusions. Finally, key information addressing the initial question and highlighting study quality and the effect of various assumptions are summarized in evidence tables.

Conclusions

CEAs are valuable tools for incorporating cost considerations into evidence-based clinical decisions. This article has outlined the USPSTF's strategy to incorporate information from CEAs into its process for recommending clinical preventive services. Through these efforts, we hope not only to provide guidance about implementing preventive services, but to identify unmet needs in economic analyses of preventive health care, illuminate some of the trade-offs in alternative approaches to delivering preventive services, and provide substrata for policy discussions and public debate over the role of cost effectiveness in allocating health care resources.

In the future, ranking of preventive services based on cost effectiveness may provide busy clinicians and their patients with some scientific basis for deciding how to best spend their limited time providing or carrying out the services that are most likely to have the greatest impact on health. At present, CEAs should be considered an important aid to decision makers striving to achieve the best possible health for a population.

Supported by contract #290-97-0018 (Task Order #2) to the Oregon Health Sciences University (SS, MH) and contract #290-97-0011 (Task Order #3) to the Research Triangle Institute/University of North Carolina (TJH, MP) from the Agency for Healthcare Research and Quality, and contract # DAMD17-94-J-4212 from the Department of the Army (JSM). The views expressed in this article are those of the authors and do not necessarily reflect those of the Agency for Healthcare Research and Quality or the Department of the Army.

We thank Vilma G. Carande-Kulis, MS, PhD; Joanna E. Siegel, ScD, RN; Dennis G. Fryback, PhD; Milton J. Weinstein, PhD; and the members of the third U.S. Preventive Services Task Force, for comments on earlier versions of this manuscript; the *Partnership for Prevention* Committee on Clinical Preventive Service Priorities and Peter J. Neumann, ScD, for sharing their work; and Kathryn Pyle Krages, AMLS, MA, Susan Wingenfeld, and Gary Miranda, MA, for administrative support and help with manuscript preparation and editing.

REFERENCES

1. Levit K, Cowan C, Lazenby H, et al. Health spending in 1998: signals of change. The Health Accounts Team. Health Affairs 2000;19:124–32.
2. Weinstein MJ, Garber AM, Fryback DG. Disease Prevention Research at NIH: An Agenda for All. Workshop J: Prevention strategies, economic realities, and identification of prevention research needs. Prev Med 1994; 23:571–2.
3. Teutsch SM, Murray JF. Dissecting cost-effectiveness analysis for preventive interventions: a guide for decision makers. Am J Manag Care 1999;5:301–5.

4. Gold M, Seigel J, Russell L, Weinstein MC. Cost-effectiveness in health and medicine. New York: Oxford University Press, 1996.

5. Gold MR, Patrick DL, Torrance GW, et al. Identifying and valuing outcomes. In: Gold M, Seigel J, Russell L, Weinstein MC, eds. Costeffectiveness in health and medicine. New York: Oxford University Press, 1996:82–134.

6. Kattlove H, Liberati A, Keeler E, Brook RH. Benefits and costs of screening and treatment for early breast cancer: development of a basic benefit package. JAMA 1995;273:142–8.

7. Prosser LA, Koplan JP, Neumann PJ, Weinstein MC. Barriers to using cost-effectiveness analysis in managed care decision making. Am J Manag Care 2000;6:173–9.

8. Mandel JS, Bond JH, Church TR, et al. Reducing mortality from colorectal cancer by screening for fecal occult blood: Minnesota Colon Cancer Control Study. New Eng J Med 1993;328:1365–71 (published erratum appears in N Engl J Med 1993 Aug 26;329[9]:672).

9. Selby JV, Friedman GD, Quesenberry CP Jr, Weiss NS. A case-control study of screening sigmoidoscopy and mortality from colorectal cancer. New Eng J Med 1992;326:653–7.

10. Winawer SJ, Fletcher RH, Miller L, et al. Colorectal cancer screening: clinical guidelines and rationale. Gastroenterology 1997;112:594–642 (published errata appear in Gastroenterology 1997;112[3]:1060 and 1998; 114[3]:625).

11. Eddy DM. Screening for colorectal cancer. Ann Intern Med 1990;113:373–84.

12. Frazier AL, Colditz GA, Fuchs CS, Kuntz KM. Cost-effectiveness of screening for colorectal cancer in the general population. JAMA 2000;284:1954–61.

13. Khandker RK, Dulski JD, Kilpatrick JB, Ellis RP, Mitchell JB, Baine WB. A decision model and cost-effectiveness analysis of colorectal cancer screening and surveillance guidelines for average-risk adults. Int J Technol Assess Health Care 2000;16:799–810.

14. Wagner JL, Tunis S, Brown M, Ching A, Almeida R. Cost-effectiveness of colorectal cancer screening in average-risk adults. In: Young GP, Rozen P, Levin B, eds. Prevention and early detection of colorectal cancer. Philadelphia: W.B. Saunders, 1996:321–56.

15. Eddy DM. Screening for cervical cancer. Ann Intern Med 1990;113:214–26.

16. Eddy DM. Screening for cervical cancer: common screening tests. Philadelphia: American College of Physicians, 1991.

17. Kerlikowske K, Salzmann P, Phillips KA, Cauley JA, Cummings SR. Continuing screening mammography in women aged 70 to 79 years: impact on life expectancy and cost-effectiveness. JAMA 1999;282:2156–63.

18. Prosser LA, Stinnett AA, Goldman PA, et al. Cost-effectiveness of cholesterol- lowering therapies according to selected patient characteristics. Ann Intern Med 2000;132:769–79.

19. Mandelblatt JS, Fahs MC. The cost-effectiveness of cervical cancer screening for low-income elderly women. JAMA 1988;259:2409–13.

20. Fahs MC, Mandelblatt J, Schechter C, Muller C. Cost effectiveness of cervical cancer screening for the elderly. Ann Intern Med 1992;117:520–7.

21. Ford D, Easton DF, Stratton M, et al. Genetic heterogeneity and penetrance analysis of the BRCA1 and BRCA2 genes in breast cancer families: the Breast Cancer Linkage Consortium. Am J Hum Genet 1998;62:676–89.

22. Burke W, Daly M, Garber J, et al. Recommendations for follow-up care of individuals with an inherited predisposition to cancer. II. BRCA1 and BRCA2. Cancer Genetics Studies Consortium. JAMA 1997;277:997–1003.

23. Schrag D, Kuntz KM, Garber JE, Weeks JC. Benefit of prophylactic mastectomy for women with BRCA1 or BRCA2 mutations. JAMA 2000;283: 3070–2.

24. Martin DH, Mroczkowski TF, Dalu ZA, et al. A controlled trial of a single dose of azithromycin for the treatment of chlamydial urethritis and 42 American Journal of Preventive Medicine, Volume 20, Number 3S cervicitis. The Azithromycin for Chlamydial Infections Study Group. New Eng J Med 1992;327:921–5.

25. Genc M, Mardh A. A cost-effectiveness analysis of screening and treatment for Chlamydia trachomatis infection in asymptomatic women. Ann Intern Med 1996;124:1–7.

26. Russell LB, Siegel JE, Daniels N, Gold MR, Luce BR, Mandelblatt J. Cost-effectiveness analysis as a guide to resource allocation in health: roles and limitations. In: Gold M, Seigel J, Russell L, Weinstein MC, eds. Cost-effectiveness in health and medicine. New York: Oxford University Press, 1996:3–24.

27. Drummond M, Torrance G, Mason J. Cost-effectiveness league tables: more harm than good? Soc Sci Med 1993;37:33–40.

28. Stone PW, Teutsch SM, Chapman RH, Bell C, Goldie SJ, Neumann PJ. Cost-utility analyses of clinical preventive services: published ratios, 1976–1997. Am J Prev Med 2000;19:15–23.

29. Neumann PJ, Stone PW, Chapman RH, Sandberg EA, Bell CM. The quality of reporting in published cost-utility analyses, 1976–1997. Ann Intern Med 2000;132:964–72.

30. Russell LB, Gold MR, Siegel JE, Daniels N, Weinstein MC. The role of cost-effectiveness analysis in health and medicine. Panel on Cost-Effectiveness in Health and Medicine. JAMA 1996;276:1172–7.

31. Brown ML, Fintor L. Cost-effectiveness of breast cancer screening: preliminary results of a systematic review of the literature. Breast Cancer Res Treat 1993;25:113–8.

32. Ubel PA, Nord E, Gold M, Menzel P, Prades JL, Richardson J. Improving value measurement in cost-effectiveness analysis. Med Care 2000;38:892–901.

33. Daniels N. Rationing fairly: programmatic considerations. Bioethics 1993; 7:223–33.

34. Klevit HD, Bates AC, Castanares T, Kirk EP, Sipes-Metzler PR, Wopat R. Prioritization of health care services: a progress report by the Oregon Health Services Commission. Arch Intern Med 1991;151:912–6.

35. Hadorn DC. Setting health care priorities in Oregon: cost-effectiveness meets the rule of rescue. JAMA 1991;265:2218–25.

36. Brown LD. The national politics of Oregon's rationing plan. Health Affairs 1991;10:28–51.

37. Coffield AB, Maciosek MV, McGinnis JM, et al. Priorities among recommended clinical preventive services. Am J Prev Med 2001. In press.

38. Harris RP, Helfand M, Woolf SH, et al. Current methods of the U.S. Preventive Services Task Force: a review of the process. Am J Prev Med: 2001;20(suppl 3):21–35.

39. Carande-Kulis VG, Maciosek MV, Briss PA, et al. Methods for systematic reviews of economic evaluations for the Guide to Community Preventive Services. Task Force on Community Preventive Services. Am J Prev Med 2000;18:75–91.

40. Drummond MF, Jefferson TO. Guidelines for authors and peer reviewers of economic submissions to the BMJ. Br Med J 1996;313:275–83. 41. Udvarhelyi IS, Colditz GA, Rai A, Epstein AM. Cost-effectiveness and cost-benefit analyses in the medical literature. Are the methods being used correctly? Ann Intern Med 1992;116:238–44.

Screening for Depression

By the U.S. Preventive Services Task Force (USPSTF)*

RECOMMENDATION

Recommendation and Rationale Statements present the current U.S. Preventive Services Task Force (USPSTF) recommendations, the rationale for the recommendations, and the supporting scientific evidence. These statements address preventive health services for use in primary care clinical settings, including screening tests, counseling, and chemoprevention.

The USPSTF recommendations are independent of the U.S. Government. They do not represent the views of the Agency for Healthcare Research and Quality (AHRQ), the U.S. Department of Health and Human Services, or the U.S. Public Health Service.

Summary of Recommendations

The U.S. Preventive Services Task Force (USPSTF) recommends screening adults for depression in clinical practices that have systems in place to assure accurate diagnosis, effective treatment, and followup.

The USPSTF found good evidence that screening improves the accurate identification of depressed patients in primary care settings and that treatment of depressed adults identified in primary care settings decreases

---

*This statement summarizes the current U.S. Preventive Services Task Force (USPSTF) recommendations for screening for depression and the supporting scientific evidence and updates the 1996 USPSTF recommendations on this topic. At that time, the USPSTF concluded that there was insufficient evidence to recommend for or against routine use of standardized questionnaires to screen for depression in primary care patients. The complete information on which this statement is based, including evidence tables and references, is available in the accompanying article, "Screening for Depression: A Summary of the Evidence for the U.S. Preventive Services Task Force" and in the Systematic Evidence Review on this topic [1], which can be obtained through the USPSTF Web site (http://www.ahrq.gov/clinic/uspstfix.htm) and in print through the AHRQ Publications Clearinghouse (call 1-800-358-9295; E-mail ahrqpubs@ahrq.gov).

Address correspondence to: Alfred O. Berg, MD, MPH, Chair, U.S. Preventive Services Task Force; c/o David Atkins, MD, MPH, Scientific and Technical Editor, U.S. Preventive Services Task Force; Agency for Healthcare Research and Quality, Center for Practice and Technology Assessment; 6010 Executive Boulevard, Suite 300; Rockville, MD 20912. (301) 594-4016, fax (301) 594-4027, E-mail: DAtkins@ahrq.gov

clinical morbidity. Trials that have directly evaluated the effect of screening on clinical outcomes have shown mixed results. Small benefits have been observed in studies that simply feed back screening results to clinicians. Larger benefits have been observed in studies in which the communication of screening results is coordinated with effective followup and treatment. The USPSTF concluded the benefits of screening are likely to outweigh any potential harms.

The USPSTF concludes the evidence is insufficient to recommend for or against routine screening of children or adolescents for depression.

The USPSTF found limited evidence on the accuracy and reliability of screening tests in children and adolescents and limited evidence on the effectiveness of therapy in children and adolescents identified in primary care settings.

Clinical Considerations

- Many formal screening tools are available (e.g., the Zung Self-Assessment Depression Scale, Beck Depression Inventory, General Health Questionnaire [GHQ], Center for Epidemiologic Study Depression Scale [CES-D])[2]. Asking two simple questions about mood and anhedonia ("Over the past 2 weeks, have you felt down, depressed, or hopeless?" and "Over the past 2 weeks, have you felt little interest or pleasure in doing things?") may be as effective as using longer instruments[3]. There is little evidence to recommend one screening method over another, so clinicians can choose the method that best fits their personal preference, the patient population served, and the practice setting.

- All positive screening tests should trigger full diagnostic interviews that use standard diagnostic criteria (i.e., those from the fourth edition of *Diagnostic and Statistical Manual of Mental Disorders* [DSM-IV]) to determine the presence or absence of specific depressive disorders, such as major depression and/or dysthymia[4]. The severity of depression and comorbid psychological problems (e.g., anxiety, panic attacks, or substance abuse) should be addressed.

- Many risk factors for depression (e.g., female sex, family history of depression, unemployment, and chronic disease) are common, but the presence of risk factors alone cannot distinguish depressed from nondepressed patients.

- The optimal interval for screening is unknown. Recurrent screening may be most productive in patients with a history of depression, unexplained somatic symptoms, comorbid psychological conditions (e.g., panic disorder or generalized anxiety), substance abuse, or chronic pain.

- Clinical practices that screen for depression should have systems in place to ensure that positive screening results are followed by accurate diagnosis, effective treatment, and careful followup. Benefits from screening are unlikely to be realized unless such systems are functioning well.
- Treatment may include antidepressants or specific psychotherapeutic approaches (e.g., cognitive behavioral therapy or brief psychosocial counseling), alone or in combination.
- The benefits of routinely screening children and adolescents for depression are not known. The existing literature suggests that screening tests perform reasonably well in adolescents and that treatments are effective, but the clinical impact of routine depression screening has not been studied in pediatric populations in primary care settings. Clinicians should remain alert for possible signs of depression in younger patients. The predictive value of positive screening tests is lower in children and adolescents than in adults, and research on the effectiveness of primary care-based interventions for depression in this age group is limited.

Scientific Evidence

Epidemiology and Clinical Consequences

Depressive disorders are common, chronic and costly. The World Health Organization identified major depression as the fourth leading cause of worldwide disease in 1990, causing more disability than either ischemic heart disease or cerebrovascular disease[5]. In primary care settings, the point prevalence of major depression ranges from 5 percent to 9 percent among adults, and up to 50 percent of depressed patients are not recognized[6,7]. Other disabling depressive illnesses include dysthymia (a chronic low-grade depression) and minor depression (an episodic, less severe illness). These two illnesses are as common as major depression in primary care settings. Depressive disorders are also relatively common in younger persons, with estimated prevalence of 0.8 percent to 2.0 percent in children and 4.5 percent in adolescents.

Accuracy and Reliability of Screening Tests

Several depression screening instruments are available; most instruments have relatively good sensitivity (80 percent to 90 percent) but only fair specificity (70 percent to 85 percent)[2]. Most instruments are easy to use and can be administered in less than 5 minutes. Shorter screening tests, including simply asking questions about depressed mood and anhedonia, appear to detect a majority of depressed patients and, in some cases, perform better than the original instrument from which they were derived[3].

Assuming optimal test performance and a prevalence of major depression of 5 percent to 10 percent in primary care settings, about 24 percent to 40 percent of patients who screen positive will have major depression. Some patients with "false positive" results on screening may have dysthymia or subsyndromal depressive disorders that might benefit from treatment or closer monitoring; others may have comorbid disorders such as anxiety disorder, substance abuse, panic disorder, post-traumatic stress disorder, or grief reactions; still others may have no disorder at all. The finding of a positive screen therefore requires further diagnostic questioning by the clinician to establish an appropriate diagnosis and initiate a plan for treatment and followup.

Screening instruments have been tested in children and adolescents, with sensitivity ranging from 40 percent to 100 percent and specificity from 49 percent to 100 percent. Because the underlying prevalence is much lower than in adults, the positive predictive value is low.

Effectiveness of Early Treatment

Effective treatments are available for patients with depressive illnesses detected in primary care settings[1,8]. Antidepressant medications for major depression, including tricyclic antidepressants (TCAs) and selective serotonin reuptake inhibitors (SSRIs), are clearly more effective than placebo. Most of the data supporting effectiveness come from structured trials with selected populations, although more recent studies using "usual care" comparison groups and real-world settings have produced similar effects. Newer agents perform similarly to older agents.

Psychosocial and psychotherapeutic interventions are probably as effective as antidepressant medications for major depression, but they are clearly more time-intensive[7]. The benefits of psychotherapy for other depressive illnesses are less well studied. Few studies have examined the effect of combining medications and psychotherapy.

No studies have examined treatment outcomes for children or adolescents identified by primary care clinicians through screening. Evidence for treating adolescents comes from school and community settings where SSRIs and cognitive-behavioral therapy, but not tricyclic antidepressants, appear to be effective. Whether these results can be generalized to primary care settings or to children is unclear.

Effectiveness of Screening

The review for the USPSTF identified 14 randomized, controlled trials that have examined the effectiveness of screening for depression in primary care settings[9]. In eight studies, the only intervention was feedback of screening results to clinicians; remaining studies combined feedback with other interventions for patients or clinicians. The trials reported various outcomes, including recognition of depression, rates of treatment, and clinical improvement among patients with depression. In seven trials, routine depression screening with feedback of screening results to providers generally increased recognition of depression, especially major depression, by a factor of 2 to 3 compared with usual care. Trials that examined the effect of feedback of screening results on the proportion of depressed patients who received treatment showed mixed results: in four fair-to-good quality trials that used feedback alone, there was no significant effect on treatment rates, but four of the five trials that combined feedback with treatment advice or other system supports reported increased treatment rates in the intervention group compared with usual care. Ten trials measured the effect of screening and feedback on depression outcomes from 1 month to 2 years after the intervention. Five of these 10 studies reported significant improvements in the clinical outcomes of depressed patients, and three others reported improvements that did not reach statistical significance.

All three trials that compared the effects of integrated recognition and management programs with usual care in community primary care practices showed significantly improved patient outcomes. Integrated programs included feedback, provider and/or patient education, access to case management and/or mental health care, telephone followup, and institutional commitment to quality improvement. One trial, which included both newly detected cases of depression and patients already under treatment, showed improvement in patient symptoms at 6 months only among patients beginning a new treatment episode. No improvement was noted among patients who had recently been treated (that is, those who would have been identified without specific screening). Two trials showed improved symptoms at 12 months; one of these also showed more employment retention in intervention compared with usual care patients. All three trials required allocation of clinic resources to detection and management programs.

On the basis of estimates from the above-mentioned trials, approximately 11 patients identified as depressed as a result of screening would need to be treated to produce one additional remission[9]. If depression (including major depression, dysthymia, and minor depression) is present in 10 percent of primary care patients, then 110 patients would need to be screened to produce one additional remission after 6 to 12 months of treatment. The number needed to treat for benefit would be smaller for patients with major depression only, but a larger group would need to be screened to identify them.

Potential Harms of Screening and Treatment

The potential harms of screening include false-positive screening results, the inconvenience of further diagnostic work-up, the adverse effects and costs of treatment for patients who are incorrectly identified as being depressed, and potential adverse effects of labeling. None of the research reviewed provided useful empirical data regarding these potential adverse effects.

Recommendations of Others

The Canadian Task Force on Preventive Health Care (CTFPHC) found fair evidence to exclude routine screening of asymptomatic individuals for depression in 1994 but suggested that clinicians maintain a high degree of clinical suspicion for depression among their patients[10]. The CTFPHC is currently revisiting this recommendation. The American College of Obstetricians and Gynecologists recommends that clinicians should be alert to symptoms of depression and question patients about psychosocial stressors and family history of depression when taking their history[11]. The American Academy of Pediatrics recommends that pediatricians ask questions about depression in routine history-taking throughout adolescence[12]. The American Medical Association recommends screening for depression among adolescents who may be at risk owing to family problems, drug or alcohol use, or other indicators of risk[13].

REFERENCES

1. Pignone M, Gaynes BN, Rushton JL, et al. Screening for Depression. Systematic Evidence Review No. 6 (Prepared by the Research Triangle Institute—University of North Carolina Evidence-based Practice Center under Contract No. 290-97-0011) AHRQ Publication. No. 02-S002. Rockville, MD: Agency for Healthcare Research and Quality, May 2002.
2. Williams JW, Hitchcock Noel P, Cordes JA, Ramirez G, Pignone M. Rational clinical examination. Is this patient clinically depressed? JAMA 2002;287:1160-7.
3. Whooley MA, Avins AL, Miranda J, Browner WS. Case-finding instruments for depression: Two questions are as good as many. J Gen Intern Med 1997;12:439-45.
4. American Psychiatric Association. Diagnostic and Statistical Manual of Mental Disorders: DSM-IV. 4th ed. Washington, DC: American Psychiatric Association; 1994.
5. Murray CJ, Lopez AD. Global Burden of Disease. Cambridge, MA: Harvard University Press; 1996.
6. Depression Guideline Panel. Depression in Primary Care: Volume 1. Detection and Diagnosis. Clinical Practice Guideline, Number 5. Rockville, MD: U.S. Department of Health and Human Services; 1993. AHCPR Publication No. 93-0550.
7. Simon GE, VonKorff M. Recognition, management, and outcomes of depression in primary care. Arch Fam Med 1995;4:99-105.
8. Mulrow CD, Williams JW Jr, Chiquette E, et al. Efficacy of newer pharmacotherapies for treating depression in primary care patients. Am J Med 2000;108:54-64.
9. Pignone MP, Gaynes BN, Rushton JL, et al. Screening for depression in adults: a summary of the evidence for the U.S. Preventive Services Task Force. Ann Intern Med 2002.
10. Canadian Task Force on the Periodic Health Examination. The Canadian Guide to Clinical Health Care. Ottawa, Ontario: Health Canada;1994:450-4.

11. American College of Obstetricians and Gynecologists. Guidelines for Women's Health Care. Washington, DC: American College of Obstetricians and Gynecologists; 2002:126-33, 235-6,79.

12. Suicide and suicide attempts in adolescents. Committee on Adolescents. American Academy of Pediatrics. Pediatrics 2000;105;871-4.

13. American Medical Association. Guidelines for Adolescent Preventive Services (GAPS): Recommendations Monograph. Chicago: American Medical Association; 1997.

ACKNOWLEDGMENTS

Members of the U.S. Preventive Services Task Force are Alfred O. Berg, MD, MPH, Chair, USPSTF (Professor and Chair, Department of Family Medicine, University of Washington, Seattle, WA); Janet D. Allan, PhD, RN, CS, Vice-chair, USPSTF (Dean and Professor, School of Nursing, University of Texas Health Science Center, San Antonio, TX), Paul S. Frame, MD (Tri-County Family Medicine, Cohocton, NY, and Clinical Professor of Family Medicine, University of Rochester, Rochester, NY); Charles J. Homer, MD, MPH (Executive Director, National Initiative for Children's Healthcare Quality, Boston, MA); *Mark S. Johnson, MD, MPH (Associate Professor of Clinical Family Medicine and Chairman Department of Family Medicine, University of Medicine and Dentistry of New Jersey-New Jersey Medical School, Newark, NJ); *Jonathan D. Klein, MD, MPH (Associate Professor of Pediatrics and of Community and Preventive Medicine, University of Rochester School of Medicine, Rochester, NY); Tracy A. Lieu, MD, MPH (Associate Professor, Department of Ambulatory Care and Prevention, Harvard Pilgrim Health Care and Harvard Medical School, Boston, MA); Cynthia D. Mulrow, MD, MSc (Professor of Medicine, University of Texas Health Science Center, Audie L. Murphy Memorial Veterans Hospital, San Antonio, TX); C. Tracy Orleans, PhD (Senior Scientist, The Robert Wood Johnson Foundation, Princeton, NJ); Jeffrey F. Peipert, MD, MPH (Director of Research, Women and Infants' Hospital, Providence, RI); Nola J. Pender, PhD, RN (Professor and Associate Dean for Research, School of Nursing, University of Michigan, Ann Arbor, MI); *Albert L. Siu, MD, MSPH (Professor of Medicine, Chief of Division of General Internal Medicine, and Medical Director of the Primary Care and Medical Services Care Center, Mount Sinai School of Medicine and The Mount Sinai Medical Center, New York, NY); Steven M. Teutsch, MD, MPH (Senior Director, Outcomes Research and Management, Merck & Company, Inc., West Point, PA); Carolyn Westhoff, MD, MSc (Associate Professor of Obstetrics, Gynecology and Public Health, Department of Obstetrics and Gynecology, Columbia University College of Physicians and Surgeons, New York, NY); and Steven H. Woolf, MD, MPH (Professor of Family Medicine, Department of Family Practice, Virginia Commonwealth University, Fairfax, VA).

*These current members were not on the Task Force at the time this recommendation was voted.

Appendix A USPSTF Recommendations and Ratings

The Task Force grades its recommendations according to one of five classifications (A, B, C, D, I) reflecting the strength of evidence and magnitude of net benefit (benefits minus harms).

A. The USPSTF strongly recommends that clinicians routinely provide [the service] to eligible patients. The USPSTF found good evidence that [the service] improves important health outcomes and concludes that benefits substantially outweigh harms.
B. The USPSTF recommends that clinicians routinely provide [the service] to eligible patients. The USPSTF found at least fair evidence that [the service] improves important health outcomes and concludes that benefits outweigh harms.
C. The USPSTF makes no recommendation for or against routine provision of [the service]. The USPSTF found at least fair evidence that [the service] can improve health outcomes but concludes that the balance of benefits and harms is too close to justify a general recommendation.
D. The USPSTF recommends against routinely providing [the service] to asymptomatic patients. The USPSTF found at least fair evidence that [the service] is ineffective or that harms outweigh benefits.
I. The USPSTF concludes that the evidence is insufficient to recommend for or against routinely providing [the service]. Evidence that the [service] is effective is lacking, of poor quality, or conflicting and the balance of benefits and harms cannot be determined.

Appendix B USPSTF Strength of Overall Evidence

The USPSTF grades the quality of the overall evidence for a service on a 3-point scale (good, fair, or poor).

Good: Evidence includes consistent results from well-designed, well-conducted studies in representative populations that directly assess effects on health outcomes.

Fair: Evidence is sufficient to determine effects on health outcomes, but the strength of the evidence is limited by the number, quality, or consistency of the individual studies; generalizability to routine practice; or indirect nature of the evidence on health outcomes.

Poor: Evidence is insufficient to assess the effects on health outcomes because of limited number or power of studies, important flaws in their design or conduct, gaps in the chain of evidence, or lack of information on important health outcomes.

Screening for Bacterial Vaginosis in Pregnancy

U.S. Preventive Services Task Force

Summary of Recommendations

- The U.S. Preventive Services Task Force (USPSTF) concludes that the evidence is insufficient to recommend for or against routinely screening high-risk pregnant women for bacterial vaginosis (BV). (See Clinical Considerations for discussion of populations at high risk.) **I recommendation.**

The USPSTF found good-quality studies with conflicting results that screening and treatment of asymptomatic BV in high-risk pregnant women reduces the incidence of preterm delivery. The magnitude of benefit exceeded risk in several studies, but the single largest study reported no benefit among high-risk pregnant women.

- The USPSTF recommends against routinely screening average-risk asymptomatic pregnant women for BV. **D recommendation.**

There is good evidence that screening and treatment of BV in asymptomatic women who are not at high risk does not improveoutcomes such as preterm labor or preterm birth.

This statement summarizes the third U.S. Preventive Services Task Force (USPSTF) recommendations for screening pregnant women for bacterial vaginosis and the supporting scientific evidence. Explanations of the ratings and of the strength of overall evidence are given in Appendix A and in Appendix B, respectively. The complete information on which this statement is based, including evidence tables and references, is available in the accompanying article Screening for Bacterial Vaginosis in Pregnancy[1] and in the Systematic Evidence Review[2] on this topic, which can be obtained through the USPSTF Web site (www.ahrq.gov/clinic/uspstfix.htm), through the National Guideline Clearinghouse (www.guideline.gov), or in print through the AHRQ Publications Clearinghouse (1-800-358-9295).

Address correspondence to: Alfred O. Berg, MD, MPH, c/o Dana Best, MD, MPH, U.S. Preventive Services Task Force, Agency for Healthcare Research and Quality, Center for Practice and Technology Assessment, 6010 Executive Boulevard, Suite 300, Rockville, MD 20912. E-mail: dbest@ahrq.gov.

Reprints are available from the AHRQ Web site at www.ahrq.gov/clinic/uspstfix.htm, through the National Guideline Clearinghouse (www.guideline.gov), or in print through the AHRQ Publications Clearinghouse (1-800-358-9295).

Clinical Considerations

- For women with a history of preterm delivery, screening for BV is an option.

  A single previous episode of preterm delivery by itself may not reliably identify a population of women who will benefit from screening and treatment. Nevertheless, screening may be appropriate in specific circumstances. Studies demonstrating a benefit of screening and treatment were performed among populations of women at especially high risk (35% to 57%) of preterm birth. Clinicians should consider previous history of preterm delivery, other risk factors, and time of presentation in making the decision whether or not to screen for BV in women at high risk.

- For clinicians electing to screen high-risk women, the optimal screening test is not certain.

  Accepted clinical criteria for BV include vaginal pH >4.5, amine odor on the application of KOH, appearance of a homogeneous vaginal discharge, and presence of clue cells on a microscopic examination of a wet mount. Presence of at least three of these four criteria is generally considered diagnostic of BV. The use of more limited criteria (e.g., clue cells alone) has not been evaluated.

- Neither the optimal time to screen high-risk pregnant women nor the optimal treatment regimen for pregnant women with BV is clear.

  The three trials that demonstrated a reduction in preterm birth screened in the second trimester (13 to 24 weeks of pregnancy) used various regimens of oral metronidazole alone or oral metronidazole and erythromycin.

- Treatment is appropriate for pregnant women with symptomatic BV infection.

  These women were excluded from most screening trials and may be at higher risk than those without symptoms. Treatment can relieve symptoms such as vaginal discharge.

Scientific Evidence

Epidemiology and Clinical Consequences

BV describes an imbalance in the normal vaginal bacterial flora characterized by a decrease in *Lactobacilli* and an increase in *Gardnerella*, *Mycoplasma*, and anaerobic bacteria. BV is a common cause of abnormal vaginal discharge and has been associated with adverse pregnancy outcomes. The true prevalence of BV in the community is not known. Studies in academic medical centers and public hospitals found that 9% to 23% of pregnant women had BV, with infection more common among African-American women than Caucasian women.

Observational studies have consistently shown an association between BV and adverse pregnancy outcomes, including preterm delivery (relative risks [RRs] ranging from 1.4 to 6.9), preterm premature rupture of membranes (RR = 52.0 to 7.3), spontaneous abortion (RR = 51.3 to 2.0), and preterm labor (RR = 52.0 to 2.6). Preterm delivery is associated with significant respiratory, neurologic, and developmental abnormalities in the newborn that might result in death or long-term disability. A short course of antibiotic therapy can alter the microflora imbalance associated with BV, but cure rates are variable and recurrences are common. Because BV may be a marker for adverse pregnancy outcomes, rather than a causative factor, controlled trials have been conducted to determine whether treating BV will also improve pregnancy outcomes.

Accuracy and Reliability of Screening Test

The screening test employed in most epidemiologic studies and treatment trials of BV has been the Gram stain of the vaginal discharge. In practice, a combination of other clinical findings is usually used (see "Clinical Considerations"). Comparisons of clinical criteria and Gram stain yield sensitivities from 62% to 97% and specificities from 66% to 95%, using the Gram stain as the standard. The use of more limited diagnostic criteria has not been evaluated in studies of adverse pregnancy outcomes.

Effectiveness of Treatment of Bacterial Vaginosis

Seven randomized controlled trials have evaluated the effect of various antibiotic treatments versus placebo on pregnancy outcomes among women with BV: Three studies enrolled only high-risk women (primarily history of prior preterm delivery), two reported results separately for women with and without a prior history of preterm delivery, and two enrolled average-risk women. Among four studies reporting results for average-risk women, there were no differences between control groups and treatment groups in rates of preterm delivery, preterm premature rupture of membranes, or delivery of low birth weight infants.

Five studies reported conflicting results among women at increased risk because of a history of preterm delivery in previous pregnancies. Oral antibiotic treatment reduced the incidence of preterm delivery before 37 weeks in three studies, which enrolled women at particularly high risk (incidence of preterm delivery in placebo groups 35% to 57%). In contrast, in a large multicenter, American trial completed in 1999, a different regimen of oral metronidazole provided no benefit for the subgroup of women who had a history of previous preterm delivery. A fifth small study reported no benefit of vaginal clindamycin among high-risk women.

Potential Adverse Effects of Screening and Treatment

Because BV is common, screening and treatment could subject a substantial number of women to the inconvenience and minor side effects (primarily nausea) of taking metronidazole and other antibiotics during pregnancy. The regimens used to treat BV are generally considered safe in pregnancy, but several studies raise the possibility of harms in some women or their infants. In two studies, a subgroup of women who did not have BV but received treatment with metronidazole or clindamycin experienced trends toward higher incidence of preterm delivery before 34 weeks gestation (12% to 13% vs 4% to 5%). In addition, neonatal sepsis was significantly increased among women receiving vaginal clindamycin.

Discussion

Epidemiologic data and some intervention trials support the hypothesis that screening for and treating BV may reduce the risk of preterm delivery among some women. Studies published to date do not suggest any benefit of treating BV among asymptomatic, averagerisk women, but additional studies of earlier intervention with different drug regimens are being conducted in these populations. At present, however, the lack of demonstrated benefit and possibility of adverse effects of treatment in women without BV suggest that routine screening of average-risk women should be discouraged outside of research protocols. For pregnant women with prior preterm delivery, the inconsistent results of well-done studies prevent a clear recommendation for or against screening. Reasons for the conflicting results are not clear but may involve differences in other risk factors for preterm delivery among enrolled women or differences in drug regimens and timing of therapy. Further studies are needed, using diagnostic criteria and treatment protocols that are representative of community practice.

Recommendations of Others

In 1998, the Centers for Disease Control and Prevention (CDC) concluded that testing for BV "may be conducted early in the second trimester for asymptomatic patients who are at high risk for preterm labor (e.g., those who have a history of previous preterm delivery). Current evidence does not support universal testing for BV."[3] Updated recommendations from

CDC are expected in 2001. A similar conclusion was reached in 1998 by the American College of Obstetricians and Gynecologists.[4] A systematic review of randomized controlled trials of BV treatment, completed in 1998 for 60 American Journal of Preventive Medicine, Volume 20, Number 3S the Cochrane Collaboration, concluded that evidence did not support screening all pregnant women but that there was some evidence of benefit for women with a history of a previous preterm delivery.[5]

Members of the U.S. Preventive Services Task Force are: Alfred O. Berg, MD, MPH, Chair, USPSTF (Professor and Chair, Department of Family Medicine, University of Washington, Seattle, WA); Janet D. Allan, PhD, RN, CS, Vice-chair, USPSTF (Dean and Professor, School of Nursing, University of Texas Health Science Center, San Antonio, TX); Paul S. Frame, MD (Tri-County Family Medicine, Cohocton, NY, and Clinical Professor of Family Medicine, University of Rochester, Rochester, NY); Charles J. Homer, MD, MPH (Executive Director, National Initiative for Children's Healthcare Quality, Boston, MA); Tracy A. Lieu, MD, MPH (Associate Professor, Department of Ambulatory Care and Prevention, Harvard Pilgrim Health Care and Harvard Medical School, Boston, MA); Cynthia D. Mulrow, MD, MSc (Professor of Medicine, University of Texas Health Science Center, Audie L. Murphy Memorial Veterans Hospital, San Antonio, TX); C. Tracy Orleans, PhD (Senior Scientist, The Robert Wood Johnson Foundation, Princeton, NJ); Jeffrey F. Peipert, MD, MPH (Director of Research, Women and Infants' Hospital, Providence, RI); Nola J. Pender, PhD, RN (Professor and Associate Dean for Research, School of Nursing, University of Michigan, Ann Arbor, MI); Harold C. Sox Jr, MD (Professor and Chair, Department of Medicine, Dartmouth-Hitchcock Medical Center, Lebanon, NH); Steven M. Teutsch, MD, MPH (Senior Director, Outcomes Research and Management, Merck & Company, Inc., West Point, PA); Carolyn Westhoff, MD, MSc (Associate Professor of Obstetrics, Gynecology and Public Health, Department of Obstetrics and Gynecology, Columbia University College of Physicians and Surgeons, New York, NY); and Steven H. Woolf, MD, MPH (Professor of Family Medicine, Department of Family Practice, Medical College of Virginia, Fairfax, VA).

REFERENCES

1. Guise J-M, Mahon SM, Aickin M, Helfand M, Peipert JF, Westhoff C. Screening for bacterial vaginosis in pregnancy. Am J Prev Med 2001;20:62– 72.
2. Guise J-M, Mahon S, Aickin M, Helfand M. Screening for bacterial vaginosis in pregnancy. Systematic evidence review. Pub. No. AHRQ01-S001. Rockville, MD: Agency for Healthcare Research and Quality, 2001.
3. Centers for Disease Control and Prevention. 1998 guidelines for treatment of sexually transmitted diseases. MMWR Morb Mort Wkly Rep 1998;47: 70–4.
4. Bacterial vaginosis screening for prevention of preterm delivery. Committee Opinion No. 198. Washington, DC: American College of Obstetricians and Gynecologists; February 1998.
5. Brocklehurst P, Hannah M, McDonald H. Interventions for treating bacterial vaginosis in pregnancy (Cochrane Review). In: The Cochrane Library, 4, 2000. Oxford: Update Software. Available at http://hiru. mcmaster.ca/cochrane

---

Appendix A Third U.S. Preventive Services Task Force (USPSTF)
                Recommendations and Ratings

The USPSTF grades its recommendations according to one of five classifications
    (A, B, C, D, or I), reflecting the strength of evidence and magnitude of net
    benefit (benefits minus harms).

A. The USPSTF strongly recommends that clinicians routinely provide [the
    service] to eligible patients. (The USPSTF found good evidence that [the
    service] improves important health outcomes and concludes that benefits
    substantially outweigh harms.)

B. The USPSTF recommends that clinicians routinely provide [the service] to
    eligible patients. (The USPSTF found at least fair evidence that [the service]
    improves important health outcomes and concludes that benefits outweigh
    harms.)

C. The USPSTF makes no recommendation for or against routine provision of
    [the service]. (The USPSTF found at least fair evidence that [the service] can
    improve health outcomes but concludes that the balance of benefits and
    harms is too close to justify a general recommendation.)

D. The USPSTF recommends against routinely providing [the service] to
    asymptomatic patients. (The USPSTF found at least fair evidence that [the
    service] is ineffective or that harms outweigh benefits.)

I. The USPSTF concludes that the evidence is insufficient to recommend for or
    against routinely providing [the service]. (Evidence that [the service] is
    effective is lacking, of poor quality, or conflicting and the balance of benefits
    and harms cannot be determined.)

Appendix B Third U.S. Preventive Services Task Force (USPSTF)
                Strength of Overall Evidence

The USPSTF grades the quality of the overall evidence for a service on a 3-point
    scale (good, fair, or poor).

Good: Evidence includes consistent results from well-designed, well-conducted
    studies in representative populations that directly assess effects on health
    outcomes.

Fair: Evidence is sufficient to determine effects on health outcomes, but the
    strength of the evidence is limited by the number, quality, or consistency of the
    individual studies; generalizability to routine practice; or indirect nature of the
    evidence on health outcomes.

Poor: Evidence is insufficient to assess the effects on health outcomes because of
    limited number or power of studies, important flaws in their design or
    conduct, gaps in the chain of evidence, or lack of information on important
    health outcomes.

Screening for Chlamydial Infection

U.S. Preventive Services Task Force

Summary of Recommendations

- The U.S. Preventive Services Task Force (USPSTF) strongly recommends that clinicians routinely screen all sexually active women aged 25 years and younger, and other asymptomatic women at increased risk for infection, for chlamydial infection (see Clinical Considerations for discussion of risk factors). **A recommendation.**

The USPSTF found good evidence that screening women at risk for chlamydial infection reduces the incidence of pelvic inflammatory disease and fair evidence that community-based screening reduces prevalence of chlamydial infection. The USPSTF concludes that the benefits of screening substantially outweigh the potential harms. (See Potential Adverse Effects of Screening for discussion of potential harms).

- The USPSTF makes no recommendation for or against routinely screening asymptomatic low-risk women in the general population for chlamydial infection. **C recommendation.**

The USPSTF found at least fair evidence that screening low-risk women could detect some additional cases of Chlamydia trachomatis, but concludes that the

This statement summarizes the third U.S. Preventive Services Task Force (USPSTF) recommendations for screening for chlamydial infection and the supporting scientific evidence, and it updates the 1995 recommendations contained in the Guide to Clinical Preventive Services, second edition[1] Explanations of the ratings and of the strength of overall evidence are given in Appendix A and Appendix B, respectively. The complete information upon which this statement is based, including evidence tables and references, is available in the accompanying article, Screening for Chlamydial Infection[2] and in the Systematic Evidence Review[3] on this topic, which can be obtained through the USPSTF Web site (www.ahrq.gov/clinic/uspstfix.htm), through the National Guideline Clearinghouse (www.guideline.gov), or in print through the AHRQ Publications Clearinghouse (1-800-358-9295).

Address correspondence to: Alfred O. Berg, MD, MPH, c/o Dana Best, MD, MPH, U.S. Preventive Services Task Force, Agency for Healthcare Research and Quality, Center for Practice and Technology Assessment, 6010 Executive Boulevard, Suite 300, Rockville, MD 20912. E-mail: dbest@ahrq.gov.

Reprints are available from the AHRQ Web site at www.ahrq.gov/clinic/uspstfix.htm, through the National Guideline Clearinghouse (www.guideline/gov), or in print through the AHRQ Publications Clearinghouse (1-800-358-9295).

potential benefits of screening low-risk women may be small and may not justify the possible harms.

- The USPSTF recommends that clinicians routinely screen all asymptomatic pregnant women aged 25 years and younger and others at increased risk for infection for chlamydial infection (see Clinical Considerations for discussion of risk factors in pregnancy). **B recommendation.**

The USPSTF found at least fair evidence that screening and treatment of women at risk for chlamydial infection improves pregnancy outcomes and concludes that the benefits of screening outweigh potential harms.

- The USPSTF makes no recommendation for or against routine screening of asymptomatic, low-risk pregnant women aged 26 years and older for chlamydial infection. **C recommendation.**

The USPSTF found fair evidence that the benefits of screening low-risk pregnant women are small and may not justify the possible harms.

- The USPSTF concludes that the evidence is insufficient to recommend for or against routinely screening asymptomatic men for chlamydial infection. **I recommendation.**

No direct evidence was found to determine whether screening asymptomatic men for chlamydial infection is effective for reducing the incidence of new infections in women. The benefits and harms of screening men cannot be determined, but the potential magnitude of benefits could be large if the effectiveness of screening men can be demonstrated.

Clinical Considerations

- Women and adolescents through age 20 years are at highest risk for chlamydial infection, but most reported data indicate that infection is prevalent among women aged 20–25.

  Age is the most important risk marker. Other patient characteristics associated with a higher prevalence of infection include being unmarried, African-American race, having a prior history of sexually transmitted disease (STD), having new or multiple sexual partners, having cervical ectopy, and using barrier contraceptives inconsistently. Individual risk depends on the number of risk markers and local prevalence of the disease. Specific risk-based screening protocols need to be tested at the local level.

- Clinicians should consider the characteristics of the communities they serve in determining appropriate screening strategies for their patient population.

More targeted screening may be indicated in specific settings as better prevalence data become available. Prevalence of chlamydial infection varies widely among communities and patient populations. Knowledge of the patient population is the best guide to developing a screening strategy. Local public health authorities can be a source of valuable information.

- The optimal interval for screening is uncertain.

For women with a previous negative screening test, the interval for re-screening should take into account changes in sexual partners. If there is evidence that a woman is at low risk for infection (e.g., in a mutually monogamous relationship with a previous history of negative screening tests for chlamydial infection), it may not be necessary to screen frequently. Re-screening at 6 to 12 months may be appropriate for previously infected women because of high rates of reinfection.

- The optimal timing of screening in pregnancy is also uncertain.

Screening early in pregnancy provides greater opportunities to improve pregnancy outcomes, including low birth weight and premature delivery; however, screening in the third trimester may be more effective at preventing transmission of chlamydial infection to the infant during birth. The incremental benefit of repeated screening is unknown.

- Screening high-risk young men is a clinical option.

Until the advent of urine-based screening tests, routine screening of men was rarely performed. As a result, very little evidence regarding the efficacy of screening in men in reducing infection among women exists. Trials are underway to assess the effectiveness of screening asymptomatic men. The choice of specific screening technique is left to clinical judgment.

Choice of test will depend on issues of cost, convenience, and feasibility, which may vary in different settings. Although specificity is high with most approved tests, false-positive results can occur with all non-culture tests and rarely with culture tests. The Centers for Disease Control and Prevention (CDC) is developing laboratory guidelines that outline the advantages and disadvantages of available tests. These guidelines will be available at www.cdc.gov in 2001.

- Partners of infected individuals should be tested and treated if infected or treated presumptively.

- Clinicians should remain alert for findings suggestive of chlamydial infection during pelvic examination of asymptomatic women (e.g., discharge, cervical erythema, and cervical friability).

- Clinicians should be sensitive to the potential effect of diagnosing a sexually transmitted disease on a couple.

To prevent false-positive results, confirmatory testing may be appropriate in settings with low population prevalence.

Scientific Evidence

Epidemiology and Clinical Consequences

Chlamydia trachomatis is the most common sexually transmitted bacterial pathogen in the United States. There are estimated to be 3 million new infections each year. Chlamydial infection can cause urethritis, cervicitis, pelvic inflammatory disease (PID), and result in ectopic pregnancy, infertility, and chronic pelvic pain in women. In men, chlamydial infection can cause nongonococcal urethritis and acute epididymitis, and result in infertility, chronic prostatitis, reactive arthritis, and urethral strictures. In pregnant women, chlamydial infection is associated with adverse pregnancy outcomes, including preterm delivery and postpartum endometritis; perinatal transmission to infants can cause neonatal conjunctivitis and pneumonia. Chlamydial infection increases the risk of acquiring HIV infection.

Seventy percent to 90% of women and a large percentage of men with chlamydial infection are asymptomatic. The prevalence of asymptomatic infection varies widely depending on the population tested and individual characteristics and risk factors, ranging from 4% to 12% among female family planning clinic patients, 9% among female Army recruits, and 2% to 7% among female college students. Significant declines in prevalence have been noted over the last 10 years in areas where screening programs have been in place.

Accuracy and Reliability of Screening Test

A number of tests are available to identify chlamydial infection that use endocervical or urethral swab specimens and urine specimens. Until recently, culture has been accepted as the most specific test but it requires specialized handling and laboratory services. Antigendetection tests (direct fluorescent antibody [DFA] assay and enzyme immunoassay [EIA]) and non-amplified nucleic acid hybridization, as well as newer technologies based on amplified DNA assays (polymerase chain reaction [PCR], ligase chain reaction [LCR], strand displacement assay [SDA], hybrid capture system [HCS] and transcription-mediated amplification [TMA] of RNA) may provide improved sensitivity, lower expense, availability, or timeliness of results over culture. New tests that use urine specimens provide a noninvasive method of screening both men and women. Self-administered vaginal and vulval-introital swabs using PCR and LCR, including submitting samples by mail, are being used in research settings. The sensitivities and specificities of nucleic acid amplification tests are all high, ranging from 82% to 100%. The sensitivity of antigen detection tests (EIA, DFA) is slightly lower (70%–80%) but specificity remains high (96%–100%).

Effectiveness of Early Detection

The strongest evidence supporting screening is a well-designed randomized trial demonstrating that screening women at risk (prevalence of infection 7%) reduced the incidence of PID from 28 per 1000 womanyears to 13 per 1000 woman-years. The prevalence of chlamydial infection has declined in populations that have been targeted by screening programs (primarily women attending family planning and other publicly funded clinics). In addition, two ecologic analyses in Europe reported reductions in ectopic pregnancy and PID with the advent of community-based screening for chlamydial infection. There is little evidence of the effectiveness of screening asymptomatic women who are not in high-risk groups.

There is fair evidence indicating that screening for chlamydial infection among asymptomatic high-risk pregnant women and subsequent treatment improves pregnancy outcomes. Two nonrandomized trial studies demonstrated improved pregnancy outcomes following treatment of chlamydial infection: less premature rupture of membranes, less low birth weight, higher infant survival, and fewer small-for-gestational age births. There is little evidence regarding the effectiveness of screening and treatment of asymptomatic pregnant women who are not in high-risk groups.

There is good evidence showing that treatment of men can eradicate chlamydial infection. Unfortunately, there are no studies describing the effectiveness of screening or early treatment of men in reducing acute infection and sequelae in men or women.

Potential Adverse Effects of Screening

No studies were identified that directly examined adverse effects of screening. Potential harms include adverse effects of both false-positive and true-positive diagnoses of an STD on patients and their partners, the inconvenience of pelvic examinations for tests employing cervical specimens, and the potential harms of adverse reactions from antibiotic treatment. There may be added cost for confirmation of positive results and testing of partners.

Practice and Policy Considerations

Evaluation of cost-effectiveness of a specific screening strategy considers test performance, cost, treatment and disease outcomes, prevalence of infection in the screened population, and other factors. The USPSTF identified eight cost-effectiveness or cost-benefit analyses that examined screening in nonpregnant and pregnant women. These analyses suggest that screening may be cost-saving when conducted among nonpregnant women who are at moderate to high risk of chlamydial infection. These studies also suggest that selective screening is more likely to be cost-effective than universal screening, and that less expensive and more sensitive DNA or RNA tests would improve cost-effectiveness when compared with culture. However, because of inconsistencies in methodology and assumptions made in these cost analyses, the USPSTF concludes that available evidence on cost-effectiveness is insufficient to guide specific screening recommendations. An interactive model that allows clinicians to compare the costeffectiveness of different screening strategies is available at www.cdc.gov/nchstp/dstd/HEDIS.htm.

Recommendations of Others

The Canadian Task Force on Preventive Health Care[4] recommends that all members of high-risk groups be screened for chlamydial infection. The CDC[5] recommends at least routine annual screening for sexually active women under age 20 and for women aged 20–24 who meet either of the following criteria: inconsistent use of a barrier contraceptive or more than one sexual partner during the last 3 months, women older than age 24 who meet both criteria of inconsistent use of a barrier contraceptive and more than one sexual partner during the past 3 months. The American College of Obstetricians and Gynecologists[6] recommends routine screening for chlamydial infection for all sexually active adolescents and other asymptomatic women at high risk for infection. In 2000, annual chlamydia screening of sexually active women between the ages of 15 and 25 years was added to the National Committee for Quality Assurance Health Plan Employer Data and Information Set (HEDIS)[7] quality measures.

Discussion

The introduction of sensitive, easy-to-use tests has increased the primary care physician's ability to incorporate screening for chlamydial infection into the routine care of younger women, and there is now good evidence that screening can produce important clinical benefits. Important gaps remain, however, in the information needed to guide screening in the primary care setting. Both benefits and cost-effectiveness of screening increase with the prevalence of infection, which varies markedly between communities. There is no agreement, however, on the precise prevalence that justifies screening. Clinical strategies to identify women at risk need to balance feasibility and specificity: more detailed risk assessments may yield more specific information but be harder to implement than asking questions about age and marital status. Moreover, better data on the prevalence and incidence of infection in community practice are needed to develop optimal strategies for screening in a general practice.

The advent of urine-based tests allows for routine specimen collection without a pelvic examination that may increase acceptability to patients and providers. Urine screening has also spurred interest in screening young men. Asymptomatic young men are an important reservoir for infection and are less likely than women to be detected in the course of usual care. Whether targeting men will be an effective and costeffective strategy for reducing the burden of disease in women will depend on additional factors that have not been adequately studied, including compliance with therapy, referral of female partners, infectivity of asymptomatic men, and rates of reinfection following treatment. Trials are underway to assess the role of screening men as one strategy for controlling chlamydial infection.

Members of the U.S. Preventive Services Task Force are: Alfred O. Berg, MD, MPH, Chair, USPSTF (Professor and Chair, Department of Family Medicine, University of Washington, Seattle, WA); Janet D. Allan, PhD, RN, CS, Vice-chair, USPSTF (Dean and Professor, School of Nursing, University of Texas Health Science Center, San Antonio, TX); Paul S. Frame, MD (Tri-County Family Medicine, Cohocton, NY, and Clinical Professor of Family Medicine, University of Rochester, Rochester, NY); Charles J. Homer, MD, MPH (Executive Director, National Initiative for Children's Healthcare Quality, Boston, MA); Tracy A. Lieu, MD, MPH (Associate Professor, Department of Ambulatory Care and Prevention, Harvard Pilgrim Health Care and Harvard Medical School, Boston, MA); Cynthia D. Mulrow, MD, MSc (Professor of Medicine, University of Texas Health Science Center, Audie L. Murphy Memorial Veterans Hospital, San Antonio, TX); C. Tracy Orleans, PhD (Senior Scientist, The Robert Wood Johnson Foundation, Princeton, NJ); Jeffrey F. Peipert, MD, MPH (Director of Research, Women and Infants' Hospital, Providence, RI); Nola J. Pender, PhD, RN (Professor and Associate Dean for Research, School of Nursing, University of Michigan, Ann Arbor, MI); Harold C. Sox, Jr., MD (Professor and Chair, Department of Medicine, Dartmouth-Hitchcock Medical Center, Lebanon, NH); Steven M. Teutsch, MD, MPH (Senior Director, Outcomes Research and Management, Merck & Company, Inc., West Point, PA); Carolyn Westhoff, MD, MSc (Associate Professor of Obstetrics, Gynecology and Public Health, Department of Obstetrics and Gynecology, Columbia University College of Physicians and Surgeons, New York, NY); and Steven H. Woolf, MD, MPH (Professor of Family Medicine, Department of Family Practice, Medical College of Virginia, Fairfax, VA).

REFERENCES

1. U.S. Preventive Services Task Force. Guide to clinical preventive services, 2nd ed. Washington, DC: Office of Disease Prevention and Health Promotion, U.S. Government Printing Office, 1996.
2 Nelson HD, Helfand M. Screening for chlamydial infection. Am J Prev Med 2001;20(suppl 3):95–107.
3. Nelson HD, Saha S. Screening for chlamydial infection. Systematic evidence review. Pub. No. AHRQ01-S003. Rockville, MD: Agency for Healthcare Research and Quality, 2001.

4. Davies HD, Wang EEL. Periodic health examination, 1996 update: 2. Screening for chlamydial infections. CMAJ 1996;154:1631–44.
5. Centers for Disease Control and Prevention. Recommendations for prevention and management of Chlamydia trachomatis infections. MMWR Morb Mort Wkly Rep 1993;42:1–39.
6. American College of Obstetricians and Gynecologists, ACOG Committee on Primary Care. Committee Opinion No. 229. Washington DC: American College of Obstetricians and Gynecologists, 1999.
7. National Committee for Quality Assurance. HEDIS 2000: The health plan employer data and information set. Volume 1: Narrative—What's in it and why it matters. Washington, DC: National Committee for Quality Assurance, 2000.

Appendix A Third U.S. Preventive Services Task Force (USPSTF) Recommendations and Ratings

---

The USPSTF grades its recommendations according to one of five classifications (A, B, C, D, or I), reflecting the strength of evidence and magnitude of net benefit (benefits minus harms).

A. The USPSTF strongly recommends that clinicians routinely provide [the service] to eligible patients. (The USPSTF found good evidence that [the service] improves important health outcomes and concludes that benefits substantially outweigh harms.)

B. The USPSTF recommends that clinicians routinely provide [the service] to eligible patients. (The USPSTF found at least fair evidence that [the service] improves important health outcomes and concludes that benefits outweigh harms.)

C. The USPSTF makes no recommendation for or against routine provision of [the service]. (The USPSTF found at least fair evidence that [the service] can improve health outcomes but concludes that the balance of benefits and harms is too close to justify a general recommendation.)

D. The USPSTF recommends against routinely providing [the service] to asymptomatic patients. (The USPSTF found at least fair evidence that [the service] is ineffective or that harms outweigh benefits.)

I. The USPSTF concludes that the evidence is insufficient to recommend for or against routinely providing [the service]. (Evidence that [the service] is effective is lacking, of poor quality, or conflicting and the balance of benefits and harms cannot be determined.)

Appendix B Third U.S. Preventive Services Task Force (USPSTF) Strength of Overall Evidence

The USPSTF grades the quality of the overall evidence for a service on a 3-point scale (good, fair, or poor).

Good: Evidence includes consistent results from well-designed, well-conducted studies in representative populations that directly assess effects on health outcomes.

Fair: Evidence is sufficient to determine effects on health outcomes, but the strength of the evidence is limited by the number, quality, or consistency of the individual studies; generalizability to routine practice; or indirect nature of the evidence on health outcomes.

Poor: Evidence is insufficient to assess the effects on health outcomes because of limited number or power of studies, important flaws in their design or conduct, gaps in the chain of evidence, or lack of information on important health outcomes.

Screening Adults for Lipid Disorders

U.S. Preventive Services Task Force

Summary of Recommendations

- The U.S. Preventive Services Task Force (USPSTF) strongly recommends that clinicians routinely screen men aged 35 years and older and women aged 45 years and older for lipid disorders and treat abnormal lipids in people who are at increased risk of coronary heart disease. **A recommendation.**

The USPSTF found good evidence that lipid measurement can identify asymptomatic middle-aged people at increased risk of coronary heart disease and good evidence that lipid-lowering drug therapy substantially decreases the incidence of coronary heart disease in such people with abnormal lipids and causes few major harms. The USPSTF concludes that the benefits of screening for and treating lipid disorders in middle-aged and older people substantially outweigh harms.

- The USPSTF recommends that clinicians routinely screen younger adults (men aged 20 to 35 years and women aged 20 to 45 years) for lipid disorders if they have other risk factors for coronary heart disease. (See Clinical Considerations for a discussion of risk factors.) **B recommendation.**

The USPSTF found good evidence that lipid measurement can identify younger people at increased risk for coronary heart disease, that risk is highest in those with

---

This statement summarizes the third U.S. Preventive Services Task Force (USPSTF) recommendations for screening for lipid disorders and the supporting scientific evidence, and it updates the 1995 recommendations contained in the Guide to Clinical Preventive Services, second edition.[1] Explanations of the ratings and of the strength of overall evidence are given in Appendix A and in Appendix B, respectively. The complete information on which this statement is based, including evidence tables and references, is available in the accompanying article Screening and Treating Adults for Lipid Disorders[2] and in the Systematic Evidence Review[3] on this topic, which can be obtained through the USPSTF Web site (www.ahrq.gov/clinic/uspstfix.htm), and in print through the AHRQ Clearinghouse (1-800-358-9295). Screening for lipid disorders in children and adolescents will be addressed in a separate statement.

Address correspondence to: Alfred O. Berg, MD, MPH, c/o Dana Best, MD, MPH, U.S. Preventive Services Task Force, Agency for Healthcare Research and Quality, Center for Practice and Technology Assessment, 6010 Executive Boulevard, Suite 300, Rockville, MD 20912. E-mail: dbest@ahrq.gov

Reprints are available from the AHRQ Web site at www.ahrq.gov/clinic/uspstfix.htm, through the National Guideline Clearinghouse (www.guideline.gov), or in print through the AHRQ Publications Clearinghouse (1-800-358-9295).

other risk factors, and that the absolute benefits of lipid-lowering treatment depend on a person's underlying risk of coronary heart disease. The USPSTF concludes that benefits of screening for and treating high-risk young adults outweigh harms.

- The USPSTF makes no recommendation for or against routine screening for lipid disorders in younger adults (men aged 20 to 35 years or women aged 20 to 45 years) in the absence of known risk factors for coronary heart disease. **C recommendation**.

The USPSTF found good evidence that lipid measurement in low-risk young adults can detect some individuals at increased long-term risk of heart disease, but the absolute reduction in risk as a result of treating dyslipidemia in most people is small before middle age. Fair evidence suggests that a substantial proportion of the benefits of treatment may be realized within 5 years of initiating therapy. The USPSTF concludes the net benefits of screening for lipid disorders in low-risk young people are not sufficient to make a general recommendation.

- The USPSTF recommends that screening for lipid disorders include measurement of total cholesterol (TC) and high-density lipoprotein cholesterol (HDLC). **B recommendation**.

The USPSTF found good evidence that measurement of HDL-C along with TC improves the identification of people at increased risk of cardiovascular disease. Good evidence from randomized trials demonstrates that people with low HDL-C without high TC benefit from treatment.

- The USPSTF concludes that the evidence is insufficient to recommend for or against triglyceride measurement as a part of routine screening for lipid disorders. **I recommendation**.

Evidence that elevated triglyceride level is an independent risk factor for heart disease is conflicting, and prospective data are lacking to determine whether including triglyceride is more effective for screening than simply measuring TC and HDL-C.

Clinical Considerations

- TC and HDL-C can be measured on nonfasting or fasting samples.

Abnormal results should be confirmed by a repeated sample on a separate occasion, and the average of both results should be used for risk assessment. Although measuring both TC and HDL-C is more sensitive and specific for assessing coronary heart disease risk, TC alone is an acceptable screening test if available laboratory services cannot provide reliable measurements of HDL. In conjunction with HDL-C, low-density lipoprotein cholesterol (LDL-C) and TC provide comparable information, but measuring LDL-C requires a fasting sample and is more expensive. In patients with elevated risk on screening results, lipoprotein analysis, including fasting triglycerides, may provide information that is useful in choosing optimal treatments.

- Screening is recommended for men aged 20 to 35 years and for women aged 20 to 45 years in the presence of any of the following:
  - Diabetes
  - A family history of cardiovascular disease before age 50 years in male relatives or age 60 years in female relatives
  - A family history suggestive of familial hyperlipidemia
  - Multiple coronary heart disease risk factors (e.g., tobacco use, hypertension)

- The optimal interval for screening is uncertain.

On the basis of other guidelines and expert opinion, reasonable options include every 5 years, shorter intervals for people who have lipid levels close to those warranting therapy, and longer intervals for low-risk people who have had low or repeatedly normal lipid levels.

- An age to stop screening is not established.

Screening may be appropriate in older people who have never been screened, but repeated screening is less important in older people because lipid levels are less likely to increase after age 65 years.

- Treatment decisions should take into account overall risk of heart disease rather than lipid levels alone.

Overall risk assessment should include the presence and severity of the following risk factors: age, gender, diabetes, elevated blood pressure, family history (in younger adults), and smoking. Tools that incorporate specific information on multiple risk factors provide more accurate estimation of cardiovascular risk than categorizations based on counting the numbers of risk factors.[4,5]

- Treatment choices should take into account costs and patient preferences.

Drug therapy is usually more effective than diet alone, but choice of treatment should consider overall risk, costs of treatment, and patient preferences. Guidelines for treating high cholesterol are available from the National Cholesterol Education Program of the National Institutes of Health.[6] Although diet therapy is an appropriate initial therapy for most patients, a minority achieve substantial reductions in lipid levels from diet alone; drugs are frequently needed to achieve therapeutic goals, especially for high-risk people. Lipidlowering treatments should be accompanied by interventions addressing all modifiable risk factors for heart disease, including smoking cessation, treatment of blood pressure, diabetes, and obesity, as well as promotion of a healthy diet and regular physical activity. Long-term adherence to therapies should be emphasized.

- All patients, regardless of lipid levels, should be offered counseling about the benefits of a diet low in saturated fat and high in fruits and vegetables, regular physical activity, avoiding tobacco use, and maintaining a healthy weight.

Scientific Evidence

Epidemiology and Clinical Consequences

Consistent evidence from long-term, prospective studies indicates that high levels of TC and LDL-C and low levels of HDL-C are important risk factors for coronary heart disease, the leading cause of mortality and morbidity in the United States. The risk for coronary heart disease increases with increasing levels of TC and LDL-C, and declining levels of HDL-C, in a continuous and graded fashion with no clear threshold of risk. According to National Center for Health Statistics data from 1988 to 1994, 17.5% of men and 20% of women aged 20 to 74 years had high levels of TC (240 mg/dL or greater).

Accuracy and Reliability of Screening Test

TC, LDL-C, and HDL-C are independent predictors of coronary heart disease risk, but considering other risk factors (age, diabetes, smoking, blood pressure) in addition to lipid levels markedly improves the estimation of risk. The ratios of TC to HDL-C (TC/HDL-C) or LDL-C to HDL-C (LDL-C/HDL-C) classify risk better than TC alone.

TC and HDL-C can be measured accurately on nonfasting venous or capillary blood samples, but LDL-C requires fasting samples for accurate measurement. At least two measurements are necessary to ensure that true values are within 10% of the mean of the measurements.

Effectiveness of Early Intervention

In four large primary prevention trials, cholesterol-lowering drug treatment for 5 to 7 years decreased risk of coronary heart disease events approximately 30% in people with high TC or average cholesterol and low HDL-C. In the one trial that included women, treatment appeared to be as effective in postmenopausal women as in men. The average benefit of treating abnormal lipids in women, however, may be smaller than in men of similar ages because of their lower rates of heart disease. Although trials have enrolled few people younger than age 45 years or older than age 65 years, the USPSTF concluded that the benefits of treatment could be generalized to older and younger people whose underlying risk of coronary heart disease is comparable to or greater than that of subjects in the existing trials (annual incidence of coronary heart disease 0.6% to 1.5% per year).

The only trials examining diet with coronary heart disease outcomes have modified diet in conjunction with interventions on other risk factors, in patients with heart disease, or using atypical institutional diets. Reducing dietary saturated fat and weight loss can lower TC and LDL-C as much as 10% to 20% in some individuals, but the average effect of diet interventions in outpatients is relatively modest (2% to 6% reduction in TC). Lipid screening does not clearly improve the effectiveness of routine diet interventions.

Potential Adverse Effects of Screening

Studies of adverse effects of screening are limited but have not found adverse psychological effects (i.e., labeling) in patients identified with abnormal lipids. Screening could subject some low-risk people to the inconvenience and expense of treatments that may offer only minimal benefits.

Discussion

The clearest benefit of lipid screening is identifying individuals whose near-term risk of coronary heart disease is sufficiently high to justify drug therapy or other intensive lifestyle interventions to lower cholesterol. Screening men older than age 35 years and women older than age 45 years will identify nearly all individuals whose risk of coronary heart disease is as high as that of the subjects in the existing primary prevention trials. In a population with a 1% risk of coronary heart disease per year, drug treatment of 67 people for 5 years is required to prevent one coronary heart disease event. Most younger people have a substantially lower risk, unless they have other important risk factors for coronary heart disease or familial hyperlipidemia.

The primary goal of screening younger people is to promote lifestyle changes, which may provide longterm benefits later in life. The average effect of diet interventions is small, however, and screening is not necessary to advise young adults about the benefits of a healthy diet and regular exercise. Although universal screening may detect some patients with familial hyperlipidemia earlier than selective screening, whether this will lead to important reductions in coronary events is not known.

Recommendations of Others

Routine measurement of nonfasting TC and HDL every 5 years is recommended by the National Cholesterol Education Program's Adult Treatment Panel II (ATP II), sponsored by the National Institutes of Health,[6] and endorsed by the American Heart Association[7] and the American College of Obstetricians and Gynecologists.[8] The American College of Physicians and American Academy of Family Physicians suggest periodic cholesterol measurement in men aged 35 to 65 years and in women aged 45 to 65 years.[9-11] In 1994, the Canadian Task Force on Preventive Health Care recommended selective case-finding in men aged 30 to 59 years, rather than routine screening.[12] The ATP II and the Canadian Task Force recommendations are currently being updated.

Members of the U.S. Preventive Services Task Force are: Alfred O. Berg, MD, MPH, Chair, USPSTF (Professor and Chair, Department of Family Medicine, University of Washington, Seattle, WA); Janet D. Allan, PhD, RN, CS, Vice-chair, USPSTF (Dean and Professor, School of Nursing, University of Texas Health Science Center, San Antonio, TX); Paul S. Frame, MD (Tri-County Family Medicine, Cohocton, NY, and Clinical Professor of Family Medicine, University of Rochester, Rochester, NY); Charles J. Homer, MD, MPH (Executive Director, National Initiative for Children's Healthcare Quality, Boston, MA); Tracy A. Lieu, MD, MPH (Associate Professor, Department of Ambulatory Care and Prevention, Harvard Pilgrim Health Care and Harvard Medical School, Boston, MA); Cynthia D. Mulrow, MD, MSc (Professor of Medicine, University of Texas Health Science Center, Audie L. Murphy Memorial Veterans Hospital, San Antonio, TX); C. Tracy Orleans, PhD (Senior Scientist, The Robert Wood Johnson Foundation, Princeton, NJ); Jeffrey F. Peipert, MD, MPH (Director of Research, Women and Infants' Hospital, Providence, RI); Nola J. Pender, PhD, RN (Professor and Associate Dean for Research, School of Nursing, University of Michigan, Ann Arbor, MI); Harold C. Sox Jr, MD (Professor and Chair, Department of Medicine, Dartmouth-Hitchcock Medical Center, Lebanon, NH); Steven M. Teutsch, MD, MPH (Senior Director, Outcomes Research and Management, Merck & Company, Inc., West Point, PA); Carolyn Westhoff, MD, MSc (Associate Professor of Obstetrics, Gynecology and Public Health, Department of Obstetrics and Gynecology, Columbia University College of Physicians and Surgeons, New York, NY); and Steven H. Woolf, MD, MPH (Professor of Family Medicine, Department of Family Practice, Medical College of Virginia, Fairfax, VA).

REFERENCES

1. U.S. Preventive Services Task Force. Guide to clinical preventive services. 2nd ed. Washington, DC: Office of Disease Prevention and Health Promotion, U.S. Government Printing Office, 1996.
2. Pignone MP, Phillips CJ, Atkins D, Teutsch SM, Mulrow CD, Lohr KN. Am J Prev Med 2001;20(3S) 75 Screening and treating adults for lipid disorders. Am J Prev Med 2001;20: 77–89.
3. Pignone MP, Phillips CJ, Lannon CM, et al. Screening Adults for Lipid Disorders. Systematic Evidence Review. Pub. No. AHRQ01-S004. Rockville, MD: Agency for Healthcare Research and Quality, 2001.

4. Wilson PW, D'Agostino RB, Levy D, Belanger AM, Silbershatz H, Kannel WB. Prediction of coronary heart disease using risk factor categories. Circulation 1998;97:1837–47.
5. Jackson R. Updated New Zealand cardiovascular disease risk-benefit prediction guide. BMJ 2000;320:709–10. Also available at: www.bmj.com/cgi/content/full/320/7236/709.
6. Summary of the second report of the National Cholesterol Education Program (NCEP) Expert Panel on the Detection, Evaluation, and Treatment of High Blood Cholesterol in Adults (Adult Treatment Panel II). JAMA 1993;269:3015–23.
7. Grundy SM, Balady GJ, Criqui MH, et al. A statement for healthcare professionals from the Task Force on Risk Reduction, Consensus Panel Statement (AHA). Circulation 1997;95:2330.
8. American College of Obstetricians and Gynecologists (ACOG), Committee on Primary Care. Primary and Preventive Care: Periodic Assessments. Committee Opinion No. 229. Washington, DC: ACOG; December 1999.
9. American Academy of Family Physicians. Clinical recommendations: 2000–2001. Leawood, KS: American Academy of Family Physicians; 2001. In press. Also available at www.aafp.org/exam/.
10. Garber AM, Browner WS, Hulley SB. Clinical guideline, Part II: cholesterol screening in asymptomatic adults, revisited. Ann Intern Med 1996;124: 518–31.
11. Garber AM, Browner WS, Hulley SB. Guidelines for using serum cholesterol, high-density lipoprotein cholesterol, and triglyceride levels as screening tests for preventing coronary heart disease in adults. Ann Intern Med 1996;124:515–7.
12. Logan AG. Lowering the blood total cholesterol level to present coronary heart disease. In: Canadian Task Force on the Periodic Health Examination. Canadian Guide to Clinical Preventive Health Care. Ottawa: Health Canada; 1994:650–69.

Appendix A Third U.S. Preventive Services Task Force (USPSTF) Recommendations and Ratings

The USPSTF grades its recommendations according to one of five classifications (A, B, C, D, or I), reflecting the strength of evidence and magnitude of net benefit (benefits minus harms).

A. The USPSTF strongly recommends that clinicians routinely provide [the service] to eligible patients. (The USPSTF found good evidence that [the service] improves important health outcomes and concludes that benefits substantially outweigh harms.)

B. The USPSTF recommends that clinicians routinely provide [the service] to eligible patients. (The USPSTF found at least fair evidence that [the service] improves important health outcomes and concludes that benefits outweigh harms.)

C. The USPSTF makes no recommendation for or against routine provision of [the service]. (The USPSTF found at least fair evidence that [the service] can improve health outcomes but concludes that the balance of benefits and harms is too close to justify a general recommendation.)

D. The USPSTF recommends against routinely providing [the service] to asymptomatic patients. (The USPSTF found at least fair evidence that [the service] is ineffective or that harms outweigh benefits.)

I. The USPSTF concludes that the evidence is insufficient to recommend for or against routinely providing [the service]. (Evidence that [the service] is effective is lacking, of poor quality, or conflicting and that the balance of benefits and harms cannot be determined.)

Appendix B Third U.S. Preventive Services Task Force (USPSTF)
Strength of Overall Evidence

The USPSTF grades the quality of the overall evidence for a service on a 3-point scale (good, fair, or poor).

Good: Evidence includes consistent results from well-designed, well-conducted studies in representative populations that directly assess effects on health outcomes.

Fair: Evidence is sufficient to determine effects on health outcomes, but the strength of the evidence is limited by the number, quality, or consistency of the individual studies; generalizability to routine practice; or indirect nature of the evidence on health outcomes.

Poor: Evidence is insufficient to assess the effects on health outcomes because of limited number or power of studies, important flaws in their design or conduct, gaps in the chain of evidence, or lack of information on important health outcomes.

Newborn Hearing Screening

U.S. Preventive Services Task Force

Summary of Recommendation

- The USPSTF concludes the evidence is insufficient to recommend for or against routine screening of newborns for hearing loss during the post-partum hospitalization. **I recommendation.**

  The USPSTF found good evidence that newborn hearing screening leads to earlier identification and treatment of infants with hearing loss. However, evidence to determine whether earlier treatment resulting from screening leads to clinically important improvement in speech and language skills at age 3 years or beyond is inconclusive because of the design limitations in existing studies.

  Although earlier identification and intervention may improve the quality of life for the infant and family during the first year of life, and prevent regret by the family over delayed diagnosis of hearing loss, the USPSTF found few data addressing these benefits. The USPSTF could not determine from existing studies whether these potential benefits outweigh the potential harms of false-positive tests that many low-risk infants would experience following universal screening in both high- and low-risk groups.

  The USPSTF found good evidence that the prevalence of hearing loss in infants in the newborn intensive care unit (NICU) and those with other specific risk factors (see "Clinical Considerations") is 10 to 20 times higher than the

This statement summarizes the third U.S. Preventive Services Task Force (USPSTF) recommendations on newborn hearing screening and the supporting scientific evidence, and it updates the 1995 recommendations contained in the *Guide to Clinical Preventive Services, second edition.*[1] Explanations of the ratings and of the strength of overall evidence are given in Appendix A and Appendix B, respectively. The complete information on which this statement is based, including evidence tables and references, is available in the article, "Universal Newborn Hearing Screening: A Summary of the Evidence"[2] and in the Systematic Evidence Review[3] and Summary of the Evidence on this topic, which can be obtained through the USP-STF Web site (www.ahrq.gov/clinic/uspstfix.htm), through the National Guideline Clearinghouse (www.guideline.gov), or in print through the AHRQ Publications Clearinghouse (1-800-358-9295).

Corresponding Author: Alfred O. Berg, MD, MPH, Chair, U.S. Preventive Services Task Force, c/o David Atkins, MD, MPH, Scientific and Technical Editor, U.S. Preventive Services Task Force, Agency for Healthcare Research and Quality, Center for Practice and Technology Assessment, 6010 Executive Boulevard, Suite 300, Rockville, MD 20852. (301) 594-4016, fax (301) 594-4027, E-mail: datkins@ahrq.gov *prevalence of hearing loss in the general population of newborns. Both the yield of screening and the proportion of true positive results will be substantially higher when screening is targeted at these high-risk infants, but selective screening programs typically do not identify all infants with risk factors. Evidence that early identification and intervention for hearing loss improves speech, language, or auditory outcomes in high-risk populations is also limited.*

Clinical Considerations

• Currently, universal newborn hearing screening (UNHS) is required by law in more than 30 states and is performed routinely in some health care systems in other states. Selective screening of infants in the NICU and those with other risk

• Risk factors for sensorineural hearing loss (SNHL) among newborns include NICU admission for 2 days or more; syndromes known to include hearing loss (eg, Usher's syndrome, Waardenburg's syndrome); family history of childhood SNHL; congenital infections (eg, toxoplasmosis, bacterial meningitis, syphilis, rubella, cytomegalovirus, herpes virus); and craniofacial abnormalities (especially morphologic abnormalities of the pinna and ear canal).

• If a program for routine hearing screening of newborns is implemented, it should include systematic education to fully inform parents and clinicians about the potential benefits and harms of the testing protocol. Most infants with positive in-hospital screening tests will subsequently be found to have normal hearing, and clinicians should be prepared to provide reassurance and support to parents of infants who need follow-up audiologic evaluation.

• If any program for newborn hearing screening is implemented, screening should be conducted using a validated protocol, usually requiring 2 screening tests. Equipment used should be well maintained, staff should be thoroughly trained, and quality control programs to reduce avoidable false-positive tests should be in place. Programs should develop protocols to ensure that infants with positive screening tests receive appropriate audiologic evaluation and follow-up after discharge.

Scientific Evidence

Epidemiology and Clinical Consequences

Each year, an estimated 5,000 infants are born in the United States with moderate, severe, or profound bilateral SNHL. The estimated prevalence of bilateral SNHL is 1–2 per 1,000 newborns in the U.S., but may be 10–20 times higher among infants in the NICU than in the healthy nursery population. Prevalence of bilateral SNHL is also increased in infants with other selected risk factors (see "Clinical Considerations").

The diagnosis of congenital hearing loss is often delayed. In one survey conducted before hearing screening was common, the median age at diagnosis was 13 months for infants with severe to profound bilateral SNHL and 17 months for those with mild to moderate hearing losses.[4]

Children with hearing loss experience delayed development in language, learning, and speech. Impairment exists as early as age 3 years and has consequences throughout life, leading to lower reading abilities, poorer school performance, and under- or unemployment.

Accuracy, Reliability, and Short-Term Impact of Screening Tests

Between 50% and 75% of infants with moderate to profound bilateral SNHL have one or more specific risk factors (see "Clinical Considerations").[5,6] Until recently, most newborn hearing screening programs in the United States focused on identifying and screening infants at risk for SNHL. However, these programs typically do not identify infants at risk for hearing loss due to failure to administer screening questionnaires or loss to follow-up, and they will miss affected infants who have no risk factors.

In the late 1990s, the development of rapid, lowcost screening tests made it feasible to implement screening programs for all newborns for congenital hearing loss during the birth hospitalization. Two types of tests are commonly used: otoacoustic emissions (OAEs) and auditory brainstem response (ABR). Typically, screening programs use a twostage screening approach (either OAE repeated twice, OAE followed by ABR, or automated ABR repeated twice). Criteria for defining a "pass" or "fail" on the initial screening test vary, and results are sensitive to equipment, the tester's training, and ongoing quality control.

The true sensitivity and specificity of newborn hearing screening are difficult to estimate from most screening programs. One large, good-quality study measured the sensitivity and specificity of OAE and ABR using an independent "gold standard," visual reinforcement audiometry, performed at 8 to 12 months.[7] One-stage screening with an ABR or OAE test can detect 80% to 95% of affected ears, depending on how an abnormal test result is defined. The two-stage protocol of OAE and ABR missed 11% of affected ears, but was more specific than testing with the ABR or OAE alone. Because the prevalence of SNHL is low, there are many more false positives than true positives, especially in lowrisk populations. Overall, 6.7% of infants who failed in-hospital screening tests were eventually diagnosed with bilateral SNHL in the best study of newborn hearing screening;

among those without risk factors for hearing loss, only 2% of those failing such screening tests were later found to have SNHL.[8]

Children who fail in-hospital screening tests are usually referred for repeat testing between 2 and 8 weeks after discharge; positive second-stage results are usually validated by a combination of otolaryngologic and audiologic consultation, diagnostic ABR testing, or other electrophysiologic testing that can be performed as early as age 3 months. Visual reinforcement audiometry cannot be performed reliably before age 8 to 9 months.

Universal newborn hearing screening reduces the age at which infants with hearing loss are diagnosed and treated. Studies of statewide universal newborn hearing screening programs in the United States have found that the mean age of identification of hearing impairment has decreased from 12–13 months before screening programs were introduced to 3-6 months since their introduction.[9,10] The mean age at which infants receive hearing aids has been reduced from 13–16 months before universal newborn hearing screening programs began to 5–7 months[9,11] following their introduction. In a large controlled study comparing in-hospital UNHS with no screening, UNHS significantly increased the number of infants with hearing loss referred to audiologists by the age of 6 months and increased the probability that infants with moderate and severe hearing loss would be diagnosed by the age of 10 months (57% vs 14%).[8] Compared with selective screening of high-risk newborns, universal screening would result in the early diagnosis (before 10 months) of one additional case for every 1,441 infants screened, and early treatment (before 10 months) of one additional case for every 2,401 newborns screened, by one estimate.[2,3]

Effectiveness of Early Intervention to Improve Language Outcomes

There are no prospective, controlled studies that directly examine whether newborn hearing screening and earlier intervention result in improved speech, language, or educational development.

Although several retrospective studies have variously concluded that infants entering treatment programs at younger ages, or infants identified in hospitals with universal screening programs, have better long-term language outcomes,[2,3] all of these studies have significant methodological flaws.

All of the available retrospective studies began with a convenience sample of children enrolled in early intervention programs, rather than with an inception cohort of children at the point of identification of hearing loss. None described loss to follow-up between enrollment in the intervention program and the age of assessment, and criteria for inclusion and exclusion were not clearly described. In most studies, early identification was not necessarily the result of screening. Therefore, underlying differences between children identified or enrolled early and those identified or enrolled late may have contributed to the observed language differences. Although some studies attempted to adjust for appropriate confounding factors, the USPSTF judged that statistical adjustment cannot compensate for the potential biases arising from unbalanced cohort selection, concluding that the studies do not establish the effectiveness of early identification and treatment.

Other Potential Benefits or Harms of Screening and Treatment

Because UNHS reduces the average age for intervention by 6 to 9 months, improved hearing or increased prelanguage stimulation over that period might, in themselves, be considered important benefits of newborn hearing screening. In addition, there might be a psychological benefit to parents or to hearing-impaired children of avoiding regret in the future due to the delayed diagnosis and treatment of hearing impairment. However, the USPSTF was unable to identify any evidence that would allow it to assess the magnitude of these potential benefits or determine whether they alone were sufficient to offset the potential harms of screening.

Because most positive screening tests are false positives, the most likely potential adverse effects of screening are parental anxiety and misunderstanding, and labeling of normal infants as hearing-impaired until the definitive diagnosis can be made months later. Even a small increased risk of these effects could have a large impact on the net benefit of a screening program. In low-risk populations, there are 25 to 50 false positives for each true case of hearing impairment.[8] In existing newborn hearing screening programs, 13% to 31% do not follow up for definitive testing, which might allay concerns about the baby's health.

Findings from studies that evaluated parental anxiety are mixed. In the largest controlled trial of screening, parents whose infants were screened had similar anxiety and attitudes as parents whose infants were not screened.[12] In another survey, 98% of parents said they would give permission for screening, 95% said they would prefer screening even if the baby failed, and 85% said that anxiety caused by failing a screening test would be outweighed by the potential benefit of early detection.[13] In other studies, false-positive results produced significant or lasting anxiety in 3% to 14% of parents, even after follow-up testing. No studies have evaluated whether parental anxiety has any long-term effect on parent-child interaction.

Because definitive diagnoses may take months to confirm, false-positive diagnosis of SNHL may occasionally lead to unnecessary intervention in an infant who hears normally. In one large screening trial, the initial audiologic diagnosis was incorrect in 2 of 27 infants diagnosed with SNHL (7%), and the infants proved to have normal hearing when reexamined at age 4 months or 10 months.[2,3]

The yield of newborn hearing screening is comparable to or higher than that of other wellaccepted newborn screening programs. To identify one infant with moderate to severe hearing loss, newborn hearing screening would require screening an estimated 600 infants. Relative to selective screening, universal newborn hearing screening requires screening an estimated 1,400 infants to identify one additional affected infant, yields that are comparable to or better than those for newborn screening programs for other disorders, including hemoglobinopathy and phenylketonuria.1 Thus, if the effects of screening and subsequent treatment on longer-term language outcomes could be confirmed, the cost-effectiveness of newborn hearing screening might be equal or superior to that of many other newborn screening services.

Recommendations of Others

The Joint Committee on Infant Hearing 2000 Position Statement, developed and approved by the American Academy of Audiology, the American Academy of Pediatrics (AAP), the American Speech-Language-Hearing Association (ASHA), the Council on Education of the Deaf, and Directors of Speech and Hearing Programs in State Health and Welfare Agencies, endorses early detection of and intervention for infants with hearing loss (early hearing detection and intervention, [EHDI]) through integrated, interdisciplinary state and national systems of UNHS, evaluation, and familycentered intervention.[5] Audiologic evaluation and medical evaluations should be in progress before 3 months of age. Infants with confirmed hearing loss should receive intervention before 6 months of age from health care and education professionals with expertise in hearing loss and deafness in infants and young children.[5,14,15]

The Centers for Disease Control and Prevention supports universal newborn hearing screening through its Early Hearing Detection and Intervention (EHDI) Program, which assists states in implementing screening and intervention programs and supports research and data collection on EHDI programs.[16] A 1993 National Institutes of Health Consensus Development Panel also recommended universal screening for hearing impairment prior to 3 months of age in order to identify and initiate treatment for all hearing-impaired infants by 6 months of age.[17] A publication promoting the early identification of hearing loss has been published by the Maternal and Child Health Bureau of the Health Resources and Services Administration (HRSA). HRSA supports universal screening and has provided funding to assist states in developing such programs.[18]

The American Academy of Family Physicians (AAFP) and the Canadian Task Force on Preventive Health Care are currently reviewing their positions on Universal Newborn Hearing Screening. The American

College of Obstetricians and Gynecologists recommends screening for hearing loss in neonates with any of the following risk factors: family history of hereditary childhood SNHL, in utero infection, craniofacial anomalies, birth weight less than 1,500 grams, hyperbilirubinemia requiring exchange transfusion, ototoxic medications, bacterial meningitis, Apgar score of 0–4 at 1 minute or 0–6 at 5 minutes after birth, mechanical ventilation lasting 5 days or longer, or stigmata or other findings associated with a syndrome known to include a sensorineural or conductive hearing loss.[19]

The British National Coordinating Centre for Health Technology Assessment supports universal neonatal hearing screening, supplemented by a targeted infant distraction test at about 7 months of age, primarily for those children not screened neonatally.[20]

REFERENCES

1. U.S. Preventive Services Task Force. Guide to Clinical Preventive Services, second edition. Washington, DC: Office of Disease Prevention and Health Promotion; 1996.
2. Thompson DC, McPhillips H, Davis RL, Lieu TA, Homer CJ, and Helfand M. Universal newborn hearing screening: summary of evidence. *JAMA*. 2001; 286.
3. Helfand M, Thompson DC, Davis R, McPhillips H, Homer CJ, Lieu TA. Newborn *Hearing Screening: Systematic Evidence Review*. Pub. No. AHRQ02-S001. Rockville, MD: Agency for Healthcare Research and Quality; 2001 (forthcoming).
4. Harrison M, Roush J. Age of suspicion, identification, and intervention for infants and young children with hearing loss: a national study. *Ear Hear*. 1996;17(1):55–62.
5. Joint Committee on Infant Hearing. Joint Committee on Infant Hearing Year 2000 Position Statement: Principles and Guidelines for Early Hearing Detection and Intervention Programs. *Pediatrics*. 2000;106(4):798–817. Available at: http://www.infanthearing.org/jcih/. (accessed October 15, 2001).
6. Fortnum H, Davis A. Epidemiology of permanent childhood hearing impairment in Trent Region, 1985–1993. *Br J Audiol*. 1997;31(6):409–46.
7. Norton SJ, Gorga MP, Widen JE, et al. Identification of neonatal hearing impairment: evaluation of transient evoked otoacoustic emission, distortion product otoacoustic emission, and auditory brain stem response test performance. *Ear Hear*. 2000;21:508–28.
8. Wessex Universal Neonatal Hearing Screening Trial Group. Controlled trial of universal neonatal screening for early identification of permanent childhood hearing impairment. Wessex Universal Neonatal Hearing Screening Trial Group. *Lancet*. 1998;352:1957–64.
9. Vohr BR, Carty LM, Moore PE, Letourneau K. The Rhode Island Hearing Assessment Program: experience with statewide hearing screening (1993–1996). *J Pediatr*. 1998;133(3):353–7.
10. Johnson JL, Kuntz NL, Sia CC, White KR, Johnson RL. Newborn hearing screening in Hawaii. *Hawaii Med J*. 1997;56(12):352–5.
11. Prieve B, Dalzell L, Berg A, Bradley M, Cacace A. The New York State universal newborn hearing screening demonstration project: outpatient outcome measures. *Ear Hear*. 2000;21(2).
12. Kennedy CR. Controlled trial of universal neonatal screening for early identification of permanent childhood hearing impairment: coverage, positive predictive value, effect on mothers and incremental yield. Wessex Universal Neonatal Screening Trial Group. *Acta Paediatr Suppl*. 1999;88(432):73–5.
13. Barringer DG, Mauk GW. Survey of parents perceptions regarding hospital-based newborn hearing screening. *Audiol Today*. 1997;9:18–19.
14. American Academy of Pediatrics. Task Force on Newborn and Infant Hearing. Newborn and infant hearing loss: detection and intervention, 1998–1999. *Pediatrics*. 1999;103(2): 527–30.
15. Pediatricians make new recommendations on hearing screening [press release]. American Academy of Pediatrics; April 5, 1999. Available at: http://www.aap.org
16. Centers for Disease Control, National Center for Birth Defects and Developmental Disabilities, Early Hearing Detection and Intervention Program. What is EHDI? Accessed at: http://www.cdc.gov/ncb-ddd/ehdi/ehdi.htm October 15, 2001.

17. National Institutes of Health. Early identification of hearing impairment in infants and young children. NIH Consensus Statement. 1993; Mar 1–3;11(1):1–24. Accessed at: http://text.nlm.nih.gov/nih/cdc/www/92txt .html

18. National Center for Hearing Assessment and Management. Early identification of hearing loss: implementing universal newborn hearing screening programs. National Center for Hearing Assessment and Management; 1997. Accessed at: http://www.infanthearing.org/ impguide/impguide.pdf

19. American Academy of Pediatrics and American College of Obstetricians and Gynecologists. *Guidelines for Perinatal Care,* 4th ed. Washington, DC: ACOG. 1997: 160–2.

20. Department of Health. Piloting the introduction of universal neonatal screening in England. Accessed at http://www.doh.gov.uk/uhnspilots/ index.htm October 15, 2001.

Appendix A U.S. Preventive Services Task Force—Recommendations and Ratings

The Task Force grades its recommendations according to one of 5 classifications (A, B, C, D, I) reflecting the strength of evidence and magnitude of net benefit (benefits minus harms):

A. The USPSTF strongly recommends that clinicians routinely provide [the service] to eligible patients. *The USPSTF found good evidence that [the service] improves important health outcomes and concludes that benefits substantially outweigh harms.*

B. The USPSTF recommends that clinicians routinely provide [the service] to eligible patients. *The USPSTF found at least fair evidence that [the service] improves important health outcomes and concludes that benefits outweigh harms.*

C. The USPSTF makes no recommendation for or against routine provision of [the service]. *The USPSTF found at least fair evidence that [the service] can improve health outcomes but concludes that the balance of benefits and harms is too close to justify a general recommendation.*

D. The USPSTF recommends against routinely providing [the service] to asymptomatic patients. *The USPSTF found at least fair evidence that [the service] is ineffective or that harms outweigh benefits.*

I. The USPSTF concludes that the evidence is insufficient to recommend for or against routinely providing [the service]. Evidence that [the service] is effective is lacking, of poor quality, or conflicting and the balance of benefits and harms cannot be determined.

Appendix B U.S. Preventive Services Task Force—Strength of Overall Evidence

The USPSTF grades the quality of the overall evidence for a service on a 3-point scale (good, fair, poor):

Good: Evidence includes consistent results from well-designed, well-conducted studies in representative populations that directly assess effects on health outcomes.

Fair: Evidence is sufficient to determine effects on health outcomes, but the strength of the evidence is limited by the number, quality, or consistency of the individual studies, generalizability to routine practice, or indirect nature of the evidence on health outcomes.

Poor: Evidence is insufficient to assess the effects on health outcomes because of limited number or power of studies, important flaws in their design or conduct, gaps in the chain of evidence, or lack of information on important health outcomes.

MEMBERS OF THE U.S. PREVENTIVE SERVICES TASK FORCE

Alfred O. Berg, MD, MPH Chair, USPSTF (Professor and Chair, Department of Family Medicine, University of Washington, Seattle, WA)

Janet D. Allan, PhD, RN, CS Vice-chair, USPSTF (Dean and Professor, School of Nursing, University of Texas Health Science Center, San Antonio, TX)

Paul S. Frame, MD (Tri-County Family Medicine, Cohocton, NY, and Clinical Professor of Family Medicine, University of Rochester, Rochester, NY)

Charles J. Homer, MD MPH (Executive Director, National Initiative for Children's Healthcare Quality, Boston, MA)

Mark S. Johnson, MD, MPH (Associate Professor of Clinical Family Medicine and Chairman, Department of Family Medicine, University of Medicine and Dentistry of New Jersey-New Jersey Medical School, Newark, NJ)

Jonathan D. Klein, MD, MPH (Associate Professor of Pediatrics and of Community and Preventive Medicine, University of Rochester School of Medicine, Rochester, NY)

Tracy A. Lieu, MD, MPH (Associate Professor, Department of Ambulatory Care and Prevention, Harvard Pilgrim Health Care and Harvard Medical School, Boston, MA)

Cynthia D. Mulrow, MD, MSc (Professor of Medicine, University of Texas Health Science Center, Audie L. Murphy Memorial Veterans Hospital, San Antonio, TX)

C. Tracy Orleans, PhD (Senior Scientist, The Robert Wood Johnson Foundation, Princeton, NJ)

Jeffrey F. Peipert, MD, MPH (Director of Research, Women and Infants' Hospital, Providence, RI)

Nola J. Pender, PhD, RN (Professor and Associate Dean for Research, School of Nursing, University of Michigan, Ann Arbor, MI)

Albert L. Siu, MD, MSPH (Professor of Medicine, Chief of Division of General Internal Medicine, and Medical Director of the Primary Care and Medical Services Care Center, Mount Sinai School of Medicine and The Mount Sinai Medical Center, New York, NY)

Steven M. Teutsch, MD, MPH (Senior Director, Outcomes Research and Management, Merck & Company, Inc., West Point, PA)

Carolyn Westhoff, MD, MSc (Associate Professor of Obstetrics, Gynecology and Public Health, Department of Obstetrics and Gynecology, Columbia University College of Physicians and Surgeons, New York, NY)

Steven H. Woolf, MD, MPH (Professor of Family Medicine, Department of Family Practice, Medical College of Virginia, Fairfax, VA)

Screening for Breast Cancer

U.S. Preventive Services Task Force

Summary of Recommendation

The U.S. Preventive Services Task Force recommends screening mammography, with or without clinical breast examination, every 1–2 years for women aged 40 and older. **B recommendation.**

The USPSTF found fair evidence that mammography screening every 12–33 months significantly reduces mortality from breast cancer. Evidence is strongest for women aged 50–69, the age group generally included in screening trials. For women aged 40–49, the evidence that screening mammography reduces mortality from breast cancer is weaker, and the absolute benefit of mammography is smaller, than it is for older women. Most, but not all, studies indicate a mortality benefit for women undergoing mammography at ages 40–49, but the delay in observed benefit in women younger than 50 makes it difficult to determine the incremental benefit of beginning screening at age 40 rather than at age 50. The absolute benefit is smaller because the incidence of breast cancer is lower among women in their 40s than it is among older women. The USPSTF concluded that the evidence is also generalizable to women aged 70 and older (who face a higher absolute risk of breast cancer) if their life expectancy is not compromised by comorbid disease. The absolute probability of bene-

---

This statement summarizes the current U.S. Preventive Services Task Force (USPSTF) recommendations on screening for breast cancer and the supporting scientific evidence, and it updates the 1996 recommendations contained in the Guide to Clinical Preventive Services, second edition.[1] Explanations of the ratings and of the strength of overall evidence are given in Appendix A and Appendix B, respectively. The complete information on which this statement is based, including evidence tables and references, will be available in the article, "Breast Cancer Screening with Mammography: Summary of the Evidence"[2] and in the Systematic Evidence Review on this topic,[3] prepared for the U.S. Preventive Services Task Force by the AHRQ-supported Evidence-based Practice Center at Oregon Health & Science University. These documents are currently undergoing final revision and will soon be accessible at the USPSTF Web site (www.ahrq.gov/clinic/uspstfix.htm), through the National Guideline Clearinghouse (www.guideline.gov), or in print through the AHRQ Publications Clearinghouse (1-800-358-9295).

To update their recommendations on screening for breast cancer, the USPSTF reviewed the evidence regarding the effectiveness of mammography, clinical breast examination, and breast self-examination in reducing breast cancer mortality. The USPSTF did not review the evidence regarding genetic screening, surveillance of women with prior breast cancer, or formal evaluation of new screening modalities that have not been studied in the general population. A meta-analysis using a Bayesian random effects model was conducted for the USPSTF to obtain a *fits of regular mammography increases along a continuum with age, whereas the likelihood of harms from screening (falsepositive results and unnecessary anxiety, biopsies, and cost) diminishes from ages 40–70. The balance of benefits and potential harms, therefore, grows more favorable as women age. The precise age at which the potential benefits of mammography justify the possible harms is a subjective choice. The USPSTF did not find sufficient evidence to specify the optimal screening interval for women aged 40–49* (see Clinical Considerations).

The U.S. Preventive Services Task Force concludes that the evidence is insufficient to recommend for or against routine clinical breast examination (CBE) alone to screen for breast cancer. **I recommendation.**

No screening trial has examined the benefits of CBE alone (without accompanying mammography) compared to no screening, and design characteristics limit the generalizability of studies that have examined CBE. The USPSTF could not determine the benefits of CBE alone or the incremental benefit of adding CBE to mammography. The USPSTF therefore could not determine whether potential benefits of routine CBE outweigh the potential harms.

The U.S. Preventive Services Task Force concludes that the evidence is insufficient to recommend for or against teaching or performing routine breast self-examination (BSE). **I recommendation.**

The USPSTF found poor evidence to determine whether BSE reduces breast cancer mortality. The USPSTF found fair evidence that BSE is associated with an increased risk of false-positive results and biopsies. Due to design limitations of published and ongoing studies of BSE, the USPSTF could not determine the balance of benefits and potential harms of BSE.

Clinical Considerations

- The precise age at which the benefits from screening mammography justify the potential harms is a subjective judgment and should take into account patient preferences. Clinicians should inform women about the potential benefits (reduced chance of dying from breast cancer), potential harms (eg, false-positive results, unnecessary biopsies), and limita-

summary of relative risk estimates of the effectiveness of screening with mammography, either alone or in combination with clinical breast examination, in reducing breast cancer mortality. Clinical studies that evaluated breast self-examination were included in the review. Sources for estimates cited in this Recommendation and Rationale statement are described in the Systematic Evidence Review on this topic (forthcoming).

Corresponding Author: Alfred O. Berg, MD, MPH, Chair, U.S. Preventive Services Task Force, c/o David Atkins, MD, MPH, Scientific and Technical Editor, U.S. Preventive Services Task Force, Agency for Healthcare Research and Quality, Center for Practice and Technology Assessment, 6010 Executive Boulevard, Suite 300, Rockville, MD 20852. (301) 594-4016, fax (301) 594-4027, E-mail: datkins@ahrq.gov.

tions of the test that apply to women their age. Clinicians should tell women that the balance of benefits and potential harms of mammography improves with increasing age for women between the ages of 40 and 70.

- Women who are at increased risk for breast cancer (eg, those with a family history of breast cancer in a mother or sister, a previous breast biopsy revealing atypical hyperplasia, or first childbirth after age 30) are more likely to benefit from regular mammography than women at lower risk. The recommendation for women to begin routine screening in their 40s is strengthened by a family history of breast cancer having been diagnosed before menopause.

- The USPSTF did not examine whether women should be screened for genetic mutations (eg, BRCA1 and BRCA2) that increase the risk of developing breast cancer, or whether women with genetic mutations might benefit from earlier or more frequent screening for breast cancer.

- In the trials that demonstrated the effectiveness of mammography in lowering breast cancer mortality, screening was performed every 12–33 months. For women aged 50 and older, there is little evidence to suggest that annual mammography is more effective than mammography done every other year. For women aged 40–49, available trials also have not reported a clear advantage of annual mammography over biennial mammography. Nevertheless, some experts recommend annual mammography based on the lower sensitivity of the test and on evidence that tumors grow more rapidly in this age group.

- The precise age at which to discontinue screening mammography is uncertain. Only two randomized controlled trials enrolled women older than 69, and no trials enrolled women older than 74. Older women face a higher probability of developing and dying from breast cancer but also have a greater chance of dying from other causes. Women with comorbid conditions that limit their life expectancy are unlikely to benefit from screening.

- Clinicians should refer patients to mammography screening centers with proper accreditation and quality assurance standards to ensure accurate imaging and radiographic interpretation. Clinicians should adopt office systems to ensure timely and adequate follow-up of abnormal results. A listing of accredited facilities is available at http://www.fda.gov/cdrh/mammography/certified.html

- Clinicians who advise women to perform BSE or who perform routine CBE to screen for breast cancer should understand that there is currently insufficient evidence to determine whether these practices affect

breast cancer mortality, and that they are likely to increase the incidence
of clinical assessments and biopsies.

Scientific Evidence

Epidemiology and Clinical Consequences

Breast cancer is the most common non-skin malignancy among women in
the United States and second only to lung cancer as a cause of cancerrelated death. In 2001, an estimated 192,200 new cases of breast cancer were
diagnosed in American women, and 40,200 women died of the disease.[4]
The risk of developing breast cancer increases with age beginning in the
fourth decade of life. The probability of developing invasive breast cancer
over the next 10 years is 0.4% for women aged 30–39, 1.5% for women
aged 40–49, 2.8% for women aged 50–59, and 3.6% for women aged
60–69.[4] Individual factors other than age that increase the risk for developing breast cancer include family history or a personal history of breast
cancer, biopsy-confirmed atypical hyperplasia, and having a first child after
age 30.[5]

Accuracy and Reliability of Screening Tests

The USPSTF examined the test characteristics of mammography, CBE,
and BSE. Precise estimates of sensitivity and specificity of screening are
made more difficult by the varied criterion standards in available studies.
Estimating the predictive value of positive and negative tests is also difficult
because studies have been conducted on populations with a widely varying
prevalence of breast cancer.

Mammography. Estimates of the sensitivity of mammography vary with
the methods used to calculate it.[2] In a good quality systematic review, the
first round of mammography detected 77% to 95% of cancers diagnosed
over the following year, but only 56% to 86% of cancers diagnosed over the
next 2 years.[6] Sensitivity is lower among women who are younger than 50
(51% to 83%), have denser breasts, or are taking hormone replacement
therapy.[3]

In screening trials, the false-positive rate of the initial round of mammography was 3% to 6% (ie, specificity 94% to 97%).[3] Specificity is
increased with a shorter screening interval and the availability of prior
mammograms.[3] In a large study in a health maintenance organization, the
rate of false-positive mammograms (those requiring some additional follow-up) was higher in women aged 40–59 (7% to 8%) than in women aged
60–79 (4% to 5%).[7]

The probability that an abnormal mammogram is due to cancer
increases with age. A large study in Northern California estimated positive

predictive values for abnormal mammograms at 2% to 4% among women aged 40-49, 5% to 9% among women aged 50–59, and 7% to19% among women aged 60 and older.[3,8] Positive predictive values were also higher among women with a family history of breast cancer in two studies.[3]

Clinical breast examination. In a recent good quality review of data from clinical trials, the sensitivity of CBE ranged from 40% to 69%, specificity from 86% to 99%, and positive predictive value from 4% to 50%, using mammography and interval cancer as the criterion standard.[9] In a large community study, only 4% of women with an abnormal CBE were subsequently diagnosed with cancer.[10]

Breast self-examination. The accuracy of BSE is largely unknown. Available evidence shows sensitivity ranging from 26% to 41% compared with CBE and mammography.[3] Specificity of BSE is largely unknown.

Effectiveness of Early Detection

The USPSTF reviewed 8 randomized controlled trials (RCTs) of mammography (4 of mammography alone and 4 of mammography plus CBE) that have reported results with 11–20 years of follow-up.[8–15] The USPSTF found important methodological limitations in each trial, but rated only one trial as "poor" based on established criteria used by the USPSTF to evaluate the quality of evidence for screening tests. The most serious problems concerned the assembly and maintenance of comparable groups, methods for ascertaining outcomes, and generalizability to routine practice. The USPSTF concluded that the flaws were problematic but unlikely to negate the reasonably consistent and significant mortality reductions observed in these trials.

Imperfections in the mammography trials have been recognized and discussed in the literature and by the original investigators for many years. Recently, a 2001 Cochrane Collaboration review of the same trials concluded that 6 of the 8 trials were "flawed" or of "poor quality" and that the pooled results from the remaining 2 better trials did not support a benefit from mammography. Although the USPSTF was concerned about many (but not all) of the flaws identified in this review, it did not consider the presence of flaws sufficient reason in itself for rejecting trial results. Instead, it examined whether observed mortality reductions in the trials were likely to be explained by the biases potentially introduced by such flaws. Studies rated to be of "fair" quality by the USPSTF contained flaws that were considered unlikely to account for observed benefits (or lack of benefits).

The trials reported mortality reductions ranging from no significant effect (the Canadian trial) to a 32% reduction in breast cancer mortality.

The metaanalysis performed for the USPSTF on the most current published data found that the pooled effect size of the combined trials was sizable and statistically significant: the summary relative risk (RR) of breast cancer death among women randomized to screening in 7 trials that included women older than 50 was 0.77 (95% CI, 0.67–0.89). Eliminating 1 trial considered to be of poor quality and 1 trial that lacked a usual care control group did not change the results (RR = 0.75, 95% CI 0.63–0.89). Similar results were observed in the 4 trials of mammography alone: RR = 0.74 (95% CI 0.59–0.93).

Earlier subgroup analyses from mammography trials raised questions about whether screening is effective in women younger than 50. Seven trials enrolled women aged 40–49. Six of these were rated by the USPSTF to be of at least "fair" quality, but only one of these was designed to specifically address the benefits of screening in this age group: it reported no reduction in breast cancer mortality with annual mammography and CBE.[17] Of the remaining 5 fair-quality trials that included women younger than 50, 2 trials have now reported significant mortality reductions with screening in this age group[12,14], 2 have reported non-significant mortality reductions[11,15], and 1 found no benefit.[13] In a meta-analysis performed for the USPSTF pooling results for women aged 40–49 in these 6 trials, the relative risk of breast cancer mortality was 0.83 (95% CI 0.64–1.04) among screened women; inclusion of the seventh, poor-quality study did not change results.[2] These results are similar to prior meta-analyses based on older data.

Because these data represent a subgroup analysis of trials not designed to test the benefits of beginning screening at a specific age, questions remain about the additional benefits of beginning screening before age 50. On average, the time until mortality benefits begin to be observed in these trials is longer in women younger than 50 than in older women (8 years vs 3 to 4 years) and some of the observed benefits could be due to screening after age 50.[3,22] Analyses of individual studies suggest that at least some of the mortality reduction is due to early detection of tumors before age 50, but definitive estimates of the proportion of benefits due to early screening cannot be made.[3, 23]

Clinical Breast Examination. No study has compared CBE to no screening. The reductions in breast cancer mortality in studies using mammography alone are comparable to those using mammography plus CBE.[3,23]

Breast Self-Examination. The role of BSE in reducing breast cancer mortality has been evaluated in 1 Chinese[24] and 1 Russian[25] RCT and 1 nonrandomized controlled trial of BSE education in the United Kingdom.[26] None of the 3 trials has demonstrated a reduction in breast cancer mortality or significant improvements in the number or stage of cancers detected, with follow-up ranging from 5 to 14 years; follow-up is continuing in 1 trial that observed a slight non-significant reduction in mortality in the BSE group at 9 years.[25] In a goodquality nested case-control analysis from a Canadian screening study, the overall practice of BSE was not associated with a reduction in mortality.[27] Although none of these studies provides support for BSE, the USPSTF concluded that these studies did not exclude a possible benefit, due to their limited duration of follow-up and questions about whether results from other countries are generalizable to women in North America.

When To Stop Screening

Although there are no trial data directly evaluating screening in women older than 74, two RCTs suggest benefits among women enrolled in screening trials up to ages 70 and 74.[14,15] Because risk of breast cancer is high after age 70, the benefits of mammography could be important. However, this is offset by the fact that some older women (especially the very old and those with comorbid illness) will die from other causes before they observe any benefits from early detection.

Screening Interval

In clinical trials, mortality reductions occurred in programs with screening intervals ranging from 12–33 months, with no clear difference due to interval.[13–21] Data suggest that breast cancer grows more rapidly in women younger than 50, and the sensitivity of mammography is lower in this age group; thus, shorter screening intervals have been advocated for women aged 40–49. Among the trials showing or suggesting a benefit of screening in women younger than 50, screening intervals that ranged from 12–33 months appeared to achieve comparable results, providing no direct evidence of incremental benefits over annual screening[13,14,16–18]

Potential Harms of Screening

Similar to other cancer screening tests, the large majority (80% to 90%) of abnormal screening mammograms or CBEs are false-positives.[3] These may require follow-up testing or invasive procedures such as breast biopsy to resolve the diagnosis, and can result in anxiety, inconvenience, discomfort, and additional medical expenses.[3] In 1 large community study, 6.5% of screening mammograms required some additional follow-up and, over a 10-year period, 23% of all women had experienced at least 1 abnormal mammogram.[7] The cumulative risk of a false-positive result after 10 mammograms was estimated to be 49%.[7] The proportion of falsepositive results that lead to biopsy varies substantially in different settings.[28] In screening trials, 1% to 6% of all women screened underwent biopsy, and the proportion of biopsies that revealed cancer ranged from 12% to 78%.[28] In two RCTs, BSE education resulted in a nearly two-fold increase in false-positive results, physician visits, and biopsies for benign disease.[24,25]

The consequences of false-positive mammograms are uncertain. Most, but not all, studies report increased anxiety from an abnormal mammogram.[2] At the same time, some studies report that women in the United States may be willing to accept a relatively high number of false-positive results in the population in return for the benefits of mammography.[2,29] Studies do not indicate that falsepositive results diminish adherence to subsequent screening.[3]

False-negatives also occur with mammograms and CBE. Although false-negative results might provide false reassurance, the USPSTF found no data indicating these led to further delays in diagnosis.[3]

Some experts view the over-diagnosis and treatment of ductal carcinoma in situ (DCIS) as a potential adverse consequence of mammography. Although the natural history of DCIS is variable, many women in the United States are treated aggressively with mastectomy or lumpectomy and radiation.[2] Given the dramatic increase in the incidence of DCIS in the past two decades (750%) and autopsy series suggesting that there is a significant pool of DCIS among women who die of other causes[3], screening may be increasing the number of women undergoing treatment for lesions that might not pose a threat to their health.

A final potential concern about mammography is radiation-induced breast cancer, but there are few data to directly assess this risk. A 1997 review, using risk estimates provided by the Biological Effects of Ionizing Radiation report of the National Academy of Sciences, estimated that annual mammography of 100,000 women for 10 consecutive years beginning at age 40 would result in up to 8 radiation-induced breast cancer deaths.[30]

Recommendations of Others

Nearly all North American organizations support mammography screening, although groups vary in the recommended age to begin screening, the interval for screening, and the role of CBE. The American Medical Association (AMA)[31], the American College of Radiology (ACR)[32], and the American Cancer Society (ACS),[33] all support screening with mammography and CBE beginning at age 40. The American College of Obstetricians and Gynecologists (ACOG)[34] supports screening with mammography beginning at age 40 and CBE beginning at age 19. The Canadian Task Force on Preventive Health Care (CTFPHC),[35] the American Academy of Family Physicians (AAFP),[36] and the American College of Preventive

Medicine (ACPM)[37] recommend beginning mammography for averagerisk women at age 50. AAFP and ACPM recommend that mammography in high-risk women begin at age 40, and AAFP recommends that all women aged 40–49 be counseled about the risks and benefits of mammography before making decisions about screening.[36,37] A 1997 Consensus Development Panel convened by the National Institutes of Health concluded that the evidence was insufficient to determine the benefits of mammography among women aged 40–49. This panel recommended that women aged 40–49 should be counseled about potential benefits and harms before making decisions about mammography.[39] In 2001, the CTF-PHC concluded there was insufficient evidence to recommend for or against mammography in women 40–49.[40]

Organizations differ on their recommendations for the appropriate interval for mammography. Annual mammography is recommended by AMA, ACR, and ACS.[31,32,33] Mammography every 1–2 years is recommended by AAFP, ACPM, and the CTFPHC.[36,37,35] ACOG recommends mammography every 1–2 years for women aged 40–49 and annually for women aged 50 and older.[34]

In their 2001 report, the Canadian Task Force on Preventive Health Care recommends against teaching breast self-examination to women aged 40–69.[41] The AMA, ACOG, ACS, and AAFP support teaching BSE.[31,34,33,36]

REFERENCES

1. U.S. Preventive Services Task Force. *Guide to Clinical Preventive Services, Second Edition.* Washington, DC: Office of Disease Prevention and Health Promotion; 1996.
2. Humphrey LL, Helfand M, Chan BKS. Breast cancer screening with mammography. Summary of the Evidence for the U.S. Preventive Services Task Force (forthcoming).
3. Humphrey LL, Chan BKS, Detlefsen S, Helfand M. Screening for Breast Cancer: Systematic Evidence Review. Rockville, MD: Agency for Healthcare Research and Quality (forthcoming).
4. American Cancer Society. Cancer facts and figures, 2001–2002. Atlanta, Georgia: American Cancer Society. (http://www.cancer.org). Accessed February 18, 2002.
5. National Cancer Institute. Surveillance, Epidemiology, and End Results Program 1995–1997. (http://www.nci.nih.gov). Accessed February 18, 2002.
6. Mushlin AI, Kouides RW, Shapiro DE. Estimating the accuracy of screening mammography: a meta-analysis. *Am J Prev Med.* 1998;14(2):143–153.
7. Elmore JG, Barton MB, Moceri VM, et al. Tenyear risk of false positive screening mammograms and clinical breast examinations. *N Engl J Med.* 1998;338(16):1089–96.
8. Kerlikowske K, Carney PA, Geller B, et al. Performance of screening mammography among women with and without a first-degree relative with breast cancer. *Ann Intern Med.* 2000;133(11):855–863.
9. Barton MB, Harris R, Fletcher SW. Does this patient have breast cancer? The screening clinical breast examination: should it be done? How? *JAMA.* 1999;282(13):1270–80.
10. Bobo JK, Lee NC, Thames SF. Findings from 752,081 clinical breast examinations reported to a national screening program from 1995 through 1998. *J Natl Cancer Inst.* 2000 Jun 21;92(12):971–6.
11. Shapiro S. Periodic screening for breast cancer: the HIP Randomized Controlled Trial Health Insurance Plan. *J Natl Cancer Inst Monogr.* 1997:27–30.
12. Bjurstam N, Bjorneld L, Duffy SW, et al. The Gothenburg breast screening trial: first results on mortality, incidence, and mode of detection for women ages 39–49 years at randomization. *Cancer.* 1997;80(11):2091–2099.

13. Frisell J, Lidbrink E, Hellstrom L, Rutqvist LE. Followup after 11 years—update of mortality results in the Stockholm mammographic screening trial. *Breast Cancer Research & Treatment*. 1997;45:263–270.

14. Andersson I, Janzon L. Reduced breast cancer mortality in women under age 50: updated results from the Malmo Mammographic Screening Program. *J Natl Cancer Inst Monogr.* 1997:63–67.

15. Tabar L, Vitak B, Chen HH, et al. The Swedish Two-County Trial twenty years later. Updated mortality results and new insights from longterm follow-up. *Radiol Clin North Am.* 2000;38(4):625–651.

16. Alexander FE, Anderson TJ, Brown HK, et al. 14 years of follow-up from the Edinburgh randomised trial of breast-cancer screening. *Lancet.* 1999;353(9168):1903–1908.

17. Miller AB, Baines CJ, To T, Wall C. Canadian National Breast Screening Study: 1. Breast cancer detection and death rates among women aged 40 to 49 years [published erratum appears in *Can Med Assoc J.* 1993 Mar 1;148(5):718]. *CMAJ.* 1992;147:1459–1476.

18. Miller AB, Baines CJ, To T, Wall C. Canadian National Breast Screening Study: 2. Breast cancer detection and death rates among women aged 50 to 59 years [published erratum appears in *Can Med Assoc J* 1993 Mar 1;148(5):718]. *CMAJ.* 1992;147:1477–1488.

19. Miller AB, To T, Baines CJ, Wall C. The Canadian National Breast Screening Study: update on breast cancer mortality. *J Natl Cancer Inst Monogr.* 1997:37–41.

20. Harris RP, Helfand M, Woolf SH, et al. Methods of the third U.S. Preventive Services Task Force. *Am J Prev Med.* 2001;20(3S):21–35.

21. Olsen O, Gøtzche PC. Screening for breast cancer with mammography (Cochrane Review), *The Cochrane Library*, issue 4, 2001.

22. Cox B. Variation in the effectiveness of breast screening by year of follow-up. *J Natl Cancer Inst Monogr.* 1997;(22):69–72.

23. Nystrom L, Rutqvist LE, Wall S, et al. Breast cancer screening with mammography: overview of Swedish randomised trials. *Lancet.* 1993 Apr 17;341(8851):973–978.

24. Thomas DB, Gao DL, Self SG, et al. Randomized trial of breast self-examination in Shanghai: methodology and preliminary results. *J Natl Cancer Inst.* 1997;89(5):355–365.

25. Semiglazov VF, Moiseenko VM, Manikhas AG, et al. Interim results of a prospective randomized study of self-examination for early detection of breast cancer. Russia/St.Petersburg/ World Health Organization *Vopr Onkol.* 1999;45(3):265–271.

26. UK Breast Cancer Detection Working Group. 16-year mortality from breast cancer in the UK trial of early detection of breast cancer. *Lancet.* 1999;353(9168):1909–1914.

27. Harvey BJ, Miller AB, Baines CJ, Corey PN. Effect of breast self-examination techniques on the risk of death from breast cancer. *CMAJ.* 1997 Nov 1;157(9):1205–1212.

28. Fletcher SW, Harris RP, Gonzalez JJ, et al. Increasing mammography utilization: a controlled study. *J Natl Cancer Inst.* 1993;85:112–120.

29. Schwartz LM, Woloshin S, Sox HC, Fischhoff B, Welch HG. US women's attitudes to false positive mammography results and detection of ductal carcinoma in situ: cross sectional survey. *Br Med J.* 2000;320(7250):1635–1640.

30. Feig SA, Hendrick RE. Radiation risk from screening mammography of women aged 40–49 years. *J Natl Cancer Inst Monogr.* 1997(22):119– 124.

31. American Medical Association. Report 16 of the Council on Scientific Affairs (A-99). Mammographic Screening for Asymptomatic Women. June 1999. (http://www.amaassn. org/ama/pub/article/2036–2346.html). Accessed January 2002.

32. Feig SA, D'Orsi CJ, Hendrick RE, et al. American College of Radiology guidelines for breast cancer screening. *Am J Roentgenol.* 1998 Jul;171(1):29–33.

33. ACS guidelines for the early detection of breast cancer: update 1997. *CA Cancer J Clin.* 1997; 47(3):150–153.

34. American College of Obstetricians and Gynecologists. Primary and preventive care: periodic assessments. ACOG Committee Opinion 246. Washington, DC: ACOG, 2000.

35. Canadian Task Force on the Periodic Health Examination. Ottawa (Canada): Health Canada; 1994. pp. 788–795 (reaffirmed by the Canadian Task Force on the Periodic Health Examination 1999). (http://www.ctfphc.org/ index.html). Accessed February 18, 2002.

36. Periodic Health Examinations: Summary of AAFP Policy Recommendations & Age Charts. (http://www.aafp.org/exam). Accessed January 2002.

37. Ferrini R, Mannino E, Ramsdell E, Hill L. Screening Mammography for Breast Cancer: American College of Preventive Medicine Practice Policy Statement. *Am J Prev Med.* 1996;12(5):340–341.

38. Early detection of breast cancer. Wellington, New Zealand: Royal New Zealand College of General Practitioners; 1999, 61 pp.

39. NIH Consensus Statement Online 1997 Jan 21–23; 15(1):1–35. (http://odp.od.nih.gov/consensus/cons/103/103_statement.htm). Accessed December 12, 2001.
40. Preventive health care, 2001 update: screening mammography among women aged 40–49 years at average risk of breast cancer. (http://www.ctfphc.org). Accessed January 2002.
41. Preventive health care, 2001 update: Should women be routinely taught breast selfexamination to screen for breast cancer? *CMAJ.* 2001;164 (3):1837–1846.

Appendix A U.S. Preventive Services Task Force—Recommendations and Ratings

The Task Force grades its recommendations according to one of 5 classifications (A, B, C, D, I) reflecting the strength of evidence and magnitude of net benefit (benefits minus harms):

A. The USPSTF strongly recommends that clinicians routinely provide [the service] to eligible patients. *The USPSTF found good evidence that [the service] improves important health outcomes and concludes that benefits substantially outweigh harms.*

B. The USPSTF recommends that clinicians routinely provide [the service] to eligible patients. *The USPSTF found at least fair evidence that [the service] improves important health outcomes and concludes that benefits outweigh harms.*

C. The USPSTF makes no recommendation for or against routine provision of [the service]. *The USPSTF found at least fair evidence that [the service] can improve health outcomes but concludes that the balance of benefits and harms is too close to justify a general recommendation.*

D. The USPSTF recommends against routinely providing [the service] to asymptomatic patients. *The USPSTF found at least fair evidence that [the service] is ineffective or that harms outweigh benefits.*

I. The USPSTF concludes that the evidence is insufficient to recommend for or against routinely providing [the service]. Evidence that [the service] is effective is lacking, of poor quality, or conflicting and the balance of benefits and harms cannot be determined.

Appendix B U.S. Preventive Services Task Force—Strength of Overall Evidence

The USPSTF grades the quality of the overall evidence for a service on a 3-point scale (good, fair, poor):

Good: Evidence includes consistent results from well-designed, well-conducted studies in representative populations that directly assess effects on health outcomes.

Fair: Evidence is sufficient to determine effects on health outcomes, but the strength of the evidence is limited by the number, quality, or consistency of the individual studies, generalizability to routine practice, or indirect nature of the evidence on health outcomes.

Poor: Evidence is insufficient to assess the effects on health outcomes because of limited number or power of studies, important flaws in their design or conduct, gaps in the chain of evidence, or lack of information on important health outcomes.

MEMBERS OF THE U.S. PREVENTIVE SERVICES TASK FORCE

Alfred O. Berg, MD, MPH Chair, USPSTF (Professor and Chair, Department of Family Medicine, University of Washington, Seattle, WA)

Janet D. Allan, PhD, RN, CS Vice-chair, USPSTF (Dean and Professor, School of Nursing, University of Texas Health Science Center, San Antonio, TX)

Paul S. Frame, MD (Tri-County Family Medicine, Cohocton, NY, and Clinical Professor of Family Medicine, University of Rochester, Rochester, NY)

Charles J. Homer, MD MPH (Executive Director, National Initiative for Children's Healthcare Quality, Boston, MA)

Mark S. Johnson, MD, MPH (Associate Professor of Clinical Family Medicine and Chairman, Department of Family Medicine, University of Medicine and Dentistry of New Jersey-New Jersey Medical School, Newark, NJ)

Jonathan D. Klein, MD, MPH (Associate Professor of Pediatrics and of Community and Preventive Medicine, University of Rochester School of Medicine, Rochester, NY)

Tracy A. Lieu, MD, MPH (Associate Professor, Department of Ambulatory Care and Prevention, Harvard Pilgrim Health Care and Harvard Medical School, Boston, MA)

Cynthia D. Mulrow, MD, MSc (Professor of Medicine, University of Texas Health Science Center, Audie L. Murphy Memorial Veterans Hospital, San Antonio, TX)

C. Tracy Orleans, PhD (Senior Scientist, The Robert Wood Johnson Foundation, Princeton, NJ)

Jeffrey F. Peipert, MD, MPH (Director of Research, Women and Infants' Hospital, Providence, RI)

Nola J. Pender, PhD, RN (Professor and Associate Dean for Research, School of Nursing, University of Michigan, Ann Arbor, MI)

Albert L. Siu, MD, MSPH (Professor of Medicine, Chief of Division of General Internal Medicine, and Medical Director of the Primary Care and Medical Services Care Center, Mount Sinai School of Medicine and The Mount Sinai Medical Center, New York, NY)

Steven M. Teutsch, MD, MPH (Senior Director, Outcomes Research and Management, Merck & Company, Inc., West Point, PA)

Carolyn Westhoff, MD, MSc (Associate Professor of Obstetrics, Gynecology and Public Health, Department of Obstetrics and Gynecology, Columbia University College of Physicians and Surgeons, New York, NY)

Steven H. Woolf, MD, MPH (Professor of Family Medicine, Department of Family Practice, Medical College of Virginia, Fairfax, VA)

Screening for Skin Cancer

U.S. Preventive Services Task Force

Summary of Recommendations

- The U.S. Preventive Services Task Force (USPSTF) concludes that the evidence is insufficient to recommend for or against routine screening for skin cancer using a total-body skin examination for the early detection of cutaneous melanoma, basal cell cancer, or squamous cell skin cancer. **I recommendation.**

Evidence is lacking that skin examination by clinicians is effective in reducing mortality or morbidity from skin cancer. The USPSTF could not determine the benefits and harms of periodic skin examination. (See Clinical Considerations for discussion of selected populations at high risk.)

Other strategies to prevent skin cancer, such as counseling to reduce risky health behaviors and performance of skin self-examination, will be addressed in a separate recommendation.

This statement summarizes the third U.S. Preventive Services Task Force (USPSTF) recommendations for screening for skin cancer and supporting scientific evidence, and updates the 1995 recommendations contained in the *Guide to Clinical Preventive Services*, second edition.[1] Explanations of the ratings and of the strength of overall evidence are given in Appendix A and in Appendix B, respectively. The complete information upon which this statement is based, including evidence tables and references, is available in the accompanying article Screening for Skin Cancer[2] and in the Systematic Evidence Review[3] on this topic, which can be obtained through the USPSTF Web site (www.ahrq.gov/clinic/uspstfix.htm), through the National Guideline Clearinghouse (www.guideline.gov), or in print through the AHRQ Clearinghouse (1-800-358-9295).

Address correspondence to: Alfred O. Berg, MD, MPH, Chair, U.S. Preventive Services Task Force, c/o Dana Best, MD, MPH, Assistant Scientific and Technical Editor, U.S. Preventive Services Task Force, Agency for Healthcare Research and Quality, Center for Practice and Technology Assessment, 6010 Executive Boulevard, Suite 300, Rockville, MD 20912. E-mail: dbest@ahrq.gov.

Reprints are available from the AHRQ Web site at www.ahrq.gov/clinic/uspstfix.htm, through the National Guideline Clearinghouse (www.guideline.gov), or in print through the AHRQ Publications Clearinghouse (1-800-358-9295).

Clinical Considerations

- Benefits from screening are unproven, even in high-risk patients.

  Clinicians should be aware that fair-skinned men and women aged >65, patients with atypical moles, and those with >50 moles constitute known groups at substantially increased risk for melanoma.

- Clinicians should remain alert for skin lesions with malignant features noted in the context of physical examinations performed for other purposes.

  Asymmetry, border irregularity, color variability, diameter >6 mm ("A," "B," "C," "D"), or rapidly changing lesions are features associated with an increased risk of malignancy. Suspicious lesions should be biopsied.

- The USPSTF did not examine the outcomes related to surveillance of patients with familial syndromes, such as familial atypical mole and melanoma (FAM-M) syndrome.

Scientific Evidence

Epidemiology and Clinical Consequences

In the United States, the lifetime risk of dying of melanoma is 0.36% among men and 0.21% among women. Between 1973 and 1995 the incidence of melanoma increased from 5.7 per 100,000 to 13.3 per 100,000. Although primary prevention efforts have focused on young people, the elderly (especially elderly men) bear a disproportionate burden of morbidity and mortality from melanoma and nonmelanoma skin cancer. Men aged >65 (5.2% of the U.S. population) are diagnosed with 22% of the new cases of malignant melanoma each year; women aged >65 (7.4% of the population) are diagnosed with 14% of new cases. In the elderly, melanoma tends to be diagnosed at a later stage and is more likely to be lethal than it is in the general population.

  Basal cell and squamous cell carcinomas, in contrast to melanoma, are very common, especially in the elderly. However, they cause limited morbidity or mortality even in the absence of formal screening.

Accuracy and Reliability of Screening Test

The most commonly advocated screening test for skin cancer is a total-body skin examination by a clinician. Although data are sparse and based entirely on studies of volunteer patients, the sensitivity and specificity of a total-body skin examination performed by a dermatologist for the diagnosis of skin cancer are reported to be high, 94% and 98%, respectively. Data regarding the accuracy of the total-body skin examination performed by nonspecialists are few, but suggest slightly lower sensitivity and much lower specificity than examinations performed by dermatologists.

Another screening strategy is to use a questionnaire or interview to assess risk factors such as family history and sun exposure and refer only high-risk patients for total-body skin examinations. Clinicians and patients can reliably measure some risk factors for melanoma, but the validity of formal risk-assessment tools to screen unselected patients in primary care has not been established.

Yield of Screening Test

While dependent on the population screened, rates of *suspected* melanoma in mass screening, case finding, and population-based screening range from 0 to 9 per 100 people screened, with the most common findings between 1 and 3 per 100. Rates of *confirmed* melanoma and melanoma in situ are commonly in the range of 1 to 4 per 1000 people screened. One to five percent of screened patients are confirmed to have nonmelanoma skin cancer.

Effectiveness of Early Detection

There are no randomized trials or case–control studies that directly examine whether screening by clinicians is associated with improved clinical outcomes such as reduced morbidity or mortality from skin cancer. The possibility that earlier treatment as a result of screening improves health outcomes must rely on indirect evidence.

Screening consistently identifies melanomas that are, on average, thinner (i.e., at an earlier stage) than those found during usual care. It is not known if this stage shift leads to decreased morbidity or mortality. A case–control study in which skin self-examination was associated with a lower incidence of lethal melanoma provides indirect evidence that the shift to earlier stages found in screening may be associated with better clinical outcomes. Evidence from studies of the consequences of delay in diagnosis is inconsistent.

Even without formal screening programs, mortality from basal cell and squamous cell carcinoma is low compared to mortality from melanoma, but early detection and treatment may reduce morbidity and disfigurement from these cancers. No studies were found that evaluated whether screening improves the outcomes of these cancers.

Potential Adverse Effects of Screening

There are no serious risks from total-body skin examination but examination may be embarrassing to some patients and inconvenient in some settings. Screening could result in unnecessary treatment, either due to misdiagnosis or to detection of lesions that might not have caused clinical consequences. Screening also detects large numbers of benign skin conditions, which are very common in the elderly and could lead to additional biopsies and unnecessary or expensive procedures.

Recommendations of Others

The Canadian Task Force on Preventive Health Care concluded that the evidence was insufficient to recommend for or against skin cancer screening for the general population, but suggests that regular total-body skin examination may be prudent for a subgroup of very high-risk individuals.[4] The American Cancer Society recommends skin examination as part of a cancerrelated checkup every 3 years for people aged between 20 and 40, and on a yearly basis for anyone aged >40.[5] The American College of Preventive Medicine recommends total-body skin examination in high-risk individuals, including those with a family or personal history of skin cancer, predisposing phenotypic characteristics, and increased occupational or recreational exposure to sunlight, or clinical evidence of precursor lesions (e.g., dysplastic or congenital nevi), but does not recommend routine screening.[6] The American College of Obstetricians and Gynecologists recommends yearly, or as appropriate, skin examination of women aged ≥13 based on risk factors (increased recreational or occupational exposure to sunlight; family or personal history of skin cancer; clinical evidence of precursor lesions).[7] A National Institutes of Health (NIH) Consensus Panel recommends screening for melanoma as part of routine primary care.[8] The Australian National Health and Medical Research Council does not recommend mass screening or screening of high-risk people for melanoma.[9] All of these organizations advise public or patient education to change behaviors that may increase the risk of skin cancer, including sun avoidance, sun protection, and skin self-examination.

Discussion

Periodic total-body skin examination can increase the detection of thin (earlier stage) melanoma; however, controlled studies are needed to determine whether early detection would actually have an important effect on mortality. Additional questions remain about the ability of primary care clinicians to perform adequate examinations in the context of usual care. Studies of skin health behaviors and studies of factors associated with advanced melanoma suggest that older persons are at high risk and are unlikely to benefit from existing skin cancer prevention efforts such as public education and clinician education efforts regarding sun avoidance and/or sun protection. While it is unproven, skin cancer screening (using a risk assessment strategy with examination or referral of high-risk patients) is the most promising strategy for addressing the excess burden of disease in older persons. Since most elderly individuals consult a clinician at least yearly, case finding by clinicians focusing on the elderly may reach vulnerable individuals who may not benefit from other approaches.

Members of the U.S. Preventive Services Task Force are: Alfred O. Berg, MD, MPH, Chair, USPSTF (Professor and Chair, Department of Family Medicine, University of Washington, Seattle, WA); Janet D. Allan, PhD, RN, CS, Vice-chair, USPSTF (Dean and Professor, School of Nursing, University of Texas Health Science Center, San Antonio, TX); Paul S. Frame, MD (Tri-County Family Medicine, Cohocton, NY, and Clinical Professor of Family Medicine, University of Rochester, Rochester, NY); Charles J. Homer, MD, MPH (Executive Director, National Initiative for Children's Healthcare Quality, Boston, MA); Tracy A. Lieu, MD, MPH (Associate Professor, Department of Ambulatory Care and Prevention, Harvard Pilgrim Health Care and Harvard Medical School, Boston, MA); Cynthia D. Mulrow, MD, MSc (Professor of Medicine, University of Texas Health Science Center, Audie L. Murphy Memorial Veterans Hospital, San Antonio, TX); C. Tracy Orleans, PhD (Senior Scientist, The Robert Wood Johnson Foundation, Princeton, NJ); Jeffrey F. Peipert, MD, MPH (Director of Research, Women and Infants' Hospital, Providence, RI); Nola J. Pender, PhD, RN (Professor and Associate Dean for Research, School of Nursing, University of Michigan, Ann Arbor, MI); Harold C. Sox, Jr., MD (Professor and Chair, Department of Medicine, Dartmouth-Hitchcock Medical Center, Lebanon, NH); Steven M. Teutsch, MD, MPH (Senior Director, Outcomes Research and Management, Merck & Company, Inc., West Point, PA); Carolyn Westhoff, MD, MSc (Associate Professor of Obstetrics, Gynecology and Public Health, Department of Obstetrics and Gynecology, Columbia University College of Physicians and Surgeons, New York, NY); and Steven H. Woolf, MD, MPH (Professor of Family Medicine, Department of Family Practice, Medical College of Virginia, Fairfax, VA).

REFERENCES

1. U.S. Preventive Services Task Force. Guide to clinical preventive services, 2nd ed. Washington, DC: Office of Disease Prevention and Health Promotion, U.S. Government Printing Office, 1996.
2. Helfand M, Mahon SM, Eden KB, Frame PS, Orleans CT. Screening for skin cancer. Am J Prev Med 2001;47–58.
3. Helfand M, Mahon S, Eden K. Screening for skin cancer. Systematic evidence review. Pub. No. AHRQ01-S002. Rockville, MD: Agency for Healthcare Research and Quality, 2001.
4. Feightner JW. Prevention of skin cancer. In: Canadian Task Force on the Periodic Health Examination. Canadian guide to clinical preventive health care. Ottawa: Health Canada, 1994;850–9.
5. American Cancer Society. Melanoma: detection and symptoms. Available at: http://www3.cancer.org/cancerinfo/Accessed February 15, 2001.
6. Ferrini RL, Perlman M, Hill L. American College of Preventive Medicine policy statement: screening for skin cancer. Am J Prev Med 1998;14:80 –2.
7. American College of Obstetricians and Gynecologists Committee on Gynecologic Practice. Primary and preventive care: periodic assessments. Committee opinion no. 246. Washington, DC: American College of Obstetricians and Gynecologists, Dec 2000.
8. NIH Consensus Development Panel on Early Melanoma. Diagnosis and treatment of early melanoma. JAMA 1992;268:1314–19.
9. National Health and Medical Research Council. Guidelines for preventive interventions in primary health care: cardiovascular disease and cancer. Report of the Assessment of Preventive Activities in the Health Care System Initiative. Canberra, Australia: National Health and Medical Research Council, Commonwealth of Australia, Dec 1996.

Appendix A Third U.S. Preventive Services Task Force (USPSTF)
Recommendations and Ratings

The USPSTF grades its recommendations according to one of five classifications
(A, B, C, D, or I), reflecting the strength of evidence and magnitude of net
benefit (benefits minus harms).

A. The USPSTF strongly recommends that clinicians routinely provide [the
service] to eligible patients. (The USPSTF found good evidence that [the
service] improves important health outcomes and concludes that benefits
substantially outweigh harms.)
B. The USPSTF recommends that clinicians routinely provide [the service] to
eligible patients. (The USPSTF found at least fair evidence that [the service]
improves important health outcomes and concludes that benefits outweigh
harms.)
C. The USPSTF makes no recommendation for or against routine provision of
[the service]. (The USPSTF found at least fair evidence that [the service] can
improve health outcomes but concludes that the balance of benefits and
harms is too close to justify a general recommendation.)
D. The USPSTF recommends against routinely providing [the service] to
asymptomatic patients. (The USPSTF found at least fair evidence that [the
service] is ineffective or that harms outweigh benefits.)
I. The USPSTF concludes that the evidence is insufficient to recommend for or
against routinely providing [the service]. (Evidence that [the service] is
effective is lacking, of poor quality, or conflicting and the balance of benefits
and harms cannot be determined.)

Appendix B Third U.S. Preventive Services Task Force (USPSTF)
Strength of Overall Evidence

The USPSTF grades the quality of the overall evidence for a service on a 3-point
scale (good, fair, or poor).

Good: Evidence includes consistent results from well-designed, well-conducted
studies in representative populations that directly assess effects on health
outcomes.

Fair: Evidence is sufficient to determine effects on health outcomes, but the
strength of the evidence is limited by the number, quality, or consistency of the
individual studies; generalizability to routine practice; or indirect nature of the
evidence on health outcomes.

Poor: Evidence is insufficient to assess the effects on health outcomes because of
limited number or power of studies, important flaws in their design or
conduct, gaps in the chain of evidence, or lack of information on important
health outcomes.

Aspirin for the Primary Prevention of Cardiovascular Events

By the U.S. Preventive Services Task Force (USPSTF)*

RECOMMENDATION

Recommendation and Rationale Statements present the current U.S. Preventive Services Task Force (USPSTF) recommendations, the rationale for the recommendations, and the supporting scientific evidence. These statements address preventive health services for use in primary care clinical settings, including screening tests, counseling, and chemoprevention.

The USPSTF recommendations are independent of the U.S. Government. They do not represent the views of the Agency for Healthcare Research and Quality (AHRQ), the U.S. Department of Health and Human Services, or the U.S. Public Health Service.

Summary of Recommendation

- The U.S. Preventive Services Task Force (USPSTF) strongly recommends that clinicians discuss aspirin chemoprevention with adults who are at increased risk for coronary heart disease (CHD) (see "Clinical Considerations"). Discussions with patients should address both the potential benefits and harms of aspirin therapy. (**A recommendation.**)

---

*This statement summarizes the current U.S. Preventive Services Task Force (USPSTF) recommendation for aspirin for the primary prevention of cardiovascular events and the supporting scientific evidence, and it updates the 1995 recommendations contained in the Guide to Clinical Preventive Services, second edition.[1] Explanations of the ratings and of the strength of overall evidence are given in Appendix A and Appendix B, respectively. The complete information on which this statement is based, including evidence tables and references, is available in the article "Asprin for the Primary Prevention of Cardiovascular Events: Summary of the Evidence."

This article first appeared in the *Annals of Internal Medicine*. Select for copyright, source, and reprint information.

Address correspondence to: Alfred O. Berg, M.D., M.P.H., Chair, USPSTF, c/o David Atkins, M.D., M.P.H., Scientific and Technical Editor, USPSTF, Agency for Healthcare Research and Quality, Center for Practice and Technology Assessment, 6010 Executive Boulevard, Suite 300, Rockville, MD 20852. Telephone (301) 594-4016, fax (301) 594-4027, E-mail: datkins@ahrq.gov.

The USPSTF found good evidence that aspirin decreases the incidence of coronary heart disease in adults who are at increased risk for heart disease. They also found good evidence that aspirin increases the incidence of gastrointestinal bleeding and fair evidence that aspirin increases the incidence of hemorrhagic strokes. The USP-STF concluded that the balance of benefits and harms is most favorable in patients at high risk of CHD (5-year risk of greater than or equal to 3 percent) but is also influenced by patient preferences.

Clinical Considerations

- Decisions about aspirin therapy should take into account overall risk for coronary heart disease. Risk assessment should include asking about the presence and severity of the following risk factors: age, sex, diabetes, elevated total cholesterol levels, low levels of high-density lipoprotein (HDL) cholesterol, elevated blood pressure, family history (in younger adults), and smoking. Tools that incorporate specific information on multiple risk factors provide more accurate estimation of cardiovascular risk than categorizations based simply on counting the numbers of risk factors (http://www.intmed.mcw.edu/clincalc/heartrisk.html).[2]

- Men older than 40 years, postmenopausal women, and younger people with risk factors for coronary heart disease (eg, hypertension, diabetes, or smoking) are at increased risk for heart disease and may wish to consider aspirin therapy. Table 1 shows how estimates of the type and magnitude of benefits and harms associated with aspirin therapy vary with an individual's underlying risk for coronary heart disease. Although balance of benefits and harms is most favorable in high-risk people (5-year risk greater than 3 percent), some people at lower risk may consider the potential benefits of aspirin to be sufficient to outweigh the potential harms.

- Discussions about aspirin therapy should focus on potential coronary heart disease benefits, such as prevention of myocardial infarction, and potential harms, such as gastrointestinal and intracranial bleeding. Discussions should take into account individual preferences and risk aversions concerning myocardial infarction, stroke, and gastrointestinal bleeding.

- Although the optimal timing and frequency of discussions related to aspirin therapy are unknown, reasonable options include every 5 years in middle-aged and older people or when other cardiovascular risk factors are detected.

- Most participants in the primary prevention trials of aspirin therapy have been men between 40 and 75 years of age. Current estimates of benefits and harms may not be as reliable for women and older men.

- Although older patients may derive greater benefits because they are at higher risk for CHD and stroke, their risk for bleeding may be higher.

- Uncontrolled hypertension may attenuate the benefits of aspirin in reducing CHD.

- The optimum dose of aspirin for chemoprevention is not known. Primary and secondary prevention trials have demonstrated benefits with a variety of regimens, including 75 mg per day, 100 mg per day, and 325 mg every other day. Doses of approximately 75 mg per day appear as effective as higher doses; whether doses below 75 mg per day are effective has not been established. Enteric-coated or buffered preparations do not clearly reduce adverse gastrointestinal effects of aspirin. Uncontrolled hypertension and concomitant use of other nonsteroidal anti-inflammatory agents or anticoagulants increase risk for serious bleeding.

Scientific Evidence

Epidemiology and Clinical Background

Cardiovascular disease, including ischemic coronary heart disease, stroke, and peripheral vascular disease, is the leading cause of death in the United States.[3] Yearly, over 1 million Americans experience new or recurrent myocardial infarction or fatal coronary heart disease. Most events occur in older people and those with recognized risk factors for cardiovascular disease, including high cholesterol, high blood pressure, diabetes, or a history of smoking.

The early-documented and clear success of aspirin in preventing further clinical disease in some patients with known heart disease (secondary prevention) raised interest in aspirin as a potential primary preventive intervention in men and women without known heart disease.[4] Two early randomized trials of aspirin had conflicting results, however, and lacked sufficient power to estimate major harms, such as gastrointestinal bleeding and hemorrhagic stroke.[5,6] Thus, the role of aspirin in primary prevention has remained controversial. The new USPSTF recommendation incorporates additional data from three recent trials and provides more reliable estimates of both benefits and harms of aspirin in patients without known heart disease.

Efficacy of Chemoprevention

Five trials have examined the effects of daily or every-other-day aspirin for the primary prevention of cardiovascular events over periods of 4 to 7 years.[5-9] Most participants were men older than 50 years. Meta-analysis of pooled data from all of the studies showed that aspirin therapy reduced the risk for CHD by 28 percent (summary odds ratio [OR], 0.72; 95 percent CI, 0.60 to 0.87). Summary estimates showed no significant effects of aspirin on total mortality (OR, 0.93; 95 percent CI, 0.84 to 1.02) and stroke (OR, 1.02; 95 percent CI, 0.85 to 1.23).

Harms of Chemoprevention

These five primary prevention trials, and a larger number of randomized controlled trials (RCTs) of secondary prevention that enrolled patients with heart disease or stroke, demonstrate that aspirin increases rates of gastrointestinal bleeding. Estimated rates of major gastrointestinal bleeding episodes are approximately 2 to 4 per 1,000 middle-aged individuals (4 to 12 for older individuals) given aspirin for 5 years.[10-12]

These controlled trials in primary and secondary prevention settings also suggest that aspirin increases rates of hemorrhagic strokes by a small amount (0–2 per 1,000 individuals given aspirin for 5 years).[5-7] Such estimates are less reliable than those of gastrointestinal bleeding because few strokes were reported in the trials.

Recommendations of Others

In 1994, the Canadian Task Force on Preventive Health Care concluded that the evidence was not strong enough to recommend for or against use of aspirin for primary prevention of heart disease in men or women and recommended that physicians and patients balance the reduced rate of nonfatal myocardial infarction against potential adverse effects.[13] In 2000, the American Diabetes Association recommended that clinicians consider aspirin for primary prevention of heart disease in diabetic patients who are older than 30 years or have risk factors for cardiovascular disease and no contraindications to aspirin therapy.[14] In 1997, the American Heart Association concluded that aspirin may be warranted for patients at high risk of myocardial infarction but that health care providers must consider a patient's particular cardiovascular risk profile, the demonstrated benefits of aspirin on reducing risk for a first myocardial infarction, and known as well an unknown side effects of aspirin.[15]

In 1998, the European Society of Cardiology recommended low-dose aspirin (75 mg) for patients with well-controlled hypertension and men at "particularly" high risk for coronary heart disease, but not for all individuals at high risk.[16]

ACKNOWLEDGMENTS

Members of the U.S. Preventive Services Task Force are Alfred O. Berg, M.D., M.P.H., Chair, USPSTF (Professor and Chair, Department of Family Medicine, University of Washington, Seattle, WA); Janet D. Allan, Ph.D., R.N., C.S., Vice-chair, USPSTF (Dean and Professor, School of Nursing, University of Texas Health Science Center, San Antonio, TX); Paul S. Frame, M.D. (Tri-County Family Medicine, Cohocton, NY, and Clinical Professor of Family Medicine, University of Rochester, Rochester, NY); Charles J. Homer, M.D., M.P.H. (Executive Director, National Initiative for Children's Healthcare Quality, Boston, MA); Mark S. Johnson, M.D., M.P.H. (Associate Professor of Clinical Family Medicine and Chairman Department of Family Medicine, University of Medicine and Dentistry of New Jersey-New Jersey Medical School, Newark, NJ); Jonathan D. Klein, M.D., M.P.H. (Associate Professor of Pediatrics and of Community and Preventive Medicine, University of Rochester School of Medicine, Rochester, NY), Tracy A. Lieu, M.D., M.P.H. (Associate Professor, Department of Ambulatory Care and Prevention, Harvard Pilgrim Health Care and Harvard Medical School, Boston, MA); Cynthia D. Mulrow, M.D., M.Sc. (Professor of Medicine, University of Texas Health Science Center, Audie L. Murphy Memorial Veterans Hospital, San Antonio, TX); C. Tracy Orleans, Ph.D. (Senior Scientist, The Robert Wood Johnson Foundation, Princeton, NJ); Jeffrey F. Peipert, M.D., M.P.H (Director of Research, Women and Infants' Hospital, Providence, RI); Nola J. Pender, Ph.D., R.N. (Professor and Associate Dean for Research, School of Nursing, University of Michigan, Ann Arbor, MI); Albert L. Siu, M.D., M.S.P.H (Professor of Medicine, Chief of Division of General Internal Medicine, and Medical Director of the Primary Care and Medical Services Care Center, Mount Sinai School of Medicine and The Mount Sinai Medical Center, New York, NY); Steven M. Teutsch, M.D., M.P.H. (Senior Director, Outcomes Research and Management, Merck & Company, Inc., West Point, PA); Carolyn Westhoff, M.D., M.Sc. (Associate Professor of Obstetrics, Gynecology and Public Health, Department of Obstetrics and Gynecology, Columbia University College of Physicians and Surgeons, New York, NY); and Steven H. Woolf, M.D., M.P.H. (Professor of Family Medicine, Department of Family Practice, Medical College of Virginia, Fairfax, VA).

REFERENCES AND NOTES

1. U.S. Preventive Services Task Force. Guide to Clinical Preventive Services. 2nd edition. Washington, DC: Office of Disease Prevention and Health Promotion, U.S. Government Printing Office; 1996.
2. Wilson PW, D'Agostino RB, Levy D, Belanger AM, Silbershatz H, Kannel WB. Prediction of coronary heart disease using risk factor categories. Circulation 1998;97(18):1837–47.
3. Hoyert DL, Kochanek KD, Murphy SL. Deaths: Final Data for 1997. National Vital Statistics Reports. Hyattsville, MD: National Center for Health Statistics; 1999.
4. Collaborative overview of randomised trials of antiplatelet therapy—I: Prevention of death, myocardial infarction, and stroke by prolonged antiplatelet therapy in various categories of patients. Antiplatelet Trialists' Collaboration. BMJ 1994;308:81–106.
5. Final report on the aspirin component of the ongoing Physicians' Health Study. Steering Committee of the Physicians' Health Study Research Group. N Engl J Med 1989;321:129–35.
6. Peto R, Gray R, Collins R, Wheatley K, Hennekens C, Jamrozik K. Randomised trial of prophylactic daily aspirin in British male doctors. Br Med J (Clin Res Ed) 1988;296:313–6.
7. Thrombosis prevention trial: randomised trial of low-intensity oral anticoagulation with warfarin and low-dose aspirin in the primary prevention of ischemic heart disease in men at increased risk. The Medical Research Council's General Practice Research Framework. Lancet 1998;351:233–41.
8. Hansson L, Zanchetti A, Carruthers SG, et al. Effects of intensive blood pressure lowering and low-dose aspirin in patients with hypertension: principal results of the Hypertension Optimal Treatment (HOT) randomised trial. HOT Study Group. Lancet 1998;280:1930–5.
9. Collaborative Group of the Primary Prevention Project (PPP). Low-dose aspirin and vitamin E in people at cardiovascular risk: a randomized trial in general practice. Lancet 2001;357:89–95.

10. Roderick PJ, Wilkes HC, Meade TW. The gastrointestinal toxicity of aspirin: an overview of randomised controlled trials. Br J Clin Pharmacol 1993;35:219–26.
11. Dickinson JP, Printice CR. Aspirin: benefit and risk in thromboprophylaxis. QJM 1998;91:523–38.
12. Stalnikowicz-Darvasi R. Gastrointestinal bleeding during low-dose aspirin administration for prevention of arterial occlusive events. J Clin Gastroenterol 1995;21:13–6.
13. Anderson G. Acetylsalicylic acid and the primary prevention of cardiovascular disease. In: Canadian Task Force on the Periodic Health Examination. Ottawa (Canada): Health Canada; 1994: 680–90.
14. Aspirin Therapy in Diabetes. American Diabetes Association. Diabetes Care 2001;24(suppl 10):S62–S63. Available at: www.diabetes.org/clinicalrecommendations/Supplement101/S62.htm. Accessed May 25, 2001.
15. Hennekens CH, Dyken ML, Fuster V. Aspirin as a therapeutic agent in cardiovascular disease: a statement for healthcare professionals from the American Heart Association. Circulation 1997;96:2751–3.
16. Prevention of coronary heart disease in clinical practice. Recommendations of the Second Joint Task Force of European and other Societies in coronary prevention. Eur Heart J 1998;19(10):1434–1503.

Appendix A Third USPSTF Recommendations and Ratings

The USPSTF grades its recommendations according to one of five classifications (A, B, C, D, or I), reflecting the strength of evidence and magnitude of net benefit (benefits minus harms).

A. The USPSTF strongly recommends that clinicians routinely provide [the service] to eligible patients. (The USPSTF found good evidence that [the service] improves important health outcomes and concludes that benefits substantially outweigh harms.)

B. The USPSTF recommends that clinicians routinely provide [the service] to eligible patients. (The USPSTF found at least fair evidence that [the service] improves important health outcomes and concludes that benefits outweigh harms.)

C. The USPSTF makes no recommendation for or against routine provision of [the service]. (The USPSTF found at least fair evidence that [the service] can improve health outcomes but concludes that the balance of benefits and harms is too close to justify a general recommendation.)

D. The USPSTF recommends against routinely providing [the service] to asymptomatic patients. (The USPSTF found at least fair evidence that [the service] is ineffective or that harms outweigh benefits.)

I. The USPSTF concludes that the evidence is insufficient to recommend for or against routinely providing [the service]. (Evidence that [the service] is effective is lacking, of poor quality, or conflicting and that the balance of benefits and harms cannot be determined.)

Appendix B Third USPSTF Strength of Overall Evidence

The USPSTF grades the quality of the overall evidence for a service on a 3-point scale (good, fair, or poor).

Good: Evidence includes consistent results from well-designed, well-conducted studies in representative populations that directly assess effects on health outcomes.

Fair: Evidence is sufficient to determine effects on health outcomes, but the strength of the evidence is limited by the number, quality, or consistency of the individual studies; generalizability to routine practice; or indirect nature of the evidence on health outcomes.

Poor: Evidence is insufficient to assess the effects on health outcomes because of limited number or power of studies, important flaws in their design or conduct, gaps in the chain of evidence, or lack of information on important health outcomes.

Mailing Registration

Neither the U.S. Public Health Service nor the U.S. Department of Health and Human Services endorses any particular organization or its activities, products, or services.

The U.S. Public Health Service currently plans to update both **the Guide to Clinical Preventive Services and the Clinician's Handbook of Preventive Services** as new preventive health data becomes available. Please register to join International Medical Publishing's mailing list for information about these updates and other public health titles.

Name: _____

Address: _____

Address: _____

Phone: _____

Fax: _____

Mail your registration to:

International Medical Publishing, Inc.
Attn: Guide
P.O. Box 479
McLean, VA 22101

Or Fax to 703-734-8987

Order Form

In addition to your address, please include an e-mail or phone number so that we might contact you with any questions about your order.

Name: _____

Address: _____

City, State, Zip: _____

Daytime phone/E-mail: _____

Please send a Personal Check or Credit Card (circle one):

Visa   Mastercard

Card Number _____ Expiration _____

Signature _____

Title	Quantity	Price	Total
Guide CPS 2nd+3rd Edition		$60.00	
	*Tax (see below)		
	**S&H (see bellow)		
	Total		

*Sales Tax 5% in VA.
**Shipping charges are $5.95 for the first book and $0.50 (50 cents) for each additional book. Please call for other rates.
Please send your order to:

International Medical Publishing, Inc.
P.O. Box 479
McLean, VA 22101

Information and ordering: (800) 530-4146   Fax: (703) 734-8987
E-mail inquiries to: orders@medicalpublishing.com
Online: www.medicalpublishing.com

Order Form

In addition to your address, please include an e-mail or phone number so that we might contact you with any questions about your order.

Name: _____

Address: _____

City, State, Zip: _____

Daytime phone/E-mail: _____

Please send a Personal Check or Credit Card (circle one):

               Visa   Mastercard

Card Number _____ Expiration _____

Signature _____

Title	Quantity	Price	Total
Guide CPS 2nd+3rd Edition		$60.00	
	*Tax (see below)		
	**S&H (see bellow)		
	Total		

*Sales Tax 5% in VA.
**Shipping charges are $5.95 for the first book and $0.50 (50 cents) for each additional book. Please call for other rates.
Please send your order to:
> **International Medical Publishing, Inc.**
> **P.O. Box 479**
> **McLean, VA 22101**

Information and ordering: (800) 530-4146   Fax: (703) 734-8987
E-mail inquiries to: orders@medicalpublishing.com
Online: www.medicalpublishing.com

Table 1. Birth to 10 Years

Interventions Considered and Recommended for the Periodic Health Examination	Leading Causes of Death
	Conditions originating in perinatal period
	Congenital anomalies
	Sudden infant death syndrome (SIDS)
	Unintentional injuries (non-motor vehicle)
	Motor vehicle injuries

Interventions for the General Population

SCREENING
Height and weight [Ch 21]
Blood pressure [Ch 3]
Vision screen (age 3–4 yr) [Ch 33]
Hemoglobinopathy screen (birth)[1] [Ch 43]
Phenylalanine level (birth)[2] [Ch 44]
T_4 and/or TSH (birth)[3] [Ch 45]

COUNSELING
Injury Prevention [Ch 57,58]
Child safety car seats (age <5 yr)
Lap-shoulder belts (age ≥5 yr)
Bicycle helmet, avoid bicycling near traffic
Smoke detector, flame retardant sleepwear
Hot water heater temperature <120–130°F
Window/stair guards, pool fence
Safe storage of drugs, toxic substances, firearms, & matches
Syrup of ipecac, poison control phone number
CPR training for parents/caretakers

Diet and Exercise
Breast-feeding, iron-enriched formula and foods (infants & toddlers) [Ch 22,56]

Limit fat & cholesterol, maintain caloric balance, emphasize grains, fruits, vegetables (age ≥2 yr) [Ch 56]
Regular physical activity* [Ch 55]

Substance Use [Ch 54]
Effects of passive smoking*
Anti-tobacco message*

Dental Health [Ch 61]
Regular visits to dental care provider*
Floss, brush with fluoride toothpaste daily*
Advice about baby bottle tooth decay*

IMMUNIZATIONS [Ch 65]
Diphtheria-tetanus-pertussis (DTP)[4]
Oral poliovirus (OPV)[5]
Measles-mumps-rubella (MMR)[6]
H. influenzae type b (Hib) conjugate[7]
Hepatitis B[8]
Varicella[9]

CHEMOPROPHYLAXIS
Ocular prophylaxis (birth) [Ch 27]

Interventions for High-Risk Populations

POPULATION	POTENTIAL INTERVENTIONS (See detailed high-risk definitions)
Preterm or low birth weight	Hemoglobin/hematocrit (HR1)
Infants of mothers at risk for HIV	HIV testing (HR2)
Low income; immigrants	Hemoglobin/hematocrit (HR1); PPD (HR3)
TB contacts	PPD (HR3)
Native American/Alaska Native	Hemoglobin/hematocrit (HR1); PPD (HR3); hepatitis A vaccine (HR4); pneumococcal vaccine (HR5)
Travelers to developing countries	Hepatitis A vaccine (HR4)
Residents of long-term care facilities	PPD (HR3); hepatitis A vaccine (HR4); influenza vaccine (HR6)
Certain chronic medical conditions	PPD (HR3); pneumococcal vaccine (HR5); influenza vaccine (HR6)
Increased individual or community lead exposure	Blood lead level (HR7)
Inadequate water fluoridation	Daily fluoride supplement (HR8)
Family h/o skin cancer; nevi; fair skin, eyes, hair	Avoid excess/midday sun, use protective clothing* (HR9)

[1]Whether screening should be universal or targeted to high-risk groups will depend on the proportion of high-risk individuals in the screening area, and other considerations (see Ch. 43). [2]If done during first 24 hr of life, repeat by age 2 wk. [3]Optimally between day 2 and 6, but in all cases before newborn nursery discharge. [4]2, 4, 6, and 12–18 mo; once between ages 4–6 yr (DTaP may be used at 15 mo and older). [5]2, 4, 6–18 mo; once between ages 4–6 yr. [6]12–15 mo and 4–6 yr. [7]2, 4, 6 and 12–15 mo; no dose needed at 6 mo if PRP-OMP vaccine is used for first 2 doses. [8]Birth, 1 mo, 6 mo; or, 0–2 mo, 1–2 mo later, and 6–18 mo. If not done in infancy: current visit, and 1 and 6 mo later. [9]12–18 mo; or older child without hx of chickenpox or previous immunization. Include information on risk in adulthood, duration of immunity, and potential need for booster doses.

*The ability of clinician counseling to influence this behavior is unproven.

HR1 = Infants age 6–12 mo who are: living in poverty, black, Native American or Alaska Native, immigrants from developing countries, preterm or low birth weight infants, or infants whose principal dietary intake is unfortified cow's milk (see Ch. 22).

HR2 = Infants born to high-risk mothers whose HIV status is unknown. Women at high risk include: past or present injection drug use; persons who exchange sex for money or drugs, and their sex partners; injection drug-using, bisexual, or HIV-positive sex partners currently or in past; persons seeking treatment for STDs; blood transfusion during 1978–1985 (see Ch. 28).

HR3 = Persons infected with HIV, close contacts of persons with known or suspected TB, persons with medical risk factors associated with TB, immigrants from countries with high TB prevalence, medically underserved low-income populations (including homeless), residents of long-term care facilities (see Ch. 25). See Ch. 25 for indications for BCG vaccine.

HR4 = Persons ≥2 yr living in or traveling to areas where the disease is endemic and where periodic outbreaks occur (e.g., countries with high or intermediate endemicity; certain Alaska Native, Pacific Island, Native American, and religious communities). Consider for institutionalized children aged ≥2 yr. Clinicians should also consider local epidemiology (see Ch. 65–67).

HR5 = Immunocompetent persons ≥2 yr with certain medical conditions, including chronic cardiac or pulmonary disease, diabetes mellitus, and anatomic asplenia. Immunocompetent persons ≥2 yr living in high-risk environments or social settings (e.g., certain Native American and Alaska Native populations) (see Ch. 66).

HR6 = Annual vaccination of children ≥6 mo who are residents of chronic care facilities or who have chronic cardiopulmonary disorders, metabolic diseases (including diabetes mellitus), hemoglobinopathies, immunosuppression, or renal dysfunction (see Ch. 66). See Ch. 66 for indications for amantadine/rimantadine prophylaxis.

HR7 = Children about age 12 mo who: 1) live in communities in which the prevalence of lead levels requiring individual intervention, including residential lead hazard control or chelation, is high or undefined; 2) live in or frequently visit a home built before 1950 with dilapidated paint or with recent or ongoing renovation or remodeling; 3) have close contact with a person who has an elevated lead level; 4) live near lead industry or heavy traffic; 5) live with someone whose job or hobby involves lead exposure; 6) use lead-based pottery; or 7) take traditional ethnic remedies that contain lead (see Ch. 23).

HR8 = Children living in areas with inadequate water fluoridation (<0.6 ppm) (see Ch. 61).

HR9 = Persons with a family history of skin cancer, a large number of moles, atypical moles, poor tanning ability, or light skin, hair, and eye color (see Ch. 12).

Table 2. Ages 11–24 Years

Interventions Considered and Recommended for the Periodic Health Examination	Leading Causes of Death
	Motor vehicle/other unintentional injuries
	Homicide
	Suicide
	Malignant neoplasms
	Heart diseases

Interventions for the General Population

SCREENING
Height & weight [Ch 21]
Blood pressure[1] [Ch 3]
Papanicolaou (Pap) test[2] (females) [Ch 9]
Chlamydia screen[3] (females <20 yr) [Ch 29]
Rubella serology or vaccination hx[4] (females >12 yr) [Ch 32]
Assess for problem drinking [Ch 52]

COUNSELING
Injury Prevention [Ch 57,58]
Lap/shoulder belts
Bicycle/motorcycle/ATV helmets*
Smoke detector*
Safe storage/removal of firearms* [Ch 50,59]

Substance Use
Avoid tobacco use [Ch 54]
Avoid underage drinking & illicit drug use* [Ch 52,53]
Avoid alcohol/drug use while driving, swimming, boating,etc.* [Ch 57,58]

Sexual Behavior [Ch 62,63]
STD prevention: abstinence;* avoid high-risk behavior;* condoms/female barrier with spermicide*
Unintended pregnancy: contraception

Diet and Exercise
Limit fat & cholesterol; maintain caloric balance; emphasize grains, fruits, vegetables [Ch 56]
Adequate calcium intake (females) [Ch 56]
Regular physical activity* [Ch 55]

Dental Health [Ch 61]
Regular visits to dental care provider*
Floss, brush with fluoride toothpaste daily*

IMMUNIZATIONS [Ch 65,66]
Tetanus-diphtheria (Td) boosters (11–16 yr)
Hepatitis B[5]
MMR (11–12 yr)[6]
Varicella (11–12 yr)[7]
Rubella[4] (females >12 yr) [Ch 32]

CHEMOPROPHYLAXIS
Multivitamin with folic acid (females planning/capable of pregnancy) [Ch 42]

Interventions for High-Risk Populations

POPULATION	POTENTIAL INTERVENTIONS (See detailed high-risk definitions)
High-risk sexual behavior	RPR/VDRL (HR1); screen for gonorrhea (female) (HR2), HIV (HR3), chlamydia (female) (HR4); hepatitis A vaccine (HR5)
Injection or street drug use	RPR/VDRL (HR1); HIV screen (HR3); hepatitis A vaccine (HR5); PPD (HR6); advice to reduce infection risk (HR7)
TB contacts; immigrants; low income	PPD (HR6)
Native Americans/Alaska Natives	Hepatitis A vaccine (HR5); PPD (HR6); pneumococcal vaccine (HR8)
Travelers to developing countries	Hepatitis A vaccine (HR5)
Certain chronic medical conditions	PPD (HR6); pneumococcal vaccine (HR8); influenza vaccine (HR9)
Settings where adolescents and young adults congregate	Second MMR (HR10)
Susceptible to varicella, measles, mumps	Varicella vaccine (HR11); MMR (HR12)
Blood transfusion between 1978–1985	HIV screen (HR3)
Institutionalized persons; health care/lab workers	Hepatitis A vaccine (HR5); PPD (HR6); influenza vaccine (HR9)
Family h/o skin cancer; nevi; fair skin, eyes, hair	Avoid excess/midday sun, use protective clothing* (HR13)
Prior pregnancy with neural tube defect	Folic acid 4.0 mg (HR14)
Inadequate water fluoridation	Daily fluoride supplement (HR15)

[1]Periodic BP for persons aged ≥21 yr. [2]If sexually active at present or in the past: q ≤ 3 yr. If sexual history is unreliable, begin Pap tests at age 18 yr. [3]If sexually active. [4]Serologic testing, documented vaccination history, and routine vaccination against rubella (preferably with MMR) are equally acceptable alternatives. [5]If not previously immunized: current visit, 1 and 6 mo later. [6]If no previous second dose of MMR. [7]If susceptible to chickenpox.

*The ability of clinician counseling to influence this behavior is unproven.

HR1 = Persons who exchange sex for money or drugs, and their sex partners; persons with other STDs (including HIV); and sexual contacts of persons with active syphilis. Clinicians should also consider local epidemiology (see Ch. 26).

HR2 = Females who have: two or more sex partners in the last year; a sex partner with multiple sexual contacts; exchanged sex for money or drugs; or a history of repeated episodes of gonorrhea. Clinicians should also consider local epidemiology (see Ch. 27).

HR3 = Males who had sex with males after 1975; past or present injection drug use; persons who exchange sex for money or drugs, and their sex partners; injection drug-using, bisexual, or HIV-positive sex partner currently or in the past; blood transfusion during 1978–1985; persons seeking treatment for STDs. Clinicians should also consider local epidemiology (see Ch. 28).

HR4 = Sexually active females with multiple risk factors including: history of prior STD; new or multiple sex partners; age under 25; nonuse or inconsistent use of barrier contraceptives; cervical ectopy. Clinicians should consider local epidemiology of the disease in identifying other high-risk groups (see Ch. 29).

HR5 = Persons living in, traveling to, or working in areas where the disease is endemic and where periodic outbreaks occur (e.g., countries with high or intermediate endemicity; certain Alaska Native, Pacific Island, Native American, and religious communities); men who have sex with men; injection or street drug users. Vaccine may be considered for institutionalized persons and workers in these institutions, military personnel, and day-care, hospital, and laboratory workers. Clinicians should also consider local epidemiology (see Ch. 66, 67).

HR6 = HIV positive, close contacts of persons with known or suspected TB, health care workers, persons with medical risk factors associated with TB, immigrants from countries with high TB prevalence, medically underserved low-income populations (including homeless), alcoholics, injection drug users, and residents of long-term care facilities (see Ch. 25). See Ch. 25 for indications for BCG vaccine.

HR7 = Persons who continue to inject drugs (see Ch. 53).

HR8 = Immunocompetent persons with certain medical conditions, including chronic cardiac or pulmonary disease, diabetes mellitus, and anatomic asplenia. Immunocompetent persons who live in high-risk environments or social settings (e.g., certain Native American and Alaska Native populations) (see Ch. 66).

HR9 = Annual vaccination of: residents of chronic care facilities; persons with chronic cardiopulmonary disorders, metabolic diseases (including diabetes mellitus), hemoglobinopathies, immunosuppression, or renal dysfunction; and health care providers for high-risk patients (see Ch. 66). See Ch. 66 for indications for amantadine/rimantadine prophylaxis.

HR10 = Adolescents and young adults in settings where such individuals congregate (e.g., high schools and colleges), if they have not previously received a second dose (see Ch. 65, 66).

HR11 = Healthy persons aged ≥13 yr without a history of chickenpox or previous immunization. Consider serologic testing for presumed susceptible persons aged ≥13 yr (see Ch. 65, 66).

HR12 = Persons born after 1956 who lack evidence of immunity to measles or mumps (e.g., documented receipt of live vaccine on or after the first birthday, laboratory evidence of immunity, or a history of physician-diagnosed measles or mumps) (see Ch. 65, 66).

HR13 = Persons with a family or personal history of skin cancer, a large number of moles, atypical moles, poor tanning ability, or light skin, hair, and eye color (see Ch. 12).

HR14 = Women with prior pregnancy affected by neural tube defect who are planning pregnancy (see Ch. 42).

HR15 = Persons aged <17 yr living in areas with inadequate water fluoridation (<0.6 ppm) (see Ch. 61).

Table 3. Ages 25–64 Years

Interventions Considered and Recommended for the Periodic Health Examination	Leading Causes of Death
	Malignant neoplasms
	Heart diseases
	Motor vehicle and other unintentional injuries
	Human immunodeficiency virus (HIV) infection
	Suicide and homicide

Interventions for the General Population

SCREENING
Blood pressure [Ch 3]
Height and weight [Ch 21]
Total blood cholesterol (men ages 35–65, women ages 45–65) [Ch 2]
Papanicolaou (Pap) test (women)[1] [Ch 9]
Fecal occult blood test[2] and/or sigmoidoscopy (≥50 yr) [Ch 8]
Mammogram ± clinical breast exam[3] (women 50–69 yr) [Ch 7]
Assess for problem drinking [Ch 52]
Rubella serology or vaccination hx[4] (women of childbearing age) [Ch 32]

COUNSELING

Substance Use
Tobacco cessation [Ch 54]
Avoid alcohol/drug use while driving, swimming, boating, etc.* [Ch 57,58]

Diet and Exercise
Limit fat & cholesterol; maintain caloric balance; emphasize grains, fruits, vegetables [Ch 56]
Adequate calcium intake (women) [Ch 56]

Regular physical activity* [Ch 55]

Injury Prevention [Ch 57,58]
Lap/shoulder belts
Motorcycle/bicycle/ATV helmets*
Smoke detector*
Safe storage/removal of firearms* [Ch 50,59]

Sexual Behavior [Ch 62,63]
STD prevention: avoid high-risk behavior;* condoms/female barrier with spermicide *
Unintended pregnancy: contraception

Dental Health [Ch 61]
Regular visits to dental care provider*
Floss, brush with fluoride toothpaste daily*

IMMUNIZATIONS [Ch 32,66]
Tetanus-diphtheria (Td) boosters
Rubella[4] (women of childbearing age)

CHEMOPROPHYLAXIS
Multivitamin with folic acid (women planning or capable of pregnancy) [Ch 42]
Discuss hormone prophylaxis (peri- and postmenopausal women) [Ch 68]

Interventions for High-Risk Populations

POPULATION	POTENTIAL INTERVENTIONS (See detailed high-risk definitions)
High-risk sexual behavior	RPR/VDRL (HR1); screen for gonorrhea (female) (HR2), HIV (HR3), chlamydia (female) (HR4); hepatitis B vaccine (HR5); hepatitis A vaccine (HR6)
Injection or street drug use	RPR/VDRL (HR1); HIV screen (HR3); hepatitis B vaccine (HR5); hepatitis A vaccine (HR6); PPD (HR7); advice to reduce infection risk (HR8)
Low income; TB contacts; immigrants; alcoholics	PPD (HR7)
Native Americans/Alaska Natives	Hepatitis A vaccine (HR6); PPD (HR7); pneumococcal vaccine (HR9)
Travelers to developing countries	Hepatitis B vaccine (HR5); hepatitis A vaccine (HR6)
Certain chronic medical conditions	PPD (HR7); pneumococcal vaccine (HR9); influenza vaccine (HR10)
Blood product recipients	HIV screen (HR3); hepatitis B vaccine (HR5)
Susceptible to measles, mumps, or varicella	MMR (HR11); varicella vaccine (HR12)
Institutionalized persons	Hepatitis A vaccine (HR6); PPD (HR7); pneumococcal vaccine (HR9); influenza vaccine (HR10)
Health care/lab workers	Hepatitis B vaccine (HR5); hepatitis A vaccine (HR6); PPD (HR7); influenza vaccine (HR10)
Family h/o skin cancer; fair skin, eyes, hair	Avoid excess/midday sun, use protective clothing* (HR13)
Previous pregnancy with neural tube defect	Folic acid 4.0 mg (HR14)

[1]Women who are or have been sexually active and who have a cervix: q ≤ 3 yr. [2]Annually. [3]Mammogram q1–2 yr, or mammogram q1–2 yr with annual clinical breast examination. [4]Serologic testing, documented vaccination history, and routine vaccination (preferably with MMR) are equally acceptable alternatives.

*The ability of clinician counseling to influence this behavior is unproven.

HR1 = Persons who exchange sex for money or drugs, and their sex partners; persons with other STDs (including HIV); and sexual contacts of persons with active syphilis. Clinicians should also consider local epidemiology (see Ch. 26).

HR2 = Women who exchange sex for money or drugs, or who have had repeated episodes of gonorrhea. Clinicians should also consider local epidemiology (see Ch. 27).

HR3 = Men who had sex with men after 1975; past or present injection drug use; persons who exchange sex for money or drugs, and their sex partners; injection drug-using, bisexual, or HIV-positive sex partner currently or in the past; blood transfusion during 1978–1985; persons seeking treatment for STDs. Clinicians should also consider local epidemiology (see Ch. 28).

HR4 = Sexually active women with multiple risk factors including: history of STD; new or multiple sex partners; nonuse or inconsistent use of barrier contraceptives; cervical ectopy. Clinicians should also consider local epidemiology (see Ch. 29).

HR5 = Blood product recipients (including hemodialysis patients), persons with frequent occupational exposure to blood or blood products, men who have sex with men, injection drug users and their sex partners, persons with multiple recent sex partners, persons with other STDs (including HIV), travelers to countries with endemic hepatitis B (see Ch. 66).

HR6 = Persons living in, traveling to, or working in areas where the disease is endemic and where periodic outbreaks occur (e.g., countries with high or intermediate endemicity; certain Alaska Native, Pacific Island, Native American, and religious communities); men who have sex with men; injection or street drug users. Consider for institutionalized persons and workers in these institutions, military personnel, and day-care, hospital, and laboratory workers. Clinicians should also consider local epidemiology (see Ch. 66, 67).

HR7 = HIV positive, close contacts of persons with known or suspected TB, health care workers, persons with medical risk factors associated with TB, immigrants from countries with high TB prevalence, medically underserved low-income populations (including homeless), alcoholics, injection drug users, and residents of long-term care facilities (see Ch. 25). See Ch. 25 for indications for BCG vaccine.

HR8 = Persons who continue to inject drugs (see Ch. 53).

HR9 = Immunocompetent institutionalized persons aged $\geq$50 yr and immunocompetent persons with certain medical conditions, including chronic cardiac or pulmonary disease, diabetes mellitus, and anatomic asplenia. Immunocompetent persons who live in high-risk environments or social settings (e.g., certain Native American and Alaska Native populations) (see Ch. 66).

HR10 = Annual vaccination of residents of chronic care facilities; persons with chronic cardiopulmonary disorders, metabolic diseases (including diabetes mellitus), hemoglobinopathies, immunosuppression, or renal dysfunction; and health care providers for high-risk patients (Ch. 66). See Ch. 66 for indications for amantadine/rimantadine prophylaxis.

HR11 = Persons born after 1956 who lack evidence of immunity to measles or mumps (e.g., documented receipt of live vaccine on or after the first birthday, laboratory evidence of immunity, or a history of physician-diagnosed measles or mumps) (see Ch. 66).

HR12 = Healthy adults without a history of chickenpox or previous immunization. Consider serologic testing for presumed susceptible adults (see Ch. 65, 66).

HR13 = Persons with a family or personal history of skin cancer, a large number of moles, atypical moles, poor tanning ability, or light skin, hair, and eye color (see Ch. 12).

HR14 = Women with previous pregnancy affected by neural tube defect who are planning pregnancy (see Ch. 42).

Table 4. Age 65 and Older

Interventions Considered and Recommended for the Periodic Health Examination	Leading Causes of Death
	Heart diseases
	Malignant neoplasms (lung, colorectal, breast)
	Cerebrovascular disease
	Chronic obstructive pulmonary disease
	Pneumonia and influenza

Interventions for the General Population

SCREENING
Blood pressure [Ch 3]
Height and weight [Ch 21]
Fecal occult blood test[1] and/or
  sigmoidoscopy [Ch 8]
Mammogram ± clinical breast exam[2]
  (women ≤69 yr) [Ch 7]
Papanicolaou (Pap) test (women)[3] [Ch 9]
Vision screening [Ch 33]
Assess for hearing impairment [Ch 35]
Assess for problem drinking [Ch 52]

COUNSELING

Substance Use
Tobacco cessation [Ch 54]
Avoid alcohol/drug use while driving,
  swimming, boating, etc.* [Ch 57,58]

Diet and Exercise
Limit fat & cholesterol; maintain caloric
  balance; emphasize grains, fruits,
  vegetables [Ch 56]
Adequate calcium intake (women) [Ch 56]
Regular physical activity* [Ch 55,58]

Injury Prevention [Ch 57,58]
Lap/shoulder belts
Motorcycle and bicycle helmets*
Fall prevention*
Safe storage/removal of firearms* [Ch 50,59]
Smoke detector*
Set hot water heater to <120–130°F*
CPR training for household members

Dental Health [Ch 61]
Regular visits to dental care provider*
Floss, brush with fluoride toothpaste daily*

Sexual Behavior
STD prevention: avoid high-risk sexual
  behavior;* use condoms* [Ch 62]

IMMUNIZATIONS [Ch 66]
Pneumococcal vaccine
Influenza[1]
Tetanus-diphtheria (Td) boosters

CHEMOPROPHYLAXIS
Discuss hormone prophylaxis (women)
  [Ch 68]

Interventions for High-Risk Populations

POPULATION	POTENTIAL INTERVENTIONS (See detailed high-risk definitions)
Institutionalized persons	PPD (HR1); hepatitis A vaccine (HR2); amantadine/rimantadine (HR4)
Chronic medical conditions; TB contacts; low income; immigrants; alcoholics	PPD (HR1)
Persons ≥75 yr; or ≥70 yr with risk factors for falls	Fall prevention intervention (HR5)
Cardiovascular disease risk factors	Consider cholesterol screening (HR6)
Family h/o skin cancer; nevi; fair skin, eyes, hair	Avoid excess/midday sun, use protective clothing* (HR7)
Native Americans/Alaska Natives	PPD (HR1); hepatitis A vaccine (HR2)
Travelers to developing countries	Hepatitis A vaccine (HR2); hepatitis B vaccine (HR8)
Blood product recipients	HIV screen (HR3); hepatitis B vaccine (HR8)
High-risk sexual behavior	Hepatitis A vaccine (HR2); HIV screen (HR3); hepatitis B vaccine (HR8); RPR/VDRL (HR9)
Injection or street drug use	PPD (HR1); hepatitis A vaccine (HR2); HIV screen (HR3); hepatitis B vaccine (HR8); RPR/VDRL (HR9); advice to reduce infection risk (HR10)
Health care/lab workers	PPD (HR1); hepatitis A vaccine (HR2); amantadine/rimantadine (HR4); hepatitis B vaccine (HR8)
Persons susceptible to varicella	Varicella vaccine (HR11)

[1]Annually. [2]Mammogram q1–2 yr, or mammogram q1–2 yr with annual clinical breast exam. [3]All women who are or have been sexually active and who have a cervix: q≤3 yr. Consider discontinuation of testing after age 65 yr if previous regular screening with consistently normal results.

*The ability of clinician counseling to influence this behavior is unproven.

HR1 = HIV positive, close contacts of persons with known or suspected TB, health care workers, persons with medical risk factors associated with TB, immigrants from countries with high TB prevalence, medically underserved low-income populations (including homeless), alcoholics, injection drug users, and residents of long-term care facilities (see Ch. 25). See Ch. 25 for indications for BCG vaccine.

HR2 = Persons living in, traveling to, or working in areas where the disease is endemic and where periodic outbreaks occur (e.g., countries with high or intermediate endemicity; certain Alaska Native, Pacific Island, Native American, and religious communities); men who have sex with men; injection or street drug users. Consider for institutionalized persons and workers in these institutions, and day-care, hospital, and laboratory workers. Clinicians should also consider local epidemiology (see Ch. 66, 67).

HR3 = Men who had sex with men after 1975; past or present injection drug use; persons who exchange sex for money or drugs, and their sex partners; injection drug-using, bisexual, or HIV-positive sex partner currently or in the past; blood transfusion during 1978–1985; persons seeking treatment for STDs. Clinicians should also consider local epidemiology (see Ch. 28).

HR4 = Consider for persons who have not received influenza vaccine or are vaccinated late; when the vaccine may be ineffective due to major antigenic changes in the virus; for unvaccinated persons who provide home care for high-risk persons; to supplement protection provided by vaccine in persons who are expected to have a poor antibody response; and for high-risk persons in whom the vaccine is contraindicated (see Ch. 66).

HR5 = Persons aged 75 years and older; or aged 70–74 with one or more additional risk factors including: use of certain psychoactive and cardiac medications (e.g., benzodiazepines, antihypertensives); use of $\geq$4 prescription medications; impaired cognition, strength, balance, or gait. Intensive individualized home-based multifactorial fall prevention intervention is recommended in settings where adequate resources are available to deliver such services (see Ch. 58).

HR6 = Although evidence is insufficient to recommend routine screening in elderly persons, clinicians should consider cholesterol screening on a case-by-case basis for persons ages 65–75 with additional risk factors (e.g., smoking, diabetes, or hypertension) (see Ch. 2).

HR7 = Persons with a family or personal history of skin cancer, a large number of moles, atypical moles, poor tanning ability, or light skin, hair, and eye color (see Ch. 12).

HR8 = Blood product recipients (including hemodialysis patients), persons with frequent occupational exposure to blood or blood products, men who have sex with men, injection drug users and their sex partners, persons with multiple recent sex partners, persons with other STDs (including HIV), travelers to countries with endemic hepatitis B (see Ch. 66).

HR9 = Persons who exchange sex for money or drugs and their sex partners; persons with other STDs (including HIV); and sexual contacts of persons with active syphilis. Clinicians should also consider local epidemiology (see Ch. 26).

HR10 = Persons who continue to inject drugs (see Ch. 53).

HR11 = Healthy adults without a history of chickenpox or previous immunization. Consider serologic testing for presumed susceptible adults (see Ch. 65, 66).

Table 5. Pregnant Women**

Interventions Considered and Recommended for the Periodic Health Examination

---

Interventions for the General Population

SCREENING

First visit
Blood pressure [Ch 3,37]
Hemoglobin/hematocrit [Ch 22]
Hepatitis B surface antigen (HBsAg)
  [Ch 24]
RPR/VDRL [Ch 26]
Chlamydia screen (<25 yr) [Ch 29]
Rubella serology or vaccination history
  [Ch 32]
D(Rh) typing, antibody screen [Ch 38]
Offer CVS (<13 wk)[1] or amniocentesis
  (15–18 wk)[1] (age ≥35 yr) [Ch 41]
Offer hemoglobinopathy screening [Ch 43]
Assess for problem or risk drinking [Ch 52]
Offer HIV screening[2] [Ch 28]

Follow-up visits
Blood pressure [Ch 3,37]
Urine culture (12–16 wk) [Ch 31]
Offer amniocentesis (15–18 wk)[1] (age ≥35
  yr) [Ch 41]

Offer multiple marker testing[1] (15–18 wk)
  [Ch 41]
Offer serum α-fetoprotein[1] (16–18 wk)
  [Ch 42]

COUNSELING
Tobacco cessation; effects of passive
  smoking [Ch 54]
Alcohol/other drug use [Ch 52,53]
Nutrition, including adequate calcium intake
  [Ch 56]
Encourage breastfeeding [Ch 22,56]
Lap/shoulder belts [Ch 57]
Infant safety car seats [Ch 57]
STD prevention: avoid high-risk sexual
  behavior;* use condoms* [Ch 62]

CHEMOPROPHYLAXIS
Multivitamin with folic acid[3] [Ch 42]

Interventions for High-Risk Populations

POPULATION	POTENTIAL INTERVENTIONS (See detailed high-risk definitions)
High-risk sexual behavior	Screen for chlamydia (1st visit) (HR1), gonorrhea (1st visit) (HR2), HIV (1st visit) (HR3); HBsAg (3rd trimester) (HR4); RPR/VDRL (3rd trimester) (HR5)
Blood transfusion 1978–1985	HIV screen (1st visit) (HR3)
Injection drug use	HIV screen (HR3); HBsAg (3rd trimester) (HR4); advice to reduce infection risk (HR6)
Unsensitized D-negative women	D(Rh) antibody testing (24–28 wk) (HR7)
Risk factors for Down syndrome	Offer CVS[1] (1st trimester), amniocentesis[1] (15–18 wk) (HR8)
Prior pregnancy with neural tube defect	Folic acid 4.0 mg,[3] offer amniocentesis[1] (15–18 wk) (HR9)

---

[1]Women with access to counseling and follow-up services, reliable standardized laboratories, skilled high-resolution ultrasound, and, for those receiving serum marker testing, amniocentesis capabilities. [2]Universal screening is recommended for areas (states, counties, or cities) with an increased prevalence of HIV infection among pregnant women. In low-prevalence areas, the choice between universal and targeted screening may depend on other considerations (see Ch. 28). [3]Beginning at least 1 mo before conception and continuing through the first trimester.

*The ability of clinician counseling to influence this behavior is unproven.

**See Tables 2 and 3 for other preventive services recommended for women of childbearing age.

HR1 = Women with history of STD or new or multiple sex partners. Clinicians should also consider local epidemiology. Chlamydia screen should be repeated in 3rd trimester if at continued risk (see Ch. 29).

HR2 = Women under age 25 with two or more sex partners in the last year, or whose sex partner has multiple sexual contacts; women who exchange sex for money or drugs; and women with a history of repeated episodes of gonorrhea. Clinicians should also consider local epidemiology. Gonorrhea screen should be repeated in the 3rd trimester if at continued risk (see Ch. 27).

HR3 = In areas where universal screening is not performed due to low prevalence of HIV infection, pregnant women with the following individual risk factors should be screened: past or present injection drug use; women who exchange sex for money or drugs; injection drug-using, bisexual, or HIV-positive sex partner currently or in the past; blood transfusion during 1978–1985; persons seeking treatment for STDs (see Ch. 28).

HR4 = Women who are initially HBsAg-negative who are at high risk due to injection drug use, suspected exposure to hepatitis B during pregnancy, multiple sex partners (see Ch. 24).

HR5 = Women who exchange sex for money or drugs, women with other STDs (including HIV), and sexual contacts of persons with active syphilis. Clinicians should also consider local epidemiology (see Ch. 26).

HR6 = Women who continue to inject drugs (see Ch. 53).

HR7 = Unsensitized D-negative women (see Ch. 38).

HR8 = Prior pregnancy affected by Down syndrome, advanced maternal age (≥35 yr), known carriage of chromosome rearrangement (see Ch. 41).

HR9 = Women with previous pregnancy affected by neural tube defect (see Ch. 42).

Table 6.
Conditions for Which Clinicians Should Remain Alert

Condition	Population	Chapter
Symptoms of peripheral arterial disease	Older persons, smokers, diabetic persons	5
Skin lesions with malignant features	General population, particularly those with established risk factors	12
Symptoms and signs of oral cancer and premalignancy	*Persons who use tobacco, older* persons who drink alcohol regularly	16
Subtle or nonspecific symptoms and signs of thyroid dysfunction	Older persons, postpartum women, persons with Down syndrome	20
Signs of ocular misalignment	Infants and children	33
Symptoms and signs of hearing impairment	Infants and young children (<3 yr)	35
Large spinal curvatures	Adolescents	47
Changes in functional performance	Older persons	48
Depressive symptoms	Adolescents, young adults, persons at increased risk for depression	49
Evidence of suicidal ideation	Persons with established risk factors for suicide	50
Various presentations of family violence	General population	51
Symptoms and signs of drug abuse	General population	53
Obvious signs of untreated tooth decay or mottling, inflamed or cyanotic gingiva, loose teeth, and severe halitosis	General population	61
Evidence of early childhood caries, mismatching of upper and lower dental arches, dental crowding or malalignment, premature loss of primary posterior teeth (baby molars) and obvious mouth breathing	Children	61